Paris . Beaujon Hosp. 19–

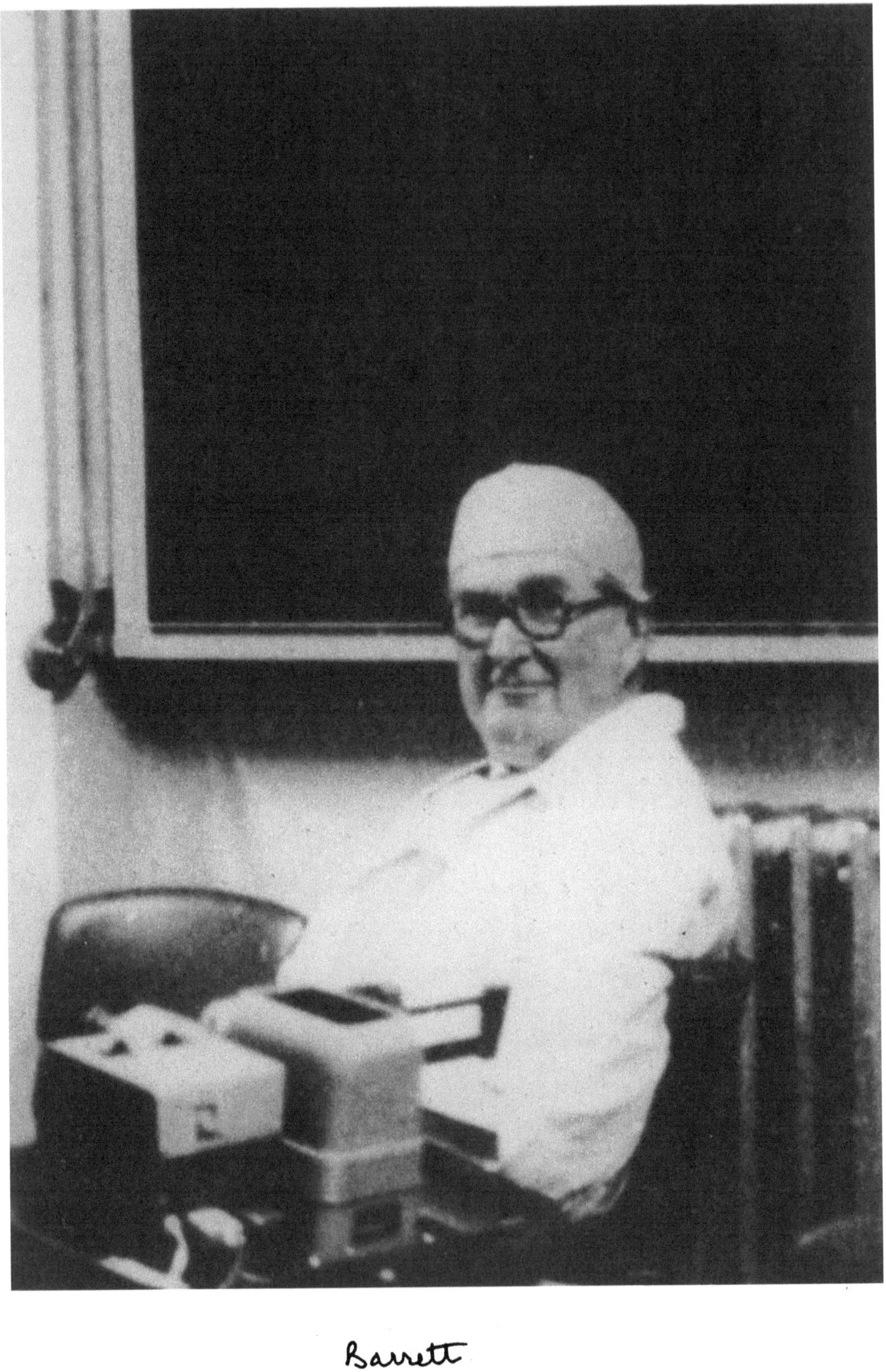

Barrett

The lower oesophagus lined
by columnar epithelium

Friendly confrontation,

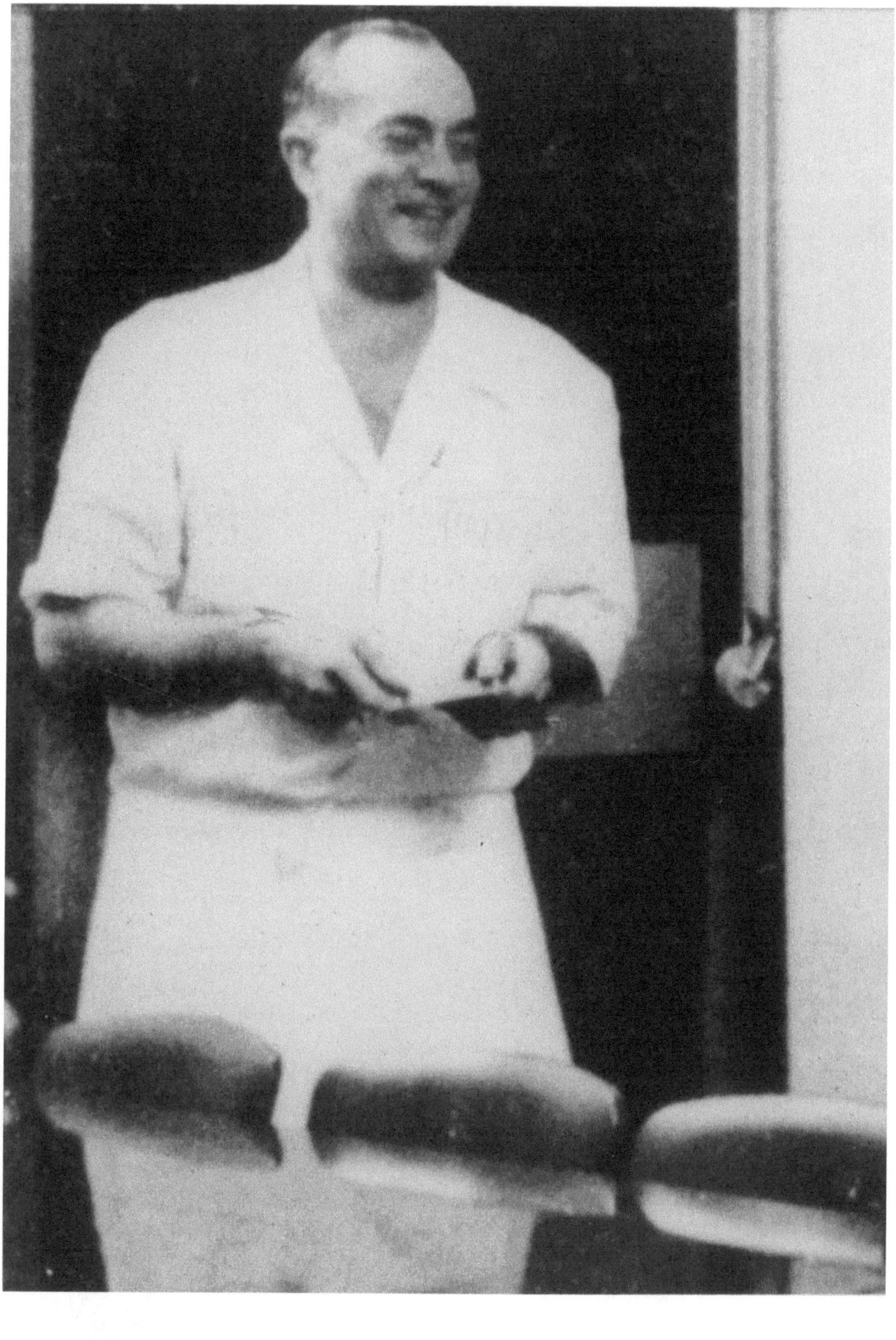

J L Lortat-Jacob

[illegible]

O.E.S.O.
Organisation internationale d'Etudes Statistiques pour les maladies de l'Œsophage
International Organization for Statistical Studies on Diseases of the Esophagus

Université de Paris 7 – Faculté Xavier-Bichat
University of Virginia School of Medicine
R. Giuli R.W. McCallum (Eds.)

Benign Lesions of the Esophagus and Cancer

Answers to 210 Questions

Springer-Verlag
Berlin Heidelberg New York
London Paris Tokyo

Robert Giuli, M. D., FACS, FCCP
Professor of Surgery
Service de Chirurgie Digestive
Hôpital Beaujon
100, Blvd. du Genéral Leclerc
F-92110 Clichy – Paris

Richard W. McCallum, M. D., FACP,
FRACP (Australia), FACG
Professor of Medicine
Chief of the Division of Gastroenterology
University of Virginia
School of Medicine
Box 145
Charlottesville, VA 22908
USA

ISBN-13:978-3-642-73057-3 e-ISBN-13:978-3-642-73055-9
DOI: 10.1007/978-3-642-73055-9

Softcover reprint of the hardcover 1st edition 1989

2127/3140/543210 – Printed on acid-free paper

Preface

J.-L. Lortat-Jacob

In 1984, OESO, under the direction and prompting of Robert Giuli, organized its first Congress devoted to cancer of the esophagus, during which 135 questions were put to several dozen teams from 23 countries. The answers given were, and continue to be, studied statistically in the optimal conditions of multicenter compilation, by members of several disciplines and according to a common protocol.
A book of over 400 pages has recorded these studies.*

Today, 3 years later, Robert Giuli has programmed and brought to fruition this new Congress, based on the same original and rigorous process, so difficult to formulate and lead to a satisfactory conclusion. This time, it is devoted to benign disorders of the esophagus, especially to their relations to malignant disease of this organ. The replies obtained to 210 questions already make it possible to define certain essential etiopathogenetic factors in this pathology, and to discern the elements of an exceptional therapeutic synthesis.

Once again, two very carefully edited volumes, one in English, one in French, sum up the results obtained, and faithfully reproduce the contributions of each participant.

These studies, in which the principle of general allocation and compilation remains the original feature of OESO, have gained much support throughout the world, and the ISDE (International Society for Diseases of the Esophagus) has joined with OESO in a voluntary association whose efficacy seems very evident to me today.

The completeness of the work so far accomplished will be found in this book. It will be seen, especially, that it contains the premises for subsequent fruitful syntheses, statistically controlled and put into practice by numerous studies that will now be undertaken on an international scale.

As Honorary President of OESO, I must especially thank those teams in the whole world that have agreed to participate in these studies, sometimes subject to demanding, but necessary, constraints. I also thank Robert Giuli and Madame Sancho-Garnier for having collected all this information, monitored its validity and ensured its publication.

I am certain that these post-congress undertakings will be epoch-making.

J.-L. Lortat-Jacob
President of Honour
of OESO

* (Cancer of the Esophagus in 1984, 135 questions. 426 pp. Maloine Publ., Paris)

Preface

K. Inokuchi

Diseases of the esophagus still remain today one of the most disappointing chapters of digestive pathology, and one where are confronted still the greatest number of contradictory opinions, even views radically opposed.

Whether it's a matter of the various medical treatments of "theoretically benign" lesions of this organ, or of the numerous operative techniques imagined, or modified, and defended by each surgical team,

whether it's a matter of the epidemiology of malignant tumors, whose incidence is currently increasing, of their early detection, or of the very conception of their treatment,

there still exist in all these areas major practical uncertainties that are, today, the source of useful and fruitful controversy.

In the heart of this debate, endoscopists and pathologists play an essential, fulcrum role, in trying to classify these problems, which are sometimes only different stages of the same evolution.

*

In 1979, when Robert Giuli created OESO, with J. L. Lortat-Jacob, there was an indisputable need for of a multicenter polydisciplinary approach, rigorously controlled by statistics, and OESO represented a concrete means to satisfying this need. At the same time, Pr. Komei Nakayama, recognized the world over as the pioneer of this pathological entity, decided to bring together all those everywhere interested in diseases of the esophagus, and founded ISDE.

This prestigious Society has today matured, and has, at the same time, become the one Society, uniting all those various Societies also interested in the same problems.

To efficiently set up randomized therapeutical trials is a highly difficult task, which is even more uncertain when it is a question of uniting different countries, and different continents.

OESO, by means of its strict organization and the motivation of its members, has managed to organize several trials, in the fields as essential as the treatment of cancer of the esophagus or the systematic detection of esophageal dysplasia.

For the purpose of efficiency, ISDE and OESO agreed to form a voluntary association, and the members of ISDE will then benefit from the statistical framework of OESO, and from the different studies, surveys and therapeutical trials which are already underway or are proposed as projects for the future.

*

For this Congress, Robert Giuli took up again the original formula used for the first Congress of the Group: he invited us all to participate in a specific focusing on those diseases, supposedly benign, but whose potential degeneration is now widely recognized.

Physiologists, epidemiologists, gastroenterologists, pathologists and, of course, surgeons, exchanged during 7 sessions sometimes quite different views, while answering 210 precise questions...

Such an approach could have legitimately seemed to be an impossible attempt, if it hadn't already been tried at the time of the first Congress of O.E.S.O.

I would stress that the format of this conference, i. e. preparing these questions in advance to have them answered in a short period of time by recognized authorities from all over the world is extremely unique and effective.

The contents of the meeting, as shown by this volume, more than adequately attests to their own depth, range, and quality.

*

Lastly, as President of the ISDE, I would like to emphasize the importance for our Society of the continued support from OESO in the field of statistical studies on diseases of the esophagus.

I am sure that our present and future cooperation will be extremely fruitful.

Professor Kiyoshi Inokuchi
President of the ISDE
International Society for Diseases of the Esophagus

Preface

F. Bonnet de Paillerets

It would not be fitting for the pediatrician that I am to judge all the value of the contributions of these past four days on the benign diseases of the esophagus, even if these contributions seem to be most important.

Something, quite evident moreover, has impressed the academic that I equally am, used to congresses, meetings, symposiums and the like, which demand our profession: that is, the richness of the methodology used.

It's true that the method chosen by Robert Giuli enhanced the efficiency of each reply, the spontaneity of the exchanges, and the effectiveness of the audio-visual techniques.

This is equally true for the method adopted for the multicentric trials of OESO: retrospective studies, whose results have yielded the objective confirmation of conclusions that only highly selected teams in the world could foresee from their own personal experience, prospectives inquiries which have already given a great deal of information, and above all, randomized therapeutical trials, now underway, that OESO alone has been able to organize on such an international scale.

*

As Dean of one of the largest Faculties of Paris, may I thank Jean-Louis Lortat-Jacob and Robert Giuli for the fervour they create and maintain for the benefit of the scientific community, and express my pride in having been associated with such a success.

François Bonnet de Paillerets
Dean of the Faculty of Medicine
Xavier Bichat

Preface

U. Veronesi

With this Second Congress on "Benign lesions of the esophagus and cancer", the OESO is moving a further step ahead in the knowledge of such an important and critical disease as esophageal cancer.

If we look back to the first Congress held in 1984, we can immediately realize that the enormous effort put into the OESO project, to concentrate all the clinical resources existing in the field, has obtained concrete and practical results.

A large international randomized trial on the efficacy of combined treatments for esophageal cancer is now running, and some 38 centres from 16 different countries are cooperating in this trial with a multidisciplinary approach.

It is already an important achievement, because we need cooperative studies in clinical oncology which are able to rise the relevant questions, but also large enough to answer them properly and in the shortest time.

Benign esophageal lesions and true precancerous conditions are another domaine where clinical investigation is needed. Early detection and chemoprevention in high risk population could well become in the near future a way to reduce cancer mortality, even in this field.

*

We wish the OESO Group and Robert Giuli, who has organized this second Congress with his usual competence and experience, the greatest success for future prospects of clinical research.

Professor Umberto Veronesi
Director of the Istituto Nazionale per lo studio
e la cura dei tumori (Milan)
President of E.O.R.T.C.

Introduction

R. Giuli

The first International Congress of the OESO Group took place in Paris in May 1984. Its very particular feature consisted of gathering together at an international assembly, then comprising 23 countries, the most important specialists in 10 different disciplines, in an attempt to reply to 135 questions formulated as regards esophageal cancer.

The general approbation evoked by this original formula among those who participated at this Congress, or who read the proceedings resulting from it, as well as the effectiveness progressively obtained in the OESO Group in the common performance of studies amenable to statistical analysis, have enabled us to pursue our plans for collective working since that date.

Within the framework of the OESO, several international groups specializing in thoracic surgery, digestive and E.N.T. surgery, endoscopy, gastroenterology, pathology, radio and chemotherapy, and epidemiology, in regular and effective collaboration, have made it possible to elaborate 3 working protocols, the details of which will be given at the end of this book: the first relates to an international therapeutic trial on cancer of the esophagus, randomized in 3 fields, for which half the necessary patients have already been collected in a little over a year, another one is a randomized trial on the treatment of esophageal dysplasias with vitamin A, and the third, an epidemiologic enquiry into caustic and peptic strictures of the esophagus.

*

At the same time, we began the preparation of our second Congress, devoted to "theoretically benign" lesions of the esophagus. As opposed to the conventional arrangements of congresses where papers are requested on a general theme chosen beforehand, the unusual form of our first Congress was maintained, offering the audience a sequence of brief replies (around 5 minutes) without repetition to a succession of precise questions whose intricate themes related to very varied fields.

The object was to attempt to follow, over 4 days, the logical steps pursued by the specialist confronted with his patient, while emphasizing especially the uncertainties he would encounter and the difficult questions he might have to ask himself.

A program was progressively drawn up and completed, that allowed recognized specialists in one discipline to express themselves with authority on a very elective aspect of their experience, at the same time allowing the others of different specialties to profit from the information thus offered to them.

Then, contact was made with all those, wherever in the world, who seemed best suited to collaborate in this difficult step, so very different from their habitual role at the congresses to which they were invited. There was no question of asking them to prepare an exhaustive or fragmentary account of their experience. On the contrary, they were asked to reflect on a very limited aspect of their work and, in order to structure their reply, to examine those features of their observations that were not necessarily obvious at the outset. Recognized specialists from Paris, from France and from 26 other countries agreed to play the unusual game I suggested to them, to reply in a few long minutes to one or more of these 210 questions, the answers to which sometimes seemed unlikely to be obtainable.

*

This synthesis has been well carried out thanks to the collective effort of all those who were so kind to respond to my request. The long list of these, in the subsequent pages of this book, will enable the reader to find there all those whose names are familiar to him, at least in his own discipline. In one way or another, each of these is the Chief of a prestigious school or his most efficient representative, and I am grateful to them for having agreed to comply with the difficult rules of this game and to contribute little by little to an overall appreciation.

*

Without any desire or ability to make a choice within the list, I nevertheless want to cite a few of these participants separately:

My teacher, Jean-Louis Lortat-Jacob first of all, honorary President of the OESO, who faithfully shares all my enthusiasms. Like all of us, he wished to supply his part of the global synthesis that is our goal, and was able to adapt to the limited time allotted him to give the principles of his own operations and the main features of the essential chapters of pathology which he has helped to describe and clarify. He well knows how much my gratitude to him is renewed at every moment of my professional life.

His friend, like him a pioneer in surgery of the esophagus, Professor Ronald Belsey, has from the outset given us the benefit of all that his powerful personality can supply. He too has complied with the same constraints as the other contributors, and it is he who gives us at the end of this book his opinions on the useful further developments he envisages for this Congress. It's little to say how thankful I am to him also for all that he contributes.

Dr Hélène Sancho-Garnier, Head of the Department of Medical Statistics at the Institut Gustave Roussy at Villejuif, has brought to our collective endeavour, since its origin in 1979, the discipline of statistics and the enlightened aid of her intelligent competence. It is she who is mainly responsible today for the analysis of the data of the OESO therapeutic trial in cancer of the esophagus, the only one of its kind in the world, and who coordinates with her team the difficult collation of information arriving from 16 countries.

I am glad to repeat here to Madame Luboinski, Dr. Sancho-Garnier's assistant, how important her aid is in this field, to ensure that the handling of the information gathered is regular, rigorous and especially without any defect in interpretation.

Professor Henry Appelman, a world-famous pathologist, has agreed to centralize in his laboratory at Ann Arbor, Michigan, all of the histologic sections obtained from each operated patient included in this trial, to interpret them himself, and to give the ultimate histologic analysis his personal guarantee of uniformity of interpretation. Rare are those who would have accepted such a burden of work with such alacrity, and the gratitude of all of us is felt equally deeply.

In addition, he has agreed to organize for this Congress an international Symposium on classification of cancer of the esophagus. Its proceedings were followed by numerous enthusiastic listeners, and the account given in this work demonstrates the personal quality of this undertaking.

The multidisciplinary nature of OESO made it necessary to devote an important part of our Congress to problems of pure physiology and gastroenterology. This was because it was necessary to take our bearings as regards the experimental basis and precise modes of action of the treatments that are now, or soon will be, offered to us for the management of reflux and peptic esophagitis.

Serge Bonfils, René Lambert and Jean-François Rey agreed to direct 2 sessions at this Congress in which, following the same procedure, many of the great names in gastroenterology, both in France and abroad, took part. Their scientific support was essential and I thank them for their contribution to the satisfactory course of this Congress.

The account given of the discussions dealing with clinical pharmacology is of particular interest to all of us: to the gastroenterologists, who are now confronted with an essential stage, constructed step by step without repetition, in the range of medical treatments currently at their disposition, and to the surgeons, who will be able to better define their operative indications and possibly take a different view of the results of their procedures.

In this same field, the presence of Professors Savary and Gardiol, Dr Ollyo, and all those working actively on Barrett esophagus with Professor Mosimann in what has been termed "the Lausanne group" was particularly effective. It will be seen that each of their contributions has been an especially clear formulation of the aspect of the problem under review, and one of the weighty arguments on the global matter being investigated.

Surgery – its techniques, indications and failures – was obviously widely considered throughout the succession of questions. 19 of the members of the American Esophagus Club, headed by Mark Orringer, have actively participated in this vast gathering and I thank them for their contributions.

Esophageal surgeons are also associated within the ISDE (International Society for Diseases of the Esophagus), presided over by Professor Inokuchi whom I thank particularly for his introduction to this book. The voluntary association between this prestigious Society and OESO, in the objective sharing the results of the studies undertaken, is already an effective source.

The presidency of the first and last sessions of this Congress by R. Siewert and D. Skinner, respectively Vice-President of the I.S.D.E., and coming President of I.S.D.E., as well as the participation of G. Castrini, Chairman of the European

Federation of I.S.D.E., is a symbol of a pooling of every effort with the sole aim of effectiveness.

*

Indeed, the future is that of our combined exertions. Before this Congress, I suggested to those who might wish to join in our studies, to put forward a research protocol capable of being brought to a successful conclusion by OESO: the 16 teams from 9 countries which replied to us, and whose projects are set out at the end of this book, now provide the most effective motivation to maintain our momentum.

Many and sincere thanks to them all.

Robert Giuli
Coordinator of OESO

Each of the contributors had the courtesy, long before this Meeting, to send me the exact text of his reply, arranged for publication, and comprising useful references. These different papers, in chronological order following the program of the Congress, make up this book.

It is divided according to the sessions, with the names of those who agreed to be Chairman or "Free Commentator"; they had the delicate role of ensuring harmonious development of the program by giving their personal impetus to each session.

*

For all that his Association contributed during the preparation of this Congress, I express to Professor Maurice Payet, President of AIRMEC, my sincere and legitimate thanks.

*

Michèle Liégeon has been the mainspring of our organization.
She continues to help us daily.
To work with her is an irreplaceable privilege.

Contents

Esophageal dysplasia

Reflux esophagitis

Physiopathology of peptic esophagitis (1)

Physiopathology of peptic esophagitis (2)

Non-surgical treatments

Medical treatments of peptic esophagitis

Conservative surgical procedures (1)

Conservative surgical procedures (2)

Surgical resections and evaluation of surgical results

Evaluation of surgical results

Barrett's esophagus (1)

Barrett's esophagus (2)

Malignant degeneration of benign lesions (1)

Malignant degeneration of benign lesions (2)

Malignant degeneration of benign lesions (3)

Symposium on the anatomic pathology of esophageal neoplasia

Squamous cell carcinoma of the esophagus

List of Senior Authors

- **Argentina**

BADALONI, Adolfo,
Vidal 1956, Piso 1°, Depto. 2, 1428 Buenos Aires, Argentina

MAMMONI, Osvaldo H.,
Diag. 73 N° 1915, 1900 La Plata, Argentina

SEINELDIN, Semy,
Avenida Francia 889, 2000 Rosario, Santa Fé, Republica Argentina

- **Austria**

FRIEHS, Gerhard,
Department of Thoracic Surgery, University Medical School, 8036 Graz, Landeskrankenhaus, Austria

- **Australia**

DENT, John,
Gastroenterology Unit, Royal Adelaïde Hospital, North Terrace, Adelaide, South Australia 5000

JAMIESON, Glyn G.,
Department of Surgery, Royal Adelaide Hospital, 5000 Adelaide, Australia

- **Belgium**

DELTENRE, Michel,
Clinique de Gastroentérologie, Hôpital Universitaire Brugmann, Place Van Gehuchten, 4, 1020 Bruxelles, Belgique

FIASSE, René,
Service de Gastro-entérologie, Cliniques Saint Luc UIL, Avenue Hippocrate, 10, B-1200 Bruxelles, Belgique

GRŬWEZ, Jacques,
Academisch Ziekenhuis, Brusselsestraat 69, 3000 Leuven, Belgique

LERUT, Toni,
Chirurgie Générale, Université de Louvain, Brusselsestraat 69, 3000 Louvain, Belgique

MARLIERE, Philippe,
Clinique des Deux Alice, Département de Gastro-entérologie, Groeselenberg 57, 1180 Bruxelles, Belgique

VANTRAPPEN, Georges,
Universitaire Zienkenhuizen, U.Z. Gasthuisberg, Herestraat 49, 3000 Leuven, Belgique

• **Brazil**

PINOTTI, Henrique Walter,
Head of Digestive Surgery Department, Medical School of University of Sao Paulo, Rua Itacolomi, 193, CEP 01239 São Paulo, Brasil

• **Canada**

BEAUCHAMP, Gilles,
Department of Surgery, Hôpital Maisonneuve-Rosemont,
5415 Boulevard de l'Assomption, Montreal, Québec H1T 2M4, Canada

HENDERSON, Robert D.,
Women's College Hospital, 76 Grenville Street, Toronto, Ontario M5S 1B2, Canada

PEARSON, F. Griffith,
Department of Surgery, Toronto General Hospital, Bell Wing 1–636, Toronto, Ontario M5G 2C4, Canada

RIDDELL, Robert H.,
Department of Pathology, Room 2N19, McMaster University Medical Center,
1200 Main Street West, Hamilton, Ontario L8N 3Z5, Canada

WATERS, Paul F.,
Mont Sinaï Hospital, 600 University Avenue, Suite 453, Toronto, M5G 1X5, Canada

• **Chile**

LIRA DEL CAMPO, Exequiel,
Surgery Oncology, Vicuna Mackenna 3 OF. 902, Santiago de Chile, Chile

• **Finland**

KIVILAAKSO, Eero,
Second Department of Surgery, Central Hospital, Haartmaninkatu 4,
00290 Helsinki, Finland

• **France**

BALMES, Jean-Louis,
Service de Gastroentérologie, Hôpital Saint Eloi, Avenue Bertin Sans,
34059 Montpellier Cedex, France

BARBIN, Jean Yves,
Chirurgie Générale et Digestive, Hôpital Guillaume et René Laënnec, B.P. 1005, 44035 Nantes Cedex, France

BAULIEUX, Jacques,
Hôpital de la Croix Rousse, 93 Grand Rue de la Croix Rousse,
69317 Lyon Cedex 04, France

BEL, André
Clinique Médicale D, Hôpital de la Croix Rousse,
93 Grand-Rue de la Croix Rousse, 69317 Lyon Cedex 04, France

BOGOMOLETZ, W. V.,
Laboratoire d'Anatomie pathologique, Institut Jean Godinot, B.P. 101,
51056 Reims Cedex, France

BOMMELAER, Gilles,
Centre d'Hépato-gastro-entérologie, Hotel Dieu, B.P. 69,
63003 Clermont-Ferrand Cedex, France

BORIES, Philippe,
Clinique Maladies Appareil Digestif, Hôpital Saint Eloi,
4, avenue Bertin-Sans, 34059 Montpellier Cedex, France

CARABALONA, Pierre,
Service de Chirurgie Générale A, Hôpital Saint-Eloi, 4 avenue Bertin-Sans,
34000 Montpellier, France

CARAYON, Pierre,
Service de Gastroentérologie, Hôpital Jean Munoz, 2 place Saint Jacques,
25030 Besançon Cedex, France

COLIN, Raymond,
Maladies de l'Appareil Digestif, Hôpital Charles-Nicolle, 1 rue de Germont,
76031 Rouen Cedex, France

COURAUD, Louis,
Service de Chirurgie, Hôpital Xaveir Arnozan, Avenue Pasteur,
33604 Pessac Cedex, France

DENIS, Philippe,
Laboratoire de Physiologie, Hôpital Charles Nicolle, 1 rue de Germont,
76031 Rouen Cedex, France

DOMERGUE, Jacques,
Service de Chirurgie, Centre Paul Lamarque, Cliniques Saint Eloi, B.P. 5054,
34094 Montpellier Cedex, France

DUPIN, Béatrice,
Service de Chirurgie Thoracique, Hôpital Salvator,
249 boulevard de Sainte Marguerite, 13274 Marseille Cedex 9, France

FAVRE, Jean-Pierre,
Service de Chirurgie III, Hôpital Général, 3 rue du Faubourg Raines,
21033 Dijon, France

FLAMENT, J. B.,
Service de Chirurgie Générale, Hôpital Robert Debré, Rue Alexis Carrel,
51092 Reims Cedex, France

FUENTES, Pierre,
Service de Chirurgie Thoracique, Hôpital Sainte Marguerite,
270 boulevard Sainte Marguerite, 13274 Marseille Cedex 9, France

GALMICHE, Jean Paul,
Clinique des maladies de l'appareil digestif, Hôpital R. G. Laennec, B.P. 1005,
44035 Nantes Cedex, France

GASTARD, Joseph,
Hepato-gastro-entérologie, Hôpital Pontchaillou, Rue Henri Le Guilloux,
35033 Rennes Cedex, France

GILLET, Michel,
Service de Chirurgie, Hôpital Jean Minjoz, 25030 Besançon Cedex, France

GIUDICELLI, Roger,
Service de Chirurgie Thoracique, Hôpital Salvator,
249 boulevard de Sainte Marguerite, 13247 Marseille Cedex 9, France

GOUTALLIER, Philippe,
Service de Chirurgie, Clinique de l'Archette, 504 avenue du Loiret, 45000 Orleans,
France

GUILLET, Jacques,
Service de Biophysique, Centre Hospitalier d'Agen, 47000 Agen, France

HEMET, Jacques,
Laboratoire d'Anatomie Pathologique, Hôpital Charles Nicolle, 1 rue de Germont,
76031 Rouen Cedex, France

LAMBERT, R.,
Service d'hépato-gastro-entérologie, Hôpital Edouard Herriot, 5 place d'Arsonval,
69374 Lyon Cedex 09, France

MAFFIOLI, Claude,
18 rue Laurent Desramez, 51100 Reims, France

MANTION, G.,
Service de Chirurgie Digestive, C.H.U. – Hôpital Jean Minjoz,
2 place Saint Jacques, 25030 Besançon, France

OTTIGNON, Yves,
Maladies de l'Appareil Digestif, 6 quai Bugnet, 25000 Besançon, France

PAPAZIAN, Arsène,
Clinique Jules Verne, 34 rue Charles Dubois, 80043 Amiens Cedex, France

REBOUD, Eugène,
Service de Chirurgie Thoracique, Hôpital Salvator,
249 Boulevard Sainte Marguerite, 13009 Marseille, France

REY, Jean-François,
Hépato-gastro-entérologie, Institut Arnault Tzanck, Avenue du Dr Maurice Donat,
06700 Saint Laurent du Var, France

RIBET, Michel,
Clinique Chirurgicale, Hôpital Albert Calmette, Boulevard du Pr. J. Leclerq,
59037 Lille Cedex, France

RICHELME, Henri,
C.H.U. Pasteur, Avenue de la Voie Romaine, B.P. 69, 06002 Nice Cedex, France

SOUQUET, Jean-Christophe,
Service d'Hépato-gastro-entérologie, Hôpital Edouard Herriot,
5, place d'Arsonval, 69374 Lyon Cedex 9, France

STOPPA, René,
Service de Chirurgie A, Centre Hospitalier Régional, Place Victor Pauchet,
80000 Amiens, France

VANKEMMEL, Michel,
Service de Chirurgie Digestive, Hôpital Claude Huriez, place de Verdun,
59037 Lille Cedex, France

VERHAEGHE, Pierre,
Clinique Chirurgicale, Hôpital Nord, B.P. 3006, 80030 Amiens Cedex, France

VEYRAC, Michel,
Clinique des Maladies de l'Appareil Digestif, Hôpital Saint Eloi, Rue Bertin Sans,
34059 Montpellier, France

VIARD, Henry,
Clinique Chirurgicale Hôpital du Bocage, 2 Bd Mal de Lattre de Tassigny,
21034 Dijon Cedex, France

VICARI, Fernand,
Centre de Physio-pathologie digestive et Nutritionnelle, 127 rue Saint Dizier,
54000 Nancy, France

- **Paris**

ALEXANDRE, Jean Henri,
Clinique Chirurgicale, Hôpital Broussais, 96 rue Didot, 75674 Paris Cedex 14,
France

BADER, Jean-Pierre,
Unité de Gastro-entérologie, Hôpital Henri Mondor,
51 av. du Mal de Lattre de Tassigny, 94010 Créteil, France

BONFILS, Serge,
Service d'Hépato-Gastro-Entérologie, Hôpital Bichat, 48, Rue Henri Huchard,
75018 Paris, France

CARGILL, Guillaume,
77 rue Vergnaud, 750 Paris, France

CHAMPAULT, Gerard,
Chirurgie Générale, Hôpital Jean Verdier, Avenue du 14 juillet, 93140 Bondy,
France

CHAPUIS, Yves Louis,
Chirurgie Générale, Hôpital Cochin, 27, rue du Faubourg Saint Jacques,
75674 Paris Cedex 14, France

CHARLEUX, Henri,
Service de Chirurgie Générale, Hôpital Bichat, 46, rue Henri Huchard, 75018 Paris,
France

GALIAN, Annie,
Service d'Anatomo-pathologie, Hôpital Lariboisiere, 2 rue Ambroisé Paré,
75475 Paris Cedex 10, France

GAYRAL, François,
Service de Chirurgie, Hôpital Antoine Béclère, 157 rue de la Porte de Trivaux,
92140 Clamart, France

GIULI, Robert,
Service de Chirurgie Digestive, Hôpital Beaujon, 92110 Clichy, Paris, France

HAUTEFEUILLE, Pierre,
Service de Chirurgie Digestive, Hôpital Lariboisière, 2 rue Ambroise Paré,
75010 Paris, France

HAY, Jean Marie
Clinique Chirurgicale, Hôpital Louis Mourier, 178 rue des Renouillers,
92701 Colombes Cedex, France

ISAL, Jean Pierre,
Groupe Pharmaceutique Astra France, 64 rue du 8 mai 1945,
92025 Nanterre Cedex, France

JIAN, Raymond,
Service de Gastro-entérologie, Hôpital Saint Lazare,
107 rue du Faubourg Saint Denis, 75475 Paris Cedex 10, France

JULIEN, Michel,
Service de Chirurgie Digestive, Hôpital Henri Mondor,
51, Avenue de Lattre de Tassigny, 94010 Creteil, France

LARRIEU, Hubert,
Service de Chirurgie, Hôpital Antoine Beclère, 157 rue de la Porte de Trivaux,
92140 Clamart, France

LAVERGNE, Anne,
Service Central d'Anatomo-pathologie, Hôpital Lariboisière, 2 rue Ambroise Paré,
75475 Paris Cedex 10, France

LE QUERLER, Yves,
Service d'Hépato-gastro-entérologie, Hôpital Bichat, 48, rue Henri Huchard,
75018 Paris, France

LEVESQUE, Marc,
Service Radiologie, Hôpital Louis Mourier, 178 rue des Renouillers,
92700 Colombes, France

LORTAT-JACOB, Jean-Louis,
14 rue Duroc, 75007 Paris, France

MALAFOSSE, Michel,
Service de Chirurgie, Hôpital Rothschild, 33 Boulevard de Pichus,
75571 Paris Cedex 12, France

MARMUSE, Jean-Pierre,
Service de Chirurgie Générale, Hôpital Bichat, 46 rue Henri Huchard,
75018 Paris

MIGNON, Michel,
Clinique Maladies de l'appareil digestif, Hôpital Bichat, 46, Rue Henri Huchard, 75018 Paris, France

MILLAT, Bertrand,
Service de Chirurgie, Hôpital Antoine Beclère, 157, rue de la Porte de Trivaux, 92140 Clamart, France

MOREAUX, Jean,
Centre Médico-Chirurgical de la Porte de Choisy, 15 avenue de la Porte de Choisy, 75634 Paris Cedex 13, France

NAHUM, Henri,
Service de Radiologie, Hôpital Beaujon, 100, Boulevard du Général Leclerc, 92118 Clichy Cedex, France

PAOLAGGI, J. A.,
Service d'Hépato-gastro-entérologie, Hôpital Beaujon,
100 boulevard du Maréchal Leclerc, 92110 Clichy, France

PARC, Rolland,
Centre de Chirurgie Digestive, Hôpital Saint Antoine,
184 rue du Faubourg Saint Antoine, 75571 Paris Cedex 12, France

PATEL, Jean Claude,
Chirurgie Générale, Hôpital Ambroise Paré, 9 Avenue Charles de Gaulle, 92104 Boulogne Cedex, France

PETITE, J. P.,
Service de Gastro-Entérologie, Hôpital Broussais, 96 rue Didot, 75674 Paris Cedex 14, France

POTET, François,
Service d'Anatomie Pathologie, Hôpital Beaujon,
100 Boulevard du Général Leclerc, 92110 Clichy, France

PREMONT, Michel,
Service de Chirurgie, Centre Hospitalier Marcelin-Berthelot, 30 rue Kilford, 92401 Courbevoie, France

RIBARDIERE, Jean-Louis,
Service de Chirurgie Digestive, 9 avenue de Paris, 94300 Vincennes, France

RICHARD, Claude A.,
Chirurgie Générale, Hôpital Saint Louis, 2, Place du Dr. A. Fournier, 75010 Paris, France

RIGNAULT, Daniel,
H.I.A. Begin, 69 avenue de Paris, 94160 Saint Mande, France

SANCHO-GARNIER, Hélène,
Statistique Appliquée à la Recherche, Institut Gustave Roussy,
39–53 rue Camille Desmoulins, 94805 Villejuif Cedex, France

SOULE, Jean-Claude,
Service Hépato-gastro-entérologie, Hôpital Henri Mondor,
51 av. Mal de Lattre de Tassigny, 94010 Creteil, France

THEODORE, Christian,
Centre Médical de Recherches et de Traitements Diététiques de Forcilles,
Férolles-Attily, 77170 Brie Comte Robert, France

VATIER, Jacques,
Service de Biochimie A, Hôpital Bichat, 46 rue Henri Huchard, 75018 Paris, France

VAYRE, Pierre,
Chirurgie Générale et Digestive, Groupe Hospitalier Pitié-Salpétriere,
47/83 boulevard de l'Hôpital, 75651 Paris Cedex 13, France

ZIELINSKI, Béatrice,
Clinique des Maladies de l'Appareil Digestif, Hôpital Bichat,
46 rue Henri Huchard, 75018 Paris, France

- **Great Britain**

BELSEY, Ronald,
Department of Surgery, University of Chicago, 5841, South Maryland Avenue, Chicago, IL 60637, USA

EARLAM, Richard John,
The London Hospital, Whitechapel, London E1 1BB, England

HOWARD, David,
The Institute of Laryngology, Royal National Throat, Nose & Ear Hospital,
330/332 Gray's Inn Road, London, WC1X8EE, England

JEYASINGHAM, Kumarasingham,
Department of Thoracic Surgery, Frenchay Hospital, Bristol BS16 1LE (0272), England

WATSON, Anthony,
Department of Surgery, Royal Lancaster Infirmary, Ashton Road,
Lancaster LA1 4RP, England

- **Greece**

MANTONAKIS, Stelios,
Service de Chirurgie Digestive, Hôpital «Asclepeion» Voulas, 166.73 Voula Attikis, Athenes, Grèce

- **Hong Kong**

WONG, John,
Department of Surgery, University of Hong Kong, Queen Mary Hospital,
Hong Kong

- **Hungary**

Csikos, Mihaly,
Oesophageal Surgery, Municipal Hospital, P.O. Box 455, 6701 Szeged, Hungary

KISS, Janos,
Postgraduate Medical School, 1st Department of Surgery, Szabolcs u. 35 – pf. 112, 1389 Budapest, Hungary

KOTSIS, Lajos,
Postgraduate Medical School, Thoracic Surgical Clinic, Pihenö ut 1, 1529 Budapest XII, Hungary

KULKA, Fred,
Postgraduate Medical School, Thoracic Surgical Clinic, Pihenö ut 1, 1529 Budapest XII, Hungary

• **India**

DESAI, P. B.,
Tata Memorial Hospital, Parel, Bombay 400012, India

• **Italy**

CASTRINI, Guido,
2 Clinica Chirurgica dell Universita di Roma, Policlinico Umberto 1, 1 Padiglione, 00161 Roma, Italia

CRESPI, Massimo,
Istituto «Regina Helena», Per Lo Studio E la Cura dei Tumori, Viale Regina Helena 291, 00161 Roma, Italia

DEL GENIO, Alberto,
Universita degli Studi di Napoli, 1 Facolta di Medicina E Chirurgia, Servicio di esofagologia Chirurgica, 1 Policlinico, Piazza Miraglia, Napoli, Italia

MASCI, Enzo,
Instituto di Medicina Interna, Via Pace, 9, 20122 Milano, Italy

MORALDI, Aldo,
Clinica Chirurgica, Dell'Universita di Roma, Policlinico Umberto 1, 00161 Roma, Italia

STIPA, Sergio,
Clinica Chirurgica, Policlinico Umberto 1, Padiglione 1, 00161 Roma, Italia

• **Japan**

BARRON, Patrick J.,
St Marianna University, 2095 Sugao-Miyamac-ku KAWASAKI KANAGAWA, Japan

ENDO, Mitsuo,
1st Department of Surgery, Tokyo Medical and Dental University, 5–45, Yushima 1-chome, Bunkyo-ku, 113 Tokyo, Japan

IDE, Hiroko,
Department of Surgery, Institute of Gastroenterology, Tokyo Women's Medical College, 8-1 Kawada-cho Shinjuku-ku, Tokyo 162, Japan

INOKUCHI, Kiyoshi,
The International Society for Diseases of the esophagus I.S.D.E., Institute of gastroenterology, Tokyo Women's Medical College, 8-1 Kawada-cho Shinjuku-Ku, Tokyo 162, Japan

KAWAURA, Yukimitsu,
Department of Surgery, Kanazawa University School of Medicine, Takaramachi-13-1, Kanazawa, 920, Japan

• **Netherlands**

MUD, Henk J.,
Ste Clara Hospital, Olympiaweg 350, 3078 Rotterdam, The Netherlands

• **People's Republic of China**

HUANG, Guo Jun,
Cancer Institute & Hospital, Chinese Academy of Medical Sciences, P.O. Box 2258 – Beijing, People's Republic of China

• **Poland**

ORLOWSKI, Tadeusz M.,
Department of Thoracic Surgery, Medical Academy of Wroclaw, 105 Grabiszynska St., 53439 Wroclaw, Poland

• **Portugal**

VEIGA-FERNANDES, Fernando,
Avenida do Brasil 200 7^0 Dto, 1700 Lisboa, Portugal

• **South Africa**

BREMNER, Cedric G.,
University of Witwatersrand, Medical School, Department of Surgery, York Road, Parktown, 2193 Johannesburg, South Africa

CONLAN, A. Alan,
University of Witwatersrand, Department Thoracic Surgery, Medical School, York Road, Parktown, Johannesburg 2193, South Africa

• **Spain**

PARIS ROMEU, Francisco,
Thoracic Surgery, Hôpital «La Fé», Avenida Campenar 21, 46009 Valencia, Espagna

SANCHO-FORNOS, Salvador,
Cirugia General y Digestiva, Ciudad Sanitaria «La Fé», Plaza de Tetuan, 6, 46003 Valencia, Espana

• **Sweden**

THOR, Kjell B. A.,
Department of Surgery, Ersta Hospital, 11635 Stockholm, Sweden

• **Switzerland**

FONTOLLIET, Charlotte,
Institut de Pathologie, C.H.U. Vaudois, Bugnon 25, 1011 Lausanne, Suisse

GARDIOL, Daniel,
Institut de Pathologie, C.H.U. Vaudois, 1011 Lausanne, Suisse

MEYRAT, B.,
Hôpital Cantonal, Clinique Chirurgicale, Rheinstrasse 26, 4410 Liestal, Suisse

MONNIER, Philippe,
Service O.R.L., C.H.U. Vaudois, 1011 Lausanne, Suisse

OLLYO, Jean B.,
Gastro-entérologie, Policlinique Médicale Universitaire, 19 rue César Roux, 1005 Lausanne, Suisse

ROSSETTI, Mario,
Hôpital Cantonal, Clinique Chirurgicale, Rheinstrasse 26, 4410 Liestal, Suisse

SAVARY, Marcel,
Clinique O.R.L., C.H.U. Vaudois, 1011 Lausanne, Suisse

• **United States**

APPELMAN, Henry D.,
Department of Pathology, University Hospitals 2G332/0054, 1500 East Medical Center Drive, Ann Arbor, MI 48109-0054, USA

BOMBECK, C. Thomas,
The Abraham Lincoln School of Medicine, Department of Surgery, P.O. Box 6998, Chicago, IL 60680, USA

CAMERON, Alan J.,
Department of Gastroenterology, WI9A, Mayo Clinic, Rochester, MN 55905, USA

CONDON, Robert E.,
Department of Surgery, Medical College of Wisconsin, 8700 West Wisconsin Avenue, Milwaukee, WI 63226, USA

CORREA, Pelayo,
Department of Pathology, LSU Medical Center, 1901 Perdido Street, New Orleans, LA 70112, USA

DAWSON, Steven L.,
Interventional Radiology, Department of Radiology, Lahey Clinic Medical Center, 41 Mall Road, Burlington, MA 01805, USA

DeMEESTER, Tom R.,
Creighton University, Department of Surgery, Suite 3740, 601 North 30th Street, Omaha, NE 68131, USA

DONAHUE, Philip E.,
Department of General Surgery, Cook County Hospital, 1835 Harrison Street, Chicago, IL 60612, USA

ELLIS, F. Henry Jr.,
Thoracic and Cardiovascular Surgery, New England Deaconess Hospital,
185 Pilgrim Road, Boston, MA 02215, USA

FERGUSON, Mark K.,
Thoracic Surgery, University of Chicago Medical Center,
5841 S. Maryland Avenue, Box 255, Chicago, IL 60637, USA

GOUGE, Thomas H.,
Department of Surgery, New York University Medical Center,
550 First Avenue – Suite 6B, New York, NY 10016, USA

HIEBERT, Clement A.,
Thoracic and Cardiovascular Surgery, 321 Brackett Street, Portland, ME 04102, USA

LITTLE, Alexander G.,
Department of Surgery, The University of Chicago, 5841 S. Maryland Avenue, Chicago, IL 60637, USA

LOW, Donald E.,
General Surgery, Health Resources Building, 909 University Street, Seattle, WA 98101, USA

MAHER, James W.,
Department of Surgery, University of Iowa Hospitals, Newton Road, Iowa City, IA 52242, USA

McCALLUM, Richard W.,
Division Gastroenterology, School of Medicine, Charlottesville, VA 22908, USA

ORRINGER, Mark B.,
The University of Michigan Hospitals Thoracic Surgery, Box 0344,
C7079 University 2/20 Taubman Center, Ann Arbor, MI 48109, USA

PAYNE, W. Spencer,
Thoracic Surgery, Mayo Clinic/W6B, 200 First Street, S.W., Rochester, MN 55905, USA

PORIES, Walter J.,
Department of Surgery, ECU School of Medicine, East Carolina University, Greenville, NC 27834, USA

ROBBINS, Alan H.,
Department of Radiology, New England Baptist Hospital, 91 Parker Hill Avenue, Boston, MA 02120, USA

SICULAR, Arthur,
Department of Surgery, Mt Sinai Medical Center, 1, Gustave L. Levy Place, New York, NY 10029, USA

SKINNER, David B.,
New York Hospital, 525 East New York, NY 10021, USA

SPECHLER, Stuart Jon,
Boston V.A. Medical Center, 150 South Huntington Avenue, Boston, MA 02130, USA

• West Germany

HERFARTH, Christian,
Klinik Allgemein. Chirurg., Heidelberg IM, Neuenheimer Feld 110,
6900 Heidelberg, Federal Republic of Germany

HOLSCHER, Arnulf H.,
Department of Surgery, Technical University of München, Ismaninger Straße 22,
8000 München 80, Federal Republic of Germany

HUSEMANN, Bernhard,
Chirurgische Klinik mit Poliklinik der Universität Erlangen-Nürnberg,
Maximiliansplatz, 8520 Erlangen-Nürnberg, Federal Republic of Germany

KOCKEL, Norbert,
Chirurgische Klinik des Krankenhauses Düsseldorf-Gerresheim, 4000 Düsseldorf,
Federal Republic of Germany

KUMMERLE, Fritz,
Klinikum der Johannes-Gutenberg-Universität, Postfach 3960, Langenbeckstraße 1,
6500 Mainz, Federal Republic of Germany

LEHNERT, Thomas,
Chirurgische Klinik, Im Neuenheimer Feld 110, Kirschnerstr. 1, 6900 Heidelberg,
Federal Republic of Germany

SIEWERT, Jörg Rüdiger,
Surgery Clinic, Poliklinik rechts der Isar der Technical University of München,
Ismaninger Straße 22, 8000 München 80, Federal Republic of Germany

ULRICH, Bernward,
Krankenhaus Düsseldorf-Gerresheim, Chir. Klinik, Gräulinger Straße,
4000 Düsseldorf-Gerresheim, Federal Republic of Germany

WEISER, H. F.,
Chirurgische Klinik und Poliklinik University of München, Ismaninger Straße 22,
8000 München 80, Federal Republic of Germany

WILLITAL, Günther H.,
Klinik und Poliklinik für Kinder, University of Münster,
Albert-Schweitzer-Straße 33, 4400 Münster, Federal Republic of Germany

• Uruguay

PRADERI, Luis Alberto,
Clinica Quirurgicà «F», Hospital de Clinicas 7° Piso, Avenida Italia s./n.,
Montevideo (Uruguay)

Statistical estimation of the prevalence and incidence of the degeneration of benign lesions

H. Sancho-Garnier (Villejuif, Paris)

As a matter of fact, Incidence and Prevalence, which both measure frequencies, are often mixed up.

Prevalence measures an instantaneous frequency of a disease in a defined population.

The interest of this index is obvious in Public Health, when planning a mass-screening program, for example.

The calculation is:

$$P = \frac{\text{Number of cases with the Disease}}{\text{Number of subjects in the studied population}} \text{ at a definite time}$$

Incidence measures a frequency in the appearance of a disease, in defined population.

This index measures a characteristic of the behaviour of the disease, and is time-dependant.

Its calculation needs a follow-up survey.

$$I = \frac{\text{Number of new cases with the Disease}}{\text{Number of subjects in the studied population}} \text{ during a given period}$$

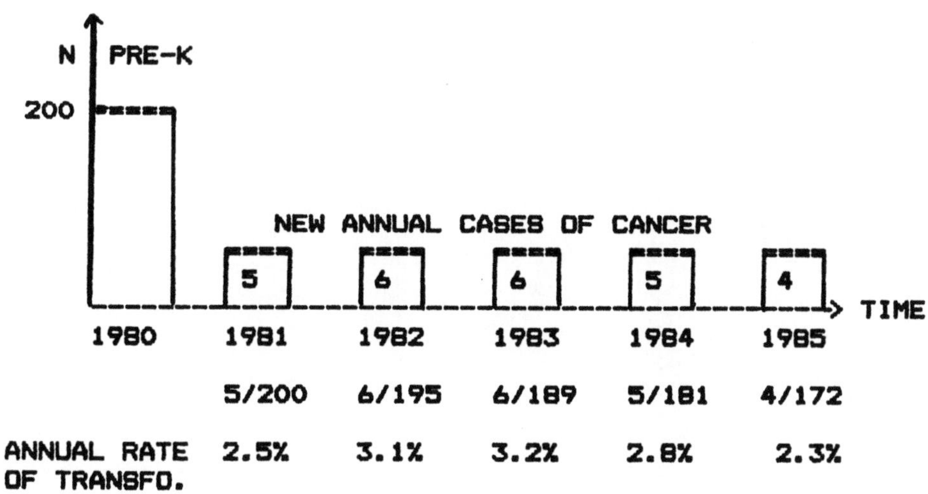

Fig. 1. Incidence of malignant transformation of pre-cancerous lesions

Annual Incidence rate: 26/937=2.8%(Hypothesis: annual rate is constant)

For example, in Calvados (France), 492 new cases of esophageal cancer in males, were observed between 1978 and 1982.

.The population of the department during these five years was: $281\,600 \times 5 = 1\,408\,000$

The annual incidence is: $\frac{492}{1\,408\,000} = 34.5/100\,000$

To measure the incidence of degeneration, it is necessary to survey, over a long period, a defined population of patients with pre-cancerous lesions and to point out all cancer cases appearing.

Fig. 1 sums up the process of calculating this incidence.

*

The terms "prevalence" and "incidence" are much used in the following pages, as they were during the Congress. We do not always agree with the exactness of their use.

Infrequent but recognized associations

President: *Jörg R. Siewert* (Munich)

Free Commentators: *A. Badaloni* (Buenos Aires)
J. A. Cameron (Rochester)
G. J. Huang (Peking)
M. Malafosse (Paris)
S. Stipa (Rome)
D. B. Skinner (Chicago)

Rare lesions

Plummer Vinson Syndrome

D. J. Howard (London)

In order to provide clarification concerning the present state of the Plummer Vinson syndrome, a review of the past literature is necessary: Patterson [1] and Brown Kelly [2] reported studies on patients with dysphagia associated with stomatitis, glossitis and hypochromic anemia, in London, in 1919. Working in America at the same time, Plummer and Vinson [3] were studying patients who suffered from what they described as hysterical dysphagia and in whom they found hypochromic anemia and they wrote their cases up in 1922. The syndrome has subsequently been most commonly known by their names. Both Patterson and Brown Kelly mention the predominance of the female sex and noted an association with post-cricoid stenosis, web formation and an increased incidence of carcinoma, but in contrast there was no mention of carcinoma in Plummer and Vinson's first publication.

During the 1920's and 1930's the incidence of post-cricoid carcinoma developing in this syndrome varied considerably, but was as high as 90% in some series reported from Europe, notably those from Sweden and Wales. This dramatic association received widespread acceptance but it is important to note that it was far from universally demonstrated and other workers reporting from Middle and Eastern Europe and, later in the 40's and 50's, from South America and other countries around the world, did not report such a high incidence and indeed the Plummer Vinson syndrome itself has not been so commonly reported around the world.

Even more modern publications in places like Africa [4] where chronic iron deficiency states are very common, remark that Plummer Vinson syndrome and hypo-pharyngeal carcinoma of the type we see are rareties. The exact association with an iron deficiency state and the presence of dysphagia, webs and subsequent carcinoma, is far from clear: simple treatment of these patient's iron deficiency does not always bring about resolution of their symptoms, nor does it correlate with the presence or absence of a web. Sometimes bougienage is also required and occasionally both treatments will not bring about resolution.

Other nutritional abnormalities have been noted in these cases with the syndrome, such as Vitamin B12 deficiency, and there is a high incidence of gastric atrophy in these patients.

So what of the relevance of the Plummer Vinson syndrome in modern practice, for indeed the literature on the subject has not been anything like so common in the last 20 years. Since 1965, we have undertaken 110 gastric pull up operations [5] on patients with hypo-pharyngeal malignancies. In 74 of these patients we believe the malignancy arose in the post-cricoid region. Just over half, i.e. 56 of these patients have been women, so the incidence amongst women is high in our series, as it is in many others. However, detailed evaluation of these patients has shown that in this time period, only 5 of the women had a definite previous history of the Plummer

Vinson syndrome and only 3 had a previous history of hypo-pharyngeal or esophageal webs. The overall incidence of the Plummer Vinson syndrome in this group is therefore 9% in women. There were no cases in men.

This series is therefore in contrast to many of the older publications on the subject and indeed gives rise to a new question – if the Plummer Vinson syndrome is not responsible for the increased incidence of carcinoma in this area in women, then there must still be other factors which require evaluation in the future.

References

1. Patterson DR (1919) Journal of Laryngology 34: 289
2. Kelly AB (1919) Journal of Laryngology 34: 285
3. Vinson PP (1922) Minnesota Medicine 5: 107
4. Trowell HC (1960) Non Infective Disease in Africa. Arnold, London
5. Harrison DFN and Thompson AE (1986) Head and Neck Surgery 8: 418

Myomas

T. Lerut, C. Aelvoet, Y. Leclef, and *J. A. Grüwez* (Leuven)

Although leiomyomas are relatively rare in the gastrointestinal tract, they still are the most frequent tumors of the digestive system. However leiomyomas of the esophagus only comprise 5–10% of all leiomyomas found throughout the entire gastrointestinal tract, the stomach being the most frequent localization. In the esophagus they account for 80% of all benign tumors [6].

It is well known that leiomyomas of the stomach, the gut, or the colon have the potential of degeneration, and differential diagnosis between benign leiomyoma and a tumor with early degeneration can sometimes be very difficult on pathologic examination [4]. In contrast, leiomyomas of the esophagus have the reputation of always being benign, but it seems logical to question whether an esophageal leiomyoma can degenerate.

The most thorough review of the world literature was done by Seremitis who collected 838 cases of leiomyoma [6].

Leiomyoma was most frequently found in the distal or middle third of the esophagus, very seldom in the upper third where the striated muscle is predominant [5]. These tumors present themselves most often as a solitary lesion. Rather exceptionally, multiple tumors are found, or one has to deal with a diffuse leiomyomatosis.

There is a high variability of size and weight with a maximum of 17 cm and 5000 gram, in all sorts of shapes [8]. These tumors are in the muscle coat and are rather mobile. A smooth intact mucosa covers the endoscopically-seen intraluminal protusion. In this regard, the question of taking a biopsy or not remains controversial, since taking a biopsy might jeopardize to some extend the enucleation of the tumor without opening the mucosa.

The treatment is surgical, being a simple enucleation of the tumor in the majority of cases. Only leiomyomas involving an important segment of the esophagus require resection and consequent reconstruction, usually a colon-interposition [6].

Only a couple of cases of malignant degeneration are documented in the literature. The best known case is that of Biasini (1949), where a leiomyoma of 4.5×6 cm was found that contained small zone of leiomyosarcoma [1].

In 1981 Christ described a case of a 70-year old man who had a big tumor in the transition zone of the middle and distal third of the esophagus [3]. The biopsy revealed a myoma. Because of mental illness of this patient, no further treatment was performed. One year later the patient was readmitted because of rapid deteriorisation of his general condition. A repeated biopsy revealed a rhabdomyosarcoma. Of course, the question remains as to whether these sarcomas originally develop from a leiomyoma.

A more recent review of the Anglo Saxon literature by Choh et al. 1986, revealed that leiomyosarcomas are very infrequent and only 45 cases were reported where it was impossible to determine whether these sarcomas were originating from degenerated leiomyomas [2].

The author describes a case of a tumor just proximal to the cardia which clinically, radiologically and endoscopically presented itself as a benign leiomyoma; after simple enucleation, on pathological examination it proved to be a grade II leiomyosarcoma. The patient was asymptomatic up to 14 months postoperatively.

In our department in the period between 1971 to 1986, 22 cases of leiomyoma were treated. All but one were enucleated successfully. One patient presented a diffuse leiomyomatosis of the distal esophagus that needed resection and colon interposition. This patient died of a postoperative complication. All surviving patients were followed up. None of them had any remaining complaints. No recurrence has been observed.

In the literature, a recurrence has been reported in only one patient requiring a second intervention 15 years after the initial intervention [7].

Recently a patient has been referred to our department for further treatment. For a few months she had been complaining of dysphagia and heartburn. The barium swallow showed a small sliding hiatus hernia, in association with a well circumscribed mass 3 cm in diameter, suggestive of leiomyoma. On endoscopy, an intraluminal protrusion with a smooth mucosa lying over it was seen. Biopsy was taken and pathological examination showed no anomalies.

Through a left thoracotomy, a longitudinal myotomy followed by enucleation of a whitish well-circumscribed mobile tumor was performed. In addition, a Belsey Mark IV antireflux procedure was performed for the associated hiatal hernia. Pathological examination revealed a low grade malignant leiomyosarcoma with focal zones of leiomyoblastoma scattered throughout areas of normal smooth muscle fibres. It is however impossible to determine whether this is a degenerated leiomyoma. Resection of the distal esophagus will be carried out in the future. Indeed, a recent study performed on 56 cases of smooth muscle tumors of the gastrointestinal tract followed-up for a minimum of 10 years, showed that even low grade malignant leiomyosarcomas have a high tendency for local recurrence (around 50%), occurring usually after several years (median interval: 4 years) [4].

This case clearly illustrates the need for caution in tumors presenting as benign, and even frozen section are not always able to disclose malignancy. Especially tumors located at the cardia require extra attention, as some of them are probably in fact leiomyomas of the stomach, with a greater potential for malignancy.

Conclusion

Leiomyomas of the esophagus are infrequent, and their degeneration appears to be very exceptional. But the fact that they may degenerate, which can only be confirmed after enucleation or resection, is itself an indication for surgery, regardless of the symptoms.

In these patients enucleation will nearly always be possible, with practically no fatal risks, as shown by Seremitis; over the past 12 years of his review, no postoperative mortality was reported [6].

References

1. Biasini A (1949) Su di un caso di fibroleiomyoma dell'esophago ipobronchiale in transformazione maligna; asportazione per via transpleuro diaframmatica e esophago-gastrostomia guarigione. Pathologica 41: 260–267
2. Choh JH, Khazee AH, Ihm HJ (1986) Leiomyosarcoma of the esophagus. Report of a case and review of the literature. J Surg Onc 32: 223–226
3. Christ F (1981) Maligne Entartung eines Ösophagus myoms. Fortschr Röntgenstr 135, 4: 449–500
4. Evans HL (1985) Smooth muscle tumors of the gastro-intestinal tract. A study of 56 cases followed for a minimum of 10 years. Cancer 56: 2242–2250
5. Piacentini L (1955) Leiomyoma of the esophagus. J Thorac Surg 29: 296–326
6. Seremetis MG, Lyons WS, De Guzman VC, Peabody JW (1976) Leiomyomata of the esophagus. An analysis of 838 cases. Cancer 38: 2166–2177
7. Standerfer RJ, Paneth M (1982) Recurrent leiomyoma of the esophagus. Thorax 37: 478–479
8. Vantrappen G, Pringot J (1974) Benign tumors and cysts of the esophagus. Diseases of the esophagus (1974) Vantrappen G, Hellemans J (eds): Springer, New York, 431–446

Diverticula

R. Giuli (Paris)

It is not uncommon to find diverticula in a cancerous esophagus, and in such cases it is obviously not possible to speak of malignant change (Figs. 1, 2). On the other hand, cases where the two processes may be causally linked are extremely rare and out of 221 diverticula resected, this possibility was considered on only two occasions: once at midthoracic level and once with an epiphrenic diverticulum (Figs. 3, 4).

This degree of rarity makes it impossible regard these cancers as the outcome of possible diverticular esophagitis, but rather as a simple coincidence.

While the discovery of neoplastic cells in a diverticulectomy specimen in very elderly subjects may suggest that the limited excision practised has been sufficient, the long and silent previous development of this lesion is often an index of inoperability.

However, the possibility of such an association must be recognized, to justify regular surveillance of a patient suffering from a diverticulum whose excision has not

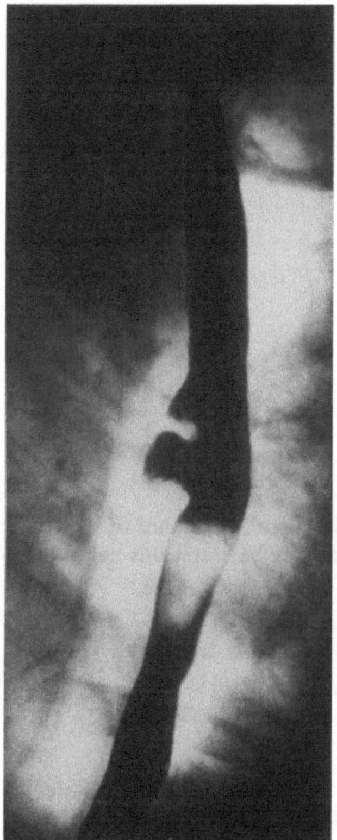

Fig. 1. Diverticulum associated with esophageal cancer

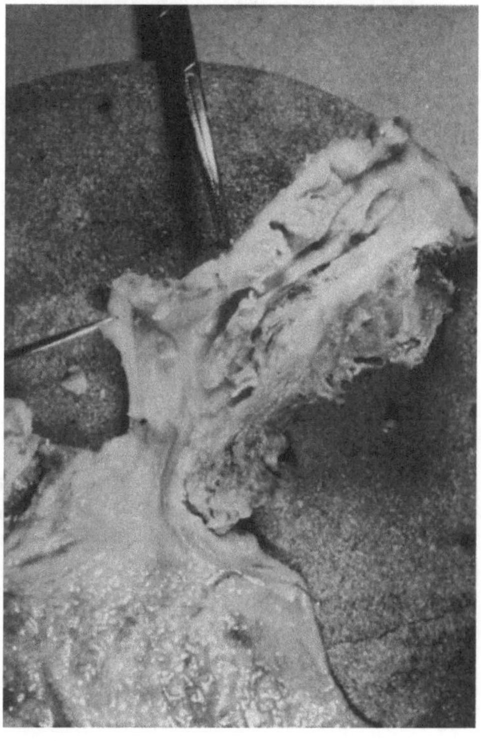

Fig. 2. Resected specimen

been considered necessary. It may happen that localized features of esophagitis produce a modification of the symptoms and very suspect appearances at endoscopy, which may, as in this patient (Fig. 5), be worsened by the biopsy.

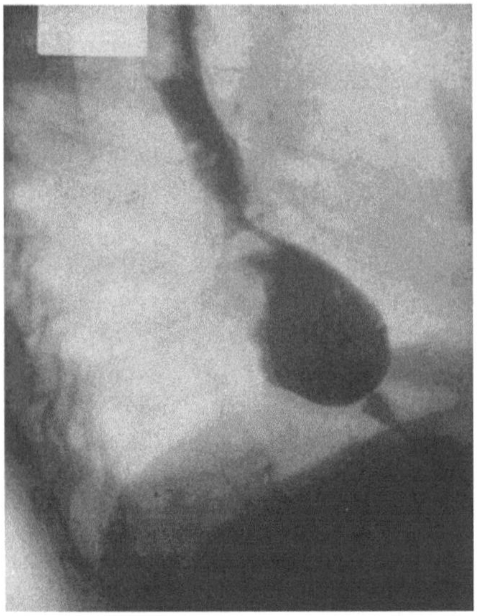

Fig. 3. Carcinoma in an epiphrenic diverticulum

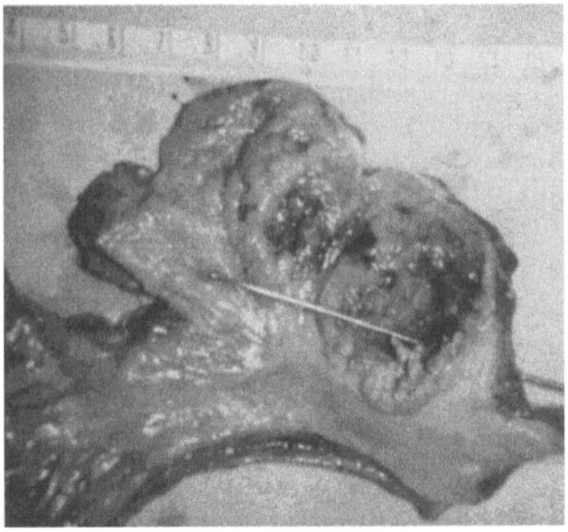

Fig. 4. Resected specimen

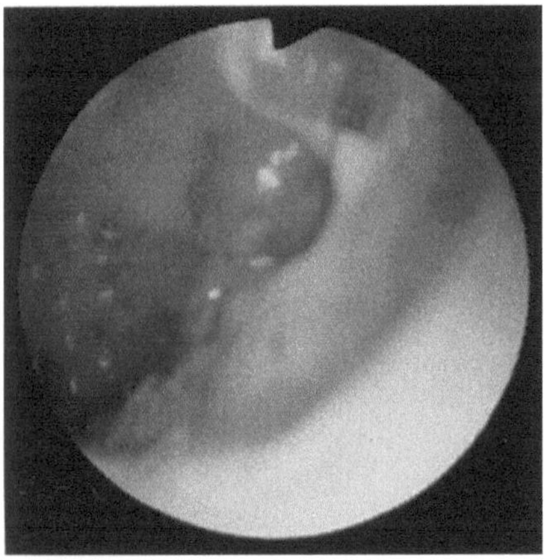

Fig. 5. The endoscopic appearance of the edge of a diverticulum may be suspicious because of esophagitis

C. A. Hiebert (Portland)

Given the probability of surface active ingested carcinogens as factors in the genesis of esophageal cancer, one would expect esophageal diverticula at any level to be targeted for malignant change. This double problem was first reported by Pitt in 1896 [1] but fewer than 50 cases have been found in the world literature in the ensuing 91 years [2]. In the Portland experience, there is but a single case for an incidence of well under 1%. These tumors are most common in Zenker's diverticula but are occasionally seen in traction or pulsion diverticula at a lower level. Translation of published anecdotes into incidence is rather meaningless; suffice it to say, the condition is rare. It is important nonetheless to be aware of the possibility during the workup and treatment of any patient with a diverticulum especially if one is performing a diverticulopexy rather than an excision [3].

References

1. Pitt GN (1896) Epithelioma and oesophageal pouch. Trans Pathol Soc Lond 47:44
2. Fujita H et al. (1980) Carcinoma within a middle esophageal (parabronchial) diverticulum: a case report and a review of the literature. JPN Surg 10:142. (Reported by Postlethwait in Surgery of the Esophagus. Second Edition, Page 145, Publisher Appleton-Century-Crofts, 1986)
3. Hiebert CA (1976) Surgery for cricopharyngeal dysfunction under local anesthesia. Am J Surg 131:423–427

T. Lerut, C. Aelvoet, Y. Leclef, and *J. A. Grüwez* (Leuven)

The increasing application of endoscopy has contributed to a great extent to the fact that the pharyngoesophageal diverticulum is being diagnosed more frequently and more accurately nowadays. The surgical treatment of this condition has become a fairly simple and safe procedure with excellent functional results.

This explains the increasing number of series published over the last two decades, and degeneration within the diverticulum has been described sporadically.

A review of the Western literature reveals about 50 cases of degeneration within the diverticulum, all of which were a spinocellular carcinoma [1–7]. The largest reported series is that of the Mayo Clinic, with 4 cases out of 549 treated between 1932 and 1982 [3].

This leads us to the conclusion that the incidence of degeneration of a Zenker's diverticulum is about one in 300 to 400 patients (0.30%–0.25%). This incidence is more than one hundred times the incidence of esophageal cancer on the whole, which is estimated to be around 3.5 per 100000 patients per year.

On careful examination some of the published cases show the tumor in the region of the cricopharygeal muscle and/or the hypopharynx, with a concomitant Zenker's diverticulum, with or without tumor invasion. It is difficult in these patients to state if the tumor developed primarily in the diverticulum or not. But in still more than half the patients, the tumor did not extend beyond the border of the diverticulum, bringing the real incidence to 1/500–1/600 cases. These cases are especially interesting since these well circumscribed tumors produce no other symptoms than the symptoms related to the diverticulum and the technical examinations will not necessarily make any contribution. A barium swallow will show only a small impression within the sac of the diverticulum, which would be very difficult to differentiate from impacted food [2].

Endoscopy offers a better way to diagnose these tumors, and requires a careful wash-out of all food remaining in the sac.

All growths within the sac are strongly suspect since almost none of these have ever been shown to be benign. All infiltrations of the wall are likewise suspect, and should be biopsied for pathological examination. However, endoscopy of a Zenker's diverticulum, with a biopsy of the mucosal lining remains potentially dangerous with special danger of perforation; this examination is therefore not accepted by everyone as a routine preoperative examination.

The diagnosis is often only made at operation, when tumor mass can be felt within the sac. The nature of the tumor is confirmed by frozen section.

In a few cases, only small lesions were present, and the diagnosis was only made postoperatively by the pathologist.

There is no clear understanding of the etiology of these degenerations. Longstanding evolution, with stagnation of food, could be a source of chronic irritation that could cause degeneration, although degeneration has been seen as early as six months after the diagnosis of a Zenker's diverticulum was made [3].

Gaillard [2] stated that irritation of the diverticulum by continuous compression against the cervical spine could be a predisposing factor. Surgical procedures vary from simple resection of the diverticulum to a pharyngo-laryngectomy, with stripping of the esophagus, with gastric pull-up or colon interposition for the reconstruction [6]. Few cases were treated with radiotherapy.

In general, the prognosis of a degenerated Zenker's diverticulum is bad. Survival of more than 2 years is seldom. Nevertheless, this bad prognosis is strongly related to the original spread into the surrounding structures, and also to the possible involvement of the lymph nodes. Two patients recently reported from the Mayo Clinic [3] showed a survival of 8 and 4.5 years after resection of the diverticulum. The first patient had a tumor of 2 cm in size, which on anatomo-pathological examination was a carcinoma in situ. A complete removal was performed. The second patient had a polyp-type lesion of $1.5 \times 1 \times 0.2$ cm. An invasive squamous cell carcinoma was diagnosed at pathological examination. A complete removal was also performed.

The question of the surgical treatment of Zenker's diverticulum arises as a consequence of these observations.

The presence of an occult carcinoma favours resection combined with a myotomy above the diverticulopexy, combined with a myotomy. In the latter method there is no opening of the lumen, avoiding the danger of fistulas and abscesses. If this method is chosen, a careful preoperative endoscopy is mandatory, together with careful palpation of the diverticulum during the operation.

In our series of 85 diverticulopexies and myotomies between 1976 and 1986, no case of carcinoma was diagnosed. All patients have been followed and up to now no degeneration was seen. This compares with the literature where no case of degeneration after diverticulopexy or endoscopic treatment was seen [7].

Conclusion

A pharyngo-esophageal diverticulum has a higher incidence of degeneration into a squamous cell epithelioma carcinoma, the incidence being higher than in the general population. However, this does not make it a real premalignant condition. Urgent diverticulectomy is not necessary for every Zenker's diverticulum.

The most important indication for surgery remains the risk of aspiration pneumonia and nutritional deficit.

Surgical treatment involving resection and myotomy, or diverticulopexy and myotomy, seems to be an effective means of preventing carcinoma.

Carcinoma is most often found in very large, longstanding diverticula.

Surgery is the preferred treatment of a degenerated diverticulum. Prognosis is related to its spread into surrounding structures and lymph node involvement.

In small tumors, resection of the diverticulum seems to be sufficient, with good chances for cure. This last observation is an additional argument to treat every Zenker's diverticulum surgically, regardless of its symptoms.

References

1. Andrieu-Guitrancourt J (1984) Cancer in pharyngo-oesophageal diverticulum. Report of 2 cases. J Fr Otorhinolaryngol 33 (4), 183–188
2. Gaillard J, Hagenauer, Pignal JL, Dubreuil C (1980) Cancérisation d'un diverticule pharyngo-œsophagien. J Fr Otorhinolaryngol 26: 400–403
3. Huang BS, Unni KK, Payne WS (1984) Long term survival following diverticulectomy for cancer in pharyngo-oesophageal (Zenker's) diverticulum. Ann Thor Surg 38: 207–210
4. Johnson JT, Curtin HD (1985) X-ray study of the *month*. Carcinoma associated with Zenker's diverticulum. Ann Otol Rhinol Laryngol 94: 324–325
5. Michot F, Liegois A, Lecomte D, Huguet D (1979) Cancérisation d'un diverticule pharyngo-œsophagien. J Chir 116: 117–118
6. Pech A, Reboud E, Cannoni M, Thomassin JM (1981) La cancérisation d'un diverticule pharyngo-œsophagien. J Fr Otorhinolaryngol 30: 113–116
7. Zonneville JA, Waldeck KJJ, Hamming JJ (1981) Carcinoma in situ in a pharyngo-oesophageal diverticulum. The Netherl J Surg, 33–2, 94–97

M. Rossetti (Liestal)

Among the 66 pharyngo-esophageal diverticula that we operated between 1960 and 1986, we met two squamous-cell carcinomas. Their diagnosis which was a pathological one, was not expected on the basis of the X-ray examination. One of them was a fungating tumor of 2 cm diameter and the other one was an early carcinoma.

One esophago-tracheal fistula with a malignant degeneration developed on a traction diverticulum among the 6 diverticula of this type that we operated because of airway fistula, perforation, or dysphagia in the middle esophagus. We did not have any cancer in our 7 epiphrenic diverticula. In summary (Table), among the 79 operated diverticula, we found 2 malignant degenerations (2.5%) and one carcinoma with a possible relationship to a traction diverticulum.

Table

79	operated diverticula (1960–87)	
66	pharyngo-esophageal	
	2	squamous-cell carcinoma:
	1	2 cm diameter
	1	early-cancer
7	epiphrenic diverticula (no cancers)	
6	traction diverticula	
	1 malignant air-ways-fistula	

J. R. Siewert (Munich)

In my experience, it is nearly not necessary to discuss the problem of cancer development in diverticula.

In our department we operated on 67 patients with esophageal diverticula during the last 5 years (50 patients with cervical diverticula, 14 patients with an epiphrenic diverticulum). No carcinoma was seen in these patients. In only one patient did we have a problem of diagnosis because of the *coincidence* between a cervical diverticulum and a cervical esophageal cancer below the diverticulum.

In the literature, there are only a few case reports dealing with this problem. This is an analysis of the publications during the last 10 years. We have found 24 case reports on cancer in cervical diverticula, 5 case reports on cancer in so-called parabronchial diverticula and 10 on epiphrenic diverticula. If we believe the data coming from the Mayo-Clinic, the frequency is 0.3% (Fig. 1).

Nevertheless, it seems that it is not necessary to consider this problem in indication of surgery of diverticula or in the choice of surgical procedure. For example it is not an argument against diverticulopexy, provided that a good endoscopy is performed preoperatively.

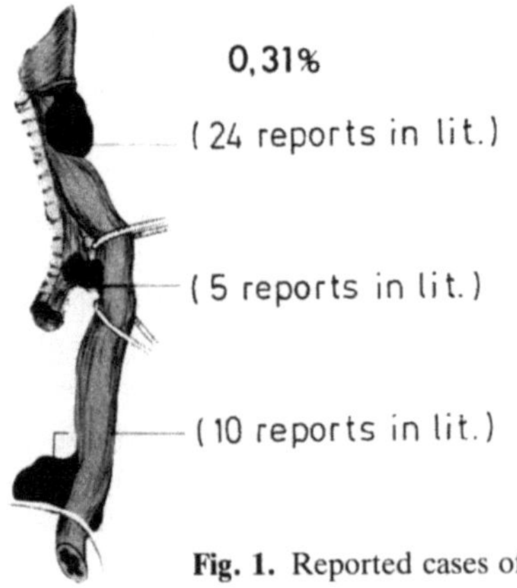

Fig. 1. Reported cases of cancers in diverticula

What is the prognostic significance of esophageal papillomas?

A. Galian, and *A. Lavergne* (Paris)

In contrast to condylomas at other localizations (skin, anogenital area), squamous cell papillomas or condylomas of the esophagus have not been frequently documented [2, 4, 6, 8]. They are rare lesions, as only about 60 cases have been reported.

Esophageal squamous cell papillomas or condylomas are presently considered as probably viral-induced lesions, due to human papilloma virus (HPV), and have definite histological criteria, which permit them to be differentiated from other esophageal lesions such as esophagitis and the common papilloma.

Clinical and fiberoptic endoscopy features

No clinical symptom calls attention to an esophageal condyloma. Fiberoptic endoscopy, generally performed for epigastralgia (gastritis, peptic ulceration, hiatus hernia), shows a prominent white esophageal lesion, 1–5 mm in diameter or simple erythema in any localization.

Histologic characters

The histologic features of these lesions have been defined by analogy to their homologues, especially in anogenital areas (uterus cervix) and show three architectural types: the flat, the papillomatous, and the inverted condylomas [6, 8] (Figs. 1, 2). It is noteworthy that the papillomatous type may only be recognized by fiberoptic endoscopy. The histologic criteria are:

a) acanthosis with hyperkeratosis and papillomatosis;
b) sharpness of the border between the deep and superficial layers of the esophageal epithelium;
c) cellular alterations, located in the superficial layers and showing a dyskeratosis of the superficial cells, single cell dyskeratosis, multinucleation and particularly koilocytosis (Figs. 3, 4).

For Syrjänen [6, 7], at least six of these parameters have to be present to make the diagnosis. However this diagnosis should not be made without the presence of koilocytosis, although this author observed poilocytosis only in 40% of supposed condylomas. The condyloma, using these histologic criteria, has to be differentiated from simple esophagitis, also showing acanthosis, papillomatosis and sometimes cellular lesions such as dyskeratosis. It is the same for the esophageal common papilloma, histologically very close to condyloma, because of the presence of acanthosis, papillomatosis, dyskeratosis and hyperkeratosis. In esophagitis and

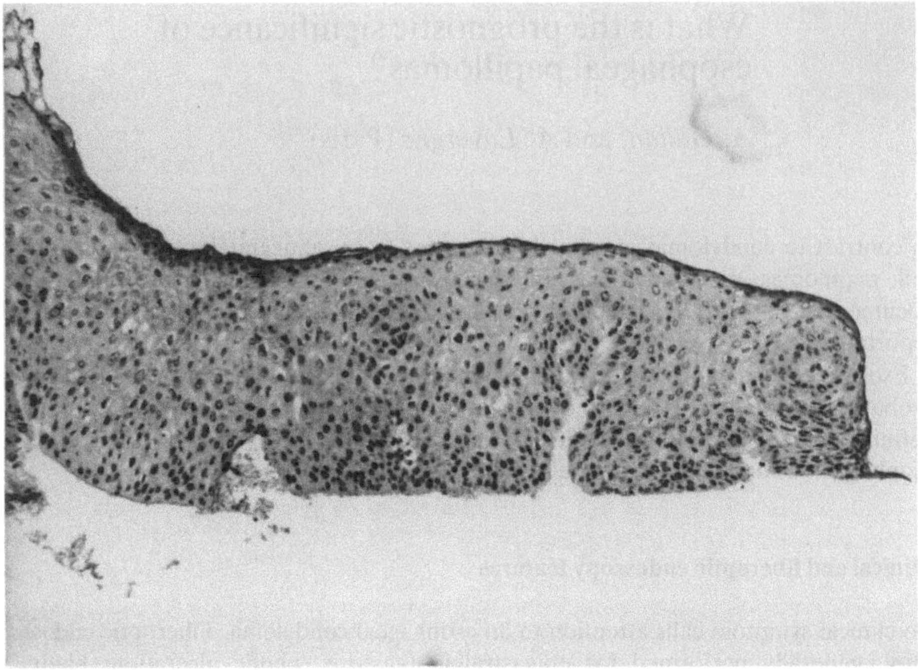

Fig. 1. A flat esophageal condyloma without papillomatosis but with acanthosis and parakeratosis (H&E×100)

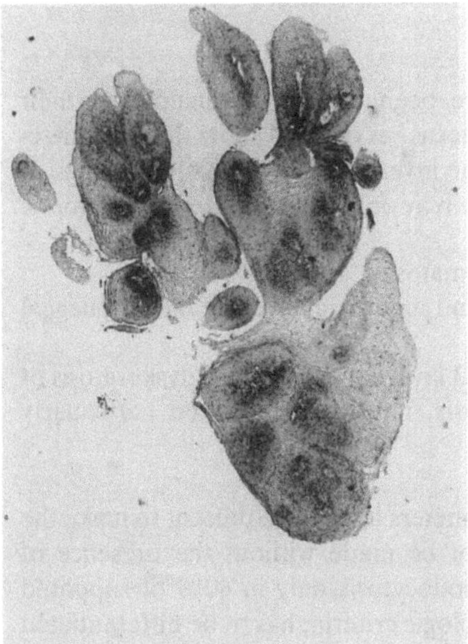

Fig. 2. A small esophageal papillomatous condyloma (H&E×45)

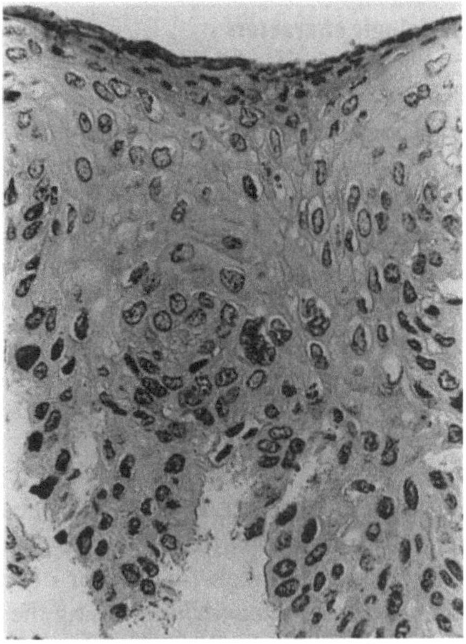

Fig. 3. The flat condyloma shows multinucleated cells, mitosis and parakeratosis (H&E×250)

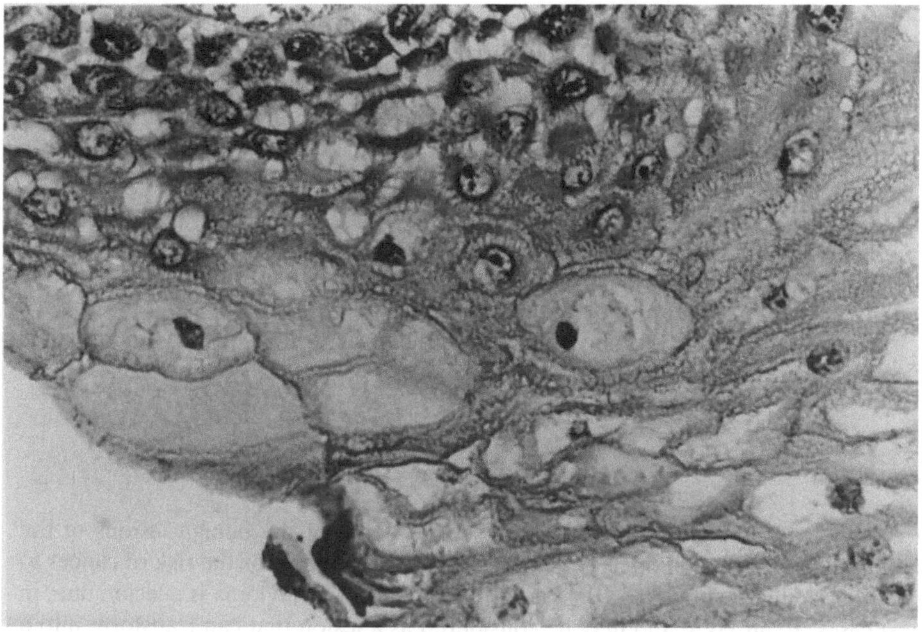

Fig. 4. The koilocytic cell shows a cytoplasmic vacuolization and a hyperchromatic pyknotic nucleus (H&E×400)

common papilloma, however, koilocytosis and multinucleated cells are not observed.

Evolutive data

It is actually well established that squamous cell carcinomas of the uterus cervix may develope in preexisting condylomas that are due to HPV [1]. Condylomas have been observed in surgical specimens of esophageal squamous cell carcinomas, in a study of 60 cases, showing 40% with condylomas [6, 8]. A connection between the two lesions has therefore been suggested. Moreover, immunologic studies, using anti-HPV or anti-bovine papilloma virus antisera, have shown the presence of intranuclear antigens in koilocytic cells and in many of the superficial dyskeratotic cells of condylomas in 30% of cases [4, 7, 8]. More recently, by the in situ DNA hybridization method, it has been demonstrated that some squamous cell carcinomas contained the HPV DNA [3], but this was not constant [5].

Future prospects

These studies are still insufficient but they allow us establishment of plan for future studies, including:

1. systematic fiberoptic endoscopy biopsy on any salient or flat esophageal lesion.
2. search for histologic criteria of condylomas on any esophageal lesion.
3. histoimmunological study of esophageal condylomas by usual method, and, if possible, by molecular probes, to prove the presence of HPV and its type or types. It has effectively been shown that HPV 16 and 18 are observed in uterine carcinomas whereas HPV 6 and 11 are only found in benign lesions [1].
4. study of the esophageal condyloma-carcinoma association on surgical samples with immunologic search for HPV.
5. complete fiberoptic endoscopy resection of any esophageal condyloma, when only partial biopsies were performed the first time.
6. regular fiberoptic endoscopy control with biopsies, in patients with previous esophageal condylomas, to detect recurrences.

Conclusion

It is actually possible to answer the question: "Some of the benign lesions of the esophagus, such as papillomas (or condylomas) are too rare for the risk of cancer to be evaluated but it should be considered." Esophageal condyloma is a lesion due, in most cases, to an HPV and may be considered as a lesion that can transform into a squamous cell carcinoma; it has to be diagnosed with precise histologic criteria. Research must be performed to be able to determine in particular the type or types of HPV implicated in the development of the condylomas and the eventual carcinoma.

References

1. Danos O (1986) Papillomavirus: Progrès récents. Path Biol 34: 971–973
2. Hille JJ, Markowitz S, Margolius K, Isaacson C (1985) Human papillomavirus and carcinoma of the esophagus. N Engl J Med 312: 1707
3. Kulski J, Demeter T, Sterrett GF, Shilkin KB (1986) Human papillomavirus DNA in oesophageal carcinoma. Lancet 11, 683–684
4. Lesec G, Gogusev J, Fermaud H, Gorce D, Lemaitre JP, Verdier A (1985) Présence d'un antigène viral de groupe "papilloma" dans un condylome oesophagien chez l'homme. Gastroentérol Clin Biol 9: 166–168
5. Ostrow RS, Manias DA, Fong WJ, Zachow KR, Faras AJ (1987) A survey of human cancers for human papillomavirus DNA by filter hybridization. Cancer 59: 429–434
6. Syrjanen KJ (1982) Histological changes identical to those of condylomatous lesions found in esophageal squamous cell carcinomas. Arch Geschwulstforsch 52: 283–292
7. Syrjanen KJ, Pyrhonen S, Aukee S, Koskela E (1982) Squamous cell papilloma of the oesophagus: a tumour probably caused by human papilloma virus (HPV). Diagn Histopathol 5: 291–296
8. Winkler B, Capo V, Reumann W, Ma A, La Porta R, Reilly S, Green P, Richart RM, Crum CP (1985) Human papilloma-virus infection of the esophagus. A clinico-pathologic study with demonstration of papillomavirus antigen by the immunoperoxidase technique. Cancer 55: 149–155

Can esophageal keratosis be considered as a precancerous lesion?

J. Gastard, J. F. Bretagne, M. Gosselin, and *M. P. Ramée* (Rennes)

Esophageal keratosis is a rare condition corresponding to a complete keratinisation of the esophageal epithelium [1, 4].

Symptoms: Heartburn, dysphagia and gastrointestinal hemorrhage may reveal hyperkeratosis, but these symptoms are related to associated conditions, mostly gastro-esophageal reflux [1–4].

Endoscopy: Hyperkeratosis corresponds to white plaques, a few millimetres up to a few centimetres in size. On close inspection, the whitish thickening shows longitudinal and transversal lines, mimicing a mosaioscopic. Treatment with 5% lugol reveals the iodonegative nature of the plaque and outlines clear cut margins [1].

Pathology: Histologic examination shows a complete keratinisation of the esophageal epithelium corresponding to orthokeratosis. Superficial epithelial cells are completely keratinisated, and do not contain cell nuclei, but keratohyalin granules. The deeper layer shows no hyperplasia or elongation of vascular papillae. There is no dysplasia or fungal hyphae.

Diagnosis: Hyperkeratosis must be distinguished from other histological entities appearing also as white plaques. These conditions may be associated with an abnormal keratinisation, most commonly parakeratosis. These entities are of diverse origin:

1. Benign lesions

White exudates of peptic and mycotic esophagitis are easily recognized. Glycogenic acanthosis [12] is the commonest cause of esophageal plaques. Histologically, the epithelium is thickened, due to an obvious increase in the glycogenfilled layer above the basal zone. Esophageal papillomas are described as lowdomed plaques, having irregular acanthosis and sometimes, perinuclear cytoplasmic vacuolation of the superficial cells. Occasionnally, keratinisation may occur [12]. Esophageal white plaques are also described in Darrier's disease.

2. Possibly precancerous lesions

An abnormal keratinisation (mostly parakeratosis) occurs frequently in some conditions, contrasting to its rarity in autopsy findings (2 p. 1000) [9].

- In alcoholic cirrhotic patients, esophageal leucoplakia occurs in 49% of the patients. In this condition, abnormal keratinisation is associated with acanthosis or atrophy, cellular atypia of the stratum spinosum, inflammatory cell infiltration of the lamina propria and elongation of the papillae.

- In esophageal squamous cell carcinomas, the adjacent mucosa frequently shows hyperkeratotic plaques. In regions with high incidence of squamous cell carcinomas, such as Guriev county, esophageal white plaques are frequently observed [10].
- In Kelly-Patterson's disease, atrophy of the mucosa and muscle is frequently associated with epithelial hyperkeratosis. This condition is frequently complicated with occurrence of squamous cell carcinoma [8].

3. Cancerous lesions

White plaques may also correspond to severe dysplastic lesions or in situ carcinomas. This endoscopic aspect represents 8.6% of the in situ carcinomas in the Wang's series [11] and was described in 3 out of 18 cases by Monnier et al [7].

Etiology: pathogenesis of esophageal keratosis is unknown. The frequently associated peptic esophagitis raises the role of a chronic irritative process.

Follow up: healing of peptic esophagitis does not change keratotic lesions [1–4). The development of esophageal carcinoma was never described.

Conclusion

Keratinisation of esophageal epithelium, corresponding to parakeratosis, is frequently observed in cancerous lesions and in populations with a high incidence of esophageal carcinomas.

Orthokeratosis is rarely described in these conditions. At this time, orthokeratosis would seem to be a benign esophageal process. Additional studies of a larger number of cases are necessary to determine the malignant potential.

References

1. Bretagne JF, Ramee MP, Gosselin M, Gastard J (1982) Kératose de l'œsophage associée à une sténose peptique. Gastroenterol Clin Biol 6: 869–871
2. Etienne JP, Delavierre P, Petite JP, Sauleau P (1969) Les leucoplasies œsophagiennes au cours des cirrhoses. Sem Hôp Paris 45: 1589–1596
3. Ferey L, Herlin, Marnay J, Jacob JH, de Raucourt D, Gignoux M, Segol P, Ollivier JM, Mandard AM (1985) Histology and ultra structure of the human esophageal epithelium; normal and parakeratotic epithelium. J Submicrosc Cytol 17, 4: 651–665
4. Herschman BR, Uppaputhangkule V, Maas L, Gelzayd E (1978) Esophageal leukoplasia: a rare entity. Jama 239: 2021
5. Larregue M, Katz M, Gasquet C, Lansmann M, Bressieux JM (1977) Localisations œsophagiennes de la dyskeratose folliculaire, maladie de Darier. Description radiologique. A propos de 4 cas. Ann Med Interne (Paris) 128: 487–492
6. Mandard AM, Marnay J, Gignoux M, Segol P, Blanc L, Ollivier JM, Borel B, Mandard JC (1984) Cancer of the esophagus and associated lesions: detailed pathologic study of 100 esophagectomy specimens. Human pathology 15, 7: 660–669

7. Monnier P, Savary M, Pasch R, Anani P (1980) Intraepithelial carcinoma of the esophagus endoscopic morphology. Endoscopy 12: s1–s7
8. Nemours-Auguste S, Barag N (1979) Le syndrome de Kelly Patterson in: l'œsophage: la déglutition. Expansion Scientifique Française, Paris: 809–816
9. Postlethwait RW, Wendelle-Musser A (1974) Changes in the esophagus in 1000 autopsy specimens. J Thorac Cardiovasc Surg 68: 953–956
10. Sakhipov N (1983) Pathomorphologic characteristics of esophageal biopsies among inhabitants of an endemic focus of cancer of the esophagus. Arch Pathol 45, 9: 48–54
11. Wang GQ (1981) Endoscopic diagnosis of early esophageal carcinoma J of the Royal Society of Medicine 74: 502–503
12. Whitehead R (1985) Esophageal plaques and miscellaneous conditions in: Mucosal biopsy of the gastro intestinal tract. Ed WB Saunders Company, Philadelphia: 22–29

What is the association between granular cell tumors of the esophagus and cancer?

J. A. Paolaggi, M. Algard, F. Ferrandi, J. Leymarios, and *G. Molas* (Paris)

Granular cell tumor of the esophagus (GCT) was first described in 1926 by Abrikossoff. It is rare and almost always benign [1]. We have recently observed five cases. They may lead, in some circumstances, to a delicate differentiation from malignant tumors.

– *Incidence*: Granular cell tumors are submucous and their usual localization is the mouth (30 to 35%), the skin and the subcutaneous tissue (20%) [5]. The gastrointestinal tract localization of GCT is rare, about 6% [10]. Localization in the esophagus is exceptional. However, among the cases of gastrointestinal tract localization, GCT of the esophagus is not rare (observed 34 times out of 75 cases by Johnston [9]). In comparison with benign tumors of the esophagus, Farrel of the Mayo Clinic [6] only found 3 Abrikossoff tumors out of 246 benign tumors.

– *Histogenesis*: This has been an object of controversy for a long time. The myogenetic theory initially expressed by Abrikossoff, as well as the histiocytary theory [12] have been abandoned. Currently, most authors agree as to a neurological origin based on the ultrastructural, histoenzymic, and cellular culture criteria [3, 7].

– *Age, Sex and Race*: Mean age of GCT discovery was 42.5 years ranging from 12 to 65 years in the 70 cases described (65 in the literature and 5 personal observations). The sex ratio (female/male) was 0.87. Black race preponderance could not be appreciated since, in many cases, race was not reported.

– *Topography*: The esophagus GCT are usually found in the lower third part. Double localization may exist (7 out of 60) as well as a triple localization. The tumor is usually unique but it may be associated with GCT located in other sites such as pharynx, trachea, pericardium, skin, bronchi, subcutaneous tissue, arytenoid cartilage [5].

– *Discovery*: GCT are often latent. They can be discovered during endoscopy or surgical intervention, or even at post mortem. Dysphagia it the most common complaint and retrosternal pain or uneasiness have been reported 11 times out of 60.
– *X-ray*: This often normal since the lesion is of submucous nature. One may however find a smooth lacunar image with a regular notch of barium or narrowing of the esophagus on profile.
– *Endoscopy*: Endoscopy is the fundamental examination since it allows biopsy. Most often the lesion is smooth, well-limited, yellowish-white or polypoid. It may also be totally submucous or have a central crater. Multiple as well as deep biopsies must be practiced because of the submucous localization of the lesion. In 80% of the cases, diagnosis is obtained from biopsy [5].
– *Histology*: The histologic aspect is identical whatever the site of the lesion. The tumor is composed of cells piled together, sometimes in rows, sometimes anastomosed. Cytoplasm is abundant and notable for granules deeply coloured by PAS. Tumors are either well-limited or badly limited and infiltrating. Surface malpighian epithelium may show a pseudo epitheliomatous hyperplasia. According to Johnston and Helwig [9] this may be responsible for interpretation errors and lead to wrong diagnosis of epidermoid carcinoma. This aspect, or an acanthosis are noted in 50% of cases. Present histologic data lead to the belief that the risk of malignant transformation is very low or exceptional [10, 13]. However, cases with node involvement have been reported. In effect, there are no histologic criteria for malignancy, and distant metastasis is the only sign permitting a diagnosis of malignancy.

– *GCT and Cancer*: The association of GCT and cancer is not exceptional and is not specific to esophagus localization. Its frequency is estimated at 10% [4]. The associated cancer is usually a bronchial, a larynx or an esophagus carcinoma. A lymphoma has been reported [4, 13]. The cancer is usually discovered after GCT of the esophagus. Owing to the low number of cases, it is difficult to establish a relationship between these two lesions. However, alcoholism and excessive tobacco consumption, frequent in these patients, must lead to a systematic search for an associated cancer.
– *Treatment, Natural History and Prognosis*: The treatment depends on the size of the tumor as well as on the clinical symptoms. When the tumor is nonsymptomatic, small, and the patient is aged, treatment is not necessary. When the tumor is small (less than 5 mm) excision at biopsy is enough. According to Bigard et al [2], endoscopic excision by diathermy is justified for tumors with diameters less than 30 mm. In the case of tumors measuring less than 20 mm, a 24 hour follow-up after endoscopic excision seems enough [2]. 8 to 10 days follow-up is necessary when the tumor is large since hemorrhages linked to scar formation have been reported [4].

Surgical excision is justified for large tumors, enucleation being the best treatment. Segment resection may be considered when enucleation seems dangerous or when inflammatory phenomena are present near the tumor. Prognosis is usually good, whatever treatment is used.

References

1. Abrikossoff AL (1926) Über Myome, ausgehend von der quergestreiften willkürlichen Muskulatur. Virchows Arch Path Anat 260:215–233
2. Bigard MA, Gaucher P, Champigneulle B, Brucker P (1983) Tumeurs à cellules granuleuses de l'œsophage. A propos de 6 cas récents. Gastroenterol clin Biol 7:1044–1045
3. Chomette G, Auriol M, Tereau Y, Guilbert F (1980) La tumeur à cellules granuleuses: schwannome granulo-cellulaire? Etude histoenzymologique et ultrastructurale. Arch Anat Cytol Path 28:365–370
4. Doffoel M coll (1983) Tumeurs à cellules granuleuses de l'œsophage. A propos d'un cas associé à un carcinome bronchique et traité par exérèse endoscopique. Gastroenterol Clin Biol: 591–595
5. Elhadad A, Piquet F, Slama JL, Godefroy Y, Paugam B (1984) La tumeur à cellules granuleuses de l'œsophage. Revue de la littérature. A propos d'un cas. Ann Chir 38:441–445
6. Farrel KH, Devine KD, Harrisson ED Jr, Ols AM (1973) Granular cell of the esophagus, incidence and surgical treatment. Ann Otol Rhinol Laryngol 82:784–789
7. Gertsch P, Mosimann R (1980) A rare tumor of the esophagus: the granular cell myoblastoma – Report of a case in review of the literature. Endoscopy 12:245–249
8. Hivet M, Roupret B, Ladouch-Badre A, De Muynck L (1980) Tumeur à cellules granuleuses de l'œsophage: tumeur d'Abrikossoff, Ann Chir 34:487–490
9. Johnston J, Helwig EB (1981) Granular cell tumors of the gastrointestinal tract and perianal region. A study of 74 cases. Dig Dis Sci 26:807–816
10. Lebas de Lacour JC, Jammet P, Christoforov B, Pequignot H (1982) Les localisations œsophagiennes du myoblastome à cellules granuleuses dites tumeurs d'Abrikossoff. Sem Hôp Paris, 383–386
11. Lehn E, Collery P, Salas H, Pluot M, Levasseur JC (1981) Association d'une tumeur à cellules granuleuses et d'un cancer de l'œsophage. J Chir Paris 118:325–329
12. Leroux R, Delarue J (1939) Sur trois cas de tumeurs à cellules granuleuses de la cavité buccale. Bull Ass Fraç Cancer 28:427–447
13. Tune JM, Bowles MH, Grunow WA, Patel GK, Texter EC Jr (1981) Granular cell myoblastoma of the esophagus. Am J Gastroenterol 75:426–430

Megaesophagus

Isn't treatment by repeated dilatations a factor of chronic mucosal irritation?

H. W. Pinotti, I. Cecconello, V. Felix, and *B. Zilberstein*
(Sao Paulo)

Hydrostatic dilatation of the cardia, when indicated in the management of megaesophagus, is performed with a rubber balloon developed in our Department [1, 2]. The distal segment of the balloon is more distensible, it is easily positioned and consequently its efficiency is increased and the risk of the procedure decreased.

The mercury tip facilitates passage of the balloon through the cardia. Following a 12 hour fast and with the patient seated, the balloon is introduced orally after topical anesthesia of the oropharynx. When the end of the balloon is felt to be in the stomach, the first 50 ml of water are introduced, distending the distal segment of the balloon. Traction on the balloon positions it adequately, and the increasing volume of water dilates the terminal esophagus until the patient complains of pain; this serves as a limit to complete the procedure. It provides a margin of safety, considerably reducing morbidity, avoiding esophageal rupture. This technique is illustrated in Fig. 1, and the results in Fig. 2.

Dilatation of the cardia is a valid method in the management of megaesophagus so long as it is indicated, and cures or alleviates dysphagia after the first or at most 2 or 3 sessions. It should not be used indiscriminately, but restricted to early cases of megaesophagus. It may even be used under special circumstances, such as to improve weight loss and malnutrition, or even during pregnancy, even in more advanced stages of the disease when the correct indication would be surgical.

In our Department, surgery is recommended when the results of two or three dilatations have not been satisfactory. In many cases, especially in young muscular men where distension of the terminal esophagus is difficult because of the rigid diaphragmatic muscles reducing the chances of effective dilatation, surgery is the treatment of choice.

A follow up of 146 cases of megaesophagus submitted to the procedure show that 45.28% were cured of dysphagia, while 54.10% required new dilatations. 3.42% (4 cases) of rupture and 2 deaths (1.37%) were reported, in spite of all precautions and attempting to stop the water flow as soon as the patient reported feeling pain.

A review of 1041 cases of Chagasic megaesophagus in the Brazilian literature (4 references) reported satisfactory results with various methods of dilatation of the cardia, but always with some morbidity and mortality. The same is true of 6637 cases of idiopathic megaesophagus (33 references) in the international literature (Table 1).

Another important point is the possibility of reflux esophagitis occurring after the procedure: in 1967 we demonstrated that dilatation can rupture the muscle at the region of the lower esophageal sphincter, lowering it's pressure. Endoscopy done immediately after dilatation was able to demonstrate erosions, small hematomas,

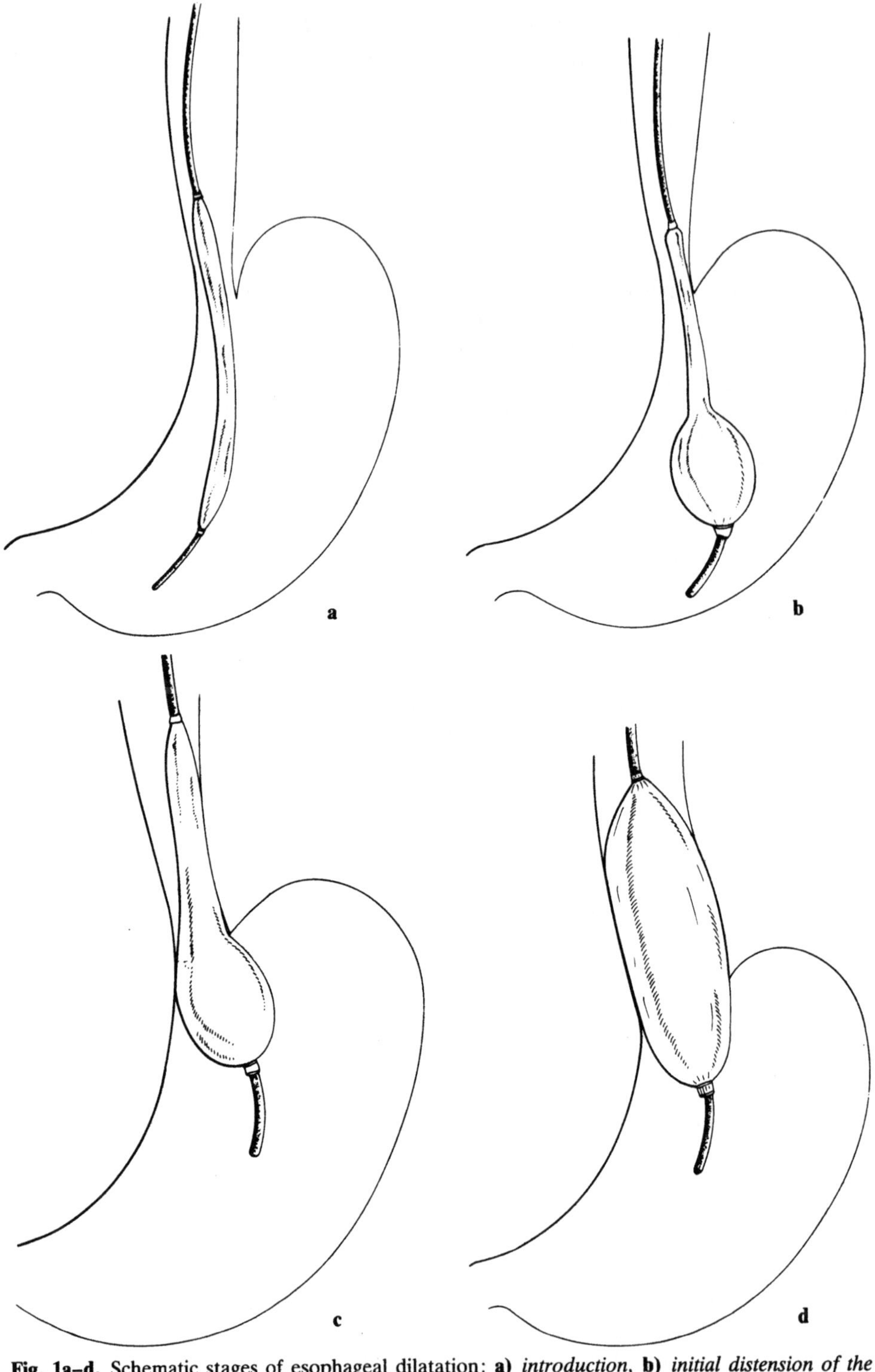

Fig. 1a–d. Schematic stages of esophageal dilatation: **a)** *introduction,* **b)** *initial distension of the balloon,* **c)** *balloon anchored at the cardia,* **d)** *forceful dilatation of the distal esophagus*

Table 1. Results of dilatation of the cardia

Megaesophagus	Cases	Good Results	Esophagitis	Perforation	Deaths
Chagasic	1041	69%	7,3%	1,2%	0,67%
Idiopathic	6637	80%	16,0%	2,0%	0,82%

These results have increased surgical indication for the treatment of megaesophagus, since esophagocardiomyectomy with fundoplication presents excellent results without mortality [3]

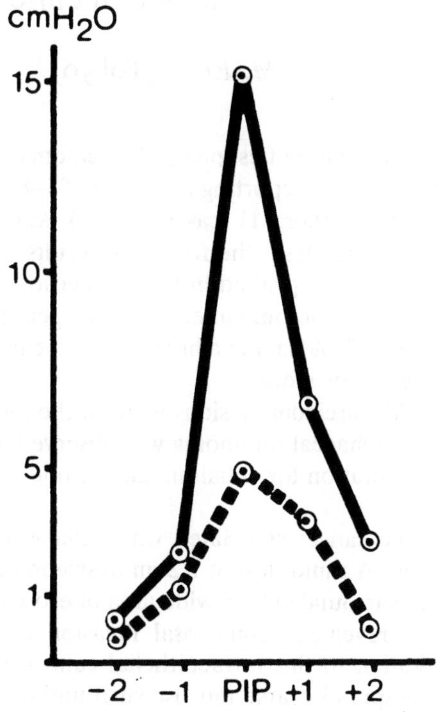

Fig. 2. The resting pressure of the lower esophageal sphincter before (full line) and after (interrupted line) dilatation. There is statistical significance between the groups

and even bleeding points in the distal esophagus. We have found that patients with ineffective dilatations of the cardia that are later operated on present periesophageal fibrosis, indicative of a previous muscular rupture followed by scarring.

However, it is more likely that chronic changes of the esophageal mucosa, when found in patients undergoing repeated dilatations, are more apt to be caused by permanent stasis or gastroesophageal reflux than by local trauma from the balloon.

References

1. Pinotti HW (1967) Megaesôfago. Motilidade do esôfago e teste do refluxo ácido, antes e após dilatação forçada da cárdia. São Paulo. Thesis – Faculdade de Medicina da Universidade de São Paulo

2. Pinotti HW (1969) Instrumento dilatador da cárdia para tratamento do megaesôfago. Amb Rev Assoc Med Bras 15: 271
3. Pinotti HW, Gama-Rodrigues JJ, Ellenbogen G, Arab-Fadul R, Raia A (1974) Novas bases para o tratamento cirúrgico do megaesôfago: esofagocardiomiectomia com esofagogastropexia. Amb Rev Assoc Med Bras 20: 331

Should the ineffectiveness of dilatations lead to suspect a cancer?

M. Endo (Tokyo)

The incidence of esophageal carcinoma accompanying achalasia is high, with various investigators reporting rates of 0.5%–8.0%. Among 153 cases of achalasia observed by the author, 11 cases (7.2%) were accompanied by esophageal carcinoma. Analyzing these, the following results were obtained:

1. Incidence peaked in the 5th decade,
2. In cases accompanied by esophageal carcinoma, the history of achalasia was long, with 70% having a history of 10 years or more, of whom 40% had a history of 30 years or more.
3. All carcinoma lesions were in the middle or upper third of the esophagus,
4. esophageal carcinoma was observed in three patients who had undergone radical operation for achalasia and in one patient in whom dilatation was performed.

The cancer associated with achalasia was commonly diagnosed at an advanced stage. A tumor lesion 1.2 cm in size in the resected specimen was found. The tumor was surrounded by a wide area of erosive and coarse mucosa. Histological examination revealed submucosal invasion of cancer in the small tumorous lesion. In addition to this intraepithelial cancer and severe dysplasia, were observed in the widespread coarse mucosa surrounding the tumor.

However, it is difficult to agree with the idea that cancer necessarily develops with a significantly greater frequency in cases in which surgical dilatations or other means to improve passage are ineffective.

The fact that esophageal carcinoma was also found in patients who had a radical operation for achalasia and in whom dysphagia had been improved, suggests that the increased risk associated with achalasia does not involve only stagnation of foodstuff or chronic stimulation. Rather, the esophageal mucosa seems to possess an inherent potential for carcinogenesis and this may in fact be nonreversible.

What are the rules to follow in the surgical treatment of megaesophagus?

A. Del Genio, N. Di Martino, G. Izzo, and *V. Maffettone* (Naples)

The aim of surgical treatment of esophageal achalasia is to remove dysphagia by means of LES activity annulment; in fact, the absence or inadequacy of LES relaxation determines the extent of dysphagia. This result is obtained by disconnecting the muscle fibers of the esophageal junction during the whole length of the high pressure zone of LES activity. This surgical procedure, which was described by Heller in 1913, and called extramucosal "cardias" myotomy, has been modified many times in recent years.

Nowadays, the rules to be followed in this operation are still a much disputed matter. An age old controversy still exists with respect to the evaluation of the surgical approach (thoracic or abdominal), although Heller used the abdominal access.

Concerning myotomy, there are many discussions about its extent: some surgeons emphasize long myotomy (above 12 cm) in order to obtain a complete myotomy. In contrast, other authors suggest a short myotomy, i.e., only on the esophageal side of the sphincter; in this way it is possible to avoid reflux, and to determine the disappearance of dysphagia.

Another point of discussion is if myotomy should be followed by an antireflux procedure: according to some authors, the incidence of esophagitis after myotomy is low, both after a short myotomy without "cardias" mobilization and after a complete myotomy. In contrast, most surgeons consider that myotomy can abolish LES activity completely, and that reflux is an ever present event, even if it does not always cause esophagitis.

The achalasic esophageal body is aperistaltic, with delayed clearing; even a poor reflux can develop esophagitis and then dysphagia, which is at first functional and then organic. Such dysphagia will determine the loss of the beneficial effects of myotomy.

The difficulty in preparing an adequate gut that will allow food to pass without peristalsis and prevent reflux adequately, is the obstacle to the use of an antireflux procedure.

A further field of discussion has been opened to those who perform an antireflux procedure (Dor, Toupet, Hill, Belsey) after myotomy. Both partial fundoplication and 360° total fundoplication (Nissen) are supported by different surgeons. The ideal operation is to create a new sphincter by antireflux technique, after the abolition of LES activity by myotomy.

According to our experience, the rules to be followed in the surgical treatment of achalasia are the following: the approach should be abdominal for these reasons: it is better tolerated by patients; it allows the operation under epidural anesthesia, which is very useful in elderly patients affected by poor general status or/and cardiopulmonary diseases; it allows an easier completion of the antireflux procedure. The thoracic approach is suggested only when myotomy must be extended to the aortic arch (as in vigorous achalasia) or when an epiphrenic diverticulum is also present. (1 case in 58 in our experience.)

It is appropriate to cut the hepatic left triangular ligament. The "pars condensa" of the gastro-hepatic omentum must not be involved, in order to avoid damage to the vagal nerves in it. The peritoneal reflection fold and the Laimer-Bertelli membrana have to be cut directly. It is necessary to mobilize mediastinal esophagus adequately. This maneuver can be obtained by blunt dissection, being careful to preserve the vagal nerves.

It is preferable to perform myotomy by means of scissors, as a good dissection level exists between the esophageal mucosa and the muscle layers. The cutting of proximal gastric muscular fibers is more difficult, because they are in close contact with the corium of the mucosa. Myotomy must be prolonged along the whole LES length.

Since February 1972, we have been using intraoperative esophageal manometry (I.E.M.) to evaluate the sphincter HPZ complete annulment. I.E.M. allows a test of total myotomy. Even a few corium mucosa adherent circular fibers, which can escape the most skillful surgeon's eye, can support a high pressure zone. This high pressure zone can be responsible for the persistence of postoperative achalasia. Furthermore, I.E.M. allows location of the site and extension of the myotomy. So we can avoid an ineffective, too short moytomy, or a too long one, which could cause pouch deformities. Postoperative dysphagia related to incomplete myotomy has never been present in our experience.

An antireflux procedure is unavoidable, as LES sphincter activity has been abolished. We utilize Nissen-Rossetti's fundoplication adequately calibrated by means of I.E.M. Fundoplication is performed using the anterior wall of the gastric fundus which is turned round the esophagus, and then sutured anteriorly by non-transfixed esophagus wall stitches.

Carrying out this maneuver, the blunt dissection of the mediastinal esophagus is increasingly useful, for it avoids fundoplication tension, as the esophagus is dropped in the abdomen. In this way, we can prevent telescopic phenomena as a postoperative complication. A continuous single stage prolene (3/0) suture of no longer than 3–4 cm is carried out. A better approach to the two edges of the wrapping-gut and an improved homogeneous junctional activity is obtained by this kind of suture.

Intraoperative manometry is used to test the antireflux procedure.

We demonstrated, by experiment and clinical observations, that higher pressure values can be reached by varying the wrapping-gut closing degree. If the pressure is too high, the wrapping-gut ist remade; on the contrary, in the presence of low pressure, the wrapping-gut is strengthened by means of a further suture.

The question to be asked is: which HPZ pressure values are to be reached intraoperatively and if those values are correlated with long-term clinical results: our 15 years' experience allows us to state that correlation is statistically significant, and the values reached are between 20–30 mmHg with respect to a length of 2–4 cm.

*

With the aim of supplying a more homogeneous survey, we are going to report our our personal experience performed just by one surgeon (Del Genio), even if we have had the possibility of examining a larger number of patients in our Surgical Department.

Fifty-eight patients have been operated on according the previously reported rules. On the basis of the intraoperative manometric Nissen values, we obtained two patients groups: In group 1 (21 patients) the intraoperative average value was 15.6±2.39 mmHg (normocalibrated Nissen). In group 2 (37 patients) the intraoperative average value was 25.2±4.51 mmHg (hypercalibrated Nissen). These patients have had a long-term follow-up, which has included clinic symptoms, manometry, pH-metry (24 hour), radiology and endoscopy.

The follow-up time varied from 6 months to 10 years. Five patients from 21 Heller and normocalibrated Nissen (23.8%) were affected by reflux esophagitis during the follow-up. In the same group, 2 patients (9.52%) had asymptomatic complications; one of them had a Nissen disruption and the other one a pouch deformity. Two out of 37 Heller and hypercalibrated Nissen patients died after operation (mortality rate: 2/58=3.4%), the first (cirrhotic) of esophageal fistula and pylephlebitis and the second of Boerhaave syndrome, which was characterized by vomiting after spontaneous and too early restoration of alimentation (12 hours after operation). Two patients (2/35) presented transitory dysphagia which disappeared spontaneously after 3 months. In only one case (1/35=2.8%), we reported a gas bloat syndrome which disappeared spontaneously. In this Heller and hypercalibrated Nissen group we never had reflux. One splenectomy was necessary (1/58=1.7%). A Mallory-Weiss syndrome occurred, and it was cured by medical therapy. One slipped Nissen and Saik I complication occurred respectively in two patients. The manometric follow-up showed a progressive pressure value drop till 50% (Table 1) which became stable within the first year. These results have justified the use of the hypercalibrated Nissen to avoid a remarkable nHPZ value decrease which is not able to protect from reflux.

With respect to the adynamic dolico-megaesophagus, we think that the most proper rule is to perform a total esophagectomy without thoracotomy, as it has been demonstrated by us and others that myotomy is unable to resolve dysphagia.

In conclusion, the use of I.E.M. which was first employed by us during both myotomy and antireflux procedure, allows us to eliminate most discussion about the

Table 1. Manometric follow-up after Heller myotomy and Nissen fundoplication for esophageal achalasia

	Preop. mmHg	Intraop. mmHg	6 Months mmHg	1 Year mmHg	5–10 Years mmHg
Heller + normo-calibrated Nissen	21.3±3.01 21 pts	15.6±2.39 21 pts	11.2±2.21 12 pts	9.44±2.61 8 pts	8.05±2.51 8 pts
Heller + hyper-calibrated Nissen	23.8±2.98 37 pts	25.2±4.51 37 pts	20.0±2.64 21 pts	17.2±2.33 12 pts	15.9±2.85 6 pts
Heller + refluxed normocalibrated Nissen	24.4±2.63 5 pts	11.3±1.55 5 pts	9.33±1.41 5 pts	8.00±1.20 3 pts	7.33±1.05 3 pts

surgical treatment of achalasic megaesophagus. Moreover, I.E.M. allows the performance of an operation which is very close to ideal. Functional disorders, which in our experience occur with a low incidence (8.5%), disappear within 6 months to one year due to the progressive nHPZ value decrease.

References

1. Amato G, Maffettone V, Landolfi V, Cosenza A, Di Martino N, Del Genio A (1985) L'endoscopia intraoperatoria in corso di reinterventi sull'esofago terminale. Chirurgia Gastroenterologica. Atti VII Congr CICD pp551–554
2. Del Genio A, Pignatelli C, Chiariello L, Maffettone F, Califano G (1968) L'elettromanometria nello studio della funzione motoria dell'esofago. Rass Med Sperim 15:58–81, suppl IV
3. Del Genio A, Pignatelli C, Lanzara A (1979) Guides to the therapy of achalasic megaesophagus in our experience. "Interdisciplinary Trends in Surgery" Xth Congress of the European Federation of the International College of Surgeons, Milan 1977, Minerva Medica Ed 259–262
4. Del Genio A (1985) Intraoperative esophageal manometry. Relazione al The inaugural Congress of the International Society for Disease of the Esophagus, Tokyo, November 1980. Giorn Ital Chir 39:3–7
5. Del Genio A, Di Martino N, Fei L, Amato G, Izzo G, Landolfi V, Maffettone V (1983) Sul ruolo della manometria intraoperatoria nell'intervento di Heller più Nissen nel trattamento chirurgico dell'acalasia: follow-up clinico, radiologico e manometrico. La Chirurgia Toracica 36:39–48
6. Del Genio A, Di Martino N, Fei L, Maffettone V, Ambrosio A (1986) L'esame manometrico intraoperatorio dell'esofago serve a migliorare l'intervento e quindi anche la prognosi dei pazienri? Relazione al 2° Congresso SIATEC, Genova maggio 1985. Acta Chirurgica Italica 42:762–769
7. Del Genio A, Di Martino N, Napolitano V, Landolfi V, Maffettone X, Ruggiero R, Fusco F (1984) Acute aperistaltic megaesophagus as a complication of Nissen fundoplication: a case report. Ital J Surg Scien 14:135–138
8. Donahue PE, Schlesinger PK, Bombeck CT, Samelson S, Nyhus LM (1986) Achalasia of the esophagus. Treatment controversies and the method of choice. Ann Surg 203:505–511
9. Duranceau A, La Fontaine ER, Valliers B (1982) Effect of total fundoplication on function of the esophagus after myotomy for achalasia. Am J Surg 143:22–28
10. Ellis FH Jr, Olsen A (1969) Achalasia of the esophagus. Philadelphia WB Saunders Co. p206
11. Heller E (1913) Extramukose Cardioplastic bei chronischen Cardiospasm mit Dilatation der Esophagus. Mitt Grenz Chir 27:141–149
12. Lanzara A (1947) Essenza e limiti del cardiospasmo. Un tentativo di definizione clinica e patogenetica della malattia. Arch Chir Tor I:55
13. Lanzara A (1983) Intraoperative esophageal manometry: ten years experience. IInd International Congress "International Society for diseases of the esophagus" Roma 1983, Abstr pA1–6. Atti del Congresso pp 25–27
14. Lanzara A (1984) Discinesie esofagee. 87° Congr Soc Ital Chir Roma pp 585–595
15. Lanzara A (1986) Modern nosologic classification of the esophageal disordered motor activity (DMA). Relazione all'International Esophageal Week, Monaco Abstr p 160 n° 234. In corso di stampa sugli atti del Congresso.
16. Lanzara A, Del Genio A (1979) La fundoplicatio sec. Nissen. Arch Atti Soc Ital Chir I: 813–829
17. Lind JF, Burns CM, Dangall TM, Winnipeg FR (1965) "Physiological" repair for hiatus hernia. Manometric Study. Arch Surg 91:233–237
18. Lind JF, Cotton DI, Blancord R, Crispin JS, Dimopolad GE (1969) Effects of thoracic displacement and vagotomy on the canine gastro-esophageal junction zone. Gastroenterology 56:1078–1085
19. Nissen R (1961) Gastropexy and fundoplication in surgical treatment of hiatal hernia. Am J Dig Dis 6:954–961

20. Orringer MB, Sloan HS (1978) Esophagectomy without thoracotomy. Thorac Cardiovasc Surg 76: 643–654
21. Rossetti M (1963) Oesophago-cardiomyotomie und fundoplicatio; Eine physiologische Operation bei Cardiospasma und Megaesophagus. J Suisse Chir 93: 925–931
22. Siewert JR, Blum AL, Waldeck F (1976) Funktionsstörungen der Speiseröhre. Springer Verlag, Berlin Heidelberg New York
23. Siewert JR, Peoper HJ, Jennewein HM, Waldeck F (1973) Die Oesophago-jejunoplicatio eine Anastolosentechnik zur Reflux, Vertintung nach totaler Gastrektomie. Der Chirurg 44: 115
24. Vantrappen G, Hellemans J (1980) Treatment of achalasia and related motor disorders. Gastroenterology 79: 144–154
25. Vantrappen G, Jansen J, Hellemans J, Coremans G (1979) Achalasia, diffuse esophageal spasm and related motility disorders. Gastroenterology 76: 450–457
26. Winans CS, Harris LD (1967) Quantitation of lower esophageal sphincter. Gastroenterology 52: 779–783

Ch. Herfarth, and *Th. Lehnert* (Heidelberg)

Achalasia of the esophagus is not a new medical problem. The first description of this emptying disorder of the esophagus was written more than 300 years ago by Thomas Willis (Oxford) in 1674. We have learned since from pathoanatomical studies that the underlying pathology of the narrowed distal esophageal segment is a degeneration or absence of the ganglion cells of Auerbach's plexus. Pathogenetic factors have not yet been identified precisely, but viral or bacterial infections as well as parasitic infestations such as in Chagas disease (Trypanosoma cruzi) all have been incriminated.

Causal treatment is, therefore not available and management of this condition must be aimed at the alleviation of the symptoms.

Clinical manifestations of achalasia include dysphagia and regurgitation of food due to the failure of the lower esophageal sphincter (LES) to relax after swallowing, uncoordinated esophageal contractility and sometimes an increased resting pressure of the LES. Gastroesophageal reflux may also be present.

Recognizing that achalasia is a progressive disease, it can be classified into three stages, according to the effectiveness of the mechanisms controlling esophageal emptying (Table 1): in grade 3 achalasia all 3 mechanisms have become ineffective;

Table 1. Pathophysiological grading of achalasia

Achalasia / Esophageal emptying	grade 1	grade 2	grade 3
LES relaxation	(+)	∅	∅
Esophageal contractility	+	(+)	∅
Hydrostatic forces	+	+	∅

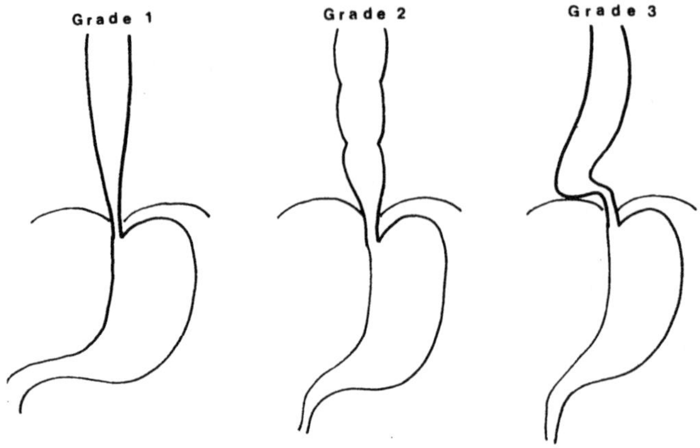

Fig. 1. Morphological features of grade 1–3 achalasia

in this final stage of the disease, the tubular esophagus has lost its contractility completely, is grossly dilated and has adopted the shape of a syphon (Fig. 1). This condition has also been designated megaesophagus for its prominent radiologic features (Fig. 2).

Techniques currently used to treat achalasia include pneumatic dilatation of the stenotic segment and cardiomyotomy which most surgeons combine with an antireflux procedure such as Nissen fundoplication. The results of both types of treatment are comparable regarding mortality (dilatation vs. myotomy 0.5 vs. 1.4 per cent),

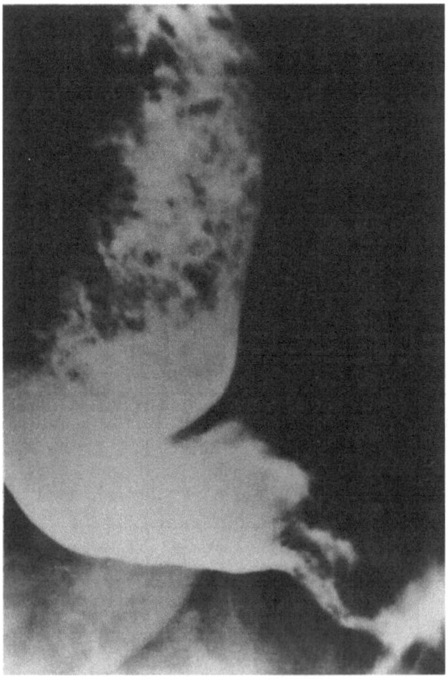

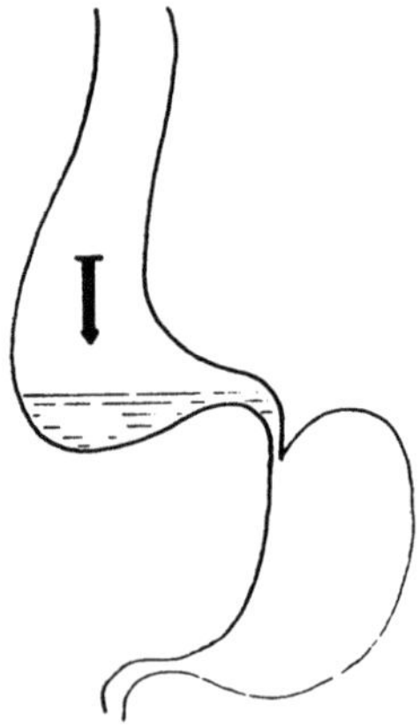

Fig. 3. Diagrammatic presentation of pathophysiological abnormalities associated with megaesophagus

Fig. 2. Radiologic features of megaesophagus

Table 2. Problem-oriented surgical approach to failed esophageal emptying

Treatment / Pathology	Dilatation	Cardiomyo-tomy	Esophagomyo-plication
Failure of LES to relax	+	+	+
Missing esophageal contractility	∅	∅	+
Misdirected hydrostatic forces	∅	∅	+

perforation (3.5 vs. 4.0 per cent) and subsequent gastroesophageal reflux (10 vs. 18 per cent). Such treatment will yield satisfactory longterm results in the majority of patients with grade 1 or 2 achalasia [1]. In grade 3 achalasia or megaesophagus, however, hydrostatic pressures are misdirected due to kinking and dilatation of the tubular esophagus (Fig. 3) and any procedure simply aimed at draining the esophagus may therefore fail to correct the situation [2].

In an attempt to restore esophageal contractility and to correct syphoning of megaesophagus we have developed a procedure designated esophagomyoplication (Table 2).

In the initial step of the operation a balloon catheter is inflated in the lower esophagus to delineate the narrowed segment precisely. Then a typical extramucous myotomy is performed which extends distally at least 1.5 cm over the stenosis. To prevent gastroesophageal reflux a semifundoplication (240° wrap) is added.

Following this, the esophageal myotomy is extended upward to the azygos vein (Fig. 4). The mucosal tube of the esophagus is then freed of its surrounding muscular layer (Figs. 5, 6) sparing the nutritional arteries from the aorta. The final step of the procedure has the dissected muscular sheath tightened around the mucosal tube in a double layer straight-jacket fashion (Fig. 7). Using a balloon catheter, the remaining esophageal lumen is adjusted to an inner diameter of 2.5 cm.

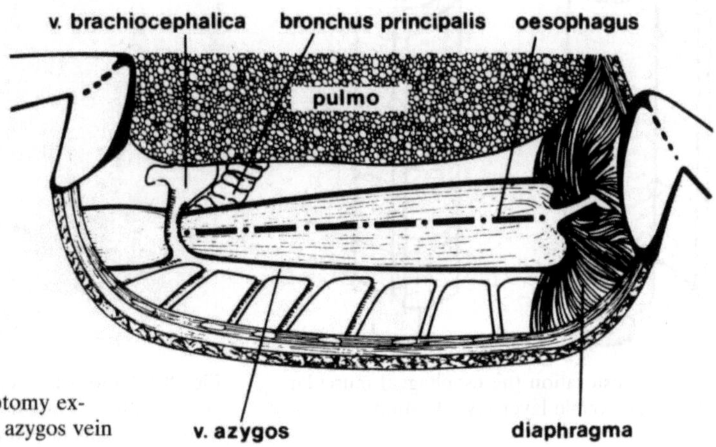

Fig. 4. Esophagomyotomy extended upward to the azygos vein

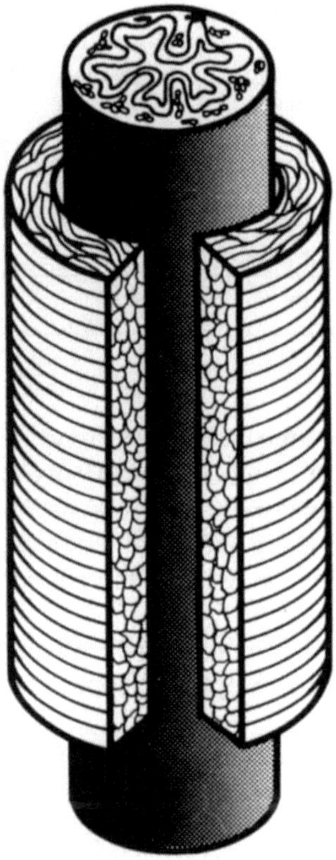

Fig. 5. Circular dissection of the muscular layer of the esophagus

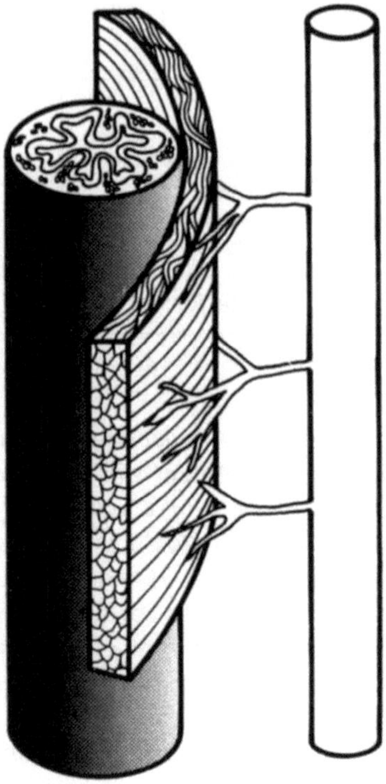

Fig. 6. Preservation of nutritional arteries originating from the aorta

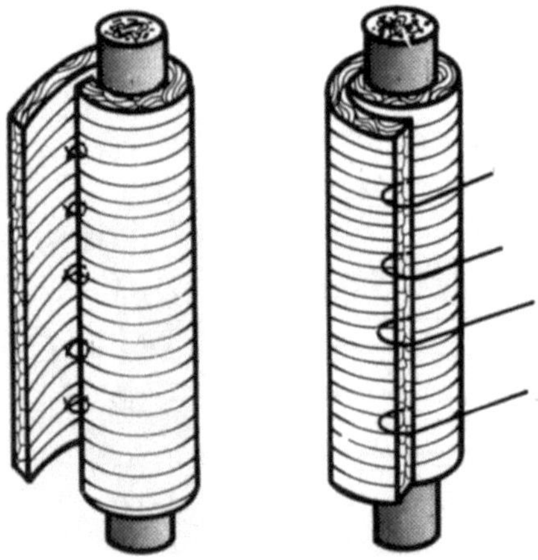

Fig. 7. Restoration the esophageal muscular sheath by double layer myoplication

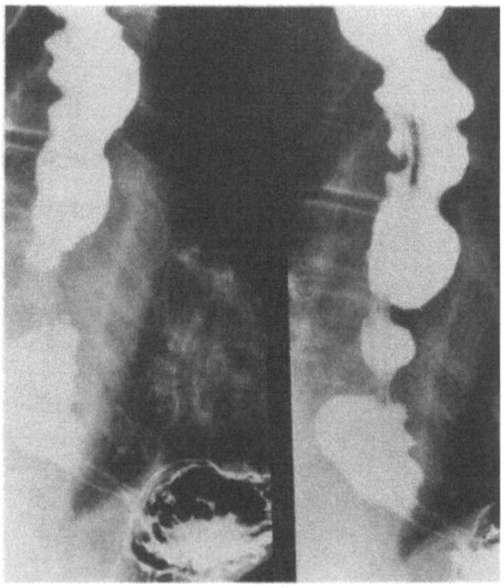

Fig. 8. Radiologic study of esophagus one year after esophagomyoplication for megaesophagus in two patients

Two patients who had this procedure have been followed-up at one year: clinically both patients were free of symptoms of dysphagia and regurgitation, although both had learned to chew solids thoroughly. No symptoms of gastroesophageal reflux could be elicited.

On endoscopy, esophageal mucosa appeared normal macroscopically, but in one patient with positive acid reflux test, signs of esophagitis were present on histologic examination of biopsy specimens. In both patients pH clearance was delayed. Manometric studies revealed uncoordinated contractions in both patients. In one patient the LES resting pressure was 8 mm Hg and no defined pressure profile could be determined in the other. X-ray examination showed that elongation, dilatation and siphoning of the esophagus had been controlled effectively in both patients (Fig. 8).

Other surgical approaches to megaesophagus include segmental [3] or longitudinal resection [4] of the tubular esophagus or esophagogastrostomy [5]. The esophagomyoplication described above for the treatment of grade 3 achalasia, or megaesophagus, has the advantage of leaving esophageal mucosa intact, thus avoiding the risk of contamination by luminal contents and anastomotic leakage. With the favourable results achieved in two patients followed-up at one year, further study and excercise of this procedure should be encouraged.

References

1. Arvanitakis C (1975) Achalasia of the Esophagus. A reappraisal of esophagomyotomy vs. forceful dilatation. Dig Dis 20: 841
2. Menguy R (1971) Management of Achalasia by Transabdominal Cardiomyotomy and Fundoplication. Surg Gynecol Obstet 133: 482
3. Ciaglia P, Segal G (1962) Segmental Esophagectomy Ancillary procedure for mega-esophagus with sigmoid elongation. J Thorac Cardiovasc Surg 44: 44
4. Malm A, Schwindt W (1969) A new surgical approach to the treatment of mega-esophagus. J Thorac Cardiovasc Surg 57: 312
5. Heyrovsky H (1927) Diagnostik und Therapie der chirurgischen Erkrankungen der Speiseröhre. Wien Med Wochenschr 77: 1649

What is the incidence of reflux in achalasia?

G. Cargill, and *M. Duché* (Paris)

Achalasia is defined as a lack of relaxation of the lower esophageal sphincter (LES). Esophageal manometry is the best test for the diagnosis of this disorder, which is found in many diseases: achalasia (megaesophagus), scleroderma, lupus, amylosis, dysautonomia, neoplasic syndroms; sphincter immaturity and iatrogenic achalasia after a Nissen procedure for example.

Reflux incidence changes according to these pathologies. In scleroderma and lupus were the lower esophageal tone is decreased, gastro-esophageal reflux is frequent, as shown in various studies; associated dysmotility is a worsening factor. Sphincter immaturity in infants may be associated with achalasia, with a slight increase in sphincter tone and paradoxical reflux observed in about 60% of cases. These rare abnormalities are associated with important fainting half the time.

Finally, if we consider clinical achalasia – classical megaesophagus - reflux incidence is very low, at least before treatment. In 8 cases studied before Heller's procedure Di Mauro never finds any reflux. For our own actual experience, we have investigated, by manometry, 784 megaesophagus cases. A gastro-esophageal reflux has been found in 12 cases (1.53%), but pHmetry was only performed in 43% of these cases.

In 9 cases, an important lower esophageal sphincter malposition (hiatus hernia) was found, associated with a normal tone or slightly decreased tone. Achalasia to swallowing is clear and corpus diskinesia is typical. pHmetry shows reflux episodes promoted by abdominal hyperpressure. These episodes are long, followed by a very low rise in pH, attesting to very bad clearance.

In 3 other cases, manometric data showed: minor malposition of the LES, high tone, inverted gastro-esophageal pressure gradient, demonstrating stasis. In these 3 patients, reflux incidence was directly linked to the absorption of calcium antagonists and/or nitrate drugs.

After treatment by pneumatic dilatation and/or surgical procedure, reflux incidence is higher. We propose a systematic pHmetry and a manometrical manometry study to try to determine LES decreased tone and/or malposition.

In our experience, the incidence of reflux is higher after dilatations (7.8%) than after a Heller procedure associated with repair of the anti-reflux mechanisms (3.7%). We have no experience of simple myotomy not associated with an anti-reflux procedure. Clearance is of poor quality in all cases, and associated with the hypoperistalsis associated with the disease. This may sometimes partially regress after surgical or instrumental treatment, but the peristaltic waves usually remain of inadequate amplitude, and are not propagated [2, 3]. It is difficult to draw any conclusion from this series in view of the marked disparity between the two groups of patients. Monitoring by pH measurement has been much more rare, though often requested because of the persistence of abnormal features after treatment, or suggestive signs in patients who have undergone dilatation.

The values we indicate here remain within the very wide range of values given in the literature. These data are in any case consistent with the pressure values obtained after treatment and reported in the literature. For instance, Seo [4], in a routine study performed in 10 children, shows that the LES pressure is significantly greater after dilatation than after myotomy (46 mm Hg as against 8 mm Hg) and that reflux is 3 times greater after myotomy than after dilatation (36% as against 12%). This short pediatric study further shows a much less satisfactory response to dilatation than that observed in adults [5, 6, 7] and may explain the higher incidence of reflux in patients who have been dilated. Guelrud [5] in a very recent study in the adult shows that the residual pressure after dilatation is of the order of 6.2 ± 0.8 mm Hg. A low pressure after a first dilatation is regarded by this author as a good prognostic factor in terms of the duration of the improvement obtained. Finally, as described by Smart [8], achalasia may develop in a patient suffering from reflux.

To sum up, it seems possible to conclude that:

1. The incidence of reflux in achalasia is small but not nil before treatment, but commoner after treatment, and may justify routine diagnosis.
2. Broadly, several types of reflux may be distinguished:
   a) After treatment, those associated with a failure in one of the parameters of continence and essentially with malposition of the sphincter, the frequency of which in the general population is such that a coincidence with a megaesophagus is possible.
   b) Iatrogenic reflux, as associated with medical treatment reducing the extent of the tonic barrier of the LES (this action may be associated with a positional defect).
   c) Reflux resulting from instrumental or surgical treatment that is potentially very dangerous to the wall in view of the associated motor disturbance.

References

1. Mauro DI (1986) Min Med
2. Lamet M et al (1985) Return of peristalsis in achalasia after pneumatic dilatation. Am J Gastroenterol 80, 8: 602–604
3. Ponco J et al (1986) Return of esophageal peristalsis after Heller's myotomy for idiopathic Achalasia. Dig Dis and Sci 31, 5: 545–547
4. Seo JK et al (1987) Esophageal Manometric and Clinical response to treatment in children with achalasia. Digestive Diseases Week Chicago
5. Guelrud M, Nath B (1987) Is lower esophageal sphincter (LES) pressure a good prognostic test after pneumatic dilatation (PN) in achalasia? Digestive Diseases Week Chicago
6. Vantrappen G, et al (1971) Treatment of Achalasia with pneumatic dilatations. Gut 12: 268–275
7. Dellipani AW, et al (1986) Pneumatic dilatation in the Management of Achalasia experience of 45 cases. Quarterly J of Med 58: 277, 253, 258
8. Smart HL, et al (1986) Achalasia following gastro-esophageal reflux. J Royal Soc Med 79, 71, 73

K. Jeyasingham, and *H. R. J. Payne* (Bristol)

Reflux in achalasia cardia can be considered under the following categories:

- Achalasia cardia co-existing with intermittent gastro esophageal reflux.
- Association of achalasia with hiatal herniation predisposing to reflux.
- Effect of medication in the treatment of achalasia cardia.
- The result of hydrostatic or pneumatic dilatation in the management of achalasia.
- Post myotomy reflux.

It might seem paradoxical that a condition that is characterised by a non-relaxing lower esophageal sphincter should at times be associated with reflux across it. The pathogenesis of achalasia in the human is not clearly understood, but it is generally agreed that there are fewer ganglion cells in the Aurbech's plexus in the esophageal wall of the tubular as well as the sphincteric portions [1]. A hypersensitivity to endogenous gastrin, vaso inhibitory peptides or exogenous nicotine, could all result in intermittent relaxation [2] leading to gastroesophageal reflux. Katz [3] in a recent communication clearly demonstrated lower esophagenal sphincter relaxation in a series of 23 patients with achalasia cardia diagnosed in clinical and radiological features. Detailed analyses of the laboratory data of these patients suggest that this may be a feature of early stage achalasia. A recent report of five patients with previously established gastroesophageal reflux developing achalasia several years after [4] again leads one to feel that achalasia does not protect a patient against gastroesophageal reflux simultaneously or in course of time.

The incidence of reflux has been estimated variously by different authors [5, 6, 7, 8, 9] at somewhere between 1.9% and 62%. The dissimilarity in the incidence of such reflux is attributable to the extent to which stringent rules regarding acid reflux were applied in each series (Table 1).

Patients undergoing medical treatment for achalasia may have reflux as a result of the medication or as a result of forcible dilatation with hydrostatic or pneumatic dilators. The incidence of reflux in patients undergoing pneumatic dilatation has again been estimated variously by different authors at one to 20% [10, 11], although no serious complications of reflux have been recorded.

The administration of calcium entry blockers such as nifedipine or diltiazem [12] can cause a 30% reduction in the resting lower esophageal sphincter tone which may contribute to reflux intermittently in patients maintained on these drugs but there again no serious reflux complications have been reported.

Although hiatal herniation does not necessarily go hand in hand with gastro esophageal reflux, the association of herniation with or without reflux should alert the unsuspecting clinician to possible reflux after therapy be it medical or surgical. The incidence of hiatal herniation associated with achalasia is estimated at 4 to 19% [5, 9, 13].

The most important category of gastroesophageal reflux associated with achalasia is that which follows a Zaaiyer modification [14] of the Heller [15] myotomy. Much has been written about the extent of the myotomy upwards, downwards, in depth and in width: those who believe that the myotomy should stop at the gastro esophageal junction and not be extended on to the anterior surface of the stomach claim that the effect of sparing the sling fibres of Helvetius ensures a competent anti-reflux mechanism, provided no disruption of hiatus is done by the dissection [16]. Atkinson demonstrated quite categorically that a lower esophageal sphincteric tone could still be measured after a modified cardiomyotomy [17], implying that the

Table 1. Reflux Following Myotomy

Clinical	– Unreliable
Radiological	– Mainstay of Diagnosis
pH Testing	– SART
	Prolonged
Incidence 0 to 56%	

Table 2. Prolonged pH testing with threshold at 4

	Total time pH<4.0	% reflux during supine period	No. reflux episodes >5 mins	Longest reflux episode
Normal (no evidence of reflux/ esophageal problems) (n=20)	0.80 ±1.02	0.22 ±0.57	<3	3.35 ±4.37
Achalasia pre-Op (n=11)	0.96 ±1.55	0.02 ±0.06	<3	3.82 ±5.36
Achalasia post-op: Heller's myotomy (n=1)	51.70	65	9	332
Achalasia post-op: modified Heller's and anti-reflux procedure (n=5)	0.58 ±1.24	0	<3	6.60 ±14.21

sphincter was not entirely disrupted at the time of surgery or that some regeneration occurs after the procedure.

Although gastroesophageal reflux associated with a hypotensive sphincter is relatively easy to diagnose, the recognition of reflux in patients with achalasia often presents problems. Clinical symptoms such as heartburn and regurgitation are unreliable [16]. The neurological status of the esophagus is such that until serious complications set in, reflux may not be evident [18]. Careful radiological screening has in the past been the mainstay of diagnosing reflux [16]. However, the practice of pH testing by the standard acid reflux test (SART) and more recently with prolonged pH monitoring (Tables 2, 3), has ensured a more accurate documentation of acid reflux provided the esophagus was not over dilated or filled with residual food and mucus.

The recorded incidence of post-myotomy reflux in the earlier years ranged from 0% to 56% [19, 20, 21]. Belsey in 1964, recording a 22% incidence of reflux after modified Heller myotomy first introduced the addition of the partial fundoplication to the modified myotomy, achieving a complete absence of reflux on clinical and radiological criteria [22]. Ellis & Cole [16], in recording reflux in 17 out of 56 cardiomyotomy patients concluded that despite adequate precautions, a small number would reflux in the period after surgery. The incidence of reflux since then has been variously recorded at one to 50%.

If the cardiomyotomy is extended to over 2 cm of the anterior surface of the stomach, reflux is produced in 100% of the patients [23], requiring some form of anti-reflux procedure if complications are to be avoided. This leads us to the three groups of surgeons in current practice. Firstly, the group who carry out an esophagomyotomy not extending more than 0.5 cm on to the stomach, inclining the incision towards the lesser curve to avoid the sling fibres of Helvetius, claiming a one to 3% reflux without recourse to an anti-reflux procedure.

Table 3. Prolonged pH testing with threshold at 5

	Total time pH < 5.0	% reflux during supine period	No. reflux episodes > 5 mins	Longest reflux episode
Normal (no evidence of reflux/ esophageal problems) (n=20)	2.12 ±2.76	0.99 ±1.54	< 10	6.96 ±7.47
Achalasia pre-Op (n=11)	9.55 ±12.24	12.20 ±26.3	< 20	39.86 ±103.9
Achalasia post-op: Heller's myotomy (n=1)	90.12	100	14	525
Achalasia post-op: modified Heller's and anti-reflux procedure (n=5)	1.83 ±1.71	1.94 ±2.16	< 3	12.80 ±17.6

The vast majority of surgeons, however, accept that such refined control of the myotomy is not always practicable and that reflux is the rule if no anti-reflux procedure is included in the surgery. Hence the second group of surgeons who carry out a cardiomyotomy extending 1 cm on to the stomach, exposing 50% of the mucosa over the myotomised narrow segment of esophagus and carrying out some form of anti-reflux repair. There is, however, a third group [9, 24] who select the patients for anti-reflux procedure if there are predisposing factors to reflux in their pre-surgery assessment.

References

1. Casella RR, Brown AL, Sayre GP, Ellis FH (1974) Achalasia of the oesophagus. Pathologic and etiologic considerations. Ann Surg 160: 474–486
2. Csendes A, Smok G, Braghetto I, Ramirez C, Velasco N, Henriquez A (1985) Gastroesophageal Sphincter Pressure and Histological Changes in Distal Esophagus in Patients with Achalasia of the Esophagus. Digestive Diseases and Sciences 30: 941–945
3. Katz PO, Richter JE, Cowan R, Castell DO (1986) Apparent Complete Lower Esophageal Sphincter Relaxation in Achalasia. Gastroenterology 90: 978–983
4. Smart HL, Mayberry JF, Atkinson M (1986) Achalasia following gastro-oesophageal reflux. Journal of the Royal Society of Medicine 79: 71–73
5. Black J, Vorbach AN, Leigh Collins J (1976) Results of Heller's operation for achalasia of the oesophagus. The importance of hiatal repair. Br J Surg 63: 949–953
6. Peyton MD, Greenfield LJ, Elkins RC (1974) Combined Myotomy and Hiatal Herniorrhaphy. Am J Surg 128: 786–790
7. Bjorck S, Dernevik L, Gatzinsky P, Sandberg N (1982) Oesophagocardiomyotomy and Antireflux Procedures. Acta Chir Scand 148: 525–529
8. Elkins (1979) in discussion following Okike et al [13]
9. Murray GF, Battaglini JW, Keagy BA, Starek PJ, Wilcox BR (1984) Selective Application of Fundoplication in Achalasia. Ann Thor Surg 37 (2): 185–188
10. Vantrappen G, Janssens J (1983) To dilate or to operate? That is the question. Gut 24: 1013–1019

11. Fellows IW, Ogilvie AL, Atkinson M (1983) Pneumatic dilatation in achalasia. Gut 24:1020–1023
12. Traube M, Hongo M, Magyar L, McCallum RW (1984) Effects of Nifedipine in Achalasia and in Patients with High-Amplitude Peristaltic Esophageal Contractions. Jama 252:1733–1736
13. Okike N, Payne SW, Neufeld DM, Bernatz PE, Pairolero PC, Sanderson DR (1979) Esophagomyotomy versus Forceful Dilatation for Achalasia of the Esophagus: Results in 899 Patients. Ann Thorac Surg 28:119–125
14. Zaaiyer JH (1923) Cardiospasm in the aged. Ann Surg 77:615–617
15. Heller E (1913) Extra mukose Kardioplastic beim chronischen Kardiospasmus mit Dilatation der Oesophagus. M & H Grenzeb Med Chir 27:141
16. Ellis F, Cole FL (1965) Reflux after cardiomyotomy. Gut 6:80–84
17. Atkinson M (1959) The oesophago-gastric sphincter after cardiomyotomy. Thorax 14:125–131
18. Orringer MB (1979) The Treatment of Achalasia: Controversy Resolved? Ann Thor Surg 25(2):100–102
19. Gertz TC (1952) Quoted by Atkinson [17]
20. Hawthorne HR, Frobesco AS, Nemir P Jr (1956) The surgical management of achalasia of the esophagus. Ann Surg 144:653
21. Acheson ED, Hadley GD (1958) Quoted by Atkinson [17]
22. Belsey R (1966) Functional diseases of the oesophagus. Thorac J & Cardiovasc Surg 52:164–187
23. Jara FM, Toledo-Pereyra LH, Lewis JW, Magilligan DJ Jr (1979) Long-term Results of Esophagomyotomy for Achalasia of Esophagus. Arch Aurg 114:935–936
24. Ellis FH, Crozier RE, Watkins E Jr (1984) Operation for esophageal achalasia. Thorac J Cardiovasc Surg 88:344–351

Is it possible not to combine an antireflux procedure with the treatment of a megaesophagus?

F. H. Ellis Jr. (Boston)

There are two controversial issues concerning therapy for esophageal achalasia. The first is whether esophagomyotomy or forceful dilation should be the initial form of therapy and the second is whether or not an antireflux procedure should be combined with esophagomyotomy. I firmly believe that esophagomyotomy is the primary treatment of choice and that excellent results can be achieved with a short myotomy without the potential dangers associated with performing an antireflux maneuver concomitantly. These brief comments are presented in support of this view.

Experimental Background

Some years ago, Dr. John McVey, working in my laboratory at the Mayo Clinic, compared the results of different types of esophagomyotomies in dogs [1]. Included in his review were three procedures:

1. the classic double Heller myotomy.
2. a long myotomy extending well on to the stomach and
3. a short myotomy limited for the most part to the distal esophagus.

Endoscopic, radiographic and pathologic evidence of reflux occurred only in those animals subjected to the more radical procedures. As a result of these findings, I have employed a short esophagomyotomy ever since and have not found it necessary to incorporate an antireflux procedure.

Surgical Technique

The technique of esophagomyotomy has been previously described [2]. It involves a left thoracotomy through which a longitudinal incision is made in the distal esophageal muscle. The incision is limited for the most part to the distal esophagus extending only a short distance (less than 1 cm) on to the stomach and is continued up on to the dilated thick walled part of the esophagus so that the total length of the myotomy is between 5 and 7 cm. About half the circumference of the esophageal mucosa is allowed to pout out through the myotomy by dissecting the muscular wall of the esophagus laterally away from the mucosa. If there is a co-existent hiatus hernia, or if the hiatus is unduly patulous allowing the esophagogastric junction to rise in the chest, the junction is repositioned intrabdominally by two non-absorbable mattress sutures through the esophageal musculature which are passed through the hiatus and secured to the undersurface of the diaphragm.

Case Material

Between January 1970 and January 1987, 149 patients underwent a 151 esophagomyotomies. Two patients required reoperation. The patients age ranged from 15 to 85 with a median age of 44. Symptoms had been present from one month to 60 years prior to operation with a median duration of 3 years. The extent of disease was classified radiographically as mild in 38% of cases, moderate in 34% and severe in 28%. Seventy-three patients had undergone treatment before being seen by us, many by a trial of bougienage, a technique of little value in this disease. Forty-eight patients had been treated on one or more occasions by forceful dilation and 25 patients including two of our own had undergone a previous operation or operations on the esophagus.

All patients underwent esophagomyotomy through a left thoracotomy. Thirty-six patients required subdiaphragmatic fixation of the esophagogastric junction by the technique described. A mucosal perforation was recognized and closed in 10 patients. Four patients required diverticulectomy of an epiphrenic diverticulum. Two patients with an associated duodenal ulcer required vagotomy and pyloroplasty and one patient with marked megaesophagus underwent a segmental resection of the redundant sigmoid shaped esophagus with end to end esophagoesophagostomy.

Results

No patients died after the operation and recovery was usually rapid and uncomplicated with postoperative hospitalization ranging from 4 to 21 days, averaging about a week. Complications arose in 13 patients (8.6%). Retained secretions required postoperative bronchoscopy in four patients and four patients had a urinary tract infection. A spontaneous pneumothorax developed in two patients. Two other patients had wound infections and a postoperative paraesophageal hernia required surgical repair in one patient.

The clinical results in some of these patients have been reported previously with an average follow-up of 6¾ years [3]. The overall improvement rate was 91% with a 94% success rate for patients undergoing primary surgery while reoperative results were less good, only 76% being improved. Of the nine patients who had poor results, 4 were reoperative cases. Gastroesophageal reflux in four patients, persistent or recurrent symptoms due to an inadequate myotomy in three an classic megaesophagus in two accounted for the nine poor results. Two of the four patients with reflux esophagitis developed strictures easily controlled by dilation. The other two were also managed medically. Follow-up of the 36 patients operated on since the original report. though admittedly of short duration, has disclosed one other example of reflux esophagitis in a complicated case operated on previously for diffuse esophageal spasm. The remaining 35 patients are currently doing well.

A comparison of pre and postoperative motility studies suggested a reason for the high success rate and low incidence of postoperative reflux. The postoperative studies were characterized by reduction in amplitude and length of the high pressure zone mainly at the expense of the supra-hiatal portion. Apparently, the subdiaphragmatic sphincteric remanent is adequate in most patients to prevent reflux but low enough that obstruction to ingested material does not occur.

These results are not unique, for a review of the literature over a recent ten year period revealed reports on more than a 1000 cases of esophagomyotomy operated on without an antireflux procedure with an overall improvement rate of approximately 90% [4]. This lends further support to the view that an antireflux procedure ist not necessary when an esophagomyotomy is properly performed. Also in support of this concept is the fact that approximately half of the patients requiring reoperation because of a failed Nissen procedure underwent reoperation because of postoperative dysphagia due in most cases to mistakenly wrapping an esophagus without peristaltic activity. This emphasizes the danger of a total wrap under these circumstances.

Summary

A short esophagomyotomy limited for the most part to the distal esophagus is the treatment of choice in the management of symptomatic patients with esophageal achalasia and should be carried out early in the course of the disease before the development of megaesophagus. When certain technical details are observed in the performance of surgery, a success rate in excess of 90% can be expected. The commonest causes of poor results are an inadequate myotomy and gastroesophageal reflux. Gastroesophageal reflux occurred in only 10% of cases and was easily managed medically without the need for a reoperative procedure.

References

1. McVey JL, Schlegel JF, Ellis FH Jr (1963) Gastroesophageal sphincteric function after the Heller myotomy and its modifications. An experimental study. Bull Soc Int Chir 22: 419–423
2. Ellis FH Jr (1983) Esophagomyotomy for achalasia of the esophagus. Modern techniques in surgery. Cardiac/thoracic surgery, installment VIII, Cohn LH (ed) Mount Kisco, N.Y., Futura Publishing Co Inc, p 57–1
3. Ellis FH Jr, Crozier RE, Watkins E Jr (1984) Operation for Achalasia. Results of esophagomyotomy without an antireflux operation. J Thorac Cardiov Surg 88: 344–351
4. Ellis FH Jr (1984) Esophageal achalasia. Is simple esophagomyotomy the treatment of choice? In: Najarian JS, Delaney JP: Advances in gastrointestinal surgery. Year Book Medical Publishers, Chicago, p 47–55
5. Leonardi HK, Ellis FH Jr (1983) Complications of the Nissen fundoplication. Surg Clin North Am 63: 1155–1165

H. W. Pinotti, C. E. Domene, I. Cecconello, and *B. Zilberstein* (Sao Paulo)

Achalasia of the esophagus of unknown etiology and that resulting from Chagas' disease are characterized by the absence of peristalsis and abnormal response of the lower esophageal sphincter (LES) on swallowing.

There is no therapy that reestablishes peristalsis, so that the objective of treatment is to destroy the sphincter mechanism of the lower esophagus to obtain better emptying of the esophageal content. In other cases, resection of the unhealthy esophagus is mandatory using the stomach or colon as a substitute.

Conservative management is possible by dilatation of the cardia with hydrostatic or pneumatic balloons that destroy the fibers of the LES. Some investigators propose this method as the initial treatment of choice in achalasia reporting good results [17, 11, 31, 25, 45]. However, comparative studies between conservative surgery and dilatation show that the former is better with less morbidity and mortality and recurrence of dysphagia and reflux esophagitis [2, 43, 12, 37, 3, 41].

Among various surgical methods for removing the obstruction in the lower esophagus the most commonly used is Heller's cardiomyotomy and its variations. Basically, isolated cardiomyotomy can be done in 4 different ways:

1. Heller's classical cardiomyotomy: 2 longitudinal incisions, one on the anterior and the other on the posterior surface, including muscles of the terminal esophagus and part of the stomach.
2. Groenveldt's modification: only one longitudinal incision on the anterior surface including esophagus and stomach.

3. Modification of Vasconcelos: myotomy performed on the right of the terminal esophagus to the lesser curvature of the stomach.
4. Variation of Ellis: anterior myotomy, including only the muscles of the terminal esophagus and a few millimeters of stomach.

Many experimental and clinical studies performed showed that classical cardiomyotomy and Groenveldt's modification are adequate for suppressing the sphincter barrier with low incidence of persistent dysphagia. However, they present significant indexes of reflux esophagitis and slightly less of recurrence of dysphagia. Ellis et al. [14], experimentally observed reflux in 5 out of 8 dogs operated on with 2 myotomies, and in 2 out of 6 dogs with only one anterior myotomy. A similar finding also in dogs, was reported by Hirao [24].

Large series of clinical studies report the incidence of gastroesophageal reflux (GER) as varying between 9.5 and 52% (Black [7]: 18%; Viard [48]: 11%; Belsey [5]: 22%; Jara [26]: 48%; Menzies-Gow [34]: 13.7%; Douglas & Nicholson [13]: 50%; Ferguson & Burford [18]: 9.5%; Barker & Franklin [4]: 35%; Jekler [27]: 15%; Acheson & Hadley [1]: 23%; Hawthorne [20]: 52%; Helsinger [22]: 16%; Boulez [9]: 17.5%; Tomlinson & Grant [44]: 30.8%).

Most authors found the incidence of this complication to be high, indicating the need for complementary measures to avoid it. The modification proposed by Vasconcelos to avoid injury to the Helvetius collar caused reflux and esophagitis in 27% of their surgical cases [10].

Ellis [15] achieved good results using his modification of short myotomy. He reported postoperative reflux as occurring in 4.4% of his cases and attributes this low incidence to non-destruction of the muscle fibers of the stomach at myotomy.

Santy et al. [42] and Pai et al. [38] also minimize the occurrence of GER after simple myotomy.

But, some studies [30, 8], showed that short myotomies cause a considerable amount of persistent dysphagia due to the non-destruction of the sphincter mechanism in all cases. For this reason, alarming indexes of postmyotomy dysphagia can be found as reported by (Black et al., [7]: 18% and Acheson & Hadley, [1]: 21%). Complete myotomy of LES can be performed more safely without injuring the gastric musculature and probably better results by using intraoperative manometry developed by Hill. However this is not possible in most medical centers.

Therefore, short myotomy for suppressing dysphagia may not present good results. On the other hand, the destruction of the sphincter mechanism is definitely followed by increased GER.

We had the opportunity of operating on 17 patients with reflux after myotomy without valve, referred to us from other services. Five of these patients already had severe esophagitis with esophageal stenosis and required resection; partial in 3 cases, transit was reestablished by interposition of a jejunal loop; subtotal in the other 2. After transmediastinal esophagectomy without thoracotomy, the stomach was interposed by esophagogastric cervical anastomosis.

Of the 12 remaining patients, 5 had severe esophagitis and substenosis; they were all submitted to cardiomyectomy and fundoplication. Followup was not possible in 9 cases. Four patients progressed well over the long term. However, those with severe esophagitis before the operation continued with persistent esophagitis and stenosis: two were treated medically and the other 3 submitted to subtotal transmediastinal esophagectomy without thoracotomy, with interposition of the stomach.

We concluded from this that in cases of postmyotomy reflux conservative surgery (cardiomyectomy and fundoplication) can be performed with good results except when partial or total stenosis of the esophagus is present. In these cases partial or subtotal resection of the organ is mandatory. If faced with the possibility of incomplete myotomy or severe esophagitis, we have resorted to large myotomies, to guarantee suppression of the LES barrier, complemented with partial fundoplication, an antireflux method.

Six hundred and twenty one patients with achalasia of the esophagus due to Chagas disease were operated on by cardiomyectomy and esophagogastro fundoplicature [39]. Followup of 227 of them for 6 months to 12 years revealed that 95.4% of the results were excellent to good.

Only 2.4% reported persistent dysphagia and 2.4% had symptoms of postoperative reflux. Our results are similar to those of others who use cardiomyotomy associated with an antireflux procedure, reporting absence of esophagitis or postoperative recurrence [36, 33, 27, 32, 40, 29, 44, 47, 16, 6, 35].

Based on what we have said, we believe that for adequate treatment of achalasia of the esophagus the following is required:

- extended myotomy, 6 cm above and 3 cm below the esophagogastric junction, to guarantee the destruction of LES and avoid incomplete myotomy.

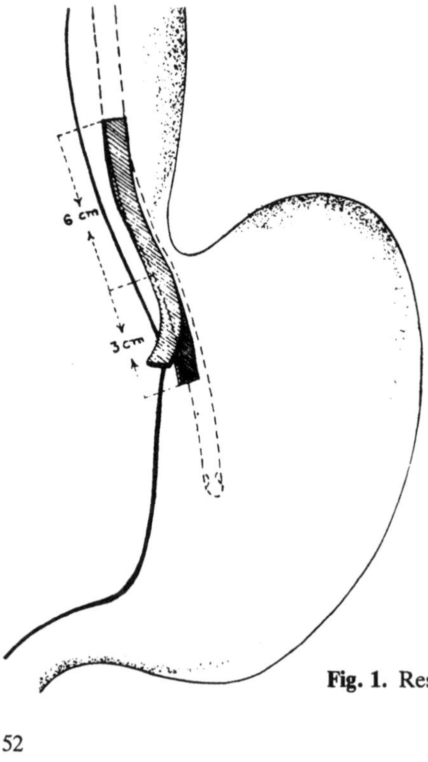

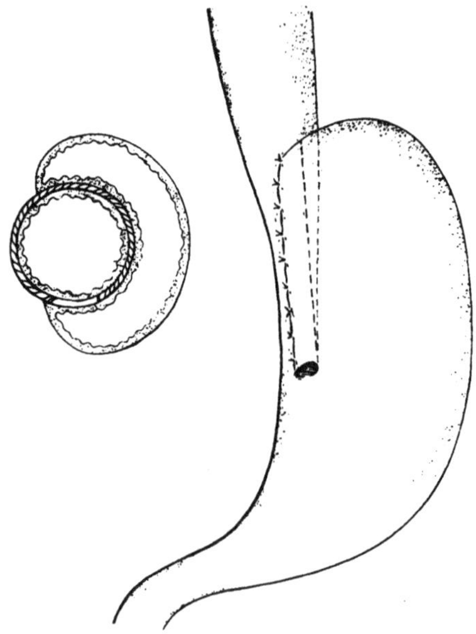

Fig. 2. Partial fundoplication

Fig. 1. Resection of a band of musculature

- resection of a band 0.5 cm in width of the incised musculature so that reapproximation of its margins and recurrence of dysphagia are more difficult (Fig. 1).
- Partial fundoplication involving ⅔ of the circumference of the anterior, left lateral and posterior surface of the esophagus. The stomach should be sutured to the margins of the myectomy in order to avoid the reapproximation of the edges and protect the exposed mucosa from possible perforations. Complete fundoplication should be avoided, for it causes postoperative dysphagia (Fig. 2).

References

1. Acheson ED, Hadley GD (1958) Cardiomyotomy for achalasia of the cardia. Brit Med J 1: 549
2. Andreollo NA, Brandalise NA, Leonardi LS (1984) Megaesôfago incipiente: dilatação ou cirurgia? Rev Ass Med Brasil 30: 4
3. Arvanitakis C (1975) Achalasia of the esophagus – A reappraisal of esophagomyotomy versos forceful pneumatic dilation. Dig Dis 20: 841
4. Barker JR, Franklin RH (1971) Heller's operation for achalasia of the cardia. A study of the early and late results. Brit J Surg 58: 466
5. Belsey R (1966) Functional diseases of the esophagus. J Thorac Cardiovasc Surg 52: 164
6. Björck S, Dernevik L, Gatzinsky P, Sandberg N (1982) Oesophagocardiomyotomy and antireflux procedures. Acta Chir Scand 148: 525
7. Black J, Vorbach AN, Collis JL (1976) Results of Heller's operation for achalasia of the oesophagus. The importance of hiatal repair. Br J Surg 63: 949
8. Borgeskov S, Nilsson T (1970) A follow-up study with pH and pressure measurements in patients treated for cardiospasm by Heller's operation. Scand J Thorac Cardiovasc Surg 4: 83
9. Boulez J, Baulieux J, Mayer B, Peix JL, Donne R, Maillet P (1981) Résultats éloignés de la myotomie de Heller dans le traitement de l'achalasie oesophagienne: à propos de 103 cas. Ann Gastro-entérol Hépatol 17: 321
10. Chaib SA, Lopasso FP, Parra OM, Saad WA, Vasconcelos E (1977) Tratamento do megaesôfago pela técnica de Heller-Vasconcelos. Experiência de 200 casos. Rev Hosp Clin Fac Med S Paulo 32: 178
11. Cohen NL, Mattel S (1983) Pneumatic dilatation as the primary treatment for achalasia. Ann Otol Rhinol Laryngol 92 :353
12. Csendes A, Velasco N, Braghetto I, Henriquez A (1981) A prospective randomized study comparing forceful dilatation and esophagomyotomy in patients with achalasia of the esophagus. Gastroenterology 80: 789
13. Douglas K, Nicholson F (1959) The late results of Heller's operation for cardiospasm. Br J Surg 47: 250
14. Ellis FH, Kiser JC, Schlegel JF, Earlam RJ, McVey JL, Olsen AM (1967) Esophagomyotomy for esophageal achalasia. Experimental, clinical and manometric aspects. Ann Surg 166: 640
15. Ellis FH Jr, Crozier RE, Watkins E Jr (1984) Operation for esophageal achalasia. Results of esophagomyotomy without an antireflux operation. J Thorac Cardiovasc Surg 88: 344
16. Espinoza FT, Lamache LI (1983) Acalasia del esófago: resultado de su tratamiento quirúrgico. Rev Gastroent Mex 48: 23
17. Fellows IW, Ogilvie AL, Atkinson M (1983) Pneumatic dilatation in achalasia. Gut 24: 1020
18. Ferguson TB, Burford TH (1960) An evaluation of the modified Heller operation in the treatment of achalasia of the esophagus. Ann Surg 152: 1
19. Groeneveldt FRB (1918) Over cardiospasmus. Ned T Geneesk 2: 1281
20. Hawthorne HR, Frobes AS, Hemir Jr P (1956) The surgical management of achalasia of the esophagus. Ann Surg 144: 653
21. Heller E (1913) Extramukose cardioplastik bein chronischen cardiospasmus mit dilatation des oesophagus. Mitt Grenzgeb Med Chir 27: 141
22. Helsinger N (1966) Gastroesophageal reflux as a complication of the Heller operation. Acta Chir Scand 356B: 96

23. Hill LD (1978) Intraoperative measurement of lower esophageal sphincter pressure. J Thorac Cardiovasc Surg 75: 378
24. Hirao T (1983) An experimental study on temporal changes of postoperative anti-reflux effect by modified Mark IV operation for esophageal achalasia. Jap Smooth Muscle Res 19: 503
25. Holloway RH, Carle DJ (1980) Pneumatic dilatation for the treatment of achalasia. Med J Aust 2: 262
26. Jara FM, Toledo-Pereira LH, Lewis JW, Magilligan Jr, DJ (1979) Long-term results of esophagomyotomy for achalasia of esophagus. Arch Surg 114: 935
27. Jekler J, Lhotka J, Borek Z (1964) Surgery for achalasia of the esophagus. Ann Surg 160: 793
28. Jekler J, Lhotka J (1967) Modified Heller procedure to prevent post-operative reflux esophagitis in patients with achalasia. Amer J Surg 113: 251
29. Lens J, Bijvoet H, Gouw GN, Wamsteker H, Belsey RHR (1980) Preliminary results of a long myotomy with antireflux procedure for achalasia of the esophagus. Netherl J Surg 32: 49
30. Malm A (1956) A 10-year report of operated achalasia of the esophagus. Gastroenterology 86: 208
31. Mandelstam P, Block C, Newell L, Dillon M (1982) The role of bougienage in the management of achalasia – the need for reappraisal. Gastrointest End 28: 169
32. Mansour KA, Symbas PN, Jones EL, Hatcher CR (1976) A combined surgical approach in the management of achalasia of the esophagus. Am Surg 42: 192
33. Menguy R (1971) Management of achalasia by transabdominal cardiomyotomy and fundoplication. Surg Gynecol Obstet 133: 482
34. Menzies-Gow N, Gummer JWP, Edwards DAW (1978) Results of Heller's operation for achalasia of the cardia. Br J Surg 65: 483
35. Murray GF, Battaglini JW, Keagy BA, Starek PJK, Wilcox BR (1984) Selective application of fundoplication in achalasia. Ann Thor Surg 37: 185
36. Olaciregui JC, Alberti JE, Covian EH (1969) Resultados del tratamiento quirurgico de la acalasia del esofago. Prensa Med Arg 56: 1021
37. Okike N, Payne WS, Heufeld DM, Bernatz PE, Pairolero PC, Sanderson DR (1979) Esophagomyotomy versus forceful dilation for achalasia of the esophagus: Results in 899 patients. Ann Thor Surg 28: 119
38. Pai GP, Ellison RG, Rubin JW, Moore HV (1984) Tow decades of experience with modified Heller's myotomy for achalasia. Ann Thorac Surg 38: 201
39. Pinotti HW, Gama-Rodrigues JJ, Ellenbogen G, Arab-Fadul R, Raia A (1974) Novas bases para o tratamento cirúrgico do megaesôfago: esofagocardiomiotomia com esofagofundogastropexia. Rev Ass Med Bras 20: 331
40. Rossetti M (1978) Achalasie des Osophagus – Operative behandlung mit abdominaler myotomie and fundoplikation. Zbl Chirurgie 103: 1180
41. Sanderson DR, Ellis Jr FH, Olsen AM (1970) Achalasia of the esophagus: results of therapy by dilation 1950–1967. Chest 58: 116
42. Santy MM (1949) Le traitement du méga-oesophage par cardiospasm A propos de 94 cas d'opération de Heller. Chirurgie 32: 804
43. Slater G, Sicular AA (1982) Esophageal perforations after forceful dilatation in achalasia. Ann Surg 195: 186
44. Tomlinson P, Grant AF (1981) A review of 74 patients with oesophageal achalasia: the results of Heller's cardiomyotomy, with and without Nissen fundoplication. Aust NZJ Surg 51: 48
45. Vantrappen G, Hellemans J, Deloof W, Valembois P, Vandenbroucke J (1971) Treatment of achalasia with pneumatic dilatations. Gut 12: 268
46. Vasconcelos E (1945) – Apud Chaib SA (1977)
47. Veiga-Fernandes F, Pinheiro MF, Guerreiro D (1981) Cardiomyotomy associated with antireflux surgery in the treatment of achalasia. World J Surg 5: 697
48. Viard H, Favre JP, Fichére JP (1983) Résultats de 90 opérations de Heller pour achalasie oesophagienne. Chirurgie 109: 479

What is the influence of the treatment of a megaesophagus on the development of a peptic esophagitis or a stenosis?

G. Castrini (Rome)

A brief introduction is necessary to discuss the influence that an esophageal myotomy may exert on the development of peptic esophagitis. First of all, we must consider the intrinsic and extrinsic mechanisms which guarantee normal gastroesophageal competence. The intrinsic mechanisms involve the lower esophageal sphincter (LES) and the mechanisms regulating it, which are either nervous (vagus nerve) or hormonal (gastrin, secretin, glucagon, CCK, and prostaglandins).

The extrinsic mechanisms are:

1. Abdominal site of distal esophagus maintained by:
   - Phrenoesophageal membrane of Leimer-Bertelli, reinforced by muscular fibers of Juvara (supradiaphragmatic) and Rouget (subdiaphragmatic).
2. Angle of His, maintained also by anchorage of cardial region by:
   - Phrenoesophageal membrane
   - Gastrophrenic ligament
   - "Pars condensa" of the small omentum
   - Left gastric artery
   - Helvetius collar
   - Oblique fibers of Willis
   - Sling of Allison (right diaphragmatic pillar).
3. Semilunar plica or valve of Von Gubaroff

The Heller-Zaaijer myotomy completely abolishes the most important among the intrinsic mechanisms, which is the LES; moreover, it deeply alters the extrinsic mechanisms due to mobilization of distal esophagus, esophagogastric junction and first portion of the stomach: a pathological gastroesophageal reflux often follows this technique [1, 2] and for this reason, it is mandatory to perform an antireflux procedure [3, 4]. In my opinion, it is not rational to abolish a high pressure zone which does not relax after swallowing and to create another high pressure zone, even if surgically calibrated by the gastric wrap doubtfully able to relax [5].

The possibility of avoiding an antireflux procedure is offered by two solutions. The first one is to leave a short subhiatal remnant of the LES, which minimizes the risk of postoperative gastroesophageal reflux, after the myotomy is performed [6]. Nevertheless, this technique could result in a residual disease because of an incomplete myotomy.

The second one is offered by our technique of esophagocardiomyotomy [7, 8], according to the following principles:

- To reestablish and to extend the length of the abdominal esophagus.
- Absolute respect of all the extrinsic anatomic components (phreno-esophageal membrane, perihiatal structures, etc.), maintaining the normal connections among esophagus, stomach and surrounding structures.

- Maintenance or increment of the His angle.
- Maintenance of the oblique fibers of the so-called "Helvetius Collar".
- Extension of the myotomy 1.5–2 cm on the gastric side.
- To fix the edges of the myotomy to the hiatus.

Such a result can be obtained performing a myotomy through a thoracic approach without opening the hiatus but doing a peri-hiatal phrenotomy in order to complete the myotomy on the abdominal side. In 39 patients followed-up of 46 operated on, we had 2.3% with pathological gastroesophageal reflux controlled by prolonged 24 hrs pH monitoring test.

Regarding the stenosis, the first physiopathological cause is a gastroesophageal reflux and the following evolutive esophagitis: we have already discussed about this problem.

Other causes can be responsible for stenosis:

- Growth of scar tissue on the myotomy or the reestablishment of the cardial muscular ring. In order to avoid that, it is necessary to make an accurate hemostasis of the breach of the myotomy and to fix the edges of the myotomy to the diaphragm to maintain the surgical esophageal breach opened because of the respiratory movements.
- An incorrect or too tight antireflux repair.

In conclusion, an antireflux repair after an esophageal myotomy for achalasia can be followed by important complications.

In our experience of 39 patients, we have not observed any esophageal stenosis. I have no statistical data from other colleagues about the incidence of stenosis following esophageal myotomy and antireflux repair.

In my personal experience I treated 9 patients operated on elsewhere for stenosis after myotomy and antireflux repair (5 Nissen, 3 Toupet, 1 Dor). We have always been obliged to perform an esophageal resection.

References

1. Nemir P Jr, Fallahnejad M, Bose B, Jacobowitz D, Frohese AS, Hawthome HR (1971) A study of the cause of failure of esophagocardiomyotomy for achalasia. Am J Surg 121: 143–149
2. Rees JR, Thorbjarnarson B, Barnes WH (1970) Achalasia. Results of operation in 84 patients. Ann Surg 171: 195–201
3. DeMeester TR, Johnson LF, Kent AH (1974) Evaluation of current operations for the prevention of gastroesophageal reflux. Ann Surg 180: 511–525
4. Stipa S, Thau A, Natale A, Giuffré L (1976) Valutazione pH-metrica del reflusso gastroesofageo dopo operazioni per acalasia. Il Policlinico Sez Chir 83: 50–57
5. Skinner DB (1977) Complications of surgery for gastroesophageal reflux. World J Surg 1: 485–490
6. Ellis FH Jr, Crozier RE, Watkins E Jr (1984) Operation for esophageal achalasia. Results of esophagomyotomy without an antireflux operation. J Thorac Cardiovasc Surg 88: 344–351
7. Castrini G (1979) Terapia chirurgica del megaesofago acalasico. Tecnica personale. Atti Soc Ital Chir 1: 716–728
8. Castrini G (1982) New approach to esophagocardiomyotomy. Report of forty cases. J Thorac Cardiovasc Surg 84: 575–578

Are there pseudo-achalasias of neoplastic origin?

G. Cargill, and *M. Duché* (Paris)

Several disorders may be associated with clinical and manometric disturbances suggestive of mega-esophagus. These include the dysautonomies, certain hormonal deficits, and especially cancers.

In fact, certain esophageal and cardiac localizations of cancer may be present with achalasia and inversion of the gastroesophageal gradient, but the clinical and/or manometric anomalies may also be associated with gastric localizations (most frequent: [1, 2, 3, 4, 6], or pulmonary [8] pancreatic or mammary [5] localizations.

Though it is difficult clinically to differentiate neoplastic from para-neoplastic achalasia, several minor signs may suggest the origin:

- the age of onset is often quite atypical (over 50 years). We may note that the incidence of discovery is maximal during the 4th and 5th decades, so that the discovery of a mega-esophagus at a later age is suggestive, the more so since, according to Barrett [10], only 15% of cases of mega-esophagus develop after the age of 60.

Loss of weight is often important and above 5 kg, where as the length of course is brief and often less than a year. Finally, the esophageal dilatation is moderate [4].

In terms of manometric presentation, the following anomalies may be noted:

- the esophageal dyskinesia is not always as great as that observed in idiopathic mega-esophagus; the peristaltic waves are of greater amplitude, less repetitive and sometimes remain propagated. The tertiary waves are rare, even absent. The disorder may be localized to that part of the esophagus situated in proximity to the inferior sphincter
- the mecholyl test is rarely positive
- the amyl nitrite test, in our experience, does not always eliminate the entire tonus of the inferior sphincter, and esophageal motility does not entirely disappear during the test. These anomalies occurred in our experience once with a gastric lesion and once with a pancreatic lesion.

However, these clinical, radiologic or manometric features are not specific or constant, and deceptive forms are numerous [7]. Localized dyskinesia may be associated with a less advanced form of mega-esophagus, as also a hardly altered aspect of this dyskinesia.

On the other hand, it is possible that the aperistalsis in the body of the esophagus may be associated with the existence of a common pressure chamber promoted by the stasis. This may also explain the polyphasic appearance of certain waves.

The mechanism of these manometric anomalies is unknown, but destruction of Auerbach's plexus is not always observed [1, 4, 6] and one may therefore routinely suspect the infiltration of the submucosa of the distal esophagus reported by some authors [9]. This may probably indicate a para-neoplastic phenomenon whose mechanism remains completely ignored to this day.

Finally, observation of this type of disorder does not allow an opinion as to the site of the neoplasia (which is usually adjacent to the cardiac region, [4].

We have not had the opportunity of monitoring the course of the initially observed esophageal kinetics after treatment of the lesion responsible for the disorder, but several authors have described a return to strictly normal motility after treatment by medical means, surgery or radiotherapy, both at the level of the inferior sphincter and in the body of the esophagus [1, 3, 8].

References

1. Menin R, Fisher R (1981) Return of esophageal peristalsis in achalasia secondary to gastric cancer. Dig Dis 26, 11: 1038–1044
2. McCallum RW (1979) Esophageal achalasia secondary to gastric carcinoma. Am J gastroenterol 71, 24: 29
3. Davis JA et al. (1975) Reversible achalasia due to reticulum cell sarcoma. N Engl J Med 293: 130–132
4. Tucker HJ et al. (1978) Achalasia secondary to carcinoma: manometric and clinical features. Ann intern Med 89: 315–318
5. Vincre G et al. (1978) Achalasia secondaria a carcinoma infiltrante l'esofago. Mia Chir 33: 1109–1114
6. Shulze KS et al. (1975) Esophageal achalasia associated with gastric carcinoma: lack of evidence for widespread plexus destruction. CMA Journal, 112: 857, 864
7. Sandler RS et al. (1982) Failure of clinical criteria to distinguish between primary achalasia and achalasia secondary to tumor. Dig Dis 27: 3, 209, 213
8. Goldin NR (1983) Secondary achalasia: association with adenocarcinoma of the lung and reversal with radiation therapy. Ann J Gastroenterol 78: 4, 203, 205
9. Kolodny M et al. (1968) Esophageal achalasia probably due to gastric carcinoma. Ann Intern Med 69: 569–572
10. Barrett NR (1964) Achalasia of the cardia: reflections upon a clinical study of over 100 cases. Br Med J 1: 1135–1140

Ch. Théodore, P.-E. Julien, G. Gargill, and *J. A. Paolaggi* (Paris)

The aim of this communication is to report an observation of an achalasia secondary to tumor and to review this disease.

Observation

A 46-year-old man was admitted to hospital because of recent onset of dysphagia, and wasting. Case history disclosed cephalic duodeno-pancreatectomy for adenocarcinoma of the Vater ampulla two years earlier. Physical examination as well as endoscopy of the cardia were normal. The esophageal manometry revealed

- hypertonicity of the lower esophageal sphincter (LOS) (80 cm of H_2O for a normal less than 35 cm);
- absence of LOS relaxation with swallowing;
- dyskinesia of the body, deglutition only producing non propagated, repetitive cupula waves. Treatment with nifedipine, followed by isosorbide dinitrate and then by pneumatic dilatation was ineffective. Exploratory laparotomy showed an abdominal esophagus *engainated* by nodes. Histology showed an adenocarcinoma.

Commentary

The clinical, radiological, endoscopic and manometric symptoms of neoplastic achalasia are those of idiopathic achalasia. The diagnosis can be considered when unusual clinical features are seen in the course of idiopathic achalasia: age older than 50 years, clinical symptoms for less than one year, important wasting, pneumatic dilatations, totally ineffective. The sensitivity of the first three signs is excellent, but their positive predictive value is small.

About a dozen observations of neoplastic achalasia have been reported, most of the time in relation to gastric adenocarcinoma; [2] cancer of the pancreas, breast, bronchus, a lymphoma, metastasis of prostatic cancer, a pleural mesothelioma [1] could exceptionally fit into the above setting. In all the cases, the neoplastic tissue is in direct contact with the esophagus.

The mechanism of neoplastic achalasia is a controversial question: the neoplastic infiltration of the esophageal submucous plexus and/or of the pneumogastrics seems insufficient to explain the manometric abnormalities; the body dyskinesia can be explained by the esophageal dilatation above the tumoral compression, dilatation can possibly induce abnormal contractions. Tomodensitometry (and may be echo-endoscopy) can give evidence of periesophageal tumoral infiltration and thus permit the limitation of exploratory thoracotomy recommended by some physicians when diagnosis of secondary achalasia is suspected.

The regression of manometric abnormalities has been seen after chemotherapy in a case of lymphoma and after resection and esogastric anastomosis in a case of cancer of the cardia.

References

1. Hostein J, Gignoux C, Roget L et al. (1984) Achalasie du sphincter inférieur de l'œsophage secondaire à un mésothéliome pleural. Gastroenterol Clin Biol 8: 880–881
2. Julien PE, Bertrand HJ, Theodore Ch et al. (1984) Achalasie d'origine néoplasique. Gastroenterol Clin Biol 8: 86–92

Caustic stenosis

Caustic Stenosis: anatomo-radiological correlations

C. G. Bremner (Johannesburg)

Lye or caustic soda (sodium hydroxide), battery acid (sulphuric), hydrochloric acid, phosphoric acid, kitchen detergents (sodium hypochlorite), potassium permanganate, iodine, creosote, lysol, paint remover, dry ice, clinitest tablets and potassium dichromate are agents ingested accidentally or in suicidal attempts, and which may cause damage to the esophagus or stomach. Caustic soda and battery acid are the two most common agents responsible in our series, and usually cause serious burns [1]. In our experience, kitchen detergents have not resulted in permanent damage. The severity of the damage to the esophagus will depend not only on the type of agents swallowed, but also on the amount and duration of contact. Caustic soda and acids are more likely to cause severe destruction and ulceration than bleaches and ammonia which usually result in mucosal edema only. Acid ingestion results in a higher prevalence of structuring and has a graver prognosis [2].

Following corrosive ingestion with liquefaction (alkaline agents) or coagulation necrosis (acid agents), the necrotic tissue will slough within several days, leaving an ulcerating surface which must heal by ingrowth of epithelium. Secondary infection with E Coli, staph, candida or klebsiella may result in further inflammation, necrosis and stricture formation. Stricture formation does not usually begin before 3 weeks, and contrast radiography at this time will provide more information than in the early stages [3]. However, the immediate burn may be serious, usually heralded by severe chest pain and sometimes shock, and in such circumstances a chest X Ray and urgent contrast study will give warning that urgent surgery is necessary.

Plain roentgenography of the chest and abdomen: These studies may give evidence of mediastinitis, peritonitis or gastric perforation. A soft tissue mass, widening of the mediastinum, mediastinal air, pleural reaction and effusion or a pneumothorax suggests serious damage.

Contrast studies: If perforation is suggested, a water soluble contrast study (Dionosil-Glaxo) should be used Fig. 1. Aspirated gastrografin causes acute pulmonary edema and barium is irritant to the mediastinum, and these agents should therefore not be used. Areas of burning or stricturing do not necessarily correspond to the areas of normal anatomical narrowing. The terminal esophagus at hiatal level is rarely involved. The region from the aortic arch to within 1–2 cm of the hiatus was the area most severely involved in Marchand's series [4].

Cine-esophagography: this is useful to demonstrate disordered motility. Kuhn and Tunell [5] have identified three distinct cine patterns of disordered motility:

1. an atonic dilated esophagus with gas trapping suggesting diffuse muscle necrosis and impending perforation,

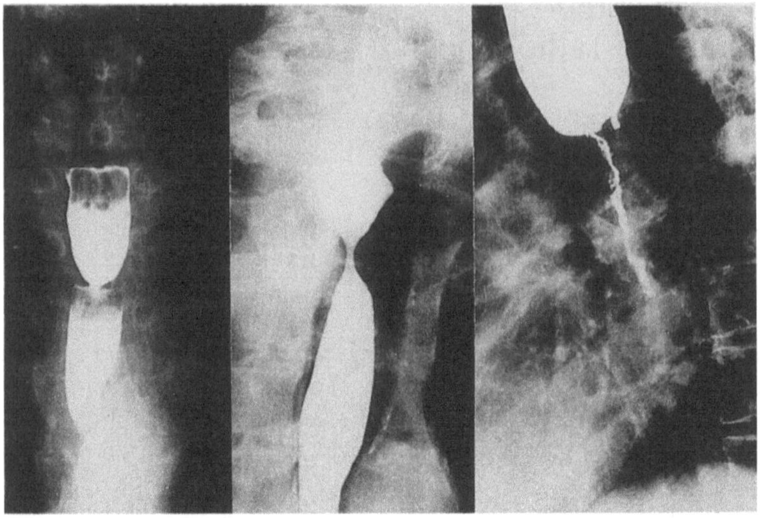

Fig. 1. Examples of strictures:
Left: a short dumb-bell stricture
Middle: a tubular stricture
Right: a densely fibrotic stricture

2. an atonic rigid narrow tube-like esophagus that invariably results in stricture,
3. an irritable esophagus where stricture formation was much less common.

Classification of corrosive burns of the esophagus (Table 1)

The degree and extent of the burn is often difficult to evaluate at the first endoscopy, and the severity of the chest and epigastric pain will also help to guide the clinician. Marchand [4] used a method of grading (Table 2) with prognostic correlates. Pharyngeal burns are difficult to assess radiologically, and are best evaluated by pharyngoscopy.

Table 1. Classification of esophageal burns, and area involved

Degree:	
First	(Mucosal) Hyperaemia, edema
Second	(Transmucosal) Ulceration
Third	(Peri-esophageal) Deep ulceration
	Mediastinal, pleural or peritoneal penetration
Area Involved:	
Oro-pharyngeal	Lips, tongue, floor of mouth, soft palate and pharynx
Laryngeal	With or without cord involvement
Esophageal	*Segmental*
	Total
Gastric	*Segmental*
	Total
Duodenal	
Jejunal	(Uncommon)

Table 2. Grading of corrosive esophageal strictures and prognosis (After Marchand)

Grade	*Features*	*Prognosis*
1	Short linear shelf strictures. Less than circumferential	No dysphagia No permanent strictures No progression
2	Short annular, circumferential strictures Minimal fibrosis	No dysphagia Occasional bolus obstruction No progression
3	Dumb-bell shape. Dense annular strictures Length 1 cm. Fibrotic wall	Fibrotic narrow stricture
4 (a)	Tubular >1 cm in length	No progressive narrowing Easy dilatation
4 (b)	Tubular >1 cm in length Densly fibrotic Narrow lumen	Difficult dilatation

Gastro-esophageal reflux following caustic injury to the esophagus

Not only does a corrosive burn heal by stricture, but the esophagus may shorten and result in a traction hiatal hernia [6]. It is our policy to do manometry and reflux tests on patients who have recovered from corrosive burns, and to advise anti-reflux measures when necessary.

Gastric burns

Severe damage to the stomach may take place in the absence of serious esophageal injury, and this pattern is said to occur more frequently with acid burns. Early contrast studies are indicated in severe burns, but may not be of value before 3 weeks after the burn. We have experienced severe gastric burns with caustic soda and acid. Antral narrowing and even complete pyloric stenosis may occur. Damage to the gastric mucosa may not be detected radiologically unless careful methods are used. Narrowing, rigidity of the gastric wall, and stenosis are not uncommon findings. Severe burning and contracture may result in diffuse gastric fibrosis. Duodenal and Jejunal fibrosis are uncommon.

Conclusions

The site of corrosive strictures is not necessarily related to anatomic segments, and are not particularly related to the cricopharyngeal or lower esophageal sphincters. The pyloric, sphincter may well protect the duodenum from burning because duodenal injuries are very uncommon. Stricture sites are unpredictable.

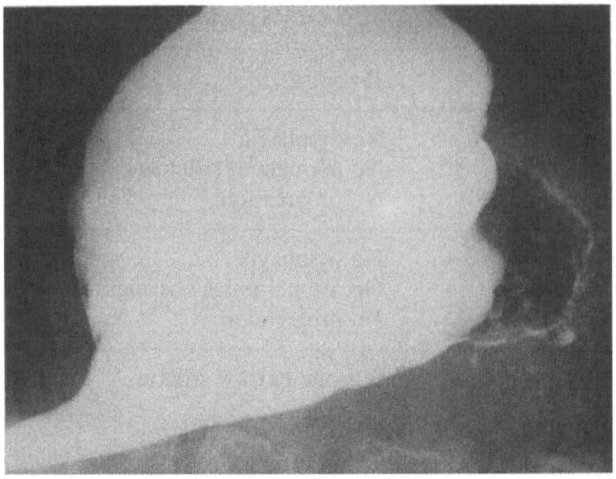

Fig. 2. Caustic antral and pyloric stenosis

References

1. Bremner CG (1986) Corrosive and Non-Reflux Oesophagitis. In Surgery of the Oesophagus. Hennessy TPJ and Cushieri A (ed). Baillière-Tindall, pp 262–285
2. Tucker JA, Yarington CT (1979) The treatment of caustic ingestion. Otolaryngology Clinics of North America 12: 345–350
3. Belsey RHR (1985) Corrosive strictures of the Esophagus. In: Esophageal Disorders. Pathophysiology and Therapy. DeMeester TR and Skinner DB (ed). Raven Press
4. Marchand P (1955) Caustic strictures of the oesophagus. Thorax 10: 171–181
5. Kuhn JR, Tunell WP (1983) The role of initial cineesophagography in caustic esophageal injury. American Journal of Surgery 146: 804–806
6. Imre J, Wooler G (1969) Peptic ulceration of the oesophagus following corrosive burns. Thorax 24: 762–764

Can early calibration with an esophageal dilator prevent the anatomic development of granulation tissue?

H. W. Pinotti, S. Ishioka, I. Cecconello, and *B. Zilberstein* (Sao Paulo)

Corrosive injury of the esophagus has attracted a great deal of attention on the part of researchers because of the potential sequelase, the most important of which is stenosis. Prophylaxis and management of these strictures seldom yields satisfactory results.

Early evaluation of changes by the use of fiberoptic endoscopy [1] has recently been advocated in an attempt to improve results. This enables us to assess the extent and depth of the injury right at the beginning and at the same time provide a more comprehensive diagnosis of gastric or duodenal damage [2].

The endoscopic examination was usually undertaken during the first 24 to 72 hours post ingestion. Contrary to the rigid endoscopes, the flexible and narrow fiberscopes are safe from risks of perforation. This early and detailed visualization of the extent of injuries is crucial and the prognosis as to possible stenosis can be made. A Maloney dilator is used beginning from the 7th to 10th post injury day in an attempt to prevent stenosis. Granulation tissue, a repair mechanism of the injured area, seems to develop from the first to second postingestion week. The use of dilators does not seem to affect this process, serving nevertheless to prevent stenosis. It depends on the depth, extent and whether half of the circumference of the esophagus is injured.

Sodium hydroxide is the most commonly used caustic agent and is responsible for about 60% of our cases. In our series of 40 patients submitted to early endoscopic evaluation, the injuries were either superficial or moderately severe in 32 cases (80%); of these, 21 (65.5%) did not develop stenosis, so that the Maloney dilator was used in only 3 (9.3%). The remaining 11 patients (27.5%) presented deeper or extensive ulcers. All were managed by dilatation for prolonged or fairly long periods. Two patients were submitted to surgery because of concomitant gastric involvement, one to antrectomy and the other to esophagocoloplasty because of the uncertain results of the dilatations.

Among the 8 patients (20.0%) with severe injuries including broad areas of necrosis of the esophageal wall, three deaths occurred from immediate complications; extensive hemorrhage, mediastinitis, and intoxication from the corrosive material. Three patients were discharged after a long period of dilatation and two underwent esophagocoloplasty.

Summarizing, in this series of 40 patients, 33 (82.5%) were discharged without stenotic sequelae, 15 (45.5%) did not require dilatation and were discharged soon after the initial endoscopic evaluation; four patients (10.0%) were managed surgically after dilatation failed to achieve lasting results. Three deaths (9.3%) resulted from the corrosive agent.

According to the endoscopic evaluation, superficial injuries such as erosions or surface ulcers, heal spontaneously without leaving sequelae or improve with a few early dilatations. Deeper ulcers and especially those effecting the circumference of the esophagus almost always progress to severe stenosis which does not always respond to dilatation. Some investigators have reported maintaining a siliconized calibrated dilator in place for about six weeks with good results [3].

Although others have reported success in the treatment of caustic stenosis using total parenteral nutrition avoiding the use of a nasogastric catheter and dilatations [4] in order not to influence the development of granulation tissue this maneuver has failed to avoid stenosis in the more severe cases.

References

1. Ortega Borjas JA, Quiros E (1973) The value of emergency endoscopy in caustic esophagogastritis. Am J Gastroenterol 60: 70–73
2. Chung RSK, DenBesten L (1975) Fiberoptic endoscopy in treatment of corrosive injury of the stomach. Arch Surg 110: 725–728
3. Wijburg FA, Beukers MM, Bartelsman JF, Heymans HS, Jager FC (1985) Nasogastric intubation as sole treatment of caustic esophageal lesions. Ann Otol Rhinol Laryngol 94: 337–341
4. Di Costanzo J, Noirclerc M, Jouglard J, Escoffier JM, Cano N, Martin J, Gauthier A (1980) New therapeutic approach to corrosive burns of the upper gastrointestinal tract. Gut 21: 370–375

What is the incidence of dysplasia associated with the regeneration of the esophageal mucosa?

M. Endo (Tokyo)

We have observed 20 patients with caustic stenosis of the esophagus who have been operated on in the last 22 years: esophagectomy was carried out in eight of the 20 cases (seven were with thoracotomy, one was without thoracotomy). A bypass operation was performed in ten of the 20 cases and other procedures were carried out in the remaining two cases.

In the resected specimens of the five cases in which histological examinations could be performed in detail, marked inflammatory changes and fibrosis were observed, but there were no signs of dysplasia.

On the other hand, in the resected specimen from a 38-year-old woman who ingested hydrochloric acid at the age of 3, cancer, dysplasia and esophagitis were recognized concomitantly as shown in Fig. 1. Cancerous invasion in this case had

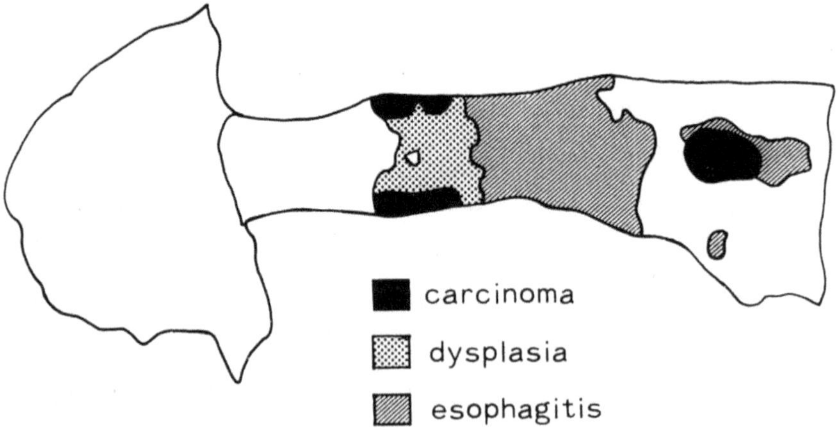

Fig. 1. Drawing of a resected specimen of a case of cancer associated with caustic stenosis

reached the muscular layer, it was histologically typed as moderately differentiated squamous cell carcinoma. In this case, the cancer was considered to be multicentric in origin. No lymph node metastasis was observed and the patient is doing well more than 3 years after operation.

There were nine cases of cancer associated with caustic stenosis of the esophagus in the Japanese literature including the one above. In these cases, cancer of the esophagus was observed 25–51 years after ingestion of a caustic substance. Dysplasia surrounding the cancer was seen in three (33%) of the nine cases.

The characteristics of caustic stenosis of the esophagus are:

- severe inflammatory changes can be seen for long periods,
- development of carcinoma was observed more than 25 years after the episode causing caustic stenosis,
- Dysplasia was not found in resected specimens from patients with only caustic stenosis; however, severe dysplasia was found in three out of nine cases of esophageal cancer associated with caustic stenosis of the esophagus.

What are the comparative late results of the different treatments?

T. Lerut, E. Lauwers, C. Aelvoet, Y. Leclef, and *J. A. Grüwez* (Leuven)

Introduction

Caustic injuries of the esophagus are a rather unusual cause of emergency in the gastrointestinal system. However, the complexity and the severity of the lesions often result in an extremely difficult therapeutic problem, even more difficult than for esophageal carcinoma or peptic stenosis.

Besides the general evaluation, it is of paramount importance to evaluate the extent of the caustic lesions. This is usually done according to the criteria Di Constanzo and Noirclerc [2]:

Stage I: Catarrhal esophagitis, confined to the mucosa,
Stage II: Whitish ulcerations, limited necrosis; small bleeding spots with lesions as deep as the muscularis,
Stage III: Extensive necrosis and bleeding; brown-black mucosa over the entire circumference of the esophagus,
Stage IV: Complete carbonization of the mucosa.

The exact determination of the depth of the lesions remains very difficult, if not impossible. Endoscopic evaluation must be done within 12 h, because thereafter the danger of perforation increases greatly. The initial treatment determines whether or not a stenosis will occur, especially in stages II and III.

Recently, mainly under the influence of the school of Marseilles [2], the therapeutic approach underwent a clear change. Except for the initial antishock therapy, a so-called therapeutic nihilism is advocated. This means, with some exceptions, that gastric lavage is not used because of the risk of exothermic reactions aggravating the condition, no nasogastric tubes, are used, and no early dilatations are performed. Emphasis is laid on giving total parenteral nutrition. This has to be continued until complete healing of the lesions as determined by endoscopy, which can take from 3 weeks for stage II to 3 months for stage III. With this regime it was possible to reduce substantially the number of stenoses.

The value of corticosteroids seems doubtful except in patients with laryngeal edema. Early surgery is indicated only if there are symptoms of free perforation, which of course requires close clinical follow-up during the first days.

Materials and Methods

Our experiences are with 35 caustic lesions of the esophagus treated between 1975 and 1986 (Table 1). Two-thirds of the patients are women and the most striking fact

Table 1. Caustic lesions of the esophagus

1975–1986		
number of patients: 35	☿ : 22 ♂ : 13	
mean age : 16.06 y.		
accidental intake: 21 patients		
mean age: 6.6 y.		19 < 15 y. 2 > 16 y.
suicidal attempt : 14 patients		
mean age: 32.3 y.		0 < 15 y. 14 > 16 y.

is the low mean age of this population (16 years) with 19 patients (54%) being under 15 years. Just over one-third of all patients and 87.5% of all patients older than 16 years were admitted after an attempt at suicide, the majority of them (86%) being women. The caustic products used were mainly alkali (71%), e.g., Destop, Calligène.

The patients can be divided into two groups: group I (20 patients) which comprises those patients who where admitted as an emergency, and group II (15 patients), those patients who were referred for further treatment on an elective basis.

Results

In group I (Table 2) there were five patients who did not require any specific treatment. Five patients with stage 2 and 3 lesions were treated conservatively.

Three of them developed a stenosis requiring dilatation, which resulted in a coloplasty in one patient. The two patients admitted last were treated with total parenteral nutrition and their lesions healed without any stenosis. Ten patients developed signs of free perforation and operations were performed immediately. They showed that there were extensive esophageal lesions in each case, and that the burns extended to other organs in eight of the ten patients. Three patients died, primarily due to extensive pulmonary lesions. As a result of the return to the use of the stripping technique in cancer surgery by Akiyama [1], we also applied this method for caustic lesions in five patients. Thus, a thoracotomy was avoided, which certainly diminished the operative trauma.

In group 2 (Table 3) were 15 patients, referred on an elective basis. Eleven were treated by dilatation, and in one patient this was followed by coloplasty. In four patients a coloplasty was performed initially, with a simultaneous or second-stage esophagectomy in three out of the four. For the whole group, 32 out of 35 patients survived (91%); (Table 4). Five patients did not require any treatment at all, and 14

Table 2. Caustic lesions of the esophagus

Group I: urgent admission: 20 patients
- 5 patients: 4 stage I
  1 stage II
  no specific treatment
- 5 patients: stage II–III
  conservative treatment and dilatation of the esophagus*
- 10 patients: stage IV associated with symptoms of free perforation
  esophagectomy** (8 associated with more extensive resections in the abdominal cavity)
  mortality 3/10

* 1 patient underwent a coloplasty later
** 5 times, a "stripping" of the esophagus was carried out

Table 3. Caustic lesions of the esophagus

Group II	elective treatment	: 15 patients
	dilatation	: 11 patients*
	coloplasty	: 4 patients

* 1 patient underwent a coloplasty later

Table 4. Caustic lesions of the esophagus

Groupe I:
emergency: 20 patients
mortality: 3

Group II:
elective: 15 patients

32 patients

- 5 patients: no treatment
- 14 patients: conservative (12 received dilatation)
- in 12 patients, 13 coloplasties were performed
- 1 jejunoplasty

patients were treated conservatively, of whom 12 (all children) required dilatation (Table 5). In 11 cases the Rehbein dilatation method was used, safely dilating the stenosis using an endless thread coming out through a gastrostomy. Dilatation was performed under general anesthesia. In one now adult patient, dilatation was performed by means of an olive dilator. Two perforations were observed that could be treated conservatively. In nine patients, treatment was complete at the time of this study. The mean number of dilatations per patient was 26, ranging from 18 to 42. The mean duration of treatment was 46 months (range 24–84). This method is thus a rather tedious and time-consuming form of treatment, especially in children, for whom general anesthesia is mandatory for each dilatation.

The follow-up revealed that three patients have occasional dysphagia, and that six children are free of symptoms. Multiple dilatations and scar-tissue formation with retraction can induce hiatal hernia and reflux. In one patient reflux has been observed and in two patients a hiatal hernia has been noticed, but no antireflux surgery has as yet been necessary. Thirteen coloplasties were performed in 12 patients (eight adults, four children; Table 6) with three short and ten long segment coloplasties. There was no postoperative mortality. All but one coloplasty were performed in an isoperistaltic manner, with the left colic artery functioning as a vascular pedicle. Necrosis developed in one case, which was cured by a second plasty using the right colon and a cervical skin tube. There were no anastomotic leaks, but there was one cervical leak at the esophageal stump after a second-stage esophageal resection following the coloplasty. This fistula was closed through a cervical approach.

Table 5. Caustic lesions of the esophagus

Dilatations
12 patients: all children
11 times Rehbein
1 dilatation with olive
Complications : 2 perforations (conservative treatment)
mortality : 0
results: 3 patients: still in treatment
9 patients: treatment completed.

Number of dilatations: mean : 26 (18 – 42)

Period: mean: 46 months (24 m. – 84 m.)

Follow-up: 9 patients
3 occasional
6 no complaints

1 gastro-esophageal reflux
2 hiatus hernia without reflux

Table 6. Caustic lesions of the esophagus

Coloplasty
13 coloplasties in 12 patients: 8 adults
4 children
3 short segment
10 long segment (1 hypopharyngeal anastomosis)
Postoperative mortality: 0
Postoperative complications : 2
1 necrosis of the interposition → iterative coloplasty + cervical skintubulus
1 fistula at the proximal esophageal stump after late resection of the esophagus surgical closure of the fistula
Late complications
- 4 strictures of the anastomosis → dilatation
- 1 "bulging" of the cervical colon → reduction by cervicotomy
- 1 stoma-ulcer at the coloduodenostomy medical treatment
- 1 redundant colon → reoperation

Follow-up: late mortality: 2 (1 anisoperistaltic colon)
8 patients: no complaint
1 patient: still being dilated
1 patient: dysphagia with solid food (cervical skintubulus)

There were seven late complications. Four anastomotic strictures were successfully treated by dilatation. It is worth while mentioning that the anastomosis often has to be carried out on scar tissue at the esophageal site, since the caustic lesions often also involve the hypopharynx and pharynx. Other complications were an unesthetic bulging of the cervical colon, a stoma ulcer at the site of a coloduodenal anastomosis and an asymptomatic redundant colon. This was in the patient in which we had to use the right colon, which due to its bulk more easily causes redundancy.

Two patients died during the follow-up period. One, a psychiatric patient, died after 3 years from an unknown cause. One patient died 1 year after coloplasty because of recurrent pulmonary infections. This was the patient who received an anisoperistaltic colon instead of the classic isoperistaltic one. One patient is still receiving dilatation treatment for an anastomotic substenosis but is doing well. Eight patients have no symptoms. Finally, in one adult geriatric patient, a jejunoplasty was performed to restore continuity.

Conclusion

Caustic injuries of the esophagus are often very severe and complex lesions also involving other organs. Emergency surgical treatment is indicated when symptoms of perforation are present. Provided there are suitable indications, coloplasty as well as dilatations give very satisfactory results, with perhaps slightly better results for coloplasty. In our experience, 78% of the patients in which the treatment for this difficult condition was completed were then free of symptoms. Patients treated with dilatation, however, have to remain under close observation because of the well-known danger of very late degeneration, after 20 or more years.

References

1. Akiyama H, Nijazumo H (1978) The use of the stomach as an oesophageal substitute. Ann Surg 188:606
2. Di Constanzo J, Noirclerc M (1980) New therapeutic approach to corrosive burns of the upper gastrointestinal tract. Gut 21:370

E. Lira (Santiago)

The question of the best treatment is almost impossible to answer exactly; there is no one treatment, whether it be mechanical dilatation or surgery that is best in all cases. The gravity of the lesions means an analysis of each case.

Our experience is based on about 400 patients who had ingested caustic substances and who came to our clinic from 1953 onwards.

The fundamental conclusion are the following. Only alkalis and inorganic acids of high concentration produce serious stenotic injuries, not only in the esophagus but also in the pharynx, stomach and duodenum (upper digestive tract). In our sample, almost all of the serious cases had ingested NaOH, KOH, H_2SO_4, $HCl_{or}HNO_3$. Around 15% died in the first few hours from multiple perforations or later of septic shock. The 85% that survived needed dilatation or surgery of the stenosis.

In this group, we must consider, in addition to the esophageal lesion, injures of the pharynx and larynx, whose treatment does not have to be surgical (except tracheostomy if necessary). Of the patients that ingested acid, 50% had a gastric compromise; half of them required gastroenterostomy, or distal, subtotal, or total gastrectomy in the acute period for hemorrhage or perforation, or later on for pyloric stenosis. Until 15 years ago, when dilatation failed or the patients were admitted to late, we practiced esophageal renoval or its derivation, with gastric, colonic, or jejunal plastic reconstruction. Now we use surgery only in exceptional cases. For 15 years the patients have been treated with direct or retrograde dilatation (through gastrostomy or jejunostomy. It is very important that the dilatation be carried out by specialists. Once an adequate lumen of the esophagus has been made the patient is taught how to autodilate and is given the appropriate olive dilator; in the beginning it is used daily, and later less frequently until cure is attained.

With this technique, practically all patients are cured. In some cases we resorted to the use of general anesthesia in the first sessions. The failures are generally in children or neurotic patients that state the intent to commit suicide. In that situation we employ surgery, generally without excision, only with derivation and visceroplastic reconstruction.

In summary, we would answer the question by pointing out that our choice is to dilate grave caustic injures from the beginning; surgery is an exceptional measure. The results obtained show that the dilatation must be done by a specialist and later by the patient, when he or she is capable of it.

We reject the use of the esophageal surgery in the acute period except when there are, complications, such as perforation or severe hemorrhage. The errors that we have seen in other institutions are almost always the same; who ever performs the procedure has to consider that the pharynx, larynx or the stomach could be injured, and make sure that the esophagus remains undamaged.

In our experience, flexible endoscopy has been a valuable tool. In the case of serious injuries, however, the endoscope can only penetrate to the point of lesion because of the danger of perforation.

Is it really possible to follow a patient for several decades?

R. Earlam (London)

Carl Linnaeus developed the original coding classification for animals and plants based on two names, the genus and species subdivisions. Thus homo sapiens has a great friend called canis familiaris.

Homo sapiens however had been identifying himself by surname or family name, and forename or christian names, for some considerable time. Canis familiaris just did not bother, except at Cruft's. The English, under the influence of their Scandinavian and German invaders had used -son, -sen, -sson or -sohn to denote the family name but this was confusing in spite of every man being the son of someone. The Scots have Mac to denote a family like Macdonald, although the etymology is complicated with MacLeod, because Leod, derives from a Norse word Leot meaning a sailor, and son of a sailor does not seem very specific.

The lesson is–first identify the patient with all his names, christian or otherwise, in the correct order, but include them all.

In the United Kingdom, there is a National Insurance number which is alphanumerical and unique. It is really only used for general practice and centrally for identifying insurance claims. It may appear on tax forms, which induces allergy, and because there is no rhyme or reason for designation of the letters and numbers, is consequently forgotten; people do not keep it in their wallet and in the UK, unlike Germany, there is no legal obligation to carry identification. If it is available, finding a death certificate becomes easier, otherwise the searcher has to go to the lower end of High Holborn in London to the Office of Population and Censuses in the Aldwych and look through the quarterly volumes, knowing the date of death, until you find the name; then, after spending two pounds and waiting two weeks, you will receive a copy of the death certificate. Is there not a better system for finding out when a patient died and from what cause?

In Sweden, where democracy is safe, they carry an identity card with a number, purely numerical. It is used for individual identification and is computerized. Tax returns have this number. So do hospitals and general practitioners; it is based on a unique event, the six figure date of birth which fixes you forever with your cohort. In

Sweden, a three figure number completes your separation from others born on that day, and in the UK, with approximately two thousand births a day it would have to be a four figure addition to make a ten figure identification of each of the 50 million inhabitants. For those interested in astrology and the effect of the phases of the moon and stars at the time of birth, a further six figure coding of the time of birth based on a 24 hour clock down to the nearest second could be added.

The British do not like illegal immigrants, nor people who claim health care without paying, but they also hate identity numbers and identity cards. They like to call the present system freedom and democracy; others would call it chaos.

One way that the English hospital system varies from the Continent is that specialists run large follow-up clinics. Is this one way of ensuring follow-up for decades? In Germany, the patients return to their general practitioner or referring doctor. In England, this does not ensure a good follow-up because the patients get bored and do not attend; additionally, patients and the administration will not carry the cost. Do not attempt this method.

The author followed up a series of duodenal ulcers who had had partial gastrectomies done many years ago by Mr Herman Taylor: such a retrospective study becomes useless statistically if too many are lost to follow up. This was no exception in spite of his very clever idea of always obtaining originally the addresses of two relatives and the bank manager (English, not his Swiss one). In this series, there was difficulty because 3% were "detained during Her Majesty's pleasure", which means they were in jail...

It did show from the death certificates that the commonest cause of death after gastric surgery was carcinoma of the bronchus, so stop them smoking.

Other methods of following-up the patients include techniques more appropriate to a private detective agency than the medical profession, and include local visits to last place of residence, telephoning the family doctor and having a drink at the local pub. But there is one new development which will help: the Post Office in the UK has put 23.5 million addresses on to a 120 mm hard disc so that you can search for names and addresses, all of which have an alphanumerical coding (the American equivalent is the ZIP code). It is an absolutely classical computerized facility because with computer graphics it could be used epidemiologically to give spatial clustering of patients with a disease, such as Crohn's disease, localised to streets where they live.

It is quite clear that central government is not using the system: In the forthcoming General Election, it has been assessed that over 2 million voters will not be voting because they are not on the list. It is possible that the banking credit card system will be the first to insist on proper identification to avoid theft and fraud. Computerized pattern recognition of photographs and finger prints is already in use, and when this technology is more advanced the uniqueness of finger printing will probably be the final method of identification. Names and written signatures are just not safe enough.

One day, the Government will insist on everybody carrying an identity card and number with preservation of privacy and secrecy of records. Until that time, doctors wishing to follow a patient for decades should use head, pencil, card index and the telephone, but do not try to follow up patients forever in a clinic.

Esophageal dysplasia and reflux esophagitis

President:	*Tom R. DeMeester* (Omaha)
Free Commentators:	*C. G. Bremner* (Johannesburg) *G. Cargill* (Paris) *G. Castrini* (Rome) *M. Endo* (Tokyo) *Ch. Herfarth, T. Lehnert* (Heidelberg) *K. Jeyasingham* (Bristol)

Esophageal dysplasia

How can esophageal dysplasia be demonstrated?

Ph. Monnier, Ch. Fontolliet, M. Savary, and *D. Gardiol* (Lausanne)

In the West, where the average incidence of epidermoid carcinoma of the esophagus does not exceed 10/1 000 000, routine detection by blind abrasive cytology is not a practical matter. Only certain very high risk groups (patients with previous otorhinological, bronchial or esophageal cancers) can justify such detection after 2 years of follow-up, provided sputum cytology and chest X-ray are combined with esophageal cytology twice a year.

In the East, it is virtually endoscopy alone that plays a real part in detection. The discovery of esophageal dysplasias is then made by chance, either during the pre-treatment assessment of otorhino–laryngologic, bronchial or esophageal cancers or during endoscopy performed to clarify symptomatology related to the upper alimentary tract [2].

Morphologic analysis of 190 intraepithelial or micro-invasive carcinomatous lesions of the upper alimentary tract (mouth, pharynx, esophagus) revealed that severe esophageal dysplasia presents rarely in the form of a leukoplakia (a white, slightly raised plaque) or a leukoerythroplakia (an association of slightly raised and depressed white and red patches). In contrast, severe dysplasias of the buccal cavity and pharynx frequently assume such an appearance [3].

In the esophagus, the severe dysplasias have an extremely low-key morphology, either of erythroplastic type (flat or slightly depressed red discoloration of the mucosa) or of occult type (invisible form without modification of the epithelial covering).

This emphasizes the importance of endoscopic vital staining to demonstrate severe dysplasias of the esophagus:

3% Lugol's iodine is a negative marker for "early" carcinomas (severe dysplasias, carcinomas in situ and micro-invasive lesions) of the esophagus. It colors the normal glycogen-rich malpighian cells brown, but does not stain the severe dysplasias, whose atypical cells have already lost their glycogen content [1, 6].

After Lugol staining, a zone of dysplasia will appear as a pale yellow patch on a brownish base. In view of the rapidity and easy performance of this vital staining (simple spray through the biopsy channel of the endoscope), this is the stain of choice for fiber-gastroscopy.

Toluidine blue (1%) is a positive marker for "early" carcinomas (severe dysplasias, in situ and micro-invasive carcinomas), which it stains purple [4, 5]. The taking-up of the stain is due to the structural disorganization of the dysplastic epithelium and the increased nucleoplasmatic content of the atypical cells (affinity of stain for RNA and DNA).

Staining is carried out in 3 stages:

1. Mucolysis with 1% acetic acid: abundant lavage of the mucosa to eliminate the excess of mucus and alimentary debris.
2. Staining with 1% toluidine blue: instillation of stain via the biopsy channel of the endoscope. Contact between the stain and the mucosa to be examined should be about a minute
3. Decoloration with 1% acetic acid: abundant lavage of the mucosa to obtain sharp definition of the blue-positive zones with suspected dysplasia, carcinoma in situ or micro-invasive carcinoma.

The possibility of mechanical cleaning with a swab impregnated with acetic acid markedly increases the production of this staining, and is the stain of choice with the rigid esophagoscope.

The efficacy of 1% toluidine blue for severe dysplasias is excellent, but it is mediocre and inconstant for slight and moderate dysplasias. In the esophagus, false-positives (generally associated with mucosal injury) are exceptional, provided one can recognize the erosive pathology of reflux esophagitis and of alimentary stasis. Falsenegatives are uniquely associated with the whitish form of "early" carcinoma, which is virtually nonexistent for severe dysplasias of the esophagus [4].

The dysplasias with cylindercell mucosa (endobrachyesophagus) do not exhibit any particular morphologic appearance at endoscopy. The vital stains mentioned above are of no value, as they are only effective in a malpighian mucosa. As a result and for the time being, only multiple staged biopsies are capable of detecting zones of dysplasia in an endobrachyesophagus. No experience in detection by ultra-violet fluorescence (after injection of a derivative of hematoporphyrin) has yet been reported.

References

1. Mandard AM, Tourneux J, Gignoux M, et al. (1980) In situ carcinoma of the esophagus: macroscopic study with particular reference to the Lugol test. Endoscopy 12: 51–57
2. Monnier Ph, Savary M, Pasche R, et al. (1981) Intraepithelial carcinoma of the esophagus: endoscopic morphology. Endoscopy 13: 185–191
3. Monnier Ph (1986) Le carcinome épidermoïde "précoce" de la voie digestive supérieure. Thèse. Faculté de Médecine de l'Université de Lausanne, Suisse
4. Monnier Ph, Savary M, Pasche R (1981) Apport du bleu de Toluidine en carcinologie bucco-pharyngo-œsophagienne. Acta Endoscopica 11: 299–310
5. Papazian A, Descombes P, Capron JP et al. (1985) Fréquence du cancer de l'œsophage synchrone des cancers des voies aéro-digestives supérieures (100 cas): intérêt des colorations vitales au Lugol et au bleu de Toluidine. Gastroentérol. Clin Biol 9, 16–22
6. Toriie S, Kohli Y, Akasaka Y et al. (1975) New trial for endoscopical observation of esophagus by dye scattering method Endoscopy 7: 75–79

Is "Asiatic" dysplasia specific?

M. Crespi, and *N. Muñoz* (Rome and Lyons)

The reply to this interesting question is firmly negative. What is specific is the uncommonly high prevalence of dysplasia in unselected population groups living in high incidence areas [1, 2] which is sharply contrasting with the low prevalence in low incidence areas within the same population and country [3].

Table 1. Endoscopic findings on precursor lesions of esophageal cancer in high-and low-risk populations

		Men			Women		
		High-risk		Low-risk	High-risk		Low-risk
Number of subjects		Iran Turkoman 218 %	China Linxian 292 %	China Jiaoxian 152 %	Iran Turkoman 212 %	China Linxian 235 %	China Turkoman 100 %
Esophagitis:	Mild	37.6	41.1	32.2	59.9	53.6	17.0
	Moderate	36.7	38.4	17.1	23.1	14.9	11.0
	Severe	11.0	8.9	1.9	4.7	1.7	0.0
	Total	85.3	88.4	50.6	87.7	70.2	28.0
Varices		13.2	7.2	1.3	18.4	9.4	2.0
Incompetent cardia		7.3	9.2	2.0	8.5	9.8	0.0
Hiatal hernia		0.9	0.7	0.7	0.9	0.0	1.0

Table 2. Histologic findings on precursor lesions of esophageal cancer in high-and low-risk populations

		Men			Women		
		High-risk		Low-risk	High-risk		Low-risk
Number of subjects		Iran Turkoman 213 %	China Linxian 292 %	China Jiaoxian 152 %	Iran Turkoman 205 %	China Linxian 235 %	China Jiaoxian 100 %
Esophagitis:	Mild	58.7	55.8	33.5	57.6	56.2	18.0
	Moderate	21.6	7.5	0.7	17.6	6.4	0.0
	Severe	2.8	1.7	0.0	1.0	0.9	0.0
	Total	83.1	65.0	34.2	76.2	63.5	18.0
Clear-cell acanthosis		66.2	80.8	82.9	64.9	72.4	85.0
Atrophy		12.7	11.6	0.7	8.3	9.8	0.0
Dysplasia		4.7	7.9	0.0	2.9	8.1	0.0

From a histologic viewpoint, the pattern of dysplasia is the usual one, characterized by enlargement and hyperchromatism of the nuclei in the middle and lower thirds of the epithelium.

An interesting histologic finding, often associated with dysplasia in these populations, is epithelial atrophy, characterized by thinning of the epithelium.

However, the characteristic endoscopic and histologic feature found in the population of Iran and China living in the high incidence areas, and never described before, was the high prevalence of a form of chronic esophagitis which was present with much lesser prevalence in the low incidence area of China (Table 1, 2).

References

1. Crespi M et al. (1979) Esophageal lesions in Northern Iran: a premalignant condition? Lancet 1:217-221
2. Munoz N et al. (1982) Precursor lesions of esophageal cancer in high risk populations in Iran and China. Lancet 1:876–879
3. Crespi M et al. (1984) Precursor lesions of esophageal cancer in a low-risk population in China: comparison with high-risk populations; Int J Cancer 34:599–602

Do the endoscopic methods and the non-endoscopic methods have the same degree of reliability?

G. J. Huang (Peking)

In China, in regions where balloon cytology has been extensively used for mass screening of esophageal carcinoma, it is found that there is a close correlation between the mortality rate of esophageal carcinoma and the incidence of esophageal dysplasia (Fig. 1). The higher the age-adjusted mortality rate of esophageal carcinoma in a region, the higher are the discovery rates of both carcinoma and severe dysplasia of the esophagus by balloon cytology (Table 1).

It is also found that the discovery rate of severe epithelial dysplasia increases with age, reaching to peak at about the age of 50 years, and declining slowly afterwards. That of esophageal carcinoma increases consistently with age, but with a slower ascent, and exceeds the peak of severe epithelial dysplasia after the age of 60 (Fig. 2). This is considered as evidence that severe esophageal dysplasia occurs about ten years prior to the development of esophageal carcinoma.

Studies have shown that severe dysplasia is an unstable intermediate or precancerous state which may regress to normal epithelium but may progress to carcinoma in a high percentage of cases. Shu[1] in a follow-up study by balloon cytology, found in a group of 530 subjects with severe dysplasia followed for 1 to 12 years, that 79 (14.9%) developed carcinoma, whereas in another group of 530 subjects with mild

Table 1. Correlation between mortality rate of esophageal carcinoma and incidence of severe dysplasia by cytological screening in selected areas in China

Area	Age adjusted mortality rate/100.000	Year	No. person screened	Results			
				Carcinoma		Severe dysplasia	
				(n)	(%)	(n)	(%)
Rencun Commune	179.84	1983	4.297	95	2.21	278	6.47
Yaocun Commune	187.85	1983	3.527	66	1.87	183	5.19
Donggang Comm.	152.23	1983	4.879	89	1.82	284	5.82
Heshun Commune	135.03	1983	4.677	79	1.69	295	6.31
Lin County	111.32	1971	7.212	78	1.08	135	1.87
Yenting County	79.00	1972	5.697	52	0.91	78	1.36
Anyang Pref.	71.12	1973	17.471	88	0.50	48	0.27
Minchong County	68.34	1975	5.169	27	0.52	16	0.31
Shanghai City	10.69	1971	878	0	0	3	0.34

(From Li JY: Advance in epidemiology of esophageal cancer)
Correlation between: Incidence of carcinoma and severe dysplasia, $r=0.901$, $p<0.001$; Mortality rate of carcinoma and severe dysplasia, $r=0.794$, $p<0.01$; Mortality rate of carcinoma and incidence of carcinoma, $r=0.939$, $p<0.001$

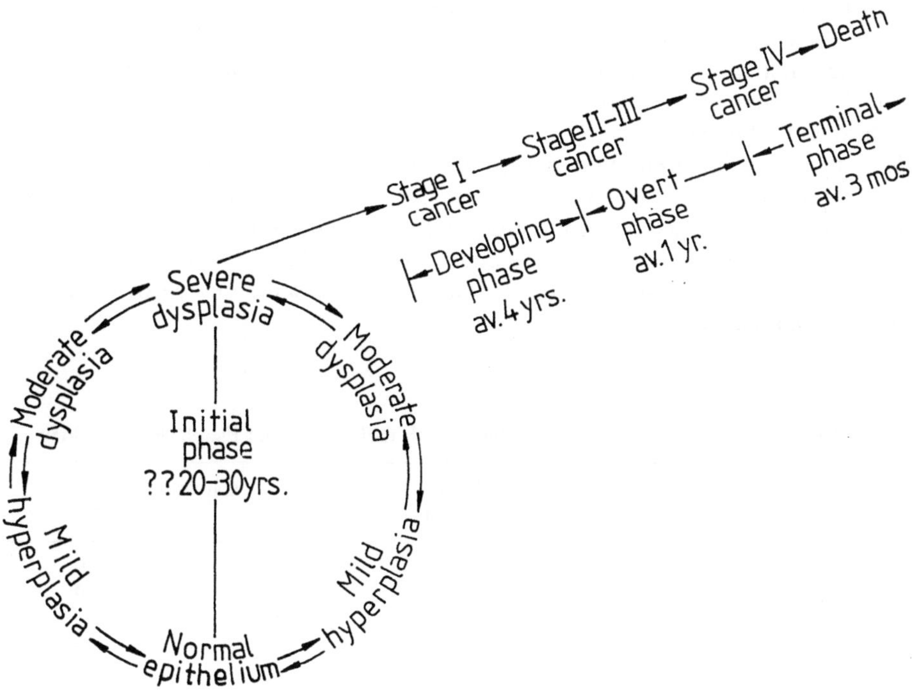

Fig. 1. Natural history of esophageal carcinoma

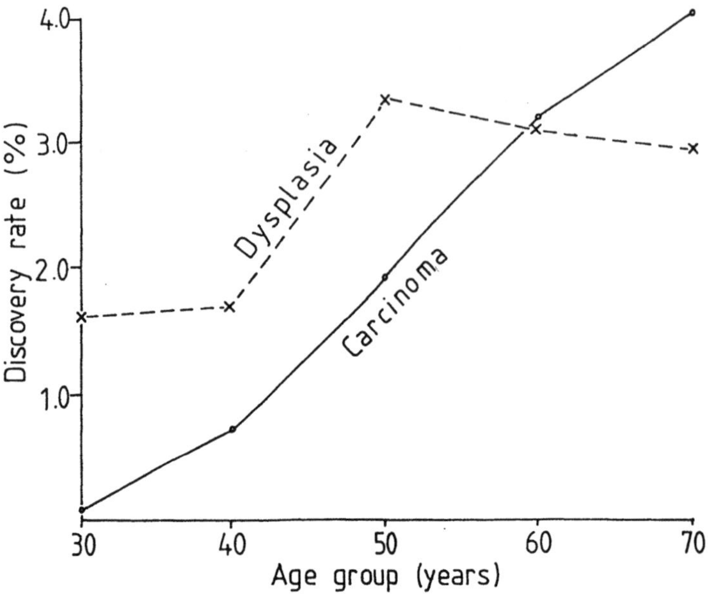

Fig. 2. Discovery rates of esophageal dysplasia and carcinoma in relation to age groups (Henan province)

hyperplasia followed for the same number of years, only 5 (0.9%) developed carcinoma, and in 477 subjects with normal cytology followed for 1 to 5 years, none had carcinoma (Table 2). Other observations have shown that severe dysplasia may return to normal epithelium after proper treatment. In an intervention treatment trial for subjects with severe dysplasia in Yaocun Commune of Linxian from 1974 to 1982, the cumulative incidence of carcinoma in the treatment group was 5.44%, while that in the nontreated group was 21.78%, a difference of high statistical significance (Table 3).

It is therefore apparent that detection and surveillance of severe esophageal dysplasia are of importance for the discovery of esophageal carcinoma at its early stage and for the evaluation of the efficacy of intervention or preventive therapy. Both balloon cytologic screening and endoscopic examination have been used for these purposes with satisfactory results and about the same degree of reliability, which is of course not 100%.

Table 2. Rate of Cancer Development in Subjects with Different Initial Esophageal Cytology

Initial cytology	No. cases	Years followed	Carcinoma No.	Carcinoma %
Marked dysplasia	530	1–12	79	14.9
Mild hyperplasia	530	1–12	5	0.9
Normal	477	1– 5	0	
	1.537		84	5.5

From: Shu YJ, et al. Chin Med J 60: 39–41, 1980

Table 3. The 8-year cumulative incidence of esophageal carcinoma in treated group and nontreated group of severe dysplasia as compared to normal subjects by case control study (Yaocun Commune, 1974–1982)

	No. persons studied	No. carcinoma	Incidence carcinoma (%)
Treated group	349	19	5.44
Control group	698	27	3.87
Results		X^2=1.38	p 0.05
Nontreated group	404	88	21.78
Control group	808	39	4.83
Results		X^2=82.55	p 0.001

(From: Li JY: Epidemiology of esophageal carcinoma)

By cytology, esophageal epithelial dysplasia may be classified into 4 grades, with early carcinoma as grade 5, according to the morphology of the cells with emphasis on the structural changes of the nuclei [2].

Grade 1 or normal epithelial cells are chiefly from the intermediate layers of the epithelium, with 10–15 % of superficial cells. Parabasal cells are rarely exfoliated and basal cells usually not.

Grade 2 is where there is mild hyperplastic change of the cells with the chromatin content of the nucleus increased and the nucleus 2 or more but less than 3 times the size of normal cells of the same layer. The chromatin granules are fine and the nuclear membrane is not thickened.

Grade 3 or severe dysplasia is characterized by the marked increase in the nuclear size of the intermediate cells, which is 3 to 4 times larger than normal. Hyperchromasia is more marked. The chromatin granules become coarse, but are rather uniform in size and even in distribution. The nuclear membrane is slightly thickened but regular. To make a diagnosis, a total of more than 3 such cells is required. Severe dysplastic cells may be subdivided into two groups according to whether their nuclear size is 3 to 4 times or over 4 times that of normal cells of the same layer.

Grade 4 or near-carcinoma cells are those with nuclei 5 or more times greater in size than normal. The chromatin granules are not as coarse as those of typical cancer cells. Near-carcinoma cells always lie in the epithelium, overlying carcinoma of the basal layers.

One grade further is early carcinoma. Typically, these cells show the diameter of their nuclei exceeding one third of their cell diameter. The chromatin granules are coarse, varied in size and uneven in distribution, with distinct malignant features.

The above morphologic criteria for classification of cells are established by visual estimation of the degree of enlargement of the nuclei, which can also be checked with a micrometer. The results of such check-ups showed that the estimation of the nuclear size has been reliable.

It is estimated that by balloon cytology the accurate diagnostic rate is over 90% for early carcinoma and severe dysplasia, and there is a false positive rate of about 1%.

Endoscopically, epithelial dysplasia per se is not perceptible, although it is often associated with esophagitis or other lesions of the esophagus such as carcinoma. It may be diffuse or discrete in distribution with normal epithelium in between, and so endoscopic biopsies may miss the dysplastic lesion and result in false negative findings. The accurate diagnostic rate of epithelial dysplasia by endoscopic brushing cytology and/or biopsies is about 85%.

It is obvious that either balloon cytology or endoscopy has its own advantages and drawbacks. Our practice is to use balloon cytology for mass screening because of its simplicity and efficiency, and to use either or both of them for periodic follow-up study in specific groups of subjects under investigation.

References

1. Shu YJ et al. (1980) Chin Med J 60: 39–41
2. Shen Q (1984) Diagnostic cytology and early detection. In: Huang GJ, Wu YK (eds) Carcinoma of the esophagus and gastric cardia. Springer-Verlag, Berlin Heidelberg New York Tokyo. p 176

How should dyplasias be followed?

A.E. Badaloni (Buenos-Aires)

Patients with moderate and severe dysplasia should be followed-up every six months, during the first two years, and subsequently, every year, if the patient's condition has improved.

That control consists of endoscopy, intravital stains, such as toluidine blue and lugol [8], multiple targeted biopsies, and detection of surface unevenness in Barrett's esophagus and brush cytology. If there isn't any evidence of suspicious lesions, multiple biopsies should be taken at one centimeter interval along the esophageal wall, as well as at the whole circumference of the squamous and columnar epithelium of the lower third of the esophagus. We use histochemical stains for the study of mucins in metaplastic (A.B, A.B-P.A.S., and H.I.D.-A.B.) [2-9], Adenocarcinomas are grouped according to Lauren's classification [3], and Morson's [5], originally for gastric dysplasias, may be applied in the esophagus too.

If there is a premalignant condition in relation to the dysplasia, we use the most successful therapeutic, including the patients in the group for control. If the multiple biopsies show severe dysplasia, we propose esophageal resection, after a detailed analysis of each case [6-7]

Material and results

Forty-four patients with Barrett's esophagus were diagnosed in Pirovano Hospital during 1980–1986. Nine adenocarcinomas where reported (20.45%; four well-differentiated, one semidifferentiated, two poorly differentiated and two undifferentiated. All of them had arisen in an intestinal metaplasia, with severe dysplasia in seven cases, and moderate in only one.

The mucin histochemistry demonstrated three cases with predominance of the incomplete intestinal metaplasia type III, which mainly secreted sulphomucins. Other three cases showed metaplasia type II, with predominant secretion of sialomucins; the rest of the cases had similar areas with metaplasia type II and III. There was no relationship between well-differentiated adenocarcinoma and intestinal metaplasia type 3.

We have seen only one case with moderate dysplasia; it originated in the metaplastic epithelium of Barrett's esophagus without neoplasm. The antireflux surgery was successful, and there were no evidence of dysplasia after three years.

Severe dysplasia was detected in the squamous epithelium of a marginal ulcer in one case, and it was resected. In three cases, moderate squamous dysplasia was found with the same localization. Two of them were treated with antireflux surgery, the other one with esophageal resection. There was no evidence of dysplasia in two patients who had been resected and in one not resected. The controls were done in each patient after four, one and four years respectively; the last one did not attend any control.

The mucin histochemistry were performed in eighteen patients with Barrett's esophagus without neoplasm. Most of them (sixteen) were studied by endoscopic biopsy, and the other two after being resected. There was a predominance of cardial metaplasia with neutral mucins, and in five cases incomplete intestinal metaplasia type 2, which mainly secreted sialomucins.

Ninety-six patients with squamous carcinoma of the esophagus underwent esophageal resection during 1980–1986. Moderate and severe dysplasia were found in twenty-one cases, and carcinoma in situ distant from the primary lesion in twelve.

Discussion

Esophagectomy should not be an absolute decision in the treatment of esophageal dysplasia, since the high morbidity and mortality oblige practising resection only with precise indication [6–7].

There was no relation between sulphomucins and the grade of tumor differentiation, despite Jaas's [2] and Riddell's [7] reports about adenocarcinomas in Barrett's esophagus.

Incomplete intestinal metaplasia type 3 was found near the adenocarcinomas of Barrett's esophagus, and it could be detected in biopsies of the metaplastic area before the histological dysplasia appeared. The secretion of sulphomucins is associated with an alteration in the intermediate cells of intestinal metaplasia type 3. It would be the earliest sign in high-risk group of patients [2]. A histochemical dysplasia? The interest in mucin studies would be based on the properties of the intermediate cells, since they present homogenous histological aspects but heterogenous histochemical morphology [4–10].

Our observation of dysplasia in the squamous epithelium in Barrett's esophagus without neoplasm (four cases), would support Haggitt's [1] hypothesis; he has reported fourteen cases of adenocarcinomas in Barrett's esophagus; two of them were adenoacanthomas which could have originated in a dysplastic squamous epithelium.

The existence of dysplasia and carcinoma in situ distant to the primary lesion, make an exhaustive preoperative endoscopic examination, necessary preferably with intravital stains. It allows the planning of adequate surgical resection avoiding other lesions remaining in the rest of the esophagus [6].

References

1. Haggitt RC, Dean PJ (1985) Adenocarcinoma in Barrett's epithelium. "Barrett's Esophagus: Pathophysiology, Diagnosis and Management". Spechler and Goyal (eds) 153–166
2. Jaas JR (1981) Mucin histochemistry of the columnar epithelium of the oesophagus:a retrospective study. J Clin Pathol 34:866–870
3. Laurèn P (1965) The two histological main types of gastric carcinoma: Diffuse and so-called intestinal-type carcinoma. Acta Pathol Microbiol Scand 64:31–49
4. Lee RG (1984) Mucins in Barrett's esophagus: a histochemical study. Am J Clin Pathol, 81:500–503
5. Morson BC, Sobinn LH, Grundmann E, Johansen A, Magayo T and Serck-Hanssen A (1980) Precancerous conditions and epithelial dysplasia in the stomach. J Clin Pathol, 33:711–721
6. Olaciregui JC, Badaloni AE y Loviscek LF (1985) Lesiones precancerosas del esófago. Consideraciones quirúrgicas. Rev Argent Cirug, 48:272–274
7. Riddell RH (1985) Dysplasia and regression in Barrett's epithelium. "Barrett's Esophagus: Pathophysiology, Diagnosis and Management". Spechler and Goyal (eds). 143–152
8. Savary M, Miller G (1978) The esophagus. Hand-book and atlas of endoscopy. Gasman Solothurn
9. Spicer SS (1965) Diamine methods for differentiating mucosubstances histochemically. J Histochem Cytochem, 13:211–234
10. Zwas F, Shields HM, Doos WG, Antonioli DA, Goldman H, Ransil BJ, Spechler SJ (1986) Scanning electron microscopy of Barrett's epithelium and its correlation with light microscopy and mucin stains. Gastroenterology 90:1932–1941

Ph. Monnier, Ch. Fontolliet, M. Savary, and *D. Gardiol* (Lausanne)

A histologic diagnosis of severe dysplasia obtained at esophageal biopsy is of little practical value unless it is integrated within the setting of its clinical context:

1. Severe dysplasia in a metaplastic columnar cell mucosa (endobrachy-esophagus) calls for immediate surgical treatment without supervisory delay, given the very high risk of associated adenocarcinoma [3]
2. Dysplasia found in a biopsy taken at the margin of an erosion or peptic ulcer in malpighian mucosa probably corresponds to the dysplasia of regenerating mucosa. It calls for simple endoscopic and biopsy monitoring after 6 weeks, with medication for the reflux esophagitis.

3. Severe dysplasia in malpighian mucosa, not associated with endoscopic signs of reflux esophagitis, calls for detailed endoscopic assessment with vital staining. The question is whether it is an isolated dysplasia or one associated with in situ or microinvasive foci of carcinoma. The initial reply to this is given by the histologic appearance [4]:

– If the lesion is of leukoplastic or leukoerythroplastic type, it is very likely that it already corresponds to a more advanced lesion than simple severe dysplasia (either a carcinoma in situ or a microinvasive carcinoma). There should then be no delay in repeating the endoscopy and biopsies under vital staining.

– If the lesion is of erythroplastic or occult type, there are two possibilities:

a) after vital staining with toluidine blue, the "blue positive" patch is solitary and of small extent (less than 1 cm^2). Biopsy using a rigid esophagoscope and a large-caliber punch forceps performs a virtual excision-biopsy, which is completed by superficial vaporization with a YAG laser. The lesion so treated should be monitored after 6 months and then annually, as the development of severe dysplasia into invasive carcinoma takes place over several years [5]. The only condition here is to have endoscopic assurance (under vital staining) that this focus of severe dysplasia is *solitary*.

b) the lesion appears *geographic and multicentric* after vital staining with toluidine blue (a zone exceeding 1–2 cm^2). There is probably a severe dysplasia associated with more advanced lesions (carcinoma in situ, intramucosal or even submucosal carcinoma). In this case, it is essential to repeat the endoscopy immediately and to perform multiple biopsies after vital staining.

Our analysis of 190 "early" carcinomas (severe dysplasias, carcinomas in situ, microinvasive and submucosal carcinomas) of the upper alimentary tract has shown that an *occult or erythroplastic lesion of less than 1 cm^2* corresponds in over 80% of cases to an intraepithelial lesion (severe dysplasia or carcinoma in situ) [2, 4]. In view of the limited extent of the lesion, biopsy with a rigid esophagoscope allows a high degree of certainty since the procedure virtually amounts to an excision-biopsy.

Once the lesion exceeds 2–3 cm^2 in surface area and assumes a multicentric appearance with toluidine blue, it is certainly associated with in situ or microinvasive foci of carcinoma. In these cases, biopsy or biopsies are only fragmentary and their degree of certainty rapidly diminishes.

If multiple biopsies reveal only a severe dysplasia at the second endoscopy, this should be repeated every 3 months, if possible with a rigid instrument and under vital staining.

Another approach is that of monitoring by blind abrasive cytology [1]. This technique is little used in the West and is certainly less effective than endoscopic monitoring.

References

1. Coordinating Group for Research on Esophageal Carcinoma, Chinese Academy of Medical Sciences and Honan Province (1973) The early detection of carcinoma of the esophagus. Scientia Sinica 16: 458–463

2. Endo M, Takeshita K, Yoshida M (1986) How can we diagnose the early stage of esophageal cancer? Endoscopic diagnosis. Endoscopy 18: 11–18
3. Hamilton SR, Smith RR (1987) The relationship between columnar epithelial dysplasia and invasive adenocarcinoma arising in Barrett's esophagus. Am J Clin Pathol 87: 301–312
4. Monnier Ph (1986) Le carcinome épidermoïde "précoce" de la voie digestive supérieure Thèse de doctorat. Faculté de Médecine de l'Université de Lausanne, Suisse
5. Yanjin M, Guangyi L, Xianzhi G et al. (1981) Detection and natural progression of early oesophageal carcinoma. JR Soc Med 74: 884–886

Do they require treatment?

R. Giuli (Paris)

Apart from the cases in which the dysplasia represents a local reaction to an actual cancer that needs to be detected, the natural history of these dysplastic lesions is poorly understood, and at the present time, we do not have sufficient data to be able to say whether such a lesion is *really reversible* and under what conditions.

Therapeutic problems are posed as soon as a dysplastic type of esophageal lesion is detected on endoscopy.

Large series in the literature (Huang, [1]) have demonstrated a *direct relationship* between the development of a malignant tumor and the pre-existence of esophageal dysplasia. *Systematic cytological screening* in a population of more than 17000 subjects revealed stage 1 or 2 dysplastic lesions in 20.6% and 5.8% of cases respectively.

Furthermore, the follow-up of 530 subjects with severe dysplasia revealed a rate of degeneration increasing from 7.9% in the first year to *66% after a period of 9 to 12 years.*

The histologic interpretation of dysplasia is based on the concepts of *disorganization of the mucosal architecture,* abnormalities of epithelial differentiation and *cellular atypia,* allowing the lesions to be classified as being mild, moderate or severe forms of dysplasia. However, the borders between these different varieties are purely subjective.

*

Moreover, when examining esophageal biopsies, that can obviously only be limited, the possibility of a *carcinoma in situ* should always be considered, as its diagnosis is often haphazard due to the difficulty of confirming the *integrity of the basement membrane* on the biopsy sample (Chomé, [2]).

In squamous mucosa, almost all early cancers are accompanied by dysplasia (Savary, [3]) which, in 90% of cases, is present in the form of satellite lesions around the principal lesion.

However, its isolated incidence, in the absence of any malignant lesions, cannot be exactly determined.

Recent epidemiologic studies have demonstrated a *correlation* between the incidence of cancer of the esophagus and certain *dietary deficiencies,* principally vitamin A (Yang, [4]). Vitamin A deficiency can be responsible for *keratosic* or dysplastic *lesions* (Chu, [5]) in the respiratory, gastrointestinal or genitourinary epithelium.

The chronic ingestion of *alcohol* can directly affect the metaolism of vitamin A (Noetzel, [6]), even in the presence of an adequate nutritional supply, by depletion of the liver stores and accentuation of the break-down phenomena of this vitamin.

Vitamin A and its analogues (retinoids) are involved in *proliferation, cellular differentiation* and *carcinogenesis* (Sporn and Roberts, [7]) and contribute to the establishement and maintenance of cellular differentiation, which can prevent the development of precancerous or malignant lesions.

Very low circulating levels of retinol (30.4 μg/dl) have been observed in a significant percentage of patients with esophageal cancer, even in the presence of a good nutritional state.

This type of study *has not been performed in patients with early cancer or dysplasia* although it would seem useful to evaluate this parameter in this type of population.

*

Some studies (Dowlatshahi, [8]) have shown that the tissue levels of *proteins bound to retinoic acid* were generally much lower than the levels observed in normal tissues, and generally close to *zero* (study conducted in 7 adenocarcinomas and 7 squamous carcinomas of the oesophagus).

It therefore seems reasonable to consider that, in contrast to other tissues, these specific proteins are a *normal constituent of esophageal tissue* and that the capacity of synthetizing this protein has been lost by the cell during its neoplastic transformation.

*

Several studies have demonstrated the *in vivo preventative effect of vitamin A* on the induction of precancerous lesions, of carcinomas, or their influence on the *regression of experimental neoplastic lesions.*

Much less experimental research has been conducted, on esophageal tumors. However, *13-cis-retinoic acid* appears to be able to decrease the tumor-related mortality in rats with a chemically induced esophageal cancer (Moon, [9]).

The therapeutic action of retinoids is evaluated by means of a *therapeutic index* which takes into account the dissociation: effectiveness and tolerance: it has been defined as the ratio between the lowest daily intra-peritoneal dose inducing a

Table 1

Compound	Doses in mg/kg inducing Hypervitaminosis A	Anti-papilloma action	Therapeutic Index
13-cis retinoic acid	400	800	0.5
Etretinate	50	25	2
Ethyl-ester arotinoid	0.1	0.25	2

hypervitaminosis A after 14 days and the weekly intra-peritoneal dose (administered for 2 successive weeks) resulting in a 50% regression in well developed papillomas (Bollag, [10], Table 1).

The O.E.S.O. Group has therefore decided to supply the main centers of alimentary endoscopy and ENT departments interested in the detection of precancerous lesions with a protocol for the routine detection of the lesions of dysplasia.

Three poles of investigation will be considered:

- Serum Vitamin A assay (retinol and retinoic esters by a fluorescent technique) in every patient and at each consultation.
- Assay of the *proteins bound to 13-cis-retinoic* acid in the tissue samples taken from the lesion and a segment of healthy esophagus.
- The treatment of dysplastic lesions by means of *retinoid substances.*

*

This protocol will be employed in two groups of patients

- Patients with *dysplasia of the esophagus* or the upper airways, without cancer, and the possibility of another lesion of the upper gastrointestinal tract: caustic esophagitis, peptic esophagitis, megaesophagus, Barrett's esophagus, and, in general, any lesion requiring pharyngoesophagoscopy.
- Patients *treated for cancer of the esophagus* or the upper airways (no longer having signs of deterioration) and with a dysplastic lesion in the esophagus or the upper airways.

Very careful examination of all the epithelial surface of the esophagus, from the top to the bottom, and then most importantly, from the bottom to the top as the endoscope is withdrawn.

The study carried out is a double-blind one, consisting on the administration of etretinate or of a placebo.

Etretinate will be prescribed at an initial dose of 50 mg per day for a period of one month (two 25 mg capsules) followed by a maintenance dose of 25 mg per day for the following 23 months, i.e. a total duration of 24 months.

Endoscopy will be performed every 4 months together with a serum vitamin A assay, in order to follow the course of the dysplastic lesions and their possible regression.

In the light of the known risks of long-term malignant change in dysplastic lesions [1] and of the constant increase in incidence of cancers of the esophagus in Western countries, if such a largescale trial were to show a real regression of the lesions of dysplasia, a possibly essential threshold will have been crossed in the field of prevention of these cancers.

References

1. Huang GJ (1984) In Cancer of the esophagus in 1984, 135 questions. First polydisciplinary International Congress of OESO. Answers compiled by R. Giuli. Paris Maloine SA Publishers, pp 320–323

2. Chomé: ibid, 334
3. Savary M, Fontolliet Ch, Monnier Ph (1982) Le problème de la dysplasie épithéliale œsophagienne in Résumés de la Réunion Internationale sur la Pathologie Œsophagienne, sous la direction de Reboud E, CHU de la Timone, Marseille: 22–23
4. Yang CS (1980) Research on esophageal cancer in China: a review. Cancer Res 40: 2633–2644
5. Chu EW, Malmgren RA (1965) An inhibitory effect of vitamin A on the induction of tumors of forestomach and cervic in the Syrian hamster by carcinogenic polycyclic hydrocarbons. Cancer Res 25: 884–894
6. Noetzel et al. (1983) Nutritional status and serum vitamin A levels in patients with esophageal cancer in Abstract of the Second International Conference on Diseases of the Esophagus, sponsored by ACCP and University of Chicago. Pritzker School of Medicine, Chicago, May 19–21
7. Sporn MB, Roberts A: Role of retinoids in differentiation and carcinogenesis. Canc
8. Dowlatshahi K, Mehta R et al: Retinoic-acid-binding protein in normal and neoplastic human esophagus. Cancer, 311
9. Moon RC, McCormick DL, Mehta RG (1982) Chemoprevention of animal tumors by retinoids. In: Meysken FL, Prasadken S, Eds Modulation and Mediation of cancer by vitamins. Basel, Switzerland: Karger AG, 44–57
10. Bollag W, Matter A (1981) From vitamin A to retinoids in experimental and clinical oncology: achievements failures, and outlook. Ann NY Acad Sci, 359: 9–23

Should severe dysplasia associated with esophagitis be resected?

G. J. Huang (Peking)

Severe non-specific esophageal dysplasia is a precancerous but reversible state which may regress to normal epithelium after appropriate intervention treatment. In such cases, it must not be treated by esophageal resection.

Severe dysplasia associated with esophagitis, which is either nonspecific or caused by either bacterial or fungal infection, or both, or by gastroesophageal reflux as a result of hiatus hernia, may be treated conservatively or by antireflux surgery such as Nissen's fundoplication, but not by esophageal resection, which may involve severe complications and even more severe postoperative reflux esophagitis.

Reflux esophagitis

When must we consider reflux esophagitis?

B. Millat, and *J. P. Pignon* (Paris)

The concept of esophagitis as a result of the digestive action of gastric juice on the esophageal mucosa was published in 1934 by Hamperl in the German literature and in 1935 by Winkelstein, a New York city physician [16, 46]. The term reflux esophagitis was introduced by Allison [1].

Fifty years later, an accurate definition is still lacking: for some authors, reflux esophagitis is considered to be present when there is an esophageal response (either subjective or objective) to injury caused by gastroduodenal contents [41]; this definition doesn't exclude patients whose symptoms are related to gastroesophageal reflux (GER) even when biopsies do not show any histologic change. Others require gross or histologic findings for a specific diagnosis of reflux esophagitis [10]. In theory, the diagnosis of reflux, the diagnosis of esophagitis and the proof of causality are all required for using the term of reflux esophagitis. A preamble on the conditions allowing the measure of the informational value of a sign is necessary: (Fig. 1)

If the sensitivity of a test evaluates its ability to detect the greater number of cases of an illness, and the specificity its ability to detect the only cases of this illness,

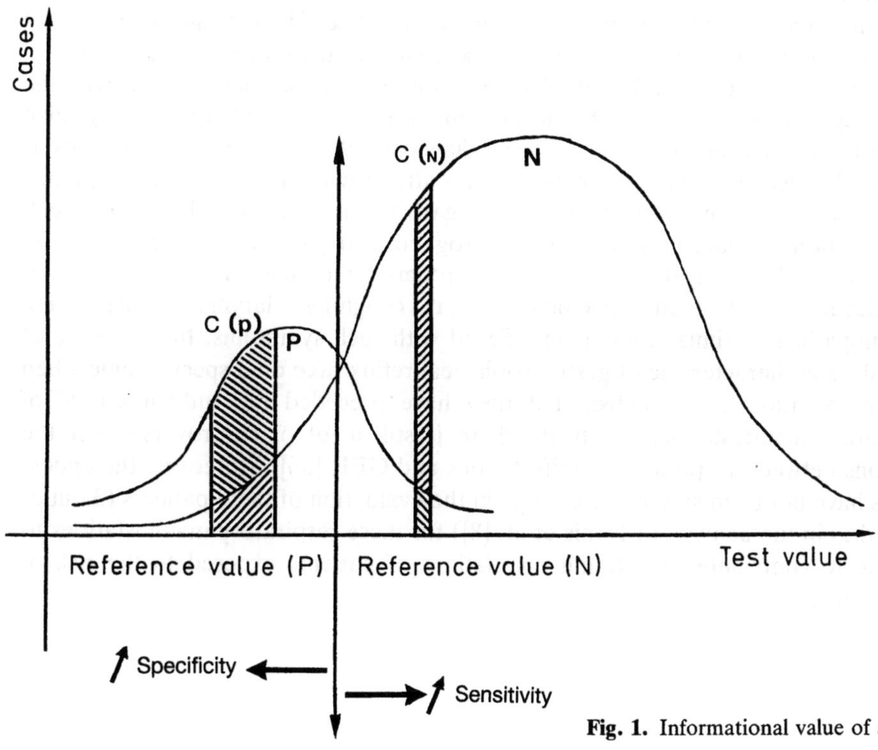

Fig. 1. Informational value of a sign

neither sensibility nor specificity can be used as prediction rules to classify patients according to the presence or the absence of the disease. Prediction rules should be evaluated only if the number of patients and controls studied are in a ratio approximating the prevalence of the disease in the general population. Actually, when the result of a test is expressed on a continuous scale, the results of patients and controls overlap. The choice of a frontier value which divides the entire population into those who have the disease and those who do not is arbitrary. Investigators can be arbitrary when there is a gold standard of the diagnosis, but not if findings are used both as predictors and as diagnostic criteria. Instead of evaluating patients representative of clinical pratice, investigators evaluate samples selected for features that might reduce the variability of the diagnostic test. Indeed, the obtained values only describe the selected group, but are devoid of clinical prediction and general applicability.

The Diagnosis of the reflux

The clinical diagnosis

No study up to this day has permitted the precise determination of the informational value of clinical signs in the course of gastroesophageal reflux. Certain ones are considered as characteristic. They are heartburn, spontaneous postprandial or nocturnal acid regurgitations, or regurgitations triggered off by forward bending (postural syndrom). These symptoms are not sufficiently sensitive to claim detection of all the subjects that present gastroesophageal reflux. Clinical signs evocative of GER may be absent in 20 to 50% of the cases, whereas the reflux is brought forward by other investigations [5, 38, 39]. The measure of their specificity clashes with the frequency of healthy subjects who, without medical inquiry, are tolerant to digestive symptoms compatible with the clinical diagnosis of reflux [31]. Esophagitis is identified in less than half the patients who attend with typical reflux symptoms. Half of the others have another pathology (gastritis, duodenitis or duodenal ulcer). Identification, by means other than interrogation, of patients considered as presenting a GER, enlarged the spectre of symptoms compatible with the diagnosis to the detriment of their specificity: night coughing, laryngitis, deglutition pneumopathies, asthma, chest pains. Faced with such symptoms, the presence of clinical signs characteristic of gastroesophageal reflux take on a special value when the interrogation can establish that they have preceded the sudden arrival of respiratory manifestations. In truth, there is still a lot of controversy over the relations between respiratory manifestations and GER [36]. Moreover, the endoscopies have not been systematic enough in the evaluation of these patients (3 out of 11 studies in the analysis of Denis et al. [8]) for these respiratory manifestations to be able to contribute to defining populations of patients exposed to the risk of esophagitis.

Direct identification of reflux

Direct identification of reflux calls for radiology, pHmetry and esophageal scintigraphy. Bernstein's test, that's to say the perfusion of acid at the level of the lower esophagus, allows the presence of an abnormal pain to ascribe the observed symptoms to the esophagus. Although it reproduces the conditions experimentally, it would be erroneous to consider it as a diagnosis test of GER.

Everything has been said about the mediocre contribution of radiology to the diagnosis of GER. Apart from the criticism we can make on this diagnosis and the doubts we can lay on its role in the reflux, we now know that the existence of a hiatal hernia doesn't allow us to forsee the existence of a reflux any more than it's absence allows us to eliminate it [24, 35]. Radiology is also an insensitive measure for direct diagnosis of reflux: less than half the patients with an esophagitis have a reflux during the X ray tests [2, 12]. The physicochemical changes of the medium used have not allowed an improvement in the sensitivity of this examination. Finally, note that the so called "siphonnage" test only serve to define the physiological relaxation of the lower esophageal sphincter (LES) during deglutition.

In the last twenty years, the principle method of recording GER was a recording of the esophageal pH using an electrode placed in the distal esophagus. The drop of the esophageal pH below four during at least 5 seconds is considered as a proof of GER. Numerous recording methods have been proposed, from a short pH measure for thirty minutes to a prolonged pH measure, eventually ambulatory for 24 hours (Table 1). A prolonged recording in the groups of patients selected by the presence of characteristic clinical signs improves the intrinsic qualities of the method, but not its sensitivity, which stays around 80% [10, 13]. The recording of the pH over 24 hours permits the analysis of the distribution of the different episodes of spontaneous reflux, as well as giving the total time the esophageal mucosa was exposed to acid pH. However there are several weak points: if a prolonged recording give a better differentiation between patients with clinically characteristic GER and those asymptomatic [7, 44, 45], it is unfortunately for them that this complementary examination is of the least practical use. Thus, we rediscover here the same reservations we put forward before:

- pH measurements demonstrate longer nocturnal acid reflux and more important post-prandial acid reflux in patients with gross esophagitis, that's to say, in practice, those identified by an endoscopy. However, neither the nocturnal pH measurment nor the post-prandial pH measurement permit us to differentiate between patients with a histologic esophagitis and those who don't have esophagitis [37].
- the electrode of the pHmetry records the pH of the liquid that is refluxed, but not its volume. The acid reflux detected could be only an indication of another noxious agent in the refluxed liquid [22, 25].
- Only an acid pH or a very alkaline pH can be detected, but not neutral refluxes or a weak alkaline reflux [33, 37].
- even though the use of ambulatory 24 hours pH measurement is becoming generalized, it would appear that depending on the type of equipement used, and the fact the ambulatory recording conditions are rarely codified, important

Table 1. Measurement of pH – values and limits

pH measurement	Specificity (Sp)	Sensitivity (Se)
30 min	0.8 (0.53–1)	0.79 (0.56–0.92)
3 hrs	1	0.86
12–24 hrs	0.98 (0.95–1)	0.82 (0.74–0.9)

Note: This is a selection of the patients studied
Other characteristics of the fluid
Variations in measurement

variations between individuals have been observed which make it difficult to interpret this type of measurement [15].

All these points show the difficulty of an exact study of the esophageal pH to define the role of reflux associated with the esophagitis lesions (Table 1).

Due to the use of an unabsorbable isotope (Tc 99^{m}), esophageal scintigraphy is a non-invasive method of research and quantification of GER [12]. The results are in the form of a reflux index which takes into account the quantity introduced into the stomach. According to the originators of the test, the diagnostic value of the scintigraphy seems to be very close to that of pHmetry. It permits direct definition of the nocturnal inhalation of gastric juice in the respiratory forms of GER [6]. Very interesting in theory for studying the mechanism of esophageal lesions, in practice the measure of reflux value comes up against problems due to the different geometry of the patient, gamma absorbtion and gastric emptying, which make scintigraphy a semi-quantitative method, rather than a true quantitative method [9]. The heavy technological investments necessary limit its frequent use.

The Diagnosis of Esophagitis

Endoscopy

In patients who have GER, the diagnostic role of endoscopy is to detect associated digestive lesions and to measure the mucosal repercussions of the GER. The existence of an esophagitis in confirmed macroscopicaly, and its intensity is measured in a semiquantative way in four grades [14].

Grade 0: no esophagitis.
Grade 1: mucosal hyperemia patchy and/or linear with (1b) or without (1a) friability and bleeding.
Grade 2: erosions, granulomatous aspect.
Grade 3: ulcer, peptic stenosis.

Erythematous esophagitis (1a) is a subjective diagnosis, and is to be classed as normal esophageal mucosa [19, 27]. On the contrary, the most severe lesions are

Table 2. Histologic diagnosis of esophagitis

Hyperplasia of basal layer	>15%	of total thickness of the epithelium
Elongation of papillae	>2/3	
- Correlation with pH value		
- Se=0.81 Sp=0.77	(Ismail-Beigi et coll. 1970)	
Technical requirements (depth and direction of biopsies)		
Areolar infiltration by neutrophil and/or eosinophil polymorphs		
- Se=0.6 Sp=0.9	(Seefeld et coll. 1977)	

quite unusual and can be completely asymptomatic, especially in old patients. Last, a macroscopic esophagitis seen during endoscopy doesn't allow us to foresee the existence of a GER (heavy smokers, alcohol drinkers), any more than its absence allows us to eliminate it. A normal endoscopy is not rare in patients whose reflux has been proved on 24 hours pHmetry [13].

Histology: (Table 2)

Histologic criteria of esophagitis have a place when macroscopic lesions are lacking. The histologic criteria for GER were proposed by Ismaïl-Beigi in 1970 with a sensitivity of 0.81, and a specificity of 0.77 [18]. That is:
- basal cell hyperplasia greater than 15% of the total thickness of the epithelium.
- and/or the extension of the papillae of the lamina propria greater than two thirds the thickness of the epithelium.

The criteria of Ismaïl-Beigi are correlated with the prolonged pH recordings, but not with the clinic, endoscopic or manometric datas [18, 20]. Suction biopsies are mandatory to give the pathologist better orientation and adequate tissue. Tolerance of suction biopsies is not perfect: fifteen per cent of patients developed chest discomfort within the first 24 hours [23]. Pinch biopsies during endoscopy are more usual, but the percentage of appropriate specimens for morphometric studies is variable; 89% rates of well oriented biopsies and 76% rates of adequate amounts of epithelium have been reported [47] but these are rather optimistic.

The diagnostic value of the Ismaïl-Beigi criteria is discussed even in the case of adequate tissue specimens [43]; these findings have been found in 57 p. cent of normal controls [45]. Furthermore, when the pathologist is unaware of the clinical or endoscopic background, agreement between observers for normal and abnormal findings is under 80%, even in Ismaïl-Beigi's own experience.

In an attempt to resolve this problem of histologic interpretation, other criteria have been proposed [43]. A polymorphonuclear neutrophil and eosinophil infiltration of the submucosa was observed more frequently in patients with an important pHmetric reflux (sensitivity=0.60) than in normal healthy subjects (specificity=0.90). Actually, histologic criteria on one hand and polymorphonuclear infiltration on the other, were seen in nearly fifty per cent of grade 1 endoscopic esophagitis patients; moreover, in the same study, these two criteria were statistically independent [47].

By supposing that at the end one has bring forward the diagnosis of reflux and that of esophagitis, is it possible to confirm the causality relationship by other examinations? Two diagnostic methods with causal ambition were recommended:
- manometry of the LES
- and esophageal clearance.

LES manometry (Table 3)

The use of esophageal manometry as a GER diagnostic test followed the recognition of the etiologic role of LES incompetence in this disease. Many works have moderated initial enthusiasm. The published results, and their interpretation are heavily influenced by the selection of the patients studied, and by the definition of the threshold values between patients and controls. One can note today [13]:
- that the clinical use of esophageal manometry is limited by numerous variability factors inherent in the technical conditions of measurement and the intrinsic variations of the LES [42]
- that if the rest pressure of the LES is indeed on average significantly lower in a group of patients with GER, the important overlap between patients and controls forbid, unless therefare extreme values, any individual predictive rule.
- that about 10 per cent of healthy subjects exhibit low basal LES pressure, so the specificity of the method is 0.90
- that important variations of sensibility have been observed ($0.20 < 0.83$), which are related to the type of patients selected. The more severe the esophagitis, the more pronounced is the hypotony of the LES.
- that for patients with symptoms and/or esophagitis, but with a normal LES resting pressure, one can observe inappropriate on manometric recordings spontaneous temporary relaxations of the LES, which could play an etiologic role [11]
- that since the tonus of the LES can restore with esophagitis recovery, the hypothesis of a consequence rather than of a causality cannot be excluded [3].

In clinical practice, except for clinical and specially surgical research protocols, one can really ask oneself if esophageal manometry is clinicaly useful. Yet, in individual patients, there is very poor correlation between a rise in LES pressure postoperatively and whether or not the reflux vanishes [4].

Table 3. Causation in relation to manometry

- Variability of measurement and intrinsic variations of LES
- No predictive value at individual level
- Se=0.55 (0.20–0.83) SP=0.89 (0.62–1)
- Transient inappropriate relaxation of LES
- Esophagitis: cause or consequence of hypotonia?

Esophageal acid clearance determination

The study of esophageal peristaltic function and esophageal acid clearance is of research relevance, however closely associated with esophagitis pathogenicity, understanding:

- evaluation of the esophageal peristaltic activity and of the number of swallows required for the return of esophageal pH above 5 [21, 29]
- ability of swallowed saliva to neutralize acid [17]
- effect of sleep on esophageal peristalsis and acid clearance [33]

Actually, the severity of esophagitis is not only related to the existence of GER, but depends also on the volume of gastric liquid able to reflux [30], on the noxious potency of the liquid [25, 28], on an enhanced esophageal mucosal contact with the noxious agents, and on the individual sensitivity of the mucosa and its ability to recover after the acid agression. Reflux is not the only pathophysiologic mechanism involved in esophagitis; in fact there is a need for a multifactorial model.

In conclusion, it is of interest to analyse what the criterias requested for inclusion in the randomized clinical trials of GER treatment were [40]. Among 52 studies requiring at least one endoscopy during the course of the trial, forty had as an aim reflux esophagitis treatment (Table 4). No patient has been included exclusively on the clinical criteria. Nine trials require only an endoscopic diagnosis, three trials require endoscopy and pinch-biopsies, 19 need clinical symptoms and endoscopy, and four the triple association of clinical symptoms and endoscopic and histologic diagnosis. Among the five remaining trials, all require clinical symptoms, but two without the confirmation of endoscopy. The Bernstein test is used as an inclusion criteria three times, manometry of the LES twice, and pHmetry only once. This study doesn't need comments. When are we allowed to speak of reflux esophagitis? More often or less often than we do in practice?

Table 4. Randomized double-blind trials: inclusion criteria

	Clinique	Endoscopy	Biopsy		Manometry	pH measurement	
9		●					
3		●	●				
19	●	●					
4	●	●	●				
1	●	●		●			
1	●	●				●	
1	●	●	or	●	or	●	
1	●			●			
1	●			●			●

References

1. Allison PR (1951) Reflux esophagitis, sliding hiatus hernia, and the anatomy of repair. Surg Gynecol Obstet 92: 419–431

2. Benz LJ, Hootkin LA, Margulies S et al (1972) A comparison of clinical measurements of gastroesophageal reflux. Gastroenterology 17: 1–5
3. Biancani P, Selling BJ, McCallum RW (1984) Effects of acute experimental esophagitis on mechanical properties of the lower esophageal sphincter. Gastroenterology 87: 8–16
4. Brand DL, Eastwood R, Martin D, Carter WB, Pope CE II (1979) Esophageal symptoms, manometry, and histology before and after anti-reflux surgery. Gastroenterology 76: 1393–1401
5. Bruley des Varannes S, Touchais JY, Weber J, Desechalliers JP, Sauger F, Denis P, Galmiche JP (1986) Oesophagite de reflux: rôles respectifs des facteurs pathogéniques œsophagiens et gastriques. Gastroenterol. Clin Biol 10: 662–668
6. Chernow B, Johnson LF, Janowitz W, Castell DO (1979) Pulmonary aspiration as a consequence of gastroesophageal reflux-a diagnostic approach. Dig Dis Sci 24: 839–844
7. DeMeester TR, Johnson LF, Joseph GJ et al (1976) Patterns of gastroesophageal reflux in health and disease. Ann Surg 184: 459–470
8. Denis P, Galmiche JP, Fouin-Fortunet H, Weber J (1984) Manifestations respiratoires associées au reflux gastro-œsophagien chez l'adulte et chez l'enfant. Gastroenterol Clin Biol 8: 758–765
9. Dodds WJ, Hogan WJ, Palmer DW (1977) Scintiscanning for gastroesophageal reflux. Gastroenterology 73: 418–419
10. Dodds WJ, Hogan WJ, Helm JF, Dent J (1981) Pathogenesis of reflux esophagitis. Gastroenterology 81: 376–394
11. Dodds WJ, Dent J, Hogan WJ, Helm JF, Hauser R, Patel GK, Egide MS (1982) Mechanism of gastroesophageal reflux in patients with reflux esophagitis. N Engl J Med 307: 1547–1552
12. Fischer RS, Malmud LS, Roberts GS, Lobis IF (1976) Gastroesophageal (GE) scintiscanning to detect and quantitate GE reflux. Gastroenterology 70: 301–308
13. Galmiche JP, Denis P, Desechalliers JP (1981) Valeur diagnostique des examens complémentaires au cours du reflux gastro-œsophagien de l'adulte. Gastroenterol Clin Biol 5: 1014–1025
14. Gibbs D (1976) Endoscopy in the assessment of reflux esophagitis. Clin Gastroenterol 5: 135–142
15. Gignoux C, Bonnet-Eymard PO, Hostein J, Fournet J (1987) Enregistrement ambulatoire du pH œsophagien pendant 24 heures dans une population de 27 témoins: analyse des facteurs techniques et méthodologiques influençant les résultats. Gastroenterol Clin Biol 11: 17–23
16. Hamperl H (1934) Peptische esophagitis. Verh Dtsch Ges Pathol 27: 208–215
17. Helm JF, Dodds WJ, Riedel DR, Teeter BC, Hogan WJ, Arndorfer RC (1983) Determinants of esophageal acid clearance in normal subjects. Gastroenterology 85: 607–612
18. Ismail-Beigi F, Horton PF, Pope CE (1970) Histological consequences of gastroesophageal reflux in man. Gastroenterology 58: 163–174
19. Johnson LF, DeMeester TR, Haggitt RC (1976) Endoscopic signs for gastroesophageal reflux objectively evaluated. Gastrointes Endosc 22: 151–155
20. Johnson LF, DeMeester TR, Haggitt RC (1978) Esophageal epithelial response to gastroesophageal reflux. A quantitative study. Am J Dig Dis 23: 498–509
21. Kahrilas PJ, Dodds WJ, Hogan WJ, Kern M, Arndorfer RC, Reece A (1986) Esophageal peristaltic dysfunction in peptic esophagitis. Gastroenterology 91: 897-904
22. Kivilaakso E, Fromm D, Silen W (1980) Effect of bile salts and related compounds on isolated esophageal mucosa. Surgery 87: 280–285
23. Knuff TE, Benjamin SB, Worsham GF, Hancock JE, Castell DO (1984) Histologic evaluation of chronic gastroesophageal reflux. An evaluation of biopsy methods and diagnostic criteria. Dig Dis Sci 29: 194–201
24. Kramer P (1969) Does a sliding hiatus hernia constitute a distinct clinical entity? Gastroenterology 57: 442–448
25. Lillemoe KD, Johnson LF, Harmon JW (1982) Role of the components of the gastroduodenal contents in experimental acid esophagitis. Surgery 92: 276–284
26. Lillemoe KD, Johnson LF, Harmon JW (1983) Alkaline esophagitis: a comparison of the ability of components of gastroduodenal contents to injure the rabbit esophagus. Gastroenterology 85: 621–628
27. Little AG, DeMeester TR, Kirchner PT, O'Sullivan GC, Skinner DB (1980) Pathogenesis of esophagitis in patients with gastroesophageal reflux. Surgery 88: 101–107
28. Little AG, Martinez EI, DeMeester TR, Blough RM, Skinner DB (1984) Duodenogastric reflux and reflux esophagitis. Surgery 96: 447–454

29. Maddern GJ, Jamieson GG (1986) Oesophageal emptying in patients with gastro-esophageal reflux. Br J Surg 73: 615–617
30. Micali B, Albanese V, Baldari S, Gogliandolo A, Gulino FM, Scarpignato C (1986) Vidange gastrique des solides au cours du reflux gastro-œsophagien. Gastroenterol Clin Biol 10: 656–661
31. Nebel OT, Fornes MF, Castell DO (1976) Symptomatic gastro-esophageal reflux: incidence and precipitating factors. Am J Dig Dis 21: 953–956
32. Orr WC, Johnson LF, Robinson MG (1984) Effect of sleep on swallowing, esophageal peristalsis, and acid clearance. Gastroenterology 86: 814–819
33. Orlando RC, Bozymski EM (1973) Heartburn in pernicious anemia: a consequence of bile reflux. N Engl J Med 289: 522–523
34. Ottignon Y, Ampelas M, Voigt JJ, Cassigneul J, Pascal JP (1984) Comparaison de trois méthodes d'enregistrement du pH œsophagien dans le diagnostic du reflux gastro-œsophagien acide. Gastroenterol Clin Biol 8: 609–615
35. Palmer ED (1968) The hiatus hernia-esophagitis-esophageal stricture complex: twenty-year prospective study. Am J Med 44: 566–579
36. Pasquis P, Tardiff C, Nouvet G (1983) Reflux gastro-œsophagien et affections respiratoires. Bull Eur Physiol-pathol Respir 19: 645–658
37. Pellegrini CA, DeMeester TR, Johnson LF, Skinner DB (1978) Alkaline gastroesophageal reflux. Am J Surg 125: 177–183
38. Pellegrini CA, DeMeester TR, Johnson LF, Skinner DB (1979) Gastroesophageal reflux and pulmonary aspiration: incidence, functional abnormality, and results of surgical therapy. Surgery 86: 110–119
39. Perrin-Fayolle M, Bel A, Kofman J, Harf R, Montagnon B, Pacheco Y, Daudet J, Nesmoz J, Perpoint B (1980) Asthme et reflux gastro-œsophagien. Résultats d'une enquête portant sur 150 cas. Poumon Cœur 36: 225–230
40. Pignon JP, Poynard T, Naveau S, Sebag G, Chaput JC Analyse critique des essais randomisés en double aveugle dans le traitement du reflux gastro-œsophagien. Gastroenterol Clin Biol Accepté pour publication
41. Pope CE II (1976) Pathophysiology and diagnosis of reflux esophagitis. Gastroenterology 70: 445–454
42. Pope CE II, Meyer GW, Castell DO (1981) Is measurement of lower esophageal sphincter pressure clinically useful? Dig Dis Sci 26: 1025–1027
43. Seefeld U, Krejs GJ, Siebenmann RE, Blum AL (1977) Esophageal histology in gastro-esophageal reflux. Morphometric findings in suction biopsies. Am J Dig Dis 22: 956–964
44. Stanciu C, Bennett JR (1973, 1974) Correlation between a physiological test of gastroesophageal reflux and sphincter squeeze. Proceedings of the Fourth International Symposium on Gastro-intestinal Motility. Banff, Alberta, Canada, Sept 6–8: 131–138
45. Weinstein WM, Bogoch ER, Bowes KL (1975) The normal human esophageal mucosa: a histological reappraisal. Gastroenterology 68: 40–44
46. Winkelstein A (1935) Peptic esophagitis: a new clinical entity. JAMA 104: 906–909
47. Zeitoun P, Pluot M, Vandromme L, Casola M (1987) Evaluation sur biopsies endoscopiques des critères histologiques d'œsophagite par reflux. Gastroenterol Clin Biol 11: 6–11

How can a normal esophago-gastric junction be defined?

B. Millat (Paris)

Like all responses that pretend to set the norm, the response must be careful.

The first response which comes up to mind leads to defining normality as being the opposite of what it is not; that is as the absence of pathological changes.

The second response would be rather doctrinal if it was realistic, and would define the normal as the gold standard, the model, reference to an esophagogastric junction in whose absence there is no digestive integrity.

The third response is more pragmatic, because of its statistical references, and leads to the consideration that an esophagogastric junction is normal if it is the same as the more usual type. Note that we would miss this normality, since it must alienate the subjects from every means of evaluation. For its appraisal we only dispose of samples of healthy volunteers whose representativity is difficult to ascertain. The fact that a "normal" subject gives his informed consent to undergo the tests necessary for the functional evaluation of his esophagogastric junction sets him definitely apart from the general population; no one however would make the hypothesis that this behaviour is related to the observed results. More uncertain are results collected from "ill" controls, that is from patients suffering from an illness presumed to be unrelated to the esophagogastric junction.

From a practical point of view, a normal EGJ can relax to allow the progression of what is swallowed, and can prevent reflux of the gastric contents into the esophagus.

From a theoretical point of view, one must define a normal EGJ as:

- clinically asymptomatic,
- without any radiological HH,
- without any pathologic pHmetric reflux,
- with a normal LES tone,
- with a normal mucosal junction.

For each test, the rate of abnormal results in a population presumed to be healthy gives a measure of its specificity. No study has evaluated these different methods of investigation in a ratio of patients to controls that allows the determination of predictive values.

Is a normal EGJ clinically asymptomatic?

The absence of any symptom suggestive of GER is generally required for the controls in the published studies. Is the absence of symptoms sufficient to ascertain the absence of reflux? Not every symptom considered to be characteristic of GER is sensitive enough to pretend to detect all patients with reflux. Characteristic clinical signs can be absent in 20 to 50 percent of cases, although the reflux is confirmed by other investigations [4, 10]. During an inquiry conducted among non-consulting subjects, 7 percent had heartburn daily and 36 percent had symptoms at least once a month [15].

Is the absence of HH required for defining normality?

HH prevalence in the general population is difficult to evaluate since an X-ray has to be requested for its detection. In the medical literature, rates from 0.8 to 2.9 percent of HH are reported durlng upper digestive tract X-ray examination whatever the prescription for radiography [16]. When the same motivation and energy are used to investigate the presence of HH in normal subjects as that in patients with symptoms of GER, rates of up to thirty three percent have been reported [9, 17]. In fact, numerous HH diagnoses have to be discussed, and the presence or the absence of HH depends to a large extent on the aggresiveness of the radiologist; when radiographic maneuvers are required to demonstrate a HH, it is estimated that only five percent of such patients have pathological GER [3].

When does a pHmetric reflux cease to be physiologic?

Results of a study indicate that on 38 individuals who did not have a HH, significant GER, that is a fall in pH below 4 not returning to neutral within 30 sec, was found in 7. Other studies have estimated the relative frequency of reflux in healthy subjects. Kantrowitz et al. [14] demonstrated that 8 out of 17 of controls who had no HH and no symptoms of reflux had minimal, and two moderate reflux. Dodds et al demonstrated 9±8 pH reductions below 4 on 10 controls with twelve hours pH recording, and Boesby with the same recording conditions from 0 to 33, pH reductions below 5 in 26 healthy subjects [2]. DeMeester et al, from 24 hours recordings, determined the percent time the pH was less than 4 in the distal esophagus; the time spent below 4 was 2.1% for 24 hours in 15 asymptomatic volunteers [7]. Actually, a pH fall is not sufficient to ascertain that a reflux is pathologic, and it is necessary to take into account the number of reflux episodes, the duration of each episode, and when they occur. Even in these conditions, discrimination may be difficult, twenty four hours pH monitoring only permits discrimination between patients with clinically characteristic symptoms of GER and asymptomatic subjects [7].

What is the normal LES tone?

The tone of the LES is a gradient of pressure between the distal esophagus and the gastric cavity. In normal subjects, mean LES basal pressure is between 15 an 20 mm Hg [2, 6]. During an abdominal compression, LES tone increases more than mechanical transmission alone would suggest, according to intrinsic LES tone properties [5, 6, 13]. An LES hypotony without pHmetric refluxes is observed in 10% of healthy subjects [10, 17]. A normal basal tone is not sufficient to define a normal esogastric junction; according to the threshold value and the selection of patients, a normal basal tone is observed in 20 to 80% of patients with pathological GER. During 12 hours esophageal manometric and pH recordings, transient complete relaxations of the LES occur, that are not related to peristaltic esophageal contractions. Reflux episodes in healthy subjects with a normal basal LES tone are caused predominantly by transient sphincter relaxations, but occur in only a third of such relaxations. Transient relaxations are less frequent and produce refluxes in healthy subjects less often than in patients with endoscopic esophagitis [8].

Where is the normal cardial mucosal junction?

The histologic cardia is the junction between the esophageal mucosa and the gastric one. Circular extension of the gastric mucosa more than 1.5 cm above the diaphragm is considered as the endoscopic definition of a HH. Except for the reservations one could have on a HH diagnosis in the endoscopic conditions of examination, an abnormal junction was observed in 42% of subjects without endoscopic esophagitis [1], this result is in accordance with the classic observation that the histologic and anatomic cardia are not superposable in a third of healthy subjects. With a potential difference (PD) definition of the transition zone from gastric to esophageal mucosa [12], an abnormal transition zone was founded in 18% of 22 of asymptomatic subjects [17]. To our knowledge no study has tried to relate the abnormalities of the PD transition zone to clinical symptoms.

The cumulative percentage of abnormality of tests in 60 normal asymptomatic individuals, was 63% [17]. Such a percentage of abnormality cast some doubt on the ability to define what is a normal esophagogastric junction, and prompt observers to be careful in the interpretation of clinical results.

Quoting off the English epidemiologist Archibald Cochrane, it is inviting to define the normality of an EGJ as the „frontier from where the medical intervention will do more harm than good".

References

1. Berstad A, Weberg R, Froyshov Larsen I, Hoel B, Hauerjensen M (1986) Relationship of hiatus hernia to reflux oesophagitis. A prospective study of coincidence, using endoscopy. Scand J Gastroenterol 21: 55–58
2. Boesby S (1975) Gastro-oesophageal acid reflux and sphincter pressure in normal human subjects. Scand J Gastroent 10: 731–736
3. Boyd DP (1964) Surgery in hiatus hernia. Surg Clin North Am 44: 597–605
4. Bruley des Varannes S, Touchais JY, Weber J, Desechalliers JP, Sauger F, Denis P, Galmiche JP (1986) œsophagite de reflux: rôles respectifs des facteurs pathogéniques œsophagiens et gastriques. Gastroenterol Clin Biol 10: 662–668
5. Cohen S, Harris LD (1971) Does hiatus hernia affect competence of the gastroesophageal sphincter? N Engl J Med 284: 1053–1056
6. Cohen S, Harris LD (1972) The lower esophageal sphincter. Gastroenterology 63: 1066–1073
7. DeMeester TR, Johnson LF, Joseph GJ, Toscano MS, Hall AW, Skinner DB (1976) Pattern of gastroesophageal reflux in health and disease. Ann Surg 184: 459–470
8. Dodds WJ, Dent J, Hogan WJ, Helm JF, Hauser R, Patel GK, Egide MS (1982) Mechanism of gastroesophageal reflux in patients with esophagitis. N Engl J Med 307: 1547–1552
9. Dyer NH, Pridie RB (1968) Incidence of hiatus hernia in asymptomatic subjects. Gut 9: 696–699
10. Galmiche JP, Denis P, Desechalliers JP (1981) Valeur diagnostique des examens complémentaires au cours du reflux gastro-œsophagien de l'adulte Gastroenterol Clin Biol 5: 1014–1025
11. Haddad JK (1970) Relation of gastroesophageal reflux to yield sphincter pressures. Gastroenterology 58: 175–184
12. Helm WJ, Schlegel JF, Code CF et al (1965) Identification of the gastroesophageal mucosal junction by transmucosal potential in healthy subjects and patients with hiatus hernia. Gastroenterology 48: 25–35
13. Janisch HD, Weirauch TR,Hampel KE (1984) Is abdominal compression a useful stimulation test for analysis of lower esophageal sphincter function? Dig Dis Sci 29: 689–695

14. Kantrowitz PA, Corson JG, Fleischli DJ et al (1969) Measurement of gastroesophageal reflux. Gastroenterology 56: 666–674
15. Nebel OT, Fornes MF, Castell DO (1976) Symptomatic gastro-esophageal reflux: incidence and precipitating factors. Am J Dig Dis 21: 953–956
16. Pridie RB (1966) Incidence and coincidence of hiatus hernia. Gut 7: 188–189
17. Venkatachalam B, Da Costa LR, Beck IT (1972) What is a normal esophagogastric junction? Gastroenterology 62: 521–527

Can clinical reflux exist together with normal esophagus?

A. Papazian (Amiens)

The relations existing between symptoms of gastroesophageal reflux (GER), hiatus hernia and peptic esophagitis are very controversial and numerous methods of studying GER have been suggested to differentiate symptomatic and asymptomatic subjects. To reply to the question whether clinically symptomatic reflux can coexist with a normal esophagus calls for a definition of the normal esophagus itself. We report here the results of two studies carried out on this subject by Johansson et al [1, 2].

The first study [1] was performed in 100 patients complaining of clinical features of GER, 24 hour pH measurement, achieved by placing the antimony electrode 5 cm above the inferior esophageal sphincter (IES) recorded acid GER (pH less than 4) during over 1% of the recording period in 77 patients and during over 4.2% of the period in 49 patients. The meals served during the day were nonacid. Thus it appears that a quarter of the symptomatic patients had episodes of acid GER for less than 1% of the recording period, which classes them with so-called "normal" subjects from this reference examination aspect.

Endoscopic examination revealed the existence of a major hiatal gap in 47 patients and of hiatus hernia in 64 patients. The degree of continence of the gastroesophageal junction thus appeared normal in almost half the patients. Further, while the esophageal mucosa appeared altered in 68 cases (erythema 17, grade 1 in 26, grade 2 in 8, grade 3 in 7 and grade 4 in 10 cases), it was macroscopically normal in 32 patients.

Histologic examination of the endoscopic biopsies looked for the classical features of peptic esophagitis according to the criteria of Ismail-Beigi et al [3]: hyperplasia of the basal epithelial layer, elongation of the dermal papillae and inflammatory infiltration. In patients with endoscopically normal mucosa, histologically abnormal findings were noted in 44% of cases.

In all patients, manometric study revealed a basal IES pressure below normal. The pressure varied according to the endoscopic staging of the esophagitis (stage A for grades 3 and 4, stage B for grades 1 and 2, stage C for normal or erythematous mucosae). On average, it was 2.4 mm (A), 5.4 mm (B) and 8.2 mm (C). There were also peristaltic disorders of the body of the esophagus in 18 patients in Group A, 26 in Group B and 35 in Group C.

Bernstein's test of acid perfusion proved positive in 76 patients. Radiologic study defined a hiatus hernia in 72 cases. Reflux provocation tests proved positive in 67 patients at pH measurement (preliminary gastric acid loading), in 48 patients at manometry (transmission of abdominal hyperpressure), and in 46 patients at radiography (barium reflux provoked by abdominal compression).

The conclusions from this first study appeared to be:

1. 49% of symptomatic patients have an endoscopically normal or simply erythematous mucosa
2. there is no statistically significant difference in the severity of pyrosis and regurgitation in terms of the normal character or degree of esophagitis of the mucosa
3. there is a significant correlation between the severity of the endoscopic esophagitis and the total duration of acid reflux, gaping of the cardia at endoscopy and incontinence of the IES at manometry.

The second study [2] was performed in similar manner in 15 patients used as controls who were completely asymptomatic.

24 hour pH measurement recorded acid GER during an average of 0.2% of the period while the sound was positioned 5 cm above the IES, and during an average of 0.1% of the period when it was positioned 15 cm above the IES.

Manometric study noted a normal IES pressure of 11.2 mm Hg for the gastric segment and of 14.7% for the esophageal segment; peristalsis of the body of the esophagus was regular, the average pressure being 77.3 mm Hg.

Endoscopic examination revealed a small hiatus hernia in one case and erythema of the lower esophagus in another.

Histologic examination showed moderate basal hyperplasia in one case and minimal leukocytic infiltration in 3.

Bernstein's test was negative in every case.

Radiologic study defined a small hiatus hernia in 4 cases.

Provocation pH, manometric and radiologic tests were negative in all cases.

It appears from this second study that, in asymptomatic subjects, structural anomalies were found only rarely and functional anomalies not at all.

At the physiopathologic level, it has been shown by Kruse-Andersen et al [4] in 26 asymptomatic subjects that simultaneous recording of acid GER and esophageal peristalsis revealed episodes of GER consecutive to reflux relaxation of the IES, this itself consecutive to the occurrence of a non-propagated contraction wave. It has long been known in human physiology that relaxation of the IES occurs reflexly in response to swallowing, so that oral-aboral peristalsis prevents the occurrence of an episode of GER. Relaxation of the IES in the absence of swallowing would explain the occurrence of GER in subjects with a normal esophagus.

To conclude, clinically symptomatic reflux can coexist with a normal esophagus, just as structural anomalies of the gastroesophageal junction and/or the esophageal mucosa may be observed in entirely asymptomatic subjects.

References

1. Johansson KE, Ask P, Boeryd B, Fransson SG, Tibbling L (1986) Esophagitis, signs of reflux, and gastric acid secretion in patients with symptoms of gastro-oesophageal reflux disease. Scand J Gastroenterol 21: 837–847
2. Johansson KE, Boeryd B, Fransson SG, Tibbling L (1986) Esophageal reflux tests, manometry, endoscopy, biopsy and radiology in healthy subjects. Scand J Gastroenterol 21: 399–406
3. Ismaïl'Beigi F, Horton PF, Pope CE 2 (1970) Histological consequences of gastroesophageal reflux in man. Gastroenterology, 58: 163–174
4. Kruse-Andersen S, Wallin L, Madsen T (1986) Acid gastro-oesophageal reflux episodes as related to the quality of preceding peristalsis. Scand J Gastroenterol, 21: 711–717

Reflux can occur without hiatus hernia: misplacement of the cardia

J.L. Lortat-Jacob (Paris)

My interest in the surgery of the esophagus goes back to 1943, to a time when occupied France was almost unaware of the techniques of modern anesthesia. Thus it was that in 1944, 6 weeks before the liberation of Paris, my friend Jean Mathey and I succeeded in performing the first resection of a cancer of the thoracic esophagus followed by gastroesophageal anastomosis, under local and regional anesthesia! At that time, esophageal reflux was poorly understood. However, the clinical and radiologic features of hiatus hernia gradually took shape and this pathology was enthusiastically welcomed by surgeons.

I thus had the opportunity to see a number of patients complaining of peculiar sensations of retrosternal burning pain ascending towards the pharynx and base of the tongue, especially in the decubitus position, although no major radiologic anomaly was noted by the radiologists. So much so that some patients, wearied by these troubles, presented as obsessives or actual psychopaths and were freely sent to consult psychiatrists.

In fact, I was able to establish that certain esophago-cardio-gastric anomalies existed that could not be described as hiatus hernia, so that the exact diagnosis was not appreciated. This led me, in 1951, to describe "cardio-fundal malpositions" characterized by shortness of the subdiaphragmatic abdominal esophagus, reduction or absence of the cardiofundal angle of His, with the fundus partly unfolded or loosely attached to the peritoneum flush with the hiatal orifice but without any hernial engagement.

Cardial malpositions are not therefore hiatus herniae, since there is no engagement of the stomach through the hiatus, but disturbances of the physiology of the cardio-hiatal region often producing severe functional symptoms, dominated by gastroesophageal reflux. These are characterized by anomalies of cardiac continence, with ascent of the cardia to the level of the hiatal orifice and accompanied by malfunction of the continence systems of the hiatal region.

It has long been known that the valvular mechanism represented by the cardio-fundal angle of His ensures continence of gastric repletion, and because of this very repletion; but this system is also involved at the level of the abdominal esophagus, because of the different pressures acting above and below the diaphragm.

The diaphragmatic orifice also plays an important role through direct compression of the cardia here and there by a pincher mechanism, while the right crus of the diaphragm, arranged like a lasso in the cardio-fundal angle, draws the lower esophagus backwards and to the right during inspiration and normally prevents any reflux.

To these two systems there is added a sphincter mechanism, postulated long ago and now confirmed by the existence of a zone of high pressure extending over a length of 3 to 5 cm up to the lower esophagus. This pressure barrier, situated on either side of the hiatus, is associated with tonic contraction of the sphincteric zone and yields during swallowing with temporary relaxation of the sphincter.

Thus, it may be imagined that modifications of the valve mechanism, relaxation of the hiatal orifice and a reduction of the pressures at the level of the lower esophagus, even when not associated, may contribute to the development of reflux even if the cardia remains in an abdominal position.

To these derangements there may be added other anatomic changes affecting essentially the tethering of the cardia:

1. a particular laxity of the phrenogastric ligament, which, at most, may become a flaccid peritoneal layer allowing easy mobilization of the gastric fundus.
2. on the other hand, the left gastric artery and the pars condensa of the lesser omentum constitute an important means of fixation of the region, yet if it is a long variant and even if the esophageal hiatus is of normal size, it can permit some ascent of the cardia with shortening and even disappearance of the abdominal esophagus.

These anatomic and physiologic considerations clearly show that, faced with a clinical reflux syndrome, the diagnosis of cardiac malposition will rest on an extremely precise interpretation of radiographs of excellent quality so as to exclude a proper diagnosis of hiatus hernia.

It has already been demonstrated, using the method of clips placed at the gastroesophageal junction, how difficult it can be to locate the esophageal hiatus radiologically with precision; the radiographic criteria of the differential diagnosis between gastric and esophageal folds is certainly not as useful and exact as some may consider it to be. Moreover, without reviving the anatomic discussion as to the existence or not of a true lower esophageal sphincter, it is acknowledged that the segment of 2–3 cm length situated between the lower esophagus and stomach, still known as the "vestibule", is capable of relaxing and lengthening quite markedly during swallowing.

When it is contracted, the exact level of the diaphragmatic hiatus in relation to the dome of the diaphragm cannot be determined very precisely. On the other hand,

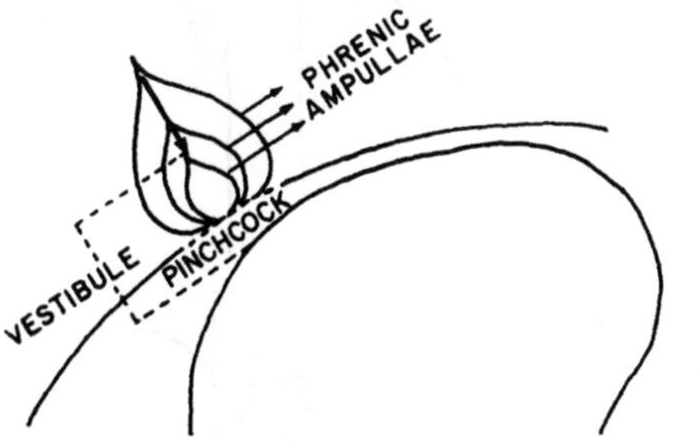

Fig. 1. Phrenic ampullae; no hernia

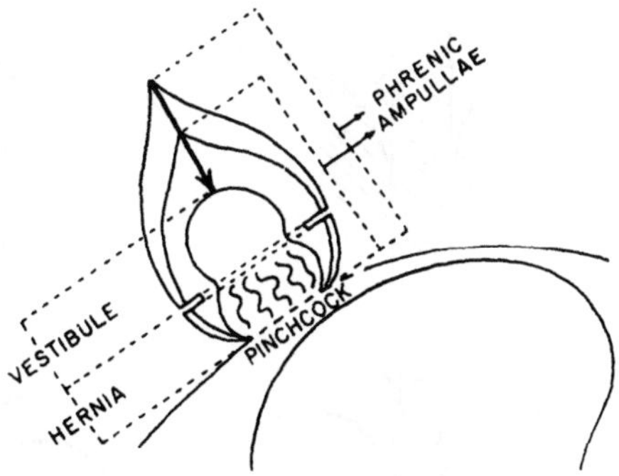

Fig. 2. Phrenic ampullae; small direct hernia

when it is relaxed, only the portion situated above the hiatus assumes a caliber wider than the rest of the esophagus; the lower portion, situated within and below the hiatus is limited in expansion by the abdominal pressure; it is therefore this lower narrow part of the vestibule that allows correct localization of the position of the esophageal orifice of the diaphragm (Fig. 1 and 2). Normally, when the pincher action of the diaphragm is effective, a piriform dilatation of decreasing girth can be seen during the progress of the barium bolus. On the other hand, in the case of cardiac incontinence, this piriform dilatation is larger in size and embodies both the esophageal vestibule and the upper part of the stomach (Fig. 3).

It is necessary, therefore, to be familiar with all these normal and subnormal appearances of the gastroesophageal junction to be in a position to make a correct diagnosis of malposition.

The radiologic projection of the esophageal hiatus varies in relation to the line of the dome of the diaphragm according to the view employed and the respiratory cycle. In strictly frontal views, the hiatus is projected above the left dome, and at the left margin of the spine at the level of D9–10 (Fig. 4a). In not very marked right anterior oblique views (those of choice for examination of the cardio-esophageal region), the hiatus is projected above the image of the left dome of the diaphragm, between dome and spine, in the clear space of the pulmonary sinus (Fig. 4b). In

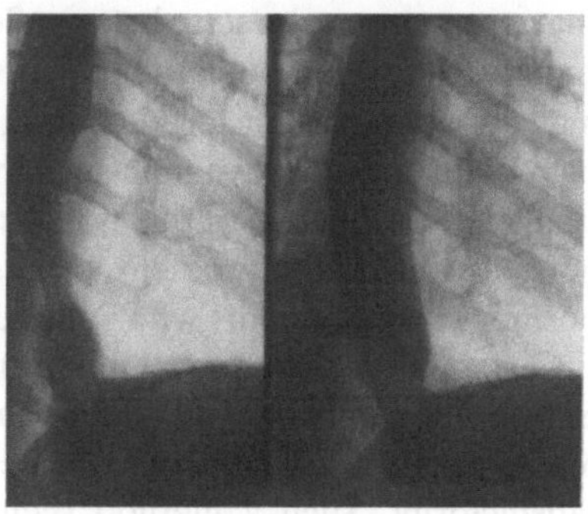

Fig. 3. Cardiac incontinence

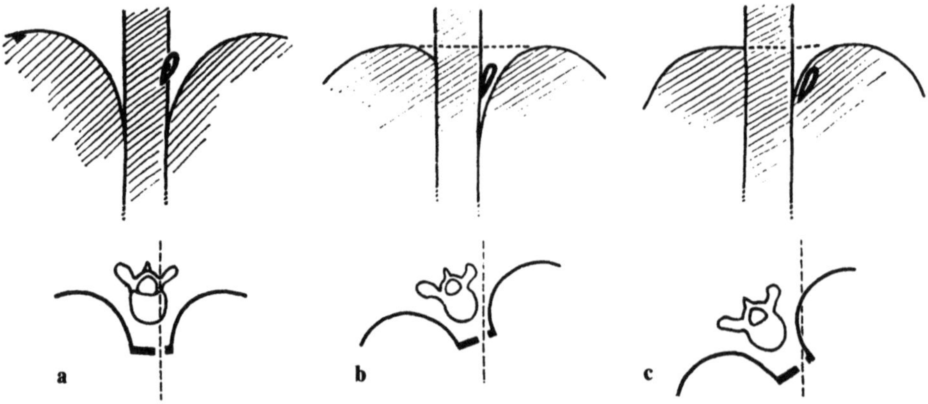

Fig. 4a–c. Different radiologic projections of the esophageal hiatus; in strictly frontal view **(a)**, in not marked right anterior oblique **(b)** view, in accentuated right oblique view **(c)**

more accentuated right anterior oblique views, it is projected at the level of, and then above, the image of the left dome of the diaphragm (Fig. 4c).

During inspiration, the contraction of the right crus of the diaphragm draws the esophagus downwards, posteriorly and to the right; the lowering of the dome is greater than that of the hiatus and the medial slope of the half-dome moves away from the spine. Thus, in an accentuated right anterior oblique view, the hiatus may be projected below the dome at the end of expiration and above it at the end of inspiration.

Usually, esophageal reflux is demonstrated without hiatus hernia, and without a gastric fold depressing the dome of the diaphragm. The interpretation of such reflux is not always simple, the more so since it may happen, after abdominal compression, that the subject exhibits either slight intermittent reflux or, more often, active regurgitation of the barium into the esophagus. If an empty swallow does not displace this barium into the stomach, the latter, in horizontal position, may remain caught up above the hiatus, very closely simulating hernial engagement of the stomach. It seems important to be familiar with such possibilities of error to be able to correctly interpret the cases in which the supposed radiographic reflux is without clinical correlation.

Moreover, in these patients it is not uncommon to observe poor gastric emptying that may amount to actual stasis. Sometimes the reflux is not demonstrated by the radiologist, even though the patients suffer from true clinical reflux. In such cases, it may be advisable not to be content with the Trendelenberg position but to get the patient to make a dynamic movement of anteflexion of the trunk, a maneuver classically productive of functional signs at clinical examination and one which often helps to localize the problem. Once initiated, the reflux continues during changes in position of the patient, who some distress in maintaining the anteflexed position.

Certainly, such a technique is not easy, particularly since the differences of translucency between the pulmonary and abdominal fields, observed simultaneously, calls for adjustments of intensity that are sometimes difficult to carry out satisfactorily. Such a method seems to have the advantage of coming closer to clinical reality, since the positions of Trendelenburg and of procubitus with compression are rarely performed in everyday life, where as anteflexion is; this may provide the reason for the major disparities that exist between the finding of radiologic reflux and the clinical symptomatology of the latter.

In every case, the importance of manometric investigation to confirm the clinical diagnosis is evident.

Treatment of these patients raises the problem of relief of a painful functional symptomatology of long standing and the prevention of the complications of esophagitis.

The immense majority of these patients will benefit from anatomic restoration of cardiac continence, as ensured by the triple procedure of Lortat-Jacob (reposition of the cardia, repair of the angle of His and closure of the crura). Suspension of the gastric fundus is an accessory maneuver which has been performed only 4 times in our series.

When performed by the abdominal route, such an arrangement is anatomically and functionally satisfactory. Only transient dysphagia during passage of large mouthfuls, disappearing spontaneously or after some dilatation sessions, and sometimes a transient trouble related to difficulty in eructation have been noted. They do not persist.

This reposition of the cardia calls for dissection of the abdominal esophagus and, by recreating an anatomic arrangement, it is usually capable of curing these patients in spectacular manner. The reflux often disappears on the very day of operation and normal life is resumed very rapidly.

Reference

1. Lortat-Jacob JL, Giuli R (1972) Les malpositions cardio-tubérositaires. Lyon Chir 68: 21–24

C. A. Hiebert (Portland)

There is general agreement that the lower esophageal sphincter is more likely to function reliably when entirely within the high pressure atmosphere of the abdomen and is more apt to fail when dislocated to the negative environment of the mediastinum. All the same, disabling reflux through a hypotensive sphincter within the abdomen can occur without radiologic evidence of a hiatal hernia.

The existence of the entity of reflux without hiatal hernia was predicted on theoretical grounds in 1954 by Barrett [1] who was evidently unaware that Belsey [2] had operated successfully on the very condition two years previously. Since then, there have been over 180 case reports of reflux without hiatal hernia identified, treated, and followed [3, 4]. Diagnosis is established by the history of posturally aggravated symptoms, the findings of a gaping lower esophageal sphincter on esophagoscopy, and by esophageal perfusion and pH studies when necessary.

Indications for antireflux surgery are the same as for patients with a radiologically demonstrable hiatal hernia and long-term results are identical. Awareness of the entity is important because the report of a "normal barium study" may lead the unwitting doctor to ascribe symptoms to angina, ulcer disease, or psychoneurosis.

References

1. Barrett NR (1954) Hiatus hernia: a review of some controversial points. Brit J Surg 42: 231–243
2. Belsey R (1952) Diaphragmatic hernia in modern trends in Gastroenterology. London. Butterworth and Company Ltd. Page 134
3. Hiebert CA, Belsey R (1961) Incompetency of the gastric cardia without radiologic evidence of hiatal hernia. J Thorac Cardiovas Surg 42: 352–362
4. Hiebert CA (1970) Primary incompetence of the gastric cardia. Am J Surg 119: 365–371.

There seems to be a total independence between the LES tonus and the existence of a hiatal hernia

B. Millat (Paris)

The question of relations between hiatal hernia (HH) and lower esophageal sphincter (LES) are only meaningful in the context of the controversy which would oppose the supporters of an anatomic, that is mechanical, theory of cardial competence and the tenants of the physiologic or functional theory.

The relations between HH and gastroesophageal reflux (GER) belong to the gastroenterological cultural inheritance. They are the result of a historical necessity and of a methodologic mistake. A historical necessity because during the first fifty years of the century, the radiology opacity was the only way to investigate the functional symptoms of the upper digestive tract. A methodologic mistake because, although radiologic observation had contributed to bringing forward positive epidemiologic relations between HH and GER, these relations did not allow the ascertaining of a causality relationship. This relation crashed when observers recognized that most patients with a HH had neither esophagitis nor GER symptoms, and that patients could have an esophagitis without any evidence of radiological HH [15, 16, 19, 25].

The existence of a LES able to maintain a pressure barrier between the esophagus body and the fundus, and to relax during swallowing, was recognized in 1950. During the following twenty years, the concept of LES incompetence as the major determinant of GER and esophagitis was widely accepted. This enthusiasm was restrained during the seventies with the publication of patients with GER and a normal LES, of low basal esophageal tonus, in nearly ten percent of healthy subjects, and generally speaking of a great overlap of basal pressures between normal controls and patients with GER. It was no more possible to establish a causality relation between LES hypotony and existence of a reflux than for HH.

Lastly, one should evoke the variability which accompanies measurement of the LES pressure and the diagnosis of HH. The basal pressure measurement for a given patient is a sum of variations inherent in the technic of recording, in the radial assymetry of the pressure and in the constantly changing tension of the sphincter [28]. These numerous parameters made a variable of sphincter hypotony which is only discriminant for extreme values, and doesn't allow discrimination in the intermediate situations of GER with or without esophagitis. On the other hand, it is now well known that it is virtually impossible to tell from radiography where the esophagus stops and the stomach begins, and exactly where the esophagus passes through the diaphragm [4]. The fact that the radiologic investigation is never conducted independently of the existence or not of GER symptoms must not be underestimated if one takes into account the influence of motivation in the research, and of subjectivity in the interpretation.

Actually HH and LES seem completely independent

Systematic surgical studies in dogs have evaluated each of the anatomic factors of possible importance to the anti-reflux function. Surgical creation of a HH failed to result in increased production of esophagitis in dogs [22], and did not result in any change in pressure at the LES [21]. Division of the phrenoesophageal membrane failed to result in changes in sphincter pressure [6]. Only when the distal esophagus or esophagogastric junction, or both, was resected did functional incompetence and lowering of pressure occur [22, 32]. The in-vitro isolated perfused esophagus and stomach of the dog contains a well-defined high pressure zone at the esophagogastric junction, even when completely removed from surrounding structures [7].

From a clinical point of view, three authors have contributed to establish the interdependence between HH and LES. In a study with 351 patients and 91 healthy volunteers, Skinner and Booth did not observe significative basal pressure differences between the groups with and without a HH, whatever the method of recording. For Haddad, there were no significant differences in esogastric pressure gradients between control and hiatal hernia patients; the differences were only significant in the group who refluxed. When Cohen and Harris compared pressure in the gastroesophageal junction of patients with no X-ray evidence of HH and no clinical evidence of reflux with that of patients with a definite HH but no symptoms of reflux, the pressures were almost identical. The patients with clinical reflux had a markedly reduced pressure at the LES, but once again mean pressure was the same for patients with and without HH [8].

Do these experimental and clinical arguments have to lead to judgment without appeal?

To tell the truth, no! The experimental studies that are referenced were performed in dogs, a species that has a true distinct anatomical sphincter identifiable anatomically in the distal esophagus. Other experiments provided results that can seem contradictory and that clarify the relations between LES and HH in a different way, at least when one implies from the existence of HH that it suppresses in part or entirely the abdominal segment of the esophagus [31]. In dogs, resection of the distal esophagus including the sphincter, and its replacement with a tube cut from the lesser curvature of the stomach, does not produce esophagitis when the neoesophageal tube is fixed so that 6 cm of the tube is within the abdominal cavity [14]. When the distal esophagus of monkeys is resected and replaced with a gastric tube of comparable diameter to the esophagus, a high pressure zone (HPZ) is recorded in the intraabdominal segment of gastric tube and a partial relaxation of this HPZ during swallowing is noted [23].

For clinical argument, it is clear that the observed results only apply to the patients selected and to the conditions of recording in the studies referred to. In Haddad's study and in Cohen's, the refluxers are easily identified by a definite basal hypotony of the LES, an event which is far from the reality in medical practice. In patients with reflux esophagitis and normal resting pressure of the LES, some authors described transient spontaneous complete relaxation of the LES [11].

It would be of interest to know if the presence of a HH is without consequences in such patients. Furthermore one would like to accept without any reservation the absence of clinical signicance of HH, that in Cohen's study the ratio of patients with HH or not, and with reflux or not, is close to the real prevalence of these both abnormalities, and especially close to the prevalence of a HH in refluxers [29].

Are there arguments in favour of a relation between HH and low resting pressure of the LES?

These arguments exist if one accepts in the definition of HH that it implies abnormal connections between the distal esophagus and the abdominal cavity. The role for the abdominal segment of the esophagus was suggested by Bombeck's human cadaver dissections where the distance from the insertion of the phrenoesophageal membrane into the esophageal wall to the flare of esophagus into the gastric pouch was measured. Evidence of esophagitis and specimens with HH were recorded. The average insertion of the membrane into the esophageal wall was 3 cm above the junction of esophagus and stomach in specimens without reflux esophagitis, and was only 0.5 cm in specimens with esophagitis. The distance was not related to the presence or absence of a HH [3].

During manometric recordings, it is possible to identify a respiratory pressure inversion point as the recording catheter tip passes from the abdominal pressure zone into the thorax. Normally, this point is located within the 3 to 4 cm of the distal esophageal HPZ. At least two centimeters of the LES lie above the inversion point. The length of the abdominal LES is related to the presence of a reflux as well as to the resting pressure of the LES [24]. During deep inhalation or abdominal wall contraction, the intragastric pressure rises as the intrathoracic esophageal pressure falls. Pressure in the thoracic portion of the HPZ also falls. Only the abdominal portion of the HPZ shows a pressure rise and protects against reflux [26]. These anatomical and physiological observations were considered to point to the importance of the abdominal segment of the distal esophagus in the control of reflux [30]. Largely speaking, the abdominal segment of the esophagus is the segment that is exposed to the abdominal pressure zone. Thus in cases of HH, the hernia sac may exert a protective role and allow transmission of abdominal pressure to the LES on condition that the insertion of the phrenoesophageal membrane, that is the upper limit of the sac, is above the sphincter [27].

The contribution of diaphragmatic muscular activity to LES pressure is circumstantial evidence in favour of relationship between HH and reflux. An experimental study in cats confirmed the hypothesis that the oscillations in LES pressure occurring synchronously with respiration result primarily from active diaphragmatic contraction [5]. In fact, only contraction of the crural part of diaphragm seems to prevent reflux, while contraction of the costal part may increase it [1, 2], although hiatal widening could influence the LES tone. A tomogram study of the diaphragm showed good correlation between a wide hiatus and a barium-demonstrable HH [12].

Although the hypothesis of the abdominal segment of distal esophagus as an essential component in the control of reflux is attractive, its importance is moderated by the observation that during a change in abdominal pressure, changes in LES pressure exceed intra-abdominal and gastric pressure increase, cannot be attributed to a passive squeeze upon the intra-abdominal segment of esophagus, and suggest the role of an intrinsic reflex mechanism for protecting the esophagus at times when the sphincter barrier might otherwise be overcome [20, 9]. The fact that both excitatory and inhibitory neural effects that may influence the response of the LES are likely to be inoperative during anesthesia suggests that studies of LES responses in the anesthetized may result in misleading conclusions [17].

Discrimination between a passive squeeze of the intra-abdominal LES and an intrinsic increase in LES tone was investigated during sustained abdominal compression (leg raising performed for the duration of a complete pull-through) and intermittent abdominal compression (leg raising for 5 sec., then the subject relaxed and the pull-through carried one sec. later). In normal persons, during IAC LES pressure exceeds a twofold resting pressure. Patients with a HH show a similar pressure rise to that of normal persons when basal LES pressure is greater than 15 mmHg, whereas in patients with HH and a low resting LES pressure, pressure rise during IAC never reaches values obtained in normal persons. Pressure recordings during SAC in patients with a HH are similar to those observed in normal persons, even in patients with resting LES pressure above 15 mmHg [18].

Are conclusions possible?

The truth is probably half way from both theories. Skinner's interesting hypothesis suggests that what is recorded as a high pressure zone in the lower esophagus is possibly not a true sphincter zone but rather the application of law of Laplace which states that the pressure required to distend a tube is inversely proportional to its diameter. Since the measurement of the esophageal HPZ is done by an infusion technique that tends to force distension of the lumen, recording of higher pressures is expected in the narrow diameter of the esophageal tube than in the large gastric pouch.

Another hypothesis is that, the transhiatal displacement of a normal EGJ which is considered as a HH, is possibly not the reality: the X-ray interpretation of an EGJ ascent may actually be the imaging of the enlarged distal esophagus. The enlargement of the distal esophagus would unavoidably result in a fall of LES tone [10]. If one considers that there is no X-ray landmark of the hiatal orifice, it is possible to imagine that two radically different situations will be described in the same manner, that is as radiological evidence of HH:

- the first is only the transhiatal ascent of a normal EGJ, that is with a normal ratio between esophageal and gastric lumen diameters without incompetence of the so call LES. Such an eventuality could be induced by powerful radiological maneuvers.
- The second would correspond to an enlargement of the distal esophagus, without any modification of the connections between EGJ and the surrounding anatomical structures. Hypotony of the LES and reflux would be expected in this case.

In conclusion, though it is clear that the relations between HH and reflux are not causality ones, the anatomical disturbances that the concept of HH implies are worth thinking over.

References

1. Altschuler SM, Boyle JT, Nixon TE, Pack AC, Cohen S (1985) Dissociation of costal and crural contractile effects on the gastroesophageal high pressure zone Gastroenterology 88: 1305 (abstract)
2. Altschuler SM, Boyle, JT, Nixon TE, Pack AC, Cohen S (1985) Electrical pacing of the cural diaphragm: a potential modality in the treatment of gastroesophageal reflux Gastroenterology, 88: 1305 (abstract)
3. Bombeck CT, Dillard DH, Nyhus LM (1966) Muscular anatomy of the gastroesophageal junction and role of phrenoesophageal ligament: autopsy study of sphincter mechanism Ann Surg 16: 643.
4. Botha GSM (1957) Radiological localization of the diaphragmatic hiatus. Lancet, 1: 662.
5. Boyle JT, Altschuler SM, Nixon TE, Tuchman DN, Pack AC, Cohen S (1985) Role of the diaphragm in the genesis of lower esophageal sphincter pressure in the cat Gastroenterology, 88: 723–730
6. Bremner CG, Schlegel JF, Ellis FH (1970) Studies of the "gastroesophageal sphincter mechanism": the role of phrenoesophageal membrane, Surgery 67: 735–740
7. Castell DO (1975) The lower esophageal sphincter. Physiologic and clinical aspects. Ann Intern Med 83: 390–401
8. Cohen S, Harris LD (1971) Does hiatus hernia affect competence of the gastroesophageal sphincter? N Engl J Med 284: 1053–1056
9. Cohen S, Harris LD (1972) The lower esophageal sphincter Gastroenterology 63: 1066–1073
10. Csendes A, Miranda M, Espinoza M, Velasco N, Henriquez A (1981) Perimeter and location of the muscular gastroesophageal junction or "cardia" in control subjects and in patients with reflux esophagitis or achalasia. Scand J Gastroent 16: 951–956
11. Dodds WJ, Dent J, Hogan WJ, Helm JF, Hauser R, Patel GK, Egide MS (1982) Mechanism of gastroesophageal reflux in patients with reflux esophagitis. N Engl J Med 307: 1547– 1552
12. Ginalski JM, Schnyder P, Moss AA, Brasch RC (1984) Incidence and significance of a widened esophageal hiatus at CT. Scan J Clin Gastroenterol, 6: 467–470
13. Haddad JK (1970) Relation of gastroesophageal reflux to yield sphincter pressures. Gastroenterology 58: 175–184
14. Henderson RD (1972) Gastroesophageal junction in hiatus hernia. Can J Surg 15: 63

15. Hiebert CA, Belsey R (1961) Incompetency of the gastric cardia without radiologic evidence of hiatal hernia. The diagnosis and management of 71 cases. J Thoracic and Cardiovas Surg, 42: 352–362
16. Hiebert CA (1970) Primary incompetence of the gastric cardia. Am J Surg 119: 365–371
17. Holloway RH, Blank E, Takahashi I, Dodds WJ, Hogan WJ, Dent J (1985) Variability of lower esophageal sphincter pressure in fasted unanesthetized opossum. Am J Physiol 248: G 398–G406
18. Janisch HD, Weihrauch TR, Hampel KE (1984) Is abdominal compression a useful stimulation test for analysis of lower esophageal sphincter function? Dig Dis Sci 29: 689–695
19. Kramer P (1969) Does a sliding hiatus hernia constitute a distinct clinical entity? Gastroenterology 57: 442–448
20. Lind JF, Warrian WG, Wankling WJ (1966) Responses of the gastroesophageal junctional zone to increases in abdominal pressure. Can J Surg 9: 32–38
21. Lind JF, Cotton DJ, Blanchard R et al (1969) Effect of thoracic displacement and vagotomy on the canine gastroesophageal junctional zone. Gastroenterology 56: 1078–1085
22. Meiss JH, Grindlay JH, Ellis FH (1958) The gastroesophageal sphincter mechanism. J Thorac Surg 36: 156–165
23. Moossa AR, Cooley GR, Skinner DB (1973) Intraluminal and intraperitoneal pressures at the cardia: effect of hormones and surgical intervention. Surgical Forum 24: 416
24. O'Sullivan GC, DeMeester TR, Joelsson BE (1982) et al Interaction of lower esophageal sphincter pressure and length of sphincter in the abdomen as determinants of gastroesophageal competence. Am J Surg 143: 40–47
25. Palmer ED (1968) The hiatus hernia-esophagitis-esophageal stricture complex. Twenty year prospective study. Am J Med 44: 566– 579
26. Pellegrini CA, DeMeester TR, Skinner DB (1976) Response of the distal esophageal sphincter to respiratory and positional maneuvers in humans. Surgical Forum 27: 380
27. Pettersson G, Bombeck CT, Nyhus L (1981) Influence of hiatal hernia on lower esophageal sphincter function: an experimental study. Ann Surg 193: 214–220
28. Pope CE 2 (1981) Is measurement of lower esophageal sphincter pressure clinically useful? Dig Dis and Sci 26: 1025–1027
29. Santos GH (1983) Is hiatus hernia responsible for reflux? Chest 84: 242–244
30. Skinner DB, Booth DJ (1970) Assessment of distal esophageal function in patients with hiatal hernia and/or gastroesophageal reflux. Ann Surg 172: 627–637
31. Skinner DB (1985) Pathophysiology of gastroesophageal reflux. Ann Surg 202: 546–556
32. Vandertoll DJ, Ellis FH, Schlegel JF et al (1966) An experimental study of the role of gastric and esophageal muscle in gastroesophageal competence. Surg Gynecol Obstet 122: 579–586

R. D. Henderson (Toronto)

This question is controversial but nevertheless very important. In my view LES tone is not directly affected by the presence of a hiatal hernia. However, the hernia produces reflux and reflux induced esophagitis causes LES hypotonia.

Several factors must be examined to evaluate this hypothesis:

- What is a hiatal hernia?
- Is a hernia necessary for reflux?
- Does a hernia produce LES hypotonia?
- What happens to the LES tone once reflux is surgically corrected?

The definition of a hiatal hernia seems simple, however mostly we refer to a hernia as a radiologically demonstrable protrusion of stomach into the chest. There are problems with this definition as the radiologic findings may vary from one study to the next.

In my opinion, intra-abdominal esophageal length is of more importance. Normally the esophagus lies 2.5 cm below the diaphragm. In all probability this intra-abdominal segment, with its exposure to intraperitoneal pressures, is vitally important in reflux control. What happens to reflux control as the length decreases to 2 cm on to 1 cm or even less? At what stage does the normal competence break down? There is some evidence to suggest that competence depends upon the combination of intra-abdominal length and LES tone; we do not have a radiologic method of quantitating the intra-abdominal esophageal length and as such do not recognize a problem until an intra-thoracic stomach pouch can be demonstrated (Fig. 1).

The next important question is whether or not a hernia is necessary for reflux to occur: again in the literature LES tone has often been regarded as the most important factor in reflux control. The major question is what cause LES hypotonia. If one examines the factors controlling reflux, it is difficult to find a cause of reflux

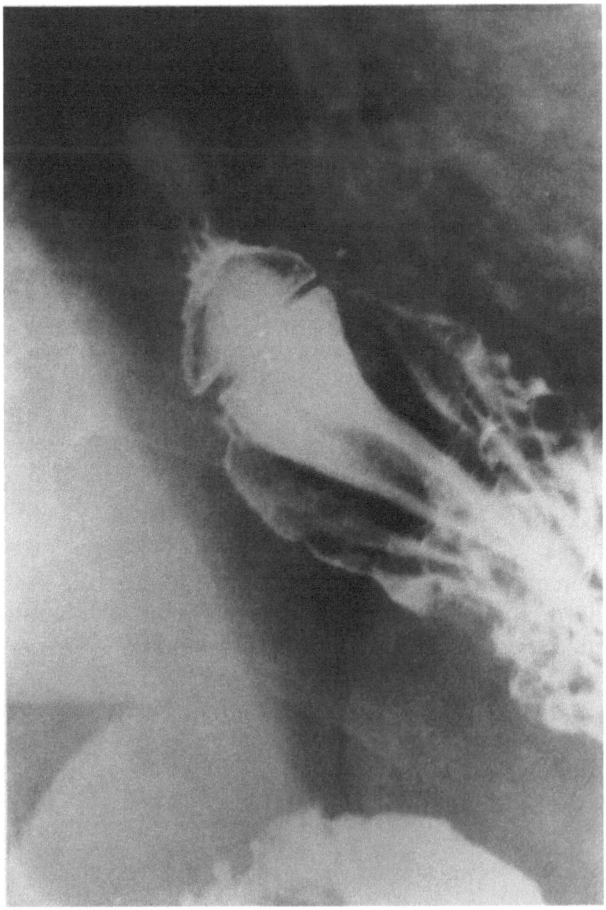

Fig. 1. Most articles refer only to the presence of an obvious hernia pouch – as illustrated. In my view a short intra-abdominal segment is equally important

other than the presence of a hernia. There is no evidence to suggest a loss of intrinsic hormone production or sensitivity and there is no evidence of a neurogenic deficit. Certainly in the experimental animal it is possible to produce esophagitis by instillation of acid and bile mixtures: in this situation, the amount of esophageal motor disorder is increased and the LES tone decreases. The motor change reverses when the infusion is stopped and the esophagus heals. This evidence suggests that reflux can lower LES tone, and healing of the reflux allows a return of tone to the normal range.

In my view the problems of incompetence are very much related to the presence of a hiatal hernia. The term "hiatal hernia" is used to cover the presence of an intrathoracic pouch of stomach, but also covers the situation where a hernia cannot be demonstrated however the intra-abdominal segment of esophagus is shortened.

– In the presence of an intra-abdominal esophagus when peritoneal pressure increases, there is increased gastric pressure and an equal transmission of pressure to the LES. Such surrounding pressure adds support to the LES, counterbalances gastric pressure increases and prevents reflux.

When the esophageal intra-abdominal length is reduced, the effectiveness of counterbalancing pressure is less pronounced and reflux is likely to be increased. These simplistic observations can be backed up by dog studies in which the LES was excised and reflux control maintain by an intrathoracic invagination esophagogastric anastomosis: In this situation, reflux control was effective when the invagination was over more than 2 cm of esophagus; less than a 2 cm invagination was associated with active reflux.

Similar studies have been conducted with inanimate latex flap valves and it can be shown that the length of exposed flap valve is important in this model in preventing reflux.

Although this concept is simple and mechanical, it is the best explanation of the value of the intra-abdominal segment of esophagus in reflux control.

– The final question which should be answered is what happens to the LES tone once reflux has been controlled: from the previous discussions the conclusion is that reflux occurs in the presence of a shortened intra-abdominal esophageal segment or hernia and the reflux then secondarily changes the esophagus and lowers LES tone. If surgical correction of reflux is effective then LES tone should recover to the normal levels.

My experience is based on 242 patients with surgical reflux control by total fundoplication gastroplasty (TFG). Each patient has a recorded preoperative LES tone and postoperative studies were conducted 3 to 5½ months postoperatively.

Preoperatively the tone varied from 0 to over 30 cm H_2O. The normal LES tone for this system ranges from 15 to 20 cm H_2O. Patient studies were grouped into those with a tone of 0–6 cm H_2O; 7–10 cm H_2O; 11–15 cm H_2O; 16–20 cm H_2O and 21 cm H_2O. The postoperative tone was then compared with the preoperative tone in each of these groups (Fig. 2).

In the 0–6 cm H_2O group there were 43 patients and the average tone increase was 240%. With a 7–10 cm H_2O tone in 70 patients the tone increase was 71.4%. In the 11–15 cm H_2O group of 60 patients the tone increase was 32% and in the 16–20 cm

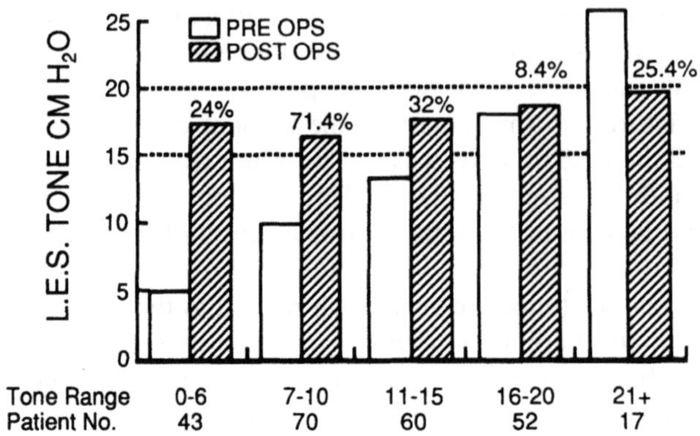

Fig. 2. In the LES, tone increases on average to create a tone which then is similar to that of a normal population

H_2O group of 52 patients the tone increase was only 8.4%. The final group of 17 patients had a preoperative tone of 21– cm H_2O. These patients were preoperatively hypertonic and postoperatively they had a tone decrease of 25.4%.

There are several points of importance: clearly, there is a wide range of preoperative tone, however, although the great majority are hypotonic, 21.5% had a normal LES tone and 7% were hypertonic. If hypotonia was the only factor in reflux, the two groups of 28.5% with normal or high LES tone would not reflux. The second factor is that LES tone rises to a normal level in all groups, regardless of the preoperative tone: this indicates that the tone increase is not directly related to the muscle tone of the fundoplication, but must instead be a result of healing in the LES with tone recovery.

*

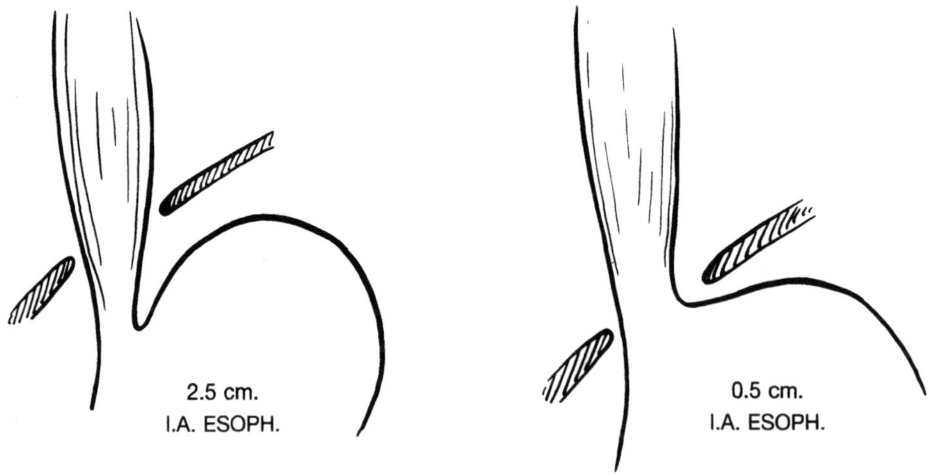

Fig. 3. The normal esophagus is 2.5 cm below the diaphgram. When the IAE is shortened, the problems of reflux are created and may well be as important as a hernia

A short intra-abdominal segment predisposes to reflux (Fig. 3); LES hypotonia is secondary to reflux injury and is not the initial cause of reflux. Once hypotonia is established, reflux will get worse. Finally, if reflux is corrected, LES tone on average will increase to a normal tone level. This tone recovery is due to esophageal healing.

References

1. Henderson RD (1983) Esophageal Manometry in Clinical Investigation. Praeger Publishers, NY
2. Code CF, Kelley ML, Schlegel JR, Olsen AM (1962) Detection of hiatal hernia during esophageal motility test. Gastroenterology 43:521
3. Henderson RD, Mugashe F, Jeejeebhoy KN, Cullen J, Szczepanski M, Boszko A, Marryatt G (1972) The role of bile and acid in the production of esophagitis and the motor defect of esophagitis. Ann thorac Surg 14:465.
4. DeMeester TR, Wang CI, Wernley JA, Pelligrini CA, Little AG, Klementschitsch P, Bermudez G, Johnson LF, Skinner DB (1980) Technique, indications and clinical use of 24-hour esophageal pH monitoring. J Thorac Cardiovasc Surg 79:656

Esophageal reflux can exist despite an elevated LES

B. Zielinski, B. Molano, T. Chevalier, and *M. Mignon* (Paris)

Episodic GE reflux is a normal phenomenon especially after eating [1, 2, 3] Different factors may contribute to the GE reflux disease and esophagitis [4, 5, 6, 7, 8, 9]:

LES pressure abnormalities

Low LES pressure: it is well known that patients with severe esophagitis have lower LES pressure [8, 9]. Yet esophageal reflux may occur when LES pressure is normal or increased [5, 6, 7]. One explanation is that LES pressure presents temporal variations and resting LES pressure (evaluated on a short period by manometry) is not necessarily representative. Other LES abnormalities may account for the development of GE reflux.

- Absence of adaptative increase in LES pressure in response to increases in abdominal pressure
- Transient spontaneous LES relaxations [4]
- Esophageal motor disorders causing delayed esophageal clearance [10, 11]
- GE reflux volume and composition [12].

Our purpose was to determine the contribution of LES pressure to the occurrence of GE reflux and the development of esophagitis.

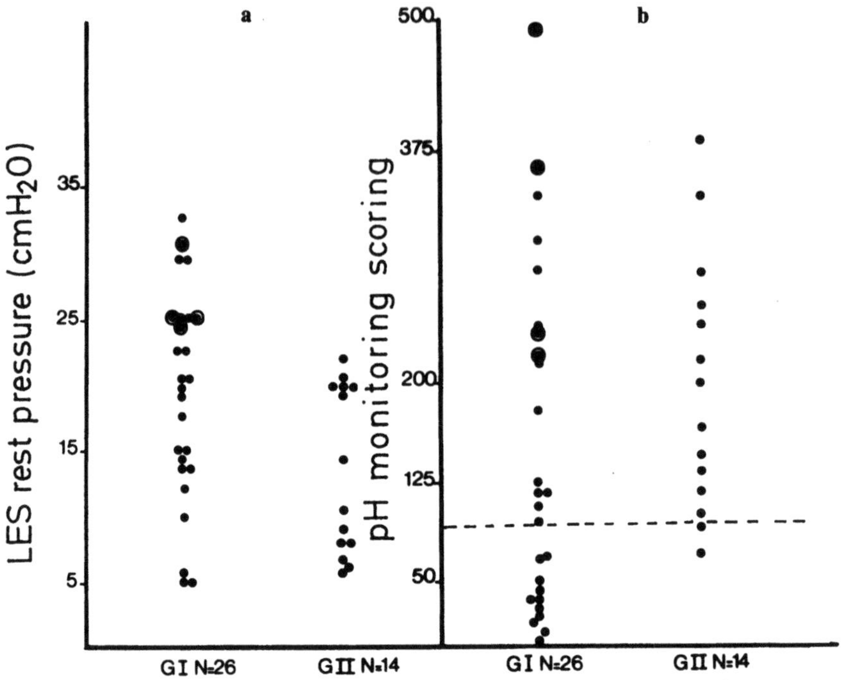

Fig. 1a, b. Individual values for: a) mean resting LES pressure; b) pH metric score according to Kaye (1) in 2 groups of patients with clinical symptoms indicative of gastroesophageal reflux: group 1 without esophagitis N=26, group 2 with grade 2–3 esophagitis N=14. Upper limit of normal for pH metric score has been indicated: Note that in 4 patients ● with pH metric score above 225 LES resting pressure lies near the upper limit of normal

Forty patients were studied. They had undergone esophageal 3 hours postprandial pH-metry, manometry and endoscopy.

Twenty-six patients (Fig.) had normal endoscopic findings or mild esophagitis (grade 1) (group 1); 14 patients had grade 2 or 3 esophagitis (group 2).

In group 1, 19 patients had esophageal symptoms typical of gastro-esophageal reflux. pH-metry Kaye score was 11–462 (median 122) (N. <90). LES pressure range was 5–32.5 cm H_2O (median 18) (N=25±9 cm H_2O). Seven patients had mild esophageal-body motor dysfunction and one had transient LES relaxations.

In group 2, pH-metry score was 69–383 (median 183). LES pressure was 6–22 (median 12). Nine patients had esophageal body motor dysfunction; one of them had achalasia, another systemic sclerosis.

In conclusion, pH-metry and manometry disturbances were associated with esophagitis severity. Yet, according to this set of data and the literature, esophageal reflux may occur in patients with normal or increased LES pressure in the resting state as measured by conventional manometry.

References

1. Kaye MD (1977) Post-prandial gastro-oesophageal reflux in healthy people. Gut 18: 709–712
2. Galmiche JP, Denis P, Desechalliers JP (1981) Valeur diagnostique des examens complémentaires au cours du reflux gastro-œsophagien de l'adulte. Gastroenterol Clin Biol 5: 1014–1025
3. Spence RAJ, Collins BJ, Parks TG, Love AHG (1985) Does age influence normal gastroesophageal reflux? Gut 26: 799–801
4. Dodds WJ, Dent J, Hogan WJ, Helm JF, Hauser R, Patel GK, Egide MS (1982) Mechanisms of gastroesophageal reflux in patients with reflux oesophagitis. N Engl J Med 307: 1547–1552
5. Code CF, Kelley ML, Schlegel JF, Olsen AM (1962) Detection of hiatal hernia during esophageal motility tests. Gastroenterology 43: 521
6. Moroz SP, Espinoza J, Cumming WA, Diamant NE (1976) Lower esophageal sphincter function in children with and without gastroesophageal reflux. Gastroenterology 71: 236
7. Henderson RD (1983) The manometric diagnosis of hiatal hernia and reflux. In: "Esophageal manometry in clinical investigation". Praeger Edit, New York, 54–75
8. Lieberman DA (1986) Chronic reflux oesophagitis: is intensive longterm medical treatment necessary? Dig Dis Sci 31: 265 (abstract)
9. Galmiche JP, Bruley des Varannes S, Colin R (1987) Les explorations fonctionnelles dans le syndrome de reflux gastrooesophagien. In: "Les troubles moteurs de l'œsophage et le reflux gastro-œsophagien. R. Colin et JP. Galmiche Editeurs, Progrès en hépatogastroentérologie, Douin Paris
10. Stanciu C, Bennett JR (1974) Oesophageal acid clearing: one factor in the production of reflux oesophagitis. Gut 15: 852–857
11. Kahrilas PJ, Dodds WJ, Hogan WJ, Kern M, Arndorfer RC, Reece A (1986) Esophageal peristaltic dysfunction in peptic esophagitis. Gastroenteroloy 91: 897–904
12. Mignon M, Bruley des Varannes S, Vallot Th, Galmiche JP (1987) Quel est le taux de la sécrétion gastrique acide chez les sujets porteurs d'une œsophagite? In: "Lésions bénignes de l'œsophage et cancer". Maloine Editeur, in press

Physiopathology of peptic esophagitis (1)

President: *Kiyoshi Inokuchi* (Fukuoka)

Free Commentators: *Ph. Donahue* (Chicago)
C. Th. Bombeck (Chicago)
G. Beauchamp (Montreal)
M. Julien (Paris)
J. Kiss (Budapest)
F. Kümmerle (Mainz)
M. Prémont (Paris)

Is stenosing esophagitis a different disease from esophagitis without stenosis?

J. B. Ollyo, J. Wellinger, M. Savary, J. J. Gonvers, (Lausanne), *T. Vallot, M. Mignon,* and *S. Bonfils* (Paris)

Opinions concerning the relationship between erosive reflux esophagitis (ERE) and reflux esophagitis with stenosis (RES) are in disagreement. Some authors [4, 9] believe that ERE and RES may be separate pathological entities for the following reasons:

1. twenty to 60% of RES appear suddenly without previous symptoms typical of gastroesophageal reflux [2, 8]. But in some patients ERE may remain asymptomatic for a long time, possibly due to a relative insensitivity of the mucosa to acid reflux [10]. Also, ERE can be unrecognized by the patient and his physician, and therefore in the absence of a diagnosis and treatment, progress to a stricture.
2. the development of a RES in a patient with ERE is rarely observed, even in the presence of gastric acid hypersecretion [4, 6]. However, it should be noted that in the majority of published series the follow-up, less than 5 years, is insufficient. It is also possible that the natural history of ERE has been modified by the wide use of UGI endoscopy (earlier diagnosis) by the inhibitors of gastric acid secretion and by efficient surgery.
3. a few small series show that the average age of the patients and the length of symptoms is the same in both groups [4, 6]. This speaks against the evolution of ERE to RES.

We believe that the 4 stages of reflux esophagitis described by Savary and Miller [7] represent stages of increasing severity of the same disease for the following reasons:

1. epidemiological data in patients with ERE and RES are approximately the same: increased incidence in the male, younger age in the male, prevalence of alcohol and tobacco abuse, frequent use of anti-inflammatory medication [4, 6];
2. at the time of diagnosis, the average age of the patients is progressively older as the stage of the lesion is more severe (Table 1). Also patients with a RES or another recognized complication of reflux disease such as ulcer, endobrachy-

Table 1. Reflux esophagitis average ages for savary's 4 grades

	Grade I n=1.564	Grade II n=420	Grade III n=160	Grade IV n=925	PS* n=324
Men (> 16 ans)	49.7	56.1	59.8	60.3	60.9
Women (> 16 ans)	56.3	62.7	63.1	64.7	63.8
Total	51.7	57.8	60.8	61.7	61.6

Chuv, Lausanne, Switzerland (01.01.1963–31.12.1986) * PS: Peptic stricture

esophagus or brachyesophagus, usually have a longer history of gastroesophageal reflux symptoms [1, 3];
3. RES is almost always associated with ERE and with one or more complications of reflux esophagitis (Table 2);
4. the progression of ERE to RES has been documented in some cases by repeated endoscopic examinations (Table 3).

In conclusion, the evolution of ERE to stricture or another complication of reflux disease (ulcer, endobrachyesophagus, adenocarcinoma) is possible and unpredictable. In all patients who are at an acceptable operative risk, we recommend surgery if the esophagitis does not heal after a treatment with inhibitors of gastric secretion for 3 to 6 months, if the esophagitis progresses in spite of this treatment, or if it recurs shortly after the end of the treatment. Indeed, surgery is the only treatment that can permanently cure gastroesophageal reflux and the earlier surgery is performed the better the results [5].

Table 2. Reflux esophagitis with stricture – endoscopic findings (Chuv, Lausanne: 1963–1986)

	Patients
Stricture + Hiatus hernia	286/324 (88%)
Cicatricial Stricture	46/324 (14%)
Stricture + Erosive Esophagitis	278/324 (86%)
Uncomplicated Stricture	92/324 (28%)
Stricture + Complications*	232/324 (72%)
– E or U or B	147/324 (45%)
– E + U or U + B or E + B	63/324 (20%)
– E + U + B	22/324 (7%)

* E: Endobrachyesophagus; U:Ulcer; B:Brachyesophagus

Table 3. Reflux esophagitis with stricture (RES) – preceded by erosive reflux esophagitis (ERE) – Chuv, Lausanne, Switzerland (1963–1986)

Adults affected by RES with a history of GER*	253/324 (78 %)
– Patients with a history of GER* Endoscoped before development of RES	42/253 (16.6%)
– Patients with ERE	27/253 (10.6%)
Time of onset of RES After diagnosis of ERE	
– Extremes (months)	2–173
– Mean (months)	37

* GER: Long-term history of gastroesophageal reflux

References

1. Ahtaridis G, Snape WJ, Cohen S (1979) Clinical and manometric findings in benign peptic strictures of the esophagus. Dig Dis Sci 24: 858–861
2. Barrett NR (1962) Benign stricture in the lower esophagus. J Thorac Cardiovasc Surg 43: 703–715
3. Benedict EB, Gillespie JE (1954) Peptic stenosis of the esophagus. Surg Gyn Obst 98: 494–502
4. Dedieu P, Gaillard F, Lavignole A et al. (1981) Œsophagites par reflux: aspects épidémiologiques, anatomo-pathologiques et évolutifs (123 cas). Gastroenterol. Clin Biol 5: 266–274
5. Ollyo JB, Savary M, Levi F (1986) Œsophagite par reflux sténosante: intérêt de l'endoscopie pour le diagnostic et la surveillance. Etude rétrospective de 305 cas. Schweiz Rundschau Med (PRAXIS) 50: 1528–1530
6. Ollyo JB (1986) L'œsophagite par reflux au cours du syndrome de Zollinger-Ellison. A propos de 33 cas. Mémoire pour le titre d'assistant étranger. Université de Paris 7, Faculté de Médecine Xavier-Bichat
7. Savary M, Miller G (1977) L'œsophage. Atlas et manuel d'endoscopie. Gassmann SA, édit Soleure
8. Savary M, Ollyo JB (10–1986) L'œsophagite par reflux et ses complications: ulcère, sténose et endobrachy-œsophage. Encycl Med Chir (Paris, France), ORL 20 822A[10], 16 p
9. Sonnenberg A (1981) Epidemiologie und Spontanverlauf der Refluxkrankheit in Blum AL, Siewert JR, Refluxtherapie. Springer-Verlag, Berlin 85–106
10. Volpicelli NA, Bedine MS, Hendrix TR (1975) Absence of acid sensitivity in patients with benign peptic esophageal strictures. Gastroenterology 68, 1007

What is the endoscopic incidence of stenosis related to reflux?

R. D. Henderson (Toronto)

Esophageal stenosis is either benign or malignant and the relative frequency of occurrence of each type will vary depending upon the national population studied. In Canada, peptic stricture is more common than malignant stricture and caustic stricture is very rare. In Japan and many parts of Africa, reflux is rare and esophageal malignancy common.

Allowing for these differences, in Canada the incidence of peptic stricture detected endoscopically will also vary with the type of population studied and the type of strictures included in the definition of peptic.

Most peptic strictures are easily defined as being reflux produced, associated with a hiatal hernia and located at the squamocolumnar junction. Variations on the standard peptic stricture must be included in any description and these are outlined in Table 1.

The standard peptic stricture has an associated hernia and reflux, varies in length and frequently has significant distortion from ulcerative esophagitis (Fig. 1).

A variation of the standard stricture is the Schatzki ring, which is a web-like narrowing at the squamocolumnar junction. The Schatzki ring is often not symp-

Table 1

Peptic Stricture
Schatzki Ring
Allison-Johnston (Barrett's)
Mid-esophageal Web
Cricopharyngeal Web
Re-activated traumatic stricture

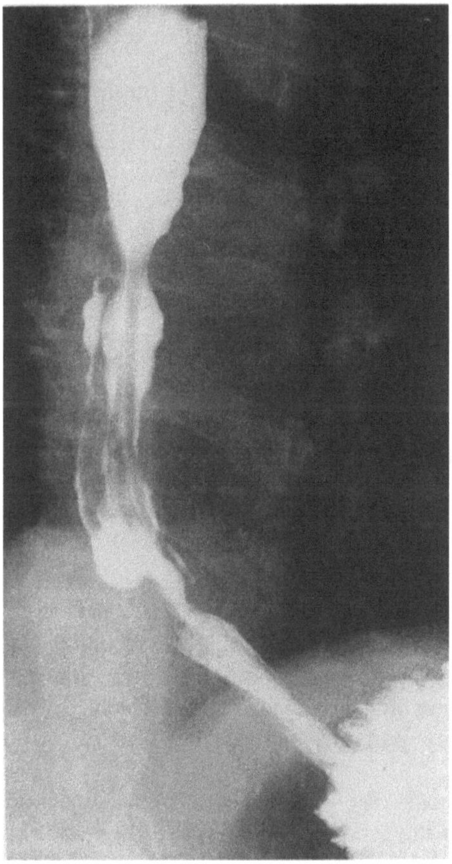

Fig. 1. In this patient, the stricture is irregular and distorted by ulceration. Malignancy cannot be radiologically excluded. This patient had a reflux induced peptic stricture

tomatic, and unlike most peptic strictures, is not necessarily associated with severe disease (Fig. 2).

The combination of standard peptic strictures and Schatzki rings account for at least 90% of reflux related esophageal strictures in the general population.

Other rarer strictures must be included for completeness: one of the most important is the Allison-Johnston stricture which occurs at the squamocolumnar junction in the mid-esophagus of patients with a gastric lined Barrett's esophagus.

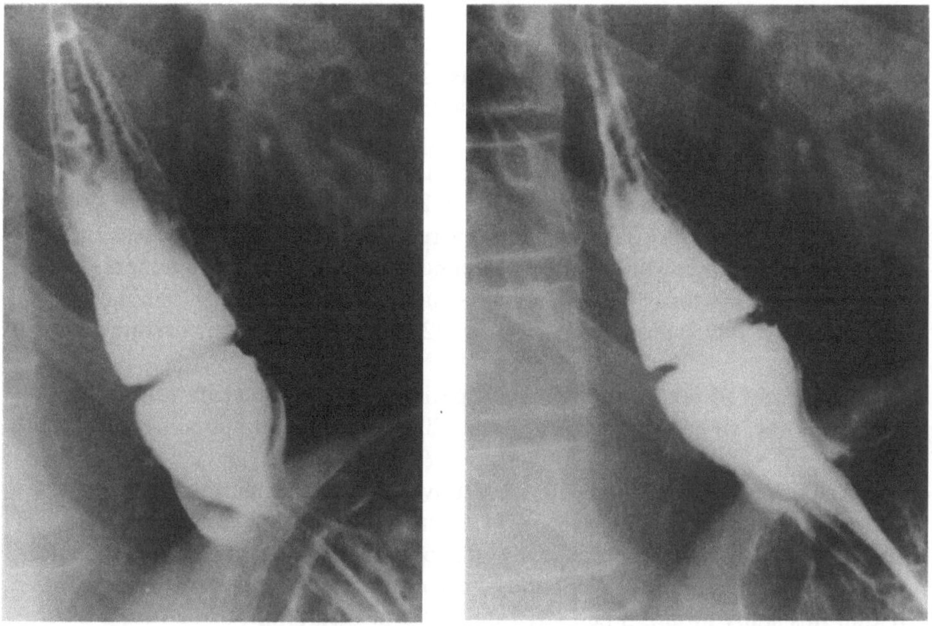

Fig. 2. The Schatzki ring is at the squamocolumnar junction. These webs are 2 mm wide with a variable luminal diameter. When the intimal lumen is less than 13 mm dysphagia may occur

Much rarer is a mid-esophageal web in the squamous lined esophagus. Occasionally also web strictures occur, secondary to reflux immediately below the cricopharyngus. The final group, included for completeness, are those produced by caustic or operative trauma which are activated or re-activated by reflux (Table 1).

Three studies will be analyzed to determine the relative incidence of esophageal peptic stricture.

- In the first group, 300 consecutive patients were evaluated for esophageal symptoms and the investigation included an endoscopic study. The overall incidence of dysphagia was 78% (234 patients); however, this dysphagia was motor in type in 69.7% (209 patients) and stricture induced mechanical dysphagia in only 8.3% (25 patients) (Table 2). This study excluded patients with a Schatzki ring.

Table 2. These symptoms were present in 300 consecutive patients with proved hiatal hernia and reflux

Heartburn	96.6%
Reflux	71.5%
Reflux & aspiration	27.6%
Nausea & vomiting	46.3%
Dysphagia total	78 %
Stricture	8.3%
Motor dysphagia	69.7%

- In the second study, 200 patients were evaluated and treated by transabdominal total fundoplication gastroplasty (TFG). Such a transabdominal surgical approach excludes patients with previous esophageal or gastric surgery, patients with severe ulcerative esophagitis or giant hernias. These exclusions affect the incidence of reported peptic stricture.
- In this study, 16% (32 patients) had a stricture. These strictures were associated with no ulceration in 4, mild ulceration in 21 and severe ulceration in 7. Within this same study group 2 patients had a Barrett's esophagus with stricture and one patient a cricopharyngeal web. In this same group there were 9 patients (4.5%) who had a Schatzke ring. Including Schatzki ring and the 1 patient with a cricopharyngeal web there were a total of 42 patients (21%) with a reflux induced stricture.

The first study of 300 are consecutive patients seen in consultation for severe reflux symptoms, while the second group of 200 were a patient population selected for surgery.

- The final group reported are 100 consecutive strictures treated by total fundoplication gastroplasty and followed 1–11.5 years. The incidence of stricture in this surgical group is 9.6% (total study group 1040 patients), however this study excludes Schatzki rings and cricopharyngeal webs.

Within this study group, 3 had strictures without ulceration, 62 had local ulceration at the site of the stricture and 35 had extensive esophageal ulceration. It is worth noting that in some patients, if the stricture is tight enough, reflux is prevented and ulceration heals.

The study group of 100 included 13 patients with scleroderma and 26 patients with previous esophageal or gastric surgery. Four of these patients had had a previous caustic injury re-activated by the development of a hiatal hernia and reflux.

References

1. Hennessy TPJD, Cuschieri A (1986) Surgery of the Oesophagus. Bailliere Tindall, London, Philadelphia, Toronto
2. Henderson RD (1980) The Esophagus: Reflux and Primary Motor Disorders. Williams and Wilkins, Baltimore/London

What is the endoscopic incidence of stenosis related to reflux and what is the incidence of recurrences of reflux stenosis?

W. S. Payne (Rochester)

J. R. Bennett of Hull, England [1] has suggested an incidence of between 20 and 40 new strictures per year per million population in the United Kingdom.

While precise epidemiologic data are lacking, a review of Mayo Clinic experience

Table 1. Esophageal endoscopies and stricture dilations. Mayo Clinic – 1985

	No. of Patients	Exams (%)	Treatment (%)
Total esophagogastroduodenoscopies/year	3.411	100	–
Total dilations performed/year	443	13	100
Indications for esophageal dilation			
Reflux strictures	310	9	70
Schatzki's ring	34	1	8
Miscellaneous (achalasia, webs, cancer, caustic, post-radiation, etc.)	99	3	22

for the year 1985 (Table 1) indicates a 9–10% prevalence of reflux-induced esophageal stenosis among 3.411 patients undergoing esophageal endoscopy. During that same year, 282.075 patients were examined at the Mayo Clinic, suggesting a prevalence among our patient population of 110–122 cases/100.000 patients, depending, of course, on one's interpretation of the etiology of Schatzki ring. These figures are probably distorted upwards since the Mayo Clinic serves as a tertiary referral center of considerable geographic scope and does not draw patients from a fixed or finite population base.

The natural history of untreated reflux-induced esophageal stenosis is unknown, though it is generally appreciated that it is capable of producing in some a slowly progressive dysphagia and esophageal retention with regurgitation of fresh, bland food and saliva with some experiencing respiratory aspiration and even nutritional depletion.

It is current clinical practice to palliate reflux-induced esophageal stenosis by performing esophageal bougienage or dilation using graduated sounds or inflated balloons of various sizes. Recent literature reaffirms the general safety and effectiveness of dilation therapy [2–7].

The typical patient coming to first dilation treatment is generally described as male and over 60 years of age. Nearly 25 percent deny current or antecedent history of gastroesophageal reflux. The response to dilation is often described as bimodal, in that nearly 50% of patients receive virtually complete and permanent relief following a single brief course of esophageal dilation. The remaining 50% follow a varied and unpredictable course despite multiple dilations and conservative medical measures. In general, the long-term response to dilation treatment can be related to the initial size of the stenosis and its pliability. There is a definite though low long-term incidence of esophageal perforation (0–7%), hemorrhage (<1%) or death (<2%). It is estimated that nearly 85–90% of patients can be maintained symptom free by dilation to 50 to 60 French size along with a vigorous antireflux medical program. Less than 10% of patients, however, come to surgical treatment for reflux-induced esophageal stenosis. This is in part related to often cited advanced age and associated cardiovascular disease of patients. It is probably equally related to physician perseverance and patient tolerance to often frequent dilation sessions over many years.

At the Mayo Clinic, nearly 85% of patients referred for surgical treatment have an esophageal stenosis which is readily dilated to 50 French and can be managed by an appropriate antireflux procedure [8, 10]. Fifteen percent, however, have stenosis which cannot be dilated above 20 to 30 French and require resection and reconstruction in a manner to prevent recurrence [10]. One hundred and one consecutive adult patients were successfully managed by a variety of techniques in a five-year period without operative deaths. Over one-third were reoperations. Swallowing was restored in all but one patient with only six percent of patients requiring one to two dilations within the first year and virtually none subsequently.

Watson [9] in a prospective randomized study of 32 patients allocated to medical-dilation therapy versus surgical antireflux procedure, concluded that surgery significantly reduced the necessity for long-term dilation.

Surgery is suggested as the treatment of choice in patients with reflux stenosis in whom there are no serious contraindications to surgery. Superior results can be anticipated when an effective antireflux procedure is accomplished at a time when esophageal stenosis is still dilatable to at least 50 French caliber.

References

1. Bennett JR (1984) Benign Oesophageal Strictures. *In* Watson A, Celestin LR (eds): Disorders of the Oesophagus: Advances and Controversies. London: Pitman Publishing, Ltd., pp 129–136
2. Patterson DJ, Graham DY, Smith JL et al. (1983) Natural history of benign esophageal stricture treated by dilatation. Gastroenterology 85: 346–350
3. Glick ME (1982) Clinical course of esophageal stricture managed by bougienage. Digest Dis 27: 884–888
4. Toledo-Pereyra LH, Michel H, Manifacio G et al. (1976) Management of acidpeptic esophageal strictures. 72: 518–524
5. Luna LL (1983) Endoscopic therapy of benign esophageal stricture. Endoscopy 15: 203–206
6. Stoddard CJ and Simms JM (1984) Dilatation of benign oesophageal strictures in the outpatient department. Brit J Surg 71: 752–753
7. Wesdorp ICE, Bartelsman JFWM, denHartog-Jager FCA et al. (1982) Results of conservative treatment of benign esophageal strictures: a follow-up study in 100 patients. Gastroenterology 82: 487–493
8. Payne WS (1984) Surgical management of reflux-induced oesophageal stenoses: results in 101 patients. Brit J Surg 71: 971–973
9. Watson A (1985) Ramdomized study comparing medical and surgical reflux control in peptic esophageal stricture treated by intermittent dilatation. Gut 26: A553–A554
10. Payne WS (1986) Reflux Oesophagitis with Stricture: Alternative methods of management. *In* Dudley H, Carter DC, Jackson JW, Cooper DKC (eds): Rob & Smith's Operative Surgery, 4th edition. London: Butterworths, pp 314–235

Is it possible to quantify reflux?

R. D. Henderson (Toronto)

The simple answer to this question is that it is not possible to quantify reflux. Despite this negative answer the question is important as if focuses attention on our methods of reflux evaluation.

Ideally we need to know the following factors:

- The total duration of reflux
- The nature of the reflux bolus
- The average frequency and duration of daily episodes of reflux.

Each method of evaluation has its advantages and disadvantages, however there is no single method which is totally effective, each method gives its own unique results, and there is a tendency to over-emphasize the importance of the data obtained.

Amongst the various methods of quantitation of reflux the following are important

- History,
- Radiology,
- Endoscopy,
- pH studies,
- Radio-isotopes.

History is important in establishing the total duration of symptoms, the progression of symptoms, frequency of reflux and the duration of episodes of heartburn. This method uses pain as an indication of reflux.

By history the nature of the refluxed bolus cannot be established. The advantage of quantitating history is that it relates episodic reflux to daily physical and dietary history. It is not possible to quantitate pain severity and directly relate this to the severity of esophageal ulceration.

Radiologic assessment has advantages and disadvantages. Since radiation exposure must be minimized it is necessary to restrict the time and frequency of examination. As part of an upper GI, reflux can be examined and the water siphon test added for a more complete study. Using radiology, minor traces of reflux are not significant. Although reflux can be referred to as moderate or severe, this is not an accurate method of quantitation. Documented reflux does not equate reliably with symptom severity, the presence of ulcerative esophagitis or with the other various methods of reflux evaluation. Radiologic evaluation has very restricted value, but is the most common method in use.

Endoscopy is not generally used as a method of quantitating reflux, but it has some significant advantages and should not be ignored. To carry out endoscopy safely the patients do not eat for several hours, but the stomach can be distended with air and the competency of the HPZ can be assessed. It is my practice to routinely document competence as:

- competent,

- minor incompetence where the HPZ relaxes and remains open longer than 10 seconds,
- total incompetence.

Other than competence one can assess gastric emptying and ulcerative esophagitis or stricture. Delayed gastric empyting is detected by retained food particles. Ulcerative esophagitis is one of the most important end points of reflux damage.

It is not possible to correlate the history of reflux, radiologic reflux, endoscopic incompetence and ulcerative esophagitis, however the presence of ulceration clearly indicates that reflux, regardless of its frequency and duration, is very important.

The measurement of esophageal pH is generally regarded as the most accurate method of quantitating reflux. Using prolonged studies and outpatient studies it is possible to document the frequency and duration of reflux and to correlate this with diet, postural change and symptoms such as chest pain or aspiration. Various formulas have been devised that allow computerization of the data. The advantage of this method is the potential to study reflux over a more prolonged period of time. There are, of course, several disadvantages.

The chief disadvantage of pH as a marker, is that heartburn can occur with reflux of food, bile or pancreatic juices and an acidic pH change is not the only component of reflux injurious to the esophagus. Bile reflux is particularly important and very difficult to detect unless pH recordings are made from the duodenum and antrum simultaneously with esophageal pH studies. Changes in pH record the change in H ion concentration, do not however indicate the volume of fluid reflux or the mixture of acid, bile and food.

Radioisotopes can be used to assess esophagogastric clearance as well as to demonstrate reflux. There are some advantages to radionucleotide assessments.

Since the amount of radioactivity is measurable it is possible to measure the percent of the swallowed bolus which refluxes. Also, the radioactivity is a marker and can be detected in the lung if the patient chokes while swallowing or aspirates at night.

The five methods of quantitating reflux have been noted. There is no single method which supplies all of the answers and as such it is not possible to quantify reflux. At this time the combination of history, radiology, endoscopy and 8–24 hour pH studies offer the best compromise. Each method has some advantage and allows assessment of reflux which is clinically relevant.

References

1. Henderson RD (1980) The Esophagus: Reflux and primary motor disorders. Williams and Wilkins, Baltimore/London
2. DeMeester TR, Johnson LF (1976) The evaluation of objective measurements of gastroesophageal reflux and their contribution to patient management. Surg Clin North America 56: 39
3. DeMeester TR, Wang CI, Wernley JA, Pelligrini CA, Little AG, Klementschitsch P, Bermudez G, Johnson LF, Skinner DB (1980) Technique, indications and clinical use of 24 hour esophageal pH monitoring. J Thorac Cardiovasc Surg 79: 656
4. Skinner DB, Belsey RHR, Hendrix TR, Zuidema GD (1972) Gastroesophageal Reflux and Hiatal Hernia. Little, Brown, Boston
5. Leisner B, Witte J, Kiefhaber P, Eder M, Pfeifer J, Lang G, Mayr B (1978) Functional scientigraphy in diagnosis of gastroesophageal reflux. Z Gastroenterol 16: 235

What are the relations between gastroesophageal reflux and pharyngoesophageal dysphagia?

T. R. DeMeester (Omaha)

Cervical dysphagia occurs in patients with documented primary gastroesophageal reflux disease and is alleviated by an antireflux repair in nearly all. Its occurrence is not associated with a motility abnormality and probably is an atypical symptom of reflux disease. The grounds for this statement are as follows.

Nine of 103 patients with gastroesophageal reflux documented by 24-hour esophageal pH monitoring had pharyngoesophageal dysphagia. On esophageal motility studies, one of the nine patients had poor pharyngeal contraction. None had a hypertensive upper esophageal sphincter pressure nor incomplete or uncoordinated relaxation of the sphincter. All but one experienced relief of dysphagia after an antireflux procedure and the exception had relief following a cricopharyngeal myotomy. Fig. 1 shows that the upper esophageal sphincter pressure was below normal in four of the nine patients. Fig. 2 shows that all but one of the nine had normal pharyngeal pressures [1].

This finding is at variance with the studies of Hunt et. al., [2] who reported an increase in upper esophageal sphincter pressure and a 36% incidence of pharyngoesophageal dysphagia in patients with reflux. A similar finding was the absence of incomplete or uncoordinated relaxation of the sphincter.

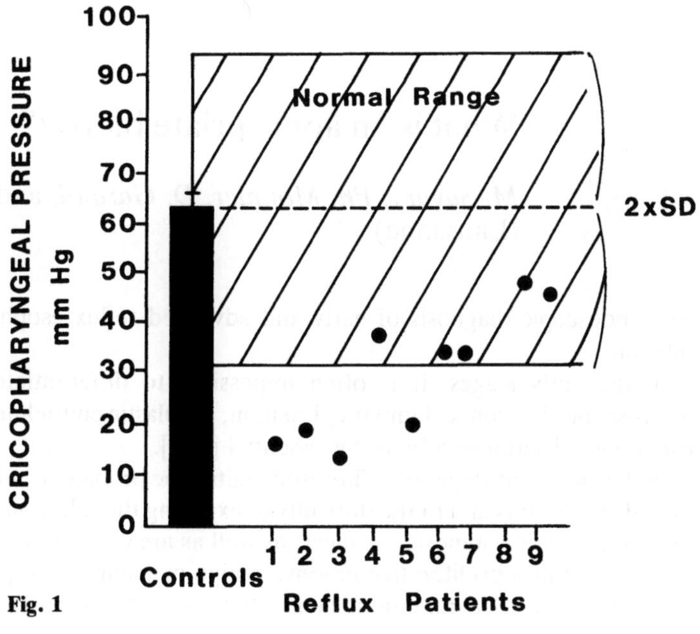

Fig. 1

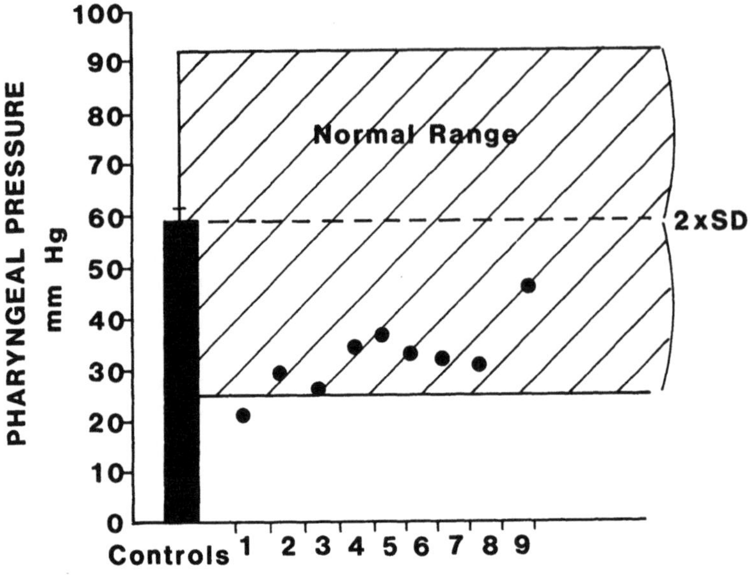

Fig. 2

References

1. Bonavina L, Khan NA, DeMeester TR (1985) Pharyngoesophageal dysfunctions: The role of cricopharyngeal myotomy. Arch Surg 120: 541–549
2. Hunt PS, Connell AM, Smiley TB (1970) The cricopharyngeal sphincter in gastric reflux. Gut 11: 303–306

What is an appropriate biopsy?

M. Savary, Ph. Monnier, D. Gardiol, and *Ch. Fontolliet* (Lausanne)

The endoscopic diagnosis of early and advanced reflux esophagitis is particularly difficult.

In the early stages, it is often impossible to differentiate reflux esophagitis macroscopically from columnar epithelium, dysplastic epithelium or even superficial carcinoma. Therefore a biopsy is essential [3, 4].

In the advanced stages of reflux esophagitis, the problem is related to the presence of multiple lesions and to the difficulty in exposing these lesions. Exudative erosions can coexist with a stenosis, an ulcer, as well as areas of columnar epithelium which can develop into proliferative lesions, benign or malignant [4]. Endoscopy is often difficult due to food retention, hemorrhage and stricture. The exploration of the esophagus distal to the stenosis is most important; a dilatation is necessarily part of a diagnostic exploration [4].

The first requirement for a biopsy is the ability to harvest a sample. This implies preparation and access procedures for the entire pathological area [2].

The second requirement is to differentiate macroscopically, in their morphology and topography, the different primary lesions which are often multiple and diverse (exudate, erosion, ulceration, stenosis, areas of columnar epithelium, polyps, buds, etc...). Vital colorations (Lugol and toluidin-blue solutions) can be of interest but never resolve the issue since they both react identically with columnar epithelium and superficial carcinoma (toluidin-blue positive and Lugol negative).

The third requirement of a biopsy is that the sampling be precise and selective. This is the fundamental requirement [2] and it implies:

- that the target lesion be exposed, clearly defined and motionless.
- that the biopsy forceps can be guided precisely and then stabilized when the lesion is seized.

These two requirements represent insurmountable technical problems with fiberoptic biopsy instruments used in the supravestibular region. The operator must aim at a target that is seen tangentially, is in motion and is occasionally optically poorly defined. Moreover, the sampling instrument is unstable and difficult to control. This explains why the histologic criteria of early reflux esophagitis remain poorly defined and change from school to school [1]. The only reliable histologic

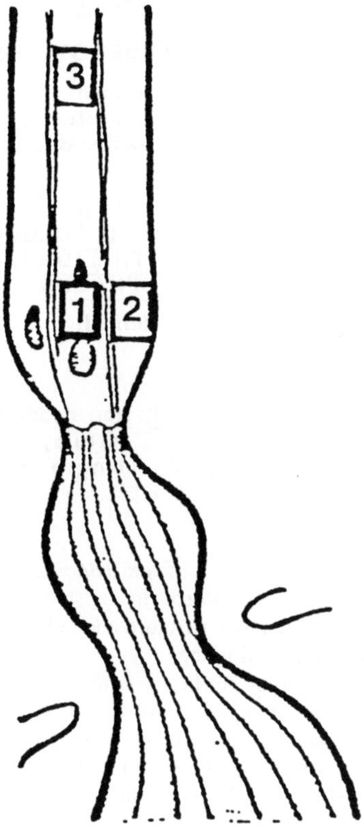

Fig. 1. *Biopsy protocol of a stage I reflux esophagitis.* Three biopsies are performed: 1. of an erythematous patch above the vestibule; 2. at the same level but of macroscopically normal mucosa; 3. at 5 cm proximal to the Z-line, of macroscopically normal mucosa

information on early reflux esophagitis available at the present time comes from the rare studies performed with biopsy forceps used with a rigid optical system. This ensures precise and selective biopsies due to the optical qualities of the instrument and above all to the stability of the contact between forceps and target [3].

The fourth requirement of a biopsy is related to the quality of the sample. Its depth should reach to the muscularis mucosae and it should be oriented correctly for microscopic examination.

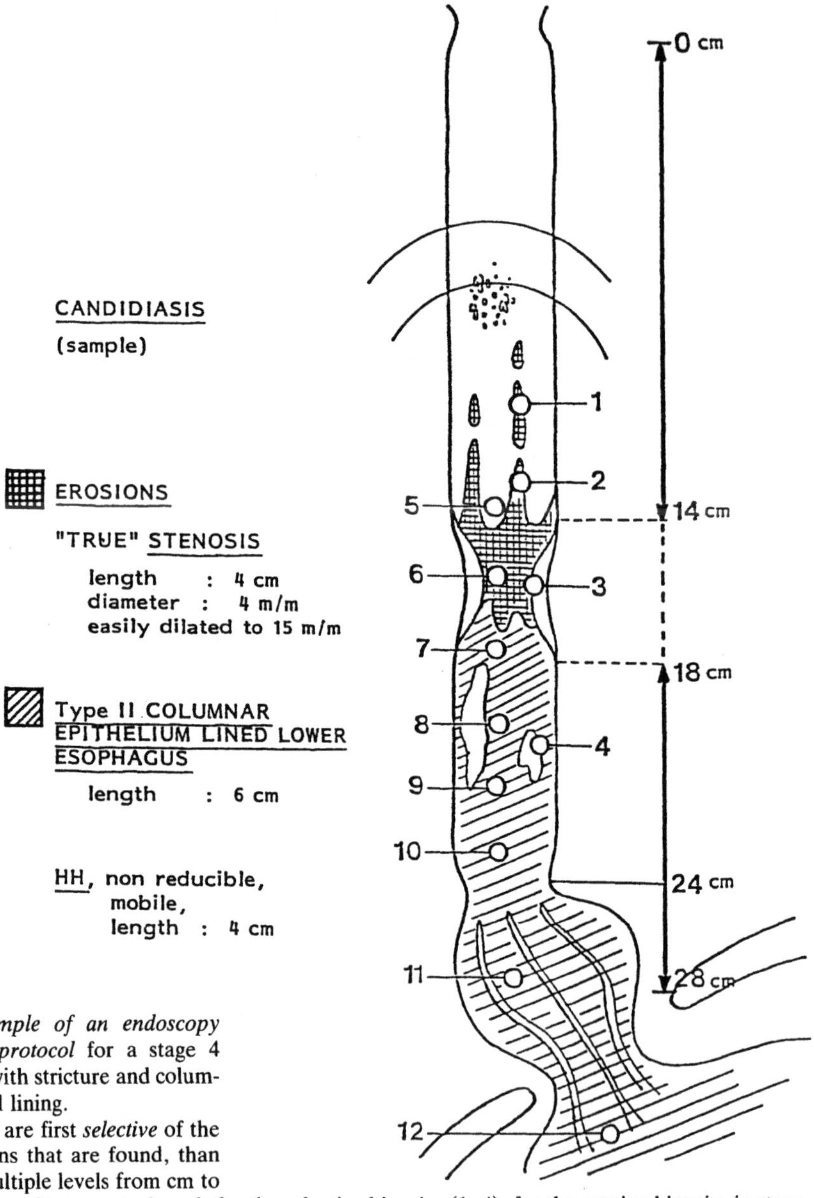

Fig. 2. *Example of an endoscopy and biopsy protocol* for a stage 4 esophagitis with stricture and columnar epithelial lining. The biopsies are first *selective* of the various lesions that are found, than *routine* at multiple levels from cm to cm. The biopsy sites are numbered: for the selective biopsies (1–4), for the routine biopsies in steps (5–12). The characteristics of the stenosis, the columnar epithelium and of a possible hiatal hernia are described

Biopsy Protocol

If biopsies are taken selectively and precisely of *early stage reflux esophagitis* (erythematous or non confluent erythematous and exudative lesions = stage I) and of healthy mucosa at the same level, we find that the disease does not involve the lower esophagus diffusely but remains localized and punctuate in the early stages (Fig. 1).

The different primary lesions *of stage 4 esophagitis* with complications (erosions, ulcers, buds, exudates) are defined after complete exploration and exposure of the entire pathological area (which usually implies a dilatation).

The first series of biopsies are selective and taken from each primary lesion.

The second series implies non selective biopsies, performed in steps from cm to cm, the most proximal being above the lesions, the most distal below the gastroesophageal vestibule.

The protocol intended for the pathologist includes the diagram of the lesions which are found as well as the sites of the various biopsies, whether selective or routine in steps (Fig. 2).

This type of protocol is particularly useful for the investigation and follow-up of cases of columnar epithelium of the lower esophagus.

References

1. Monnier Ph, Savary M (1987) "New Endoscopic Techniques" In: International Trends in General Thoracic Surgery, Vol 3 Benign Esophageal Disease. Ed DeMeester TR, Matthews HR. Mosby Company, St-Louis, Minn (in Press)
2. Savary M, Miller G (1977) "L'œsophage: manuel et atlas d'endoscopie" Ed Gassmann, Soleure
3. Savary M, Monnier Ph (1980) "Le reflux gastro-œsophagien: l'apport de l'endoscopie dans l'indication opératoire et les contrôles post-opératoires" Helv Chir Acta 47:693–706
4. Savary M, Ollyo JB (1986) "L'œsophagite par reflux et ses complications: ulcère, sténose, endobrachy-œsophage" Encycl Med Chir (Paris), Otorhinolaryngologie, 20822 A^{10}, 10, 16 p

W. V. Bogomoletz (Reims)

An adequate biopsy is a biopsy which allows the pathologist to perform proper microscopic examination and to reach correct diagnosis. Such a biopsy should be correctly orientated (vertical orientation) and should contain full-thickness mucosa (all layers of squamous epithelium as well as a sufficient amount of underlying lamina propria).

Proper orientation can be achieved by identifying the submucosal side of the biopsy and placing it on a small card, filter paper or nylon mesh square. Another method is to mount the biopsy on gel foam. These methods are easier to carry out with suction biopsy specimens than with forceps biopsies. Immediate fixation of biopsies is mandatory. Orientation of biopsies can also be obtained by using a dissecting microscope, either before or after fixation, but this is more time-consuming. Adequate paraffin embedding and careful microtomy cutting of biopsy specimens are also important to maintain proper orientation (specially assigned technician?). Serial or semi-serial sections should also be obtained.

Accepted histological criteria of reflux esophagitis include elongation of the subepithelial papillae, increased height of the epithelial basal layer and the presence of inflammatory cells in the lamina propria. These criteria can only be assessed provided that a proper orientation and full-thickness mucosa are obtained.

What are the limitations of the histological interpretation of a biopsy taken from the area of esophagitis?

C. G. Bremner (Johannesburg)

Prior to 1970, the histologic diagnosis of reflux esophagitis was poorly defined as a neutrophil infiltrate in the lamina propria.

In 1970, Ismail-Beigi et al [1] correlated gastroesophageal reflux with basal zone hyperplasia and an increase in the height of the vascular papillae. They found polymorphonuclear leukocytes in the lamina propria in only 18% of specimens from patients with gastroesophageal reflux. In 1974 the same authors studied multiple suction biopsy specimens taken from the lower 8 cm of the esophagus, and found that the abnormal changes were constant over this area [2]. Weinstein et al [3] later demonstrated that 57% of biopsies from asymptomatic patients taken in the distal 2,5 cm of the esophagus, and 19% of biopsies above 2,5 cm had elongated papillae and basal cell hyperplasia. Their patients did not have reflux tests performed, and had experienced heartburn on rare occasions. Since then, numerous studies have evaluated Ismail-Beigi's and others criteria (Table 1) [1–7].

A summary of the results of a survey appears in Table 2 [8–15], and there is obviously disagreement about the efficacy of biopsy interpretation of reflux. Several of the studies selected patients on symptoms of reflux only, and even normal controls did not have reflux excluded on pH testing. For such studies to be accurate, it would be necessary to document gastroesophageal reflux preferably by ambulat-

Table 1. Esophagitis: histologic criteria

1. Basal cell zone [1, 2, 3]	:	Thickness increased
2. Vascular papillae [1–5]	:	Height increased
		Number increased
		Transverse diameter increased
3. Neutrophils [1]	:	Increased
4. Eosinophils [6]	:	Increased
5. Capillaries [5, 7]	:	Ingrowth into epithelium
6. Langerhans cells and T Lymphocytes [5, 7]	:	Increased

Table 2. Basal cell hyperplasia and papillosis in gastroesophageal reflux

Author and Date			*Correlation*
Ismail-Beigi et al.	(1)	1970	+
Ismail-Beigi et al.	(2)	1974	+
Behar and Sheahan	(8)	1975	–
Weinstein et al.	(3)	1975	–
Seefeld et al.	(9)	1977	–
Johnson and DeMeester	(10)	1978	+
Leape et al. (children)	(11)	1981	+
Biller et al. (children)	(12)	1983	+
Collins et al.	(13)	1985	+
Kaul et al.	(14)	1986	+
Funch-Jensen et al.	(15)	1986	+

ory pH monitoring. Quantitative reflux studies would best be used to compare histological changes.

Some of the studies took biopsy material from areas within 2,5 cm of the gastroesophageal junction, and in the light of Weinstein's studies [3], their conclusion should be disregarded. Biopsy material may be inadequate from some models of fibre-optic endoscopic forceps, and some authors have found suction biopsy material to be preferable. Correct orientation of the material is important. Johnson and DeMeester [10] established reflux by pH monitoring, and their comparison with histological findings in these cases is meaningful. Eosinophilic infiltration into the esophageal wall has also been reported to be a good predictor of reflux esophagitis [6] but Collins et al [13] found eosinophils in only 52% of their reflux patients (Table 3).

We have made a study in the experimental reflux baboon model [7]. In the acid reflux model, not only did the vascular papillae increase in height, but they increased in number as well (8 per low power field increasing to 12.7 per low power field $p<0.01$). In the bile-acid reflux model the number increased from 8 to 22.1 ($p<0.001$) over a 12 month period. The distribution of the increase was seen throughout the length of the esophagus. Our studies suggest that the number of papillae should also be taken into account.

We have also examined biopsies from patients with achalasia and have found similar changes to those described by Ismail-Beigi et al. These changes are therefore not specific for reflux esophagitis but represent a hyperregenerative response to irritation.

Table 3. Intraepithelial eosinophilic granulocytes as a reflux marker

			Result	*Reflux Assessment*
Winter 1982 (infants)	(6)		+	pH probe (overnight)
Janish 1984	(16)		–	Endoscopic
Shub 1985 (infants)	(17)		+	pH probe (overnight)
Collins 1985	(13)	52%	+	Symptomatic and Endoscopic

Conclusion

Histologic changes seen on biopsy specimens from patients with reflux esophagitis are not specific to reflux, but represent a hyper-regeneration response to irritation. The changes are not sufficiantly sensitive to be of value in the diagnosis of reflux, but can be used as an adjunct to other tests for reflux.

The limitations of assessing histologic changes also depend on the site of the biopsy, the number of biopsies taken, and the method and orientation of the biopsies. Factors which may influence the histologic changes are age, alcoholism, smoking and esophageal stasis. These factors have not been adequately evaluated.

Studies used to correlate histology and reflux are valueless unless reflux is first established by a reliable method such as ambulatory pH recording. Furture studies may well consider the use of multivariant analyses of all histologic changes related to quantitative reflux results.

References

1. Ismail-Beigi F, Horton PF, Pope CE (1970) Histological consequences of gastroesophageal reflux in man. Gastroenterology 58: 163
2. Ismail-Beigi F, Pope CE (1974) Distribution of the histological changes of gastroesophageal Reflux in the distal esophagus in man. Gastroenterology 66: 1109–1113
3. Weinstein WM, Bogoch ER, Bowes KL (1975) The normal human esophageal mucosa. A histological reappraisal. Gastroenterology 68: 40–47
4. Bremner CG (1977) Reflux esophagitis in the Baboon. Significance of the number of vascular papillae. Gastroenterol 73: 1463
5. Geboes K, Haot J, Mebis J, Desmet VJ (1983) The histopathology of reflux esophagitis. Acta Chir Belg 83(6): 444–448
6. Winter HS, Madera JL, Stafford RJ et al. (1982) Intraepithelial eosinophilis. A new diagnostic criterion for reflux esophagitis. Gastroenterol 83: 818
7. Geboes K, De Wolf-Peeters C, Rutgeerts P, Janssens J, Vantrappen G, Desmet V (1983) Lymphocytes and Langerhans cells in the human esophageal epithelium. Virchows Arch 401(1): 45–55
8. Behar J, Sheahan D (1975) Histologic abnormalities in reflux esophagitis. Arch Pathol 99(7): 387–391
9. Seefeld V, Krejas GJ, Siebenmann RE, Blum AL (1977) Esophageal histology in gastroesophageal reflux. Morphometric findings in suction biopsies. Dig Dis 22: 956–64
10. Johnson LF, DeMeester TR, Haggitt RC (1978) Esophageal epithelial response to Gastroesophageal Reflux. Dig Dis 23: 498–508
11. Leape LL, Bhan I, Ramenofsky ML (1981) Esophageal biopsy in the diagnosis of reflux esophagitis. J Pediatr Surg 16(3): 379–384
12. Biller JA, Winter HS, Grand RJ, Allred EN (1983) Are endoscopic changes predictive of histologic esophagitis in children? J Pediatr 103(2): 215–218
13. Collins BJ, Elliott H, Sloan JM, McFarlane RJ, Love AH (1985) Esophageal histology in reflux esophagitis. J Clin Pathol 38(11): 1265–1272
14. Kaul B, Halvorsen T, Grette K, Petersen H, Myrvold HE, Fjosne U (1986) Gastroesophageal reflux disease. Scintigraphic, endoscopic and histological considerations. Scand J Gastroenterol 21(2): 134–138
15. Funch-Jensen P, Kock K, Christensen LA, Fallingborg J et al. (1986) Microscopic appearance of the esophageal mucosa in a consecutive series of patients submitted to upper endoscopy. Scand J Gastroenterol 21(1): 65–69
16. Janisch HD, Pfannkuch F, Von Kleist D, Degenhardt U, Bauer E, Hampel KE (1984) Histologic abnormalities on routine biopsies of patients with esophagitis and different gastric acid secretion. Appl Pathol 2(5): 272–276
17. Shub MD, Ulchen MH, Hargrove CB, Siegel GP, Groben PA, Askin FB (1985) Esophagitis: a frequent consequence of gastroesophageal reflux in infancy. J Pediatr 107(6): 881–884

K. Jeyasingham (Bristol)

Although the association of peptic and acid reflux with esophagitis was first noted as long ago as the last century [1], the histologic diagnosis of esophagitis based on the cardinal features of acute, sub-acute and chronic inflammatory cellular infiltration, posed a difficult problem until recent years [2].

The classical features of esophagitis were studied initially from autopsy specimens [3, 4, 5]. With the advent of esophageal surgery for benign conditions, histologic material became available from grasp biopsy forceps via the rigid esophagoscope [6, 7, 8] and from resected specimens [6, 7]. It soon became clear that although neutrophilic and eosinophilic cellular infiltration was a feature of moderate and severe esophagitis, the presence of round cell infiltration of the lamina propria was not necessarily indicative of inflammation, as mononuclear cells are a normal component of the lamina propria [8]. We are indebted to Ismail-Beigi, Horton and Pope [9] for the currently accepted criteria for the diagnosis of esophagitis based on

- basal cell hyperplasia, and
- location of the papillae close to the surface of the epithelium (Table 1).

A basal cell zone in excess of 15% of the thickness of the epithelium is abnormal. Papillae extending more than two thirds of the way to the surface of the epithelium indicate inflammation. In concluding that if these features were present in two biopsies the diagnosis of esophagitis was confirmed, and if present in one the epithelium is deemed abnormal, the authors conceded that the correlation between reflux and histology might possibly be greater if more than two biopsies were obtained.

Behar and Sheahan [10] modified these criteria by saying that in multiple biopsies over the lower 10 cm of the esophagus, the co-existence of basal zone hyperplasia to greater than 15% and papillary height greater than 50% of the mucosal thickness, in at least two biopsy specimens, was diagnostic of esophagitis. It is, however, worth noting that despite the above classical histologic concept of esophagitis, Sladen and his colleagues [11] in a retrospective assessment of 71 patients for esophageal symptoms concluded that endoscopy and biopsy added little to the information obtained from the acid perfusion test. They reserved biopsy to patients with special problems such as blood loss and dysphagia, or when a radiologic lesion needed clarification.

Yardley's concept [2] of a "vascularized epithelium" was composed of

- a basal zone greater than 15%,

Table 1. Criteria for diagnosis of peptic esophagitis

Basal Zone	>15%
Papillae	>66%
	Number of biopsies
	in one: abnormal (Ismail-Beigi et al. 1970)
	in two: diagnostic
	Location
	Multiple biopsies over 10 cm from LES (Behar & Sheahan 1975)

Table 2. Yardley's *"vascularized epithelium"* (Yardley 1972)

Basal zone	>15%
Papillae	>66%
Cellular infiltration of lamina propria	
Vascularized core of papillae	
Erosion, ulceration & fibrosis (in late stages)	

- papillae taller than 66% of epithelial thickness,
- increase in the number of vascular papillae in the field,
- neutrophil and eosinophil infiltration of the lamina propria (Table 2).

In the later stages of esophagitis, to the above criteria should be added the erosion, ulceration and fibroblastic proliferation [12]. In a morphometric assessment of reflux esophagitis by examination of biopsy specimens, Jarvis et al. [13] found that the most important parameters were

- number of intermediate layer nuclei per square mm
- mean intermediate layer nuclear area
- number of nuclei per mm of base epithelium, all these features suggesting an increased cell turnover of the nonulcerated epithelium before treatment.

Collins and his colleagues [14] in a well planned study to assess the specificity of the classical criteria, the sensitivity, agreement between two pathologists and the reproducibility of interpretation by any one pathologist confirmed that Ismail Beigi's criteria stood up to the tests most reliably, but their accuracy was enhanced if multiple biopsies were examined.

Apart from the histologic criteria, there are other technical factors that may contribute to difficulties in interpretation of the histology. Until the advent of the fibreoptic endoscope, esophageal epithelial biopsies were obtained by rigid grasp forceps through the rigid esophagoscope or by the Quinlon-Rubin hydraulic suction tubes. In recent years, however, most endoscopists obtain biopsy tissue with the grasp forceps of a flexible fiberoptic endoscope. The size of the cups of the forceps determine the size of such specimens and the trauma associated with the procurement. Such specimens are difficult to orientate and add to the difficulties of interpretation. Suction biopsies, however, are easily orientated, and produce thick tissue with very little trauma. However, as they are obtained "blind", their exact localization in relation to the esophago gastric junction is difficult to determine. Endoscopic biopsy, however, overcomes this factor as well as the discrepance associated with erosions, ulcerations, presence of mucus, blood or air from the stomach.

My personal routine is determined by whether the endoscopic biopsy is on the initial examination or on subsequent follow-up examinations. On the first endoscopic examination, quadrantic biopsies 2 cm proximal to the esophagogastric junction with a minimum of four specimens are obtained. On subsequent examinations, a minimum of two biopsies are obtained, unless the initial examination had revealed dysplasia, or suspicious mucosa, in which case quadrantic biopsies are repeated [15].

References

1. Quincke H (1879) "Ulcus oesophagii ex digestione". Deutsch Arch Klin Med 24: 72–(quoted by Sandry)
2. Yardley JH, Skinner DB, Belsey RHR, Hendrix TR, Zuidema G (1972) "Gastroesophageal reflux and hiatal hernia". Little Brown & Co, Boston 52–58
3. Lodge KV (1955) "The pathology of non specific oesophagitis". J Path Bact 69: 17–24
4. Peters PM "The pathology of severe digestion oesophagitis". (1955) Thorax 10: 269–286
5. Palmer ED (1955) "Subacute erosive oesophagitis". Arch Pathol 59: 51–57
6. Sandry RJ (1962) "The pathology of chronic oesophagitis". Gut 3: 189
7. Sandry RJ, (1972) Skinner et al. "Gastroesophageal reflux and hiatal hernia". ibid., 43–52
8. Siegel CI and Hendrix TR (1963) "Esophageal motor abnormality induced by acid perfusion in patients with heartburn". J Clin Investig, 42: 686
9. Ismail-Beigi F, Horton PF, Pope CE (1970) "Histological consequences of gastroesophageal reflux in man". Gastroenterology 58: 163–174
10. Behar J, Sheahan DC (1975) "Histologic abnormalities in reflux esophagitis". Arch Pathol 99: 387–391
11. Sladen GE, Riddell RH, Willoughby JMT (1975) "Oesophagoscopy, biopsy and acid perfusion test in diagnosis of "Reflux oesophagitis". Brit Med J 1: 71–76
12. Geboes K, Haot J, Mebis J, Desmet VJ (1983) "The histopathology of reflux oesophagitis". Acta Chir Belg 83: 444–448
13. Jarvis LR, Dent J, Whitehead R (1985) "Morphometric assessment of reflux oesophagitis in fibreoptic biopsy specimens". J Clin Pathol 38: 44–48
14. Collins BJ, Elliott H, Sloan JM, McFarland RJ, Love AHG (1985) "Oesophageal histology in reflux oesophagitis". J Clin Pathol 38: 1265–1272
15. Reilly MK and Jeyasingham K (1984) "A Modified Pearson Gastroplasty" (Thorax 39: 67–69

In what proportion of cases are there poor quality biopsies?

W. V. Bogomoletz (Reims)

It is difficult to define what is precisely meant by inadequate or "poor quality biopsies. Firstly, such biopsies could include all those which show failure of proper orientation or which don't contain full thickness mucosa. On the other hand, de spite clinical symptoms and endoscopic evidence of gastroesophageal reflux or esophagitis, some biopsies simply don't show pathological changes and are reported as normal. Should the latter category also be considered as "inadequate"? Furthermore, even biopsies which have been properly orientated and carefully cut, may show crushing artefacts which make histologic assessment difficult. Finally, the way in which biopsies are obtained at endoscopy, i.e. by forceps or suction, probably also affects the overall quality of biopsy material.

To my knowledge, there have been no published studies where the number or the relative proportion of inadequate biopsies has been specifically correlated to the above "technical" parameters and compared with satisfactory biopsies.

What is the role of a decrease in the peristalsis secondary to esophagitis linked disorders?

M. Veyrac, P. Bories, P. Chardon, J. Du Cailar, and *H. Michel* (Montpellier)

Esophageal motility is controlled by two types of peristalsis [3]: primary peristalsis, studied by esophageal manometry, corresponding to monophasic contractile propulsive waves excited by swallowing, and secondary peristalsis determined by distension of the body of the esophagus. The latter can be studied by acid clearance of the esophagus without swallowing [2]. The aim of this study was to investigate the role of disordered secondary peristalsis of the esophagus in resuscitation patients with or without esophagitis.

Patients and methods

14 patients (11 men, 3 women) of mean age 55 years, without history of digestive disorder, hospitalized for chest injuries and fed by intestinal tube, were divided into 2 groups (Fig. 1) of equal size according to the presence or absence of esophagitis, correlated with their duration of stay in the resuscitation unit.

Group 1 included 7 patients (5 men, 2 women–mean age 53 years) hospitalized for

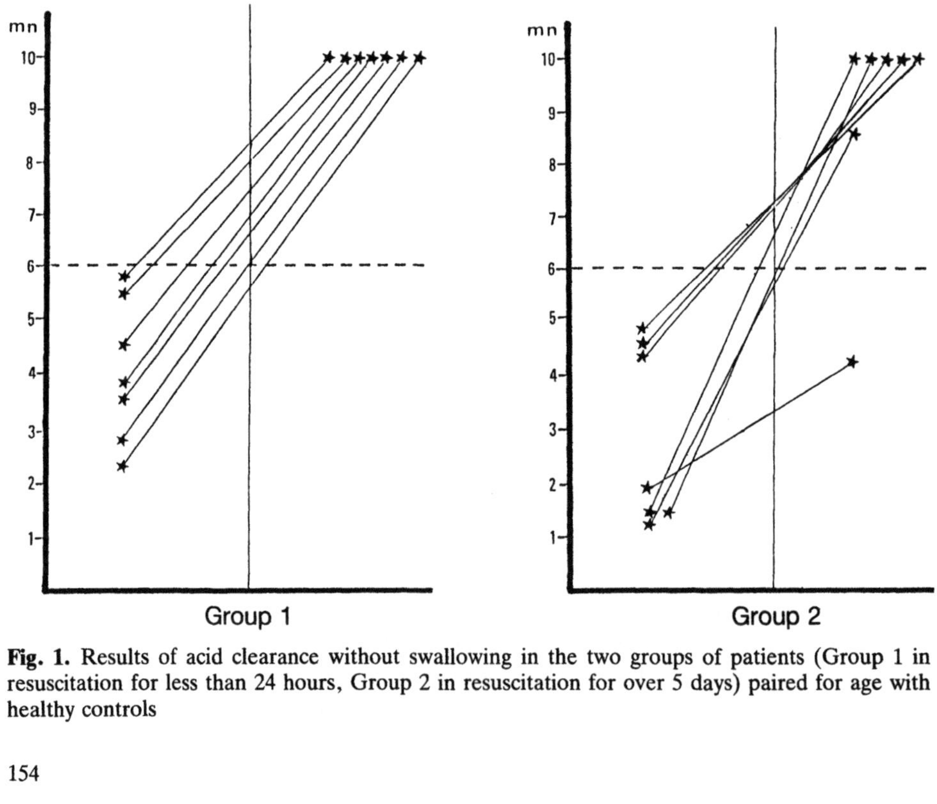

Fig. 1. Results of acid clearance without swallowing in the two groups of patients (Group 1 in resuscitation for less than 24 hours, Group 2 in resuscitation for over 5 days) paired for age with healthy controls

less than 24 hours and without esophagitis verifiable by endoscopy and histology. Group 2 comprised 6 men and 1 woman, mean age 55 years, hospitalized for over 5 days, all with esophagitis (3 of grade III and 4 of grade II). These patients were compared with two groups of 7 controls–volunteers free from esophageal symptoms-paired for age with the patients.

All the subjects (patients and controls) were submitted to a study of esophageal clearance, which measures the time required for the esophagus to empty 15 ml of 1/10 normal HCl instilled 15 cm above the cardia. This measurement of the time taken for restoration of an esophageal pH above 5 was studied by pH measurement 5 cm above the cardia in the absence of swallowing to constitute a test of acid clearance without swallowing [2]. In 5 of the 7 patients of Group 2 the test was repeated after removal of the enteral nutrition tube.

Results

In the controls the acid clearance without swallowing was 238±94 seconds, consistent with data in the literature. In the patients of Group 1 acid clearance without swallowing was significantly prolonged (600 seconds, $p < 0.01$) compared to paired controls (261±82 seconds). In Group 2, acid clearance without swallowing and with tube in place (528±124 seconds) differed significantly (p 0.01) from the controls (215±106 seconds). After removal of the tube, non-significant shortening of the esophageal clearance time without swallowing was observed (484±143 seconds)

Comments

In ventilated patients under intensive care, fed by nasogastric tube, the study of acid clearance without swallowing demonstrated disturbed secondary peristalsis of the esophagus. This disturbance was independent of the existence of an esophagus, which was itself correlated with the duration of hospitalization. On the other hand, the tube did not appear to modify the degree of the motor disorder significantly.

The conditions in which this study was performed could be factors favoring the development of esophageal motor disorder.

The consequence of this disturbance of esophageal emptying is to prolong the time of contact of an aggressive fluid with the mucosa, bringing about the onset of esophagitis. This would suggest another mechanism [1] than that of gastroesophageal reflux in the genesis of esophagitis.

References

1. Baccino E, Boles JM, Le Guillou M, Gier B, Garo B, Robaszkiewicz M, Cleuziou A (1987) Tentative de traitement préventif des œsophagites sur sonde en réanimation Gastroenterol Clin Biol 11: 24–28
2. Leveque AM, Lampert R, Minaire Y (1980) La clairance acide de l'oesophage au cours du reflux gastro oesophagien et chez des témoins étudiée par deux méthodes dont une originale Gastroenterol Clin Biol 4: 226 A
3. Minaire Y, Lambert R (1976) in Physiologie humaine. La digestion. ed Simep 206: 220

Can the role of esophageal clearance disorders be defined?

D. E. Low, and *L. D. Hill* (Seattle)

Introduction

The multifactorial nature of esophageal reflux disease has become generally accepted by both surgical and gastroenterological physicians. Esophagitis can result from uncontrolled gastroesophageal reflux or impaired acid clearance or a combination of both [1, 2]. In general, the process of lower esophageal acid clearance entails two separate and distinct steps. The first consists of an initial peristaltic wave which virtually empties the acid from the lower esophagus leaving only a residual film which maintains a low pH [3, 4]. In the second step of esophageal clearance, the residual acid film is neutralized by swallowed saliva. Thus, the general process of acid clearance may be prolonged by either abnormal esophageal emptying or impaired salivation.

The extent and severity of the esophageal damage due to reflux can be related not only to the amount and concentration of the refluxed material but also to the duration of contact between the refluxed bolus and the esophageal mucosa. Abnormal esophageal clearance likely does not figure in the majority of patients with symptomatic reflux esophagitis; however, its presence undoubtedly contributes to the severity of both the symptomatic and pathologic presentation. Initial speculation that impaired salivary flow and variation in salivary content might contribute to abnormal acid clearance in patients with reflux esophagitis has been shown to be incorrect, although the salivary response to esophageal acid perfusion has been shown to decrease with age, suggesting that elderly patients may be at increased risk for serious problems when exposed to esophageal reflux [5].

In the normal peristaltic response to a large acid bolus introduced into the lower esophagus, the residual volume of the retained acid can be reduced to 1 ml or less by one peristaltic wave [6]. The remaining neutralization of the residual acid film is effected by bicarbonate-containing saliva carried down the esophagus in subsequent swallows. We agree with others [7], who feel that the primary peristaltic mechanism remains the most important component. The initial peristaltic response to reflux must reduce the acid volume sufficiently to allow this secondary neutralization to be effective.

Acid clearance efficiency may vary in patients with gastroesophageal reflux but overall is seen to be impaired in up to 50% of patients studied [8, 9]. We believe that in a significant portion of these patients, the underlying abnormality may be a preceding, although associated, abnormality in intrinsic esophageal peristalsis. Some authors have proposed that the abnormality in peristalsis may be caused by the esophagitis produced by gastroesophageal reflux [8, 10]. However, we, along with others, suspect that these motor abnormalities precede the manifestations of the actual reflux but are a major contributor to its serious side effects [11].

Radionuclide Studies and Esophageal Clearance

In our laboratory, the initial identification of a subgroup of patients with symptomatic reflux was found during examination of patients with gastroesophageal reflux and healthy controls using esophageal scintigraphy [11]. We found that by plotting a time-activity curve of the lower esophagus after placing 1 mc of 99^{m} Technetium sulfur colloid into the stomach that we could identify not only the presence of gastroesophageal reflux but could also identify a subpopulation of patients who had poor lower esophageal clearance of the reflux material.

In our controls, we could not identify reflux either spontaneously or with induced measures. However, in the refluxing population, reflux episodes were seen spontaneously and with Valsalva. In most of these patients, the reflux episodes were seen to rapidly clear (Fig. 1). However, in 3 out of 28 patients in this group, an elevated count rate over the esophagus was maintained, even in the presence of repeated swallows. Count rates were seen to drop after each peristaltic wave only to reappear promptly to their previously high level (Fig. 2). Retention of the reflux bolus was seen to exceed several minutes, which is markedly prolonged over the generally accepted clearing time (10 to 15 seconds) for the majority of reflux episodes.

However, when the clearance time in these patients was compared with pH probe monitoring, the retention time measured with scintigraphy was seen to be less than that measured with the pH probe. This is an expression of the fact that radionuclide measurement of lower esophageal clearance examines only the peristaltic component of lower esophageal acid clearance whereas pH probe measurement looks at the combined efficiency of both the peristaltic and salivary neutralizing effects.

This initial work supports the observations made by Helm [4], which show that under normal circumstances the majority of a reflux bolus is promptly returned to the stomach by the next peristaltic wave. In addition, it provides a method to easily and noninvasively identify patients who not only have significant reflux but whose situation was complicated by impaired lower esophageal acid clearance.

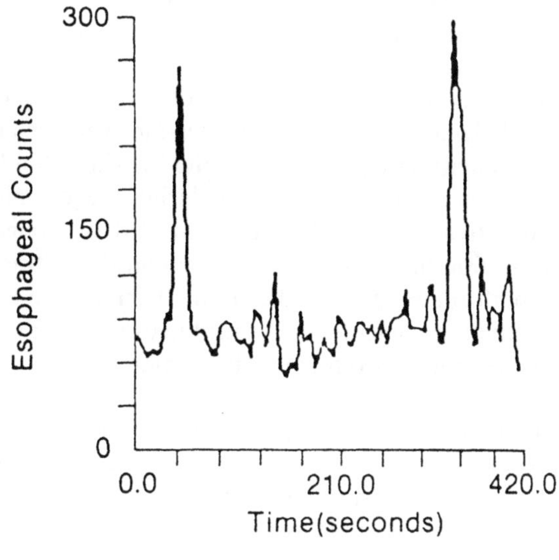

Fig. 1. Reflux episodes in a symptomatic patient. A timeactivity plot of counts recorded from the esophageal area of interest shows two bursts of reflux, one in a basal condition and one following a Valsalva maneuver at the end of the study period

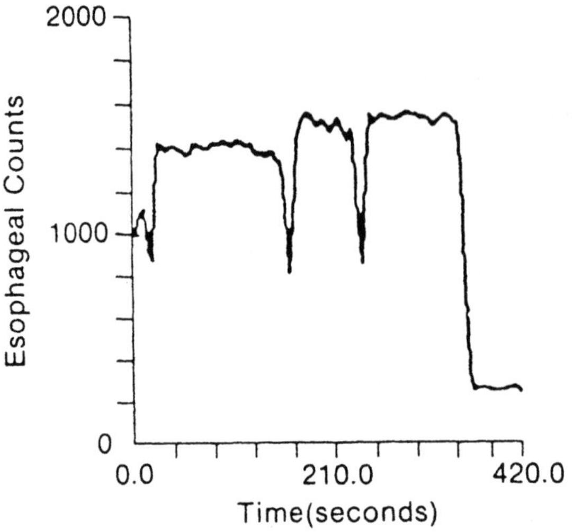

Fig. 2. Persistence of radioisotope in the esophagus of a patient with severe reflux. The esophageal counts remain high, dropping only briefly during swallows. The count rate immediately rises after the swallow as more material is refluxed

In an attempt to further identify, quantify, and study these esophageal motor disorders, our laboratory introduced a method of measuring radionuclide esophageal transit. [13, 14]. This was done utilizing a standard homogeneous bolus of ^{99}Technetium sulfur colloid in water which was swallowed in the supine position under the collimator of a gamma camera linked to a microprocessor. Ten normal volunteers and 30 subjects with dysphagia not related to mechanical obstruction were studied utilizing this technique. We found that this examination was not only more sensitive than manometry or radiology in detecting the presence of an esophageal motor abnormality but could also be utilized to provide a reasonably accurate, definitive description of the functional problem in many of the cases of patients presenting with dysphagia in the absence of mechanical obstruction.

Radionuclide transit was measured after giving a 10 ml homogeneous bolus of H_2O plus 250 mc of ^{99}Technetium sulfur colloid. This wet swallow was followed 30 seconds later by a dry swallow. Aspects of bolus transit were assessed by measuring the esophageal transit time, i.e., the time from initial entry of the bolus into the esophagus until total clearance of the esophagus was achieved. In addition, the actual dynamics of bolus progression were examined by analyzing the levels of radioactivity independently in the proximal, middle, and distal esophagus at frequent time intervals (0.4 sec) during the examination. By subsequently plotting radioactivity against time for each of these areas, the resulting graphs provided a description of bolus transit throughout the entire length of the esophagus (Fig. 3). By performing these studies in the fasting state and monitoring the radioactivity in the stomach coincidentally with the esophageal measurements, any artefacts due to gastroesophageal reflux can be minimized.

Our initial studies using these techniques examined patients with obvious motility disorders, including achalasia, scleroderma, and diffuse esophageal spasm [13]. However, the most interesting portion of this study was the significant prevalence of radionuclide transit abnormalities (64%) detected in the group that was seen to have

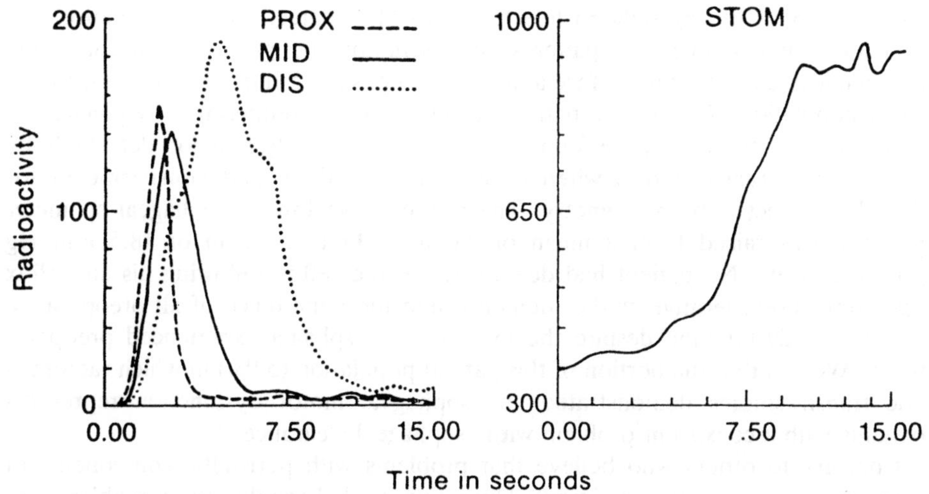

Fig. 3. Radionuclide transit graph from normal volunteer. Vertical axes represent the radioactivity in each area and the horizontal axes the time in seconds. Note sequential peaks in proximal, middle, and distal esophagus indicating smooth passage of the bolus in an aboral direction with early and complete entry into the stomach

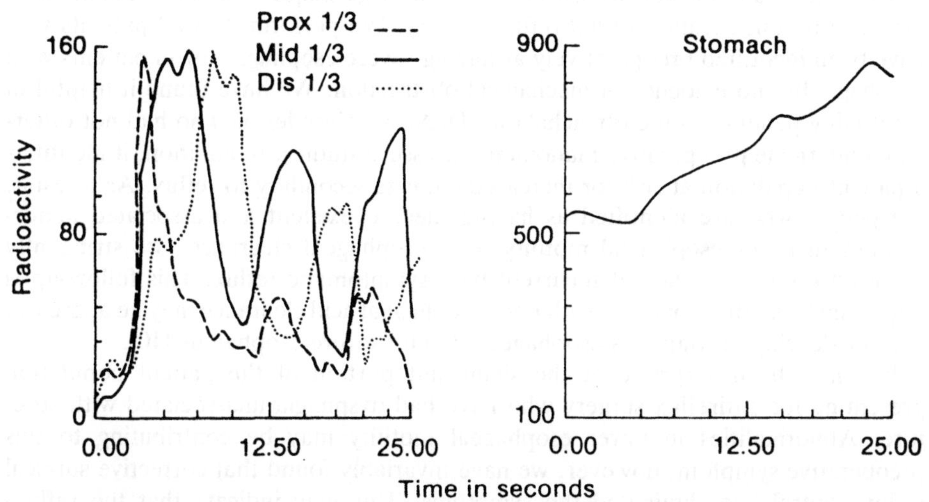

Fig. 4. Radionuclide transit graph from a patient with normal manometry. Vertical axes and horizontal axes are radioactivity and time in seconds respectively. Note multiple peaks of activity representing disorganized bolus transit. Some of the bolus, however, reached the stomach within the 25 second time period shown

otherwise normal manometric findings (Fig. 4). The abnormalities that were detected involved problems with incoordinated transit in all 9 of the cases studied.

Utilizing this technique, we began to study patients who complained of dysphagia associated with symptomatic gastroesophageal reflux but had no evidence of peptic stricture [15]. Utilizing radionuclide transit (RT) to detect esophageal motor dysfunction, we examined 29 patients with symptomatic gastroesophageal reflux uncomplicated by stricture before and three months after antireflux surgery. In our study population, 73% of the patients complained of preoperative dysphagia. Of these, 52% of the total were found to have esophageal dysfunction detectable by radionuclide transit studies whereas only 18% of these had nonspecific motor disorders detected by manometry. The preoperative lower esophageal sphincter pressure was raised from a mean of 8.6 mm Hg to a mean of 18.5 mm Hg postoperatively. No patient had demonstrable free reflux following his antireflux operation. Postoperative studies demonstrated the persistence of all preoperative esophageal dysfunction despite the loss of the dysphagia experienced preoperatively. We feel that the portion of this patient population (52%) in which radionuclide transit studies demonstrated an esophageal motor dysfunction represents patients with a coexistent problem with esophageal clearance.

Contrary to others who believe that problems with peristaltic components of esophageal clearance may be initiated by reflux, we believe that these problems are preexistent and continuing. In this population, antireflux surgery does not correct the problem of impaired acid clearance; however, it can interrupt reflux, thereby minimizing the importance of the associated peristaltic abnormality.

We utilize radionuclide transit studies in a large majority of our patients who present for consideration of antireflux surgery. We perform it in all patients who have been identified preoperatively as having severe esophagitis or in patients with dysphagia but no evidence of mechanical obstruction. We have found it helpful in identifying patients with early achalasia, DES, or scleroderma who had not otherwise undergone preoperative manometric pressure studies. In addition, it identifies a patient population at risk for increased damage secondary to reflux. As a result, the people who are identified as having these coexistent and associated abnormalities in lower esophageal motility, i.e., esophageal clearance, are stringently followed up for evidence of recurrent but asymptomatic reflux. This follow-up is important since these patients with poor esophageal acid clearance may be at greater risk for developing Barrett's esophagus [16] and severe esophagitis [10].

We have been surprised at the significant portion of the patient population presenting for antireflux surgery who have had dysphagia unassociated with stricture. Abnormalities in lower esophageal motility may be contributing to this preoperative symptom, however, we have invariably found that corrective surgical reflux control has eliminated the symptoms. This may indicate that the reflux-induced esophagitis is allowing episodes of solid food dysphagia to be detected whereas when the esophagus heals this sensory capability disappears.

Generally speaking, studies utilizing radionuclide transit have allowed us to identify subtle motor abnormalities associated with impaired esophageal clearance. These abnormalities are not always evident on routine x-ray or manometric studies. Further examination of these patients will help identify a specific role in esophageal reflux pathogenesis. In the interim it is apparent that these patients can be adequately and effectively treated with antireflux surgery.

References

1. DeMeester TR, Johnson LF, Guy JJ, Toscano MS, Hall AW, Skinner DB (1976) Patterns of gastroesophageal reflux in health and disease. Ann Surg 184: 459–470
2. Johnson LF, DeMeester TR (1981) Evaluation of elevation of the head of the bed, bethanechol, and antacid foam tablets on gastroesophageal reflux. Dig Dis Sci 26: 673–680
3. Helm JF, Dodds WJ, Riedel DR, Teeter BC, Hogan WJ, Arndorfer RC (1983) Determinants of esophageal acid clearance in normal subjects, Gastroenterology 85: 607–612
4. Helm JF, Dodds WH, Pelc LR, Palmer DW, Hogan WJ, Teeter BC (1984) Effect of esophageal emptying and saliva on clearance of acid from the esophagus. N Eng J Med 310: 284–288
5. Sonnenberg A, Steinkamp U, Weise A (1982) et al. Salivary secretion in reflux esophagitis. Gastroenterology 83: 889–895
6. Helm JF, Dodds WJ, Hogan WJ (1982) et al. Acid neutralizing capacity of human saliva. Gastroenterology 83: 69–74
7. Ferguson MK, Ryan JW, Little AG, Skinner DB (1985) Esophageal emptying and acid neutralization in patients with symptoms of esophageal reflux. Ann Surg 201: 728–735
8. Stanciu C, Bennett JR (1974) Oesophageal acid clearing: one factor in the production of reflux esophagitis. Gut 15: 852–857
9. Boesby S (1977) Gastroesophageal sphincter pressure, motility, and acid clearing. Scand J Gastroenterol 12: 407–416
10. Kahrilas PJ, Dodds WJ, Hogan WJ, Kern M, Arndorfer RC, Reece A (1986) Esophageal peristaltic dysfunction in peptic esophagitis. Gastroenterology 91: 897–904
11. Helm JF (1986) Esophageal acid clearance. J Clin Gastroenterol 8 (Suppl 1): 5–11
12. Velasco N, Pope CE, Gannan RM, Roberts P, Hill LD (1984) Measurement of esophageal reflux by scintigraphy. Dig Dis Sci 29: 977–982
13. Russell COH, Hill LD, Holmes ER, Hull DA, Gannan R, Pope CE (1981) Radionuclide transit: a sensitive screening test for esophageal dysfunction. Gastroenterology 80: 887–892
14. Russell COH, Pope CE, Gannan RM, Allen FD, Velasco N, Hill LD (1981) Does surgery correct esophageal motor dysfunction in gastroesophageal reflux? Ann Surg 194: 290–296
15. Russell COH, Gannan R, Coatsworth J et al. (1983) Relationship among esophageal dysfunction, diabetic gastroenteropathy and peripheral neuropathy. Dig Dis Sci 28: 289–293
16. Karvelis KC, Drane WE, Johnson DA, Silverman ED (1987) Barrett's esophagus: decreased esophageal clearance shown by radionuclide esophageal scintigraphy. Radiology 162: 97–99

A. G. Little, M. K. Ferguson, and *D. B. Skinner* (Chicago)

There are three interrelated but separate factors which must be considered in understanding the pathophysiology of reflux esophagitis. First, the lower esophageal sphincter (LES) or cardia must be incompetent and allow reflux of gastroduodenal contents into the lower esophagus. Secondly, the severity of injury is in part determined by the resistance of the esophageal mucosa to injury. Finally, the ability of the esophagus to clear refluxed contents will influence the duration of mucosal exposure to the potentially injurious contents and thereby affect the degree of injury. Clearly, then, the role of disordered esophageal clearance in patients with gastroesophageal reflux disease (GRD) is important and should be defined. The focus of this paper will be on techniques utilized to investigate esophageal clearance with discussion of the pros and cons of each technique.

Manometry

Manometric examinations are performed using either water-perfused catheters or catheters containing peripheral pressure measuring devices. What is determined from these investigations is the intraluminal effect of muscular esophageal contractions. Although useful, this investigation is not a primary investigation but is a secondary one. Using manometry, one can compare the findings to normal standards with regards to the pattern of contractions i.e., whether they are peristaltic or simultaneous, repetitive or spontaneous. Also one can quantitate the magnitude and duration of the contractions. This provides interesting information but unfortunately does not correlate with the actual ability of the esophagus to clear material.

For example, it has been shown that many patients with GRD have abnormal motility patterns and that these patterns tend to persist following successful antireflux operations even though radionuclide measures of esophageal clearance do show postoperative improvement [1]. It seems that the motility tracing itself is not a completely accurate representation of the efficacy of esophageal contractions.

Acid Clearance Test

The Acid Clearance Test (ACT) is carried out by monitoring esophageal pH with a transnasal pH probe placed five cm proximal to the manometrically determined upper border of the LES. With the patient supine, 15 cc of 0.1N HCL are introduced into the esophagus through another tube placed 10 cm proximal to the pH probe. Intraesophageal pH is monitored and the patient swallows at 30-second intervals. The end point of the test is the number of swallows required to elevate the pH above 5.0. In a series of investigations [2, 4] it was found that 10 swallows constituted a watershed number. All normal volunteers tested were able to raise their esophageal pH above five with 10, or less, swallows. In contrast, 62% of patients with hiatal hernias had positive tests and 68% of patients with typical reflux symptoms had positive ACTs. Finally 86% of patients with abnormal pH reflux tests had a positive ACT. This suggested that the ACT was very specific and at least moderately sensitive for identification of patients with pathologic GER. Perhaps more importantly, however, was the finding that of all the esophageal function tests analyzed, including manometry, acid perfusion (Bernstein Test) the Standard Acid Reflux Test and the ACT, the greatest discrimination between reflux patients with or without endoscopic esophagitis was achieved by the ACT.

Seventy percent of the former patients and only 36% of the latter had abnormal acid clearing, a difference which approached statistical significance.

In other words, the ACT was the indirect evaluation which had the strongest correlation with the presence of esophagitis. When correlated in light of the observation that the refluxers with and without esophagitis had similar LES characteristics, these data were interpreted to mean that refluxers with esophagitis differed from refluxers without esophagitis by having deficient esophageal body function and the inability to clear reflux material.

Esophageal clearance and/or neutralization of intraluminal acid is a complex process and the ACT is overly simplistic in that the assumption on which it is based –

that an abnormal ACT is produced solely by deficient esophageal peristalsis – is incomplete. For example, one reason for delayed acid clearance in patients with hiatal hernias is acid reflux from the hernia sac [5]. This was shown by performing simultaneous ACTs and radionuclide studies in three populations: refluxers with and without hiatal hernias and nonrefluxers with hiatal hernias. In all hernia patients, swallows resulted in an initial fall in pH which was followed by a rise. This biphasic response was not seen in those without hiatal hernias. The radionuclide studies explain this phenomenon by showing reflux of the isotope-labeled acid into the esophagus, followed by clearance, following swallows in 15 of the 20 hernia patients.

These results suggest that the ACT is not determined solely by delayed clearance per se but also, in hernia patients, is prolonged by repeated episodes of acid reflux of acid caught in the hiatal hernia.

A second consideration in interpretation or understanding of the ACT is the importance of the role of alkaline saliva in neutralization of intraesophageal acid. When saliva is aspirated from the mouth and thereby diverted from the esophagus, esophageal acid clearance as measured by the pH probe is prolonged; conversely, when salivary secretion is stimulated then clearance is accelerated [6]. This suggests that a part of what is being measured by the ACT is salivary neutralization of acid. Radionuclide imaging studies using radiolabeled acid in conjunction with manometry during the ACT have confirmed this by showing that the majority of the acid bolus instilled into the esophagus is cleared into the stomach with the first or second peristaltic wave which follows the acid instillation [7]. However, the esophageal pH electrode continues to register in the acid range until swallows begin and alkaline saliva is transported into the distal esophagus.

Radionuclide Isotope Swallow analysis

Radioisotope swallow analysis (RIS) (Table 1) is a relatively new method for the study of esophageal clearance. With the understanding of the limitations of manometry and the ACT, our group addressed the question of the role of esophageal clearance disorders with an investigation which compared ACT results with RIS in patients [8]. The RIS was performed from the posterior view using a gamma camera with data acquired into a computer. After an overnight fast, 15 cc of water containing 150–200 μCi of Tc-99m sulfur colloid were placed in the mouth of the patient who then swallowed every 15 seconds until clearance was achieved. From this data, patterns of clearance and esophageal transit times were derived.

Twenty-six symptomatic patients were studied, eight of whom had GRD as defined by esophageal pH monitoring, as were 15 control, asymptomatic volunteers. ACT was abnormal in five of the controls, 17 of the 26 patients and all eight of the GRD patients. RIS was abnormal (either prolonged transit time or delayed isotope clearance) in none of the controls, eight of the 26 patients and seven of the eight GRD patients.

This suggests that, in fact, it is delayed esophageal bolus emptying or clearance and not deficient acid neutralization by saliva that is the important abnormality in GRD patients.

Table 1. Radioisotope swallow (RIS)

1. Technique:
   A. 15 cc radiolabeled H_2O or 0.1N HCl
   B. Swallows every 15 to 30 seconds
2. Results:
   A. Helm et al.:
      1. Simultaneous ACT, RIS and manometry in normal volunteers
      2. Virtually all acid volume is cleared from the esophagus by one or two peristaltic sequences, leaving a minimal residual amount which sustains a low pH
      3. Residual acid is neutralized by swallowed saliva
   B. Ferguson et al.:

	ACT	*RIS*
Normal volunteers	5/15	0/15
Symptomatic patients	17/26	8/26
Refluxers	8/8	7/8
Sensitivity	100%	87.5%
Specificity	50%	88.9%
Accuracy	65.3%	88.5%

References

1. Russell CO, Pope CE, Gannon RM, Allen NV, Velasco N, Hill LD (1981) Does surgery correct esophageal motor dysfunction in gastroesophageal reflux. Ann Surg 194:290–296
2. Booth DJ, Kemmerer WT, Skinner DB (1968) Acid clearing from the distal esophagus. Arch Surg 96:731–738
3. Booth DJ, Kemmerer WT, Skinner DB (1969) Clearing of alkali and acid from the distal esophagus: Current Topics in Surgical Research. Chicago, IL, Year Book Medical Publishers Vol. 1, pgs 263–269
4. Skinner DB, Booth DJ (1970) Assessment of distal esophageal function in patients with hiatal hernia and/or gastroesophageal reflux. Ann Surg 172:627–637
5. Mittal RK, Lange RC, McCallum RW (1987) Identification and mechanism of delayed esophageal acid clearance in subjects with hiatus hernia. Gastroenterol 92:130–135
6. Helm JF, Dodds WJ, Riedel DR, Teeter BC, Hogan WJ, Arndorfer RC (1983) Determinants of esophageal acid clearance in normal subjects. Gastroenterol 85:607–612
7. Helm JF, Dodds WJ, Pelc LR, Palmer DW, Hogan WJ, Teeter BC (1984) Effect of esophageal emptying and saliva on clearance of acid from the esophagus. N Engl J Med 310:284–288
8. Ferguson MK, Ryan JW, Little AG, Skinner DB (1985) Esophageal emptying and acid neutralization in patients with symptoms of esophageal reflux. Ann Surg 201:728–735

What are the troubles of gastric emptying of solid food which most often causes an esophagitis? Disorders of the proximal tonus, Disorders of antrum motility

G. G. Jamieson (Adelaide)

When the gastric emptying of a solid meal of ground beef is measured, using a radioactive marker, it is found that there is a variable period of time before any food leaves the stomach. This is called the lag period of gastric emptying, and in normal controls we found it to vary between 9 and 69 minutes [1]. The lag period is made up of two stages. The first is a "reservoir stage", during which food is received into the gastric fundus and body; and remains there until the second stage commences. This is the "trituration stage" during which food is moved from the reservoir into the antral mill, where breakdown in particle size occurs. When food particles reach 1 mm in diameter, gastric emptying commences. The food then leaves the stomach at approximately a linear rate of 1.25% per minute (range 0.7%–2.3%). If there is more than 65% retention of the beef in the stomach 100 minutes after ingestion, then gastric emptying for solids is regarded as delayed [1].

It has been established that some patients with gastroesophageal reflux disease (GERD) have delayed emptying of solids although the proportion of patients varies in different series – probably as a result of methodological differences in studying gastric emptying. We found that 44% of 72 patients with GERD had delayed emptying of solids. The delay was due both to a prolonged lag period and a slow rate of emptying [1].

In 64 GERD patients assessed endoscopically, there were 36 who were diagnosed as having esophagitis and 47% of these patients had delayed gastric emptying of solids. In 28 patients without endoscopic esophagitis, 18% had delayed gastric emptying of solids ($p < 0.005$). A similar relationship between delayed emptying of solids and endoscopic esophagitis was shown by Little et al. in a group of 50 GERD patients [2].

At the present time, it is not known where the abnormality lies in gastric emptying in these patients. Current thinking places the main control of gastric emptying of solids with the antrum [3]. Behar et al. [4] documented antral dysmotility in a small group of patients with GERD, and Fink et al. [5] showed antral gastritis associated with delayed emptying in GERD patients. The role of the fundus and body of the stomach and of the pylorus, in the control of gastric emptying of solids has been ignored somewhat in recent years.

Currently we are studying gastric emptying in closer detail in patients with GERD. Our first approach is to segment the stomach regions of interest into proximal (fundus/body) and distal (antrum) to determine the relative role played by each of these areas in the retention of solid food within the stomach. Our second approach is to carry out gastro-pyloroduodenal manometry using a catheter with perfused sideholes in the stomach and duodenum and a pressure sensor sleeve, which is maintained across the pylorus. This assessment is carried out at the same time as a radionuclide assessment of the emptying of solids.

These methods will allow us to define whether it is the proximal stomach, the antrum, the pylorus or combinations of all three, which are responsible for disordered gastric emptying in patients with GERD.

References

1. Maddern GJ, Chatterton BE, Collins PJ, Horowitz M, Shearman DJC, Jamieson GG (1985) Solid and liquid gastric emptying in patients with gastro-oesophageal reflux. Br J Surg 72:344–347
2. Little AG, DeMeester TR, Kircher PT, O'Sullivan GC, Skinner DB (1980) Pathogenesis of esophagitis in patients with gastroesophageal reflux. Surgery 88:101–107
3. Kelly KA (1980) Gastric emptying of liquids and solids: Roles of proximal and distal stomach. Editorial Review, Am J Physiol G 71–76
4. Behar J, Ramsby G (1978) Gastric emptying and antral motility in reflux esophagitis. Gastroenterology 74:253–256
5. Fink SM, Barwick KW, Deluca V, Sanders FJ, McCallum RW (1984) The association of histologic gastritis with gastroesophageal reflux and delayed gastric emptying. J Clin Gastroenterol 6:301–309

What is the incidence of alkaline reflux in patients suffering from esophageal reflux?

Ph. Marlière, and *A. Gulbis* (Brussels)

The causal link between gastroesophageal reflux (GER) and esophagitis is known. The correlation between the frequency and duration of episodes of acid reflux, on the one hand, and the severity of the esophageal lesions on the other, is not complete. Animal in vitro and in vivo experiments have demonstrated the cytotoxicity of biliary-pancreatic secretion towards the esophagus. Therefore, the reflux of fluid containing strong concentrations of bile acids ought to be recognized.

One way of approach is by combined pH measurement in the esophagus and stomach, in which the gastric electrode is situated in the antrum and reacts to changes in pH due to any episodes of duodenogastric reflux (DGR). This method allows detection of "mixed" GER, i.e. reflux of fluid of pH between 4.5 and 5.5, which would be due to buffering of normally acid gastric secretion by biliary-pancreatic secretions and not just the GER of gastric juice in a hypochlorhydric patient. This method was described by Puccini et al (148 observations) and showed 75% of acid reflux, 25% of mixed reflux, and negligible alkaline reflux in a population excluding scleroderma and post-Polya cases.

This method is easy to use and, by detecting the subjects with mixed reflux, would make it possible to lessen the number of false-negatives in classic pH measurement, i.e. those presenting with esophagitis and in whom classic pH measurement is normal. However, there seem to exist (Collins et al) GER fluids with concentrations of bile acids regarded as cytotoxic to the esophagus, despite a pH below 3.5; further, there may exist causes other than reduced gastric clearance for the presence of bile acids in quantity in the stomach. Thus, it may be rather the presence of these bile acids in the stomach than reduced gastric clearance that should be investigated by chemical analysis of the fluid.

In conclusion, the incidence of alkaline GER is negligible, but hypoacid GER is important because they are common and also sometimes cytotoxic, when they correspond to a mixture of acid gastric secretions and alkaline biliary secretions and not to purely gastric, but hypochlorhydric, secretions. Though combined esophageal and gastric pH measurement may not reveal all these "mixed" refluxes, it remains an elegant method for improving the score of pH measurement in the investigation of reflux esophagitis.

What is the underlying mechanism of the toxicity of biliary acids?

A. Papazian (Amiens)

Various animal experimental studies have been performed to understand the intimate mechanism of the toxicity of the bile acids (BA) towards both the gastric and the esophageal mucosa. Their toxicity could be associated with their ability to solubilize the lipids of the cell membrane. In the concentrations usually observed in man, the dihydrozyl BA increase retrodiffusion of the H+ ions in significantly greater fashion than the trohydroxyl BA in the gastric mucosa of the dog, whether ischemic or nonischemic. As the dihydroxyl BA are more lipophile, it has been suggested that they produce more extensive membranous solubilization [1].

This hypothesis is reinforced by the studies of Duane and Wiegand [2] on the gastric mucosa of the dog.

1. A mixture of six conjugated BA reproducing the proportions observed in human bile produces rupture of the gastric mucosal barrier (GMB) as indicated by increased movements of H+ and Na+ ions and increased efflux of cholesterol and lecithin.
2. Saturation of the micellae of BA by cholesterol and lecithin prevents rupture of the GMB.
3. Tauro-dihydrocholate, a bile salt that does not form micellae, does not produce increases in the movements of H+ and Na+ ions or of cholesterol and lecithin.

These studies suggest that the micellar solubilization of the lipids of the cell membrane is the intimate mechanism of toxicity of the BA towards the GMB.

The static and sweep electron microscopic studies on the esophageal mucosa of the rabbit performed by Salo, Lehto and Kivilaakso [3] have suggested that the toxic effect of the different components of the reflux fluid may be differentiated. The proteolytic enzymes (gastric pepsin and pancreatic trypsin) produce destruction of the intercellular substance and detachment of the surface cells. The BA produce selective destruction of the cell membranes and organelles, and only bring about detachment of the mucosal cells later.

The intimate mechanism of toxicity of the BA at the esophageal mucosa remains hypothetical. The detergent action of deoxycholate, which provokes extraction of lipids from the cell membranes, has been experimentally demonstrated and the hypothesis postulated for the GMB by Duane and Wiegand [2] is supported for the esophageal mucosa by Salo et al [3].

References

1. Ritchie WP Jr, Felger TS (1981) Differing ulcerogenic potential of dihydroxy and trihydroxy bile acids in canine gastric mucosa. Surgery 89: 342–347
2. Duane WC, Wiegand DM (1980) Mechanism by which bile salts disrupt the gastric mucosal barrier in the dog. I Clin Invest 66: 1044–1049
3. Salo JA, Lehto VP, Kivilaakso E (1983) Morphological alterations in experimental esophagitis Light microscopic and scanning and transmission electron microscopic study. Dig Dis Sci 28: 440–448

There is no demonstrated correlation between the severity of esophagitis and the concentration of biliary salts in the reflux fluid

E. Kivilaakso (Helsinki)

Bile salts are alleged to be injurious to the esophageal mucosa and to promote esophagitis when refluxed into the esophagus. Especially the secondary bile salt, deoxycholate (DOCA), and in particular in its deconjugated form, has been incriminated, since DOCA is a highly potent detergent with widespread cytotoxic effects. It remains, however, obscure whether there is any correlation between bile salts in the reflux material and esophagitis. The present paper compares the contents of bile salts as well as bile salt composition in the reflux fluid with the severity of esophagitis, paying special emphasis to DOCA. The results are based on data published earlier [1].

Patients and methods

Twelve patients (7 men, 5 women, mean age 59 years) who had undergone total or subtotal gastrectomy with loop esophagojejunostomy reconstruction for gastric carcinoma 1–8 years earlier were evaluated in terms of severity of the esophagitis and bile salt determination from esophago-jejunal aspirates. The severity of symptoms (heart burn + regurgitation) and esophagitis (endoscopic + histologic) was graded from none to severe. The concentration of bile salts as well as proportional composition of individual bile salt moieties in the esophago-jejunal aspirates was determined by gaschromatography.

Results

Four patients had no esophagitis and they also had no measurable amounts of bile salts in their esophageal aspirates. The remaining 8 patients had esophagitis ranging from mild to severe and they all also had bile salts in their esophageal aspirates, total bile salt concentration ranging from 46 to 3020 μg/ml. However, there was no correlation between the severity of esophagitis and total bile salt concentration ($r=0.19$, $p>0.2$).

As regards individual bile salt moieties, free DOCA had the strongest tendency towards significant correlation with the severity of esophagitis ($r=0.58$, $p\sim0.1$), but with the other bile salts studied (conjugated DOCA, conjugated free cholate and deoxycholate) the correlation was weaker ($r=0.2–0.5$, $p>0.1$).

Conclusion

The data indicate that there is no demonstrated correlation between the severity of esophagitis and the concentration of bile salts in the reflux fluid in patients with alkaline reflux esophagitis.

Reference

1. Matikainen M, Laatikainen T, Kalima T, Kivilaakso E (1982) Bile acid composition and esophagitis after total gastrectomy. Am J Surg 143: 196

Physiopathology of peptic esophagitis (2)

President: *Serge Bonfils* (Paris)

Free Commentators: *A. A. Conlan* (Johannesburg)
A. Del Genio (Naples)
E. Kivilaakso (Helsinki)
O. H. Mammoni (Buenos Aires)
J. Cl. Patel (Paris)

The physiology of the LES is now well-known

P. E. Donahue, C. T. Bombeck, and *L. M. Nyhus*
(Chicago)

Several discoveries during the past 15 years have led to insights into the antireflux mechanisms between the stomach and the esophagus. Taken as a group, these discoveries have clarified many of the traditional questions regarding the function of the lower esophagus and proximal stomach. However, there are many other variables which require further definition before we can claim that the function of the LES is "well-known." We quickly point out that part of the mystery is beginning to disappear, as the following examples illustrate.

Since the association between pathologic reflux and inflammation of the esophagus was first hypothesized we have experienced a revolution in the manner in which gastrointestinal disease is diagnosed and the manner in which responses to therapy are gauged; the most obvious example of this fact is shown by the interdependence of digestive surgeons with endoscopes (hopefully held in their own hands).

Simply stated, it is no longer possible to categorize someone as a victim of pathologic reflux without being aware of the endoscopic appearance of the esophageal mucosa; on the other hand, for many years there was a big problem with the correct evaluation of those patients with severe subjective complaints and minimal to absent objective evidence of reflux esophagitis. Luckily for all concerned, the development of the 24-hr pH recording devices clarified many of the issues surrounding these complex patients. Also, the ability of chest physicians and cardiologists to make more precise diagnosis has contributed to the fortunate circumstance that the "problem" patient is less and less commonly found. On the other hand, it is always appropriate and necessary to view the diagnostic tests in light of their proven sensitivity and specificity, none of which are equal to 100%.

With respect to the genesis of reflux episodes in normals without esophagitis as well as those with unequivocal pathologic reflux esophagitis, there is some evidence that transient relaxations occur in the lower esophagus sphincter (TLESR's) allowing gastric contents to flow upstream by a simple pressure gradient mechanism [1]. On the other hand, the concept of mechanical failure of the lower esophageal sphincter complex has been reinforced by several laboratory models demonstrating the vicious cycle of reflux esophagitis which causes serious weakening of the antireflux mechanism at the lower end of the esophagus. We subscribe to the concept of "mechanical" LES failure which views a pathologic reflux event as a combination of factors which include but are not limited to the LES pressure and the length of the sphincter. Several investigators have shown that the strength of the LES alone is not a sensitive indicator of pathologic reflux (unless it is zero); in fact, several groups including our own have shown that effective anti-reflux operations do not create extremely high pressures in the LES and that the degree of elevation of the LES is not considered a sensitive predictor of the efficacy of an anti-reflux operation [2].

In this context, the recent work on newer techniques for defining the motility of the lower esophagus are of interest, since there is some evidence suggesting that the new technique can distinguish between those patients with failure of the LES as opposed to those with less severe degrees of dysfunction [3].

One of the disappointing features of conventional esophageal motility studies is that there is too much overlap between the results in normal versus symptomatic patients with pathologic gastroesophageal reflux. Therefore, esophageal motility studies are used primarily to exclude certain dysmotility syndromes prior to the performance of anti-reflux surgical procedures.

Of course, this disappointing feature has been a problem with virtually every diagnostic methodology applied to the study of patients with reflux symptoms. The astute clinicians have recognized that there is likely to be a constant need for experienced clinical judgement in the reflux clinic, while the students of physical science have longed for a means for refining the available diagnostic tools. The recent advent of computerized manometric techniques, and the ability of microcomputers to assist in the genesis of complex data analyses suggests that we may be witness to a new era in medical testing. Bombeck et al. have presented evidence that, with respect to the lower esophageal anti-reflux mechanisms, that the use of computerized axial manometry may provide a mechanism for distinguishing between the groups referred to previously [3].

References

1. Dent J, Dodds WJ, Friedman RH, Sekiguchi T, Hogan WJ, Arndorfer RC, Petrie DJ (1980) Mechanism of gastroesophageal reflux in recumbent asymptomatic human subjects. J Clin Invest 65: 256–264
2. Donahue PE, Samelson S, Nyhus LM, Bombeck CT (1985) The Floppy Nissen Fundoplication – Effective long-term control of pathologic reflux. Arch Surg 120: 721–730
3. Bombeck CT, Vaz O, DeSalvo J, Donahue PE, Nyhus LM (1987) Computerized axial manometry of the esophagus: a new method for the assessment of anti-reflux operations. Presented at the American Surgical Association Meeting.

The essential anatomical features of peptic stenosis are quite accurate

J. Baulieux, and *P. Maillet* (Lyons)

The first characteristic of a peptic stricture is to size at the limit of a portion with a gastric mucosa and a portion with squamous mucosa.

a) The fundamental lesion is one of the submucosa. The association of inflammatory infiltration and edema gives it a sometimes undesirable thickening.
   The mucosal lesions are these of esophagitis as described by endoscopists: congestive appearance, edematous, fungating, pseudo-membranous or ulcero-hemorraghic. The mucosal lesions of peptic stricture are usually of the major ulcero-hemorraghic type. Numerous excavated ulcerations, filled with granula-

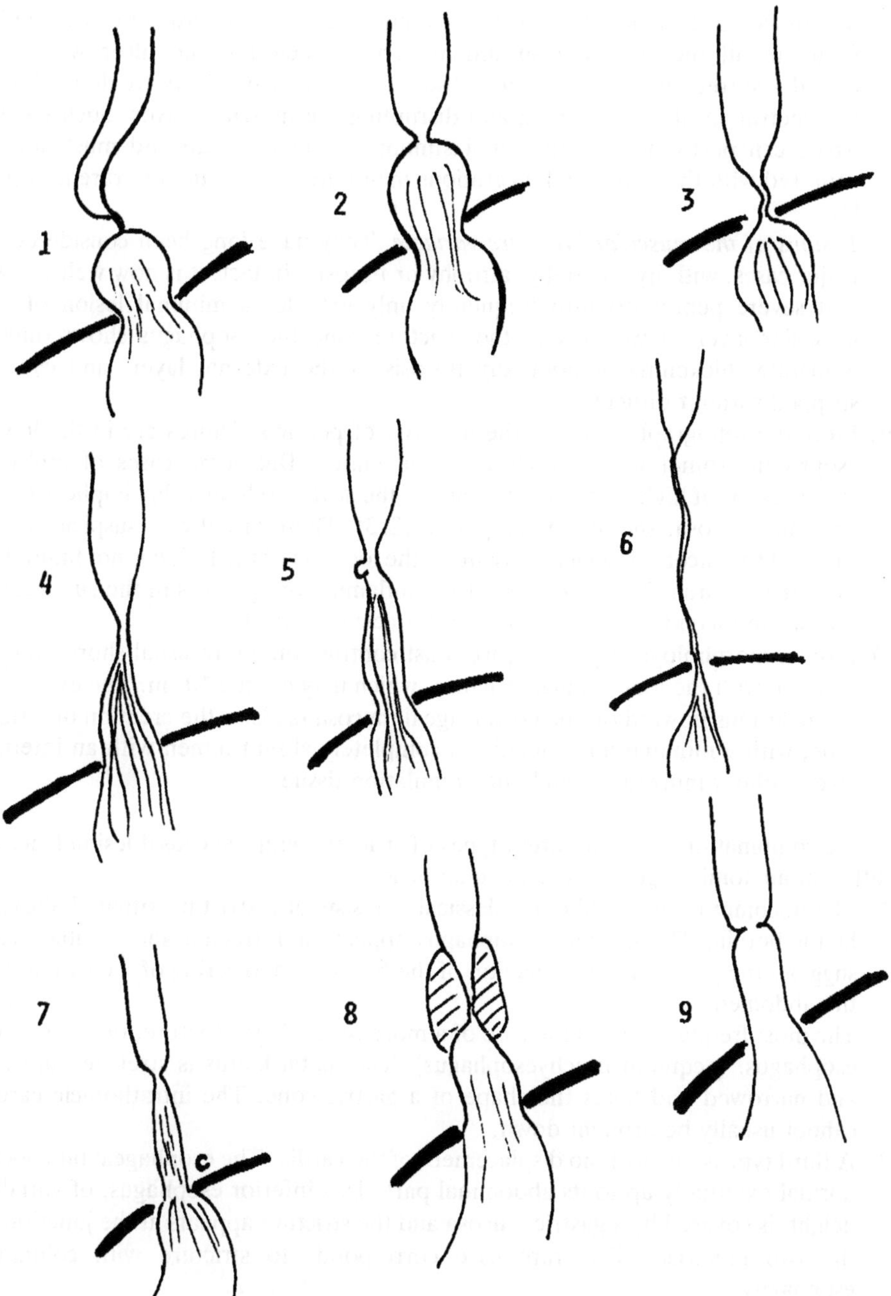

Fig. 1. Different anatomic types of peptic strictures: 1=Peptic stricture above hiatus hernia with reducible cardia; 2=Peptic stricture on hiatus hernia with brachyesophagus; 3=Low peptic stricture; 4=Peptic stricture with hernial cone and brachyesophagus; 5=Peptic stricture with true ulcer; 6=Long filiform stricture; 7=Stricture on endobrachyesophagus; 8=Pseudotumoral stricture; 9=Annular appearance (Schatzki)

tion tissue, give the jonction of the two mucosae a serrated aspect which can be found in all the resection specimens. The existence of an ulcer was once considered frequent, but this is not always the case if true ulcers are defined only as penetrating ulcers, reaching and disrupting the muscular layer. Such ulcers, which can perforate into the mediastinum, are in fact rare and must not be confused with the superficial ulcerations mentioned above and are rare as a rule [1].

Lesions of the muscular layer are variable. They have long been considered as major cases, with hypertrophy, atrophy or fibrosis. In fact, it is now well-known that severe peptic stricture frequently only includes a minimal lesion of the muscular layer, if we look at the stricture zone the esophagus shows only a moderate thickening without any fibrosis of the external layer, and can be stripped without difficulty.

b) From the topographic aspect, the majority of peptic strictures are in the lower esophagus, sometimes very close to the hiatus. But some cases of multiple strictures, or of high strictures at or above the aortic arch, possibly implicating an aberrant mucosa, should be recognized [2,3]. These are always suspicious and can lead to cancer. One fact is essential: the location of the lesion is not limited to the stricture area. The extension of the inflammatory process in the submucosa follows an ascending route along the thoracic esophagus.

c) From a morphologic aspect, [3] we must contrast the more usual short annular stricture with the long tubular stricture, which may exceed 10 cm. The extension of the lesions upward on the eosophageal mucosa leads to the creation of a rigid tube, with a minimal and sometimes completely absent lumen with an internal layer without mucosa, resembling granulation tissue.

The combination of the different types of stricture with the causal lesion leads to different anatomic types of very unequal incidence.

1. The uncommon type, although classical, consists of a stricture situated above a hiatus hernia. The proximal esophagus appears unretracted and flexible. This suggests the possibility of reduction of the hernia and lowering of the cardia into the abdomen.
2. The most frequent type is the case of a more or less high stricture, on a retracted esophagus. (acquired brachyesophagus). The hiatal hiatus is stretched upward and narrowed and takes the shape of a gastric cone. The intrathoracic cardia cannot usually be brought down.
3. A third type is one with no displacement of the cardia. The esophageal tube looks normal externally up to its abdominal part. This inferior esophagus, of variable height, is covered by a gastric mucosa and the stricture appears at the junction of the two mucosae. This rare case corresponds to stricture with columnar esophagus.

d) From a practical point of view, we must distinguish between strictures which are still reversible and easily dilatable, and tight fibrous strictures which are irreducible. Such a contrast is too inflexible, for all intermediate grades exist between the two extremes. Some fibrous strictures, even tight, can be submitted to dilatation.

As regards esophageal transit, peptic strictures vary considerably: at maximum intensity, we can find some translayer esophagitis and pseudo-neoplasia with inflammatory tumors, causing varying blockage due to a peri-oesophagitic reaction. At the minimum, some strictures become like a thin diaphragm. The lesion considered as congenital by Schatzki and Gary is, in fact, usually a preliminary stage of peptic stricture of a particularly favorable outcome (Fig. 1).

References

1. Butterfield WC (1971) Current hiatal hernia repairs, similarities, mechanisms and extended indications. An autopsy study. Surgery 69: 910
2. Maillet P, Baulieux J, Boulez J (1977) Les sténoses peptiques de l'œsophage. Lyon Méd 238: 35–42
3. Safaye-Shirazi S, Zike WL, Mason CC (1975) Esophageal stricture secondary to reflux oesophagitis, Arch Surg 110: 629

The concordance between endoscopy and histology seems good in certain types of esophagitis

Ph. Monnier, Ch. Fontolliet, M. Savary, and *D. Gardiol* (Lausanne)

Despite the precision introduced by Savary into the endoscopic description and classification of the lesions of reflux esophagitis [4], total imprecision persists as regards the histology of the first stages of supravestibular peptic damage.

The endoscopic lesions of reflux esophagitis are perfectly well defined. Edema, redness and/or mucosal friability of the lower esophagus are *in no way* suggestive of reflux esophagitis.

The fundamental lesion corresponds to an epithelial erosion, the lesional topography of which is also well-defined. The lesions are distributed in asymmetric and non uniform manner over the lower esophagus, the lesional geography being influenced by the mucosal folds; hence the linear and longitudinal nature of the lesions, their parallelism and eventually their star-shape in the advanced stages [3].

Many authors still maintain the idea of diffuse supravestibular histologic lesions, preceding the endoscopic appearance of erosive lesions of reflux esophagitis. No consensus has ever been arrived at on the subject of the histologic criteria of these initial peptic changes [1, 2, 5].

Some authors consider that granulocytic infiltration of the lamina propria represents the first sign of reflux esophagitis [5], others give this as elongation of the connective tissue papillae and hyperplasia of the basal layers of the malpighian epithelium [4]; others still speak of a combination of the different signs listed above [5].

This situation, born of errors in clinical observation and of methodology in the removal of histocytologic specimens, has engendered such confusion that no pathologist at the present time knows what histologic criteria to employ to characterize supravestibular peptic disorder when examining a biopsy. The answer to this question can never be given by the pathologist himself, who is subject to the clinical information and the quality and situation of the supravestibular biopsies provided by the endoscopist.

In order to define the histology of the first stages reflux esophagitis, we examined 56 cases of esophagitis grade 1, 39 by fiberoscopy and 17 by rigid esophagoscopy. 2 or 3 biopsies were made routinely [3]: the first on the supravestibular red patch; the second at the same level, but on an endoscopically normal zone of mucosa; possibly a third, 5 cm above the Z-line, likewise on an apparently normal mucosal area.

The asymmetric nature of the topography of the peptic lesions in the lower esophagus evident macroscopically was confirmed by photography with the operating microscope of the biopsy specimens performed simultaneously at the same level. The histology also confirmed the asymmetry of the lesional geography, since the first specimen removed from the red patch generally corresponded to an epithelial erosion associated with inflammatory infiltration of the lamina propria, whereas the reference biopsy at the same level revealed a strictly normal mucosa without traces of inflammation.

If no typical endoscopic lesion exists, there can be no question of making a diagnosis of reflux esophagitis from supravestibular biopsies taken at random, the more so since current histologic criteria are doubtful and disputed. Too many patients are currently being "benefited" by anti-H_2 treatment based on a simple supravestibular biopsy "compatible with signs of reflux esophagitis" but whose histologic criteria are far from clear.

In all the cases in our series, where the samples were taken in hyper-selective fashion from the supravestibular erosion and from the macroscopically normal adjacent mucosa (rigid esophagoscope), the histology has always revealed an epithelial erosion associated with inflammatory reaction in the lamina propria in the erythematous zone and a strictly normal mucosa (epithelium + chorion) in the reference biopsy performed at the same level.

With the fiberscope, correlation between the endoscopic and histologic diagnoses was poor in 2/3 of the cases. 9 times out of 39, an erythematous patch judged erosive by the endoscopist proved to be a cylindercell epithelium. 17 times out of 39, biopsy performed deliberately on an erosion proved absolutely normal. These findings simply stress the *extreme difficulty* of *hyper-selective* supravestibular biopsy with the fiber gastroscope, as well as the inability of the endoscopist to distinguish clearly between a tongue of cylinder-cell metaplasia and an erosion not clothed with fibrin.

The histologic picture of initial supravestibular peptic changes corresponds to an epithelial erosion associated with inflammatory infiltration of the chorion.

There does not exist any diffuse microscopic lesional state of the supravestibular mucosa preceding the appearance of the endoscopically recognizable lesion [3].

References

1. Ismail-Beigi F, Pope CE (1970) Histological consequences of gastro-oesophageal reflux in man. Gastroenterology 58: 163
2. Kobayashi S, Kasugai T (1974) Endoscopic and biopsy criteria for the diagnosis of oesophagitis with the fiberoptic oesophagoscope. J Digest Dis 19: 345
3. Monnier Ph, Savary M (1984) Contribution of Endoscopy to Gastro-Oesophageal reflux Disease. Scand J, Gastroenterol 19, 106: 26–44
4. Savary M, Miller G (1977) L'oesophage. Manuel et Atlas d'Endoscopie. ed Gassmann AG Solothurn Suisse
5. Seefeld U, Krejs GJ, Siebenmann RE et al. (1977) Esophageal histology in gastro-esophageal reflux. Am J Digest Dis 22: 956

A methodology and a precise histological technique actually often enable a good concordance between clinical symptoms, endoscopy and histological alterations

W. V. Bogomoletz (Reims)

Unfortunately, satisfactory correlations between clinical findings, endoscopy and histologic changes are not always obtained, even if an adequate biopsy technique is used. Several factors may be responsible.

Firstly, clinico-pathologic correlations differ depending on the use of forceps or suction biopsies. Knuff et al. [1] have recently shown that in routine forceps biopsies of patients with a long history of esophageal reflux, 59% of these biopsies were uninterpretable. Moreover, the subjective assessment of some of the accepted histologic criteria of reflux esophagitis – elongation of the papillae and increased height of the basal layer – are fraught with difficulty. Even the presence of intraepithelial eosinophils as a diagnostic feature of reflux esophagitis is still a controversial issue [2].

The answer may lie in setting up multifactorial and double-blind studies of different types of biopsies, associated with esophageal function studies (manometry, acid reflux test and pH monitoring).

References

1. Knuff TE, Benjamin SB (1984) Histologic evaluation of chronic gastro-esophageal reflux. An evaluation of biopsy methods and diagnostic criteria. Digestive Diseases and Sciences 29, 3: 194–201
2. Barwick KW, Santag SJ (1987) The significance of intra-epithelial eosinophils in the histologic diagnosis of gastro-esophageal reflux. Am J of Clinical Pathology 87, 1: 43–49

Transit with Technetium-99 enables to detect motility disorders unnoticed by usual means

G. G. Jamieson (Adelaide)

Much of the work with esophageal transit has been undertaken using radionuclide labelled liquids with the patient swallowing the liquid while lying in the supine position. We have used a different technique, which involves the emptying of a radionuclide labelled solid bolus from the esophagus with the patient in the sitting position. The patient chews and swallows a 10 gm disc of Technetium-99^m labelled hamburger. This is swallowed when the patient is ready and then swallowing takes place every 15 seconds on command, until 95% of the radio – activity has been cleared from the esophagus into the stomach. If this is not achieved in 30 swallows the test is stopped at that point.

In 73 patients with objectively documented gastro-esophageal reflux disease (GERD) the median number of swallows to clear the esophagus was five (range 1–30+), compared to a median of two swallows for 33 control subjects (range 1–13 swallows) [1]. Routine esophageal manometry was normal in each of these patients and no stricture was demonstrable either on barium meal and/or endoscopy.

In the total group of patients there were 38 who had experienced no dysphagia, and esophageal emptying in all of these patients fell within the normal range. In 33 patients who had experienced dysphagia, 14 patients had abnormally prolonged esophageal emptying ($p < 0.001$).

We have used this test also to examine the effect of fundoplication on esophageal emptying in 36 patients. Fundoplication alleviated the symptoms of dysphagia, if present pre-operatively in all patients, and yet there was no significant difference between esophageal emptying pre-operatively and at six months post-operatively. Furthermore we have followed a further 17 of these patients, and repeated the test 3 years after fundoplication and again we were unable to demonstrate any significant difference between the pre-operative and the 3 years post-operative values.

We have studied a separate group of 32 patients who presented with recurrent reflux disease, after previous anti-reflux surgery. When this patient group is compared with the 36 patients tested at six months after successful antireflux surgery or the 17 patients tested at three years after successful antireflux surgery, then esophageal emptying is found to be significantly slower in the failed group.

These studies suggest that poor esophageal emptying may be a primary factor in the development of reflux disease.

Reference

1. Maddern GJ, Jamieson GG (1986) Oesophageal emptying in patients with gastro-oesophageal reflux. Br J Surg 73: 615-617

B. Dupin, J. Pasquier, F. Fincker, P. Fuentes, R. Giudicelli, R. Sauvan, and *E. Reboud* (Marseilles)

During the last three years, we have performed in each patient considered for an anti-reflux procedure a triple functional esophageal examination: manometry, prolonged pH monitoring and scintigraphic study to compare the findings of these tests and to assess the usefulness of each examination.

We performed a comparative study, manometry versus scintigraphic transit, in 61 patients with gastroesophageal reflux considered for anti-reflux procedure.

Methods

All patients were submitted to

1. Manometric examination (ME): we used a low compliance pump from MUI with a four lumen tube (perfusion rate 0.6 ml/mn). Study was focused on peristaltic waves and specially low amplitude waves and simultaneous waves.
2. Scintigraphic transit study (TS): it is the first phase of esophageal scintigraphy. We used the method from Tolin [1] modified by Russell [2, 3]. TS is performed in the supine position for 10 minutes after a single swallow of one millicurie Technetium (Tc) 99 sulfur colloid in 3 ml of water, followed by dry swallows. Esophagus is divided into 3 equal areas of interest. According to Russell, normal TS is less than 15 seconds.

Results

The following table shows the comparative results between ME and TS findings.

	ME pathologic	ME normal	Total
TS > 15s	23	10	33
TS ≤ 15s	5	20	25
Total	28	30	58

In 25 cases, TS findings were normal whereas ME showed dysmotility in 5 patients. In 33 patients, TS findings showed delayed transit time whereas ME was normal in 10 patients in the same group.

Comments

In this group of patients, the frequency of delayed TS is high: 57% (33/58) perhaps because these patients were candidates for an anti-reflux procedure and had a severe GER. On the other hand, ME showed dysmotility only in 48% of cases (28/58). Since the false negatives with TS 5/28 (18%) are less than the false negatives with ME 10/33 (30%), TS seems more sensitive than ME in detecting esophageal motility disturbances.

Conclusion

Our study [4] assesses that TS is superior than ME in the study of esophageal clearance in patients with GER. Indeed, TS allows a quantitative study of esophageal transit whereas ME is a qualitative study which simply indicates the existence of motility disorders but not the presence of clearance defect.

Lastly, scintigraphic study, non-invasive test, although less sensitive than prolonged pH monitoring for the diagnosis of GER, has the advantage of allowing in the same examination, gastroesophageal reflux research and clearance study.

References

1. Tolin RD and Coll (1979) Esophageal scintigraphy to quantitate esophageal transit. Gastroenterology, 76: 1402-1408
2. Russell COH and Coll (1981) Radionuclide transit: a sensitive screening test for esophageal dysfunction. Gastroenterology, 80: 887-892
3. Fischer RS, Malmud LS (1986) Scintigraphic techniques for the study of gastrointestinal motor function. Adv Intern Med, 31: 395–418
4. Dupin B, Pasquier J, Fuentes P, Giudicelli R, Sauvan R, Reboud E (1986) Scintigraphy versus manometry and prolonged pH monitoring for assessment of esophageal function. International Esophageal Week, Munich, September 14–19

J. Guillet, C. Role, C. Billeaud, Y. Imbert, P. Ducos, E. Dupont, M. Joussein, M. Franck, and *A. Richard* (Agen)

Although the transit of a radiotracer through the esophagus after deglutition was first described in 1972 this technique has not been generally applied on a large scale to pediatrics, nor has it been developed as a routine or outpatient procedure. By means of cine-esogastro scintigraphy (CEGS) the passage of radiolabelled milk or water through esophagus and also stomach and small intestine has been studied and gastroesophageal reflux detected. Its use has also been extended to detect aspiration of swallowed liquids. Further, this powerful method allows quantitation and there are no age limits on its use. Dosimetry results are also very favourable.

Our experience after 3354 CEGS studies routinely performed for 3000 patients is described in this report.

Material and Method

The indications for this study in terms of age are given in Table 1. A contrast medium radiological study was also performed for 39% of the children.

CEGS was performed on fasting patients using a gamma camera coupled to a computer.

Table 1. Indications for, and results of CEGS in terms of patient age and degree of observed GER (++ severe, + minor, 0 absent or physiological) for 2500 pediatric patients

Age range	0–1 month			1–4 months			4–12 months			1–4 years			4–8 years			8–16 years			0–16 years		
Degree of reflux	0	+	++	0	+	++	0	+	++	0	+	++	0	+	++	0	+	++	0	+	++
Chronic or repetitive respiratory problems	1		10	5	4	41	69	5	51	139	50	191	148	95	257	133	30	185	495	184	735
Episodes of apnea or cyanosis, false passage or risk of SIDS	90	10	190	99	109	161	90	15	45	10		16		1	4				189	135	416
Vomiting, epigastric pain, haematemesis	20	4	36	16	6	21	25	1	12	5	6	22			18		1	6	66	18	115
Repeat CEGS after medical treatment for observed GER	8			29		9	99	5	10	50		2	7		1	31	2	1	224	7	23
Surgical problems pyloric stenosis esophageal atresia achalasia of the cardia severe GER after surgery			6	4	1			1	4	6		19		1	3		3	7	10	6	39
other indications				1	1				1	1									2	1	2
Totals	119	14	242	154	121	232	283	27	123	211	56	250	155	97	283	164	36	200	1086	351	1330
Grand totals 2767 studies in 2500 patients		375			507			433			517			535			400			2767	

Data acquisition

- Esophageal transit. This was observed with images on films and in the computer memory (each 500 ms). A neonate or bottle fed infant drank a few ml of formula marked with $99^{m}Tc$ sulphocolloid, using 2 µCi (74 kBq) for each ml of the usual feed volume, up to a maximum of 300µCi (11.1 MBq). The patient was held in this mother's arms next to the camera, with a lateral view. The remainder of his feed containing no radiotracer was then consumed, until the baby was replete.

Older children under 5 years of age were erect and drank a few ml of radiolabelled water against the camera, submitting a lateral view. The total activity was 300µCi (11.1 MBq) plus 20 µCi (0.74 MBq) for each year of age, but if there was growth retardation, the swallowed dose was 440 µCi (16.3 MBq) per m^2 of body surface area. Older children and adults drank supine, beneath the camera. Activity was up to 700 µCi (25 MBq).

- Detection of Gastro Esophageal Reflux (GER). The patients were supine beneath the camera. Images were recorded by computer, every 12.5 s. No unphysiologic maneuver, in an attempt to increase sensitivity, was employed during the 30 min of this part of the study. If a GER was observed with a duration greater than 10 min, the rest of the examination was performed in the seated or erect position. All events, such as coughs, dyspneic or cyanotic episodes and sudden pallor, which occured during GER were noted.
- Search for Pulmonary Contamination. Immediately after the previous part an anterior thoracic view was recorded by computer.

Two hours after ingestion of the tracer, a similar image was recorded. A careful search for pulmonary contamination by the radionuclide was made, and in the case of the slightest doubt, views from different directions, with and without markers were obtained.

- Measurement of gastric emptying. An anterior view showing activity in the gastro intestinal tract was recorded by computer 30 and 120 min after ingestion of the tracer.

Data reduction

- Esophageal transit. Two areas of interest were selected in the cervical an distal esophagus. Each area provided a time-activity curve with a prominent peak and the esophageal transit time was taken as the interval between the peaks.

The curves also allowed examination of the distal esophageal emptying. When the radiotracer remained in contact with the esophageal wall; as was seen in some forms of esophagitis, another area of interest was selected which included this zone to measure the results of a "rinsing" by the unmarked liquid.

- Search for GER. Three regions of interest were selected to include the complete esophagus, small gut and stomach. Each region provided a time-activity curve. In this way, for each episode of GER the time after ingestion, duration of the reflux, and the level to which the reflux mounted were obtained.

Also, the integrated esophageal contamination could be obtained. The quantity of activity refluxing during the most significant episode was derived as a percentage of the gastric activity and the esophageal back-ground activity present before the reflux.

Episodes of GER were classified into three main groups, depending on the highest level reached by the refluxing liquid.

We consider that any regurgitation confined to the distal 2 or 3 cm of the oesophagus and difficult to differentiate from gastric activity is physiological. A minor reflux will mount higher and if it reaches the cervical esophagus or buccal cavity it is classified as a major reflux.

- Gastric emptying: gastric emptying is given in terms of percentages of the total activity in stomach and gut, noted 30 and 120 min after ingestion of the radiotracer.

Results

The results of searches for GER are given in Table 1 in terms of age and indications for the study. About half of the CEGS were requested for repeated pulmonary problems, and a third because of the danger of the sudden death infant syndrome. Neonates or young infants were the subject of 58% of our studies. Major (51%) or minor (14%) GER were observed in 65% of the first studies performed on our patients (Table 2) while only 20% of follow up examinations during medical treatment of a previously observed GER again demonstrated reflux.

For those patients who were examined by both radiologic and isotopic means, 81% were shown to have GER. Of them, 98% were demonstrated by CEGS, and 48% by radiology, but 2% were detected by radiology alone.

A reflux was detected by both techniques in 46% of the studies, yet the maximum height of the regurgitated liquid and the duration of the reflux were greater when observed by CEGS in 57% of these cases.

An analysis of the time of occurrence of reflux demonstrated by CEGS shows that in 90% of the cases, the first GER occurred in the first 15 min after ingestion. Both the total time during which there is esophageal activity and the esophageal transit time increase as the maximum height of regurgitant liquid increases. When reflux reaches the cervical esophagus the mean duration of GER increases with patient's age (Table 3, 4).

Gastric emptying is faster in the older child than in the neonate or young infant for whom milk is used. It is faster too, in adults, when water is used instead of milk.

As the refluxing level increases and the last observed GER is delayed, gastric emptying is slowed (Table 5, 6).

Activity is rarely detected in the trachea and distal respiratory system. Three false passages were detected by radiological examinations during deglution and also seen with CEGS. Pulmonary contamination was observed immediately following reflux in five cases and was noted only on the images recorded 120 min after ingestion for 52 patients, of whom only 45 demonstrated a GER. The remaining 7 were seen to have only delayed gastric emptying. There were no correlations between these observations and abnormalities on chest radiograph. For five patients, inhalation of the tracer initiated an episode of coughing.

Dyspnoea, coughing or respiratory difficulties were noted in coincidence with 7% of the GER occurring in patients aged under 2 years who suffered from chronic or repeated respiratory problems, and in 2% in older patients.

Table 2. The distribution of episodes of GER in the first 30 min of the study which detected 2077 refluxes in the 576 patients who were first examined before treatment. The duration of the longest GER and the maximum period observed without GER is also included

Age range (years)	0		(261 patients)				1 year	1		315 patients				16 years
Number of episodes of GER	857							1220						
Time range (min)	0–2	3–5	6–9	10–14	15–19	20–24	25–30	0–2	3–5	6–9	10–14	15–19	20–24	25–30
Number of GER	13	16	18	17	13	12	11	16	16	14	17	14	11	12
First GER %	46	28	11	8	2	2	3	44	23	13	10	4	3	3
Last GER %	7	3	11	13	12	12	43	5	7	4	14	17	13	40
Duration of the Longest GER	75	14	3	2	1	3	2	73	13	3	3	2	4	2
Maximum interval between sequential GER %	26	24	22	9	13	3	3	24	25	23	10	12	3	3

Table 2. (continued) adults. (mean age: 68 years SD: 9)

Age range (years)	17 years			208 patients			86 years
Number of episodes of GER				238			
Time range (min)	0 2	3 5	6 9	10 14	15 19	20 24	25 30
Number of GER %	13	17	18	15	14	14	9
First GER %	49	23	12	8	3	3	2
Last GER %	0	1	6	17	20	22	34
Duration of the Longest GER	36	17	11	11	9	8	7
Maximum interval between GER	39	25	22	10	1	1	1

Table 3. The mean duration of the reflux ($\bar{t}$ in seconds) in terms of the patient's ages and the greatest height reached by the radiotracer (n: Number of patients SD standard deviation of $\bar{t}$)

Age range (years)	0	–	1	I	–	3	4	–	7	8	–
Maximum level attained by GER	n	$\bar{t}$	SD	n	$\bar{t}$	SD	n	$\bar{t}$	SD	n	$\bar{t}$
Buccal	44	260	479	11	421	475	20	453	624	4	1575
Cervical	35	268	467	13	162	259	32	173	348	16	270
Thoracic	41	41	82	9	30	18	11	30	19	5	620

Table 4. Mean esophageal transmit time ($\bar{t}$ in seconds) in terms of range and maximum level reached by regurgitant liquid. Significance levels from students test (denoted by ... p, 0.001 .. p, 0.005 and . p, 0.05) after comparison with cases where no reflux is present are indicated

Age range (years)	0		1	1		3	4		7	8		16
Maximum level attained by GER	n	$\bar{t}$	SD	n	$\bar{t}$	SD	n	$\bar{t}$	SD	n	$\bar{t}$	51
Buccal, cervical	41	5.2...	1.8	20	4.6.	1	9	6.1.	2.2	8	7.2...	4.2
Thoracic	20	4	1.7	19	4.2	1.3	11	5.3	1.3	4	4.9	1.5
No GER	37	3.8	1.3	24	3.8	1.4	21	4.8	1.1	13	4.6	1.9

Table 5. Gastric emptying; greatest height of reflux and patients' ages. SD, n and significance are as defined above

Maximal level of GER			Buccal		Cervical		Thoracic		No	GOR
	age range (years)	time after ingestion								
Gastric Contents As % of	0–1	30 min	31	77±11	33	76±10	16	73±12	58	73±10
		120 min	27	44±18	33	46±17	14	35±15	59	35±14
Ingested Activity SD	1–16	30 min	12	72±13	26	71±13	17	64±13	36	57±13
		120 min	12	37±19	26	28±19	17	27±24	36	12±11

Table 6. Gastric emptying as a function of time of onset of the last observed GER and age range. Ingestion of radiotracer is at time zero and n, SD and significance are as above

Time of onset (min) or last GER			0		9 10		19 20		30 No	GER
	age range (years)	time after ingestion	n		n		n		n	
Gastric Contents As % of	0–1	30 min	32	75±11	26	75±13	28	78±11	41	71±10
		120 min	30	40±18	25	44±20	27	47±18	35	35±13
Ingested Activitiy ±SD	1–16	30 min	20	67±14	13	74± 9	26	68±14	36	57±13
		120 min	20	22±21	17	32±20	27	36±23	36	12±11

Among the surgical indications for this examinations, there were 4 post operative cases of esophageal atresia, in which both a short esophageal transit time and severe GER were noted. The gastric emptying was also delayed in 3 of the 4.

In the 2 patients with achalasia of the cardia, there was a clearly observed hold up of the tracer proximal to the stenosis. The esophageal transit was slowed in the cases of scleroderma and in esophageal dysfunction. This was especially evident in the distal part. Also, a severe GER and slowed gastric evacuation were noted.

Discussion

The low irradiation resulting from CEGS (200 to 300 mrads or 2 to 3 mGy) in the proximal small gut which is the target organ, and its hight sensitivity in detecting GER justifies its use in the youngest pediatric patients.

There are clear advantages in comparison to radiologic investigations notably the sensitivity in detection and evaluation of the severity of a GER, which are fourfold better for CEGS. However, radiologic examinations are often requested by our pediatric colleagues, if the GER is shown by CEGS to be resistant to medical treatment in order to investigate the possibility of anatomical anomalies such as pyloric stenosis, hiatal hernia, or atonia of the cardia.

Studies using pH measurements in the esophageal lumen have comparable sensitivity to those using radioisotopes, for detection of GER. In fact pHmetry is considered a reference standard. However there are fundamental differences between the two methods.

Use of radioisotopes allows detection of reflux of swallowed liquids or solids, whereas pHmetry detects regurgitation of digestive secretions, mainly acids; Reflux of an alkaline compound could remain undetected if accompanied by some gastric acid. Also pHmetry requires an intraluminal electrode which, especially in the youngest patients, can modify the foregut function significantly.

Other useful information is available from CEGS. When refluxes are associated with pathological gastric emptying their severity tends to increase with slower evacuation of gastric contents.

A few patients demonstrated repeated GER with normal or even accelerated gastric emptying. The problem of dyspepsia coupled to GER is raised.

Valuable additional information is available from a study of esophageal transit in the presence of esophagitis, achalasia of the cardia or scleroderma. The transit is slower and rinsing with unmarked liquid is less effective.

If the study is performed in the supine position both the sensitivity and detail demonstrated are increased, but this is often impractical for a young child.

A GER was associated with respiratory signs and symptoms or aspiration of the tracer in 7 and 3% respectively of those patients referred for investigation because of respiratory problems. Pulmonary contamination by the radionuclide was detected in 4% of those in danger of the sudden death infant syndrome (SIDS). Thus CEGS provided direct proof of an association between reflux and SIDS. The two hour interval between ingestion and the last attempt to detect pulmonary activity is somewhat short, especially for those children whose stomachs have not been emptied in this time. It is preferable to obtain thoracic images 3 or 4 hours after tracer deglutition. If a longer time elapses, respiratory tract activity may be removed by the mucociliary mechanism.

The CEGS is a simple examination and can be performed wherever a gamma camera and computer are available. The child's parents should be encouraged to attend to promote understanding, although patient cooperation has never been a problem. We believe CEGS should be the investigation of choice whenever there is any suspicion of foregut transit problems. This remains true even when the signs and symptoms arise from another system, as with repeated or chronic respiratory infections. Further applications to the monitoring of relevant medical and surgical treatment and providing information, possibly of overwhelming importance, for babies at risk of SIDS underline its wide applicability.

Conclusion

When morphological information is required, radiologic investigations cannot be replaced by CEGS. But the patient's absorbed radiation if far less with the latter, so allowing a much longer examination. The technique is non invasive, a particular advantage in comparison with pHmetry which however has a comparable sensitivity.

The reliability, sensitivity adaptability to routine outpatient use, low levels of patient irradiation and wealth of resulting information are characteristics of CEGS that give it a uniquely valuable place in pediatric and adult patients.

References

1. Guillet J, Lambert B, Wynchank S (1984) Gastro intestinal tract function in paediatrics using cine-esophagogastroscintigraphy. 1st Amersham Büchler award. Soc Nucl Med Europe in: Nuklearmedizin – pp LXXXI-XCIII-Schmidt – Adam ed Stuttgart – N York
2. Guillet J (1985) Exploration isotopique de la motricité digestive Ciné œsogastroscintigraphie. Les cahiers pratiques de Médecine Nucléaire. Mallinckrodt. Le Mée/Seine

Radioisotopes techniques do not seem to be able to replace pH measurement

G. Beauchamp, and *R. Taillefer* (Montreal)

As interest in esophageal investigation increases, the investigator must select the appropriate test to elucidate the problem he is dealing with.

Radionuclide esophageal transit studies are now used to evaluate the esophageal motility and gastroesophageal reflux [1, 2]. Radionuclide was previously identified as a test that could be suitable to screen esophageal motor disorders [3]. It is a non invasive test with a small degree of body radiation and causes minimal discomfort. It was also felt to be as sensitive as manometry in the detection of motility disorders [4]. In a more recent experience, radionuclide transit identified abnormalities not detected by manometry, and manometry was abnormal in a group of normal radionuclide studies. The authors concluded that the radionuclide transit measurement provides additional information to complement esophageal manometry [5].

In studying esophageal phenomena, isotope techniques can use non acid liquids as well as semisolid and solid food material at varying pH. When scintigraphy is performed with acidified liquid this can increase significantly the recognition of gastroesophageal refluxers, especially in grade 1 esophagitis [6]. In animals, we have previously shown the use of scintigraphy in the recognition of morphologic changes of the mucosa [7].

Depending on what the investigator is looking at, the radioisotope can be superior to 24-hour pH monitoring. This has been shown in the evaluation of postprandial gastroesophageal reflux event, frequency and clearance. Scintigraphy has discerned the postprandial reflux events better [8]. Compared to other techniques, such as acid clearance tests, the radioisotope swallow study also appears to be superior [9].

Radionuclide studies appear to be superior to barium studies in the evaluation of gastroesophagal reflux, and equal to pH studies [10, 11].

Other radionuclide studies are used to evaluate esophageal problems. They are the radionuclide gastroesophageal reflux study and the use of 99m Tc-pertechnitate to detect the Barrett's esophagus. Radionuclide gastric emptying studies are also pertinent to the evaluation of gastroesophageal reflux and cannot be replaced by 24-hour pH monitoring [12].

The 24-hour pH studies require much less equipment than the radionuclide studies. But if they are done in the hospital setting, they are more costly. In the ambulatory setting, it can be cheaper than the laboratory setting of the radionuclide studies. 24-hour pH monitoring appears to be more physiologic and may correlate better with markers of gastroesophageal reflux disease such as esophagitis, stricture and pulmonary aspiration [13].

24-hour pH monitoring objectively determines the presence of gastroesophageal reflux. The test is effective in evaluating a variety of clinical problems related to gastroesophageal reflux such as atypical gastroesophageal reflux symptoms, respiratory problems, chest pain and other gastrointestinal symptoms suggestive of gastroesophageal reflux. The test is also useful in patients with gastroesophageal symptoms and normal endoscopy, indicating the superior sensitivity in detecting reflux [14]. In addition, the 24-hour pH allows the surgeon to identify which type of refluxer he is dealing with. The supine and combine refluxer will do well with surgery, while the upright refluxer should probably not have an antireflux procedure.

Since its description, the test has attracted much enthusiasm because of its high sensitivity and specificity. However, a more critical look at the test has shown some limitations. In a study, 24-hour pH monitoring was normal in half of the individuals presenting with reflux symptoms and in 29% of the patients with erosive esophagitis. The insensitivity of the test may be related to the manner in which the study is performed in hospital [15]. To obviate the problem of lengthy studies and insensitivity in the hospital setting, some workers have made a reassessment to shorten it, and simplified the scoring system [16].

24-hour pH monitoring will have certainly a continuing role in the research of gastroesophageal reflux. However, 12-hour pH monitoring is a highly accurate test that can be adapted to the patient's work schedule. Simplification by evaluating the postprandial period may be more practical and less expensive than prolonged 24-hour pH monitoring [17].

From 1981 to 1985, we have used the radionuclide esophageal transit study in the preoperative evaluation of our patients. The information obtained allows us to measure the transport of liquids and solids more exactly.

24-hour pH monitoring has been done in 209 patients during the period of 1981 to 1985. The test has allowed us to improve our decision in selecting surgical therapy for some 80 patients. It has also helped in deciding which antireflux procedure to perform.

The radionuclide studies and the 24-hour pH monitoring have distinct advantages. They are not comparable in term of sensitivity and specificity, because one measures the motility of the body of the esophagus and the other the effect of the stomach content on the esophagus.

References

1. Tolin RD, Malmud LS, Reilley J, Fisher RS (1979) Esophageal scintigraphy to quantitate esophageal transit (quantitation of esophageal transit). Gastroenterology 76: 1402–1408.
2. Taillefer R, Beauchamp G (1984) Radionuclide esophagogram. Clin Nucl Med 9: 465–483
3. Russell COH, Hill LD, Holmes ER, Hull DA, Cannon R, Pope CE (1981) Radionuclide transit: A sensitive screening test for esophageal dysfunction. Gastroenterology 80: 887–892
4. Blackwell JN, Hannan WJ, Adam RD, Heading RC (1983) Radionuclide transit studies in the detection of esophageal dysmotility. Gut 24: 421–426
5. De Caestecker JS, Blackwell JN, Adam RD, Hannan WJ, Brown J, Cheading R (1986) Clinical value of radionuclide oesophageal transit measurement. Gut 27: 659–666
6. Kaul B, Petersen H, Grette K, Erichsen H, Myrvold HE (1985) Scintigraphy, pH measurement, and radiography in the evaluation of gastroesophageal reflux. Scand J Gastroenterol 20: 289–294
7. Beauchamp G, Taillefer R, Devito M, Levasseur A, Lamoureux C (1985) Radionuclide esophagogram in the evaluation of experimental esophagitis: Manometric and histopathologic correlations. In Esophageal disorders: Pathophysiology and therapy. Edited by DeMeester TR and Skinner DB, Raven Press, New York. 77–81
8. Shay S, Eggli D, Maydonovitch C, Johnson L (1986) Postprandial gastroesophageal reflux event frequency and clearance: A simultaneous comparison of scintigraphy vs pH monitoring. Gastroenterology 90(5): 1630
9. Ferguson MK, Ryan JW, Little AG, Skinner DB (1985) Esophageal emptying and acid neutralization in patients with symptoms of esophageal reflux. Ann Surg 201: 728–735
10. Velasco N, Pope CE II, Cannan RM, Roberts P, Hill LD (1984) Measurement of esophageal reflux by scintigraphy. Dig Dis Sci 29: 977–982
11. Seibert JJ, Byrne WJ, Euler AR, Latture T, Leach M, Campbell M (1983) Gastroesophageal reflux – the acid test: Scintigraphy or the pH probe? Am J Radiol 140: 1087–1090
12. McCallum RW, Berkowitz DM, Lerner E (1981) Gastric emptying in patients with gastroesophageal reflux. Gastroenterology 80: 285–291
13. Johnson LP, DeMeester TR (1974) Twenty-four-hour pH monitoring of the distal esophagus. A quantitative measure of gastroesophageal reflux. Am J Gastroenterol 62: 325–332

14. DeMeester TR, Wermly JA, Little AG, Bermudez G, Skinner DB (1980) Technique, indications, and clinical use of 24-hour esophageal pH monitoring. J Thorac Cardiovasc Surg. 79:656–670
15. Schlesinger PK, Donahue PE, Schmid B, Layden TJ (1985) Limitations of 24-hour intraesophageal pH monitoring in the hospital setting. Gastroenterology 89:797–804
16. Choinière L, Miller L, Ilves R, Cooper JD (1983) A simplified method of esophageal pH monitoring for assessment of gastroesophageal reflux. Ann Thorac Surg 36:596–603
17. Fink SM, McCallum RW (1984) The role of prolonged esophageal pH monitoring in the diagnosis of gastroesophageal reflux. JAMA 252:1160–1164

M. K. Ferguson, A. G. Little, and *D. B. Skinner* (Chicago)

Introduction

The criteria for diagnosing pathologic gastroesophageal reflux (GER) are somewhat controversial, as evidenced by the variety of techniques currently employed to demonstrate its existence. Over 25% of patients with typical symptoms of reflux have no evidence of GER on any objective investigation. Quantitative and semiquantitative tests exist purported to improve diagnostic accuracy, including fluoroscopic examination for reflux, the acid perfusion (Bernstein) test, the standard acid reflux test (SART), the Tuttle test, the water siphon test, and the phenol red reflux test.

The two most widely accepted means of diagnosing pathologic gastroesophageal reflux are esophagoscopy and extended esophageal pH monitoring. While each is regarded by some as the gold standard for the diagnosis of reflux, they both have certain drawbacks which prevent their unqualified acceptance. Esophagoscopy, when used as the sole means of identifying pathologic GER, must rely on either visual or histologic identification of esophagitis. Esophagitis is not always specific for GER, and may be a response to alcohol ingestion, certain medications, monilial or herpetic infections, and caustic agents. There is considerable interobserver variation in the visual assessment of the esophageal mucosa, and esophagitis is not always histologically documented even when it is distinctly evident visually. In addition, certain round cells mistakenly interpreted as representing inflammatory cells are normally present on histologic sections of the normal esophagus. These sometimes lead to the misdiagnosis of esophagitis. Finally, pathologic GER need not necessarily be accompanied by esophagitis, particularly in those patients who have normal distal esophageal clearance [4].

Extended esophageal pH monitoring, while minimally invasive, has other drawbacks. Probe placement may be difficult or inaccurate in patients with strictures or large sliding hiatal hernias. Since acid is used as the marker for reflux, the test may not detect abnormal reflux in patients who are achlorhydric, hypochlorhydric, or who have alkaline reflux. It can be time consuming to perform, usually requiring 8 to 24 hour test periods. While esophageal pH monitoring is usually accurate in the diagnosis of GER, it is only marginally quantitative. Only a mild correlation between severity of reflux score and degree of esophagitis has ever been demonstrated [5].

Because of these shortcomings, other techniques have been sought to assess esophageal function and quantitate gastroesophageal reflux, including esophageal scintigraphy and gastroesophageal scintigraphy.

Esophageal scintigraphy was originally introduced by Kazem in 1972 for the evaluation of motility by quantitating esophageal transit [14]. Subsequent studies confirmed its usefulness in the evaluation of primary esophageal motility disorders [19]. Others found that scintigraphic measurement of esophageal transit time disclosed motility disorders in patients with GER which were undetected by standard manometric techniques [17]. One study demonstrated a close correlation between abnormal esophageal emptying and GER [6]. Fisher first employed gastroesophageal scintigraphy to quantitate the reflux of tracer material from the stomach into the esophagus [7]. Other investigators subsequently adopted this technique to evaluate GER [15].

Esophageal scintigraphy

Technique

Fasted patients are imaged from the posterior view supine or upright with data acquired into a computer. Fifteen cc's of water containing 150 μCi of ^{99m}Tc-sulfur colloid are instilled into the patient's mouth, and a swallow is initiated on command, followed by dry swallows at 15 second intervals. Count rates over the entire esophagus and over the lower third of esophagus are generated each 0.15 second. The time for isotope clearance is calculated as:

$$IC_t = \frac{E_{max} - E_t}{E_{max}} \times 100$$

where IC_t represents per cent esophageal clearance of isotope at time "t", E_{max} represents maximum count rate in the esophagus, and E_t represents esophageal count rate at time "t". The transit time is the interval from initial bolus entry into the esophagus to the maximum isotope clearance from the esophagus in one swallow [6].

Techniques of esophageal scintigraphy vary among institutions. Some scans are performed from the anterior aspect, which results in diminished counts from the distal esophagus due to the intervening heart. Most authors rely on esophageal transit time as the measure of normality, although the use of esophageal emptying may have more relevance to the study of reflux pathology. Finally, the emptying of acidic material is not tested, although acidification of esophageal contents may prolong esophageal transit time.

Results

To rely on esophageal scintigraphy to diagnose GER, one must assume that most patients with GER have detectable abnormalities of esophageal transit and/or

Table 1. Esophageal scintigraphy for diagnosing gastroesophageal reflux in adults

Source	*Year*	*Patients*	*Accuracy (%)*	*Standard*
Russell [17]	1981	29	58.6	pH monitoring, Endoscopy
van Heukelem [20]	1985	23	17.4	pH monitoring
Ferguson [6]	1985	26	88.5	pH monitoring
	Total	78	56.4	

clearance, and that these abnormalities are constant, not episodic. This does not appear to be the case. A summary of results of esophageal scintigraphy in patients with GER is found in Table 1. All studies were well controlled with pH monitoring serving as the reference standard. A wide range of variability is seen in the accuracy of these tests. The greatest accuracy occurred in a study in which abnormalities of transit time and/or clearance were accepted as pathologic [6]. The other reports relied on increases in transit time alone to diagnose pathology [17, 20]. The overall results are quite poor, with a combined accuracy of only 56.4%.

Gastroesophageal scintigraphy

Technique

Patients are fasted overnight and positioned supine under the collimator of a gamma camera connected to a digital computer for acquisition. About 300 μCi of ^{99m}Tc sulfur colloid in 300 ml of acidified orange juice is ingested. Abdominal pressure is applied using an abdominal binder inflated at 20 mm Hg increments to 100 mm Hg. Thirty-second images are obtained at each pressure gradient. A reflux episode is identified when radioactivity is detected cephalad to the gastroesophageal junction [7]. Quantitation of reflux is also possible by measuring the activity in the esophagus and comparing it to residual activity in the stomach: $R = (E_t - E_B)/G_0 \times 100$, where R=% gastro-esophageal reflux, E_t=esophageal count at time t, E_B=esophageal background count and G_0=gastric count at the beginning of the study. Gastroesophageal reflux is identified when 4% or more of the tracer is refluxed [9].

To suggest that gastroesophageal scintigraphy is a standardized method of evaluating esophagogastric function would be a mistake. Virtually every institution employing this test has developed its own modifications for its performance and interpretation, making comparisons and a final assessment of its validity difficult. These include the amount of ^{99m}Tc used, the quantity of fluid in which it is diluted, the means of transporting that fluid into the stomach (swallowing or tube instillation), acidification of the fluid, the use of manual compression or a pneumatically inflated abdominal binder to increase abdominal pressure, and the position used for scanning (prone, supine or upright). As will be seen below, considerable discrepancy exists in the accuracy of this test for diagnosing GER.

Results

Summaries of results of gastroesophageal scintigraphic assessment of GER in adults and the pediatric population are found in Tables 2 and 3. Two points are immediately evident. First, endoscopy was used as at least one of the reference standards in six of the twelve studies cited. The use of endoscopic criteria to establish the diagnosis of reflux preselects a group with more severe reflux, falsely elevating the accuracy of any diagnostic test under investigation. Second, the use of the standard acid reflux test as a reference standard was common, particularly in the pediatric age group. This test has inadequate controls in the pediatric age population and is the least quantitative of the tests used.

The accuracy of gastroesophageal scintiscans in the diagnosis of reflux is 75% in the pediatric population and 73% in the adult population. The overall accuracy is 74% which is not sufficiently high for a diagnostic test, particularly when compared to the 96% accuracy of extended esophageal pH monitoring in adults [8].

Table 2. Gastroesophageal scintigraphy for diagnosing gastroesophageal acid reflux in adults

Source	*Year*	*Patients*	*Accuracy (%)*	*Standard*
Fisher [7]	1976	30	90	SART
Velasco [21]	1984	54	74	Endoscopy
Fung [9]	1985	48	14.6	Endoscopy
Kaul [13]	1985	69	85.5	Endoscopy, SART
Kaul [12]	1986	101	86.1	Symptoms, endoscopy
	Total	302	72.8*	

* Accuracy was 83.8% excluding data from Fung et al.

Table 3. Gastroesophageal scintigraphy for diagnosing gastroesophageal acid reflux in infants and children

Source	*Year*	*Patients*	*Accuracy (%)*	*Standard*
Devos [5]	1979	8	100	Endoscopy
Heyman [10]	1979	39	59	Contrast radiography
Rudd [16]	1979	25	80	SART
Arasu [1]	1980	30	57	SART, endoscopy
Blumhagen [2]	1980	65	75	SART
Jona [11]	1981	125	77	Symptoms
Seibert [18]	1983	47	87.2	pH monitoring
	Total	339	74.9	

Discussion

There are potential benefits of using scintigraphy rather than extended esophageal pH monitoring for the diagnosis of GER. Scintigraphy is noninvasive and may be performed using standard equipment. The lack of an indwelling esophageal catheter allows a more physiologic esophageal function. There are drawbacks, however, which may prevent scintigraphy from becoming a screening or diagnostic test for GER. While the amount of radioactivity used to perform the tests is scant, the need for a radioactive tracer is nonetheless potentially hazardous, particularly in the pediatric population. Because the tests are performed over a relatively short period of time, quantitation of multiple episodes of reflux or detection of episodic motility disturbances may not always be possible. Indeed, the most troublesome types of reflux occur during sleep [3], a period which is never assessed by usual scintigraphic techniques. Finally, the use of abdominal compression, common in most gastroesophageal scintigraphic tests for reflux, is not physiologic and may produce episodes of reflux where none normally exists.

Conclusion

In its present state of development, esophageal scintigraphy is not able to replace extended esophageal pH monitoring in the diagnosis of pathologic gastroesophageal acid reflux. Esophageal scintigraphy detects only abnormalities of clearance from the distal esophagus. These abnormalities do bear some relation to GER, but there is a wide range of variability in the results of this test. Its overall accuracy of 56% makes it a poor substitute for extended esophageal pH monitoring.

Gastroesophageal scintigraphy also has major drawbacks. It does not provide estimation of reflux occurring over extended periods of time and is not physiologic when used in conjunction with abdominal binders. In some institutions gastroesophageal scintigraphy is used to document only the presence of reflux episodes, rather than their frequency or severity. When quantitation is attempted, a volume of tracer refluxed is measured, which may or may not be related to actual acid exposure to the esophagus.

The combination of these factors has led to an inadequate accuracy of this technique in diagnosing pathologic reflux. Nevertheless, if gastro-esophageal scintigraphy can be sufficiently standardized and its results compared to extended esophageal pH monitoring, it may ultimately become a valuable screening test for GER, particularly in the pediatric population and in those patients where medical therapy is indicated.

References

1. Arasu TS, Wyllie R, Fitzgerald JF, Franken EA, Siddiqui AR, Lehman GA, Eigen H, Grosfeld JL (1980) Gastroesophageal reflux in infants and children comparative accuracy of diagnostic methods. J Pediatr 96: 798–803
2. Blumhagen JD, Rudd TG, Christie DL (1980) Gastroesophageal reflux in children: radionuclide gastroesophagography. AJR 135: 1001–1004

3. DeMeester TR, Johnson LF, Joseph GJ, Toscano MS, Hall AW, Skinner DB (1976) Patterns of gastroesophageal reflux in health and disease. Ann Surg 184: 459–470
4. DeMeester TR, Wang C-I, Wernly JA, Pellegrini CA, Little AG, Klementschitsch P, Bermudez G, Johnson LF, Skinner DB (1980) Technique, indications, and clinical use of 24 hour esophageal pH monitoring. J Thorac Cardiovasc Surg 79: 656–667
5. Devos PG, Forget P, De Roo M, Eggermont E (1979) Scintigraphic evaluation of gastroesophageal reflux (GER) in children. J Nucl Med 20: 636–637
6. Ferguson MK, Ryan JW, Little AG, Skinner DB (1985) Esophageal emptying and acid neutralization in patients with symptoms of esophageal reflux. Ann Surg 201: 728–735
7. Fisher RS, Malmud LS, Roberts GS, Lobis IF (1976) Gastroesophageal (GE) scintiscanning to detect and quantitate GE reflux. Gastroenterology 70: 301–307
8. Fuchs K, DeMeester TR, Albertucci M: Specificity and sensitivity of objective diagnosis of gastroesophageal reflux disease. Surgery, in press
9. Fung WP, Van der Schaaf A, Grieve JC (1985) Gastroesophageal scintigraphy and endoscopy in the diagnosis of esophageal reflux and esophagitis. Am J Gastroenterol 80: 245–247
10. Heyman S, Kirkpatrick JA, Winter HS, Treves S (1979) An improved radionuclide method for the diagnosis of gastroesophageal reflux and aspiration in children (milk scan). Radiology 131: 479–482
11. Jona JZ, Sty JR, Glicklich M (1981) Simplified radioisotope technique for assessing gastroesophageal reflux in children. J Ped Surg 16: 114–117
12. Kaul B, Halvorsen T, Petersen H, Grette K, Myrvold HE (1986) Gastroesophageal reflux disease. Scand J Gastroenterol 21: 134–138
13. Kaul B, Petersen H, Grette K, Erichsen H, Myrvold HE (1985) Scintigraphy, pH measurement, and radiography in the evaluation of gastroesophageal reflux. Scand J Gastroenterol 20: 289–294
14. Kazem I (1972) A new scintigraphic technique for the study of the esophagus. AJR 115: 681–688
15. Menin RA, Malmud LS, Petersen RP, Maier WP, Fisher RS (1980) Gastroesophageal scintigraphy to assess the severity of gastroesophageal reflux disease. Ann Surg 191: 66–71
16. Rudd TG, Christie DL (1979) Demonstration of gastroesophageal reflux in children by radionuclide gastroesophagography. Radiology 131: 483–486
17. Russell COH, Pope CE II, Gannan RM, Allen FD, Velasco N, Hill LD (1981) Does surgery correct esophageal motor dysfunction in gastroesophageal reflux? Ann Surg 194: 290–296
18. Seibert JJ, Byrne WJ, Euler AR, Latture T, Leach M, Campbell M (1983) Gastroesophageal reflux the acid test: AJR 140: 1087–1090
19. Tolin RD, Malmud LS, Reilley J, Fisher RS (1979) Esophageal scintigraphy to quantitate esophageal transit (quantitation of esophageal transit). Gastroenterol 76: 1402–1408
20. Van Heukelem HA, Blom H, Camps JAJ, Gooszen HG, Pauwels EKJ, Biemond I: Assessment of esophageal motility by radionuclide transit studies in patients with reflux esophagitis and a pathologic 24-hour pH study. In: Esophageal Disorders: Pathophysiology and Therapy, DeMeester TR, Skinner DB (eds), Raven Press, New York (1985) pp 83–86
21. Velasco N, Pope CE II, Gannan RM, Roberts P, Hill LD (1984) Measurement of esophageal reflux by scintigraphy. Dig Dis Sci 29: 977–982

The increase of intra-parietal esophageal collagen could provide elements in the evaluation of motor disorders associated with esophagitis

H. J. Mud (Rotterdam)

A factor of prime importance in the development of reflux-esophagitis is the prolonged presence of damaging gastric contents in the esophageal lumen. Gastro-esophageal reflux as such is a physiological event, the refluate is removed from the esophagus passively by gravity in the upright patient, and actively by secondary peristalsis or, most frequently, after swallowing. During sleep the only available clearing mode is secondary peristalsis.

In many patients with reflux-esophagitis the response to reflux of gastric contents is altered and acid clearance from the esophagus often delayed. Manometric studies of the body of the esophagus show abnormalities in a large proportion of patients with reflux-esophagitis.

Already many years ago Henderson [1] has shown that there is a distinct correllation between the degree of esophagitis and the degree of esophageal motor abnormalities in patients with severe ulcerative esophagitis or with a reflux-related esophageal stricture.

Also, there is evidence, that, in patients with altered esophageal motor function, such as progressive systemic sclerosis, there is an increased risk for the development of severe reflux esophagitis and the formation of reflux-related strictures.

What I would like to comment on is that it is just possible that the delayed clearance of gastric contents by the esophagitis could be caused by changes in the esophageal wall.

Esophageal wall changes are most evident in panmural esophagitis. We find a dense inflammatory infiltrate and often fibrosis, this however is the result of longstanding gastroesophageal reflux. In these patients a very low LES pressure and esophageal motor disorders are common findings [2].

In Rotterdam, we have studied panmural esophagitis in a rat model. Reflux was induced by performing an esophagojejunostomy (Fig. 1). We sequentially measured esophageal collagen content after the induction of reflux esophagitis (Fig. 2).

The results show an early increase of collagen in the esophageal wall after only 7 days of reflux. After 42 days of reflux the increase in collagen content of the esophageal wall reached statistical significance when compared to nonrefluxing controls.

While by no means wanting to extrapolate these results directly to the human situation, they might indicate what is happening in severe reflux-esophagitis in man.

Apart from the inflammatory infiltrate which has been demonstrated in mucosal biopsies from patients with esophagitis, fibrotic changes might occur in deeper levels

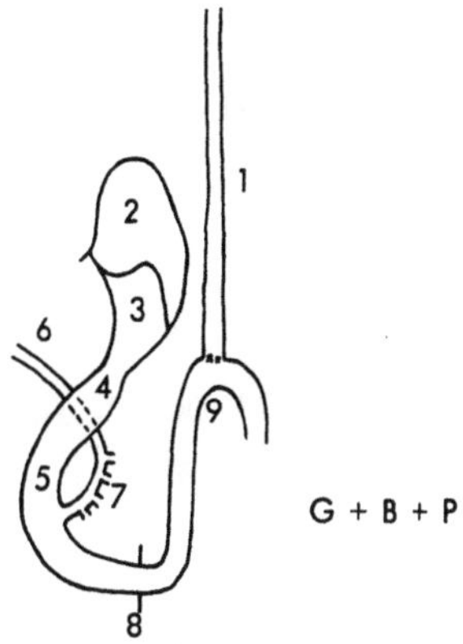

Fig. 1. Experimental induced esophagitis (rat model)

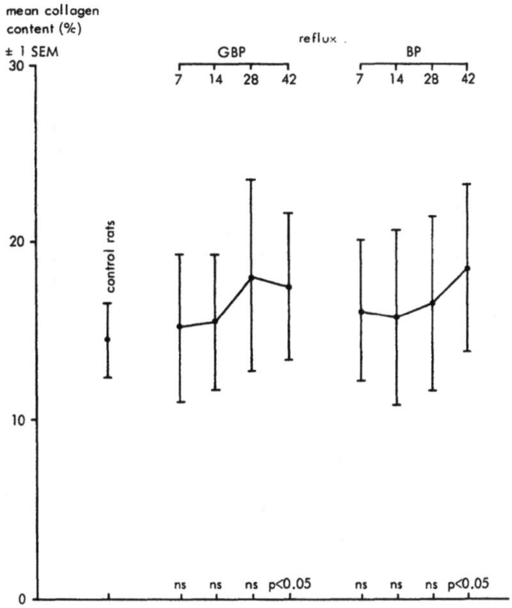

Fig. 2. Induced reflux esophagitis. Esophageal collagen content

of the esophageal wall. For obvious reasons we have not been able to demonstrate this phenomenon in man. However the residual motor abnormalities after endoscopic healing of esophagitis that have been demonstrated by several authors [3, 4, 5] could be due to the supposed increase of collagen in the esophageal wall.

In conclusion the following scenario could be imagined (Fig. 3):

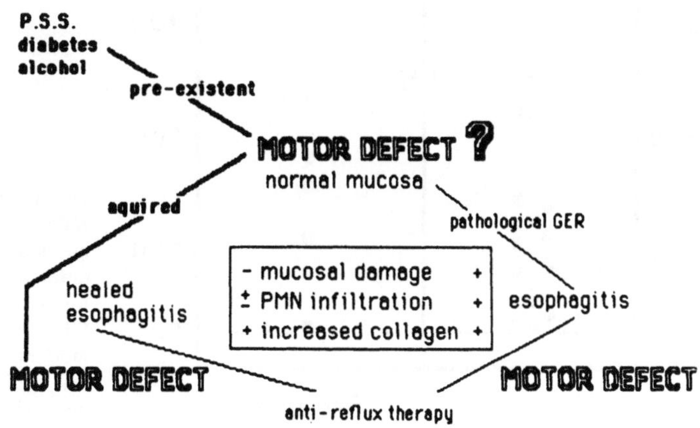

Fig. 3

References

1. Henderson RD, Pearson FG (1976) Preoperative assessment of esophageal pathology. J thorac Cardiovasc Surg 72: 512–517
2. Ahtaridis G, Snape WJ, Cohen S (1979) Clinical and manometric findings in benign peptic strictures of the esophagus. Dig Dis Sci 24: 858–861
3. Brand DL, Eartwood IR, Martin D, Carter WB, Pope CE II (1979) Esophageal symptoms, manometry and histology before and after anti reflux surgery. Gastroenterology 76: 1393–1401
4. Russell COH, Pope II CE, Gannan RM, Allen FD, Velasco N, Hill LD (1981) Does surgery correct esophageal motor dysfunction in gastroesophageal reflux? Ann Surg 194: 290–295
5. Sonnenberg A, Lepsien G, Muller-Lissner SA, Koelz HR, Siewert JR, Blum AL (1982) When is esophagitis healed? Dig Dis Sci 27: 297–302

Does the determination of an acid reflux score enable a better classification of the disease in question?

Y. Ottignon, J.P. Deschamps, and *P. Carayon* (Besançon)

Among the different techniques designed to investigate gastro-esophageal reflux (GER Fig. 1), measurement of esophageal pH is currently the method of choice [3], permitting direct measurement of the GER and quantification of the reflux phenomenon. Its use over 3 hours in the postprandial period certainly represents an excellent compromise between the diagnostic value of the test and its acceptability

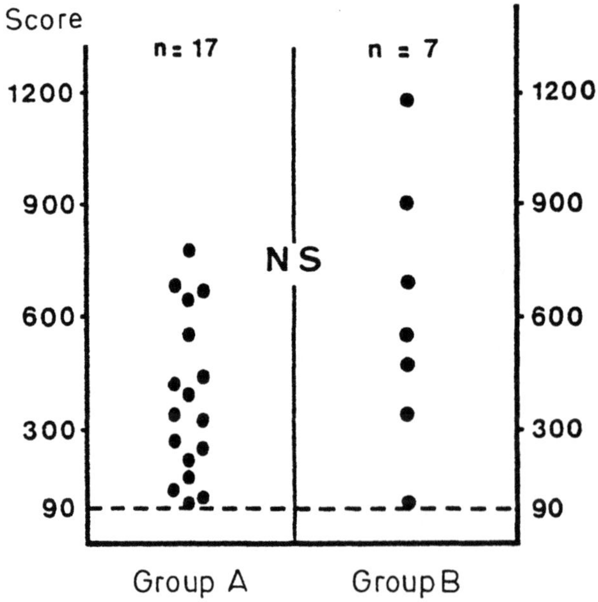

Fig. 1. Values of scores of acid reflux calculated by Kaye's method [4] related to two groups defined by their clinical symptomatology, Group A: typical GER expressed in episodic and moderate fashion; Group B: typical GER causing major interference with patient's activities

Table 1. Diagnostic value of 3-hour postprandial pH measurement in 47 patients with suspected gastroesophageal reflux

	Total no. of reflux episodes (pH<5)	Mean duration of reflux episodes (min)	No. of prolonged reflux episodes (>5 min)	Duration of the longest reflux episode (min)	No. of very acid reflux episodes (pH<2)	Duration of reflux episodes %	Score
Sensitivity	0.41 (13/32)	0.62 (20/32)	0.53 (17/32)	0.69 (23/32)	0.19 (6/32)	0.91 (29/32)	0.91 (29/32)
Specificity	0.87 (12/15)	0.87 (13/15)	0.87 (13/15)	0.80 (12/15)	0.93 (14/15)	0.80 (12/15)	0.80 (12/15)

The sensitivity and specificity were calculated for each parameter on the basis of the classification established by nocturnal pH measurement taken as the reference test for the diagnosis of GER. The upper limit of normal for each variable was fixed at m – 2 DS, calculated from recordings obtained in 15 controls

by the patient [5, 7]. Calculation of the Kaye score [4] (in terms of the duration of the episodes of acid reflux and their severity) is customarily employed for analysis of the recordings, but the variable total duration of reflux episodes below pH 5 is a simpler calculation allowing very comparable analysis [7]. Thus, in 47 patients with suspect GER, using prolonged pH measurement as a reference method, these two parameters have been shown to possess identical diagnostic value (Table 1).

The need to resort to quantification of acid reflux follows from several considerations:

- GER is above all a physiologic phenomenon which occurs orthostatically as well as in decubitus, even if it is commoner after meals, and whose chief characteristic is that of always being limited in duration [5]. Its very existence determines this need for quantification of the reflux phenomenon, an indispensable preliminary to sound discrimination between physiologic and pathologic GER.
- the therapeutic approach to GER, in particular the decision to operate, is a tricky problem in the absence of objective data. Similarly the need for better assessment of the efficacy of different medical or surgical treatments implies the use of a method quantifying the reflux
- the absence of a relation between the severity of the clinical features and the degree of reflux (Fig. 1) is well established [1, 6], so that interrogation alone is inadequate in the assessment of the reflux phenomenon. Similarly the existence of endoscopic lesions of esophagitis does not allow an opinion on the severity of GER. Even though some studies find a significant difference between the mean scores of patients with severe esophagitis and those of patients without esophagitis [2] there exists at individual level a wide scatter of results which very probably indicates the multifactorial nature of the lesions of esophagitis.

Thus a quantitative approach to the reflux phenomenon is essential (Fig. 2). It permits a better classification of the disorder in terms of reflux as measured by pH, and appears complementary and not redundant to the clinical approach and to the lesional approach to the pathology of gastroesophageal reflux.

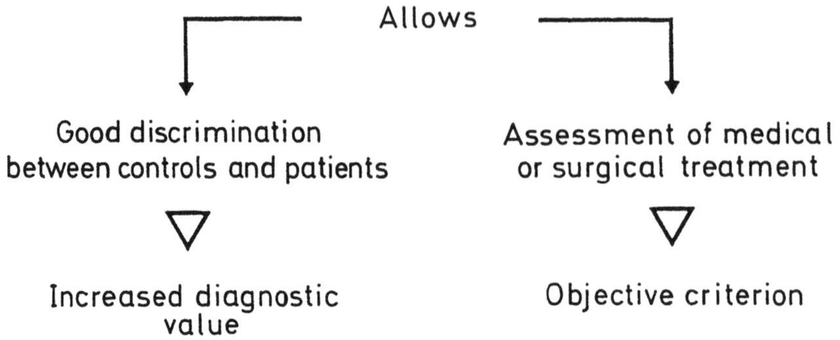

Fig. 2. Quantification of acid reflux

References

1. Atkinson M, Van Gelder A (1977) Esophageal intraluminal pH recording in the assessment of gastro-esophageal reflux and its consequences. Am J Dig Dis 22: 365–370
2. Galmiche JP, Guillard JF, Denis P, Boussakr K, Lefrancois R, Colin R (1980) Etude du pH oesophagien en période post-prandiale chez le sujet normal et au cours du reflux gastro-œsophagien. Intérêt diagnostique d'un score de reflux acide. Gastroentérol Clin Biol 4: 531–539
3. Galmiche JP, Denis P, Desechalliers JP (1981) Valeur diagnostique des examens complémentaires au cours du reflux gastro-œsophagien de l'adulte. Gastroentérol Clin Biol 5: 1014–1025
4. Kaye MD (1977) Post prandial gastro-esophageal reflux in healthy people. Gut, 18: 709–712
5. Mc Callum RW, Fink SM (1984) The role of prolonged esophageal pH monitoring in the diagnosis of gastroesophageal reflux. JAMA 252: 1160–1164
6. Ottignon Y, Deschamps JP, Voigt JJ, Cassigneul J, Lassegue A, Pascal JP, Carayon P (1983) pH-métrie œsophagienne: confrontation avec les données cliniques, endoscopiques et histologiques. Presse Med 12: 2249–2452
7. Ottignon Y, Ampleas M, Voigt JJ, Cassigneul J, Pascal JP (1984) Comparaison de trois méthodés d'enregistrement du pH œsophagien dans le diagnostic du reflux gastro-œsophagien acide. Gastroentérol Clin Biol 8: 609–615

When are motility tests indicated for the choice of treatment?

G. Friehs, P. Kohek, F.M. Jüttner, and *P. Rehak* (Graz)

The diagnosis of gastroesophageal reflux (GER) can be confirmed by a variety of different diagnostic procedures. Though the boundaries between physiologic and pathologic reflux are floating the accuracies of the tests are different. Esophageal radiography, which documents only the consequences of GER and secondary sicknesses, does not allow any essential statements about GER. The diagnosis of reflux esophagitis by X-ray is difficult and only effective at a progressive stage or if there are any complications of GER like ulcer, stenosis or Barrett's Syndrome.

Endoscopy and biopsy facilitate the evaluation of structural damage to the esophagus. For diagnosis of reflux esophagitis and for the exclusion of the diagnosis of esophageal carcinoma this procedure is indispensible. Endoscopic macroscopic staging according to Savary Miller only has an informal value.

GE scintiscan allows quantification of GER by use of a gamma camera with a computer system after application of a small amount of 99^{m}Tc DTPA. Being a short term analysis with high accuracy no association with patients subjective symptoms are possible.

Esophageal-manometry is a unique procedure in the diagnosis of esophageal disorders. It is the only procedure that allows direct assessment of the mechanical function of the esophagus and the exact location and length of the lower esophageal sphincter (LES).

24 hour long term pH monitoring of the esophagus allows first of all differentiation between physiological and pathological reflux. Furthermore it gives us the ability to study the esophageal clearance, to document day and night reflux episodes with subjective clinical symptomatic under almost physiological conditions.

Methods

If clinical symptoms (due to DeMeester's HRD score) lasted longer than 14 days or GER was pointed out by other investigations (X-ray, scintiscan, endoscopy), manometry and 24 hour pH monitoring was performed, obligatory esophageal-manometry was done using a gas-perfused catheter system. The system consists of three tubes located in a catheter with 5 mm outer diameter. Three measuring sites are placed along the catheter axis 5 cm apart according to the standard 3 point configuration. The catheter is connected to a pressure recording system. Helium is chosen as the gas because of its low effect on the patients comfort. Three point and rapid pullthrough manometry were performed to investigate mechanical function of the LES, plus length and exact location.

24 hour long-term pH monitoring was performed using a pH meter (Radiometer PHM 75) and a combined pH reference electrode (Radiometer GK 2801 C) connected to a computer (Epson HX 20).

The pH monitoring system is programmed to perform real-time analysis of the course. Computed data are shown in part on HX 20 display during the monitoring procedure to allow supervision; at the end of the measurement the results are printed out immediatelly. An optional graphic print-out of the pH course is used to compare reflux episodes with clinical symptoms noted by the patient. The evaluation is done by classification of number and duration of the pH being below pH 4 and according to the total time the pH was below pH 4 expressed in % of the investigation time.

Results

From 1984–1986 we have treated 134 patients (85 males, mean age 52,8 y, 49 females, mean age 46.0 y) with GER in the Department for Thoracic and Hyperbaric Surgery, University Medical School Graz, Austria. The pretherapeutic evaluation consisted of clinical symptoms, esophageal radiogram, endoscopy and biopsy, scintimetry, 24 hour pH monitoring and esophageal manometry. Clinical symptoms were registered according to DeMeester's device (HRD). 24 patients (17.9%) had no complaints. Heartburn was observed to be the most of all the single symptoms. The combination of heartburn and regurgitation led the group of combined complaints. 14 patients (10.4%) were suffering from heartburn in conjunction with regurgitation and dysphagia respectively (Table 1).

Reflux esophagitis, verified by histology, was found in 67 patients. While stage 1 and 2 of Savary Miller's fluoroscopic classification (S. M) of reflux esophagitis was observed in both symptomatic and asymptomatic patients, all patients in stages 3 and 4 were suffering from GER symptoms (Fig. 1).

Table 1. Clinical symptoms (HRD) (acc. to DeMeester) n=134

H=0 R=0 DO	24	17,9%
H	24	17.9%
R	4	3.0%
D	21	15.7%
H + R	31	23.1%
H + D	9	6.7%
R + D	7	5.2%
H + R + D	14	10.4%

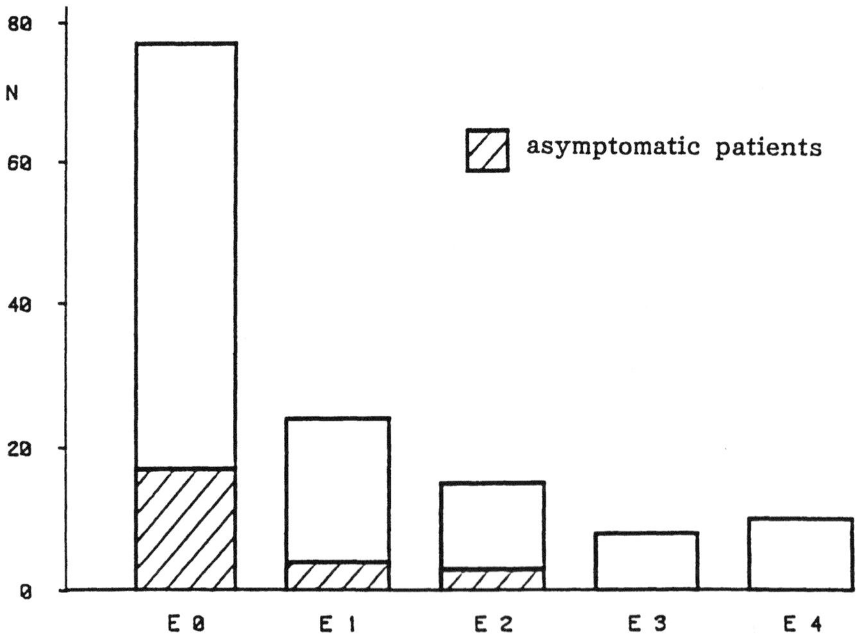

Fig. 1. Esophagitis S.M. stage

The pressure of the lower esophageal sphincter (LES) and the LES activity representing the antireflux mechanism is documented by manometry.

24 hour long term pH monitoring gives us a deep insight into the acid clearing time or esophagus clearance. Different standards are described by different investigators. Most of them consider only the time of each reflux episode (pH below pH 4). In addition so that, we introduce the Clearance Index (Koheh & Rehak-Index), which considers the reflux time between pH 4 and 5, and pays attention to the subsequent slope of the pH. This index consists of the difference from the time of pH 5 and 4 in % of the investigation-time divided by the numbers of reflux-episodes expressed in minutes (Table 2). A prolongation of the CI (Clearance Index) was seen in patients with reflux esophagitis (Fig. 2).

We compared 24 hr pH monitoring and esophageal manometry to other measures. Manometry showed good correlation to pH metry (Table 3).

Table 2. 24 h pH monitoring

Esophagitis S. M. stage		N	pH 4 % of RT	CI: pH 5–pH 4 in min. / numbers of ref.-episodes
E	0	77	4.9%	6.4 min/Episode
E	I	24	10.9% (I–II)	7.9 min/Episode
E	II	15		
E	III	8	11.7% (III–IV)	12.2 min/Episode
E	IV	10		

Table 3. GER. Diagnostic value of different tests compaired to 24 h pH monitoring

	>4,2% of RT			>2% of RT		
	f. Positiv %	=%	f. negativ %	f. Positiv %	=%	f. negativ %
Manometry n: 106=100%	12.3	67.1	23.6	17.9	65.1	17.0
LES pressure (<12 mmHg) n: 106	34.9	51.9	13.2	27.4	54.7	17.9
Scintiscan n: 38	13.1	42.2	21.1	10.5	60.6	28.9
X Ray n: 124	20.2	63.7	16.1	15.3	62.1	22.6

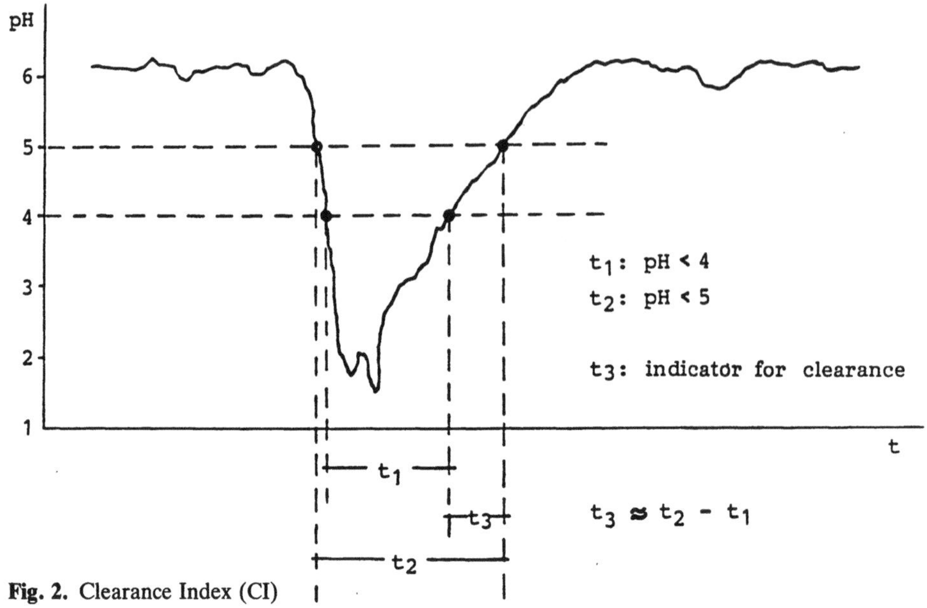

Fig. 2. Clearance Index (CI)

Therapeutic Consequences

To establish an adequate therapeutic approach manometry and 24 hour pH monitoring and endoscopy with biopsy are indispensible.

In cases without esophagitis, conservative therapy was started with mucosal protective agents, metoclopramide was added if manometry suggested an insufficient LES or if prolonged esophageal clearance (Clearance-Index) was documented by 24 hr pH monitoring.

After 12 weeks, the therapeutic effects were evaluated and in therapeutic inefficency conservative treatment was prolonged with H2 antagonists.

In cases with reflux esophagitis, conservative treatment was started primarily with H2 antagonists combined with metoclopramid according to LES pressure and clearance. If conservative procedures did not improve GER clinically or in endoscopic, manometric or pH metric re-evaluation, fundoplication according to Nissen-Rossetti was performed. This operative procedure was necessary in only 9 patients. All of them remained free of symptoms after the operation.

Conclusion

We conclude that esophageal motility tests are required in every case of GER, to establish an adequate therapeutic approach. Our data confirm the findings of other authors, proving a good correlation of data from manometry and 24 hour pH monitoring. Although manometry is a reliable method it is only valid in combination with other mandatory diagnostic procedures such as endoscopy and 24 hour pH monitoring.

A. Moraldi, C. Iascone, M. Zerilli, P. Ginevri, and *S. Stipa*
(Rome)

From 1972 to 1986 we have observed 626 patients with symptoms of gastroesophageal reflux; (Table 1) 109 patients, that is 17.4% have been submitted to surgery after failure of medical treatment. 80% of patients underwent standard manometry and during the last years we introduced the study of esophageal transit and gastric emptying by radioisotope technique; 110 cases have been studied by both methods. 63 patients have been operated on in our Department and 46 underwent preoperative manometry.

Table 1. Gastroesophageal reflux (1972–86)

Patients observed	626	
Patients operated	109	(17.4%)
Patients operated in our dept.	63	
Manometry	46	

Table 2. Gastroesophageal reflux manometry (46 Pts.)

	LES length	LES amplitude
Normal	2.5 cm	9.4 mmHg
Abnormal	2.5 cm	6.9 mmHg

N.V. (normal value) length >3 cm; amplitude >10 mmHg
p=n.s.

Table 3. Gastroesophageal reflux failures (9 Pts.)

Normal manometry	2/30	(6.6%)	p=0.05
Abnormal manometry	* 5/16	(31%)	
2/17 in Pts. not submitted to manometry			

* 3 Pts. with scleroderma

According to manometric findings patients were divided into normal (30) and abnormal (16), indicating as abnormal those patients whose esophageal body presented non-specific motor disorders like spontaneous, simultaneous or repetitive contractions or decreased amplitude of peristaltic waves, regardless of the characteristics of the lower esophageal sphincter (LES).

As far as LES (Table 3) is concerned it is interesting to note that patients with normal manometry showed mean values of length and amplitude similar to those of our normal controls (length 2.5 cm N.V. >3 cm; amplitude 9.4 mmHg N.V. >10 mmHg), whereas patients with abnormal manometry showed a mean amplitude of 6.9 mmHg; no differences were observed in terms of length (Table 2).

We have had 9 recurrences: 2 out of 17 in the group of patients who did not undergo esophageal manometry, 2 out of 30 (6.6%) in patients with normal manometric findings and 5 out of 16 (31% $p<0.05$) in patients with abnormal manometry (Table 3); 3 of these 5 patients had scleroderma and the absence of peristaltic waves may be the cause of recurrence. These three female patients presented with dysphagia and heartburn that remained unchanged, shortly after the operation.

The other four recurrences, two with normal and two with abnormal manometry, did not show any particular motor abnormality, compared to patients of the same group; that could explain why surgery failed. Unfortunately among patients submitted to surgery, only a very small group has been studied with both radioisotopic gastric emptying and esophageal transit. Therefore we cannot assess whether abnormalities of gastric emptying (which were present in 50% of our patients with proven gastroesophageal reflux) associated or not with motor dysfunction of the body of the esophagus, could influence the results of surgical treatment. At present we also do not know in which way the severity of motor abnormalities detected by the radionuclide transit will correlate with a correct indication and the results of the operation.

Are motility tests useful for the choice of treatment? There is no doubt that motility tests are essential for several reasons:

1. to make a correct diagnosis and exclude an underlying disease. Bombeck et al. [1] report 5 failures out of 22 Nissen fundoplications; these 5 patients exhibited spontaneous activity that was significantly higher than in both normal subjects and patients who were cured; these motility characteristics and the presence of much higher than normal esophageal peristaltic pressure, primary peristaltic wave longer in duration, and a higher than normal LES pressure, led the authors to conclude that these patients had a coexisting diffuse esophageal spasm that was the cause of the unsuccessful surgical treatment.
2. to assess the motility of the esophagus and the sphincter manometrics. Patients with adequate contractility of the esophageal body and manometrically deficient LES (sphincter pressure of 6.0 mmHg or less and overall sphincter length of 2.0 cm or less) should probably have the best results [2] even though this is not the rule in clinical practice. In fact in our group 3 out of 5 recurrences with abnormal manometry presented with scleroderma and severe abnormalities of motor activity.
3. to investigate a gastric pathology. In some patients gastric disease can cause reflux through a normal sphincter. Correction of reflux, in such patients may cause other complaints such as gas bloat syndrome.

A delayed gastric emptying has been often associated with gastroesophageal reflux [5]; it has been suggested that this delay plays a role in the etiology of the disease and if not corrected may permit gastroesophageal reflux to reoccur [3].

This is a controversial point that not everybody accepts; in fact in another series of patients gastric emptying abnormalities were present before and after surgical correction of reflux, but patients did well and became asymptomatic without the necessity for a gastric emptying procedure at the time of antireflux surgery [6].

Mattioli et al. [4] have studied 16 patients with gastroesophageal reflux and esophagitis and all 16 showed delayed gastric emptying; twenty four hour pH-monitoring of the gastric antrum was also investigated and in 14 patients an abnormal duodenal-gastric reflux was present. Manometry revealed an incoordination of antral-pyloric-duodenal motility with incoordinated motor duodenal hyperactivity.

For this reason, the Authors suggest performing an extramucosal duodenal myotomy in such patients together with fundoplication. Patients so treated and followed-up are doing well and are asymptomatic without recurrence of reflux.

Surgery does not correct esophageal motor dysfunction and the results are often unrelated to the presence or not of motor abnormalities; motility tests may not provide sufficient information for the choice of treatment but at least may be of value in predicting patients likely to have poor out-comes.

References

1. Bombeck CT, Battle WS, Nyhus LM (1973) Preoperative manometry in the choice of operations for gastro-esophageal reflux. Am J Surg 125: 99
2. DeMeester TR, Bonavina L, Albertucci M (1986) Nissen fundoplication for gastroesophageal reflux disease. Evaluation of primary repair in 100 consecutive patients. Ann Surg 204: 9
3. Maddern GJ, Jamieson GG, Chatterton BE, Collins PJ (1985) Is there an association between failed antireflux procedures and delayed gastric emptying? Ann Surg 202: 162
4. Mattioli F, Pandolfo N, Nebiacolombo C (1982) Aspetti correlativi della motilita' esofagea e gastroduodenale Min Chir 37: 261
5. Moraldi A, Iascone C, Caputo V, Ziparo V, Zerilli M, De Vito G, Camerino C (1985) The role of radioisotopic gastric emptying in patients with gastroesophageal reflux. Esophageal Disorders. Pathophysiology and therapy edited by Skinner DB and DeMeester TR: 87-90, Raven Press NY
6. Velasco N, Hill LD, Gannan RM, Pope CE (1982) Gastric emptying and gastroesophageal reflux. Effects of surgery and correlation with esophageal motor function. Am J Surg 144: 58

Non-surgical treatments

Is the dilatation of tight esophageal stenosis a therapeutic procedure?

S. L. Dawson (Burlington)

My answer must take into consideration the reason for the dilatation, as well as the means used for the procedure.

If a patient refuses surgery, or is not a surgical candidate, then esophageal dilatation serves to provide the only non-operative means of ensuring adequate nutritional intake to maintain life. If we frame the question in terms of whether esophageal dilatation is a curative procedure, then my answer would be more qualified, for it is only in those few cases of esophageal webs or post-surgical anastomotic strictures that we will provide immediate complete relief of the patient's problems. For those patients with strictures due to reflux esophagitis, caustic ingestion, carcinoma or radiation induced stricture, we should consider the procedure as temporary palliation, a maneuver which can be performed repeatedly with very little morbidity in order to relieve the patient's symptoms and allow continued eating.

Esophageal bougienage is a time-honored method of maintaining a lumen large enough to permit continued oral intake. Bougienage has the advantage of being able to be performed at home by the patient. In our institution, the patient is bougienaged up to a 36 French size, and is then sent home with the bougie to use on a routine basis to maintain a 12 mm esophageal lumen, sufficient to allow eating soft foods.

My particular interest, however, is in those patients in whom the esophagus has narrowed to less than 10 mm. Below this size, all patients will have dysphagia, and bougienage will not succeed in dilating the lumen, because a bougie this slender cannot exert enough downward force to enlarge the lumen. In these patients, balloon catheter dilatation of the esophagus can quickly, safely, and easily open a lumen of sufficient size to permit home bougienage. In our institution, patients with an esophageal stenosis 10 mm or smaller are referred to radiology where a 7 French balloon dilatation catheter is placed into the stenosis over a guidewire. The balloon is then inflated with contrast medium under direct fluoroscopic vision, and a direct radial pressure is therefore exerted on the stenosis, opening the lumen to the same size as the balloon. The esophageal lumen often enlarges to 18–20 mm immediately, equivalent to 54–60 French size, and bougienage is then performed to maintain the lumen's size.

This technique is especially valuable in patients who have a tortuous esophageal stricture or redundancy of the esophagus proximal to a stenosis. Also, patients with an esophageal ulcer-stricture complex are most safely dilated with this method. In these patients, bougienage can fail or cause perforation of the esophagus because of the entry of the bougie tip into the ulcer. When downward force is exerted on the bougie, the tip perforates the wall. Because balloon dilatation is performed over a guidewire which has been placed into the stomach under fluoroscopic guidance, the balloon catheter cannot perforate the esophagus.

Because the balloon exerts its force directly outward on the strictured segment, the greatest dilating force is applied to the narrowest segment of the esophagus. The balloon is not moved during the dilatation period. Unlike bougienage, which relies on exerting its outward force by pushing downward, balloon dilatation is a very gentle, controlled, firm expansion of the lumen. Patients are given intravenous sedation before the procedure, and local anesthesia is given to the pharynx to allow passage of the catheter. The actual dilatation is usually painless in benign disease, but may cause a temporary chest pain in cases of stricture due to irradiation. In these cases, intravenous analgesia is also used.

A secondary procedure which can be performed after balloon dilatation is placement of a silastic esophageal prosthesis. In patients with recurrent stricture, or in those patients where there is esophageal perforation but surgery cannot be performed due to poor overall condition, the initial balloon dilatation is followed by insertion of a silastic prosthesis, using the balloon catheter to carry the prosthesis into the stricture. Once in place, the balloon is deflated and the guidewire is removed, leaving the prosthesis in place.

We have performed esophageal balloon dilatation on over 120 patients, for both benign and malignant disease, at all levels from the cricopharyngeus to the phrenic ampulla. There have been no major complications and only one minor perforation of the upper esophagus when a resident tried to pass a guidewire without fluoroscopic guidance. Our goal has been to allow bougienage to be performed on an out patient basis and this has been successful in all patients who have left the hospital. Four patients, expired in-hospital, from causes related to the primary disease, not to the esophageal dilatation procedure.

In closing, then, I can say very firmly that, yes, esophageal dilatation of tight esophageal strictures is indeed a therapeutic procedure, but its limitations must be recognized. We cannot cure the problems of the patient whith stricture due to malignant disease but we can palliate this patient and allow the psychological benefits of continued oral alimentation, which most of us would prefer over a gastrostomy. And for the patient with benign esophageal stricture, we can use balloon dilatation to eliminate the stricture completely or allow outpatient therapy with bougienage.

S. Sancho-Fornos, C. Magallon, J. Gomez, J. Pallas, J. Botella, and *J. Segui* (Valencia)

Dilatation of peptic esophageal strictures can in our opinion be the only treatment when surgery is contraindicated. We think that bougienage in severe strictures has to be done before surgery; in all cases during surgery and in some patients after surgery.

Among 46 cases of peptic stenosis treated between 1975–1983 only five patients were not operated and managed with medical care and a non-standardized bougienage schedule with Maloney bougies. Four were men, and surgery was not proposed for the following reasons:

- Renal failure-2 patients
- Cardiac insufficiency-2 patients
- Cor pulmonale bronchiectasis-1 patient

All of them were dilated under general anesthesia the first time. 60 Fr. Maloney bougie was achieved in 3 sessions in 3 patients and 2 patients needed 4 sessions.

There was not a standardized schedule: the patient should be seen at regular intervals and questioned carefully with regards to recurrence of symptoms, with bougienage repeated at the earliest sign of return of dysphagia.

Nevertheless there are some patients that are difficult to dilate; in this cases we prefer a weekly bougienage until a size 48–50 Fr. bougie is reached, the patients were then discharged, with dietary restrictions, antacids, and postural treatment.

Monthly control, and repeated dilatation twice a year in the first year was done in four patients. One died two months after dilatation (cardiac infart) and two patients during the second year. We have only two patients with a 3 and 5 year follow-up: In our experience the Rx diameter tends to decrease and there is a tendency for the constriction to recur without complaints of heartburn.

After dilatation reflux is not supressed with medical therapy, we only reduce the gastric acid contents in periods between meals, but during meals, as is shown by 24 pH monitoring evaluation (7 cases treated with dilatation and surgery, and 3 cases only with medical treatment) reflux was the rule.

Our manometric findings in 31 cases show a non-existent or very depressed HPZ in the thoracic position, called by DeMeester "absolute mechanical failure".

As an aid to surgical treatment dilatations have an important place.

We have considered bougienage in two groups: one includes dilatations performed before and during surgery. In this group the aim is the dislaceration of an organized stricture. The second group are dilatations after surgery that try to calibrate the esophagus.

Among our 41 operated strictures with follow-up 3–10 years, we had 37 cases with one stenosis. The remaining were double (2 patients) or diffused. In 23 cases the strictures were localized to the lower third, 9 in the middle and 5 in the upper third.

We consider stricture to be severe when the internal diameter is less than 9 mm and as moderate when the adult endoscope cannot cross the stricture. The others are the mild type. We had 13 severe strictures, 16 moderate and 12 mild cases.

Before opening the abdomen we do an endoscopy and place a Maloney bougie without forceful dilatation.

Moderate and mild strictures were all dilated only during surgery and when the abdomen was open, to control the dilators (Maloney bougies) and to carry out forceful dilatation.

The postoperative bougienage was unnecessary in nearly 50% of our patients. 18 patients needed one dilatation to reach 60 Fr. bougie. 9 patients were dilated twice and 2 patients 3 times. General anesthesia is not mandatory and is used only in special patients.

We consider the dilatations to be an important step within surgical treatment, that need serious training. We had two perforations at surgery (before using Maloney bougies) and both cases were not carried out by the surgeon who is responsible for this work.

J. B. Ollyo, M. Savary, Ph. Monnier, J. Wellinger, and *J. J. Gonvers* (Lausanne)

When the endoscope cannot be passed through a peptic stricture (196/345 in our series) we use Savary-Gilliard dilators [2, 5]. The stricture is dilated up to a diameter of 15 mm. This important procedure enables the operator to do the following:

1. evaluate the superficial or transmural nature of the fibrosis by the resistance to the dilator. The dilator must be advanced in a slow, smooth and continuous movement.
2. examine the lumen of the stricture which is usually short and covered with a squamous epithelium. It may show an ulcer, an inflammatory or adenomatous polyp, columnar epihtelium or an adenocarcinoma.
3. perform multiple biopsies of the stricture and epithelium below it, especially when the surface is irregular.
4. determine if the segment below the stricture, which should be always biopsied, is part of an endobrachyesophagus (tubular aspect) or a hiatal hernia (saccular aspect, Fig. 1).

The dilatation of a stricture is a necessary part of a complete diagnostic endoscopic examination as well as a fundamental therapeutic procedure. Indeed the current treatment of peptic stricture consists of antireflux surgery. In itself this treatment has no direct effect on the stricture and should always by associated with preoperative, operative and/or postoperative dilatations (Table 1). Dilatations associated with a medical treatment (such as inhibitors of gastric secretion, sodium alginate, sucralfate, dietary recommendations) are usually recommended for old or inoperable patients and have good results (Table 2). For Loygue et al. [4] as well as for us, endoscopic dilatations are the treatment of choice for postoperative peptic strictures. The long term results are excellent.

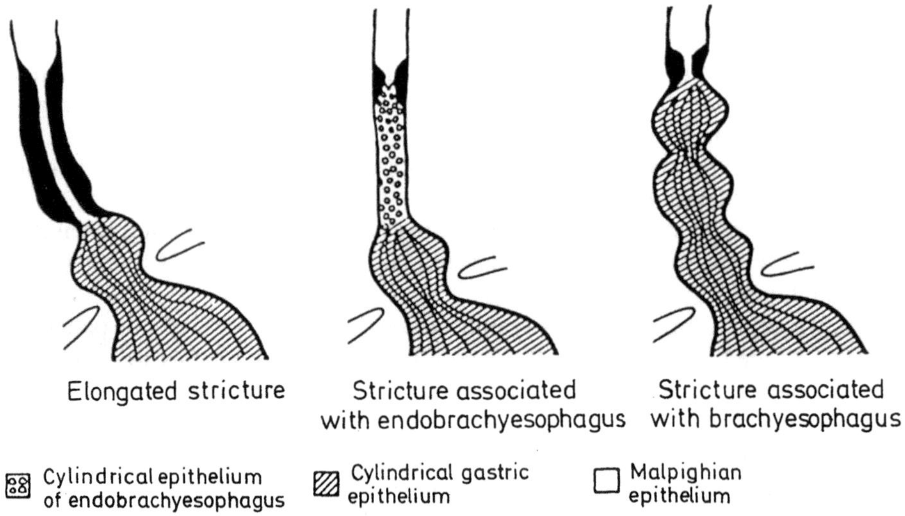

Fig. 1. Differential diagnosis of reflux esophagitis with stricture situated at the upper or middle thirds of the esophagus

Table 1. Tight peptic strictures: value of endoscopic dilatation

dilatation for diagnostic purposes	: 182/196 (92.8%)
therapeutic dilatation	
– as sole treatment	: 87/196 (44.4%)
– plus Nissen procedure	: 95/196 (48.4%)
not dilated	: 14/196 (7.2%)
(resection of stricture)	

Chuv, Lausanne, Switzerland (01. 01. 1963–31. 12. 1986)

Table 2. Late results of treatment of tight peptic strictures by dilatation

Author Reference	Number of Patients	Results				
		good	poor	unknown	perforation	deaths
Benedict E. B. [1]	133	113 (85%)	20 (15%)	0	?	2 (1.5%)
Lequerler Y. [3]	256	110 (43%)	69 (27%)	77 (30%)	0	0
Patterson D. J. [6]	127	87 (68%)	16 (13%)	24 (19%)	3 (2.3%)	0
Savary M. (*)	87	56 (64%)	18 (21%)	13 (15%)	1 (1.2%)	1 (1.2%)
Watson A. [7]	78	71 (91%)	7 (9%)	0	2 (2.5%)	0
Wesdorp I. C. [8]	68	60 (88%)	8 (12%)	0	5 (7.3%)	0

* Unpublished findings (CHUV, Lausanne, Switzerland: 01. 01. 1963–31. 12. 1986)

References

1. Benedict EB (1966) Peptic stenosis of the esophagus. A study of 133 patients treated with bougienage, surgery or both. Am J Dig Dis 11: 761–769
2. Dumont JF, Meric B, Sivak MV, Fleischer D (1985) A new method of esophageal dilatation using Savary-Gilliard bougies. Gastrointest Endosc 31: 379–382
3. Lequerler Y (1983) Traitement médical instrumental des sténoses peptiques de l'oesophage. Actualités Digestives 7: 296–298
4. Loygue J, Parc R, Letoublon C et al. (1980) Traitement des sténoses peptiques de l'œsophage. A propos de 40 cas. Chirurgie 106: 636–643
5. Monnier P, Hsieh V, Savary M (1985) Traitement endoscopique des sténoses œsophagiennes par les bougies de Savary-Gilliard: nouveautés techniques. Acta Endoscopica 15: 119–129
6. Patterson DJ, Graham DY, Lacey Smith J et al. (1983) Natural history of benign esophageal stricture treated by dilatation. Gastroenterology 85: 346–350
7. Watson A (1984) The role of antireflux surgery combined with fiberoptic endoscopic dilatation in peptic esophageal stricture. Amer J Surg 148: 346–349
8. Wesdorp ICE, Bartelsman JF, den Hartog Jager FCA, Huibregtse K, Tytgat GN (1982) Results of Conservative treatment of benign esophageal strictures: a follow up study of 100 patients. Gastroenterology 82: 487–493

What is the risk of declining results when a peptic stenosis is treated by dilatation?

Y. Lequerler (Paris)

The various studies of the outcome of dilatation in treatment of benign stenosis of the esophagus are unanimous about the immediate results. Indeed, good short-term results have been found in 75%–85% of cases.

It is much more difficult, to determine the long-term results. First follow-up reports after a period of 5 years or longer are very rare. As we shall see, recurrences do happen throughout the 5 years following the first dilatation (Fig. 1). Second, most authors include all benign stenoses (caustic stenosis, anastomotic stenosis, peptic stenosis) in the same study. Finally, the groups studied include aged subjects with or without other disorders; the latter explains the high percentage of subjects lost to observation, which is slightly more than 30%.

The present study was done on 455 patients suffering from peptic stenosis of the esophagus confirmed by endoscopy and biopsy. These cases have been followed up for a period of 1–3 years. For dilatations the Eder Puestow dilatator and in the past few years, a candle similar to that of Savary have been used. Both are very safe to use.

In 52% of cases, relapses occur during the first year. The reappearance of dysphagia with a stenosis whose diameter determined by endoscopy is less than 12 mm indicates relapse, and hence the necessity of repeating dilatation.

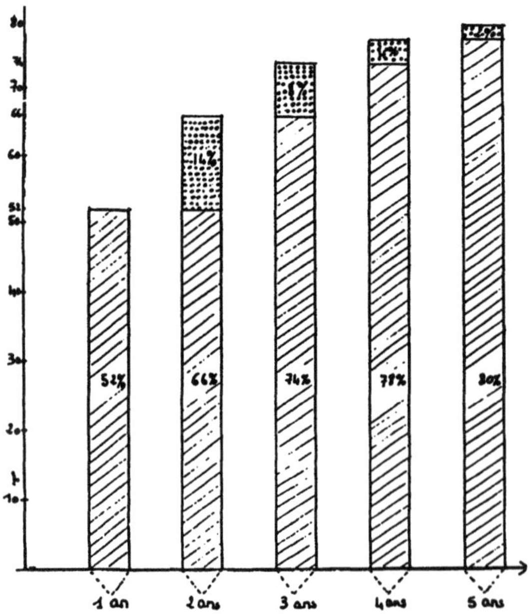

Fig. 1. Relapses with time after dilation. *Dotted areas* indicate new relapse

As shown in the Fig. 1, it can be seen that relapses become less and less frequent from a peak of 14% 2 years after the operation, to 8% after 3 years, 4% after 4 years, and 2% in the 5th year. There were no further relapses after 5 years. A second point deserves to be mentioned; is has been observed that the later the relapses occur, the smaller the number of dilatation sessions necessary. Three or four sessions are required per year in the 1st or 2nd year, but one observes that only one or two additional sessions suffices when a relapse has occurred later. In summary, we can conclude that 80% of patients treated by dilatation have a relapse in the following 5 years. The number of relapses decreases with time and less and less dilatation sessions are needed.

These results must be interpreted in the light of the subject ages (30% over 60 years; 25% over 70 years old) and the fact that they could not be treated surgically.

References

1. Baulieux J, Boulez J, Donne G, Rigollet G, Maillet P (1981) Le traitement des sténoses œsophagiennes peptiques de l'adulte. Gastroenterol Clin, Bio, 5, 1169–1175
2. Castro R, Dupin B, Lienne P: Techniques des dilatations de l'œsophage. Expérience personnelle et revue de la littérature. Acta endoscopica vol. 16 n°2 – 1986
3. Celestin LR, Campbelle WB (1981) A new and safe system for œsophageal dilatation. Lancet, I, 74
4. Daxson SL, Mueller PR, Ferrucci JT, Richter JP, Schapiro RH, Bucht RJ, Simeone JF (1984) Severe esophageal strictures: indications for balloon catheter dilatation. Radiology, 153, 631
5. Dumon JF, Castro R, Meric B, Hancy A, Dupin B, Experience of 1 100 esophageal dilatations. Book of abstracts: IVe Symposium international d'endoscopie digestive, Paris 8., 9., 10., 11. Mai 1984
6. Leichtmann GA, Novis BH, Samara M (1984) Dilatation instrumentale des sténoses œsophagiennes et gastriques à l'aide du cathéter de Gruntzig et du dilatateur de Celestin. Gastroenterol Clin Biol, 8, 616–620
7. Lequerler Y (1980) Traitement par dilatations (Eder Puestow) des sténoses peptiques serrées de l'œsophage. Ann Chir, 34, 377–378
8. Lindor KD (1985) Balloon dilatations of upper digestive tract strictures – Gastroeenterology, 89
9. Ogilvie AL, Ferguson R, Atkinson M (1980) Outlook with conservative treatment of peptic œsophageal stricture. Gut, 21, 23–25
10. Patterson D, Graham DY, Smith L, Schwartz JT, Alpert E, Lanza F, Cain D (1983) Natural History of benign Esophageal strictura treated by dilatation. Gastroenterology, 85

Medical treatments of peptic esophagitis

Presidents:	*R. Lambert* (Lyons)
	J. F. Rey (St.-Laurent-du-Var)
Free Commentators:	*A. Bel* (Lyons)
	M. Deltenre (Brussels)
	J. Dent (Adelaide)
	J. P. Galmiche (Nantes)
	M. Mignon (Paris)
	G. Vantrappen (Leuven)

Introduction

R. Lambert (Lyons)

The texts gathered in this section under the stimulus of Robert Giuli are nearly all devoted to the treatment of peptic esophagitis. At first sight, the fragmentation of the therapeutic aspects in multiple brief accounts may seem opposed to the development of a synthesis. In fact the repetition for each drug of rational bases for their prescription, degree of efficacy, limitations and tolerance, provides a more objective view and will allow each reader to form his own opinion on the basis of these references.

Two preliminary remarks are justified:

1. peptic esophagitis represents only a narrow fringe of the pathology of esophageal reflux, usually benign.
2. the large number of medicaments put forward and the absence of a single treatment program reflect both the limits of efficacy and the extent of innovation in the field of medication.

Confining ourselves to more recent history three periods may characterize treatment programs for esophageal reflux and peptic esophagitis.

The first period was completed rather more than 10 years ago with the advent of the H2 receptor antagonists. The antacids were then the main treatment as agents well adapted to the relief of reflux symptoms but virtually ineffective against esophageal lesions. The contribution of agents with a pharmacologic action on digestive motility appeared nil or even harmful (cf. atropine).

During the second period over the last 10 years the H2 receptor antagonists have brought undeniable progress. The extent of this is not as great as that observed in gastroduodenal ulcer, but its characteristics are similar: safety in use ensured by several years' experience in study of tolerance which is excellent; simplicity of prescription; rational basis of action determined by control of acidity; and objective measurement of efficacy and its limitations by endoscopic monitoring of the lesions. The different molecules currently available differ markedly at the pharmacological level but in terms of practical prescription the H2-receptor antagonists may be regarded as a single family of agents with very similar properties. Their efficacy is entirely satisfactory if one abides by the symptomatic criteria: the relief of signs of reflux. Their combination with antacid agents allows balancing up of daily and nocturnal treatment. The limits of efficacy appear in the very narrow band of patients with peptic esophagitis as the healing of ulcerative lesions is delayed and incomplete except when it is a matter of simple erosions. Likewise maintenance treatment does not effectively prevent the recurrence of ulceration. These observations illustrate the limits of efficacy of these medicaments but should not obscure their effectiveness and their excellent tolerance in the much more frequent cases of simple esophageal reflux.

The third period in therapy has now begun and therapeutic trials open attractive perspectives in the very near future. Secretory inhibition takes a forward leap in pharmacology with the appearance of the benzimidazoles (Omeprazole), agents capable of blocking acid secretion almost completely. The endoscopic cure of the ulcerations of peptic esophagitis becomes possible with these products. Nevertheless as in the case of the H2-receptor antagonists, their limitations alternate with surgical treatment, which represents a logical solution when the ulcerated peptic esophagitis is chronic.

Agents with a pharmacologic effect on esophageal motility have proved their efficacy as adjuncts to secretory inhibition particularly as regards two products: metoclopramide and cisapride.

Finally, while it is still too soon to assess objectively the efficacy of the agents which act by reinforcing mucosal protection (sucralfate, prostaglandins), the potential development of this therapy should not be underestimated.

Is esophageal reflux always symptomatic?

R. Lambert (Lyons)

Despite the absence of rigorously constructed epidemiologic studies, many arguments confirm that esophageal reflux is often asymptomatic.

Study of prevalence of symptoms in terms of severity

Castell [1] suggests a pyramidal representation of the frequency of reflux symptoms, with a very wide base corresponding to symptoms that are very moderate in intensity and frequency. These occur in patients who resort to self-medication and do not consult the doctor. The percentage of such cases is over 80% and medically speaking it is logical to regard them as asymptomatic.

The second stage of pyramid corresponds to patients with symptoms severe or frequent enough for medical consultation but not reaching the clinical grade of

Table 1. Symptomatic gastro-esophageal reflux in control subjects (385)

Heartburn	(%)
Daily	7
Weekly	14
Monthly	15
Total	36

Nebel, 1976

Table 2. Symptomatic gastro-esophageal

– Heartburn, Daily –	
Medical in-patients	14%
G I out-patients	15%
Obstetrical	21%

Nebel, 1976

severity. The third level of the pyramid very narrow, concerns patients with severe clinical manifestations of esophageal reflux.

This pyramidal presentation was suggested following an enquiry by Nebel [2] in 1976 into the medical and paramedical staff of two American hospitals (Table 1 and 2). This enquiry showed that in the control group considered asymptomatic interrogation revealed the presence of reflux in 36% of cases. This enquiry was limited to the clinical expression of reflux in the form of pyrosis. As regards frequency, daily symptoms of reflux were noted in 7% of subjects questioned, weekly symptoms in 14% and monthly symptoms in 15%.

Prevalence of atypical reflux symptoms

Respiratory symptoms – night cough, asthma, emphysema – form part of the extra-alimentary picture of esophageal reflux; the relation of cause and effect is very difficult to establish since it may be unrecognized on the one hand, or overestimated on the other. In fact, objective signs of reflux at diagnostic testing in the absence of any esophageal symptoms are found more often in around 20% of cases in patients suffering from asthma or bronchitis; but this usually relates to pharmacologic data without practical bearing. Finally, the clinical relation between esophageal reflux and pharyngeal symptoms – pharyngitis, tonsilitis, odynophagia, salivary hypersecretion – can be regarded as established in only a small proportion of cases.

Esophageal reflux revealed at the stage of complications

Some personal observations confirm the clinical latency of major esophageal reflux over a long period when the first symptomatic manifestation reveals the existence of a structural complication, e.g. dysphagia indicating peptic stricture. This is also true for the discovery of a Barrett's epithelium of acquired type clothing the lower ⅔ of the body of the esophagus in a patient who has never exhibited clinical symptoms of reflux, whereas the relation between Barrett's epithelium and esophagitis is well established.

Table 3. Pain induced by esophageal acid perfusion (25 patients with G.E.R.D.)

pH	
1.0–1.5	100%
2.0	80%
2.5–6.0	50%

Graham, 1987

Sensitivity of the esophageal mucosa to pH in gastroesophageal reflux

This relation has recently been explored by Graham [3] (Table 3), using Bernstein's acid perfusion test with solutions of pH varying from 1 to 6. This trial was made in patients with symptomatic esophageal reflux. Acid perfusions at very low pH – 1 or 1.5 – provoked pain in every patient, solutions of pH 2 provoked pain in 80% of patients and solutions of pH 2.5 to 6 in only 50% of patients. Thus acid solutions of pH above 2 do not regularly elicit pain. This may explain the disparity observed between the symptomatic relief usually afforded by H2-receptor antagonists and the continued development of structural lesions.

Recording of esophageal reflux

Spreading the recording of esophageal pH over 24 hours in diagnostic tests of reflux reveals frequent discordance between the timing of the symptomatic episodes recorded by the patient and the episodes of confirmed reflux. Naturally, the frequency of discordance varies with the threshold of intraesophageal pH chosen to signify the reflux episode (pH below 4.3 or 2).

References

1. Castell DO, Wu WC, Oh DJ, Gastroesophageal reflux disease. 1 vol Futura publ Mount Kisco. NY
2. Nebel OT, Fornes MF, Castell DO (1984) Symptomatic gastroesophageal reflux: incidence and precipitating factors. Dig Diseases Sciences 21: 953–956
3. Graham DY, Larkai E, Opekun AR, Smith JL (1987) Sensitivity of the esophageal mucosa to pH in gastroesophageal reflux. Gastroenterology 92: 1412 (abstr)

Is the underlying mechanism of LES insufficiency known? Can there be some independence between the value of LES and the existence of a hiatal hernia?

J. P. Galmiche, and *S. Bruley des Varannes* (Nantes)

15 years ago Cohen and Harris [1] published a study that showed that there was no relationship between the presence or absence of a hiatus hernia and the existence of symptomatic reflux (Fig. 1). On the other hand, the resting pressure of the LES, when below 10 mm Hg, very clearly separates these two populations and they concluded that in fact there was independence as regards hiatus hernia but not as regards hypotonia of the LES.

The results of this study have been much debated in subsequent years and a recent study by Kahrilas et al. [2] shows the extraordinary overlap that exists between the individual values measured in normal subjects, in subjects with reflux but not esophagitis, and in those with variable degrees of esophagitis. There exists a significant reduction of resting pressure at pathologic group level but a very considerable overlap of individual values and an attempt should be made to explain this apparent inconsistency.

Dent et al. [3] and Dodds et al. [4] are to be commended for having described a device permitting continuous recording of the tone of the LES. In a study which compares 10 control subjects with 10 subjects affected by esophagitis, they demonstrated the variability in time of LES tonus in relation to the values measured before meals, with a fall immediately after meals, followed during the night by a return to values higher than the pre-prandial values (Fig. 2). A single measurement of the

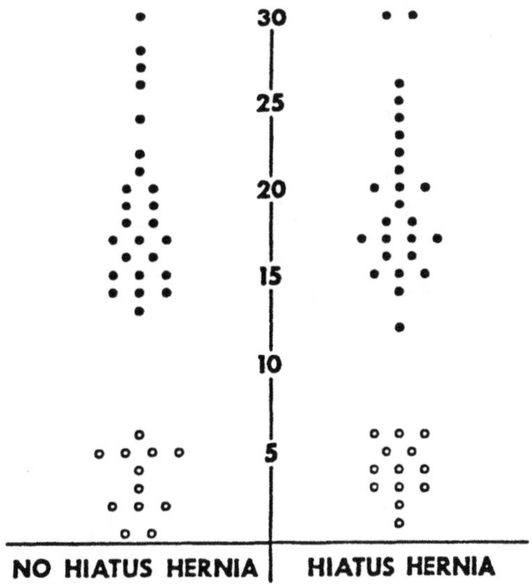

Fig. 1. Mean LES Pressures (in Millimeters of Mercury) of all patients at Rest or Base Line. The open circles represent values obtained from patients with symptomatic reflux. LES pressure did not correlate with presence or absence of hiatus hernia, but there was clear separation of symptomatic and asymptomatic patients (Cohen, Harris, 1971)

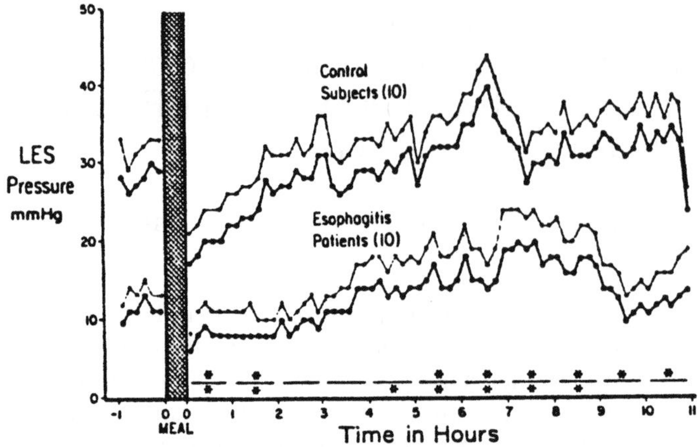

Fig. 2. Lower Esophageal Sphincter (LES) pressure during 12 hours of recording in 10 control subjects and 10 patients with reflux esophagitis
LES pressure is plotted as mean ±1 S.D. for each hour. The shaded areas represent 1 S.D. For each hour of recording, LES pressure in the patients was significantly lower than in the controls ($P<0.05$). For both patients and controls LES pressure decreased significantly (asterisks) below the respective before-meal values for two or three hours after the meal and increased significantly (asterisks) above before-meal control values during the night (Dodds et al, 1982)

resting pressure is therefore of no value and this fact doubtless explains the inconsistencies observed between the early and later studies.

On the other hand, during the course of these studies [3, 4] three mechanisms capable of producing acid reflux were demonstrated (Fig. 3) as well in normal subjects (physiologic reflux) as in those suffering from reflux:

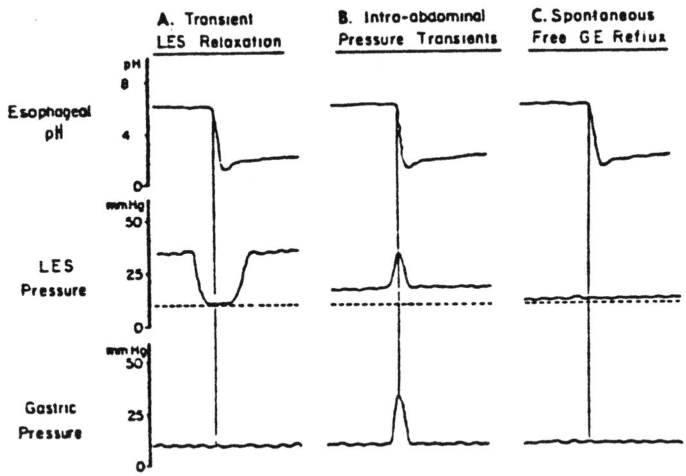

Fig. 3. Schematic representation of three different mechanisms of Gastroesophageal (GE) Reflux. Gastroesophageal reflux (shown as vertical lines) may accompany a transient lower esophageal sphincter (LES) relaxation (A), develop as stress reflux during a transient increase in intra-abdominal pressure that overcomes LES resistance (B), or occur as spontaneous free reflux across an atonic sphincter (C) (Dodds et al, 1982)

- the first of these is transient relaxation of the LES. This phenomenon is called inappropriate as it is not preceded by deglutition (Fig. 4); accompanied by a fall in pH chiefly in normal subjects with physiologic reflux.
- the second mechanism is characterized by an increase in intragastric pressure which, as it were, prevails against the possible resistance of the LES and again leads to acid reflux; (Fig. 3)
- the third mechanism is free spontaneous reflux without increase in the intragastric pressure but with permanent hypotonia of the LES, (Fig. 3) followed by a peristaltic sequence which progressively restores the pH to near-normal values.

A comparison of the distribution of these three mechanisms in a population of subjects with gastroesophageal reflux and one of control subjects shows that this transient relaxation phenomenon occurs in about 95% of cases in healthy subjects as against 65% in sick persons, the other mechanisms being equally distributed between transient increase of intra-abdominal pressure and free spontaneous reflux (Table 1). A study by Boyle et al. [5] restored to favor the role of the diaphragm. This study on the cat shows that the oscillations of LES pressure are temporally correlated with the myoelectric activity of the diaphragm. In cases of apnea there exists an interruption of myoelectric activity and a parallel stabilization of the LES pressure at the value observed at the end of expiration.

To conclude, it may now be said that hiatus hernia is neither a necessary nor a sufficient condition for observing gastroesophageal reflux. It is common during esophagitis, since it is observed in 80 to 90% of cases of esophagitis or in reflux without esophagitis, but it is also observed in 30 to 40% of cases in healthy subjects. As a recent study of pH measurement [6] has shown the incidence of hiatus hernia increases with age whereas on the contrary that of gastroesophageal reflux does not increase with age.

It is true that the correlation of LES-reflux is better than the correlation of hiatus hernia-reflux, and this has been shown both in studies in man and in experimental

Table 1. Mechanisms responsible for episodes of Gastroesophageal Reflux in 10 controls and 10 patients with reflux esophagitis (Dodds et al, 1928)

	Mechanisms of Gastroesophageal Reflux			Total no. of Reflux Episodes
	Transient LES relaxation	Transient intra-abdominal pressure increase	Spontaneous free reflux	
		number (per cent)		
Controls	84 (94)	4 (5)	1 (1)	89
Patients	228 (65)*	59 (17)*	65 (18)*	352*

* Significantly different from controls ($p < 0.01$).

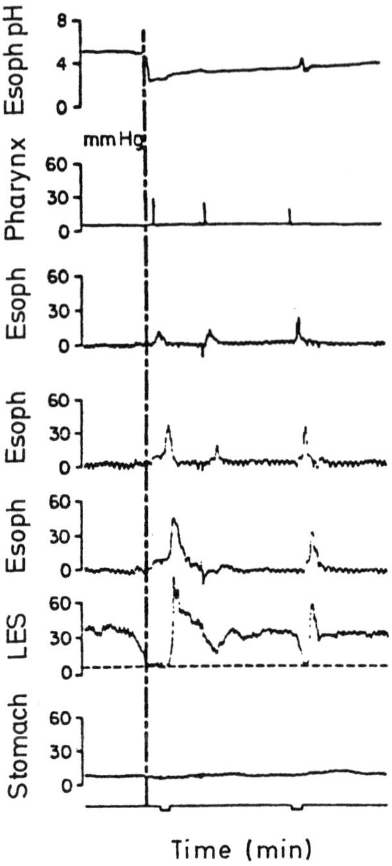

Fig. 4. Gastroesophageal Reflux associated with a transient Lower Esophageal Sphincter (LES) relaxation in a patient with reflux esophagitis (Dodds et al, 1982)

animal models, notably in the dog. However, it is legitimate to link sphincteric and anatomic factors. In fact it is established that the position of the LES in the abdomen locates it in a zone of positive pressure which contributes to impermeability of the cardiac region, the diaphragm playing an important part, and attention has recently been drawn to the possibility of anomalies of clearance in subjects with hiatus hernia.

References

1. Cohen S, Harris LD (1971) Does hiatus hernia affect competence of the gastroesophageal sphincter. N Engl J Med 284: 1053–1056
2. Kahrilas PJ, Dodds WJ, Hogan WJ, Kern M, Arndorfer RC, Reece A (1986) Esophageal peristaltic dysfunction in peptic esophagitis. Gastroenterology 91: 897–904
3. Dent J, Dodds WJ, Friedman RH et al (1980) Mechanism of gastroesophageal reflux in recumbent asymptomatic human subjects. J Clin Invest 65: 256–267

4. Dodds WJ, Dent J, Hogan WJ et al (1982) Mechanisms of gastroesophageal reflux in patients with reflux esophagitis. N Engl J Med 307: 1547–1552
5. Boyle JT, Altschuler SM, Nixon TE, Tuchman DN, Pack AI, Cohen S (1985) Role of the diaphragm in the genesis of lower esophageal sphincter pressure in the cat. Gastroenterology 88: 723–730
6. Spence RAJ, Collins BJ, Parks TG, Love AHG (1985) Does age influence normal gastroesophageal reflux? Gut 26: 799–801

Can the natural history of reflux esophagitis be defined?

G. Bommelaer, A. Abergel, S. Ajmi, M. Dapoigny, and *R. Tournut* † (Clermont-Ferrand)

As far back as the last century, when the peptic ulcer condition of the esophagus was firstly described by Quincke [13], and still in the 40's when Allison [2] picked up again its description, the theory of a peptic disease of the esophagus, linked to hiatus hernia, and whose course led from the erosive esophagitis to stricture of the esophagus was built up. Since then, numerous authors, particularly Savary, have perfectly illustrated the affiliation which exists between gastroesophageal reflux, erosive esophagitis, ulcer and stricture of the esophagus, the appearance of a columnar epithelium in the lower esophagus and the double risk of an ulcer in the Barrett's epithelium or of an adenocarcinoma [3, 5, 14, 16].

Without disputing the concept of a link between these various conditions, for which several proofs will be briefly recalled, we would like to focus on some recent data from the literature, which show that:

- lesions can heal spontaneously
- there is no parallelism between the evolution of symptoms and lesions
- it is possible to alter the natural history of reflux esophagitis.

The various grades of esophagitis correspond to various degrees of increasing severity and chronology

Arguments for this statement are numerous, we shall take most of them from Savary's papers [16].

At the time of diagnosis, the older the patients the more severe were the lesions: 50, 56, 60 and 62 years old respectively for the grades 1, 2, 3 and 4 of Savary's endoscopic classification [15]. The history of symptomatic reflux was longer in patients with a stricture of the esophagus, as compared to patients with ulcers of the esophagus [1]. The course of reflux esophagitis exhibits a marked tendency towards ulceration, parietal fibrosis responsible for the esophageal stricture, and regeneration of the esophageal epithelium into a columnar type leading to "Barrett's esophagus" [16]. So, the strictures of the esophagus occured preferentially at the 4th grade of reflux esophagitis. In the same way, the maximal incidence of Barrett's esophagus occured during the 7th decade, with a respective incidence of 6%, 1.9% and 50% in grades 1.2 and 3 of Savary's classification [16]. Finally the incidence of adenocarcinoma of the esophagus was statistically correlated to the presence of a Barrett's esophagus: 31 cases in a series of 284 Barrett's esophagus, that is almost 10%, with a mean age of 65.6 years in this survey [16].

These few data are in complete agreement with the theory of a disease with stages of increasing severity from esophagitis with erosions until Barrett's esophagus, a real preneoplastic lesion.

The spontaneous evolution of reflux esophagitis does not necessarily lead to a constant and progressive increase in the severity of the lesions

From a follow-up of 142 patients suffering from reflux esophagitis without stricture over 1 to 108 months, Palmer reported that the endoscopic lesions worsened in 28% of the patients, persisted in 20%, decreased in 17% and disappeared in 35% without any treatment [14]. Therefore, according to Palmer, the course of reflux esophagitis is totally unpredictable.

Other workers like Dedieu [9] and Behar [5], on the basis of retrospective epidemiological studies, reported two kinds of evidence against a direct line between erosive esophagitis, ulcerous esophagitis and esophageal stricture: in their experience the mean age of occurence of the three forms of esophagitis was the same and the change of an esophagitis with ulcers to an esophageal stricture was never observed in 13 cases followed for 30 months [9]. These conclusions are in accordance with data obtained in the control groups of several recent double-blind randomized therapeutic studies on reflux esophagitis: under placebo, lesions cleared in 30 to 50% of the patients [4, 6, 7, 11, 12, 18, 19]. The worsening of the lesions was seldom seen, namely in 10 to 15% of the patients. However, in this kind of study, the follow-up was short, lasting no more than 6 or 8 weeks. The major cause for a stricture to occur would be the existence of mechanisms peculiarly responsible for this course, such as a decreased lower esophageal sphincter pressure or a lack of peristalsis of the lower esophagus, rather than a delay in the course of the reflux [1]. Moreover, the incidence of malignant transformation of the esophagus, which theoretically represents the ultimate risk in esophagitis, was not statistically correlated to the prevalence of esophagitis in the survey reported by Savary [16]. Within 20 years, among 3000 esophagitis that he observed, he found only 31 adenocarcinomas, each one occuring in a Barrett's epithelium.

The natural course of symptoms correlates poorly with the course of the lesions

According to Palmer, the majority of the esophagitis, 75% out of 413, were asymptomatic when they were not associated with stricture, and for Dedieu, patients were more frequently asymptomatic when they had an ulcerous esophagitis (11%) than when they only had an erosive esophagitis (0%) [9, 14].

Therefore, an improvement of the symptoms could very well be associated with a worsening of the endoscopic lesions. Such a discrepancy in the course of symptoms and lesions was particularly frequent in the therapeutic trials with H2-inhibitors, which were generally reported as very efficient on symptoms but without any effect on the lesion score [6, 18]. In the same way, the symptoms of gastroesophageal reflux were less frequent in esophageal strictures than in erosive or ulcerous esophagitis, when dysphagia was more frequent, namely 50% of the patients according to Dedieu [9]. Nevertheless, dysphagia was in no way specific of the stricture since it was observed in 30% of erosive esophagitis and 28% of esophagitis with ulcers [9, 14, 17].

So, clearly there is a dissociation between the nature and the intensity of the symptoms on one hand and the severity of the endoscopic lesions on the other, so that estimation of the course of the lesions from the course of the symptoms alone is extremely hazardous. It is possible that a difference in esophageal sensitivity from one person to another, as can be evaluated by a Bernstein test, could explain the differential course of symptoms and lesions [6], as stated by Behar [6]. It remains to be established whether a decreased sensitivity of the esophagus could be the cause or the consequence of a more severe esophagitis.

How can the natural course of reflux esophagitis be modified?

On average, the natural course of reflux esophagitis begins at the age of 55 [9,16]. We have previously shown the crucial role of age in the natural course of the disease in the adult, the more severe lesions being generally found in older subjects. In the new-born, ageing usually leads to maturation of the lower esophageal sphincter competence, which should prompt the physician to be conservative when dealing with a reflux esophagitis in early life [8].

Chronic alcoholism, smoking and NSAID have been incriminated as causal factors in the epidemiology of esophagitis [9]. The question as to whether discontinuing these drugs could lead to an improvement of the lesions of esophagitis remains open.

No one study has shown so far that medical treatment when discontinued could alter the main mechanisms responsible for the genesis of reflux esophagitis, either lower esophageal pressure or peristalsis of the lower esophagus. Experimental data on animals suggest that healing of esophageal lesions could restore a normal lower esophageal peristalsis, restoring a normal esophageal clearance, which could provide the esophagus with a better defence mechanism against acid reflux [10].

On the other hand, surgical treatment, whatever it is, clearly modifies the natural course of the disease, by increasing the lower esophageal sphincter pressure, even if several neural pathways involved in its regulation are not restored [4].

In conclusion, many uncertainties remain about the natural course of reflux esophagitis. It is clear, however, that even in the absence of any treatment, esophagitis can clear or recur intermittently and unpredictably. The epidemiology of the disease is still too poorly known to propose definite exogenous factors that can interfere with its natural course. Surgery alone appears at this moment likely to alter the pathophysiological determinants of the reflux esophagitis in a durable way.

References

1. Ahtaridis G, Snape WJ, Cohen S (1979) Clinical and manometric findings in benign peptic strictures of the oesophagus. Dig Dis Sciences 24: 858–861
2. Allison PR (1948) Peptic ulcer of the oesophagus. Thorax 3: 20–42
3. Barrett NR (1950) Chronic peptic ulcer of the oesophagus and oesophagitis. Br J Surg 38: 175–182
4. Behar J, Sheahan DG, Biancani P, Spiro HM, Storer EH (1975) Medical and surgical management of reflux esophagitis. A 38-month report on a prospective clinical trial. N Engl J Med 293: 263–268
5. Behar J (1976) Reflux esophagitis. Pathogenesis. Diagnosis. Treatment. Arch Int Med 136: 560–566
6. Behar J, Brand DL, Brown FC, Castell DO, Cohen S, Crossley RJ, Pope CE II, Winans CS (1978) Cimetidine in the treatment of symptomatic gastroesophageal reflux. Gastroenterology 74: 441–448
7. Berstad A (1981) Overview of ranitidine in reflux oesophagitis: its effect on symptoms, endoscopic appearance and histology. In: The clinical use of ranitidine, Misiewicz JJ and Wormsley KG (eds), Medicine Publishing foundation, Oxford pp 297–304
8. Boix-Ochoa J, Casasa JM, Gil Vernet JM (1985) Gastroesophageal reflux in pediatrics: experience in 2000 cases. In: Esophageal disorders: pathophysiology and therapy, DeMeester TR and Skinner DB (eds), Raven Press, New York 459–468
9. Dedieu P, Gaillard F, Lavignolle A, Sugier H, Gibon M, Daveluy P, Perrin D, Miniconi P (1981) Oesophagites par reflux: aspects épidémiologiques, anatomo-pathologiques et evolutifs (123 cas). Gastroentérol Clin Biol 5: 266–274
10. Eastwood GL, Castell DO, Higgs RH (1975) Experimental esophagitis in cats impairs lower esophageal sphincter pressure. Gastroenterology 69: 146–153
11. Graham DY, Patterson DJ (1983) Double-blind comparison of liquid antacid and placebo in the treatment of symptomatic reflux esophagitis. Dig Dis Sciences 28: 559–563
12. Koelz HR, Birchler R, Bretholz A, Bron B, Capitaine Y, Delmore G, Fehr HF, Fumagalli I, Gehrig J, Gonvers JJ, Halter F, Hammer B, Kayasseh L, Kobler E, Miller G, Münst G, Pelloni S, Realini S, Schmid P, Voirol M, Blum AL (1986) Healing and relapse of reflux esophagitis during treatment with ranitidine. Gastroenterology 91: 1198–1205
13. Quincke H (1879) Ulcus oesophagi ex digestione. Deutsch Arch Klin Med 24: 72–74
14. Palmer ED (1968) The hiatus hernia-esophagitis-esophageal stricture complex. Am J Med 44: 566–579
15. Savary M (1971) L'expression endoscopique de l'œsophagite par reflux. International broncho-oesophagological Society. XII Congress, Simep Edit Villeurbanne 101–118
16. Savary M, Ollyo JB (1986) L'œsophagite par reflux et ses complications: ulcère sténose, endobrachyœsophage. Encycl Med Chir (Paris, France). Oto-rhino-laryngologie, 20822 A10, 10: 16 p.
17. Skinner DB (1966) Symptomatic esophageal reflux. Am J Dig Dis 11: 771–778
18. Soule JC, Pariente EA, Moschoutis P (1982) Cimétidine et reflux gastro-œsophagien. Gastroentérol Clin Biol 6: 662–668
19. Wesdorp ICE, Dekker W, Klinkenberg-Knol E (1981) Evaluation of ranitidine in the treatment of reflux oesophagitis. In: The clinical use of ranitidine, Misiewicz JJ and Wormsley KG (eds) Medicine Publishing foundation, Oxford, pp 293–296

What is the rate of gastric acid secretion in patients with esophagitis?

M. Mignon, S. Bruley des Varannes, Th. Vallot, and *J. P. Galmiche* (Paris and Nantes)

Among the multiple factors involved in the pathogenesis of reflux esophagitis, 2 are directly connected with the secretory and motor patterns of the stomach:

a) volume and agressivity of the refluxed gastric content, especially in the case of acid reflux.
b) alteration in the pressure-gradient between stomach and esophagus mainly when some degree of gastric empyting impairment exists, the latter being itself susceptible to causing increased gastric secretion in response to a meal.

Much controversy exists concerning the gastric acid secretory status of patients with peptic esophagitis and secretion was found increased, unchanged or decreased in respectively five, two, and one studies [1]. Most of these studies, however, dealt with small series of patients so that sampling hazard cannot be excluded.

Two very recent studies deserve further attention:

1. Using the Fordtran and Walsh intragastric titration technique as adapted in our laboratories, to measure gastric acid response to food, Bruley des Varannes et al. [1] simultaneously assessed acid secretion and liquid protein meal emptying: acid secretory status did not differ between a control group and patients with reflux esophagitis whatever the degree of severity of the esophageal lesions (Fig. 1).

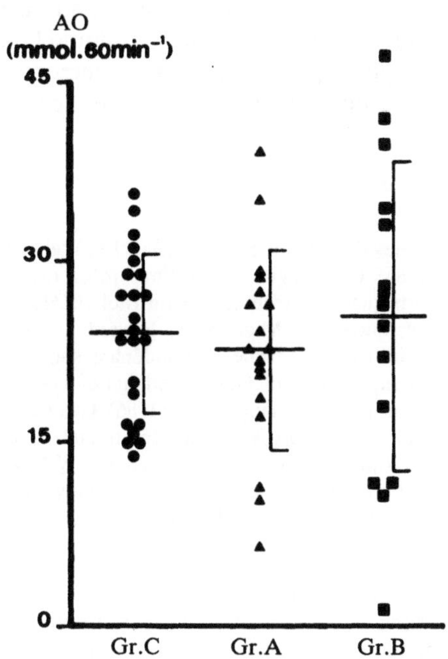

Fig. 1. Individual values for acid output after intragastric introduction of 400 ml liquid protein meal. Gr. C: control; Gr. A: grade 2–3 esophagitis; Gr. B: grade 0–1 esophagitis

No correlation was found between secretory data and the score of a 3-hour-postrandial esophageal pHmetry. However, in patients with severe esophageal lesions, a linear negative correlation was noted between half-time for gastric emptying and the resting pressure of the lower esophageal sphincter.

2. Diverging results are reported by Johansson and Tibbling [3]: according to these authors, 76% of patients with reflux esophagitis secreted an excessive amount of acid in response to maximal histamine stimulation. The relatively low specificity of the reference values used, however, decreases the relevance of Johansson and Tibbling findings [3].

An extremely important observation was reported, nevertheless, by the same authors: it was demonstrated that in patients responding (symptomatic response) to Ranitidine (150 mg twice day/8 weeks) the reduction in basal and histamine stimulation was greater than in non-responders; furthermore, in the responders there was no longer any period of acid reflux in the supine position (data from 24 hour esophageal pH-monitoring).

In summary, gastric acid secretion probably varies greatly in patients with reflux esophagitis whatever the parameter studied [1, 3, 5, 6]. It is satisfying, however, to note that the most drastic reduction in acid secretion suppresses esophageal acidification in the supine position and concurrently renders patients symptom free.

Accordingly,

a) gastric antisecretory treatment is justified in patients with reflux esophagitis and increased posology mandatory provided that acid reflux has been documented in patients with incomplete symptomatic response;
b) acid secretion is undoubtedly pathogenetic for esophageal mucosa, together with other gastric factors such as liquid [1–5] or solid [7] emptying impairment and/or esophageal factors such as decreased lower esophageal sphincter pressure or reduced esophageal acid clearance.

References

1. Bruley des Varannes S, Touchais JY, Weber J, Desechalliers JP, Sauger F, Denis P, Galmiche JP (1986) Œsophagite par reflux: rôles respectifs des facteurs pathogéniques œsophagiens et gastriques. Gastroenterol Clin Biol 10: 662–668
2. Merrouche M, Mignon M, Rigaud D, Accary JP, Chayvialle JA (1985) Conséquences de l'acidification antrale et duodénale sur le débit acide, la réponse gastrinique et la vidange gastrique chez l'ulcéreux duodénal et le sujet normal. Gastroenterol Clin Biol 9: 902–910
3. Johansson KE, Tibbling L (1986) Gastric secretion and reflux pattern in reflux oesophagitis before and during ranitidine treatment. Scand J Gastroenterol 21: 487–492
3. Blackman AH, Lambert DL, Thayer WR, Martin HF (1970) Computed normal values for peak acid output based on age, sex and body weight. Am J Dig Dis 15: 783–809
5. Baldi F, Corinaldesi R, Ferrarini F, Stanghellini V, Miglioli M, Barbara L (1981) Gastric secretion and emptying of liquides in reflux oesophagitis. Dig Dis Sci 26: 886–889
6. Boesby S (1977) Relationship between gastroesophageal acid reflux, basal gastroesophageal sphincter pressure and gastric acid secretion. Scand J Gastroenterol 12: 547–551
7. Micali B, Albanese V, Baldari S, Cogliandolo A, Gulino FM, Scarpignato C (1986) Vidange gastrique des solides au cours du reflux gastro-œsophagien. Gastroenterol Clin Biol 10: 656–661

What factors intervene in the genesis of esophageal mucosal lesions caused by reflux?

A. Papazian (Amiens)

Some clinical and experimental studies have demonstrated the noxious effect on the esophageal mucosa of hydrochloric-peptic gastric secretions and of bilio-pancreatic secretions. Esophagitis may develop after total gastrectomy in 0 to 50% of cases, depending on the type of restoration of continuity. This esophagitis has been termed "alkaline" although it is not the alkalinity of the reflux fluid that is responsible, but its content of known toxic substances such as bile acids (BA), lysolecithin and pancreatic trypsin.

Experimental data

These are set out in Table 1: it seems that in different animal species, hydrochloric acid, gastric juice, bile, bile acids and pancreatic juice may produce esophagitis. It is important to note that a combination of these various factors is more harmful than of any one factor.

Table 1. Esophageal toxicity of gastroduodenal reflux: experimental data

year	author	subject	results
1951	Cross [1]	cat dog	bile → esophagitis pancreatic juice → esophagitis
1962	Lambert [2]	rat	pancreatic juice alone and pancreatic + gastric juice → more severe esophagitis than with bile alone
1972 1975	Henderson [3] Safaie-Shirazi [4]	dog dog	bile + acid → esophagitis bile or acid alone → 0 bile increases mucosal permeability to H+ ions
1981	Hopewood [5]	man	bile acids at high concentration → lesions at all pH values bile acids at low concentration → lesions only at acid pH values

Clinical data

Some clinical findings, set out in Table 2, demonstrate the noxious effect of bilio-pancreatic secretions on the esophageal mucosa in man. In particular, patients affected by Biermers' disease, and therefore completely deprived of acid secretion may suffer from pyrosis and exhibit esophagitis at endoscopy [6]. A positive correlation has been shown between the presence or absence of pyrosis on the one

Table 2. Esophageal toxicity of gastroduodenal reflux: clinical data

year	author	results
1973	Orlando, Bozymski [6]	pyrosis and esophagitis in patients with Biermer's disease
1974	Kaye, Showalter [7]	positive correlation between gastric concentration of BA and pyrosis
1974	Stol et al. [8]	positive correlation between gastric concentration of BA and hiatus hernia
1977	Himal [9]	esophagitis after operation reducing or abolishing gastric secretion
1981	Papazian, Minaire, Moulinier, Lambert [10]	positive correlations between pyrosis, esophagitis and esophageal lesions due to BA after gastrectomy

hand and the presence or absence of esophagitis on the other, including the intensity of esophagitis due to bile acids in gastrectomized patients [10].

Interrelations of different factors

While the 3 primary secretions: gastric (hydrochloric acid pepsin), biliary (bile acids) and pancreatic (lysolecithin, trypsin), are noxious to the esophageal mucosa, this damage may vary with their combination. Lillemoe et al [11] have shown that the combination of tauro-deoxycholate and pepsin in acid medium produces mucosal aggression as quantified by a parametric score that is less severe than the application of pepsin alone in the rabbit's mucosa. Salo and Kivilaakso [12, 13] have shown that, in the rabbit mucosa, a chelate and taurocholate mixture produce no aggression; trypsin is aggressive, increased by the addition of chelate; a mixture of taurocholate and pepsin is not aggressive and the addition of hydrochloric acid to the mixture of taurocholate and pepsin produces aggression.

This synergy of the noxious effects of the different constituents of the duodeno-gastro-esophageal fluid may explain the varied lesions observed in different patients, depending on the qualitative and quantitative amounts of each constituent.

References

1. Cross FS, Wangensteen OH (1951) Role of bile and pancreatic juice in production of esophageal erosions and anemia. Proc Soc Exp Biol Med 77: 862–866
2. Lambert R (1962) Relative importance of biliary and pancreatic secretions in the genesis of esophagitis in rats. Am J Dig Dis 7: 1026–1033
3. Henderson D, Mugashe F, Jeejeebhoy KN, Cullen J, Szezepanski M, Boszko A, Marryatt G (1972) The role of bile and acid in the production of esophagitis and the motor defect of esophagitis. Ann thoracc Surg 14: 1465–1472

4. Safaie-Shirazi S, DenBesten L, Zike WL (1975) Effect of bile salts on the ionic permeability of the esophageal mucosa an their role in the production of esophagitis. Gastroenterology 68: 728–733
5. Hopewood D, Bateson MC, Milne G, Bouchier IA (1981) Effects of bile acid and hydrogen ion on the fine structure of esophageal epithelium. Gut 22: 306–311
6. Orlando RC, Bozymski EN (1973) Heartburn in pernicious anemia. A consequence of bile reflux. N Engl J Med 289: 522–523
7. Kaye MD, Showalter JP (1974) Pyloric incompetence in patients with symptomatic gastroesophageal reflux. J Lab Clin Med 83: 198–200
8. Stol DW, Murphy GM, Leigh Collis J (1974) Duodeno-gastric reflux and acid secretion in patients with symptomatic hiatal hernia. Scand J Gastroenterol 9: 97–101
9. Himal HS (1977) Alkaline gastritis and alkaline esophagitis: a review. Can J Surg 20: 403–412.
10. Papazian A, Minaire Y, Lambert R, Moulinier B (1981) Esophageal bile reflux after gastric surgery. Scand J Gastroenterol 16: 177
11. Lillemode KD, Johnson LF, Harmon JW (1985) Tauro-deoxycholate modulates the effects of pepsin and trypsin in experimental esophagitis. Surgery 97: 662–667
12. Salo JA, Kivilaakso E (1982) Role of luminal H+ in the pathogenesis of experimental esophagitis. Surgery 92: 61–68
13. Salo JA, Kivilaakso E (1984) Contribution of trypsin and cholate to the pathogenesis of experimental alkaline reflux esophagitis. Scand J Gastroenterol 19: 875–881

Can the brief duration of action of antacids enable them to practically decrease nocturnal acidity?

J.-C. Soulé, and *L. Stanescu* (Paris)

Antacid administration after a meal raises intragastric pH. The magnitude and duration of this rise depends on: the antacid potency (neutralizing and buffering capacities) of the preparation used, the amount given and the timing of administration, the gastric secretory response to eating and the rate of gastric emptying, which varies in different patients and with meal content. Fordtran et al [1] have shown that in duodenal ulcer patients the administration of 30 ml of a liquid antacid (Maalox; neutralizing capacity 78 mEq) one hour after a light meal induced a 50% mean reduction in gastric acidity 2 hours later. With a 60 ml dose, a fivefold reduction was achieved in most patients and a 10-fold reduction in approximately half of them. However, the response of individual patients to antacid therapy varied widely. In contrast, in "hyposecretors" a 30 ml dose of Maalox invariably induced acidity 3 hours after the end of the meal.

The reduction of postprandial intragastric acidity after antacid ingestion should normally result in a decrease in acid gastroesophageal reflux (GER) during the same period, especially as it increases lower esophageal sphincter pressure [2]. Behar and Bianconi [3] have shown that, in patients with GER and normal gastric acid secretion, a 30 ml dose of liquid Aluminium-Magnesium hydroxide given immediately after the meal reduced GER in the 30–150 min postprandial period but not later on.

These results obtained despite faulty methodological conditions allow us to assume that antacids given in optimal conditions should be very efficient. This was confirmed by Desechalliers et al [4]: in 15 patients, the administration of a 70 mEq dose of a liquid antacid 1 hour after a standardized meal was found to reduce postprandial GER, the mean Kaye score [5] decreasing from 283 to 107.

Contrary to their prolonged effect on intragastric pH when given 1 hour after a meal, antacids have a short duration of action when ingested in the fasting state. Administration of a 15 ml dose of Maalox in the fasting state was found to maintain intragastric pH above its initial value for no longer than 70 minutes [6, 7] and above 3 and 3.5 for 51 minutes [7] and 38 minutes [6] respectively.

So it seems unlikely that administration of an antacid at bedtime will be able to control nocturnal GER.

This presumption must however be critically reviewed as antacid efficiency may be influenced by several factors:
- The beginning and duration of the nocturnal period taken into account, particularly the delay between meal and bedtime,
- The dosage schedule of the antacid,
- The rate of gastric emptying,
- The times at which GER occurs during the night.

1. Some people go to bed early after dinner. If we consider that the nocturnal period starts with bedtime, part of the postprandial period during which GER should be controlled will be included in the nocturnal period.

2. Repeated antacid ingestion 3 hours after dinner will extend and reinforce the effect of the first ingestion (1 hour after meal) and should decrease GER for one more hour at least (since a 39 mEq dose of Maalox ingested in the fasting state raises intragastric pH above 3 for one hour), especially as an ingestion 3 hours after a meal cannot be compared to one in the fasting state.

3. The rate of gastric emptying of a meal varies widely in different patients and is greatly influenced by its content [8]. The increase in the protidic and the caloric content of the meal (whether from glucidic or lipidic sources) [10] and alcohol ingestion [11] slacken gastric emptying dramatically. Three hours after the ingestion of a 800 ml meal containing 880 Kcalories, intra gastric percentages of ingested liquids and solids exceeded 50% [10]. Moreover a delayed gastric emptying has been observed in almost half of the patients with GER [12].

   So it can be expected that ingestion of a high dose of antacid 3 hours after a meal will be able to neutralize intragastric acid and decrease GER for a period far exceeding one hour.

4. Among patients with GER, about 60% reflux during both day and night and 20% during the night only [13, personal results], To our knowledge, repartition of the reflux episodes in the night has not been studied.

With this object, we have reexamined the 24 hour esophageal pH recordings performed in our 21 last patients with typical reflux symptoms and a GER assessed on a DeMeester score [14] exceeding 18 (2 standard deviations above the mean in control volunteers).

Thirteen refluxed during both day and night and 4 during the night only. We have considered 3 periods: the post-dinner; period (PDP) including the 3 hours following dinner; the initial nocturnal period (INP) corresponding to the first 3 hours of the night after PDP; the total nocturnal period (TNP) between the end of PDP and getting up from bed. Nineteen of the 21 patients refluxed during PDP. Twelve of the 17 patients with a nocturnal reflux (70%) refluxed solely (10 patients) or mainly (2 patients) during INP.

Antacid administration 3 hours after dinner should permit control of nocturnal reflux in those patients whose reflux occurs solely in the first part of the night, i.e. in about half of the patients.

The effect of antacids on nocturnal GER has been evaluated by a single study which concluded their inefficiency: reduction of the number of reflux episodes without any reduction of their duration [4]. However, this conclusion cannot be accepted without reservation mainly because the patients were not their own controls.

We therefore decided to carry out a new study. Esophageal pH monitoring was performed in each patient on 2 consecutive days. The content and the timing of the meals were identical in both days. The patients ingested 30 ml of water 1st day) or 30 ml of Maalox (2nd day) 1 H½ and 3 H after each meal.

The duration of reflux (percentage of time above pH4) in the previously defined periods under each regimen were compared. Only 4 patients with a nocturnal reflux have been studied as yet. In 3, nocturnal reflux was limited to the INP. They all had an important reflux in the PDP.

Under Maalox treatment, GER:

a) in the PDP was suppressed in 3 patients and remained unchanged in the 4th;
b) in the INP was suppressed in 2 patients, slightly decreased in 1 and increased in the last;
c) in the TNP was suppressed in 2 patients and increased in the other 2.

Although no definite conclusions can be drawn considering the small number of patients studied these results suggest, that antacids, given in optimal conditions, have no reproducible effect on nocturnal GER, and that they even may be inefficient in patients whose reflux is limited to the first part of the night.

The short duration of action of AA, but also individual factors and particularly the changing pattern of reflux episodes along the night may explain these results.

References

1. Fordtran JS, Moravoski SG, Richardson CT (1973) In vivo and in vitro evaluation of liquid antacids. N Engl J Med 288: 923–928
2. Cargill G, Onorati CL (1985) Effets comparés d'un anti-acide fort et des alginates sur la pression sphinctérienne inférieure de l'œsophage étudiée par manométrie. Med Chir Dig 14: 81–84
3. Behar J, Bianconi P (1976) Effect of oral metoclopramide on gastroesophageal reflux in the post-cibal state. Gastroenterology 70: 331–335
4. Desechalliers JP, Galmiche JP, Touchais JY, Denis P, Colin R (1984) Ranitidine, Cimetidine, Antacids and gastro-oesophageal reflux: Results of a 20-hour oesophageal pH study. Int J Clin Pharm Res 4: 217–222
5. Kaye MD (1977) Postprandial gastro-oesophageal reflux in healthy people. Gut 18: 709–712

6. Bergmann JF, Isal JP, Caulin C, Simoneau G, Segresta A (1987) Mesure du Ph intragastrique chez l'homme après ingestion d'antiacide en comprimés. Gastroenterol Clin Biol 11:35 A
7. Monges H, Hancy A, Rouison D, Chabaud M (1971) Etude comparative de l'action des antiacides sur le pH gastrique. Mesure in situ par télémétrie. Bulletin de la Société de Gastroentérologie du Littoral Méditerranéen, (sept), Tome VII
8. Minami H, McCallum RW (1984) The physiology and pathophysiology of gastric emptying in humans. Gastroenterology 86:1592–1610
9. Ruskoné A, Cosnes J, Vidon N, Gouzigou P, Bernier JJ (1980) Secretion et vidange gastriques après différents repas homogénéïsés chez l'homme. Gastroenterol Clin Biol 4:777–785
10. Jian R, Ruskone A, Filali A, Ducrot F, Rain JD, Bernier JJ (1986) Effet de l'augmentation de la charge calorique d'un repas sur la vidange gastrique de ses phases solide et liquide. Gastroenterol Clin Biol 10:831–836
11. Jian R, Cortot F, Ducrot F, Jobin G, Chayvialle JA, Modigliani R (1986) Effect of ethanol ingestion on postprandial gastric emptying and secretion, biliopancreatic secretions and duodenal absorption in man. Dig Dis Sci 31:604–614
12. McCallum RW, Berkowitz DM, Geier E (1981) Gastric emptying in patients with gastroesophageal reflux. Gastroenterology 80:285–291
13. Le Guillou M, Robaszkiewicz M, Geier B, Cauvin JM, Le Roux G, Gouerou M (1986) Reflux gastro-œsophagien acide. Intérêt de la pH-métrie ambulatoire de longue durée. Gastroenterol Clin Biol 10:183 A
14. Johnsson LF, DeMeester TR (1974) Twenty-four hour pH monitoring of the distal esophagus, a quantitative measure of gastroesophageal reflux. Am J Gastroenterol 62:325–332

Is the use of antacids justified in biliary reflux?

A. Papazian (Amiens)

Duodenal reflux of biliary-pancreatic secretions (DGR) has been incriminated in a certain number of acute and chronic disorders of the stomach and esophagus [1]. The general principles of treatment of DGR and/or its consequences are:

- to reinforce antro-pyloric tonus and resist the motor phenomenon of reflux
- to protect the gastric or esophageal mucosal barrier
- to neutralize the aggressive agents in the reflux fluid, particularly the bile acids (BA).

No controlled study has so far proved the efficacy of any drug in the treatment of DGR and/or its consequences. Only certain special experimental and clinical studies have dealt with one or other aspect of treatment. In this context, it may seem useful to know whether so-called "antacid" drugs may be of value for apart from their antacid action based on their neutralizing and/or buffer effect(s) the AA are also endowed with rheologic properties useful in explaining the "dressing" effect empirically acknowledged for these agents. These rheologic properties may vary from one drug to another and with the environmental pH; in vitro aluminium phosphate has proved the most effective AA drug from this aspect [2]. These AA drugs directly protecting the gastric and esophageal mucosal barrier by their "drewsing" action, are also endowed with a chelating power as regards BA.

Selective studies

Clain et al [3] in 1977 showed in vitro that pure aluminium hydroxide was a chelating agent for BA, with an efficacy comparable to that of cholestyramine. This chelation was better for dihydroxyl BA than for trihydroxyl BA and better for glyo conjugated BA than for tauroconjugated BA. In their experiments the pH during incubation varied between 6.8 and 10 depending on the combination of BA and AA used. They did not feel it possible to reproduce the conditions of gastric pH (acid) as the pH obtained by acidification of the medium was unstable and promoted the precipitation of the glyco-conjugated BA and it was difficult then to distinguish chelation from precipitation. The study was made with tauro-deoxycholate, which like all the tauro-conjugated BA, remained soluble at acid pHL; chelation did not then appear modified.

Malaga et al [4] in 1979 showed in vivo that pure aluminium hydroxide and cholestyramine reduced the gastric concentrations of BA as effectively as the Roux-en-Y procedure if the gastrectomized patients suffering from so-called "alkaline" gastritis. Cousar and Gadacz [5] in 1984 showed in vitro that the hydroxysulfates of aluminium and magnesium chelated dihydroxyl BA at pH 7 as effectively as cholestyramine, the other AA tested exhibiting less effectiveness.

Vatier's study [6]

Vatier in 1986 studied in vitro the chelating power of cholestyramine (Questran), aluminium phosphate (Phosphalugel), hydroxides of aluminium and magnesium (Maalox) and the hydroxysulfates of aluminium and magnesium (Riopan). The originality of this study lay in the fact that it was performed in kinetic fashion by measuring the percentage of chelation after 0, 10, 30 and 60 minutes incubation, and that it involved separately a mixture of dihydroxyl BA and a mixture of trihydroxyl BA. The results of this study are summarized in Tables 1 and 2. These show that:

Table 1. Fixation (%) of Dihydroxyl BA (GDC + TDC)

	Time (min)	cholestyramine	PO_4Al	AlMgOH	magaldrate
pH 1.8	0	65	52	62	11
	10	56	40	71	22
	30	47	49	85	41
	60	66	36	80	17
pH 3.5	0	66	47	40	15
	10	91	22	15	20
	30	78	48	40	22
	60	62	70	27	26
pH 6	0	94	42	48	8
	10	74	21	42	22
	30	88	3	18	28
	60	93	4	38	11

* Unpublished results

Table 2. Fixation (%) of trihydroxyl BA (C + Tc)

	Time (min)	cholestyramine	PO_4Al	Al Mg OH	magaldrate
pH 1,8	0	42	55	48	12
	10	64	20	61	16
	30	73	60	46	32
	60	37	26	44	36
pH 3,5	0	42	45	30	11
	10	42	68	47	17
	30	57	67	36	26
	60	52	68	28	10
pH 6	0	50	40	44	12
	10	65	66	50	18
	30	77	59	43	25
	60	62	59	41	14

unpublished results

1. Phosphalugel and Maalox are markedly superior to Riolan, both for dihydroxyl BA and for trihydroxyl BA
2. Compared with Questran, Maalox chelates bihydroxyl BA best at pH 1.8; Phosphalugel chelates trihydroxyl BA as well at pH 1.8 and best at pH 3.5.
3. Compared with each other, Phosphalugel and Maalox differ according to the pH involved and the BA solution. For dihydroxyl BA, Maalox chelates best at pH 1.8 and Phosphalugel at pH 3.5. For trihydroxyl BA, Phosphalugel chelates best at pH 1.8 to 3.5

3 in practice, it would seem useful in treatment to employ cholestyramine, often taken as a reference agent in vitro. The animal in vivo studies are inconsistent [in 1] and its ineffectiveness against symptoms of alkaline gastritis have been demonstrated in man [6]. Cholestyramine does not bind to the BA in molecular form; at a gastric pH less than the pKa of the BA the latter are arranged in molecular form. Hence it seems preferable to use the AA in therapy since their efficacy in chelation of BA has at least been proved in vitro. Controlled studies in man certainly seem necessary.

References

1. Papazian A, Nguyen-Phuoc BK (1982) Le reflux duodéno-gastrique: mise en évidence, affections associées, conséquences, traitement. Gastroenterol Clin Biol 6: 1020–1028
2. Papazian A, Vatier J, Bossert J, Capron JP, Boisrame B (1986) Comment choisir un bon topique digestif? Nouvelles bases rationnelles du choix thérapeutique. Entretiens de Bichat, Thérapeutique, 1 octobre 1985 – Paris Société Nationale Française de Gastro-entérologie, 12 mars 1986 – Nice, Congrès Mondial de Gastro-entérologie, 12 sept 1986 – Sao Paulo
3. Clain JE, Malagelada JR, Chadwick VS, Hofmann AF (1977) Binding properties in vitro of antacids for conjugated bile acids. Gastroenterology 73: 556–559
4. Malagelada JR, Phillips SF, Higgins JA, Shorter RG, Van Heerden JA, Adson MA (1979) A prospective evaluation of alkaline reflux gastritis: bile acid binding agents and Roux-Y. Diversion. Gastroenterology 76: 1192

5. Cousar GD, Gadacz TR (1984) Comparison of antacids on the binding of bile salts. Arch Surg 119: 1018–1020
6. Vatier J Résultats personnels. Non encore publiés.
7. Meshkinpour H, Elashoff J, Stewart H, Sturdevant RA (1977) Effect of cholestyramine on the symptoms of reflux gastritis. Gastroenterology 73: 441–443

Is the antalgic effect of antacids on reflux pain linked with a neutralizing action? (Comparison with placebo)

F. Vicari (Nancy)

Yes:

- The antacids (A.A.) act in neutralizing the H^+ ions of stomach and of the liquid flowing back into the esophagus whose pH they increase significantly.
- The AA induce a reactional hypergastrinemia by alkalinisation leading to an increase in the pressure of the inferior sphincter of the esophagus.
- The alginates, which are not antacids, are nevertheless classified with medications of this group. If they do not modify the gastric acidity, they are able to reduce the esophageal acidity due to reflux, by both an anti-reflux mechanical action and by local antacid action in the esophagus in case of severe reflux, when alginate flows back before the gastric contents.

No:

- The AA also have a local role. A topical remedy with a non-antacid compound (Polysilane gel) also gives positive results on pyrosis of the GER.

This last point indirectly answers the possible comparison of an AA with a placebo. Contrary to what has been done for anti-H2 authoritative works about AA versus placebo have not been carried out in GER, at least so far as we know.

What is the effectiveness of antacids on the healing of esophageal lesions?

R. Colin, and *E. Lerebours* (Rouen)

For many years, the antacids have represented the mainstay of the medical treatment of gastroesophageal reflux (GER). The effectiveness of antacids against the symptoms of GER and particularly on pyrosis has been demonstrated [4, 6], but the few controlled studies [1, 5, 6] evaluating the effect of antacids on the lesions of esophagitis and in a general way on the natural history of esophagitis causing symptoms have given negative results. These disappointing results raise three questions:

- Are the published controlled studies altogether reliable as regards methodology?
- Are the antacids really ineffective?
- Are further controlled studies evaluating the effect of antacids on esophagitis desirable?

Three controlled studies have assessed the action of antacids on esophagitis in acute treatment [5,6] or in long-term treatment [1] by comparing them with a placebo [5, 6], ranitidine [6] or surgery [1]. These.studies exhibit one or more methodologic defects: a small number of patients incurring a Beta risk (e.g. 10 subjects in the study of Graham and Patterson); a short duration of acute treatment (5–6 weeks); doubtful selection for inclusion (exclusion of subjects responding symptomatically to a weak antacid in the study of Graham and Patterson, and selection of severe and long-standing cases in the study of Behar et al.

The negativity of the results of controlled studies of esophagitis does not allow us to conclude that antacids are ineffective. These agents neutralize the H^+ ions present in the stomach and so reduce their concentration in the reflux fluid. Under the influence of antacids in the usual dosages, long-term measurements of pH show in subjects with acid reflux a significant reduction in the proportion of time spent under each level of acid pH; this decrease is no different from that obtained with cimetidine lg/day but less than that obtained with ranitidine 300 mg/day, especially as regards the lowest levels of pH [2]. This neutralizing action probably accounts for the favorable effects of antacids on pyrosis.

Their apparent ineffectiveness for the lesions of esophagitis may be associated with an insufficient reduction of H^+ ions and a limited action in time because gastric emptying temporarily leaves the mucosa of the esophagus in contact with an aggressive medium. The favorable results in esophagitis reported with powerful antisecretory agents of long action argue in support of this hypothesis. It is possible that in certain cases factors other than chlorhydropeptic aggression may be involved in the genesis and maintenance of the lesions of esophagitis; such factors are not combated by antacid treatment.

The initiation of new controlled studies evaluating the therapeutic action of antacids on the lesions of esophagitis may appear inopportune at a time when several recent studies (reported in other sections of this work) have revealed the real efficacy of treatment based on a powerful and prolonged antisecretory effect. The motivation of such an undertaking rests on a possible improvement of the cost-benefit relationship which might support the use of antacids, either alone or in combination. It should probably be reserved for symptomatic esophagitis with minor lesions (grade 1 in Savary's classification).

References

1. Behar J, Sheahan DG, Biancani P et al (1975) Medical and surgical management of reflux esophagitis. N Engl J Med 293: 263–268

2. Desechalliers JP, Galmiche JP, Touchais JY, Denis P, Colin R (1984) Ranitidine, Cimétidine and gastro-oesophageal reflux: results of a 20-hour oesophageal pH study. Int Clin Pharm Res 4: 217–222
3. Graham DY, Lanza F, Dorseh ER (1977) Symptomatic reflux esophagitis: a double blind controlled comparison of antacids and alginate. Curr Ther Res 22: 653–658
4. Graham DY, Smith JL (1981) Why are some apparently healthy people heavy antacid users? Gastroenterology 80: 1161
5. Graham DY, Patterson DJ (1983) Double blind comparison of liquid antacid and placebo in the treatment of symptomatic reflux esophagitis. Dig Dis Sci 28: 559–563
6. Grove O, Bekker C, Jeppe-Hansen MG et al (1985) Ranitidine and high-dose antacid in reflux oesophagitis. A randomized, placebo controlled trial. Scand J Gastroenterol 20: 457–461

What is the effect of alginates on acid neutralization and on LES pressure?

J. Vatier, and *M. T. Vitré* (Paris)

Introduction

The physicochemical modifications of alginic acid in an acid medium result in the formation of a gel capable of floating on top of the acid fluid level. This property is used in the treatment of gastroesophageal reflux, as the gel obtained isolates the gastric and esophageal mucosae from the aggressive effect of the gastric contents, in particular hydrochloric acid and pepsin. Topaal (Laboratoires Sinbio), a treatment for gastroesophageal reflux, contains, in addition to alginic acid, substances with an antacid activity.

The evaluation of the in vitro pharmacological properties of this drug must answer the following questions: is the drug able to reduce the aggressive acid content of the stomach and therefore exert an antacid activity, and most importantly, can a pH gradient be created between the intragastric contents and the surface of the gel in contact with the mucosa?

In order to answer these questions, we investigated and quantified the antacid effect, determined the pH gradient under various conditions of acidity in a static medium, and evaluated the antacid capacity and the variations of the pH gradient between the liquid phase and the gel in a dynamic system, i.e. in a model simulating acid secretion and gastric emptying.

Material and Methods

1. Study

The study was conducted with Topaal, tablet and powder form (alginic acid, colloidal aluminium hydroxide, silica and magnesium carbonate); the tablet form contains half as much alginic acid (200 mg) as the powder form (400 mg).

2. *Techniques used*

a) Investigation and quantification of an antacid effect

The techniques used have been published previously [1] and their principles are recalled. They are based on the evaluation of the antacid activity in a static medium, as they do not take into account the effect of gastric emptying. The antacid mechanism of action was evaluated by continuous titration of a therapeutic unit of the drug against a 0.1 N hydrochloric acid solution. The titration curve, a graphic expression of the variation in pH as a function of the acid content, is able to demonstrate neutralization, characterised by a concomitant variation in pH with the addition of acid, and the buffer property which, conversely, is characterised by the absence of modification of pH despite the addition of acid.

The antacid capacities were measured by intermittent titration of a unit dose of the drug against a 0.1 N hydrochloric acid solution over a sufficiently long period of time to allow liberation of all of the H^+ ions binding sites, as recommended by Fordtran [2]. The titrations were performed from the spontaneous pH of the aqueous suspension of the drug up to levels of pH compatible with gastric secretion, i.e. with values for pH at the end of titration of pH 3.0, pH 2.0 and pH 1.0.

b) Investigation of the pH gradient between the liquid phase and the supernatant

This was performed by adding test doses of the drug corresponding to 500 mg of alginic acid to volumes of hydrochloric acid solution of different concentrations and by recording the variations in pH by means of two combined electrodes, one immersed in the liquid phase and the other immersed in the gel.

The test dose of 500 mg of alginic acid was placed in contact with 25, 50 and 100 ml of 100 mmol/l HCl and with 50 and 100 ml of 130 mmol/l HCl, i.e. with 2.5, 5.0, 6.5, 10.0 and 13.0 mmol of acid the pH values were measured over a period of 15 minutes.

c) Evaluation of the antacid capacity and the variations in pH gradient in a dynamic system

The model used [3] consisted of a reservoir into which a flow was introduced, simulating acid secretion, and from which part of the liquid content was extracted by a flow simulating gastric emptying. The reservoir contained 100 ml of 0.1 N HCl (pH 1.0) subjected to moderate agitation (20 r.p.m.); the secretion flow of 0.1 N HCl was constant at 3 ml/min and the emptying flow was variable: 3.0 or 4.5 ml/min, corresponding to a rate of emptying equal to the rate of secretion and greater than the rate of secretion. The combined electrodes were immersed in the contents of the reservoir in the liquid phase and in the supernatant gel. They were connected to a pH measuring and recording system. The tests were conducted with the equivalent of 500 mg or 1.000 mg of alginic acid. This protocol was used to evaluate the variations in pH gradient and the antacid capacities in response to permanent modifications in acidity and drug concentrations.

Table 1. Results of the evaluation of the antacid capacities of Topaal tablet and Topaal powder in a static system

	mmol H^+ bound per therapeutic unit or per gram of drug			
	Topaal tablet		Topaal powder	
	1 tab	g	1 sachet	g
pH 3.0	1.07	0.63	2.75	0.83
pH 2.0	1.60	0.94	3.73	1.13
pH 1.0	2.95	1.74	5.00	1.50

	Potential therapeutic capacity mmol H^+ bound per therapeutic unit	
	Topaal tablet	Topaal powder
from pH 1.0 to pH 2.0	1.35	1.27
from pH 1.0 to pH 3.0	1.88	2.25

Results

Antacid action: mechanism and antacid capacity

The mechanism of action of Topaal in the closed system essentially consisted of a neutralization effect due to the presence of silica and magnesium carbonate. The specific activity of aluminium hydroxide, normally responsible for a buffer action at pH of about 1.3–1.5, was masked by the neutralization.

The antacid capacities, expressed in mmol of acid bound per therapeutic unit or per gram of drug, measured from the spontaneous pH to pH 3.0, 2.0 and 1.0, are shown in Table 1. When expressed per gram of drug, they were essentially identical for the powder and the tablet forms; however, the differences observed were due to the varying degrees of dispersion of these two pharmaceutical forms. These titration values were used to calculate the potential therapeutic capacities [4], i.e. the number of mmol of acid consumed to raise the pH from 1.0 to 2.0 or to 3.0, i.e. to reduce the acid concentration by 90% or by 99%. It should be noted that the formation of gel was only observed at titrations at pH 1.0. The antacid activity was released during the first ten minutes, corresponding to a rapid kinetic.

Measurement of the pH gradient in a static medium

The addition of test doses equivalent to 500 mg of alginic acid to acid solutions induced a rise in the pH of the acid phase (from pH 0.9 or 1.0 at time 0 to pH 1.2 or 2.1, depending on the acid solutions used) and the formation of gel with a higher pH than that of the acid phase, increasing with time to reach a maximal value after 6 minutes (Table 2) and then remaining constant at this level between the 6th and the 15th minute. The pH of the liquid phase and of the gel decreased as a function of the initial quantity of acid to reach a constant pH level. Fig. 1 shows the variation in pH in the presence of 500 mg of alginic acid, which was identical for the two forms of

Table 2. pH values of the liquid phase and the gel under different conditions of acidity in response to the equivalent of 500 mg of alginic acid of Topaal after 6 minutes' contact. The pH values of the gel were measured at two sites: on the surface and above the liquid phase

Experimental conditions	Topaal tablet liquid	Topaal tablet gel	Topaal powder liquid	Topaal powder gel
25 ml of 100 mmol/l HCl	3.3	4.6–4.3	2.7	3.7–3.0
50 ml of 100 mmol/l HCl	1.5	4.0–3.6	1.5	3.4–3.0
50 ml of 130 mmol/l HCl	1.4	3.0–2.7	1.2	3.0–2.7
100 ml of 100 mmol/l HCl	1.5	3.6–3.2	1.2	3.8–3.0
100 ml of 130 mmol/l HCl	1.5	3.0–2.7	1.0	3.2–3.0

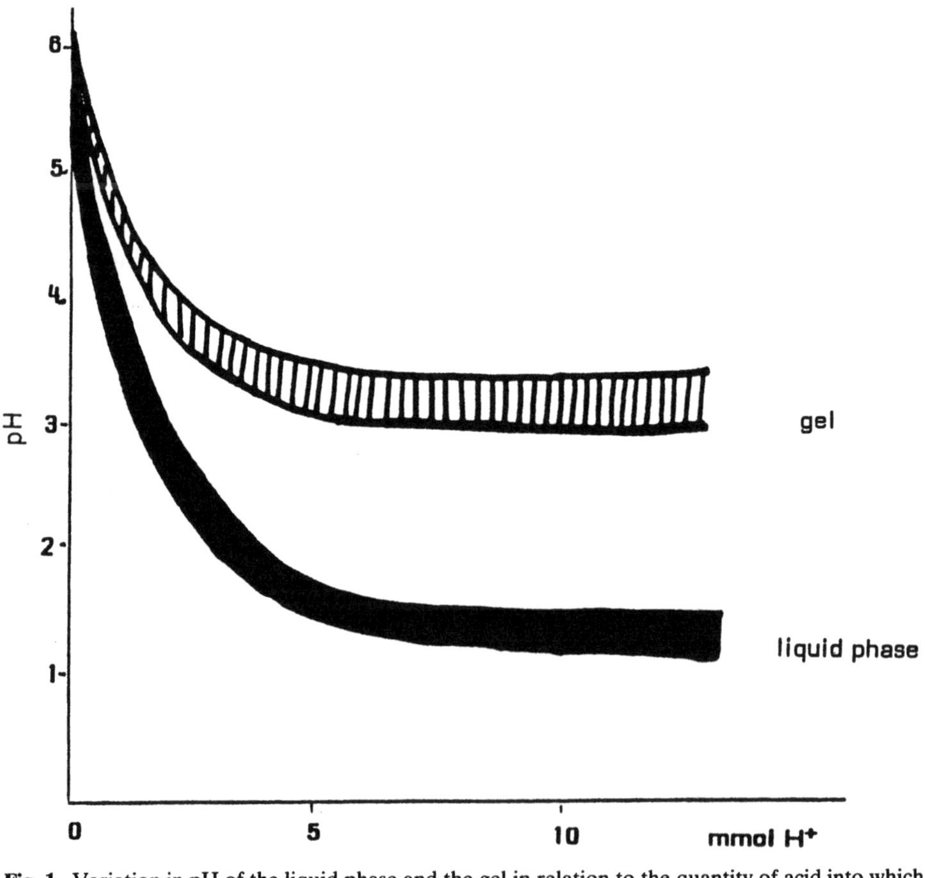

Fig. 1. Variation in pH of the liquid phase and the gel in relation to the quantity of acid into which the drugs are placed. Tests with Topaal tablet and powder. The quantity of acid, expressed in mmol, are plotted on the abscissae and the pH values are plotted on the ordinates

Topaal. These results demonstrate the existence of a pH gradient between the liquid phase and the gel, which remains at a pH greater than 3.0. The rise in pH of the acid phase is an argument in favour of the antacid activity.

Results of the dynamic study (Fig. 2, 3)

In response to the emptying flow rate of 3 ml/min, 500 mg of alginic acid induced pH levels in the gel of between pH 2.0 and 2.5, while the pH of the liquid phase, which reached pH 1.3, subsequently decreased and reached pH 1.0 between the 35th and 40th minutes. Double test doses of Topaal (1.000 mg of alginic acid) maintained the pH of the gel at a level higher than pH 3.0 for more than 30 minutes with a maximum of pH 4.2, while the pH of the liquid phase was identical to that obtained with 500 mg of alginic acid.

In response to the emptying flow rate of 4.5 ml/min, 500 mg of alginic acid induced a return to pH 1.0 in the liquid phase in less than 25 minutes, while the pH of the gel was higher than with an emptying rate of 3 ml/min for Topaal tablet and stayed around pH 2.0 with Topaal powder.

The quantity of acid consumed to reach pH 1.0 was calculated on the basis of the fact that the drugs were placed in contact with 10 mmol of acid at time 0 and that the secretion flow introduced 0.3 mmol of acid/min. At the emptying flow rate of 3 ml/min, the equivalent of 500 mg of alginic acid of the tablet and powder forms of Topaal consumed 17.5 and 19 mmol of acid, respectively; a dose of 1.000 mg consumed 22 mmol of acid. At an emptying flow rate of 4.5 ml/min, the antacid capacities were identical equal to 17.5 mmol of acid.

Discussion

Regardless of the technical modalities used, the results of this study provide two arguments in favour of the protective effect of Topaal in gastroesophageal reflux: firstly, Topaal possesses an antacid activity and secondly, in an acid medium, it induces the formation of a gel which constitutes a barrier to the diffusion of H^+ ions, by creating a pH gradient. The antacid activity can be justified on the basis of the following arguments:

1. The static evaluation of the antacid activity which revealed an antacid property based on neutralization effects, the intensity of which was relatively modest compared with that of classical antacids. For one therapeutic unit, this activity at pH 1.0 was 2.95 and 5.00 mmol of acid for Topaal tablet and Topaal powder, respectively.
2. A rise in pH of the acid solutions was observed with 100 and 130 mmol/l acid solutions; the pH of the liquid phase was increased from pH 0.9 or 1.0 to pH 1.2 and 2.1.
3. In the dynamic model, a large quantity of acid was consumed in order to return to the initial pH: between 17.5 and 22 mmol, depending on the emptying flow rate.

The differences in the results in the static and dynamic experimental models are related to the presence or absence of a permanent variation in the concentrations of

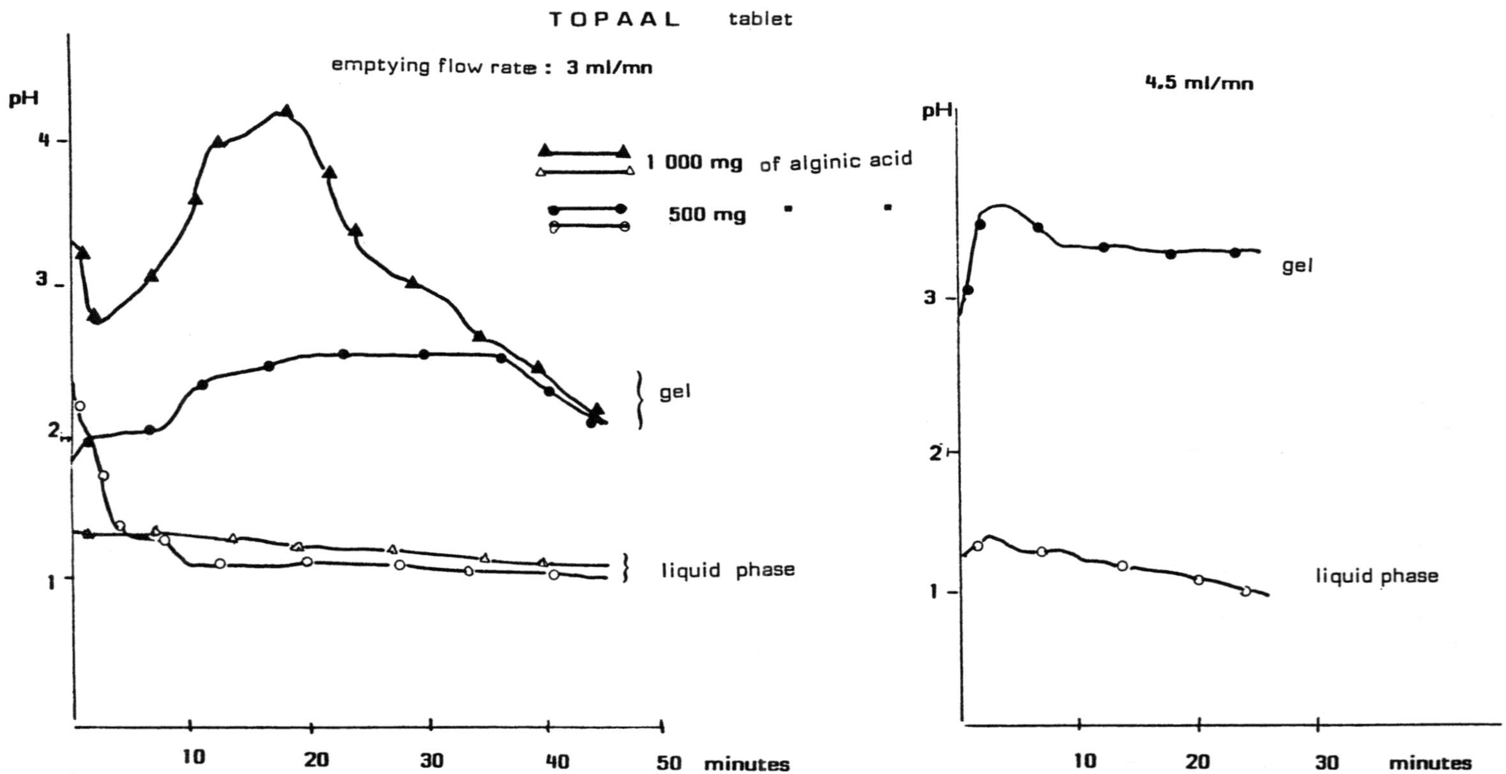

Fig. 2. pH metry recordings of the acid phase and of the gel in response to 500 mg of alginic acid contained in a Topaal tablet, as a function of the emptying flow rates of 3.0 and 4.5 ml/min. A test with 1.000 mg of alginic acid was performed with an emptying flow rate of 3.0 ml/min. The time in minutes is plotted on the abscissae and the pH values are plotted on the ordinates

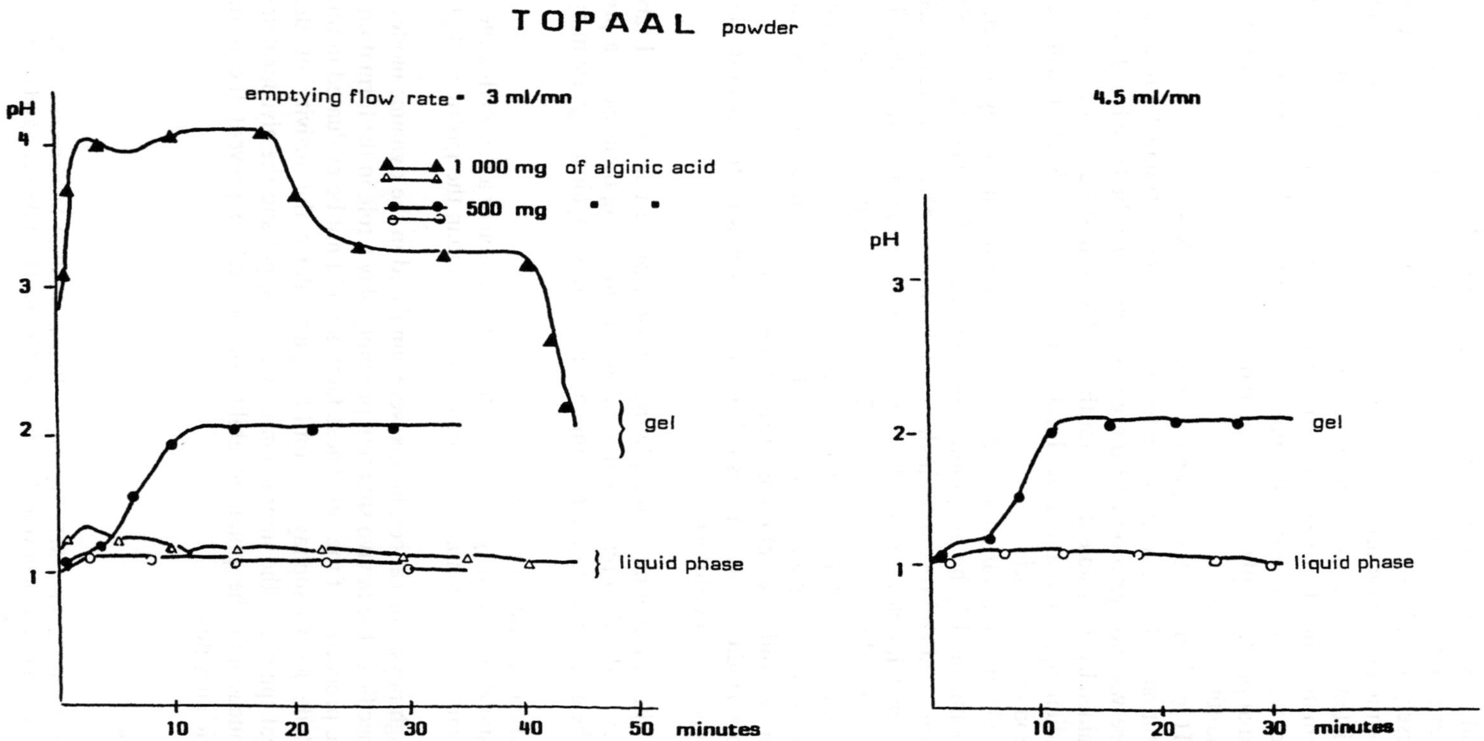

Fig. 3. pH metry recordings of the acid phase and of the gel in response to 500 mg of alginic acid contained in Topaal powder, as a function of the emptying flow rates of 3.0 and 4.5 ml/min. A test with 1.000 mg of alginic acid was performed with an emptying flow rate of 3.0 ml/min. The time in minutes is plotted on the abscissae and the pH values are plotted on the ordinates

the antacid constituents and acid. By simulating physiological acid secretion [5] and by using an emptying flow rate compatible with in vivo conditions [6], the dynamic model closely resembles physiological conditions, suggesting that, under conditions of therapeutic use, these drugs are able to exert a more potent antacid effect than that predicted on the basis of the results obtained in the static medium.

The formation and the role of the protective gel barrier warrants a few comments.

1. The gel was only formed in the presence of acid at pH of about 1.0; it was not formed at pH 3.0 or pH 2.0. It appeared and became more consistent the greater the quantity of acid.
2. The pH gradient created depended on several factors:
   a) agitation of the medium; in the test with 100 and 130 mmol/l solutions of HCl, there was no agitation and the gel was not disturbed: high pH levels were attained by the gradient (greater than pH 3.0). In the dynamic system, the pH gradient appeared at a lower level, around pH 2.0–2.5 for the same concentration of alginic acid.
   b) the pH gradient varied according to the concentration of alginic acid; in the dynamic model, the pH gradient was between pH 2.0 and 2.5 with 500 mg of alginic acid and rose to as high as pH 4.0 with 1.000 mg of alginic acid.
   c) the emptying flow rates influenced the antacid capacity and modified the pH gradient, which reached higher pH values in response to an emptying rate of 4.5 ml/min than for an emptying rate of 3 ml/min, at least for Topaal tablet. This may be explained by the fact that the acid phase is "emptied" more rapidly; while the gel tends to resist this flow.
   d) a pH gradient was established within the gel with the highest pH values recorded at the surface.

The in vitro evaluation of the pharmacological properties of Topaal tablet and powder revealed a dual pharmacological action, justifying their use as a protective agent of the gastric and esophageal mucous membranes against aggression by gastric acidity:

- an acid concentration reducing effect and
- the installation of a pH gradient due to the formation of a gel, so that the mucous membranes are in contact with higher pH levels than the gastric acid phase.

Although physiological conditions were simulated in the dynamic model, certain factors specific to the in vivo situation probably play a role in the formation and the protective properties of the gel. These factors could not be evaluated in this study; they include gastroesophageal motility, particularly the activity of the lower esophageal sphincter, the interaction between the gel and the glycoproteins of the gastric mucus and the potential ability of the gel to prevent the diffusion of proteolytic enzymes.

References

1. Vatier J, Vallot T, Vitré MT, Mignon M, Bonfils S (1983) Médicaments antiacides: étude critique de l'appréciation in vitro de la fixation des ions H^+ et de leur classification. Gastroentérol Clin Biol 7: 573–579

2. Fordtran JS, Morawski SG, Richardson CT (1973) In vivo and vitro evaluation of liquid antacids. N Engl J Med 288: 923–928
3. Vatier J, Lionnet F, Vitré MT (1987) Un modèle d'estomac artificiel pour l'étude des antiacides: application au gel phosphalugel. Gastroentérol Clin Biol 11,2 bis, 81 A
4. Vatier J (1985) Pharmacologie des antiacides. La Vie Médicale 11: 515–522
5. Bernier JJ, Vidon N, Mignon M (1973) Intérêt d'une étude coopérative multicentrique en vue d'établir une table des valeurs normales de la sécrétion gastrique acide en fonction du sexe, de l'age et du poids. Gastroentérol Clin Biol 6: 287–296
6. Etienne A, Rigaud D, Accary JP, Mignon M (1982) Comportement sécrétoire, moteur et hormonal, de l'estomac pendant une alimentation élémentaire continue, instillée en site gastrique à différents débits chez le sujet normal. Gastroentérol Clin Biol 6: 628–637

What is the action of sucralfate in the treatment of peptic esophagitis?

S. Bonfils, and *M. Dubrasquet* (Paris)

Sucralfate is a basic saccharose sulfate of aluminium whose mode of action should prove of therapeutic value in reflux esophagitis with ulcerated lesions. It has been shown that this agent forms a complex with the proteins exposed by ulcerated gastric lesions, thereby adhering locally and constituting an effective barrier to the aggressive action of acid, pepsin and bile-salts.

Experimentally, different animal models of esophagitis have been tested. In the rabbit [6], in a model of esophagitis using acid, pepsin and taurocholic acid, the simultaneous administration of sucralfate significantly decreased the severity of the esophagitis and its resultant complications; effectiveness was less against the lesions produced by taurocholic acid. In the rat [4], in a model of chronic esophagitis produced by surgical means, and although it was impossible to prove prolonged fixation of the sucralfate on the esophagus, the beneficial effect observed was equally marked but statistically significant only during the first week of treatment.

In man, in a group of 6 patients, studies with sucralfate combined with albumin labelled with technetium-99m [3] showed that adherence to the lower esophagus was observable during nearly 3 hours in subjects with actual esophageal ulceration, but only to slight and inconstant extent in patients showing only congestive esophagitis [3] suggesting that the beneficial effect observed under therapeutic conditions cannot be simply attributed to the mechanism observed in gastroduodenal ulcer.

Positive clinical results have been reported by several teams since the 1981 report of Berges [1]. More recently, in 1985, Laitinen [5] studied the effect of sucralfate against alginate in a controlled trial in 68 patients (36 sucralfate and 32 alginate + antacid). Symptomatic improvement was noted in 68% of patients in both groups, but statistically endoscopic healing of the esophagitis was seen more often with sucralfate (53% as against 34%). This puts sucralfate within the range of treatments effective against reflux esophagitis [2–7].

In our own experience in an unpublished controlled trial sucralfate was as effective as alginate in the treatment of erosive or ulcerated esophagitis. In the treatment of very severe esophagitis with evident reflux (Kaye over 150), combination of sucralfate with an anti-H_2 drug (ineffective by itself) produced undeniable therapeutic benefit.

References

1. Berges W, Sonnenberg A, Wienbeck M (1981) Sucralfat bei Reflux-osophagitis. Dtsch Med Wschr 106: 853–854
2. Elsborg L (1987) Oesophageal reflux disease: diagnosis, pathophysiology and treatment with special reference to the role of sucralfate. Scand J Gastroenterol 22 (supp 127): 101–109
3. Goff JS, Adcock KA, Schmelter R (1986) Detection of esophageal ulcerations with technitium-99m albumin sucralfate. J Nulc Med 27: 1143–1146
4. Kosawa K, Louineau F, Dubrasquet M, Bonfils S (1985) Effet du sucralfate sur l'évolution des lésions d'une œsophagite expérimentale chez le rat. Gastroenterol Clin Biol 9: 111 A (résumé).
5. Laitinen S, Stahlberg M, Kairaluoma MI, Kiviniemi H, Paakkonen M, Lahtinen J, Poikolainen E, Aukee S (1985) Sucralfate and alginate/antacid in reflux esophagitis. Scand J Gastroenterol 20: 229–232
6. Schweitzer EJ, Bass BL, Johnson LF, Harmon JW (1985) Sucralfate prevents experimental peptic esophagitis in rabbits. Gastroenterology 88: 611–619
7. Weiss W, Brunner H, Büttner GR, Gabot M, Miederer S, Mittelstaedt A, Olbermann M, Schwamberger K, Witzel L (1983) Therapie der Refluxösophagitis mit Sucralfat. Dtsch Med Wschr 108: 1706–1711

J. P. Galmiche, D. Cloarec, and *S. Bonfils* (Nantes and Paris)

Sucralfate is an octo-sulfated salt of sucrose which has the property of polymerizing in an acid medium to form a viscous and extremely adherent gel. By using technetium-labelled sucralfate it can be shown that 2 hours after ingestion of a suspension of sucralfate there is very good adhesion of the product at the site of esophageal ulceration [1, 2]. However, this quality of adhesion does not exhaust the pharmacologic properties of sucralfate, which is also capable of absorbing bile acids in vitro and in vivo, of absorbing pepsin and – perhaps equally in the esophagus and in the stomach – exerting local cytoprotective properties [3].

The experimental basis for treatment of esophagitis with sucralfate is derived from a study by Schweitzer et al [4]. This deals with the effect on the rabbit's esophagus of perfusion with hydrochloric acid alone, hydrochloric acid and pepsin, pepsin-hydrochloric acid and sucralfate, taurocholate and taurocholate with sucralfate (Fig. 1). The results were expressed in macroscopic and histologic indices of esophagitis and the permeability of the esophageal mucosa to different molecules was also studied.

The administration of sucralfate significantly diminished the indices of esophagitis caused by both pepsin and taurocholate to an equal degree.

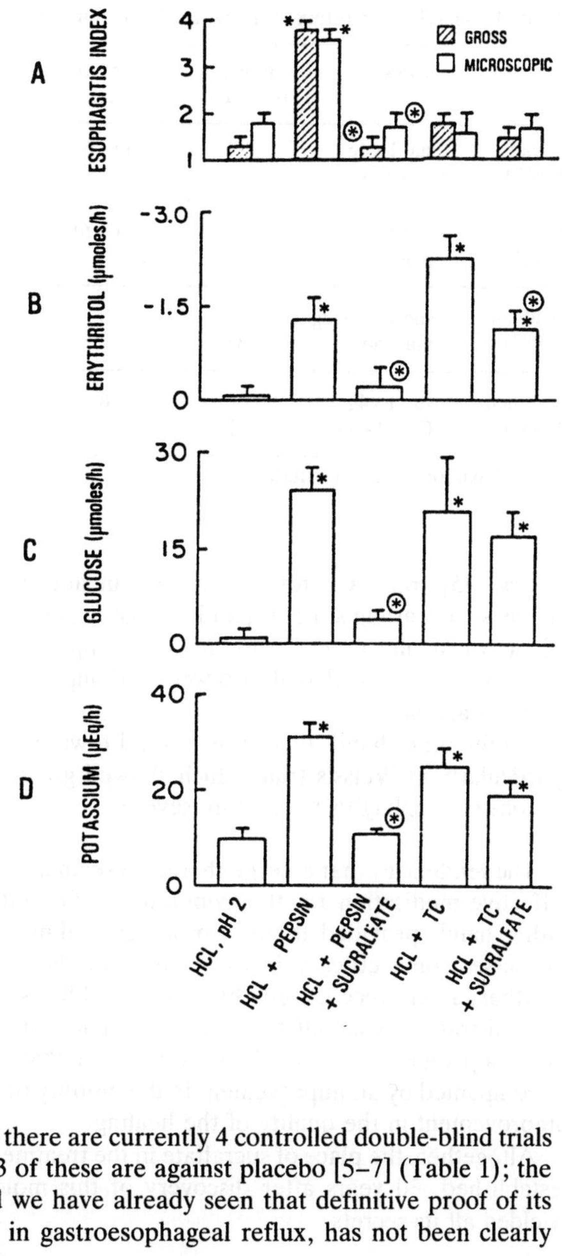

Fig. 1. Degree of esophageal injury in the initial in vivo experiments. A. Gross and microscopic esophagitis indices. B. C. and D show fluxes of erythritol, glucose, and potassium, respectively. * Significantly different from HCl at pH 2: O. Significantly different from same damaging agent but with no treatment (Schweitzer et al, 1985)

As for actual therapeutic trials, there are currently 4 controlled double-blind trials but it should be stated that only 3 of these are against placebo [5–7] (Table 1); the last is against Gaviscon® [8], and we have already seen that definitive proof of its efficacy in esophagitis, and even in gastroesophageal reflux, has not been clearly demonstrated by controlled trials.

Two of the 3 trials against placebo have been published only in summary form. These trials have generally used a dose of 4g of sucralfate suspension, except that of Williams et al [7] who used a double dose on retiring at night. The number of patients included is generally relatively few, expect in Carling's trial [6] with over 50 subjects in each group. The period of administration was 6 to 12 weeks and the course was generally assessed by the symptoms, together with endoscopic assessment of the lesions. As to the symptoms, no significant difference was seen in

Table 1. Sucralfate in reflux esophagitis: double-blind trials [5–8]

	drugs	number of patients	duration (weeks)	symptoms	lesions 6w	(% improved) 8w	12w
Weiss (1983)	suc 1×4g	22	6 (+6)	ns	45		72
	placebo	25		(+ antac)	28		40 $p<0.05$
Carling (1987)	suc 1×4g	66	6 (+6)	$p<0.002$	42		54
	placebo	61			35		41 ns
Williams (1987)	suc 1×3 + 2g	31	8	ns		81	
	placebo	37				59 ns	($p=0.007$)
Laitinen (1985)	suc 1×4g	36	6	69	53		
	Gav 2×4g	32		66 ns	34 ns		

Gav=Gaviscon® suc=sucralfate

Weiss's [5] trial save for a reduction in antacid intake; there was a significant decrease in Carling's trial [6] and no significant difference in the other two trials [7, 8] of which one used Gaviscon® for comparison. Endoscopically, no significant difference was recorded after 6 weeks, though a tendency in favor of sucralfate did seem to appear.

On the other hand, there was a trend towards significance after 8 and 12 weeks, particularly in Weiss's trial, which showed greater efficacy of sucralfate when the lesions of esophagitis were more severe.

The tendencies that emerge therefore seem as follows: this is certainly not a very effective medication for the symptoms in the initial period of treatment. On the other hand, provided there is prolonged administration, it seems that sucralfate possesses some efficacy in the healing of the endoscopic lesions of esophagitis. Further, a very recent study by Elsborg [9] has shown that after 8 and 12 weeks of administration of sucralfate there was a significant improvement in acid clearance by the esophagus (Fig. 2). Thus, it may be · that healing of these lesions is also accompanied by an improvement in the motility of the esophagus, which adds to the improvement in the quality of the healing.

Altogether, the place of sucralfate in the treatment of esophagitis is not yet clearly established. 30 years after discovery of this molecule, this product had still not yielded all its secrets.

References

1. Brooks WS (1985) Sucralfate: non ulcer uses. Am J Gastroenterol, 80: 206–209
2. Goff JS, Adcock KA, Schmelter R (1986) Detection of esophageal ulcerations with technetium 99m albumin sucralfate. J Nucl Med, 27: 1143–1146
3. Orlando RC (1987) Cytoprotection by sucralfate in acid-exposed esophagus: a review Scand J Gastroenterol, 22 suppl 127: 97–100

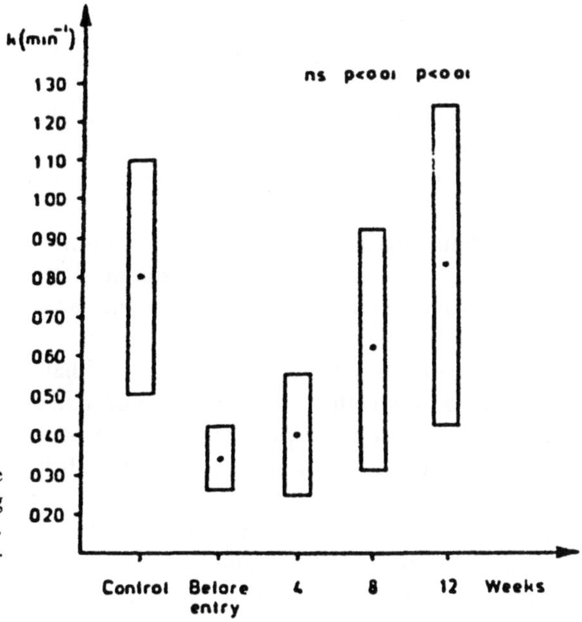

Fig. 2. Acid clearing rate from the distal esophagus before and during 12 weeks' treatment with sucralfate. Range for the reference material indicated
(Elsborg, 1987)

4. Schweitzer EJ, Bass BL, Johnson LF, Harmon JW (1985) Sucralfate prevents experimental peptic esophagitis in rabbits. Gastroenterology 88: 611–619
5. Weiss W, Brunner H. Buttner G, Gabor M (1983) Therapie der reflux ösophagitis sucralfat. DMW 108: 1706–1711
6. Carling L, Gronstedt J, Kagevi I et al. (1987) Sucralfate (suc) vs placebo in reflux esophagitis (RE). A double blind study. Gastroenterology 92: 1338 (abstr)
7. Williams RM, Orlando RC, Bozymski EM et al. (1987) Multicenter trial of sucralfate suspension in the treatment of reflux esophagitis. Gastroenterology 92: 1696 (abstr)
8. Laitinen S, Stahlberg M, Kairaludma MK et al. (1985) Sucralfate and alginate/antacid in reflux esophagitis. Scand J Gastroenterol 20: 229–232
9. Elsborg L (1987) Oesophageal reflux disease Scand J Gastroenterol 22 suppl 127: 101–109

Metoclopramide has an effect on LES pressure, esophageal contractions and gastric acid secretion

A. Bel (Lyons)

Metoclopramide (MCP), after oral or parenteral administration has no significant effect on gastric acid secretion (volume, pH, acid output, pepsin) or on serum levels of gastrin. Thus this drug without effect on gastric secretory activity is effective in peptic esophagitis in other ways, namely a pronounced effect upon esophageal and gastroduodenal motility demonstrated many years ago [3, 8].

The elevation in lower esophageal sphincter (LES) pressure after MCP is very significant, smaller in cases of reflux than in normal subjects [1, 10, 11, 4]. Intravenous or oral administration of MCP (10 or 20 mg single dose) results in an average pressure increase of 16,9 mm Hg in healthy volunteers and 10,9 mm Hg in patients with gastro-esophageal reflux [1, 2]. Healthy subjects exhibit a 100% increase of normal LES pressure. In case of hypotonic LES, pressure rises to normal level.

After administration, the onset of elevation in LES pressure begins in 2 to 5 minutes, reaches a peak in 10 to 20 minutes, and this effect lasts for at least 90 minutes. With oral administration, the values are respectively, 10 to 20 minutes, 40 minutes and 2 hours.

In the lower third of the esophagus, MCP enhances average pressure of peristaltic waves. This positive effect is more pronounced in cases of hypomotility. Sometimes, MCP was shown to cause pressure waves in patients with aperistalsis. Thus MCP accelerates clearance of the refluxed material from the oesophagus [9].

The stimulation of gastric emptying by MCP adds its own effect to those related to esophageal motility: MCP administration strongly increases the amplitude of gastric contractions, and regulates antropyloro-duodenal coordination. MCP also enhances the amplitude of duodenal contractions and induces a propulsive activity front (phase 3 of migrating motor complex) [5, 7]. These factors are necessary for evacuation of the chyme from the stomach into the duodenal bulb. This improvement of gastric emptying has been confirmed in healthy subjects, in post-vagotomy patients and in patients with diabetic gastroparesis [6].

Thus MCP, a prokinetic agent for esophagus, stomach and duodenum, is effective in the treatment of gastroesophageal reflux and peptic esophagitis.

References

1. Baumann HW, McCallum RW, Sturdevant RAL (1976) Metoclopramide – A possible antagonist of dopamine in the oesophagus of man. Gastroenterology 70: 862
2. Behar J, Ramsby G (1978) Gastric emptying and antral motility in reflux oesophagitis. Effect of oral metoclopramide. Gastroenterology 74: 253–256
3. Cohen S, Morris DW, Schoen HJ, Di Marino (AJ (1976) The effect of oral and intravenous metoclopramide on human lower oesophageal sphinter pressure. Gastroenterology 70: 484–487
4. McCallum RW, Ippoliti AF, Cooner C, Sturdevant RAL (1977) A controlled trial of metoclopramide in symptomatic gastroesophageal reflux. New England Journal of Medicine 296: 354–357
5. Malagelada JR, Rees WDW, Mazzotta LJ, Go VLW (1980) Gastric motor abnormalities in diabetic and post-vagotomy gastroparesis. Effect of metoclopramide and bethanechol. Gastroenterology 78: 286–293
6. Millar JW, Heading RC, Campbell IW, Ewing DJ, McLoughlin GP, Clarke BF (1980) Metoclopramide in diabetic gastric atony. Scottish Medical Journal 25: 176
7. Perkel MS, Hersh T, Moore C, Davidson EO (1980) Metoclopramide therapy in 55 patients with delayed gastric emptying American Journal of Gastroenterology 74: 231–236
8. Pinder RM, Brogden RN, Sawyer PR, Speight TM, Avery GS (1976) Metoclopramide – A review of its pharmacological properties and clinical use. Drugs 12: 81–131
9. Ramirez-Mata M, Ibanez G, Alarcon-Segovia D (1977) Stimulatory effect of metoclopramide on the oesophagus and lower oesophageal sphincter of patients with PSS. Arthritis and Rheumatism 20: 30–34

10. Stanciu M, Bennett JR (1973) Metoclopramide in gastro-oesophageal reflux. GUT 14: 275
11. Winnan J, Avella J, Callachan C, McCallum RW (1980) Double-blind trial of metoclopramide versus placebo-antacid in symptomatic gastro-oesophageal reflux. Gastroenterology 78: 1292

Doesn't metoclopramide allow a significant decrease in antacid consumption?

G. Cargill (Paris)

Metoclopramide, by its action on the inferior esophageal sphincter, and on the motility of the lower esophagus, decreases the incidence of gastroesophageal reflux. It is therefore logical to think that this substance may permit reduction in the intake of antacids.

This reduction is mentioned by McCallum in 1977 [1], in a trial of metoclopramide in symptomatic GER published in the New Eng. J. Med., which reported in a trial against placebo that the intake of antacids was the same during the two courses of treatment when patients received metoclopramide before the placebo but that it decreased significantly when the reverse order applied. The average daily dose was, in fact, 1.1 for patients on metoclopramide and 2.6 for those on placebo. Moreover, Bright-Asare, in 1980 [2], in a study comparing cimetidine, metoclopramide and placebo, showed that there was a significant reduction of antacid intake under treatment of the same order as that produced by cimetidine. This intake was 171 ml a week in the placebo group, 116 ml weekly in the cimetidine group and 114 ml weekly in the metoclopramide group.

In sum, it is therefore possible to affirm that metoclopramide reduces antacid intake in quite significant fashion.

Reference

1. McCallum RW et al. (1977) A controlled trial of Metoclopramide in symptomatic gastroesophageal reflux. New Engl J Med 296, 7: 354–357
2. Bright-Asare P, El Bassoussi M (1980) Cimetidine, Metoclopramide or placebo in the treatment of symptomatic gastroesophageal reflux. J Clin Gastroenterology, 149–156

Is the effect of metoclopramide on the healing of the lesions of esophagitis different from that of cimetidine?

G. Cargill (Paris)

Cimetidine is an inhibitor of H2 receptors that acts on esophagitis by means of changes it produces in the level of acid secretion. The latter is rendered less "toxic" by treatment, thus permitting healing of the esophagitis. Cimetidine has no effect on the tone of the LES, as shown by such studies as those of Freeland [1] and Carter [2].

Metoclopramide does not modofy gastric secretion, but it does alter the tone of the LES, thus participating in the restoration of an anti-reflux barrier between stomach and esophagus. Further, the modifications of motility in the lower esophagus, accompanied by improved clearance, permit an reduced contact time between the refluxing gastric content and the mucosa.

Bright Asare [3] has compared the effects of cimetidine and metoclopramide in a short term double blind study in 50 patients, 20 on metoclopramide and 10 on placebo. An assessment comprising endoscopy, study of esophageal sensitivity by Bernstein's test and a manometric study was performed before and after the 8 weeks' period of treatment.

After this period, the percentage of patients showing endoscopic improvement was slightly higher in the series treated with metoclopramide (82%) compared with other series (78% for cimetidine and placebo). The reduction in antacid intake was greater in the series treated with metoclopramide and in the cimetidine series than in the control group (114 ml – 116 ml – 171 ml per week respectively: p. 0.05). The proportion of patients with total disappearance of pain was 37% for cimetidine and 41% for metoclopramide after one week of treatment, a percentage that increased regularly up to the 8th week (80% for metoclopramide and 70% for cimetidine). The only really differing parameter between metoclopramide and cimetidine in this study was the existence of more numerous side-effects with metoclopramide.

This study resembles that of Janisch [4] comparing the efficacy in treatment of Cisapride and ranitidine for esophagitis (see Gastroenterology, 1986). Like the former, our study showed comparable efficacy of the two xenobiotics in the treatment of esophagitis.

In sum, therefore, metoclopramide and cimetidine have very different actions on reflux, one modifying gastroesophageal motility, the other the quality of the reflux, but much the same efficacy.

Reference

1. Freeland GR et al. (1977) Lower esophageal sphincter response to oral administration of Cimetidine in normal subject. Gastroenterology 72 (1): 28–30
2. Carter DC et al. (1977) Effect of Cimetidine on lower esophageal sphincter pressure. Experta Med 135–144
3. Bright-Asare P, El Bassoussi M (1980) Cimetidine, Metoclopramide or placebo in the treatment of symptomatic gastroesophageal reflux. J Clin Gastroenterol 2: 149–156
4. Janisch HD et al. (1986) A double blind multi center trial to compare the efficacy of Cisapride (Cis) and Ranitidine (Ran) in the acute treatment of gastroespohageal reflux. Gastroenterology 90

What effective dosage to propose for metoclopramide?

G. Cargill (Paris)

Metoclopramide, a substituted benzamide, is a distant cousin of Sulpiride, which acts centrally essentially as an antagonist to dopaminergic and tryptaminergic neurotransmission. Schulze-Delrieu [1], in his very complete review of this xenobiotic (Gastroenterology 1977) gives the usually administered dose as 10 mg 3–4 times a day, a dose advised in the great majority of articles in the literature.

However, doses of 60 mg/day have been suggested by S. Cohen [2] for the treatment of esophagitis. The studies of Bateman [3, 4, 5] on bioavailability of metoclopramide and those of Cohen [6], which clearly show a dose-dependent effect on the inferior sphincter, tend to suggest considerably higher dosages.

However, Schulze-Delrieu reports a 10% incidence of side-effects in adults at a dose of 10 mg 3–4 times daily. This incidence may be an overestimate and mainly concerns reactions, such as drowsiness and lassitude. But these side-effects may rarely and particularly in children, assume a much more alarming turn with dystonic reactions of the type of trismus, facial spasm, opisthotonus and oculogyric crises. These phenomena cease when treatment is stopped or the suggested doses are modified. These side-effects may be potentiated by the phenothiazines, MAOI, tricyclic antidepressants and the sympathomimetics. Finally there is a marked individual sensitivity.

Altogether, in view of the dose effect, the proportional effect on sphincteric pressure at basal pressure and the side-effects described, it seems that the dosage to be suggested is of the order of 10 mg 3–4 times daily in the adult with a preference for the oral route which allows a more prolonged action.

In children, the former dosage of 1 mg/kg/day is the source of a certain number of side-effects and a dosage of 0.5 mg/kg/day is not very effective against reflux. Our manometric and pH studies indicate that a dose of 0.8 mg/kg/day gives a proper relation between efficacy and safety and this is therefore the dose we suggest.

References

1. Schulze-Delrieu K (1979) Metoclopramide. Gastroenterology 77: 768–779
2. Harrington RA, Hamilton CW, Brogden RW, Linkewitch JA, Romankiewicz JA, Yeel RC (1983) Metoclopramide. An update review of its pharmacological properties and clinical use. Drugs 25: 451–494
3. Bateman DN, Davies DS (1979) Pharmacokinetics of Metoclopramide. Lancet I, 166
4. Bateman DN et al. (1978) Pharmacokinetic and concentration effect studies with intravenous Metoclopramide. Br J Clin Pharm 4: 640
5. Bateman DN et al. (1979) Concentration effect studies with oral Metoclopramide. Br J Clin Pharm 8: 179–182
6. Cohen S et al. (1976) The effect of oral and intravenous Metoclopramide on human lower esophageal sphincter pressure. Gastroenterology 70: 484–487

Domperidone: is its effect different from that of metoclopramide?

E. Masci (Milan)

Domperidone is a dopaminergic antagonist with antiemetic properties similar to those of metoclopramide and certain neuroleptic drugs.

The structural formula of domperidone, that is related to butyrrophenone, is different from that of metoclopramide, a procainamide derivate (Fig. 1). However, both drugs have similar effects on the motor function of the gut.

Metoclopramide increases the LES resting pressure in both (Fig. 2–3) healthy subjects and in patients with gastroesophageal reflux [1]. Single intravenous doses of domperidone increase LES pressure in healthy subjects [2], but controversial results have been reported in reflux esophagitis patients [3–4] and after oral administration [5] (Fig. 4).

As regards peristaltic activity of the esophageal body, metoclopramide was reported to increase the height and duration (Fig. 5) of esophageal contractions in both normal subjects [2] and in patients with reflux esophagitis [1].

The acid clearance of the body (Fig. 7) of the esophagus was significantly better after i.v. administration of metoclopramide [1]. However, these effects were not confirmed by another study in which no changes in the amplitude of esophageal peristaltic waves were observed after metoclopramide 10–20 mg, given orally [6].

Valenzuela et al., after domperidone 10 mg iv., did not observe a significant change in the mean amplitude of the esophageal peristaltic contractions in patients

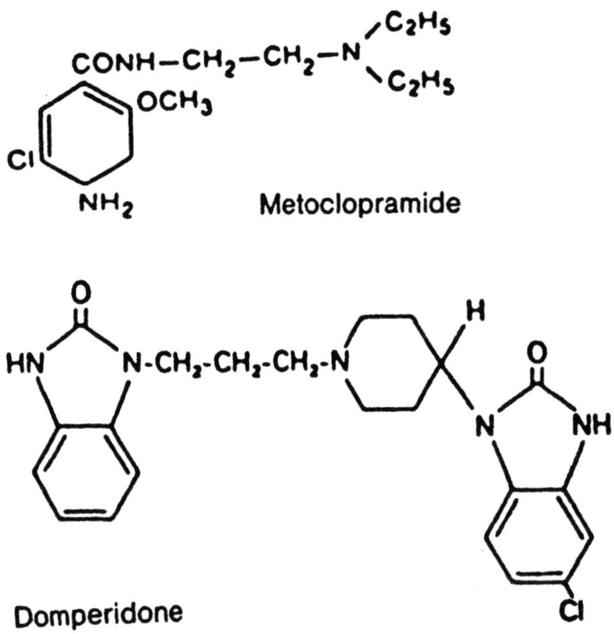

Fig. 1. Structural formula of Metoclopramide and Domperidone

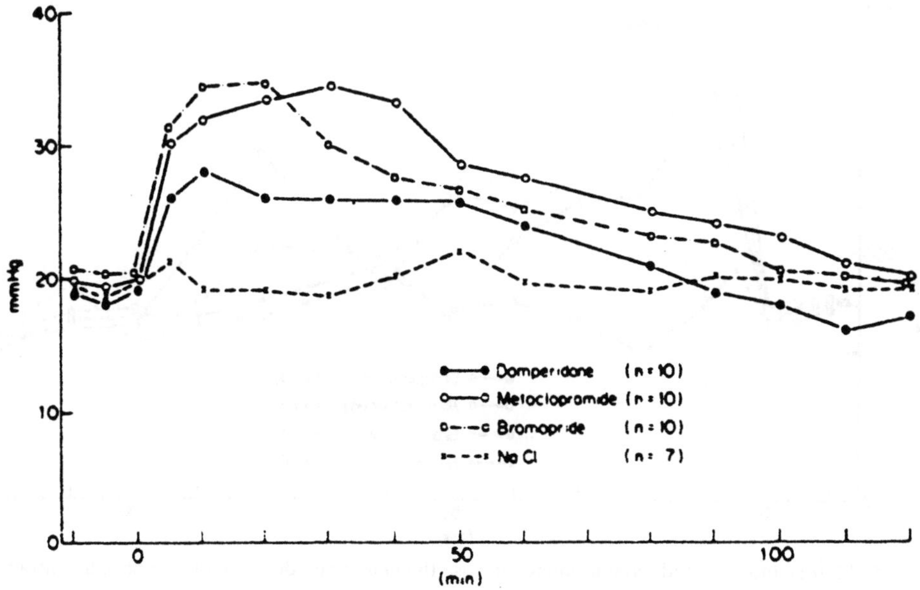

Fig. 2. Metoclopramide and Domperidone increase LES resting pressure in healthy volunteers

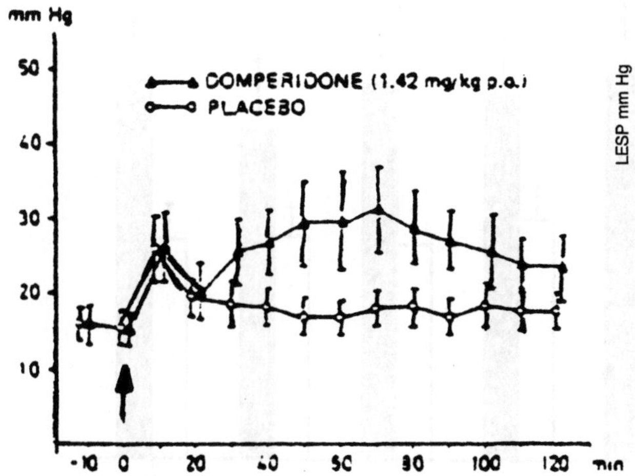

Fig. 3. LES pressure in patients with symptomatic gastro-esophageal reflux and hiatal hernia

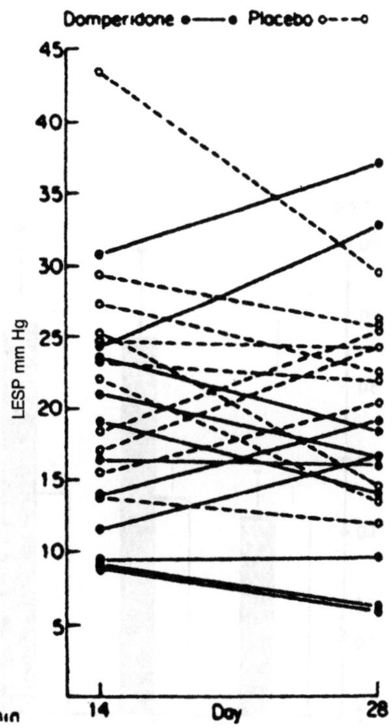

Fig. 4. No significant effects were observed on LES pressure after oral administration for 2 weeks in patients with peptic esophagitis

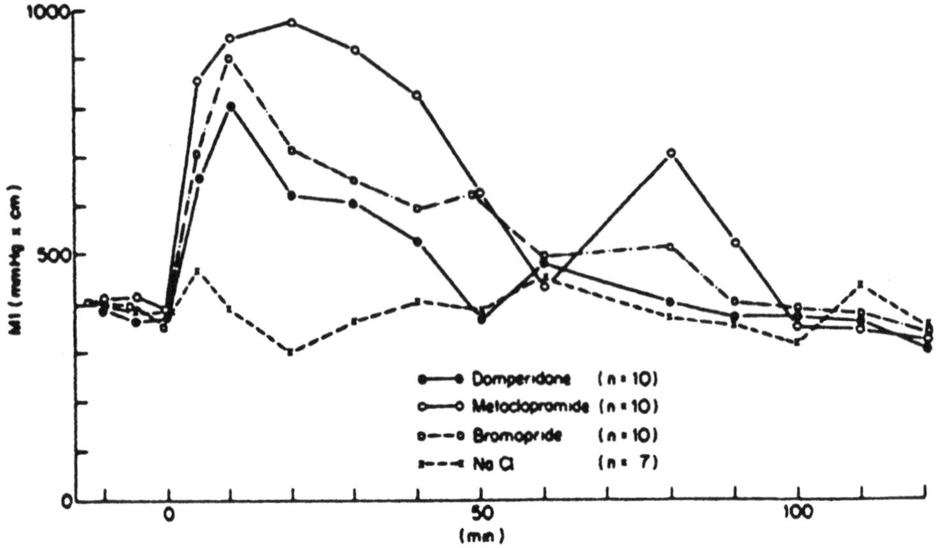

Fig. 5. Metoclopramide and Domperidone increase the height and duration of esophageal contractions

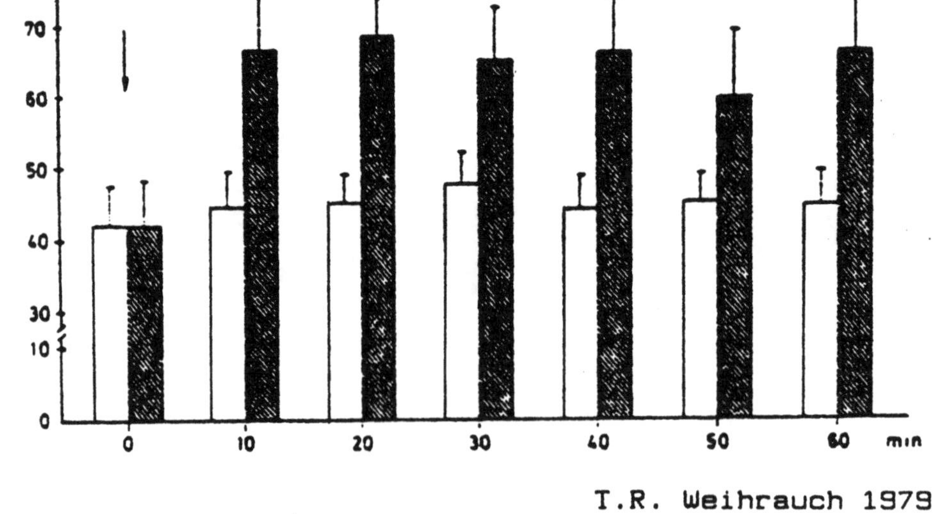

Fig. 6. Effect of Domperidone i.v. on esophageal contraction amplitudes

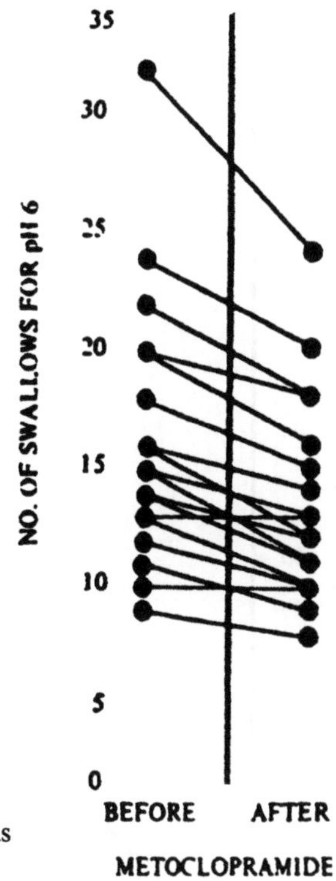

Fig. 7. The acid clearing test of the body of the esophagus was significantly better after metoclopramide administration

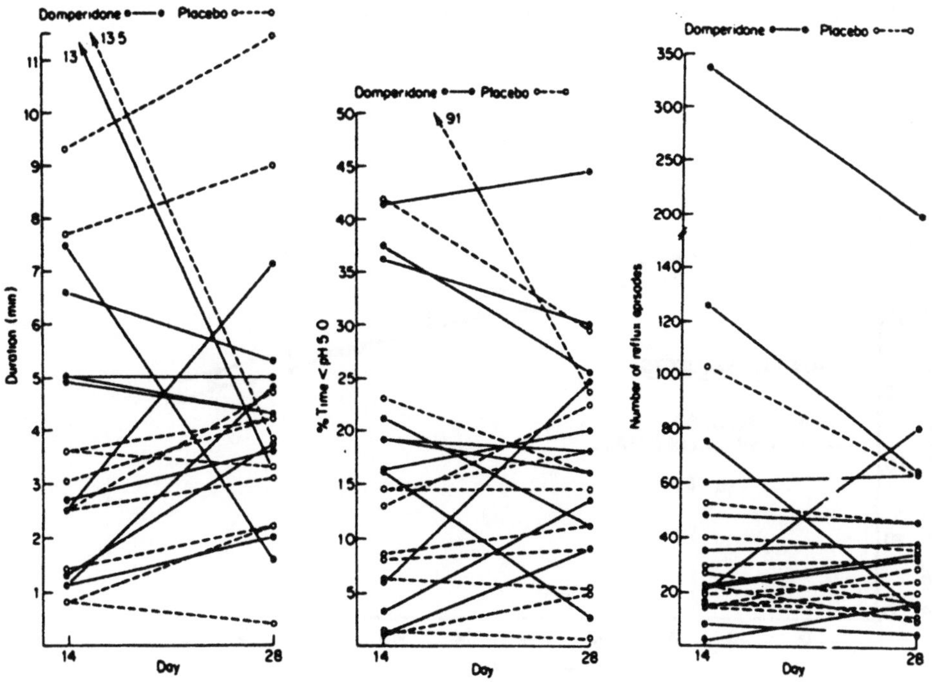

Fig. 8. No significant effect on gastro-esophageal reflux was observed after oral administration of domperidone

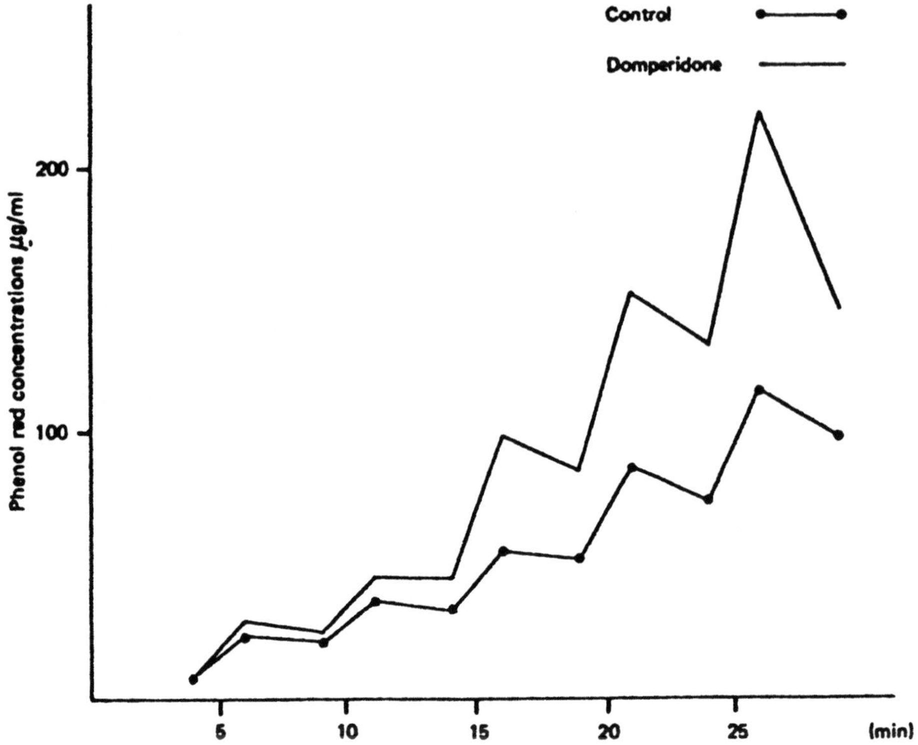

Fig. 9. Effect of domperidone i.v. on gastric emptying (liquid meal)

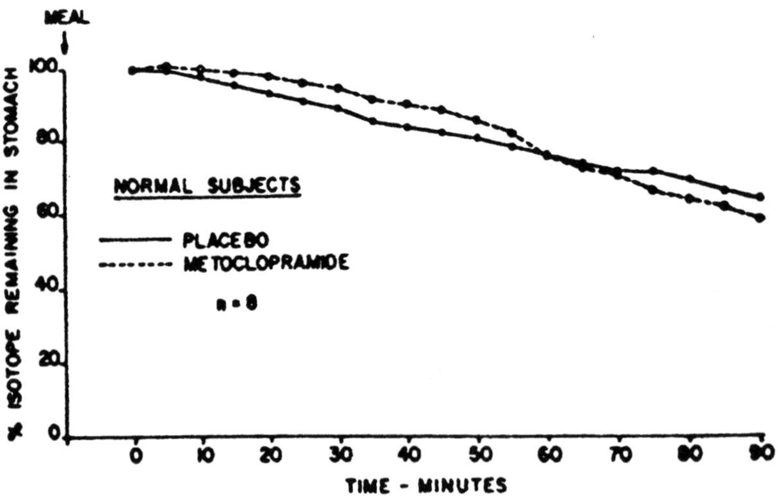

Fig. 10. No effect on gastric emptying of solid was observed in healthy subjects after Metoclopramide

with reflux esophagitis [7], but in another study a significant increase was reported (Fig. 6), [3]. No differences between domperidone and placebo were observed in gastro-esophageal reflux during a pH-metric study [5], (Fig. 8).

Different results were reported on gastric emptying when liquid or solid emptying times were studied.

With a liquid meal, domperidone showed a significant effect both in healthy volunteers and in patients with delayed gastric emptying [8], (Fig. 9). On the other hand domperidone 20 mg i.v had no significant effect on delayed gastric emptying of a radiolabelled solid meal in patients with reflux esophagitis [9]. Metoclopramide failed (Fig. 11) to modify gastric emptying of a solid meal in healthy volunteers (Fig. 10), but was significantly, effective in patients with postsurgical delayed gastric emptying [10], (Fig. 11). Both drugs were effective in conditions associated with delayed gastric emptying, such as diabetic gastroparesis or postvagotomy.

Domperidone and metoclopramide were also effective in increasing the frequency, amplitude and/or duration of antral and duodenal contractions. A better coordination between antral and dudenal contractions was observed after metoclopramide i.v. [11] and in an elegant experiment by Van Nueten et al. performed in vitro on a gastroduodenal preparation, after domperidone administration [12].

In the treatment of reflux esophagitis, despite a number of conflicting results for metoclopramide, both drugs were reported to be effective agents in the treatment of symptoms of gastroesophageal reflux (Fig. 12, Table 1).

In our experience, domperidone was also effective in promoting histological disappearance (Fig. 13–14) or improvment of esophagitis [13], whereas metoclopramide was unable to achieve similar results [14], (Table 1). In short, the main difference between metoclopramide and domperidone is that domperidone does not readily cross the bloodbrain barrier and therefore produces less extrapyramidal side-effects.

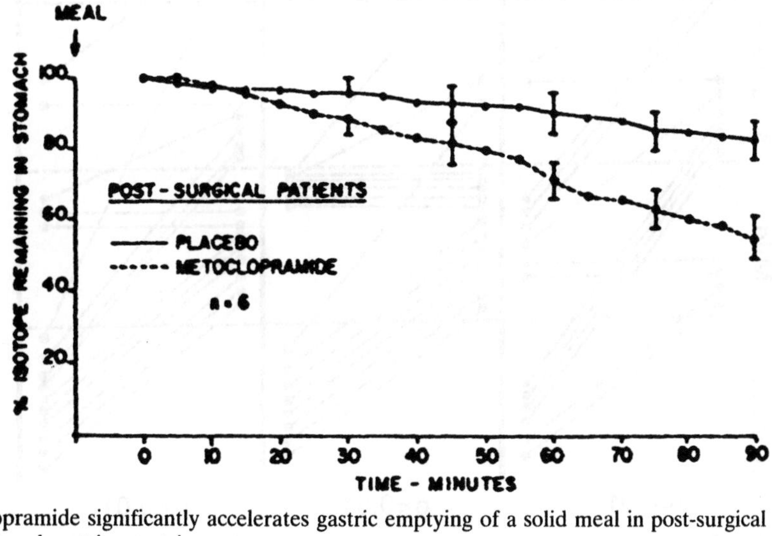

Fig. 11. Metoclopramide significantly accelerates gastric emptying of a solid meal in post-surgical patients with delayed gastric emptying

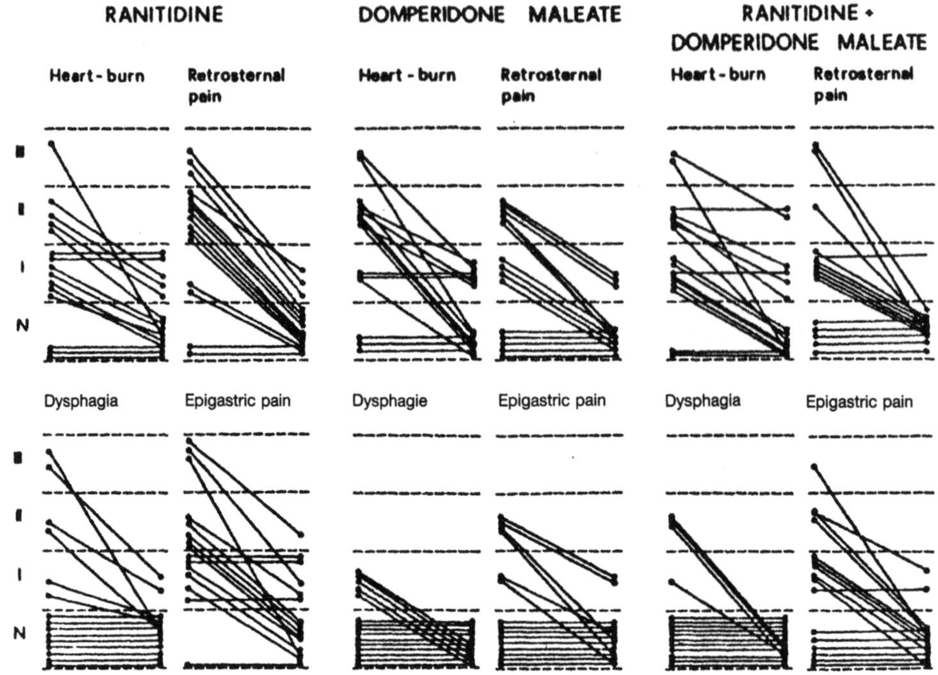

Fig. 12. Effect on clinical symptoms

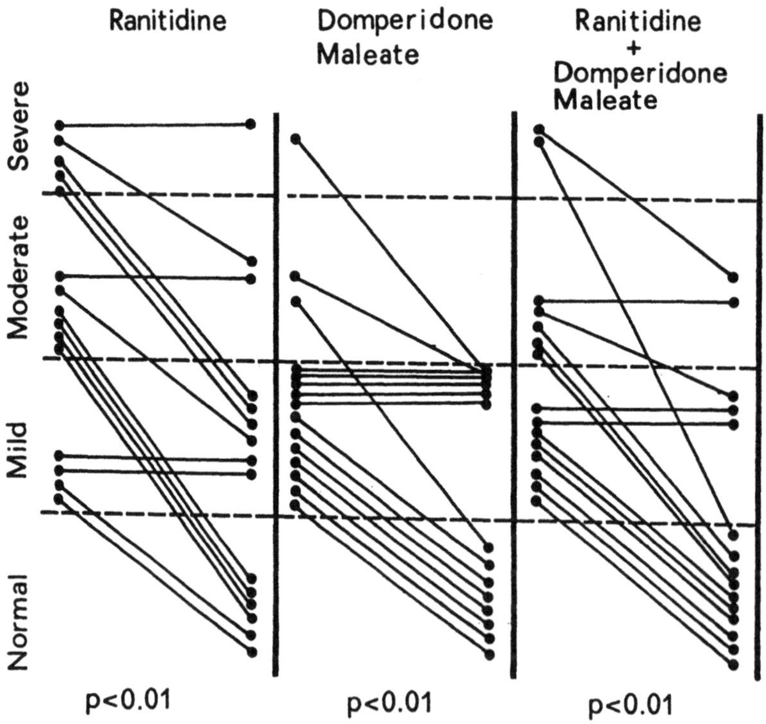

Fig. 13. Endoscopic appearance before and after the different treatments

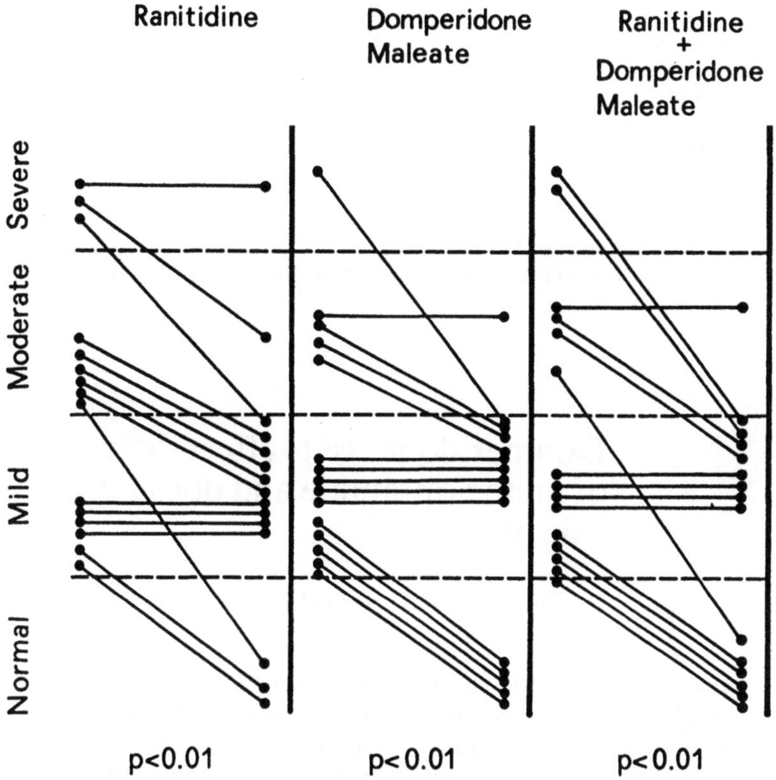

Fig. 14. Histological features before and after the different treatments

Table 1. Ranitidine vs. metoclopramide in the treatment of reflux esophagitis (6 weeks)

	Reduction of symptoms		Endoscopy		Histology	
Ranitidine 150 mg b.i.d.	$p<0.01$		$p<0.01$		$p<0.01$	
		N.S.		$p<0.05$		$p<0.05$
Metoclopramide 10 mg t.i.d.	$p<0.01$		$p<0.01$		N.S.	

References

1. Stanciu C, Bennett JR (1973) Gut 14:275–279
2. Lux G, Engel H, Rosh W (1981) Royal Society of Medicine International Congress and Symposium Series 36:29
3. Weihrauch TR, Forster CF, Krieglstein J (1979) Postgraduate Medical Journal 55 (suppl 1):7–10
4. Valenzuela JE, Defilippi C, Gutierrez F (1980) Digestive Disease and Science 25 (9):716
5. Blackwell JN, Heading RC, Fettes HR (1981) Royal Society of Internal Medicine International Congress and Symposium Series 36:57

6. Wallin L, Boesby S, Madsen T (1979) Scandinavian Journal of Gastroenterology 14: 923–927
7. Valenzuela JE (1981) Royal Society of Internal Medicine International Congress and Symposium Series 36: 51–56
8. Broekaert A (1979) Postgraduate Medical Journal 55 (suppl 1): 11–14
9. Valenzuela JE, Miranda M, Anson AN, Lim BR (1981) AGA Meeting
10. Metzger WH, Cano R, Sturdevant RAL (1976) Gastroenterology 71: 30–32
11. Johnson AG (1969) British Journal of Surgery 56: 969
12. Schruurkes JA, Van Nueten JM (1981) Gastroenterology 19: 444–445
13. Masci E, Testoni PA, Passaretti S, Guslandi M, Tittobello A (1985) Drugs under Experimental and Clinical Research 11 (10): 687–692
14. Guslandi M, Testoni PA, Masci E, Passaretti S, Tittobello A (1983) Hepato-Gastroenterology 3 (30): 96–98

Domperidone: is its effect different from that of metoclopramide and does it have central side effects?

P. Denis, C. Tardif, and *J. Weber* (Rouen)

Two reviews on domperidone and metoclopramide have recently been publsihed [1, 2]. The efficacy of the two drugs is identical for improving symptoms of dyspepsia and for preventing postoperative vomiting or that induced by chemotherapy, but there is a difference in terms of gastroesophageal reflux. Most pharmacodynamic results agree in showing that the acute intravenous or oral administration of metoclopramide (Table 1) increases the resting lower esophageal sphincter pressure (LES P) in both normal subjects and in patients with gastroesophageal reflux. However, the effect of metoclopramide is more clearcut in healthy volunteers than in patients, and the degree of the response depends on the basal LES P, on the dose and on the route of administration.

Domperidone increases the LES P in volunteers, but has no effect in reflux patients. While the increased LES P appears to be the main element in the efficacy of metoclopramide on reflux, the symptomatic improvement by domperidone in reflux patients is not accompanied by an increase in LES P [4]. These results suggest that the mechanisms of action of the two drugs for improving reflux are different.

Table 1

Pharmacologic Study Healthy volunteers LES pressure		
	Metoclopramide	Domperidone
	10–20 mg	8–16 mg
IV	↗ 3 to 34 mmHg	↗ 15 to 20 mmHg
Oral	↗	unchanged

Most therapeutic trials have indicated a symptomatic efficacy of metoclopramide [1] (Table 2) which is less well established for domperidone [4–5–6] (Table 3).

Endoscopic healing of esophagitis with metoclopramide remains to be confirmed and to be demonstrated for domperidone [1, 2]. Finally, the frequency of occurrence of extrapyramidal manifestations is higher in metoclopramide-treated patients than in those receiving domperidone (Table 4), probably because of the primarily peripheral action of the latter. This drug is effective for correcting the digestive disorders accompanying the administration of antiparkinson drugs without inducing extrapyramidal signs.

Table 2. Clinical studies metoclopramide (MCP) – results

		N° patient	Dose (mg. j)	Duration (weeks)	Pyrosis	Esophagitis
Johnson	1971	47	30	6 to 8	MCP > P	ND
Venables	1973	15	30	6 to 8	MCP > P	
Paull	1974	31	40	6 to 8	MCP > P	
McCallum	1977	31	40	6 to 8	MCP > P	ND
Bright-Asare	1980	50	40	6 to 8	MCP = CIM > P	MCP = CIM = P
Winnan	1980	19	40	6 to 8	MCP > P + Antacids	ND
Cohen	–	33	60	12	MCP > P	MCP > P

P: Placebo, ND: not done, CIM: Cimetidine

Table 3. Clinical studies – domperidone (D)

		N° patient	Dose (mg. j)	Duration (weeks)	Pyrosis	Esophagitis
Blackwell	1981	22	80 + antacid and alginate	2	D = P antacid intake reduced with D.	ND
Englert	1979	48	30	4	D > P	–
Schulze-Delrieu	1981	15	60	8	D = P no effect on intake of antacid	–
Valenzuela	1981	23	80	8	D = P decrease in severity of regurgitations	D = P

P: Placebo, ND: not done

Table 4. Central effects of domperidone

1. Distribution: systemic injection
   - increased concentrations in the peripheral tissues
   - weak concentrations in pericentral foci
2. Incapable of displacing the bond with haloperidol in the dopaminergic areas of the rat brain
3. Systemic injection of Domperidone does not increase the plasma concentrations of homovanillic acid (dopamine catabolite), unlike metoclopramide
4. Intracerebral administration of Domperidone is as effective as that of haloperidol in antagonizing the effects of intracerebral administration of dopamine
5. Effective in parkinsonians (n=13) without provoking extrapyramidal signs
6. Extrapyramidal symptoms produced by metoclopramide and domperidone are rare, and rarer with domperidone

References

1. Harrington RA, Hamilton CW, Brogden RW, Linkewich JA, Romankiewicz JA, Yeel RD (1983) Metoclopramide. An updated review of its pharmacological properties and clinical use. Drugs 25: 451–494
2. Brogden RN, Carmine AA, Heel RC, Speight TM, Avery GS (1982) Domperidone. A review of its pharmacological activity, pharmacokinetics and therapeutic efficacy in the symptomatic treatment of chronic dyspepsia. Drugs 24: 360–400.
3. Durazo F, Gramisu M, Valenzuela JE (1987) Effect of metoclopramide (MTC) on the mechanisms of gastroesophageal reflux (GER). Gastroenterology 92: 1378 (abstract).
4. Valenzuela JE Effects of domperidone on the symptoms of reflux esophagitis. Progress with domperidone: Royal Society of Medicine, International Congress and symposium series n° 36. Academic Press Inc (London).
5. Blackwell JN, Heading RC, Fettes HR Effects of domperidone on lower esophageal sphincter pressure and gastroesophageal reflux in patients with peptic esophagitis. Progress with domperidone: Royal Society of internal Medicine, International Congress and Symposium Series n° 36: 57. Academic Press Inc (London).
6. Grill BB, Hillemeier AC, Semerano LA, McCallum RW, Gryboski JD (1985) Effects of domperidone therapy on symptoms and upper gastrointestinal motility in infants with gastroesophageal reflux. J Pediatr 106: 311–316.

Bethanechol: is its association to antacid therapy advantageous for the healing of esophagitis lesions?

G. Vantrappen (Leuven)

Bethanechol is a cholinergic agent which has been shown to increase the lower esophageal sphincter pressure in adults [1, 4] as well as in children [9, 5].

Bethanechol may also decrease the number of reflux episodes per 24 hours [4] and improve clearance of acid from the esophagus in adults [3] and in children [9]. Two mechanisms may have a role in the improved acid clearance of the esophagus by bethanechol i.e. more effective propulsion due to stronger contractions progressing at a slower speed down the gullet [2, 6, 9] and stimulation of (alkaline) saliva secretion.

The effect of bethanechol on the healing of esophagitis has not been studied extensively.

In a double-blind placebo controlled trial Thanik [10] studied a group of 44 patients. Both the control group with reflux esophagitis and the bethanechol group received, together with the study compounds, high doses of antacids. The bethanechol group comprised 4 patients with grade 2, 13 patients with grade 3 and 5 patients with grade 4 esophagitis. In the placebo group there were 8 patients with grade 2, 7 with grade 3 and 7 with grade 4 esophagitis. After 2 and 4 weeks, improvement of both the endoscopic lesions and the symptoms was significantly better in the bethanechol group as compared to the placebo group. Complete healing of the lesions was observed in 40% of the bethanechol group and in 13% in the placebo group.

These results could not be confirmed in an other, similarly designed study [7], in which antacids were given to both the bethanechol group and to the placebo group. After 8 weeks the symptomatic improvement was similar in both groups, although at the interim evaluation at 2 and 4 weeks, the placebo group did better. Endoscopic healing was better in the placebo group than in the bethanechol group. Complete healing was observed in 35% of the placebo group as compared to 20% of the bethanechol group.

A last study [10] compared bethanechol + antacids with cimetidine + antacids in 43 patients with esophagitis grade 2 or more. After 6 weeks a similar degree of improvement of both the symptoms and the endoscopic lesions was obtained in the two groups. Complete healing was observed in 70% of the cimetidine group as compared to 50% in the bethanechol group.

From these observations it may be concluded that the questionable benefits of adding bethanechol to antacids or H_2 blockers, does not add much to the efficacy of the treatment.

Moreover, it does not seem to be logical to treat a disease in which acid plays such an important role by giving a drug that stimulates acid secretion.

References

1. Farrell RL, Roling GT, Castell DO (1973) Stimulation of the incompetent lower esophageal sphincter. A possible advance in therapy of heartburn. Am J Dig Dis 18: 646–650
2. Humphries TJ, Castell DO (1981) Effect or oral bethanechol on parameters of esophageal peristalsis. Dig Dis Sci 26: 129–132
3. Johnson LF, DeMeester TR (1981) Evaluation of elevation of the head of the bed, bethanechol, and antacid foam tablets on gastroesophageal reflux. Dig Dis Sci 26: 673–680
4. Miller WN, Ganeshappa KP, Dodds WJ, Hogan WJ, Barreras RF, Arndorfer RC (1977) Effect of Bethanechol of gastroesophageal reflux. Am J Dig Dis 22: 230–234

5. Orenstein SR, Lofton SW, Orenstein DM (1986) Bethanechol for pediatric gastroesophageal reflux: a prospective, blind, controlled study. J Pediatr Gastroenter Nutr 5: 549–555
6. Phaosawasdi K, Malmud LS, Tolin RD, Stelzer F, Applegate G, Fisher RS (1981) Cholinergic effects on esophageal transit and clearance. Gastroenterology 81: 915–920
7. Saco LS, Orlando RC, Levinson SL, Bozymski EM, Jones JD, Frakes JT (1982) Double-blind controlled trial of bethanechol and antacid versus placebo and antacid in the treatment of erosive esophagitis. Gastroenterology 82: 1369–1373
8. Sondheimer JM, Arnold GL (1986) Early effects of Bethanechol on the esophageal motor function of infants with gastroesophageal reflux. J Pediatr Gastroenterol Nutr 5: 47–51
9. Sondheimer JM, Mintz HL, Michaels M (1984) Bethanechol treatment of gastroesophageal reflux in infants: effect on continuous esophageal pH records. J Pediatr 104: 128–131
10. Thanik KD, Chey WY, Shah AN, Gutierrez JG (1980) Reflux esophagitis: effect of oral bethanechol on symptoms and endoscopic findings. Ann Intern Med 93: 805–808
11. Thanik K, Chey WY, Shah A, Hamilton D, Nadelson N (1982) Bethanechol or cimetidine in the treatment of symptomatic reflux esophagitis. A double-blind control study. Arch Intern Med 142: 1479–1481

Does the eso-gastric prokinetic action of cisapride play a role in the treatment of esophagitis?

G. Vantrappen (Leuven)

Cisapride is a new prokinetic agent that acts by stimulating the release of acetylcholine in the myenteric plexus. As other prokinetic agents, cisapride increases the tone of the lower esophageal sphincter, improves esophageal acid clearance and accelerates gastric emptying. Theoretically a drug with these characteristics should be useful in the treatment of reflux esophagitis.

What do the clinical trials show?

In 1986 the results of 5 clinical trials on the efficacy of cisapride in the treatment of reflux esophagitis were presented.

Hütteman et al. [3] performed a placebo controlled study on the effect of cisapride on symptoms in 39 patients with esophagitis (35 grade 1 Savary, 4 grade 2). After six weeks the symptomatic improvement in the cisapride group was superior to that in the placebo group.

In a Belgian multicenter trial [5] in 19 patients with erosive or ulcerative esophagitis, the effect of cisapride was compared to that of placebo in a double blind controlled study lasting 8 to 16 weeks. Cisapride was found to be superior to placebo in improving symptoms as well as in healing the endoscopic lesions. Complete healing was observed in 72% of the cisapride treated patients as compared to 12 in the placebo group.

In an Italian multicenter placebo controlled double blind trial Baldi et al. [1] studied 40 patients with esophagitis (12 without and 28 with erosive lesions) for a period of 12 weeks. Symptomatic and endoscopic improvement was significantly superior in the cisapride group as compared to the control group. Complete healing was observed in 63% of the cisapride-treated patients and in only 14% of the placebo-treated patients.

A German multicenter study [4] compared cisapride and ranitidine in a double blind controlled trial in 36 patients. The cisapride group comprised 17 patients (14 grade 1 Savary, 3 grade 2). The ranitidine group was composed of 19 patients (11 group 1, 8 group 2). After 6 to 12 weeks, the symptomatic and endoscopic improvement in the 2 groups was not significantly different. After 12 weeks complete healing was obtained in 94% of the cisapride treated patients and in 73% of the ranitidine group.

A French-Austrian multicenter trial [2] studied the effect of adding cisapride to cimetidine on the healing of reflux esophagitis. Fourty seven patients were included in the double blind controlled study. The cisapride + cimetidine group comprised 17 patients with esophagitis grade 2 (Savary) and 6 grade 3. The placebo + cimetidine group was composed of 18 patients with grade 2 and 6 with grade 3 esophagitis. The cimetidine + cisapride group showed significantly greater improvement in symptoms and lesions as compared to the cimetidine + placebo group. After 12 weeks complete healing was observed in 69% of the patients in the cimetidine + cisapride group as compared to 45% in the cimetidine + placebo group.

Although these results have only been published in abstract form and the number of patients included in each of the studies is limited, it seems as if cisapride may have a role in the treatment of reflux esophagitis.

References

1. Baldi F, Bianchi Porro G, Iascone C, Sabbatini F, Tittobello A, Verme G, Lobello R, Dobrilla G (1986 November) Placebo controlled study of the effect of cisapride on the lesions and symptoms of reflux oesophagitis. Lecture held at the symposium "Progress in the treatment of gastrointestinal motility: the role of cisapride." Frankfurt
2. Galmiche JP, Brandstätter G, Evreux M, Hentschel E, Kerstan E, Kratochvil P, Reichel W, Schütze K, Soule JC, Vitaux J (November 1986) Control of severe reflux oesophagitis with combined cisapride-cimetidine treatment. Lecture held at the symposium "Progress in the treatment of gastrointestinal motility: the role of cisapride." Frankfurt
3. Hütteman W (November 1986) Cisapride in the treatment of oesophagitis. A placebo-controlled trial. Lecture held at the symposium "Progress in the treatment of gastrointestinal motility: the role of cisapride." Frankfurt
4. Janisch HD, Bouzo MH, Hütteman W, Kleinert J, Pfeiffer H, Eisenhardt W, von Radetzky E (November 1986) Double-blind comparison of cisapride and ranitidine in the treatment of reflux oesophagitis. Lecture held at the symposium "Progress in the treatment of gastrointestinal motility: the role of cisapride", Frankfurt
5. Lepoutre L, Bollen J, Vandewalle N, Laukens P, Cabooter M, Vanderlinden I (November 1986) Therapeutic effects of cisapride in reflux oesophagitis. A double-blind, placebo-controlled study. Lecture held at the symposium "Progress in the treatment of gastrointestinal motility: the role of cisapride." Frankfurt

What are the indications of pirenzepine?

C. Maffioli (Reims)

At the parietal gastric cells where hydrochloric acid is secreted there are cholinergic receptors, particularly muscarinic receptors. Pirenzepine is a pyridobenzodiazepine which blocks the Ml muscarinic receptors of the gastric wall exerting a selective antimuscarinic action. This produces an inhibition of acid gastric secretion which is greater and more prolonged than with traditional anticholinergics. It is this action against acid secretion that has led to pirenzepine being proposed for the treatment of gastroesophageal reflux as it combats the noxious effect of the acidity of the reflux fluid.

Several studies have shown the effectiveness of pirenzepine against the clinical symptoms of gastroesophageal reflux and on the endoscopic lesions of esophagitis. In 1984 Evreux et al. [3] made a crossover double-blind study against placebo in 50 patients. In 1986, Niemela et al. [7] also studied the action of pirenzepine against placebo in a double-blind study in 47 patients. These two studies showed significant superiority of pirenzepine to that of placebo at both the clinical and the endoscopic level. Finally, still in 1986, Gouerou et al. [4], did a comparative study with cimetidine in 306 patients. The good clinical results were slightly inferior for gastrozepine (79.7% against 84.1% for cimetidine), though the good endoscopic results were identical.

However it is known that anticholinergics in classical antisecretory doses are contraindicated in cases of gastroesophageal reflux. They reduce the pressure of the inferior esophageal sphincter; they decrease esophageal contractions, thus increasing the period of contact between the reflux fluid and the mucosa and diminishing esophageal clearance; and they decrease the response of the LES to the administration of pentagastrin.

Several studies have been made of the action of pirenzepine on the esophagus and LES: Denis (1982 [2]), Kohek (1984 [5]), Minaire (1985 [6]), Cecconello (1986 [1]).

The conclusions from these studies are as follows:

Pirenzepine does not modify the resting pressure of the LES; on the contrary it increases it in patients with low pressure.

It does not modify peristalsis or the velocity of contractions in particular. It therefore maintains esophageal clearance.

It does not modify sphincter response to pentagastrin and retards supramaximal inhibition.

In conclusion, pirenzepine, because of its antisecretory action to acid in the stomach and the absence of inhibitor effects on the LES, forms part of the therapeutic possibilities available to practitioners dealing with acid gastroesophageal reflux.

References

1. Cecconello I, Zilberstein B, Pinotti M, Pollara WM, Pugliese V, Nasi A, Pinotti HW (1986) Treatment of reflux œsophagitis with pirenzepin. Symposium 8ème Congrès Mondial de Gastroentérologie. Sao Paulo
2. Denis P, Galmiche JP, Gibon JF, Colin R, Pasquis P, Lefrancois R (1982) Effet du pirenzepin sur la motricité œsophagienne chez l'adulte sain. Gastroenterol Clin Biol 6: 27–31
3. Evreux M, Jacquet N (1984) La pirenzepine dans le traitement de l'œsophagite. Rev Fr Gastroenterol 20 (204): 18–21
4. Gouerou H (1986) Etude multicentrique pirenzepine versus cimetidine dans le traitement du reflux gastro-œsophagien. Rapport d'expertise clinique
5. Kohek PH, Rehak PH, Friehs GB (1984) Effet de la pirenzepine sur le sphincter inférieur de l'œsophage. Medwelt 35: 943–945
6. Minaire Y (1985) Etude de l'effet de la pirenzepine chez des patients porteurs d'une hypotonie du sphincter inférieur de l'œsophage. Rapport de pharmacologie clinique
7. Niemela S, Lehtola J, Krekela I, Jaaskelainen T, Martikamen J, Sarna S, Sarelin H (1986) Pirenzepin in the treatment of reflux œsophagitis: a placebo-controlled double-blind study. Symposium. 8ème Congrès Mondial de Gastroentérologie. Sao Paulo

What are the effects of H_2-receptor-antagonists on esophageal burns, on esophagitis lesions and on the evolution of peptic stenosis?

J. F. Rey, and *M. Greff* (St Laurent du Var)

Numerous papers compared the effects of Cimetidine and Ranitidine on gastroesophageal reflux. No control studies have been published on the most recent H_2 blockers, famotidine and nizatidine.

Effect on esophageal pain

Many clinical trials compared the efficacy of H_2 blockers in reducing esophageal symptoms. Discrepancy appeared due to differences in evaluation of the pain (number of days or nights without symptoms, number of reflux symptoms during treatment, importance of severity of the reflux (Fig. 1)), differences between treated groups at the time of entry, differences of duration and amount of drug in treated groups. These discrepancies are more frequent in the literature about cimetidine [2, 4, 12] than on ranitidine which draw benefice from previous studies [6, 10].

Cimetidine was used at different doses from 1,6 g, 4 times per day draw to 800 mg twice a day. Duration of treatment was from 6 to 12 weeks. Relief of retrosternal pain and regurgitation on cimetidine was significantly more frequent in most of the

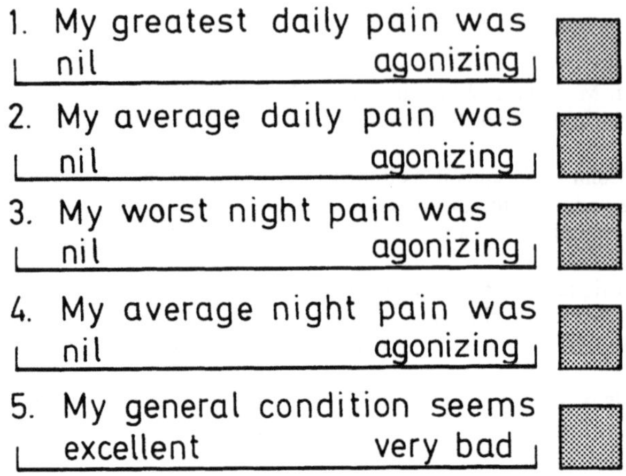

Fig. 1. Differences between studies are related to variable inclusion criteria, especially as regards assessment of symptomatology. Example of an analog scale allowing assessment of severity of symptoms, taken from Behar (1978). The scale was converted into numerical values (millimeters)

studies recorded by Soule et al. [11]. Impairment of retrosternal pain occurred in the first week of the treatment. In a study without statistically significant response, a clinical improvement was observed. Since 1978, Behar et al. [1] showed a clinical improvement in 45 patients treated with cimetidine compared to 41 patients who were given a placebo (Fig. 2). Patients on cimetidine treatment reported less regurgitation per night after 6 and 8 weeks of treatment (Fig. 3). All esophageal symptoms were notably reduced especially occurrence of retrosternal pain at night. Studies on Ranitidine included patients with symptomatic reflux, endoscopically proven esophagitis with epithelial defects on biopsy (Fig. 4). Patients received

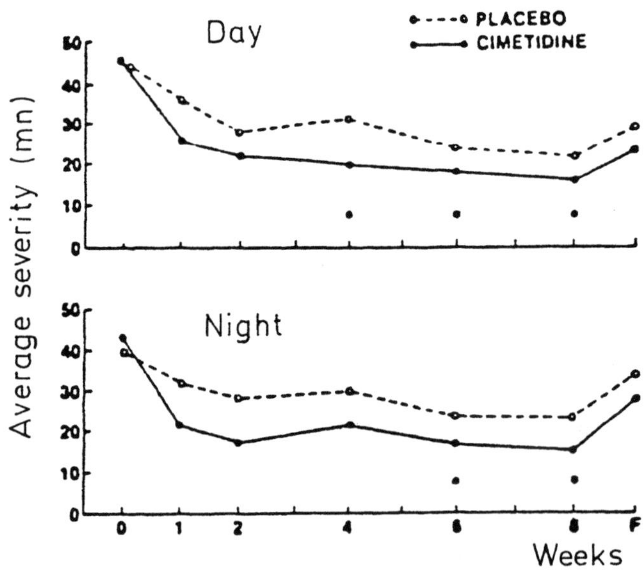

Fig. 2. Results of Behar's double-blind study of 94 patients: efficacy of cimetidine on average severity of pyrosis

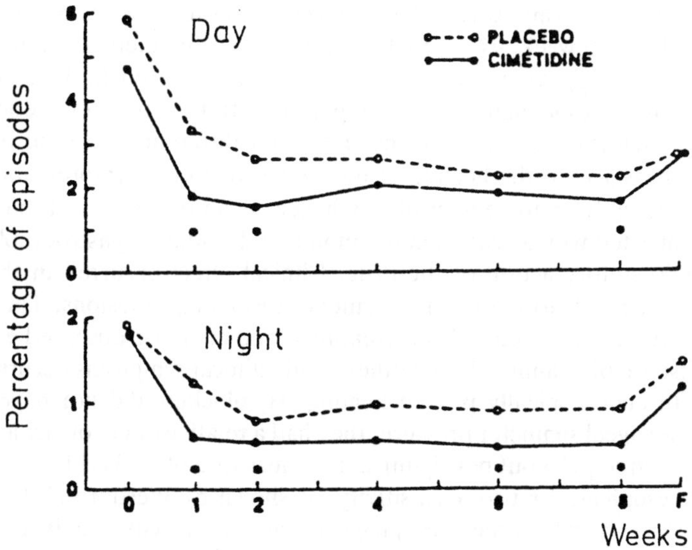

Fig. 3. Efficacy of cimetidine on average number of episodes of pyrosis by day and night

• $p < 0.05$

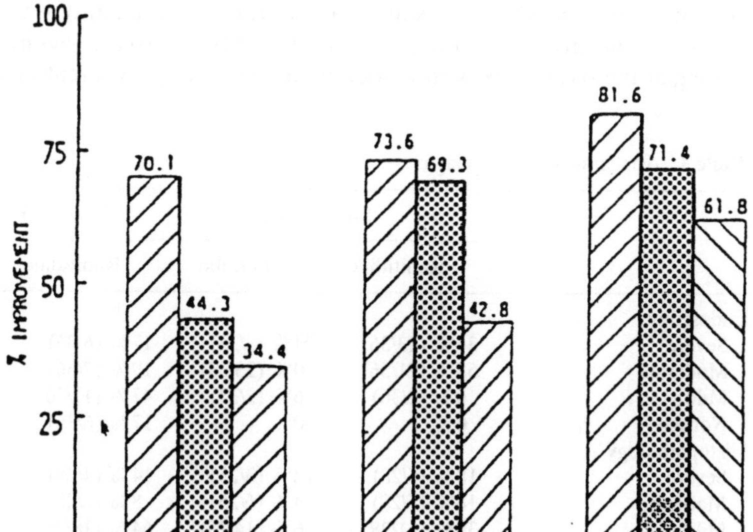

Fig. 4. Effect of ranitidine on 20 patients (300 mg three time a day). Improvement of clinical symptoms (S), endoscopic aspects (E) and histological lesions (H)

ranitidine 150 mg twice a day. Koelz [6] reported a series of 108 patients; at the end of the sixth week, 47% of all patients were completely asymptomatic. On the other hand, disappearance of all symptoms was reported in 41% of the patients with persistant esophagitis. In a comparative study between cimetidine and ranitidine, Himmig [5] did not show any significant difference between the two drugs either with respect to the healing of the lesions or to the symptomatic improvement.

Probably improvement of esophageal symptoms under H_2 blocker treatment was connected with a reduction of amount and acidity of gastroesophageal reflux by the antisecretory action of the drug. Clinical effect occurred in the first week of the treatment, before any improvement of esophageal lesions. This effect disappeared shortly after the end of this treatment and could be observed even in patients with absence of healing. On the other hand, clinical symptoms occurred in some patients with endoscopically proven healing. H_2 blockers did not have any effect on low esophageal sphincter pressure, they had a relative effect on acide reflux significant at measured pH 5 but not significant at measured pH 4. H_2 blockers should act directly on esophageal mucosa sensitivity, as shown by Wesdorp [12], with Bernstein test, after a short treatment esophageal mucosa sensivity was increased even complete healing of esophagitis.

Effect on esophagitis

Differences in the endoscopically evaluated group of patients lead to discrepancy between different studies. Cimetidine was usually more potent than placebo [2]. For trial, histologic grading was difficult due to the poor quality of biopsy specimens. The effect of cimetidine was statistically significant in a study where patients with severe esophagitis were induced. Hine et al. [3] reported a significant endoscopic healing at the sixth week with moderate histologic improvement (Table 1). Patients

Table 1. Appearance of Esophagus

	Study Entry		After 6 Weeks Treatment	
	Ranitidine	Placebo	Ranitidine	Placebo
Endoscopy				
Severe	36% (13/36)	24% (8/33)	17% (6/36)	12% (4/33)
Moderate	58% (21/36)	70% (23/33)	19% (7/36)[a]	52% (17/33)
Mild	6% (2/36)	6% (2/33)	47% (17/36)[a]	27% (9/33)[b]
Normal	0%	0%	17% (6/36)	9% (3/33)
Histopathology				
Severe	18% (5/28)	12% (3/25)	14% (4/28)	4% (1/25)
Moderate	18% (5/28)	24% (6/25)	8% (2/28)	32% (8/25)
Mild	39% (11/28)	56% (14/25)	64% (18/28)	52% (13/25)
Normal	25% (7/28)	8% (2/25)	14% (4/28)	12% (3/25)

[a] $p<0.001$, ranitidine at study entry versus ranitidine after 6 weeks treatment
[b] $p<0.05$, placebo at study entry versus placebo after 6 weeks treatment
– Effect of ranitidine on esophageal lesion. Improvement of endoscopic aspects in case of mild or moderate esophagitis

without endoscopic improvement after 6 weeks did not draw any benefit from a 3 month treatment [6]. Ranitidine effects seem more efficient on esophagitis than cimetidine in the Wesdorp study [12]. 75% of treated patients had endoscopic healing and 70% had histologic improvement compared to 45% patients who were given placebo.

The effect of H_2 receptor antagonists on esophagitis is real but moderate. The relative inefficiency was due to the leak of effect on the lower esophageal sphincter, on esophageal motility and absence of cytoprotection effects. The more powerful antisecretory action of ranitidine could explain some results on endoscopy healing and histological improvements.

Prevention of peptic stricture

Peptic stricture occurred in 2.1% of a 1661 group of patients with esophagitis reported by Zeitoun et al. [13]. No control study showed a significant benefit of treatment [3]. However, patients had strictures on presentation, sometimes induced by anti-inflammatory drugs. H_2 blockers which relieved pain and histological lesions could heal Barrett' ulcers, but did not improved endobrachy-esophageal mucosa. In one case, Saltzmann [9] described the occurrence of peptic stricture on cimetidine.

Conclusion

- H_2 receptor antagonists relieved esophageal pain. There is no correlation between effect on pain, the importance of lesions, and healing with treatment.
- H_2 blockers are more potent in severe esophagitis than in mild or moderate endoscopically proven lesions.
- H_2 blockers may prevent the development of peptic stricture but no control study has yet been published on that topic.

What are the side effects

Side-effects after H_2-receptor antagonists are well known as cimetidine has been used clinically since 1977. Cimetidine could lead to minor symptoms (diarrhea, muscular pain, erythema), moderate side-effects (gynecomastia, confusion, bradycardia) and rare severe adverse reactions such agranulopenia and pancytopenia. Drug interactions were report with propranolol and theophylline. These side-effects were also noticed but with a less extensive range with ranitidine (confusion, diarrhea, abdominal discomfort, leukopenia). We should quote the small number of cases compared to the large amount of H_2 blockers prescribed.

If you look at the side-effects during treatment for esophagitis, they appear in long term treatment or in cases of drug association. Lieberman [7] quoted one confusion and some minor troubles in patients with cimetidine and metoclopramide. Koelz [6] reported 10 cases of moderate side-effects in a 108 patient group; none were withdrawn from this ranitidine therapy. Sherbaniuk [10] observed 14% of minor adverse reactions in both placebo and ranitidine treated patients. We could conclude that adverse reactions are unusual; except in case of drug association.

References

1. Behar J, Brand DL, Brown FC, Castell DO, Cohen S, Crossley RJ, Pope CE, II, Winans CS (1978) Cimetidine in the treatment of symptomatic gastroesophageal reflux: A double-blind controlled trial. Gastroenterology 74: 441–448
2. Bennett JR, Buckton G, Martin HD (1983) Cimetidine in gastro-oesophageal reflux. Digestion 26: 166–172
3. Hine KR, Holmes GKT, Melikian V, Lucey M, Fairelough PD (1984) Ranitidine in reflux oesophagitis. A double-blind placebo-controlled study. Digestion 29: 119–123
4. Kaul B, Petersen H, Erichsen H, Myrvold HE, Grette K, Halvorsen T, Fjosne U: Gastroesophageal reflux disease. Acute and maintenance treatments with cimetidine
5. Kimmig JM (1984) Cimetidine and ranitidine in the treatment of reflux esophagitis. Z Gastroenterol 22: 373–378
6. Koelz HR, Birchler R, Bretholz A, Bron B, Capitaine Y, Delmore G, Fehr HF, Fumagalli I, Gehrig J, Gonvers JJ, Halter F, Hammer B, Kayasseh L, Kobler E, Miller G, Munst G, Pelloni S, Realini S, Schmid P, Voirol M, Blum AL (1986) Healing and relapse of reflux esophagitis during treatment with ranitidine. Gastroenterology 91: 1198–1205
7. Lieberman DA, Keefe EB (1985) Double-blind controlled trial of metoclopramide and cimetidine versus placebo and cimetidine in the treatment of severe reflux esophagitis. Gastroenterology 88: 1476
8. Pop P (1982) In: The clinical use of ranitidine. Proceedings of a symposium held in Amsterdam, 14–15 May 1982. Baskerville publishers Ltd Guildford 35–41
9. Saltzman M, Barwick K, McCallum RW (1982) Progression of cimetidine-treated reflux oesophagitis to a Barrett's stricture. Dig Dis Sci 27: 181–186
10. Sherbaniuk R, Wensel R, Bailey R, Trautman A, Grace M, Kirdeikis P, Jewell L, Pare P, Levesque D, Farley A, Archambault A, Thomson ABR (1984) Ranitidine in the treatment of symptomatic gastroesophageal reflux disease. J Clin Gastroenterol 6: 9–15
11. Soule JC, Pariente EA, Moschoutis P (1982) Cimétidine et reflux gastro-œsophagien. Gastroenterol Clin Biol 6: 662–668
12. Wesdorp E, Bartelsman J, Pape K, Tytgat GN (1978) Oral cimetidine in reflux esophagitis. A double-blind controlled trial. Gastroenterology 74: 821–824
13. Zeitoun P (1985) Place de l'endoscopie dans le diagnostic et la surveillance de l'œsophagite. Med Chir Dig n° spécial 4–7

Is healing of esophagitis lesions possible with this treatment? What is the optimal daily dosage? Is maintenance treatment necessary?

R. Lambert (Lyons)

While the antagonists to the H_2-receptors effectively relieve the symptoms of reflux esophagitis, and in particular pyrosis, their effectiveness in healing ulcerated esophageal lesions is less and certainly not comparable to that described for gastroduodenal ulcer. The characteristics of the healing process may be summarized as follows: *slow action*, manifested only after 6 week's treatment, *partial action*, the proportion of patients exhibiting complete healing falling rapidly in relation to the degree of severity of the ulcerations, *dose-dependent action* with increase of the percentage of healing when the daily dosage is higher than is proposed for gastroduodenal ulcer.

The dosage of antagonists to H_2-receptors in the patient suffering from an ulcerated esophagitis must be adapted to the severity of the lesions. If there is a simple erosive esophagitis a daily dose identical to that employed in the treatment of gastroduodenal ulcer may be laid down but should be divided into morning and evening fractions. If the ulcerations are large or confluent healing generally requires recourse to higher doses (×1.5 or 2, divided into two or four daily fractions). These dose relations apply to cimetidine, ranitidine and famotidine. The length of such treatment required for healing varies from 6 to 12 weeks according to the severity of the ulcerations. Prolongation of this attack treatment does not succeed in reducing the rate of non-responders to a negligible level.

The incomplete efficacy (Table 1) of antacid treatment does not justify maintenance treatment for the prevention of recurrences after healing as an alternative to surgical treatment. On the other hand when the patient is inoperable the conduct of maintenance treatment in responsive patients generally ensures reasonably effective control of the anatomic course, as recurrent ulceration is of moderate severity. This

Table 1. Esophagitis and H_2 antagonists – healing of ulcers –

Efficacy of H_2 antagonists
– delayed, partial, dose-related
Posology of H_2 antagonists
– b.i.d. q.i.d.
Maintenance therapy
– half/full dose
– poor efficacy

Table 2. Esophagitis healing rate – ranitidine 300 mg

	6 w	12 w
Global rate	50%	75%
Isolated erosions	78%	
Confluent longitudinal erosions	38%	
Confluent circumferential erosions	23%	

Koelz, 1986

maintenance treatment should be administred under the same conditions as antacid treatment in the form of two daily doses.

These propositions are illustrated by the recent study by Koelz in 1986 (Table 2). Patients with lesions of ulcerated esophagitis were treated with ranitidine (300 mg daily in one or two doses). The global rate of healing at the sixth week was 50%, close to the global rate of symptomatic relief (47%), but without precise correlation between symptoms and endoscopic findings. The rate of healing depended on the severity of the lesions of esophagitis, reaching 78% in patients with an isolated erosion, 38% in patients with confluent ulcerations in the longitudinal plane and 23% in those with circumferential confluent ulcerations. Continuation of initial treatment up to 12 weeks produced a global healing rate of 75%. Maintenance treatment with a half-dose of ranitidine (150 mg daily (Table 3)) extended for 6 months had no effect on the recurrence rate (42%) compared with the placebo group.

Further, a recent study by Collen (Table 4) has shown a correlation between the effect of Ranitidine (300 mg daily) on the healing of lesions of esophagitis and the

Table 3. Esophagitis recurrence rate – ranitidine 150 mg (maintenance 6 m)

Ranitidine	42%	NS
Placebo	36%	

Koelz, 1986

Table 4. Response to standard anti-H_2 therapy in G.E.R. – total reflux time pH 4 (%) –

	Responders 9	Non-responders 7
Control	30%	56%
ran. 300 mg	6%	33%
ran. 1240 mg	–	14%

Collen, 1987

esophageal pH. This study was made on 16 patients. In the 9 positive responders the global reflux time (below pH 4) only reached 30% of the 24-hour period. In the 7 non-responders it stayed at 56%. Increase of dosage (1240 mg of ranitidine daily) succeeded in reducing this proportion to 14% and in obtaining healing of the lesions. Under these circumstances, it would appear that inadequate control of acidity accounts for the failure of healing in patients treated with the usual dosage of an H_2-receptor antagonist.

References

1. Koelz HR, Birchler R, Bretholz A et al. (1986) Healing and relapse of reflux esophagitis during treatment with ranitidine. Gastroenterology 91: 1198–1205
2. Collen MJ, Ciarleglio CA, Stanczak YJ, Benjamin SB (1987) Esophageal pH monitoring, gastric acid output and gastric volume output in patients with GERD unresponsive to standard antisecretory therapy. Gastroenterology 92: 1350 (abstr)

Can Omeprazole allow healing of certain ulcerated esophagitis?

J. Dent (Adelaide)

The potential of omeprazole for the therapy of peptic esophagitis has been investigated in three separate studies conducted within Australia. The minimum criterion for enrolment of patients in these studies was erosive peptic esophagitis. This was graded in severity according to the extent and appearances of ulceration in the distal 5 cm of the esophageal mucosa as follows: grade 2, less than 10% ulceration: grade 3, from 10 to 50% ulceration, and grade 4 more than 50% ulceration, or a deep chronic appearing ulcer, regardless of the area of ulceration. The first study performed was an open therapy pilot study on eight patients who were treated with omeprazole 30 mg daily for 8 weeks. Prior to this, simultaneous 3 hour post prandial recordings of esophageal motility and esophageal and gastric pH were made. These measurements were repeated during the 7th week of therapy with omeprazole. Macroscopic ulceration had healed in 7 of 8 patients after 8 weeks therapy. The esophageal pH recordings made during therapy showed abolition of all episodes of exposure of the esophagus to a pH of less than 4. This effect was dependent upon the very effective antisecretory action of omeprazole, since gastric pH was also maintained above 4. The motility recordings showed no detectable effect of omeprazole on patterns of lower esophageal sphincter and esophageal body motor function. In particular, the frequency of gastro-esophageal reflux episodes, as determined by manometric indices of reflux, was unchanged by omeprazole therapy. From this study we concluded that omeprazole has a very substantial influence on patterns of esophageal acid exposure through its effect on the composition of gastric juice, rather than any direct effect on patterns of motility or reflux.

The second study was a randomized double blind trial performed on 63 patients, half of whom were treated with placebo and half of whom were divided between treatment with omeprazole 20 or 40 mg daily. Endoscopy was performed at 4 weeks. Unhealed patients were treated for a further 4 weeks and then re-endoscoped. After 4 weeks of treatment the healing rate of esophagitis with placebo was 6%, and with omeprazole 81% (p. 0.0001). Heartburn also showed a striking response in the omeprazole treated patients which was significantly greater than the modest improvement seen in placebo treated patients. Twenty four patients in whom esophagitis had healed during this study were followed for up to 6 months after cessation of therapy. Endoscopic and symptomatic relapse had occurred in 17 patients (79%) after 2 months, and only one patient remained healed after 6 months of observation.

In the third study, the efficacies of 20 and 40 mg of omeprazole daily were compared in 164 patients. This includes data from the 31 omeprazole treated patients of the placebo controlled study. The patients were treated for 4 weeks and then endoscoped. If unhealed, therapy was continued for a further 4 weeks when endoscopy was repeated. At 4 weeks the healing rate was 70% with 20 mg and 82% with 40 mg (p.=0.05). The cumulative healing rate at 8 weeks was 79% for 20 mg and 85% for 40 mg (p.=0.1). Both doses resulted in excellent symptom responses.

These studies indicate that omeprazole both 20 and 40 mg daily is a highly effective therapy for severe peptic esophagitis, since over 50% of our patients had grade 3 or 4 esophagitis. Physiological measurements suggest that omeprazole acts primarily through reduction of the aggressiveness of refluxed gastric juice to the esophageal mucosa. Major relapse of esophagitis occurs within a few weeks of cessation of omeprazole therapy.

G. Vantrappen (Leuven)

The efficacy and safety of omeprazole, 40 mg once daily for 4 to 8 weeks of treatment, were studied in 61 patients with ulcerative reflux esophagitis. A double-blind controlled study design was used and the patients were randomly allocated to treatment with either omeprazole 40 mg once daily or ranitidine 150 mg twice daily. Endoscopy was performed prior to inclusion into the study, after 4 weeks and, if unhealed, again after 8 weeks. Healing of esophagitis was defined as complete disappearance of all esophageal ulcerations. Symptoms were recorded before entry, after 4 weeks and again after 8 weeks in unhealed patients.

Fifty-one patients were included in the per-protocol analysis at day 29, and 50 patients at day 57. The healing rate after 4 weeks of treatment was 22 out of 26 patients (85%) treated with omeprazole and 10 out of 25 patients (40%) treated with ranitidine (p. < 0.001). The corresponding figures after 8 weeks were 24 out of 25 (96%), and 13 out of 25 (52%), p. < 0.001.

These results were confirmed in the alternative analysis according to the "intention-to-treat" approach. Patients treated with omeprazole showed a significantly faster and more profound relief in heartburn than patients treated with ranitidine: 85% had no heartburn after 4 weeks of treatment with omeprazole compared to 24% in patients treated with ranitidine (p. $= 0.00007$). The percentage of patients who were free of all reflux symptoms was significantly greater in the omeprazole-treated group as compared to the ranitidine-treated group (62% and 12% resp.; p. $= 0.001$). There were no clinically significant changes in laboratory values in any of the treatment groups. Adverse events were few and mainly mild and transient.

J. P. Isal (Paris)

Introduction

Omeprazole, the new proton pump inhibitor, has been shown to be superior to ranitidine in reflux esophagitis, at doses of 40 mg [1] and 60 mg [2] daily. The aim of this study was to define if a lower dose of omeprazole (20 mg o.m.) would be efficacious in this indication.

Patients and methods

From may 86 to april 87, 19 hospitals (3 Belgium and 16 French) participated in this randomized double-blind study, in which patients were treated daily with either omeprazole 20 mg in the morning, or ranitidine 150 mg morning and evening.

157 patients were included in this study. All were symptomatic and had an esophagitis grade 2, 3 or 4 endoscopically proven during the week preceding the inclusion. Endoscopic appearance was graded as follows:

Grade 0: normal mucosa.
Grade 1: erythema.
Grade 2: not circumferential round and linear erosions.
Grade 3: confluent circumferential erosions.
Grade 4: complicated esophagitis: erosions plus Barrett's esophagus and ulceration.

Healing was defined as complete resolution of all erosive/ulcerative lesions. Treatment lasted 1 month (or 2 months in case of unhealing at day 29). Macroscopic healing and severity of symptoms were compared for day 29 and 57 respectively.

Results

131 patients completed the study in accordance with the protocol on day 29, and 122 on day 57.

Healing rates are given below:

	D 29	D 57
Omeprazole (20 mg)	81% (50/62)	95% (58/61)
Ranitidine (150 mg)	45% (31/69)	65% (40/61)
	p<0.001	p<0.001

The statistical assessment was based on the Mantel-Haenszel test with stratification to the pre-entry esophagitis grade. Healing rates after two months are given below:

	Esophagitis grade pre-entry		
	Grade 2	Grade 3	Grade 4
Omeprazole (20 mg)	98% (43/44)	82% (9/11)	100% (6/6)
Ranitidine (150 mg)	73% (32/44)	50% (6/12)	40% (2/5)

At day 29, relief of symptoms was obtained in 76% of the cases in the omeprazole group against 33% in the ranitidine group, (p. <0.001). Heartburn, the most common symptom reported at the pre-entry visit, resolved completely within 4 weeks, in 94% of the patients receiving omeprazole, compared with 45% in the ranitidine group (p. <0.001).

Conclusion

In reflux esophagitis, omeprazole (20 mg o.m.) is found superior to ranitidine (150 mg twice daily) with regard to healing of lesion and relief of symptoms.

References

1. Blum AL, Riecken EO, Dammann HG (1986) Comparison of omeprazole and ranitidine in the treatment of reflux esophagitis. N Engl J Med 314: 716
2. Klinkenberg-Knol EC, Jansen JBMJ, Festen HPM (1987) Double-blind multicentre study comparison of omeprazole and ranitidine in treatment of reflux esophagitis. Lancet 1: 349–351

Can Omeprazole be efficient in cases that do not heal under H_2-receptor blockers?

J. C. Souquet (Lyons)

H_2-receptor antagonists improve some but not all reflux esophagitis [1, 2]. Omeprazole, actually the strongest inhibitor of gastric acid secretion [3], appears to be superior in ulcerative reflux esophagitis [4, 5]. The aim of this open study was to determine the efficacy of omeprazole for the healing of ulcerative reflux esophagitis and for the maintenance of healing for a period up to 1 year.

Study design (Table 1)

Patients were included if they had a reflux esophagitis (endoscopic stage 3 or 4) that did not heal after at least two months of full dose regimen H_2-receptor antagonists (800 mg cimetidine, 300 mg ranitidine). After acceptance of the protocol, patients were given daily 40 mg omeprazole for 4 weeks. If not healed at this time (Endoscopic stage 0 or 1), they were treated again for 4 weeks. Then in healed patients, omeprazole was given at the posology of 20 mg/d for one year with evaluation every 3 months.

Table 1. Study design

Reflux esophagitis endoscopic stage III, IV after anti-H_2 for at least 2 months
Omeprazole 40 mg/d 4 or 8 weeks
After healing, maintenance treatment
Omeprazole 20 mg/d

Patients (Table 2)

9 patients (6 male, 3 female, median age 47 yrs–19 to 85) were included for a reflux esophagitis stage 3 [1] or 4 [8] that did not responded to cimetidine or ranitidine given for a median period of 10 months (2 to 48). All patients also had antacids and 4 sucrafalte. Mean duration of esophagitis was 4 to 5 yrs. 5 patients had unsuccessful previous anti-reflux surgery.

Table 2. Patients. 9 patients (M:6, F:3) 47 yrs (19–85)

Esophagitis III	1
Esophagitis IV	8
Previous surgery	5/9
Mean duration of anti-H_2 treatment	10 months

Table 3. Esophagitis healing. 9 patients

Healing (Stage 0 or 1 at Endoscopy)	
4 weeks	5
8 weeks	7
Symptomatic improvement	9

Table 4. Maintenance treatment. 8 patients

One recurrence -------→ 40 mg
7 no recurrence
no clinical side-effects
no biochemical abnormalities
no fundic endocrine hyperplasia

Results (Tables 3, 4)

5/9 patients had complete healing at the end of 4 weeks; two more healed after 8 weeks (total healed patients: 78%). One patient had at this time a slight erosion (stage 2). Another had unexplained abdominal pain that ceased after the dose of omeprazole was reduced to 20 mg daily. With this regimen, there was an endoscopic improvement to stage 2; this patient was not included in the maintenance treatment.

All patients showed dramatic symptomatic improvement. 8 patients were given maintenance treatment, the patient with a slight erosion was clinically improved and was treated with 20 mg (and therefore included) because of hypergastrinemia under 40 mg omeprazole. One patient showed an endoscopic and clinical recurrence 3 weeks later; he healed again after omeprazole was given at 40 mg. The 7 others had no clinical or endoscopic worsening for periods of 3 to 12 months.

The only clinical side-effects was a weight gain in 2 patients. There was no significant change in the labarotory screen. Blood gastrin did not increase under this 20 mg regimen. There was no hyperplasia of fundic endocrine cells in the 4 patients who completed the one year study.

Conclusion

Omeprazole appears highly effective in promoting endoscopic healing and in relieving symptoms in patients with reflux esophagitis who did not respond to H_2-receptor antagonists. A 20 mg daily schedule prevented recurrence in all but one patient for periods up to 1 year and was well tolerated.

The physicians who participated in this study were: Drs Bauret (Montpellier), Bonfils (Paris), Carayon (Besançon), Doll (Le Chesnay), Goldfain (Dreux), Moulinier (Lyon), Rotenberg (Dreux), Veyrac (Montpellier).

References

1. Behar J, Brand DL, Brown FC et al. (1978) Cimetidine in the treatment of symptomatic gastroesophageal reflux Gastroenterology 74: 441–448
2. Koelz HR, Birchler R, Bretholz A et al. (1986) Healing and relapse of reflux esophagitis during treatment with ranitidine. Gastroenterology 91: 1198–1205
3. Clissold SP, Campoli-Richards DM (1986) Omeprazole. A preliminary review of its pharmacodynamic and pharmacokinetics properties, and therapeutic potential in peptic ulcer disease and Zollinger-Ellison syndrome. Drugs 32: 15–47
4. Klinkenberg-Knol EC, Jansen JMBJ, Festen HPM (1987) Double blind multicenter comparison of omeprazole and ranitidine in the treatment of reflux oesophagitis. Lancet i, 349–351.
5. Dent J, Hetzel DJ, Reed WD et al. (1986) Healing of peptic esophagitis with omeprazole. Gastroenterology 88: 1363

Do we know the effect of inhibitors in the synthesis of prostaglandins (indomethacin) in the treatment of esophagitis?

Y. Ottignon, A. Dorgan-Dagaeff, J. P. Deschamps, and *P. Carayon* (Besançon)

Studies dealing with the effect of inhibitors of prostaglandin synthesis in the treatment of esophagitis are very few and mainly of an experimental nature.

In animals (Table 1), the different studies carried out argue in favor of a beneficial effect of indomethacin in the treatment of esophagitis. Thus in the opossum [4] the subcutaneous injection of indomethacin in a dose of 2 to 4 mg/kg/day during one week succeeded in preventing or reducing the lesions of irradiation esophagitis in dose-dependent fashion. Similarly in the cat [2] the mucosal lesions provoked by hydrochloric acid disappear after i.v. injection of indomethacin. This lesional improvement is also accompanied by a return of the inferior esophageal sphincter pressure to normal values which suggests a potential action of indomethacin on both the esophageal mucosa and on the sphincteric zone.

In man (Table 2) the effect of inhibitors of prostaglandin synthesis in the treatment of esophagitis is unknown, but certain studies provide the basis of a reply:

Table 1. In animal

– Indomethacin diminishes or prevents lesions of irradiation esophagitis (opossum)
– Indomethacin diminishes the lesions of peptic esophagitis and increases the LES pressure (cat)

Table 2. In man

	– LES pressure increased by indomethacin (200 mg by rectal route in healthy subjects)	
	but	
	LES pressure is not modified by	
▼	▼	▼
Aspirin (1 g peros)	5 ASA (2 g peros)	Indomethacin (75 mg peros)
Concentrations of PGE2 very elevated in the lesions of esophagitis (mediation of inflammation?)		

- in the healthy volunteer the administration of 200 mg indomethacin by the rectal route produces a marked increases in LES pressure [1]. The hypothesis advanced is that of an inhibition of the synthesis of PGs of type E which possess an inhibitory action on the sphincter tonus. However these results have not been found with indomethacin administered orally in a dose of 75 mg [3] nor with other inhibitors of prostaglandin synthesis (Fig. 1) such as aspirin in a dose of 1 g by mouth and 5-aminoacetylsalicylic acid in a dose of 2 g by mouth (personal unpublished work)
- in patients with reflux esophagitis, the tissue concentrations of PGE 2 in the esophagus are raised within the lesions of the esophagitis but are near normal in the healthy mucosa [5] (Table 3). These results suggest that, in the esophagus as in the colon and rectum the PGs result in mediation of the inflammation. Were this hypothesis to be confirmed it would justify the use of inhibitors of prostaglandin synthesis in the treatment of the lesions of esophagitis.

In conclusion, in animals the efficacy of indomethacin in the treatment of esophagitis now appears well established. In man, this efficacy, though potential, remains to be demonstrated.

Table 3. Tissue concentrations in vivo of PGE2 (in ng/g of fresh tissue) in the body of the esophagus at 5 and 15 cm from the mucosal junction, in healthy mucosa and within the lesions of esophagitis

	Control subjects n=9	Patients with esophagitis n=8	
5 cm	39.1+6.5		comparison
15 cm	41.7+9.3	34.3+ 9	with other
lesion		290.4+45.7*	values *p< 0.001

The values given correspond to means+standard deviation

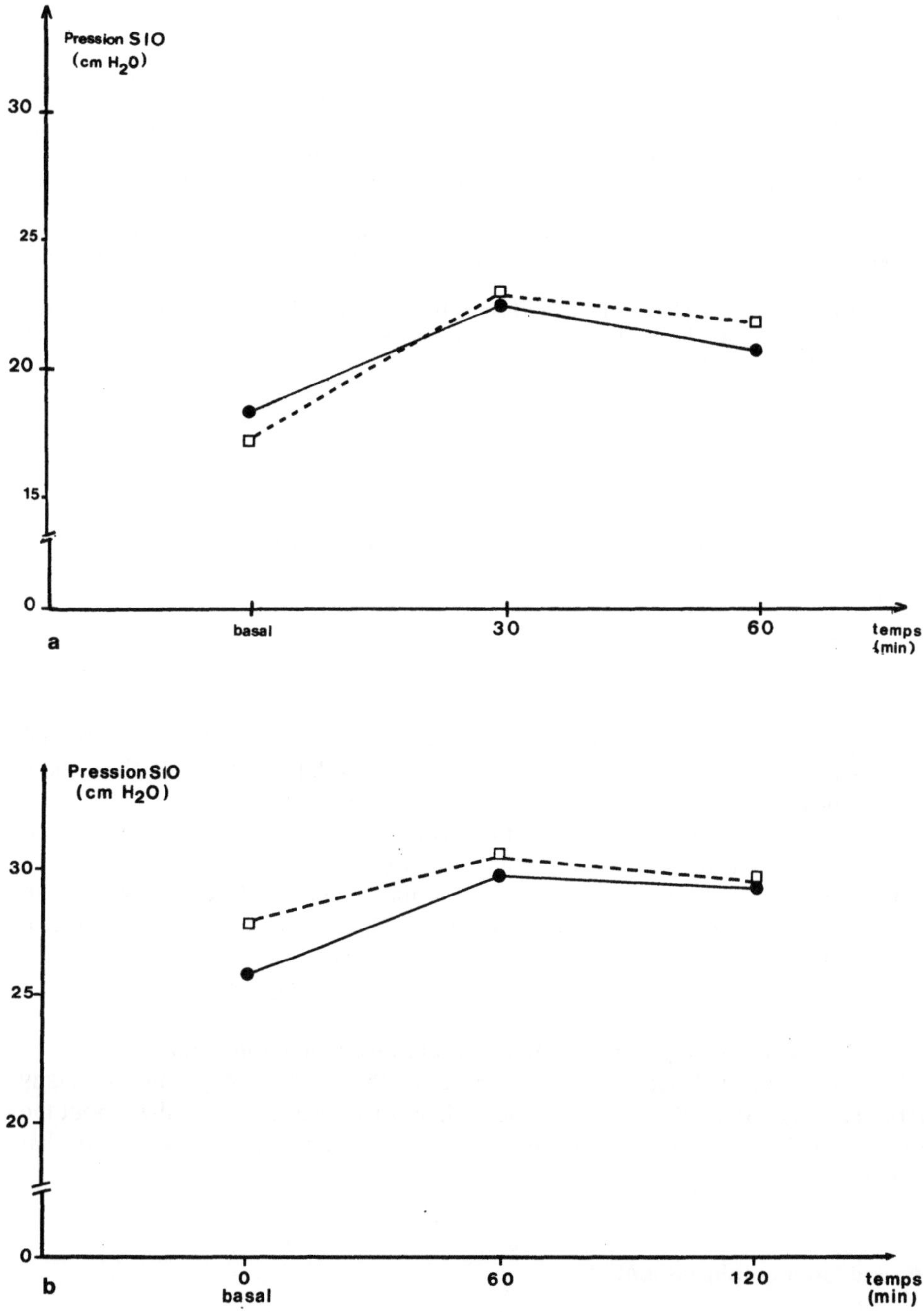

Fig. 1a, b. a) Means of pressures of inferior esophageal sphincter in basal period, 30 minutes and 60 minutes after ingestion of aspirin (continuous line) and placebo (interrupted line) in 6 healthy volunteers
b) Means of pressures of inferior esophageal sphincter in basal period, 60 minutes and 120 minutes after ingestion of 5-aminoacetylsalicylic acid (continuous line) or placebo (interrupted line) in 10 healthy volunteers

References

1. Dilawari JB, Newman A, Poleo J, Misiewicz JJ (1975) Response of the human cardiac sphincter to circulating, prostaglandins F2 et E2 and to anti-inflammatory drugs. Gut 16: 137–143
2. Eastwood GL, Beck BD, Castell DO, Brown FC, Fletcher JR (1981) Beneficial effect of indomethacin on acid-induced esophagitis in cats. Dig Dis Sci 26: 601–608
3. Kruidinier J, Tao P, Wilson DE (1978) The role of prostaglandins in lower esophageal sphincter pressure in man. Clin Res 26: 663 (Res)
4. Northway MG, Libshitz HI, Osborne BM, Feldman MS, Mamel JJ, West JH, Szwarc IA (1980) Radiation esophagitis in the opossum: radio-protection with indomethacin. Gastroenterology 78: 883–892
5. Ottignon Y, Alber D, Moussard C, Deschamps JP, Carayon P, Henry JC (1987) Esophageal mucosal prostaglandin E2 levels in health and in gastroesophageal reflux disease. Prostagland Leuk and Med in press

Can peptic esophagitis be healed by prostaglandins?

J.-P. Bader (Paris)

The logic of this question comes from the knowledge of the three essential pathophysiological data about reflux esophagitis (R. E) To each of these data corresponds potential pharmacological effects of prostaglandins (PG).

1. R. E is mostly related to the contact of gastric acid with the esophageal mucosa:
   - many PGs have an inhibitory effect on gastric acid secretion.
2. Gastroesophageal reflux (G.E.R.), a determining factor of R. E, is related to an impairment of the lower esophagus motility: hypotony of the lower esophageal sphincter (LES) and bad clearance of the lower esophagus:
   - some PGs have a prokinetic action on parts of the digestive tract.
3. R. E is an inflammatory process:
   - many PG have a protective effect on digestive mucosa inflammation.

The first point will not be discussed here, as the antisecretory action of many natural and synthetic PG is well documented. We will focus on the studies about the effects of PG on lower esophagus motility and the inflammatory processes in that region.

PG and lower esophagus motility

Animal studies (Tables 1, 2)

G. Coruzzi et al. noted that PGE_1 exerted a relaxant effect on isolated rat LES preparations, while a PGE_1 analog, 16-methyl-16 methoxy PGE_1, induced LES contraction at doses higher than 10 ng/ml [1].

Table 1. PG and esophageal motility in animals (1)

	Type of PG	Experimental animal	Route of admin.	Pressure of LES	Peristalsis
G. Coruzzi et al.	PGE_1 16 methyl 16-methoxy PGE_1	rat Isolated LES idem	"in vitro" idem	↘ ↗	
D. R. Sinar et al.	PGE_1	cat	IV infusion	↘	↘ amplitude
D. R. Sinar et al.	PGE_1	baboon	IV infusion		↘ duration amplitude

Table 2. PG and esophageal motility in animals (2)

	Type of PG	Experimental animal	Route of admin.	Pressure of LES
R. K. Goyal	PGE_1	opossum	IV	↘
et al.	PGE_2	opossum	IV	↘
J. W. Maher	15-méthyl PGE_2	dog	perfusion IV	↗
N. Iwai	$PGF_{2\alpha}$	dog	perfusion IV	↗

In cats, D. R. Sinar et al. showed a reduction of LES pressure and of the amplitude of peristaltic contractions with PGE_1 [13].

The same author observed a 77% reduction of the amplitude of peristaltic contractions and a decrease in the duration of the waves in the distal esophagus in baboons given a continuous infusion of 5 ng/kg/min PGE_1. However, the effect on the distal esophagus was much weaker [14].

A similar reduction of LES pressure was obtained by R. K. Goyal et al. in opossums with PGE_1 and PGE_2 [4].

J. W. Maher (Fig. 1) et al. using an i.v. bolus of 0,5 mcg/kg 15-methyl PGE_2 in dogs, showed an increase in LES pressure similar to that obtained with gastrin, but without any rise in its plasmatic levels [7].

N. Iwai et al., studying the effects of Nissen fundoplication in dogs, showed that the preoperative LES pressure was markedly increased by a continuous i.v infusion of 1.5 r/kg/min $PGF_{2\alpha}$ [6].

Human studies (Table 3)

R. K. Goyal (Fig. 2) investigated in 12 normal volunteers the effect of a continuous i.v infusion of PGE_2 [4]. He found similar results as in opossums, i.e, a dose-dependent reduction of the LES pressure, beginning with a dose of 0.05 ng/kg/min and maximum (a 60% reduction) with a dose of 0.4 ng/kg/min [4]. A decrease in the amplitude of peristaltic contractions on the distal esophagus was also observed [4].

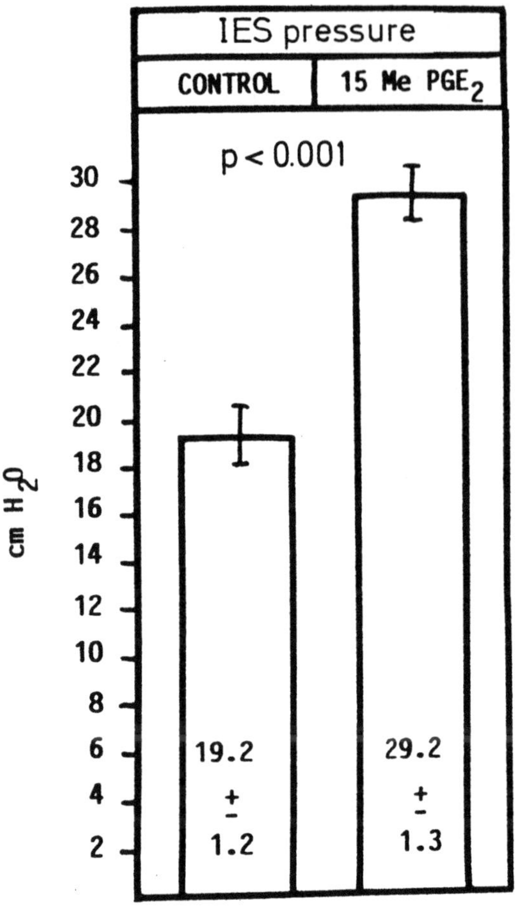

Fig. 1. Action of 15-methyl PGE_2 on LES pressure in the dog (after Maher)

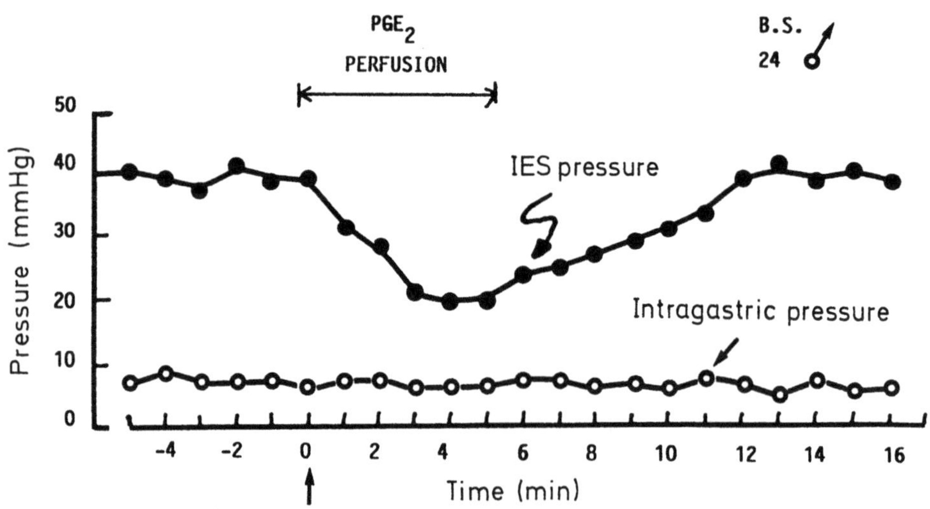

Fig. 2. Action of PGE_2 on LES pressure in the healthy man (after Goyal)

Table 3. PG and esophageal motility in man (3)

	Type of PG	Subject	Route of administr.	Pressure of LES	Peristalsis
R. K. Goyal	PGE_2	VS	IV inf.	$\searrow$	
J. B. Dilawari	PGE_2	VS + GER	IV inf.	$\searrow$	
–	$PGF_{2\alpha}$	idem	idem	$\nearrow$	
G. J. Schwartz	Trimoprostil Trimethy-Desoxy PGE_2	VS	oral	=	=

In 41 subjects (8 normal volunteers and 33 presenting with G.E.R. with or without R.E), J. B. Dilawari et al. confirmed the inhibitory effect of PGE_2 given a 0.08 mcg/kg/min continuous i.v infusion on the LES pressure [2]. In the same subjects, they showed the stimulatory action of PGF_2 on LES with doses from 0.05 to 0.8 mcg/kg/min (Fig. 3). In addition they showed that indomethacin known as an inhibitor of some endogen PG synthesis, has a stimulatory effect on LES pressure when administered intrarectally in a dose of 200 mg.

Little information is available about the effects of the analogs of PG used at present in gastroenterology on distal esophagus motility.

However, G. J. Schwartz et al. compared trimoprostil, a trimethyldesoxy PGE_2, administered orally at doses of 0.75 mg and 1.5 mg with placebo in 12 healthy volunteers. No significant difference was observed, thus no effect of the drug on LES pressure and esophageal peristaltic waves was found [12].

PG and lower esophagus normal or inflammatory mucosa

Animal studies

Most of experimental works show a worsening of experimental esophagitis lesions with the administration of PG and, conversely, a protective effect of indomethacin [3, 5, 9].

Human studies (Table 4)

The main study was reported by Y. Ottignon (Fig. 4) et al. [10]: PGE_2 levels in esophageal mucosa were measured in 9 healthy volunteers, 11 patients presenting

Table 4. PGE_2 content of the esophageal mucosa (mcg/g)

			Esophagitis	
	healthy volunteers	GER	non inflammatory zones	inflammatory zones
Y. Ottignon	41±9	37±11	34±9	290 + 45
S. Pugh	96±40		39±4	

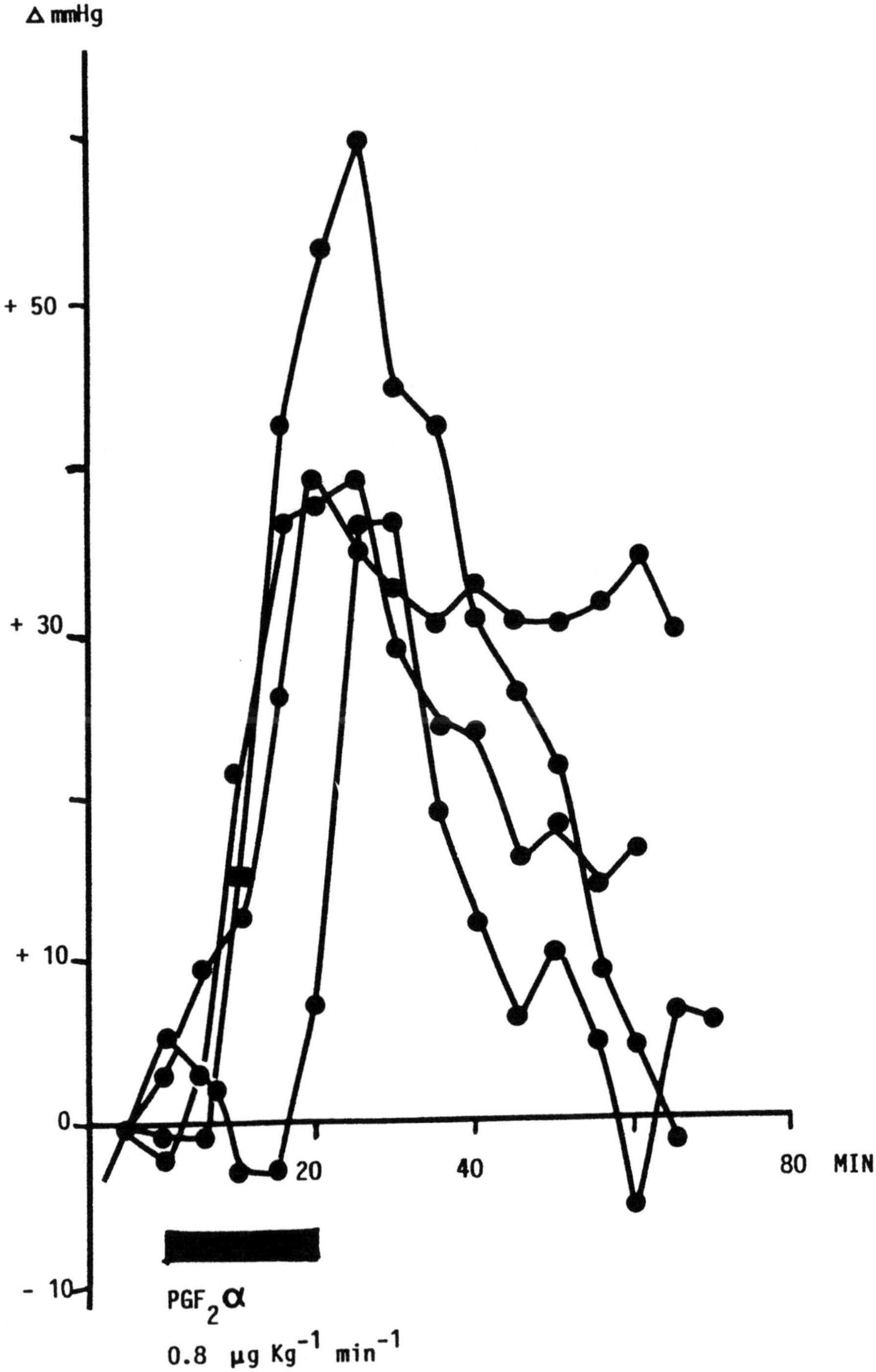

Fig. 3. Action of PGE_2 on LES pressure (after Dilawari)

with G.E.R without R.E and 8 patients with R.E. A marked increase in PGE_2 levels in the inflammatory tissue of patients with R.E (290.4±45.7 ng/g) was found as compared to all other samples: healthy volunteers (41.7±9.3 ng/g), G.E.R (37.8±11.2 ng/g) and R.E within normal mucosa (34.3±9.0 ng/g).

Thus, the presence of an inflammatory process seems to be correlated with high levels of PGE_2. In contrast, no correlation was found between local concentration of PGE_2 and basal pressure of LES.

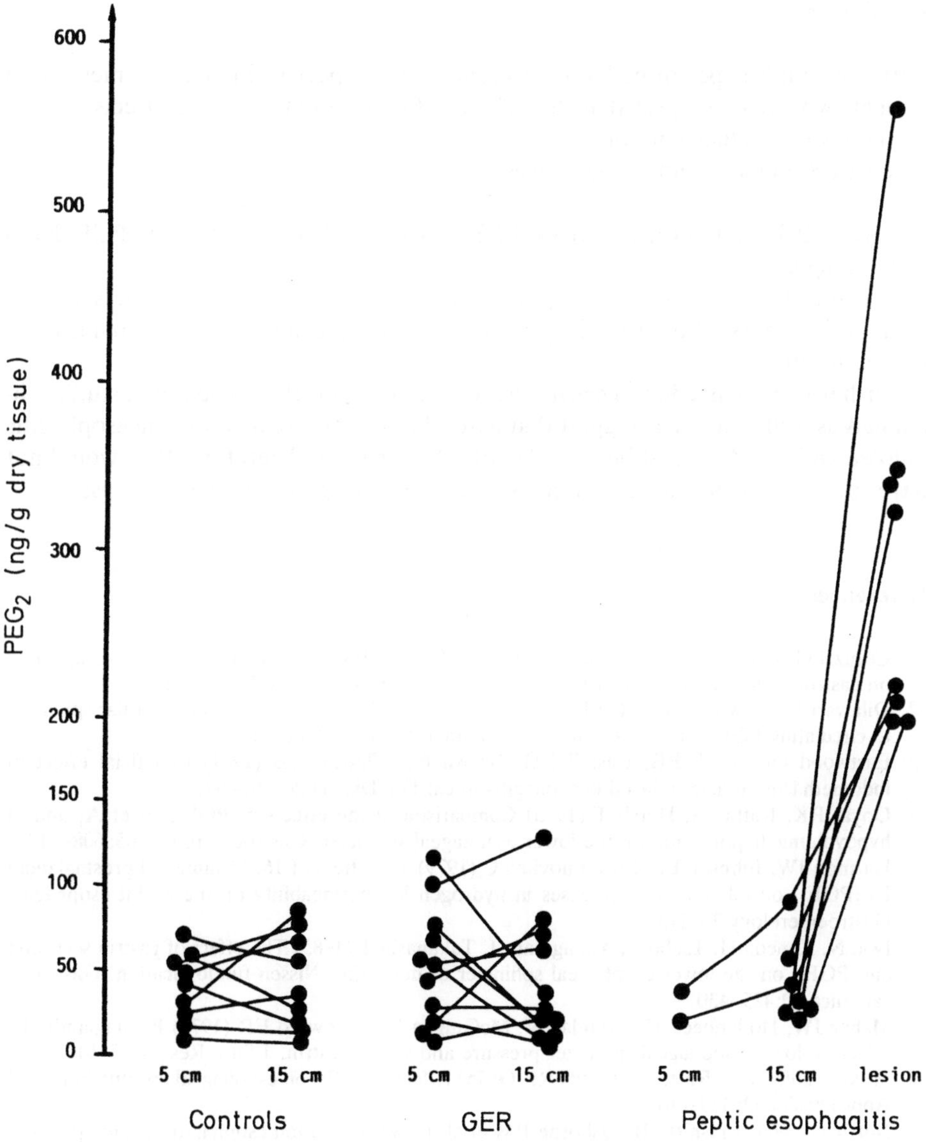

Fig. 4. PGE_2 content of esophageal mucosa in man (after Ottignon)

However, S. Pugh, another investigator who also studied PGE_2 concentration in lower esophageal mucosa in 10 healthy subjects and 8 patients with R.E found opposite results:

- normal esophageal mucosa: 96.8±40.6 pg/mg
- R.E mucosa: 39.4±15.1 pg/mg

A comparison of both methods would be necessary to appreciate these contradictory results.

Conclusion

Different studies performed on different animal species, in healthy men or in patients with R.E, suggest that the different PG have not the same effects:

- on lower esophagus motility
- on LES pressure and on peristalsis.

Natural PGE_1 and PGE_2 decrease LES pressure and peristalsis, while PGF_2 has a stimulating effect.

In contrast, the action of PGE_1 and PGE_2 can be reversed with some synthetic analogs. The possibility of developing new PG acting against G.E.R remains open for the future.

Further work is needed to clarify the action of PG on R.E. The initial studies, in animals as well as in men, suggest that natural PG levels are increased in esophagitis mucosa and could at least be an index of inflammation. Therefore, they would not have the same cytoprotective effect as they have on gastroduodenal mucosa.

References

1. Coruzzi G, Poli E, Adami M, Bertaccini G. Effect of MDL 646 a new synthetic prostaglandin on gastroesophageal motility in the rat. Il Farmaco Ed Sc 38 (fasc 2): 121–127
2. Dilawari JB, Newman A, Poleo J, Misiewicz JJ (1975) Response of the human cardiac sphincter to circulating $PGF_{2\alpha}$ and E_2 and to antiinflammatory drugs. Gut 15: 137–143
3. Eastwood GL, Beck BB, Castell RO, Brown FC, Fletcher JB (1981) Beneficial effect of indomethacin on acid induced oesophagitis in cat Dig Dis Sci 26: 601–608
4. Goyal RK, Rattan S, Hersh T (1973) Comparison of the effects of PGE_1, E_2 et A_2 and of hypovolumic hypotension on the lower esophageal sphincter. Gastroenterology 65: 608–612
5. Harmon JW, Johnson LF, Maydonovitch C (1979) The effect of 16, 16-dimethyl prostaglandin E_2 (PGE_2) on bile-induced increases in hydrogen ion permeability on the rabbit esophagus. Gastroenterology 76: 1151
6. Iwai N, Kaneda H, Tsubo T, Yanagihara J, Takahashi T (1985) The effect of gastrin secretion and $PGF_{2\alpha}$ on the lower esophageal sphincter of dogs after Nissen fundoplication. Gastroent Japonica 20:425–430
7. Maher JW, Hollenbeck JI, Crandall V, McGuigan J, Woodward ER (1978) Prostaglandin E_2 effect on lower esophageal sphincter pressure and serum gastrin. J Surg Res 24: 87–91
8. Mukhopadhyay A, Rattan S, Goyal RK (1975) Effect of PGE_2 on esophageal motility in man. J Appl Physiol 39: 479–487
9. Northway MG, Libshitz HI, Osborne BM et al. (1980) Radiation esophagitis in the opossum: radioprotection with indomethacin. Gastroenterology 78: 883–892

10. Ottignon Y, Alber D, Moussard C, Deschamps JP, Carayon P, Henry JC. Esophageal mucosa PGE_2 levels in health and in gastroesophageal reflux disease (to be published in "Prostaglandins and Medicine")
11. Pugh S, Williams SE, Lewin MS, Barton TP, Salmon PR, Clark CG (1985) Prostaglandin E_2 in normal and abnormal upper GI endoscopic biopsies. Gut 26: 560A–561A (abstract)
12. Schwartz GJ, Levine RA, Sondheimer JB, Petokas S, Gallo-Torres HE, Scheinbaum HL (1985) Effect of trimoprostil, a PGE_2 analog on esophageal motility in man. Gastroenterology 88: 1577 (abstract)
13. Sinar DR, Fletcher JR, Castell DO (1981) Prostaglandins E_1 effect on resting and cholinergically stimulated lower esophageal sphincter pressure in cats. Prostaglandins 21: 581–590
14. Sinar DR, Cordova CM, Fletcher JR, Castell DO (1982) Decreased esophageal peristaltic amplitude in response of Prostaglandin E_1 and prostacyclin in the bàboon. Dig Dis Sci 27: 1067–1072

M. Deltenre, C. Jonas, E. De Koster, M. van Gossum, and *B. Ramdani* (Brussels)

When considering therapeutic possibilities of prostaglandins, clinicians must be aware that actually available drugs are prostaglandins (PGs) analogues, which had to be developped mainly because of bioavailability problems and might greatly differ from endogenous PGs and 'natural' PGs, largely investigated in animal models.

Up till now, experience with both natural PGs and analogue components in physiology of the esophagus and gastroesophageal reflux is rather poor. In fact, when reviewing possible factors involved in harmful G.E.R., there are few theoretical reasons for designing therapeutic trials with PG analogues:

1. PGEs induce relaxation of circular smooth muscle of the gastro-intestinal tract and are reported to decrease LES pressure [11]:
2. Impaired esophageal acid clearance (primary or secondary to acid-induced esophageal lesions) is usually considered as an important factor in G.E.R: possible action of PG's on lower esophagus motility has not been investigated to our knowledge.
3. Theoretically, esophageal mucosal resistance for various aggressive agents (including acid) depends on appropriate submucosal blood flow. Once more, although beautiful data have confirmed PG's protective action against senescence of human gastric mucosa [8, 25], NSAI drugs [4, 9, 16, 24], which are now well known to be potent inhibitors of gastric endogenous PG's synthesis [21], and smoking [15, 20], no evidence about such positive action of PG's for the esophagus has been published. Moreover, some papers described a good (or even better) protective effect of ranitidine against aspirin induced gastric lesions [14, 19].

   Even if such a positive action of PG's exists for the esophagus, no systemic action of PG's analogues can be conceived (this is a large part of their safety in GD ulcer's treatment) and the duration of close contact between esophageal mucosa and orally given PG is too short to hope topical action, which seems to be efficient in the stomach [1].

4. Delayed gastric emptying [5] and to a lesser degree, duodeno-gastric reflux, may play a role in peptic esophagitis: endogenous PG's may accelerate gastric clearance of fluids [23] but PGE_1 analog showed no influence in gastric emptying in clinical human experiments [18]. Moreover, PGs seem to favorize duodenogastric reflux [7].
5. Finally, just as in peptic ulcer disease [2, 6, 10], the main potential therapeutic action of PG analogues is inhibition of acid secretion. Results obtained with potent acid secretion inhibitors in terms of esophagitis' healing rate are rather deceiving (except perhaps for omeprazole).

However there is no clear reason to prefer PG analogues to anti-H_2: ranitidine was proved to be superior to enprostil for treatment of duodenal ulcer (with less side effects [17]) and even to promote endogenous secretion of gastric PGs, at least in DU patients [22]. Moreover, ranitidine was reported to have no action on LES pressure [26].

In the interim report on 107 patients included in a multicentric, parallel, double blind, placebo-controlled study of Enprostil in management of reflux esophagitis (grade 0 to 3), Knauer et al. [13], found a difference in relief of nocturnal symptoms and also, numerous patients with side effects (even in placebo group; see Table 1).

Despite discouraging and non significant results in terms of improvement and healing, this study revealed that a PG analog regimen had to reach acid inhibition doses to hope some therapeutic effect in peptic esophagitis: a prospective open study using misoprostol (Cytotec R) 5×200 μg was initialized by our group in patients with peptic esophagitis grade 2 or 3. Postural precautions and diet were given. 5 informed patients were included within 1 month and all dropped out (see Table 2).

Table 1

		Enprostil 35 μg bid	7 μg bid	Placebo
*Improvement	Week 4	48%	44%	43%
	Week 8	53%	42%	38%
	Week 12	76%	48%	41%
Healing rate	Week 4	9%	18%	8%
	Week 8	31%	21%	16%
	Week 12	45%	30%	22%
Diarrhea		31%	24%	28%

* at least one grade

Table 2

Patient	Drop out delay	Cause of drop out
Male 42y	5 days	Heartburn unchanged, diarrhea, dizziness
Female 39y	7 days	Majored heartburn and epigastric pain
Male 70y	7 days	Nausea, abdominal cramps
Female 61y	7 days	Majored heartburn, diarrhea, dizziness
Female 64y	10 days	Majored heartburn, dizziness (with rechallenge)

The study was discontinued: as attempted, no improvement was found at endoscopy when patients dropped out. Despite the fact that single dose of misoprostol was reported to have no cardiovascular effect [3], a systemic effect of this PGE_1 analogue could be suspected among our patients. Diarrhea, reported in 13% of patients included in large clinical trials [12], was not the main cause for treatment's discontinuation.

From both theoretical and clinical points of view, there is no indication for available PG-like synthetic derivates in the management of peptic esophagitis in 1987. Prostaglandins did not fulfil their promise in GD ulcer's treatment [10], no benefit can be conceptually attempted in peptic esophagitis.

In the future, some studies might show some benefit in prevention of esophageal lesions after radiotherapy or NSAID-induced esophagitis but no animal studies may actually lead to undertake clinical trial in that field.

References

1. Agrawal NM, Godiwala T, Arimura A, Dajani EZ (1986) Cytoprotection by a synthetic prostaglandin against ethanol induced gastric mucosal damage. A double blind endoscopic study in human subjects. Gastrointest Endosc 32: 67–70
2. Brand DL, Roufail WM, Thomson ABR, Tapper EJ (1985) Misoprostol, a synthetic PGE_1 analog, in the treatment of duodenal ulcers: A multicenter double-blind study. Dig Dis Sci 30: 147S–158S
3. Brecht TH (1986) Circulatory parameters after administration of misoprostol Dig Dis Sci 31
4. Cohen MM, Clark L, Armstrong L et al. (1985) Reduction of aspirin-induced fecal blood loss with low-dose misoprostol tablets in man. Dig Dis Sci 30: 605
5. Collins BJ, McFarland RJ, O'Hare MMT et al. (1986) Gastric emptying of a solid-liquid meal and gastro-intestinal hormone responses in patients with erosive oesophagitis. Digestion 33: 61
6. Deakin M, Ralage J, Paul A et al. (1986) Effect of Enprostil, a synthetic prostaglandin E2 on 24 hour intragastric acidity, nocturnal acid and pepsin secretion. Gut 27: 1054
7. Dooley CP, Bao BCH, Mello WD et al. (1985) Effects of aspirin and prostaglandin E2 on interdigestive motility complex and duodenogastric reflux in man. Dig Dis Sci 30: 513–521
8. Fich A, Arber N, Sestieri M et al. (1985) Effect of misoprostol and cimetidine on gastric cell labelling index. Gastroenterology 89: 57
9. Gilbert DA, Surawicz CM, Silverstein FE et al. (1984) Prevention of acute aspirin-induced gastric mucosal injury by 15-R-15 methyl prostaglandin E2: an endoscopic study Gastroenterology 86: 339
10. Hawkey CJ, Walt RP (1986) Prostaglandins for peptic ulcer: a promise unfulfilled. Lancet 2: 1084–6
11. Herman AG (1986) Les prostaglandines: une nouvelle catégorie de médicaments? Actuel, Nov 86: 2–7
12. Herting RL, Clay GA (1985) Overview of clinical safety with misoprostal. Dig Dis Sci 30: 11 185S–193S
13. Knauer CM, Archambault A, Bynum TE, Chey WY, Gregory P, Hirschowitz BI, Navert H, Robinson M, Sutherland L, Thomson ABR, Bynum L (1985) The efficacy of Enprostil in reflux esophagitis (Interim report) Proceedings of 'Enprostil symposium', Toronto
14. Konturek SJ, Kwiecien NK, Obtulowicz W et al. (1983) Comparison of prostaglandin E2 and ranitidine in prevention of gastric bleeding by aspirin in man. Gut 24: 89
15. Lam SK, Lau WY, Choi TK et al. (1986) Prostaglandin E1 (misoprostol) overcomes the adverse effect of chronic cigarette smoking on duodenal ulcer healing. Dig Dis Sc 31 nr2 68S
16. Lanza FL (1986) A double-blind study of prophylactic effect of misoprostol on lesions of gastric and duodenal mucosa induced by oral administration of tolmetin in healthy subjects. Dig Dis Sci 31 nr2 131S

17. Lauritsen K, Laursen LS, Havelund TA et al. (1986) Enprostil and ranitidine in duodenal ulcer healing: Double blind comparative study. Br Med J 292: 864–866
18. Moore JG, Alazraki N, Clay GD (1986) Effect of synthetic prostaglandin E1 analog on gastric emptying of meals in man. Dig Dis Sci 31: 16
19. Muller P, Damman HG and Simon B (1986) Acute acetylsalicylic acid-induced gastric mucosal injury/An endoscopic comparative study in man with oral prostaglandin analogues, omeprazole and ranitidine. Drug Res 36: 265–268
20. McCready DR, Clark L, Cohen MM (1985) Cigarette smoking reduces human gastric luminal prostaglandin E2. Gut 26: 1192–1196
21. McCready DR, Wallace JL, Cohen MM (1984) Prostaglandin biosynthesis by gastric mucosa. 2. Studies in man. Can Clin Biochem 17: 183–187
22. Rachmilewitz D, Ligumsky M, Ficha A et al. (1986) Role of endogenous gastric prostanoids in the pathogenesis and therapy of duodenal ulcer. Gastroenterology 90: 963–969
23. Sanders KM (1984) Role of prostaglandins in regulating gastric motility. Am J Physiol 247: G117
24. Silverstein FE, Kimmey MB, Saunders DR et al. (1986) Gastric protection by misoprostol against 1300 mg of aspirin. Dig Dis Sci 31 nr 2 137S
25. Tytgat GNJ, Offerhaus GJA, van Minnen AJ et al. (1986) Influence of oral 15(R)-15 methyl prostaglandin E2 on human gastric mucosa. Gastroenterology 90: 1111
26. Wallin L, Madsen T, Boesby S (1983) Gastro-oesophageal function in normal subjects after oral administration of ranitidine. Gut 24: 154

Y. Ottignon, D. Alber, C. Moussard, J. C. Henry,
and *P. Carayon* (Besançon)

The action of the prostaglandins on the esophageal mucosa is not well known as little work has been done on this. In animals, both direct and indirect arguments suggest that the PGs have no cell-protective action at esophageal level. Thus, in the rabbit [3] 16,16-dimethyl PGE_2 in a dose of 2.4 mg/kg/h by i.v. injection increases the permeability of the esophageal mucosa to H+ ions during perfusion with a biliary acid. Further, in different animal species [2] the administration of PGE_1 or PGE_2 diminishes the pressure of the inferior esophageal sphincter in dose-dependent fashion. Conversely, in the cat [1] the i.v. injection of inhibitors of PG synthesis causes the disappearance of the esophageal mucosal lesions provoked by hydrochloric acid while restoring a normal sphincteric pressure.

In man, the effect of PGs on the lesions of peptic esophagitis is unknown. Several therapeutic trials of synthetic PGs of the E series in the treatment of esophagitis with reflux are currently in progress but so far without available results. However, certain studies suggest that the PGs would not have a beneficial effect on peptic esophagitis, but on the contrary an exacerbational effect: In the healthy volunteer the administration of PGE_1 or PGE_2 [5, 7] decreases the pressure of the inferior esophageal sphincter in dose-dependent fashion, which has led several authors to consider their use in achalasia. Contrary to what is observed with natural PGs, the administration of 16,16-dimethyl PGE_2 [4] does not seem to modify the basal pressure of the inferior esophageal sphincter; on the contrary it produces inhibition of the sphincter response to pentagastrin and arouse fears of a poor adaptation of sphincter function under PGs.

In patients with reflux esophagitis [6], the esophageal tissue concentrations of PGE_2 are very much increased within the lesions of esophagitis, whereas they are normal at a distance from these lesions and in patients with uncomplicated gastroesophageal reflux (Fig. 1, 2). Thus, in the esophagus the PGs (or at least PGE_2) may be implicated in the pathogenesis of the inflammation (as in the colon and rectum) and may not have the same cell-protective function as in the stomach or duodenum.

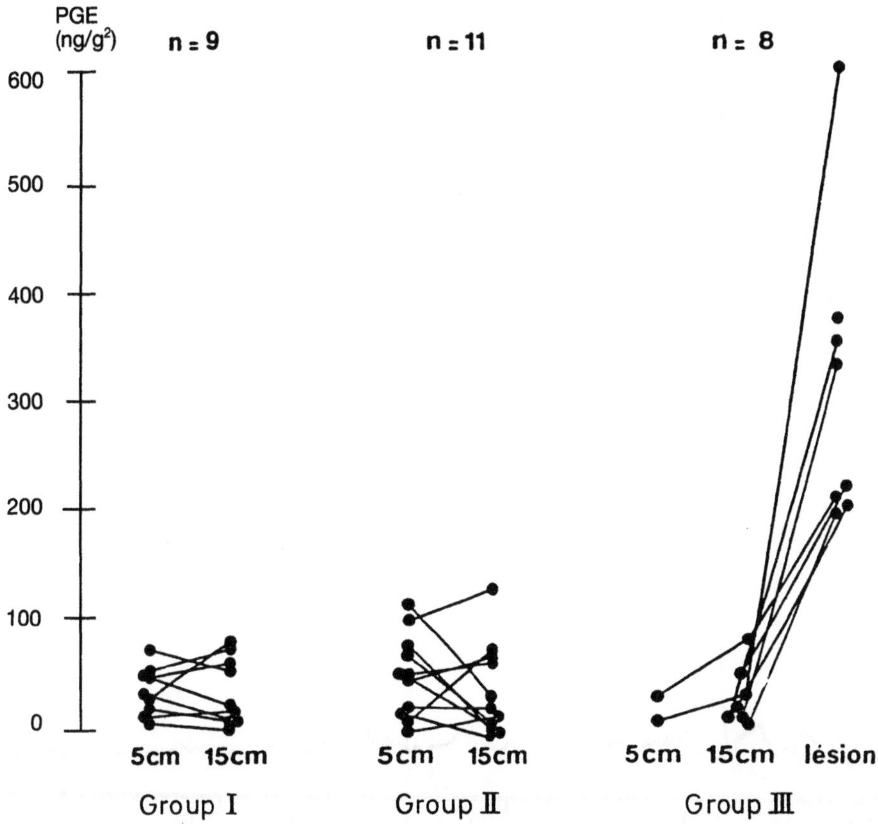

Fig. 1. Tissue concentrations of PGE2 in vivo obtained from biopsy specimens of esophageal mucosa performed at 5 and 15 cm from the mucosal junction and within the lesions of esophagitis in the control subjects (Group 1, n=9) and in patients with uncomplicated gastroesophageal reflux (Group II, n=11) or with reflux esophagitis (Group III, n=8)

References

1. Eastwood GL, Beck BD, Castell DO, Brown FC, Fletcher JR (1981) Beneficial effect of indomethacin on acid-induced esophagitis in cats. Dig Dis Sci 26: 601–608

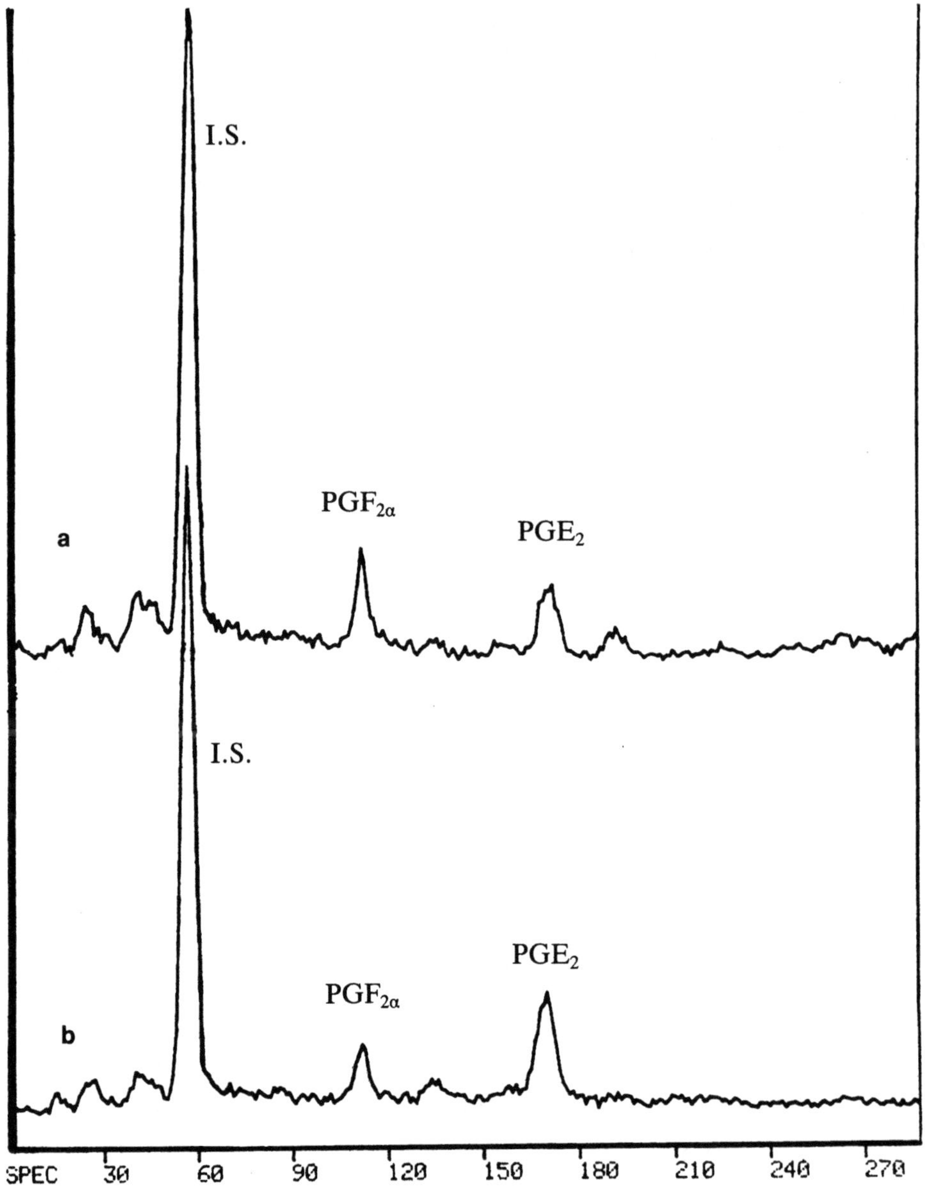

Fig. 2a–c. In vitro byosinthesis of prostanoids in human esophageal mucosa: quantitative profiling obtained by capillary column gas chromatography mass spectrometry. **a)** Healthy mucosa; **b)** Gastro esophageal reflux but apparently healthy mucosa; **c)** Reflux esophagitis lesion (I.S. = Internal Standard)

2. Goyal RK, Rattan S (1973) Comparison of the effects of PGE1, E2, A2 and of hypovolumic hypotension on the lower esophageal sphincter. Gastroenterology 65: 608–612
3. Harmon JW, Johnson LF, Maydonovitch C (1979) The effect of 16-16 dimethyl prostaglandin E2 (PGE2) on bile induced increases in hydrogen ion permeability on the rabbit esophagus. Gastroenterology 76: 1151 A

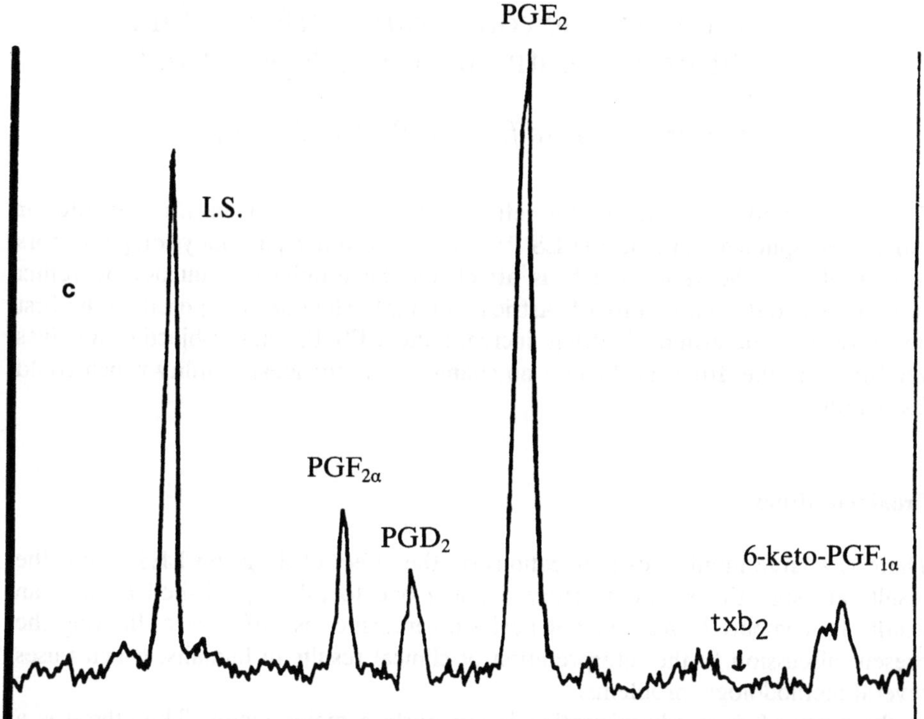

Fig. 2c

4. McCallum RW, Ippoliti AF, Sturdevant RAL (1975) Effect of oral 16-16 dimethyl prostaglandin E2 on the LES in man. Gastroenterology 68: 949 A
5. Mukhopadhyay AK, Rattan S, Goyal RK (1975) Effect of prostaglandin E2 on esophageal motility in man. J Appl Physiol, 39: 479–481
6. Ottignon Y, Alber D, Moussard C, Deschamps JP, Carayon P, Henry JC (1987) Esophageal mucosal prostaglandin E2 levels in health and in gastroesophageal reflux disease. Prostagland Leuk and Med in press
7. Sorensen HR, Boesby S, Pedersen SA (1974) The effect of prostaglandin E1 on resting gastroesophageal sphincter pressure in normal human subjects. Scand J gastroenterol, 9–29

What are the comparative effects of the different treatments on LES pressure?

P. Denis, C. Tardif, and *J. Weber* (Rouen)

The aim of medical treatment for reflux is the correction of insufficient inferior esophageal sphincter pressure (LES P), and of the other pathophysiologic factors responsible for the reflux (such as attack on the esophageal mucosa by reflux substances and decreased rate of gastric emptying). The question posed by the first objective is to determine if drugs increase the LES P, while objective involves verifying that the drugs used cause no changes in esophageal motility which could favor reflux.

Prokinetic drugs

There is a large number of publications on the effect of drugs on LES P, but the results are sometimes contradictory, leading one to ask if published results can validly be compared. We will not deal with interspecies differences, limiting the present discussion to the interpretation of clinical results in humans, which raises several methodologic problems:

a) the route of drug administration is obviously a major factor. Thus there is a clearcut increase in LES P when domperidone is given I.V. [1], while the same drug given orally has no effect [2] (Table 1);
b) the recording techniques may suggest a different effect in the same subject given the same drug [3] (Table 2);

Table 1. Comparative effects of different medical treatments on LES pressure

	Route of administration Example: domperidone		
	Dose	Route	LES P
Weihrauch 1979	8 mg	I.V.	Increased
Wallin	20 mg	Oral	Unchanged

Table 2. Comparative effects of different medical treatments on LES pressure

	Recording technique Example: atropine	
	The same volunteer subjects:	
Cohen, 1972 The same results as Cohen		Jensen, 1978 The same results as Jensen

Table 3. Comparative effects of different medical treatments on LES pressure

	Measurement of LES P (cm H_2O) (Pozzessere 1982)	
Mean of 3 methods of recording	Control 16.8±2.4	Drug 19.8.±2.7
	N. S.	
Highest value with one of the 3 routes	22.4±3.4	29.9±3.8
	$p < 0.05$	

c) measurement of the LES P itself must be taken into account. Thus, the pressure may be significantly increased or remain unchanged in the same subject, depending on whether we consider the mean value of the LES P or its maximum level [4] (Table 3);
d) the pressure may be increased between meals but not soon after meals [5] (Fig. 1), explaining why the period of the 24 cycle during which measurements are carried out is important;
e) finally, results in healthy subjects and in reflux patients may differ, as in the case of metoclopramide [6] (Fig. 2).

The difficulties listed above render the comparison of different drugs very difficult. Furthermore, the effect of these drugs on the LES P in patients with an incompetent sphincter cannot be determined from the effect observed in healthy subjects. In these conditions, it appears that domperidone has little or no effect on LES P in reflux patients. Urecholine, metoclopramide and cisapride increase the LES P in patients with gastroesophageal reflux [6–9].

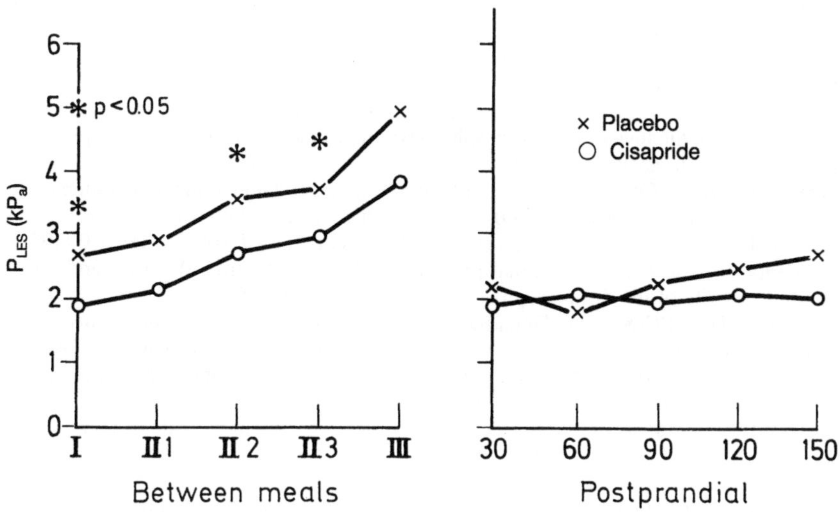

Fig. 1. Comparative effects of different medical treatments on LES pressure

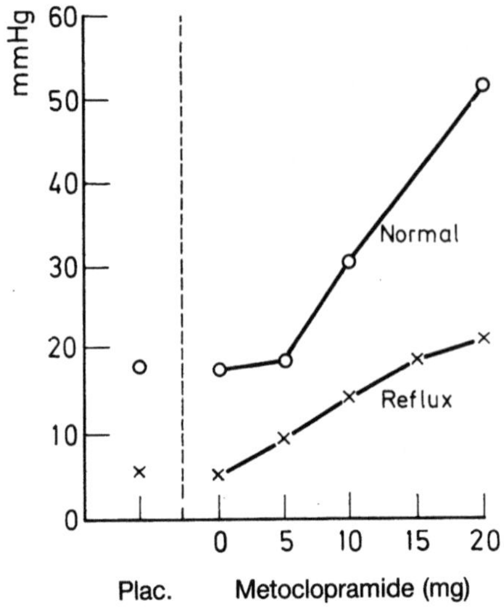

Fig. 2. Comparative effects of different medical treatments on LES pressure

Other drugs

Among the other drugs that can be used for the medical treatment of reflux, it is admitted that the LES P is unchanged by antacids, cimetidine [10], ranitidine [11], omeprazole [12] and sucralfate [13]. The question of anticholinergics remains controversial, though pirenzeprine does not appear to have an effect on the LES P in therapeutic doses [14].

References

1. Weihrauch T, Forster ChF, Krieglstein J (1979) Evaluation of the effect of domperidone on human esophageal and gastroduodenal motility by intraluminal manometry. Postgrad Med J 55 (suppl 1): 7–10
2. Wallin L, Madsen T, Boesby S (1985) Effect of Domperidone on gastroesophagel function in normal human subjects. Scand J Gastroenterol 20: 150–154
3. Ndjitoyap C, Lerebours E, Weber J, Galmiche JP, Denis Ph (1987) Anticholinergic pharmacological studies of the lower esophageal sphincter: importance of the technique of pressure recording. Int J Clin Pharm Res 7: 89–93
4. Pozzessere C, Materia E, Corazziari E, Anzini F (1982) Effects of Domperidone on esophageal motor activity and gastro-esophageal reflux. Ital J Gastroenterol 14: 159–161
5. Smout AJPM, Bogaard JW, Grade AC, Ten Thije OJ, Akkermans LMA, Wittebol P (1985) Effects of cisapride, a new gastrointestinal prokinetic substance, on inter-digestive and postprandial motor activity of the distal esophagus in man Gut 26: 246–251
6. Cohen S, Morris DW, Schoen HJ, Dimarino AJ (1976) The effect of oral and intravenous metoclopramide on human lower esophageal sphincter pressure. Gastroenterology 70: 484–487
7. Behar J, Biancani P (1976) Effect of oral metoclopramide on gastroesophageal reflux in the post-cibal state. Gastroenterology 70: 331–335
8. McCallum RW, Kline MM, Curry N, Sturdevant RAL (1975) Comparative effects of metoclopramide and bethanechol on lower esophageal sphincter pressure in reflux patients. Gastroenterology 68: 1114–1118
9. Janssens J (1986) Effect of cisapride on esophageal motility. Progress in the treatment of gastrointestinal motility disorders: the role of cisapride. Symposium Frankfurt Novembre

10. Goodall RJ, Temple JG (1980) Effect of cimetidine on lower esophageal-sphincter pressure in esophagitis. Br Med J: 611–612
11. Denis Ph, Galmiche JP, Ducrotte Ph, Colin R, Pasquis P, Lefrancois R (1981) Effect of ranitidine on resting pressure and pentagastrin response on human lower esophageal sphincter. Dig Dis Sci 26: 999–1002
12. Dent J, Downton J, Heddle R, Buckle PJ, Toouli J, Mackinnon A, Wyman JB (1986) Effects of omeprazole on peptic esophagitis and esophageal motility and pH. Scand J Gastroenterol 21 (suppl 118): 181
13. Leport J, Bloch F, Petit JP (1985) Etude de l'activité du sucralfate sur la motricité oesophagienne chez le sujet sain Rev Med Int 6: 327–328

Comparative effects of the treatments on esophageal motricity and esophageal clearance

G. Cargill, and *M. Duché* (Paris)

We limit this brief discussion to a certain number of prokinetic treatments which modify the motility of the lower esophagus by direct action on this region, an indirect action being possible either by modification of the inferior esophageal sphincter pressure or by modifying, in reflux cases, the quality and/or quantity of reflux fluid. According to Eckardt [1], this motor improvement during the treatment of reflux does not exist when the disorder of motility is secondary to ulcerative esophagitis.

We have deliberately excluded substances such as the anticholinergics, nitrated derivatives and calcium-antagonists which reduce the motility of the lower esophagus and which may be grouped with many agents (theophylline . . .)

Many agents act on the lower esophagus, including:

- metopimazine (Vogalène)
- metoclopramide (Primpéran, Anausin, Reglan)
- metobutapride
- clebopride
- eserine (Vagoserine)
- domperidone (Motilium, Peridys, Peridon)
- cisapride
- bethanechol (Urécholine)

It is difficult to make a comparative analysis of the effects of these different xenobiotics on esophageal motility since some of them have been compared with the reference substance – usually metoclopramide – but not with the other agents on this list.

Very little information is available as regards metopimazine, and we are unaware of any study of the effects of this substance on the lower esophagus.

Metoclopramide, on the other hand, is the reference substance in this field and possesses an action on the entire upper alimentary tube. Its action on the inferior sphincter and lower esophagus is well documented.

This xenobiotic reduces the frequency and duration of reflux, but it is difficult to determine whether this action is associated with a true decrease in the occurrence of reflux or an increased capacity of the esophagus to get rid of the acid (Stanciu) [2]. This effect on esophageal motility has not been found by every author (Behar) [3], though it is obvious in other studies, both in healthy subjects where the mean amplitude of the peristaltic waves exceeds 33.08±2.2 mm Hg in basal conditions at 51.33±3.2 mm Hg after metoclopramide, and also in sufferers from reflux. An increase in the speed of propagation of the peristaltic waves has been reported by some authors, but this is less definite than the other effects and has been disputed in some studies.

In our own experience, conducted in a series of 10 healthy volunteers, by means of a manometric study using the classic technique of catheter perfusion, we have found that metoclopramide has a significant effect on the amplitude of the peristaltic waves which is maximal at 50 minutes, exceeding 81.94±9.85 cm H20 to 103.5±12.95 cm H20, the maximal effect on velocity being obtained at the 36th minute after administration on average.

Metobutapride, like metoclopramide, is a substituted benzamide not currently commercially available. In a study performed in November 1984, we compared the effects of this xenobiotic with those of metoclopramide in a population of 10 healthy volunteers in a cross-over double-blind study performed using kinetic manometry. After verifying the absence of any effect of order or interaction, no difference was found between the two products either as regards inferior sphincteric function or the amplitude of the peristaltic waves or their velocity of propagation.

Clebopride, another substituded benzamide, seems to possess an effect on the LES and the motility of the lower esophagus close to that of metoclopramide, but we have found no controlled study directly comparing the two products, either on inferior sphincteric action or on the amplitude or velocity of propagation of the peristaltic waves.

Eserine, through its action on acetylcholine metabolism, has an action on the tone of the LES and lower esophageal motility, as we showed in a study vs placebo in 10 healthy volunteers. This marked effect is significant and begins rapidly, to continue for at least 90 minutes. However, we know of no study comparing this xenobiotic with the other agents listed here.

Domperidone, which differs from metoclopramide by the absence of central action, also possesses an action of the tone of the LES and on motility of the lower esophagus. This action was compared with that of metoclopramide by Lux [4], who found the effect of domperidone inferior to that of metoclopramide and that of bromopride, the duration of action of these three products being relatively similar and short and of the order of 50 minutes.

Cisapride, a product currently under development, also modifies the motility of the lower esophagus. Its action on the symptoms of reflux is similar to that of domperidone (Verhaegen [5]). Its action on the reflux is of the same type and order as that of metoclopramide, and its effect on motility of the lower esophagus is stated to be equal or slightly superior. Weiser [6] finds that the two drugs have equal efficacy on acceleration of esophageal clearance in healthy subjects.

Bethanechol also has an effect on the LES and lower esophagus. In a dose of 25 mg, its sphincteric action was of the same order as that of 10 mg of metoclopramide in 15 patients with low LES pressure (MacCallum [7]) but his study did not compare effects on the lower esophagus or on clearance.

To sum up, numerous substances affect the lower esophagus and induce increased amplitude of the peristaltic waves at this level. This phenomenon generally corresponds to an increase in local clearance. The available studies suggest that this effect is much the same between the different products. However, it is difficult to make a comparison between these products because of the small number of controlled studies dealing with this subject.

References

1. Eckardt VF (1987) Does healing of esophagitis improve esophageal motor function. Digestive disease week, Chicago, May 10–13
2. Stanciu C, Bennett JR (1973) Metoclopramide in gastro-œsophageal reflux. Gut 14: 275
3. Behar J et al. (1976) Effect of oral Metoclopramide on gastro-œsophageal reflux in the post cibal state. Gastroenterology, 70 (3): 331–335
4. Lux G et al. (1981) The stimulation of esophageal motility with Bromopride, Domperidone and Metoclopramide. Roy Soc Med ICSS 36: 29–36
5. Verhaegen H (Nov. 1985) Treatment of chronic dyspepsia with Cisapride and Domperidone. In: Cisapride Investigational New Drug Brochure, Fifth Edition, Janssen Ed
6. Weiser HF et al. (1984) Influence of Cisapride on esophageal acid clearance. In: Chirurgisches forum 84 F. Experium U klinische forschung. Ed L Koslowski Springer Berlin p 131–134
7. McCallum RW et al. (1975) Comparative effects of Metoclopramide and Bethanechol on lower esophageal sphincter pressure in reflux patients. Gastroenterology 68: 1114–1118

Comparative effects of the treatments on duodeno-gastric reflux

J. P. Petite, P. Loison, and *Ph. Guincestre* (Paris)

Duodeno-gastric reflux is often implied in acute or chronic gastric ailments. It appears to have a negative effect on the esophagus in case it is associated with a gastroesophageal reflux.

There are three ways of antagonizing the noxious impact of duodeno-gastric reflux:

- stimulation of gastro-intestinal motility
- chelation (of biliary acids)
- cytoprotection.

Through one or the other of these actions, gastroesophageal reflux active drugs can counter duodeno-gastric reflux.

Gastro-duodenal motility stimulating agents

Stimulation of gastro-duodenal motility leads to a decrease in the number and duration of duodeno-gastric reflux episodes. It thus minimizes contact with gastric and esophageal mucosae.

Dopaminergic antagonists

The leading drug is metoclopramide, followed more recently by Domperidone, which has a specific action on peripheric dopaminergic receptors.

Metoclopramide stimulates gastric emptying in patients in which it is reduced for solids as well as for liquids. It leads to a better synchronization of gastro-intestinal motility and increases both gastric motility wave frequency and intensity [9].

It reduces pyloric basal activity [8].

Domperidone has similar effects; scintigraphic studies have shown a significant reduction of duodeno-gastric reflux [11, 13].

However, clinical improvement of dyspeptic patients is not obvious [8].

Cisapride

Cisapride is a new motility agonist with no dopaminergic action.

It is a more potent stimulant of antro-pyloric and duodenal motility than metoclopramide.

It increases gastric emptying either given as a bolus or regularly.

Chelating agents

Although chelation does not reduce the amount of duodenogastric reflux, it minimizes its consequences by neutralizing the noxious effects of biliary acids.

Antacids

The chelating power of antacids may vary. Aluminium hydroxyde has the highest chelating power, in aqueous solution as well as toward bile [3]. That chelating activity of Aluminium hydroxyde is saturated but at high concentration.

Magnesium hydroxide and aluminium phosphate have a slightly lesser chelating power [3]. The chelating action is greater for dihydroxylated biliary acids than for trihydroxylated ones, and for glycuroconjugated biliary acids than for tauroconjugated ones [3]. However, clinical studies on post-surgical biliary gastritis have failed to demonstrate any clinical efficiency with antacids [17].

Sucralfate

Sucralfate has a chelating power on all biliary acids. It is most efficient at a pH between 2 and 3 [23]. Here again, there is no well documented clinical effect.

Cytoprotective agents

Prostaglandins

Although theoretically all prostaglandins seem able to protect gastric mucosa against biliary aggression, results vary according to the methods and prostaglandins: in animals, 16,16 dimethyl PGE2 reduces cellular injury caused by 10 mM of taurocholate [25]. In man, the taurocholate-induced fall in transmucosal potential difference is limited after giving 16,16 dimethyl PGE2 [20]. PGF2 also has a cytoprotective action toward biliary acids. PGI2 seems to have no effect [25].

Misoprostol, a synthetic derivative of PGE1 could not bring any improvement either on variations of potential difference or on histological cellular injuries after taurocholate [5, 19].

Given at non-antisecretory doses for 6 weeks, PGE2 didn't improve post-gastrectomy gastritis [21].

Sucralfate

In animal, the taurocholate-induced fall of potential difference is limited by Sucralfate [10]. In man, 1 g of Sucralfate also reduces the fall of potential difference induced by 10 mM of glyco-cholate [2].

That cytoprotective action is lower at a very low pH [2].

Sucralfate given (6 g daily) in post-surgical alkaline reflux gastrites reduced cellular injury but failed to show any action on symptoms [1].

Anti-secretory Agents

AntiH_2 drugs

The Action of anti H2 agents on duodenogastric reflux is not clear. An effect on the volume of duodenogastric reflux is discussed. According to Soulé, cimetidine does not modify duodenogastric reflux [24], as for Melville, an intravenous bolus of 200 mg of Cimetidine significantly *increases* duodenogastric reflux [18].

On the contrary, 200 to 400 mg daily of ranitidine given intravenously reduces duodeno-gastric reflux by some 50% [5].

No study has shown any action of cimetidine on pyloric activity or on gastric emptying speed. A dose of 200 mg of cimetidine given intravenously cannot modify the Na+ flux induced by 5 mM of taurocholate, as could have been suggested when using inhibitors of H1 and H2 receptors [16].

In a study on rats with a tied-up pylorus, cimetidine was shown to be active in protecting the gastric mucosa against taurocholate 40mM. This protective action only appears at doses of 10 or 25 mg/kg, i.e. with an anti-secretory action. However, doses of 2mg/kg without anti-secretory effect, and 50mg/kg, with maximal anti-secretory action, are not active [27].

Omeprazole

Omeprazole does not alter gastric emptying or pyloric activity. On rats with a tied pylorus, it was unable to modify the 40mM taurocholate-induced gastric mucosal injuries [23].

Conclusion

Most drugs active on gastroesophageal reflux seem able to reduce experimentally the volume or noxiousness of the duodeno-gastric reflux.

Yet most clinical studies have so far failed to show any benefit.

References

1. Buch KL, Weinstein WM, Hill TA, Elashoff JD, Reedy TJ, Ippoliti AF, Tedesco FJ, Singh M (1985) Sucralfate therapy in patients with symptoms of alkaline reflux gastritis. A randomized, double-blind Study. Am J Med 79, Suppl 2c, 49–54
2. Caspary WF (1981) The influence of glycocholic acid and sucralfate on transmural potential difference of the human stomach. In: Duodenal ulcer – Gastric ulcer: Sucralfate, a new therapeutic concept. Ed Caspary WF, Baltimore 22–27
3. Clain JE, Malagelada JR, Chadwick VS, Hofmann AF (1977) Binding properties in vitro of antiacids for conjugated bile acids. Gastroenterology 73: 556–559
4. Corinaldesi R, Stanghellini W, Raiti C, Rea E, Salgemini R, Barbara L (1987) Effect of chronic administration of cisapride on gastric emptying of a solid meal and on dyspeptic symptoms in patients with idiopathic gastroparesis. Gut 28: 300–305
5. Dammann HG, Kruger HJ, Simon B, Begemann R (1982) Effect of ranitidine on duodenogastric reflux and nocturn gastric acid secretion in man. In Clinical use of ranitidine, Medecine publishing fondation symposium. Series 5: 109–113
6. Fimmel CJ, Muller-Lissmer SA, Blum AL (1984) Bile salt induced, acute gastric mucosal damage in man: time course and effect of misoprostal, a PGE1 analogue. Scand J Gastroenterol 19 (suppl 92) 184–188.
7. Fournet J, Hostein J (1987) Reflux duodenogastrique. Bases pharmacologiques d'un traitement médical. Gastroentérol Clin Biol 11: 158–164
8. Goldstein F, Thornton JJ, Abramson J, Mac Groarty DJ, Kline IK (1981) Bile reflux gastritis and oesophagitis in patients without prior gastric surgery with pilot study of the therapeutic effects of metoclopramide. Am J Gastroenterol, 76: 407–411
9. Hancolk BD, Bowenjones E, Dixon R (1974) The effect of metoclopramide on gastric emptying of solid meals. Gut 15: 462–467
10. Harrington SJ, Schlegel JF, Code CF (1981) The protective effect of sucralfate on the gastric mucosa of rats. J Clin Gastroenterol 3: 129–134
11. Hordijk ML, Van Roon F, Silberbusch J (1986) Domperidone reduces duodenogastric reflux in patients with chronic gastritis. Neth J Med 29: 144

12. Jian R, Ducrot F, Piedeloup, Mary JY, Najean Y, Bernier JJ (1985) Measurement of gastric emptying in dyspeptic patients, effect of a new gastrokinetic agent (cisapride). Gut 26: 352–358
13. Johnson AG, Eyre-Brook IA, Holroyd AM, Smallwood M (1983) Antroduodenal coordination and duodenogastric reflux in man: a preliminary report. Clin Res Reviews, 3: 81–90
14. Konturek JJ, Brzozowski I, Piastucki I, Radecki T, Dembienskakiel A (1983) Role of prostaglandin and thromboxane biosynthetis in gastric necrosis produced by taurocholate and ethanol. Dig Dis Sci 28: 154–160
15. Lederer PC, Ellermann A, Ludwif S, Lux G (1985) Effect of cisapride and metoclopramide on antroduodenal motor activity in man. Gastroenterology 88: 1468 (Abstr)
16. Lewi HJEE, Carter CD (1983) Bile salt-induced gastric mucosal damage and histamine receptor antagonists. Gut 24: 33–37
17. Mann NS (1976) Bile induced acute erosive gastritis: Its prevention by antiacids, cholestyramine and prostaglandin E2. Am J Dig Dis 21: 89–92
18. Melville RJ, Suleiman SI, Whitfield PF, Parkin JV, Nwabunike TO, Hobjley M (1985) Effect of cimetidine on gastric secretion and duodenogastric reflux. Gut 26: 766–769
19. Monk JP, Clissold SP (1987) Misoprostol: a preliminary review of its pharmacodynamic and pharmacokinetic properties, and therapeutic efficacity in the treatment of peptic ulcer discase. Drugs 33: 1–30
20. Muller P, Fischer N, Damann HG, Kather H, Simon B (1981) Cytoprotective effect of 16 di CH3 PGE2 on gastric mucosal lesion produced by bile salts. Br J Clin Pharmacol 12: 253–254
21. Nicolai JJ, Van De Stadt J, Tytgat GNJ (1986) Double-blind crossover trial of PGE2 in postgastrectomy reflux gastritis. Dig Dis Sci 31: 1281–1286
22. Papazian A, Nguyen-Phoc BK (1982) Le reflux duodénogastrique: mise en évidence, affections associées, conséquences, traitement. Gastroentérol Clin Biol 6: 1020–1028
23. Soule JC (1985) Cytoprotection gastrique et duodénale: prostaglandines et autres cytoprotecteurs. J Pharma Clin 4: 61–82
24. Soule JC, Pariente EA, Moschoutis P (1982) Cimétidine et reflux gastroœsophagien. Gastroentérol Clin Biol 6: 662–668
25. Terano A, Ota S, Mach T, Hiraishi H, Stachura J, Tarnawski A, Ivey KJ (1987) Prostaglandin protects against taurocholate induced damage to rat gastric mucosal cell culture. Gastroenterol 92: 669–677
26. Thomforde GM, Zzynsmeister AR, Brown ML, Malagelada JR (1985) Effect of cisapride and metoclopramide on gastrointestinal motility and transit in a chronic dog model. Gastroenterology 88: 1613 (Abstr)
27. Utley RJ, Salim ASM, Carter DC (1985) Effect of cimetidine and omeprazole on aspirin and taurocholate induced gastric mucosal damage in the rat. Gut 26: 770–775

Comparative effects of the treatments on the volume and the number of bouts of reflux

J. P. Petite, and *P. Loison* (Paris)

Objective evaluation of the efficicacy of a therapy for gastroesophageal reflux requires assessing the various parameters of that reflux: number, duration and acidity level of the reflux episodes.

24 hour pHmetry seems to be the most adequate method [3, 5], but few studies have so far evaluated 24 hour pHmetry modifications induced by drugs recommended in gastroesophageal reflux.

Only Desechalliers et al [2] have compared the action of cimetidine (1 g daily), ranitidine (300 mg daily), and antacids (60 ml daily), using 3 hour and later 20 hour pHmetry (Tables 1 and 2): during 3 hour pHmetry, the number of reflux episodes is

Table 1. Results of 3 hour pHmetry in 4 groups

		Score de Kaye	Number of episodes	Mean duration (mn)
Non treated (n=43)		196 (92–848)	15 (4–34)	4.8 (1.6–23.4)
Cimetidine (n=15)	BT	208 (101–389)	17 (11–31)	3.6 (1.5–11.1)
	AT	73* (1–514)	10* (1–32)	1.6 (0.3– 2.5)
Ranitidine (n=15)	BT	190 (98–763)	10 (4–34)	8 (0.9–28)
	AT	57* (0–154)	8 (10–32)	1.5* (0–21.4)
Antacids (n=15)	BT	283 (167–604)	12 (4–24)	6.2 (2.3–19.9)
	AT	107* (0–550)	8 (0–39)	3.8 (1.0–22.6

BT, before treatment; AT, after treatment

* p=0.05

Table 2. Results of 20 hour pHmetry in 4 groups

	Number of episodes	Mean duration (mn)
Non treated (n=43)	75 (9–289)	4.5 (1.4 –13.5)
Cimetidine (n=15)	46* (18–86)	3.6 (1.3 –35.5)
Ranitidine (n=15)	23* (0–111)	3.8 (0.19– 9)
Antacids (n=15)	41* (0–131)	5 (0 –28.4)

* p=0.05

reduced in all 3 groups compared to pre-treatment findings, but the difference is significant in the cimetidine group only. The mean duration of reflux episodes is also reduced in all 3 groups, but only the ranitidine group shows significant values.

20 hour pHmetry shows a significant reduction of the number of reflux episodes in all 3 groups. However the mean duration of the episodes is not statistically modified.

These findings suggest that gastric acidity active drugs also act in gastroesophageal reflux by reducing the number of reflux episodes. However publications are too few and furthermore fail to compare various antiH_2 agents.

References

1. April N (1979) Quantitative reduction of gastroesophageal acid reflux by Cimetidine; Gastroenterology 76: 1092–1097
2. Desechalliers JP, Galmiche JP, Touchais JY, Denis P, Colin R (1984) Ranitidine, Cimétidine, antacids and gastroesophageal reflux: results of a 20 hours oesophageal pH study. Int J Clin Pharm Research 4: 217–222
3. Euler AR, Byrne WJ (1981) Twenty four hours oesophageal intraluminal pH probe testing a comparative analysis. Gastroenterology 80: 957–961
4. Frasse R, Hanin C, Dive C (1980) Controlled trial of Cimetidine in reflux oesophagitis. Dig Dis Sci 25: 750–755.
5. Kaye MD (1977) Post prandial gastroesophageal reflux in healthy people. Gut, 18: 709–715.
6. Wesdorp CE, Dekker W, Klinkenberg-Knol E (1982) Evaluation of Ranitidine in the treatment of reflux oesophagitis. In Misiewicz JJ, Wormsley KG Eds "The Clinical use of Ranitidine" Oxford. The Medicine Publishing Fondation 293–296

Effects of the different treatments on the acidity of reflux

E. Masci (Milan)

It has been reported that most patients with reflux esophagitis have a pathologically increased gastric acidity [1], (Table 1) although these data are not confirmed by all authors. However, even if the pathogenesis of reflux esophagitis is multifactorial, gastric acid is probably the most important factor in developing esophageal mucosal lesions

Therefore, it is very important to compare the effects on gastric acid secretion of the different drugs, employed in the treatment of reflux esophagitis. The antisecretive action of H_2-blockers is widely known: gastric acid secretion in basal conditions and after pentagastrin stimulation has been studied before and after ranitidine treatment in patients with reflux esophagitis [2] (Table 2). Gastric secretory rate was significantly lower during ranitidine treatment, than before treatment and in comparison with placebo. Basal and stimulated acid secretion were also more markedly reduced during treatment in patients healed with ranitidine in comparison with non-responders (Table 3).

Table 1. Gastric secretory activity (mean±SD) in 17 esophagitis patients and 10 controls

	Esophagitis	Controls	P
BAO (mEq/hr)	4.26± 3.95	2.01± 0.65	<0.05
MAO (mEq/hr)	17.89±10.48	13.53± 4.06	NS
Basal volume (ml/hr)	127.3 ±57.25	88.50±41.17	=0,05
Maximal volume (ml/hr)	242.1 ±82.87	176.7 ±39.65	<0,01
Basal [H+] (mEq/liter)	34.35±21.20	25.00± 9.09	NS
Maximal [H+] (mEq/liter)	87.17±31.12	90.50±26.31	NS

Note: Patients with reflux esophagitis have a pathologically increased gastric acidity, also if this data are not confirmed by other authors

F. Baldi et al. 1981

Table 2. Effects of ranitidine and placebo on gastric secretion in patients with reflux esophagitis

	Ranitidine, n=32		Placebo, n=30	
	Before treatment	During treatment	Before treatment	During treatment
BAO, mmol/h	3.7± 3.8	0.8±1.7***	3.4± 3.8	2.6± 2.2
MAO, mmol/h	22.0± 9.9	10.2±6.5***	20.6±11.0	20.1± 8.5
PAO, mmol/h	27.6±11.4	13.5±7.7***	26.3±11.2	26.3±11.2
GSR				
Basal, ml/min	1.4± 0.7	0.9±0.5***	1.3± 0.7	1.2± 0.7
Stimulated, ml/min	3.7± 1.3	2.2±0.9***	3.5– 1.5	3.5± 1.2

*** $p<0.001$

K. E. Johansson and L. Tibbling 1986

Table 3. Effects of ranitidine on gastric secretion in non-responders

	Before trial		Ranitidine	
	NR, n=23	R, n=17	NR, n=17	R, n=15
BAO, mmol/h	2.8± 3.5	3.9± 3.6	1.4±2.2	0.2±0.3*
MAO, mmol/h	20.2±10.0	21.5±10.0	13.3±6.8	6.6±4.0**
PAO, mmol/h	25.8±12.0	27.0±11.7	15.6±8.8	9.7±4.9***
GSR				
Basal, ml/min	1.3± 0.6	1.3± 0.7	1.1±0.6	0.6±0.3*
Stimulated, ml/min	3.4± 1.2	3.6± 1.5	2.7±0.9	1.7±0.5***

* $p<0.05$, ** $p<0.01$, *** $p<0.001$

Note: Gastric acidty was more reduced in patients healing with ranitidine in comparison with non-responders

K. E. Johansson and L. Tibbling 1986

These data raise the question of the relation between the healing rate of esophagitis and antisecretory activity of the different drugs; although in clinical studies ranitidine showed better results than cimetidine, because of the different periods of treatment, comparisons are different.

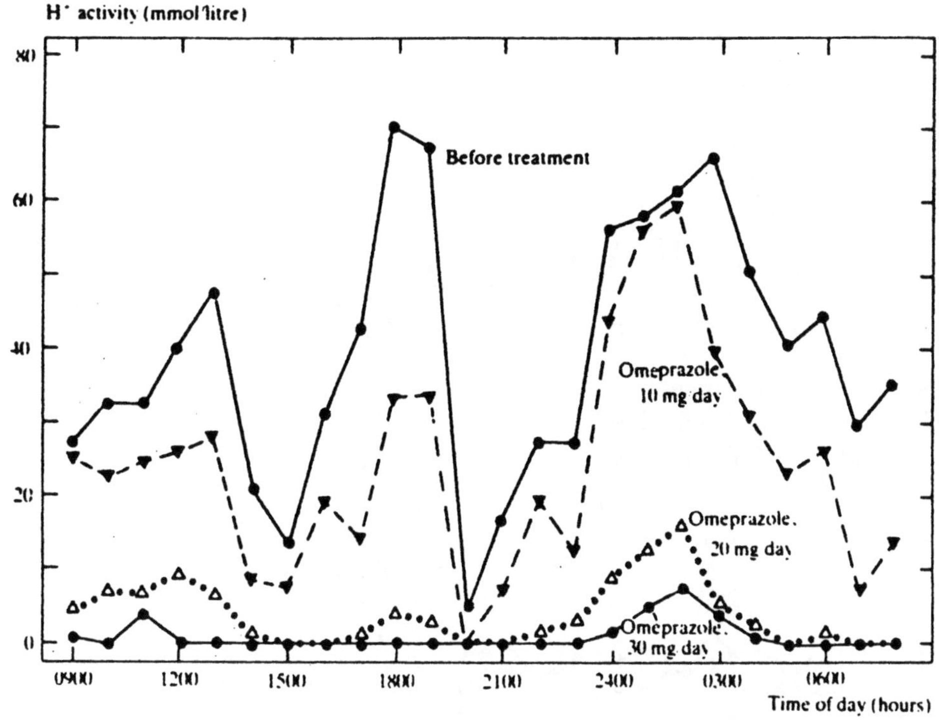

Fig. 1. Omeprazole at a dose of 20–60 mg once daily reduces gastric acidity up to 99% in healthy subjects

Not yet available, but with a strong antisecretory action is omeprazole, a new gastric acid inhibitor that specifically blocks the gastric proton pump in the parietal cells. In doses of 20–60 mg once daily, it reduces 24 hours gastric acidity up to 99 % in healthy subjects [3] (Fig. 1).

This strong antisecretory effect seems to be important in healing reflux esophagitis, since a controlled trial showed a significantly higher healing rate after 4 and 8 weeks with omeprazole than with ranitidine [4], (Table 4). The safety of the drug, however, requires further evaluation.

Table 4. Macroscopic healing (shift to grade 1 or normal by endoscopy after 4 and 8 weeks' treatment)

	No healed					
Pretreatment grade of esophagitis	Omeprazole			Ranitidine		
	n	4 wk	8 wk	n	4 wk	8 wk
2	12	8	10	11	7	8
3	13	11	12	15	0	2
Total	25	19	22	26	7	10

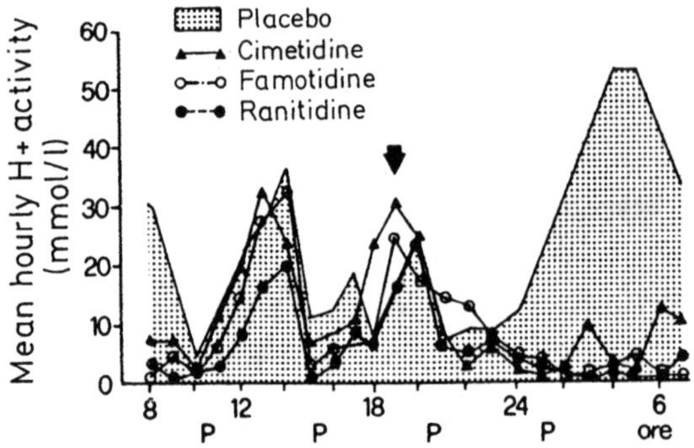

Fig. 2–3. The evening dose of H_2 Blockers, as employed in peptic ulcer therapy, because of the pH fall during evening, may not even be the best dosage in reflux esophagitis

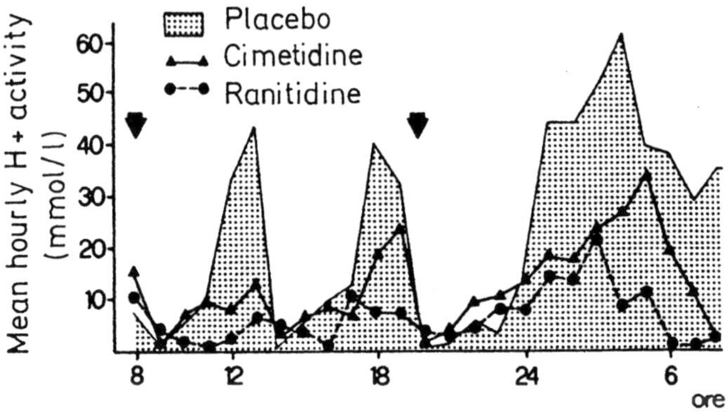

Fig. 3

Using antisecretory drugs, another important question is when the drug must be administered: although, on my knowledge, controlled trials are not available, the evening dose, as employed in peptic ulcer therapy, may not ever be the best dosage in reflux esophagitis (Fig. 2, 3).

Probably, in the treatment of esophagitis, the best dosage must be scheduled on the basis of patients' symptoms and on the results of pH-metric studies; in fact an antisecretory drug given at night will not heal esophagitis and reduce symptoms in patients with gastro-esophageal reflux during the day.

A weak but well established antisecretory effect is reported with the administration of pirenzepine, a selective anticholinergic drug. Because of its selective

Table 5. Effect of domperidone 20 mg i.v. on basal and pentagastrin (0,25 ng kg^{-1} h^{-1}) stimulated gastric acid output and juice volume in healthy subjects (mean±s.e. mean)

Number of subjects	Drug	Acid output (mmol/h) Basal	Acid output (mmol/h) Stimulated	Volume (ml/h) Basal	Volume (ml/h) Stimulated
12	Placebo	4.66±0.4	22.21±2.4	73±7.1	205±8.1
12	Domperidone 20 mg	4.91±0.5	22.01±2.5	70±4.6	209±6.9

Note: No effects were observed on gastric acid secretion after domperidone i.v. [6]

action on gastric secretion, with no effects on LES pressure and gastro-esophageal motility, it is the only anticholinergic drug, that can be used in the treatment of reflux esophagitis.

On the contrary, no antisecretory effect has been observed with antidopaminergic drugs.

In a study performed by our group, testing basal and pentagastrin-stimulated gastric secretion, no effect was observed after domperidone i.v. administration [6], (Table 5). Also no effects were observed with other antidopaminergic drug as

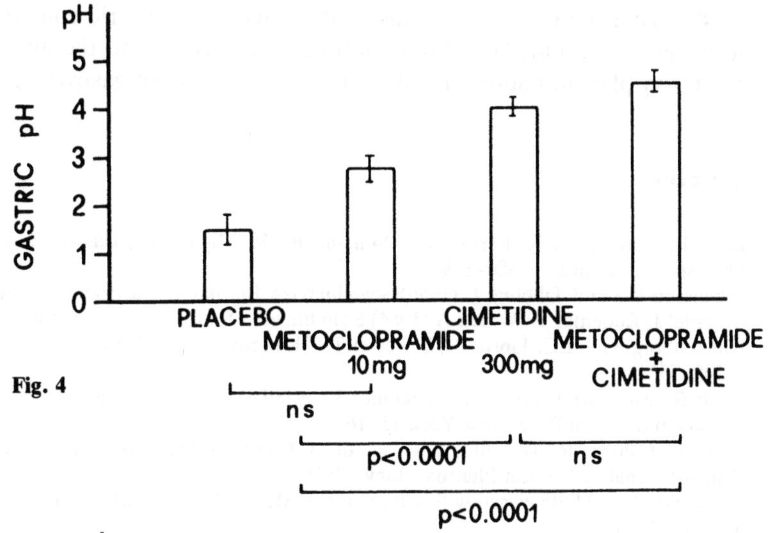

Fig. 4

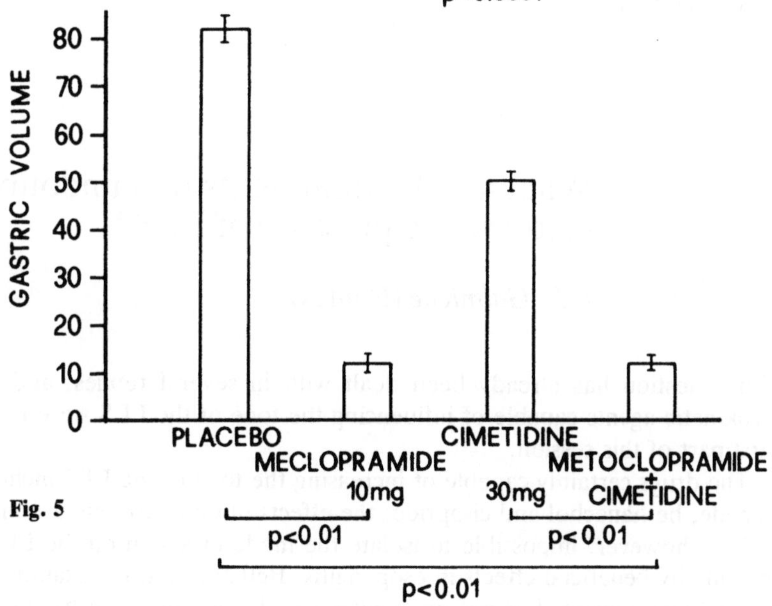

Fig. 5

Fig. 4–5. Metoclopramide has no effect on gastric pH, but significantly better reduces, in comparison with cimetidine, the volume of gastric content; the amount of gastric content may play an important role in the pathogenesis of GER metoclopramide, valopride and sulpiride. Also cisapride, a new prokinetic drug, is devoid of effects on gastric acid secretion.

However, interesting data are reported in a recent study comparing the effect of metoclopramide and cimetidine on gastric secretory volume [7] (Figs. 4, 5). Although metoclopramide has no effect on gastric pH, it has been observed, after administration of the drug, a significantly better reduction of the volume of gastric content in comparison with cimetidine.

Therefore, although metoclopramide and antidopaminergic drugs have no effects on gastric acid secretion, by means of their action on gastric emptying, they may reduce gastric content, better than antisecretory drugs, and the amount of gastric content may play an important role in the pathogenesis of gastroesophageal reflux.

References

1. Baldi F, Corinaldesi R, Ferrarini F, Stanghellini V, Miglioli M, Barbara L (1981) Digestive Disease and Science 26:886–889
2. Johansson KE and Tibbling L (1986) Scandinavian Journal of Gastroenetrology 21:487–492
3. Naesdel J, Bodemar G, Walen A (1984) Scandinavian Journal of Gastroenterology 19:916–922
4. Klinkenberg-Knol EC, Jansen JHB, Festen HPH, Menwissen SGM, Lamers CBH (1987) Lancet 1:349–351
5. Cheli R, Molinari F (1986) Pirenzepine: knowledge and new trend – Cortina International Verona and Raven Press New-York 15–16
6. Masci E, Caldara R, Testoni PA, Guslandi M, Cambielli M, Passaretti S, Tittobello A (1984) British Journal of Clinical Pharmacology 17:588–590
7. Tadikonda LK, Madhavareddy S, Chinthagada M, Adel A, Anesthesia and Analgaesia (1984) 63:1014–1016

What are the treatments that undoubtedly increase the pressure of LES?

J. P. Galmiche (Nantes)

This question has already been dealt with in several replies, and the different prokinetic agents capable of influencing the tone of the LES were reviewed in the first part of this session.

The drugs certainly capable of increasing the tone of the LES include metoclopramide, bethanechol and cisapride; the effects of domperidone are more variable.

It is, however, impossible to isolate the mode of action on the LES from other potentially beneficial effects in esophagitis. Bethanechol, for example (Fig. 1) acts as prokinetic agent, but not exclusively so. If acid clearance by the esophagus is measured independently of action on esophageal peristalsis, it is seen that the aspiration of saliva prolongs this clearance, whereas administration of Bethanechol decreases clearance time. If the saliva is aspirated at that time, this same drug no longer has the effect of improving acid clearance by the esophagus.

It should also be remarked that drugs other than specifically prokinetic agents are capable of influencing the LES. Apart from the antacids, which certainly do affect the LES, but at very high pH levels above 6, mention may be made of

a) the beta-adrenergic antagonists, and
b) possibly certain H_2-receptor antagonists such as Ranitidine, which may have an effect of cholinergic nature.

Nevertheless, in our own experience, Ranitidine, by both the intravenous and the oral route, does not modify LES pressure.

In terms of the question posed, drug prescription does not refer only to medication as such; while some medication increases the resting pressure of the LES, some factors also decrease it, notably certain nutritional habits, smoking and alcohol consumption. Therefore, the drugs employed must be integrated with general management including added advice on hygiene and diet which reinforces the anti-reflux barrier and has a parallel effect on esophageal acid clearance (for a general review of these effects, see Scarpignato [1]).

Reference

1. Scarpignato C (1987) Bases pharmacologiques du traitement du reflux gastro-œsophagien et de l'œsophagite peptique in Collin R et Galmiche JP "Les troubles moteurs de l'œsophage. Le reflux gastro-œsophagien". Doin Publ Paris (under press)

Can continuous administration of antacids be considered?

F. Vicari (Nancy)

1. Common sense or practice shows that antiacids (a. a.) are often prescribed by the general practitioner before any endoscopic examination and stopped in case of success or possibly given again in case of recurrence.
   Once the endoscopy has been carried out with if necessary esophageal pH metry and manometry, the a. a. are prescribed if mild esophagitis is discovered (grade 1). Otherwise, preference is given to anti-H_2 even at this stage.
   If in mild forms, a. a. happen to be inefficient after a 15-day or 1-month treatment, they are replaced by anti-H2, the modifiers of LES tonus and of esogastric kinesis being most often directly associated.
   So if efficient, the a. a. are stopped when clinical and if possible endoscopic recovery is obtained. If they need to be given again, there is no continuity in the prescription. If they are inefficient, they are rapidly replaced by anti-H2 or according to the stage by surgery.

When relief is obtained by a. a. in a patient who cannot be submitted to surgery and who does not tolerate anti-H_2, then continuous a. a. treatment can be envisaged but this is the exception proving the rule.

2. Even if a. a. could be prescribed continuously most of them have pharmacological limits.
   As a matter of fact, if magnesium compounds are laxative, aluminium compounds have the opposite effect and especially a sustained treatment (except for alumina phosphate) can expose to the risk of osteoporosis by lack of phosphate (elimination of these salts in stools under the form of insoluble phosphate).
   Moreover risks of encephalopathy are increased for patients with chronic renal insufficiency.
   At least if it is not possible to pertinently answer the question: "Aluminum factor of senile dementia?" it is still to be considered. Let us hope that the actual interest taken by searchers worldwide in Alzheimer's disease will soon allow to answer it.

After interruption of the treatment, is the risk of recurrence elevated, and what other factors could be implicated in the determinism of reflux to avoid an indefinite intake of antacids?

J. L. Balmes (Montpellier)

This reply is necessarily rapid in view of the form taken by the symposium and the first question is very difficult to answer for several reasons: when speaking of the risk of recurrence, what are the criteria chosen: clinical, endoscopic, histologic, pH measurement, manometry, scintigraphy? Which of these criteria are observed when initiating treatment, and what type of treatment?

Moreover, several factors are involved in the population studied:

1. the major factor is the decreased tone of the inferior esophageal sphincter, which may be primary or secondary to esophagitis or other causes (drug problems, smoking, dietetic errors). In these cases of secondary loss of tone of the inferior esophageal sphincter, the phenomenon may be reversible if the esophagitis does not exceed grade 2
2. the presence or not of abnormal clearance of the esophagus which may be deranged by esophagitis [1, 10] or by swallowing without a bolus of saliva [13]
3. the laws of gastric emptying
4. the actual nature of the reflux: acid, peptic, biliary, pancreatic
5. the length of the abdominal segment of the inferior esophageal sphincter.

Added to these different parameters are the presence or absence of a hiatus hernia and the difficulty of determining prevalence in a population where the clinical features of gastroesophageal reflux are considered as normal by 5% of persons. There is also the frequency of atypical clinical forms.

There are few studies dealing with long-term follow-up of these types of pathology. These studies mainly compare groups of patients submitted to different treatments [5, 9, 11, 17, 19, 20) versus placebo, showing a more or less constant range of recurrence. At 6 months, this is of the order of 50% for active drug treatment and 60% for placebo, and at 1 year it is of the order of 60 % for antacids and 70% for placebo. Thus it may be said that, out of 100 patients treated for 6 months, at least 60% will relapse during the year with or without treatment by anti-$H_2$2 drugs.

What are the risk factors?

Personal analysis of a short series of patients followed up for 2 years (89 cases, mean age 55.7 years, range 22–86 years, 42 men, 47 women, distribution: 8 grade III, 42 grade II, 29 grade I and 10 grade 0) virtually confirms the data in the literature.

The grade III cases were not improved by medical treatment. In grades 0, I, and II, 50% were stabilized by medical treatment and this very rapidly (10–15 days). 50% were only temporarily improved. Among the 50% improved cases, 75% in grade I and 40% in grade II no longer had histologic evidence of esophagitis.

Among the various prognostic factors considered we may say that we found that age had no influence, the presence of hiatus hernia as well as the length and therefore the extension in the level of ulceration in grade II cases were indicative of poor prognosis [2, 12, 15], and the presence of a factor involved in decreasing the pressure of the inferior esophageal sphincter was on the contrary favorable, provided it could be eliminated (smoking, dietetic errors, drugs).

It is relatively easier to answer the second question: what other factors may be involved in determining reflux so as to avoid the indefinite prescription of antacids.

1. A certain number of drugs which produce decreased tonus of the inferior esophageal sphincter should be given in reduced dosage or in interrupted courses. These include progesterone, theophylline, anticholinergics (except pirenzepine), beta-adrenergic agonists, alpha-adrenergic antagonists, dopamine, diazepam, calcium inhibitors, meperidine and prostaglandins E2, E1, A2.
2. Tobacco [3, 7]: twenty minutes after smoking two cigarettes the tone of the inferior esophageal sphincter decreases by 50%. Further, in smokers the action of anti H_2 drugs on nocturnal secretion is diminished, the decrease being only 38% instead of 86% in the nonsmoker. There should be no smoking after taking the night's medication.
3. Alcohol [18] has a controversial action: some consider that it decreases the tone of the superior esophageal sphincter and that of the inferior sphincter as well as primary peristalsis. Others believe that its main action is directly on the mucosa.
4. Dietetic error may be influential, either by decreasing the tone of the inferior esophageal sphincter as do fats, or in a more complex manner as with chocolate, which contains methylxanthine in addition to its large fat content. This inhibits

phosphodiesterase, which produces cyclic accumulation and therefore relaxation. The effects of substances such as lemons, tomatos and coffee are probably exerted by direct action (physical, osmotic or pH-dependent effects) [14].

5. With regard to the problem of gastric distension [4, 7], there seems to be no relation between gastric emptying and the presence of reflux. On the contrary, when the stomach is full the periods of relaxation of the inferior esophageal sphincter are longer. Therefore gastroesophageal reflux occurs more readily after meals.
6. Loss of weight in obese individuals is one of the traditional elements in treatment but is based on empiric data. Recent studies have not confirmed a decrease in tonus of the inferior esophageal sphincter in the obese [16].
7. Elevation of the head of the bed [6]. In subjects with gastroesophageal reflux clearance approaches that in normal subjects sleeping horizontally but remains greater than in asymptomatic volunteers placed in the same conditions.

References

1. Baldi F, Ferrarini F, Balestra R, Borioni D, Longanesi A, Miglioli M, Barbara L (1985) Oesophageal motor events at the occurrence of acid reflux and during endogenous acid exposure in healty subjects and in patients with oesophagitis. Gut 26: 336–341
2. Berstad A, Weberg R, Larsen IF et al. (1986) Relationship of hiatus hernia to reflux oesophagitis. A prospective study of coincidence, using endoscopy. Scand J Gastroenterol 21/1: 55–58
3. Boyd EIS, Wilson JA, Wormsley KG (1983) Smoking impairs therapeutic gastric inhibition Lancet 1: 95–97
4. Bruley des Varannes S, Touchais JY, Weber J, Desechalliers JP, Sauger F, Denis P, Galmiche JP (1986) Œsophagite de reflux: rôles respectifs des facteurs pathogéniques œsophagiens et gastriques Gastroentérol. Clin Bio 10: 662–668
5. Castell DO (1986) Reflux esophagitis: new frontiers. J Clin Gastroenterol, vol 8 suppl 1
6. DeMeester TR, Johnson LF, Guy JJ (1976) Pattern of gastroesophageal reflux in health and disease. Ann Surg 1984: 457–470
7. Denn SH GW, Castell DO (1971) Inhibitory effect of smoking on the lower esophageal sphincter. N Engl J Med 284: 1136–1137
8. Holloway RJ, Hongo M, Berger K, McCallum RW (1985) Gastric distention: a mechanism for post prandial gastro-oesophageal reflux. Gastroenterology 89: 779–784
9. Johansson KE, Tibbling L (1986) Maintenance treatment with ranitidine compared with fundoplication in gastro-oesophageal reflux disease. Scand J Gastroenterol 21: 779–788
10. Kahrilas PJ, Dodds WJ, Hogan WJ, Kern M, Arndorfer PC, Reece A (1986) Esophageal peristaltic dysfunction in peptic esophagitis. Gastroenterology 91: 897–904
11. Kaul B, Petersen H, Erichsen H, Myrvold HE, Grette K, Halvorsen T, Fjosne U (1986) Gastroesophageal reflux disease. Acute and maintenance treatments with cimétidine. Scand J Gastroenterol 21: 139–145
12. Koelz HR, Birchler R, Bretholz A, Bron B, Capitaine Y et al. (1986) Healing and relapse of reflux esophagitis during treatment with ranitidine. Gastroenterology 91: 1198–1205
13. Kruse-Andersen S, Wallin L, Madsen T (1986) Acid gastro-oesophageal reflux episodes as related to the quality of preceding peristalsis. A study in normal subjects. Scand J Gastroenterol 21: 711–717
14. Llyod DA, Borda IT (1981) Food induced heartburn: effect of osmolarity. Gastroenterology 80: 740–741
15. Mittal RK, Lange RC, McCallum RW (1987) Identification and mechanism of delayed esophageal acid clearance in subjects with hiatus hernia. Gastroenterology 92: 130–135

16. O'Brien TF, Stroop EM (1980) Lower esophageal sphincter pressure and esophageal function in obese humans. J Clin Gastroenterol 2: 145–147
17. Sherbaniuk R, Wensel R, Bailey R (1984) Ranitidine in the treatment of symptomatic gastrooesophageal reflux. J Clin Gastroenterol 86: 1179
18. Silver LS, Worner TM, Korsten MA (1986) Esophageal function in chronic alcoholics Am J Gastroenterol 81: 423
19. Sontog S, Vlahavic ZR, Orr W (1985) Ranitidine versus placebo in long term of gastroesophageal reflux. Gastroenterology 88: 1595
20. Wesdorp ICE (1984) Oesophagitis and its complication. Medical treatment. Scand J Gastroenterol 19, Suppl 106: 87–97

What are the factors that play a role in the genesis of esophagitis and on which ones do antacids react?

T. Chevalier, and *S. Bonfils* (Paris)

Esophagitis is the chief complication of gastroesophageal reflux. It is the outcome of the attack of the gastric reflux fluid on the malpighian mucosa of the esophagus. Its occurrence depends on the severity of the reflux (frequency and duration of episodes of reflux) and also on the nature of the reflux and resistant capacity of the esophageal mucous membrane.

As the esophagitis is a complication of the gastroesophageal reflux each of the factors involved in the pathogenesis of the reflux disorder may determine the onset of esophagitis. The continence of the inferior esophageal sphincter (LES) and the capacity for esophageal clearance, i.e. its ability to empty itself (which depends on peristalsis and the swallowing of saliva) determine the frequency and duration of episodes of reflux and their possible consequences for the esophageal mucosa.

However not all subjects with reflux develop esophagitis, which implies that certain adjuvant factors are necessary for the development of the lesions. Incontinence of the LES and disorders of peristalsis in the body of the esophagus exert an overall bad effect on the prognosis in reflux disease with a positive correlation between the severity of the esophagitis and the existence of dyskinesia. A raised pH measurement in relation to these various factors must in principle cause apprehension that the reflux disorder will progress to esophagitis.

However, other factors are concerned in provoking the lesions and this accounts for certain disparities (raised pH values without esophagitis) and the poor predictive value of motor disorders at individual level.

The development of esophagitis is also influenced by the resistance of the mucosa and the aggressivity of the reflux fluid. The phenomena of cell protection are poorly understood in the esophagus, even if it is acknowledged that the resistive capacity of the malpighian mucosa is less than that of the gastric mucosa. As for the nature of the reflux fluid, this is acid in the great majority of cases, Theoretically there is no reason why there should not be an alkaline reflux but its frequency as a primary pathogenic factor is difficult to assess in practice in the absence of a satisfactory method of investigation. Its practical importance is limited to the problems of certain surgical procedures.

From the physiopathologic aspect the use of antacids might be expected to have a beneficial effect in the treatment of gastroesophageal reflux and its complication of esophagitis. Reduction of the aggressivity of the reflux fluid towards the esophageal mucosa could result not only from the direct intragastric neutralizing action, but also from the inactivation of pepsin, the enzymatic activity of which is maximal at acid pH.

However, controlled trials have not demonstrated the therapeutic efficacy of antacids, either alone or combined with an antisecretory agent. Comparison of the pH measurements with antacids and antisecretory agents suggests that the differences in efficacy of treatment in the two cases are associated with a less marked and less prolonged reduction of esophageal acidity with the antacids than with the antisecretory drugs.

Reference

1. Dodds WJ, Hogan WJ, Helm JF, Dent J (1981) Pathogenesis of reflux esophagitis Gastroenterology 81: 376–394

At what time must medical treatment give way to surgical indication in erythematous esophagitis

M. Savary, J. B. Ollyo, Ph. Monnier, J. Wellinger, J. J. Gonvers, and *Ch. Fontolliet* (Lausanne)

Some authors consider that localized or diffuse erythema of the lower esophagus is the initial stage of reflux esophagitis [2, 3, 6]. We believe that the initial lesion of reflux esophagitis is epithelial erosion [4]. The endoscopic image is an exudate that can be separated from the underlying hyperemic and hemorrhagic mucosa [5].

In the presence of erythematous areas without an exudate the diagnosis of stage 1 esophagitis requires a biopsy of that precise area. Indeed in the lower esophagus an erythematous area can correspond to any of the following histologies: acquired or congenital columnar epithelium, epithelial dysplasia, in situ or microinvasive carcinoma, epithelial erosion.

From a histologic point of view, the initial peptic lesion, whether erythematous or exudative, is defined by our stage 1 as a complete or incomplete epithelial erosion with an inflammatory infiltrate of the lamina propria [5]. Other histologic criteria are debatable and non specific. A diagnosis of reflux esophagitis cannot be made on their basis alone: epithelial changes such as elongation of conjunctive papilla and hyperplasia of the basal layer, inflammatory changes such as infiltration of the lamina propria with lymphocytes and plasmocytes or presence of eosinophils and/or PMN's, vascular changes such as dilatation of superficial veins, proliferation of capillaries, disappearance of endothelial cells [1, 2, 7].

All erythematous lesions of the lower esophagus should be biopsied. If the histology shows erosions, the treatment should be the same as for erosive reflux esophagitis. In the absence of macroscopic or histologic erosions, no medical or surgical treatment is required in our opinion.

References

1. Geboes K, Desmet V, Vantrappen G, Mebis J (1980) Vascular changes in esophageal mucosa. An early histologic sign of esophagitis. Gastrointest Endosc 26: 29–32
2. Meier RF, Sieber R, Bauerfeind P, Blum AL (1986) Endoscopy as final arbiter in controlled clinical trials in peptic disorders. Clin Gastroenterol 15: 377–391
3. Mounier-Kuhn P, Gaillard J (1968) La pathologie du reflux gastro-œsophagien Œsophagites et sténoses peptiques. Arnette, édit, Paris
4. Savary M, Miller G (1977) L'œsophage. Manuel et atlas d'endoscopie. Gassmann SA, édit, Soleure
5. Savary M, Ollyo JB (1986) L'œsophagite par reflux et ses complications: ulcère, sténose, endobrachy-oesophage. Encycl Med Chir (Paris, France) ORL; 20822 A[10]; 10: (16 p.)
6. Skinner DB, Belsey RHR, Hendrix TR et al (1972) Gastroesophageal reflux and hiatal hernia. Boston, Little, Brown and Co
7. Tummala V, Barwick KW, Sontag SJ, Vlahcevic RZ, McCallum RW (1987) The significance of intraepithelial eosinophils in the histologic diagnosis of gastroesophageal reflux. Am J Clin Pathol 87: 43–48

Surgical indication in erosive esophagitis

J. B. Ollyo, J. J. Gonvers, J. Wellinger, M. Savary,
and *Ph. Monnier* (Lausanne)

A few studies [2, 4, 5] have shown that 6 to 12 weeks of treatment with antacid medication such as cimetidine, ranitidine or omeprazole heals the majority of stage 1–3 erosive reflux esophagitis of the Savary-Miller classification [7]. The other drugs, such as antacids, sodium alginate, sucralfate, metoclopramide, domperidone and bethanechol chloride do not seem to work as well as H_2 blocking agents or omeprazole [3, 8]. They are not used alone.

The value of medical treatment is limited by the risk of recurrence when the medication is stopped. A recent study [5] has shown that the recurrence rate is not influenced by 150 mg of ranitidine a day. Consequently it becomes necessary to continue the treatment on a long term basis with therapeutic doses to prevent a recurrence. Otherwise one must treat each episode of esophagitis as it occurs and accept the risk of developing a complication such as ulcer, stenosis, endobrachy-esophagus or adenocarcinoma.

Surgery should be discussed, if the patient is an acceptable operative risk, in the following situations:

1. persistence or progression of erosive reflux esophagitis (e.g. progression from stage 1 to stage 2–3, appearance of a complication) after initial treatment for a minimum of 3 to 6 months with full therapeutic doses.
2. presence of a combined acid and alkaline gastroesophageal reflux, either diagnosed by gastric and esophageal pH measurements [6], or suspected because of progression of esophagitis during the treatment [1]. Indeed, no medical treatment is specific or effective for combined reflux esophagitis.
3. presence of a primary disturbance of esophageal motility, specific or not.
4. frequent bouts of esophagitis of increasing intensity, with probable evolution towards a complication.

In our experience, there is a relationship between the presence of erosive esophagitis and the risk of developing a complication (stenosis, ulcer, columnar epithelium). The principal arguments in favor of this evolution are:

- the age of the patients is progressively more as the reflux lesions are more advanced (Fig. 1). This may mean that the 4 stages of reflux esophagitis described by Savary and Miller [7] are stages of increasing severity of the same disease.
- the appearance of a complication in 2% of our 3069 patients with reflux esophagitis. The average time interval between the endoscopic documentation of esophagitis and the complication is 56 months.
- the presence of a history of chronic reflux symptoms (> 6 years) in 76% of our 925 patients with a complication of reflux.

Surgery continues to be of value in the treatment of erosive reflux esophagitis. Its main role is determined by the failures and inherent limitations of medical treatment.

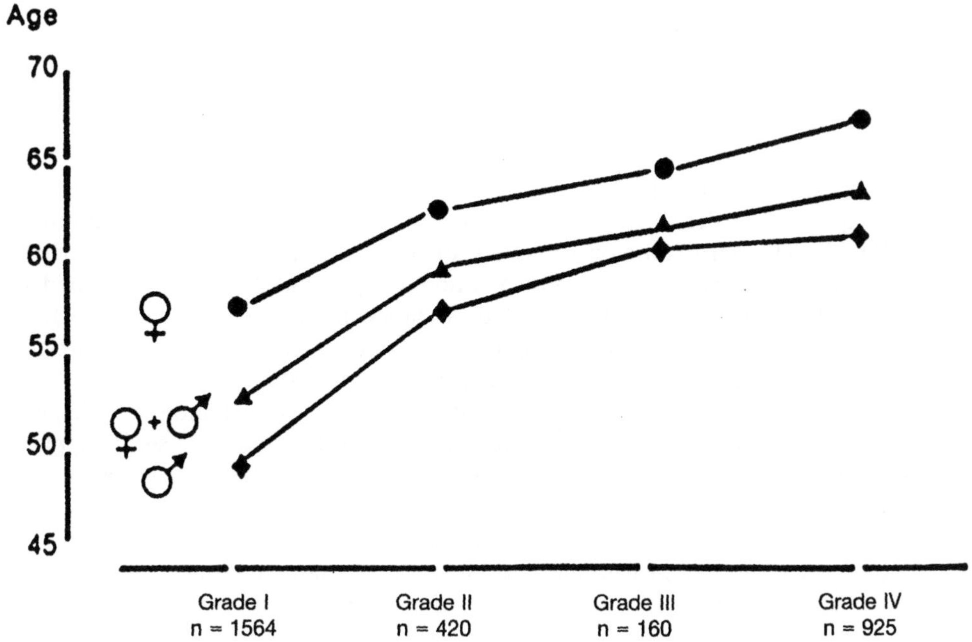

Fig. 1. Reflux esophagitis: mean age according to the Savary-Miller classification

References

1. Audebert M, Huguier M (1984) La cimétidine peut-elle favoriser l'apparition d'une œsophagite? Gastroenterol Clin Biol 8: 198–199
2. Damman HG, Blum AL, Lux G et al (1986) Unterschiedliche Heilungstendenz der Reflux-ösophagitis nach omeprazol und rantinidin. Dtsch Med Wschr 111: 123–128
3. Elsborg L, Beck B, Stubgaard (1985) Effect of sucralfate on gastroesophageal reflux in esophagitis. Hepato-Gastroenterol 32: 181–184
4. Goy JA, Magnard JH, McNaughton M, O'Shea A (1983) Ranitidine and placebo in the treatment of reflux oesophagitis. A double blind radomized trial. Med J Aust 2: 558–561
5. Koelz HR, Birchler R, Bretholz A et al (1986) Healing and relapse of reflux esophagitis during treatment with ranitidine. Gastroenterology 91: 1198–1205
6. Pucciani F, Marcuzzo G, Cortesini C (1985) La pH-metria combinata esofagea e gastrica nello studio della malattia da reflusso gastro-esofageo Clin Ter 112: 3–8
7. Savary M, Ollyo JB (1986) L'œsophagite par reflux et ses complications: ulcère, sténose, endobrachy-œsophage. Encycl Med Chir (Paris, France) ORL 20822 A10, 10 (16 p)
8. Wesdorp ICE (1984) Oesophagitis and its complications: medical treatment. Scand J Gastroenterol 19; suppl 106: 87–95

Surgical indication in Barrett's esophagus

H. Richelme, and *D. Benchimol* (Nice)

It is acknowledged that in the great majority of cases endobrachyesophagus (EBE) is an acquired disorder secondary to severe and prolonged gastroesophageal reflux (GER) [6]. The very common discovery of an adenocarcinoma within an EBE makes this entity a true precancerous condition [6, 8]. Medical treatment is aimed at reducing the harmfulness of the GER thus stabilizing the development of EBE. Surgery may be indicated to treat a GER or for the excision of EBE with malignant degeneration (actual or suspected) or for certain complicated forms of EBE.

The demonstration of the existence of EBE calls for complete esophageal investigation in every case, to be repeated during the subsequent course. It supplies information essential in the choice of treatment. The investigational aspects are as follows:

1. Clinical: symptoms of GER, dysphagia, recent change in symptomatology.
2. Manometry and pH measurement to assess the position and tone of the inferior esophageal sphincter and the severity, duration and nature of the GER.
3. Endoscopy to assess the extent of the EBE, the type of mucosal junction and possible presence of proximal heterotopic islets and the existence of complications (Barrett or Savary ulcers, adenomas, strictures, endoscopically suspect zones).
4. Histologic: multiple, staged and directed biopsies provide actual cartography of the EBE. They identify the nature of the metaplastic mucosa, whether gastric, junctional or intestinal. Histochemical studies are essential to study the type of intestinal metaplasia and to investigate for secretion of abnormal mucins (sulfomucins). Finally and chiefly histologic study makes it possible to detect the lesions of dysplasia which is graded as absent, moderate, severe or indeterminate.

In every case histology is the key factor in deciding the form of treatment.

The histology is unfavorable

There may be an adenocarcinoma in EBE found at initial presentation or during the course of treatment. Immediate excision is indicated after assessment of operability and resectability.

There may be lesions of severe dysplasia either at the outset or appearing secondarily. Such severe dysplasia must be now regarded more as an index of adenocarcinoma situated within the EBE than as a precancerous lesion [5, 10].

There may be intestinal metaplasia of type II B (incomplete metaplasia with secretion of abnormal mucins). This may be regarded as a precancerous condition [7, 10].

The last two cases relate to patients who either actually have an adenocarcinoma or are susceptible to developing it. Therefore the only logical treatment after endoscopic and histologic study is an excisional operation [9] especially when there are also cocarcinogenic factors (especially smoking). We consider the method of choice to be the Lewis-Santy operation which gives an excision of adequate extent in breadth and height and provides good digestive comfort at the price of an acceptable mortality and morbidity. The only imperative here is not to leave in place any islet of heterotopic mucosa in the proximal esophagus.

The histology is favorable

Dysplasia is absent or moderate; metaplasia is of cardiac, fundal or intestinal type, but complete and/or without secretion of abnormal mucins. Management will be determined by the symptomatology, endoscopy and the manometric and pH measurement findings.

The EBE is uncomplicated

If there is no GER, all that is required is endoscopic monitoring to detect any histologic changes.

If the existence of GER is verified, the persistence of symptoms or extension in the level of the EBE despite medical treatment are the indications for surgery. An anti-reflux procedure is logical in view of its virtually constant efficacy in this type of indication [6]. The Nissen-Rossetti procedure seems to us to be the best technique. Apart from radical treatment of the GER the aim of this operation is the stabilization and even in rare cases the regression of the EBE [1]. Of course postoperative pH monitoring of the efficacy of the surgical set-up is essential. Regular endoscopic and histologic surveillance remains necessary to ensure the arrested development of the EBE, as adenocarcinoma developing after anti-reflux procedures have been described [2, 3, 6, 11].

The EBE is complicated

a) Ulcers are present, of Barrett or Savary type. In themselves they are not an indication for surgery, as regression under medical treatment is usual [4]. However they are indicative of the progressive nature of the EBE and of the severity of the underlying GER. Their resistance to a short well-managed course of medical treatment should make it imperative to consider an anti-reflux procedure.
b) There is a stricture within the EBE. It is always difficult to confirm that this is benign despite multiple biopsies after dilatation and this doubt should lead to consideration of excisional surgery.

Conclusion

It is difficult to lay down guidelines for treatment in the presence of an EBE. The demonstration of an EBE should always arouse suspicion of an adenocarcinoma at the time of diagnosis or during progress under treatment.

The existence of sound markers (severe dysplasia, intestinal metaplasia of type II B should permit its detection and treatment at a "useful" stage. On the other hand, in the presence of non-suspect EBE, its extension under well-managed medical treatment and/or the severity of the underlying GER are the factors that should lead to anti-reflux surgery.

References

1. Brand DL, Ylvisaker JT, Gelfand M, Pope CE, (1980) Regression of columnar esophageal (Barrett's) epithelium after anti-reflux surgery. N Engl J Med 302: 844–848
2. Cameron AJ, Ott BJ, Payne WS (1985) The incidence of adenocarcinoma in columnar-lined (Barrett's) esophagus. N Engl J Med 313: 857–859
3. Hamilton SR, Hutcheon DF, Ravich WJ, Cameron JL, Paulson M (1984) Adenocarcinoma in Barrett's esophagus after elimination of gastroesophageal reflux. Gastroenterology 86: 356–360
4. Henrion J, Heller F (1983) Endobrachy œsophage (œsophage de Barrett). Etude clinique et endoscopique de 22 cas. Acta gastro-ent belg 46: 207–219
5. Kalish RJ, Clancy PE, Orringer MB, Appelman HD (1984) Clinical, epidemiologic and morphologic comparison between adenocarcinomas arising in Barrett's esophageal mucosa and in the gastric cardia. Gastroenterology 86: 461–467
6. Naef AP, Savary M, Ozello L (1975) Columnar-lined lower esophagus: an acquired lesion with malignant predisposition. Report of 140 cases of Barrett's esophagus with 12 adenocarcinomas. J Thorac Cardiovasc Surg 70: 826–834
7. Potet F, Peuch Maur M (1984) Etude histochimique des mucines dans l'endobrachyœsophage. Arch Anat Cytol Path 32: 59
8. Sarr MG, Hamilton SR, Marrone GC, Cameron JL Barrett's esophagus: its prevalence and association with adenocarcinoma in patients with symptoms of gastroesophageal reflux
9. Saubier EC, Gouillat C, Sanianiego C, Guillaud M, Moulinier B Adenocarcinoma in columnar-lined Barrett's esophagus. Analysis of 13 esophagectomies
10. Schmidt HG, Riddell RH, Walther B, Skinner DB, Riemann JF (1985) Dysplasia in Barrett's esophagus. J Cancer Res Clin Oncol 110: 145–152
11. Starnes VA, Adkins RB, Ballinger JF, Sawyers JL (1984) Barrett's esophagus. A surgical entity. Arch Surg 119: 563–567

Surgical indication in peptic esophagitis in children

J. B. Ollyo, D. Berger, M. Roulet, J. Wellinger, and *M. Savary* (Lausanne)

Reflux esophagitis is rarely diagnosed in patients under 16 years old (Table 1). In our experience children under 2 years old with stage 1–3 erosive reflux esophagitis (Savary-Miller classification) almost always respond to simple medical treatment such as postural positioning, thick and frequent meals, metoclopramide and antacids. H_2 blocking agents [4] and constant flow enteric feeding may be used if the child has severe vomiting or is severely malnourished, but are not often required.

Table 1. Spread of reflux esophagitis according to the Savary-Miller endoscopical grading

	children < 16 years	adults > 16 years
N° of Patients	1015	25 948
Hiatal hernia	183	8 650
reflux esophagitis	101	3069
– Stage I – Stage II – Stage III – Stage IV	51 8 3 39	1564 420 160 925

Chuv, Lausanne, Suisse (01. 01. 1963–31. 12. 1986)

The medical treatment of erosive reflux esophagitis in the child who has acquired the erect position is usually the same as for the adult (H_2 blocking agents) and has similar results [9].

Regardless of the child's age, surgery should be discussed in the following situations:

1. persistence or progression of erosive lesions after optimal medical treatment [12] for at least 3 months,
2. reflux esophagitis complicated by a peptic stenosis [7, 10, 11] a junctional or Barrett's ulcer [10] or an acquired endobrachyesophagus [5, 8] which may have a malignant evolution even in the child [6],
3. presence of primary disturbance of esophageal motility [1, 13] which may be in part responsible for the reflux esophagitis [12],
4. association of reflux esophagitis with other anatomic anomalies such as fixed hiatal hernia, paraesophageal hernia or diaphragmatic hernia,
5. recurrent respiratory infections resistant to treatment or failure to thrive due to reflux [2, 3].

References

1. Arana J, Tovar JA, Garay J (1986) Abnormal preoperative and postoperative esophageal peristaltis in gastroesophageal reflux. J Ped Surg 21: 711–714
2. Berger D, Bischof-Delaloye A, Landry M, Roulet M, Micheli JL (1986) Bronchopulmonary aspiration syndrome and gastroesophageal reflux in infants and children. Pediatr Surg Int 1: 168–171
3. Byrne WJ, Euler AR, Ashcraft E et al (1982) Gastroesophageal reflux in the severely retarded who vomit: criteria for and results of surgical intervention in twenty-two patients. Surgery 91: 95–98
4. Cucchiara S, Staiano A, Romaniello G et al (1984) Antacids and cimetidine treatment for gastroesophageal reflux and peptic oesophagitis. Arch Dis Child 59: 842–847
5. Dahms BB, Rothstein FC (1984) Barrett's esophagus in children: A consequence of chronic gastroesophageal reflux. Gastroenterology 86: 318–323
6. Fekete F, in Potet F (1983) Aspects anatomo-pathologiques de l'endobrachy-œsophage. Actualités digestives 7: 285–291

7. Genton N, Savary M, Pippa R (1974) Hernies hiatales et sténoses peptiques chez l'enfant. JF ORL 23: 151–154
8. Hassal E, Weinstein WM, Ament ME (1985) Barrett's esophagus in childhood. Gastroenterology 89: 1331–1337
9. Koelz HR, Birchler R, Bretholz A et al (1986) Healing and relapse of reflux esophagitis during treatment with ranitidine. Gastroenterology 91: 1198–1205
10. Monereo J, Cortes L, Blesa E (1973) Peptic esophageal stenosis in children. J Ped Surg 8: 475–478
11. Nihoul-Fekete C, Mitrofanoff P, Lortat-Jacob S (1978) Les sténoses peptiques de l'œsophage chez l'enfant. Etude de 59 cas. Ann Chir 32: 657–663
12. Savary M, Ollyo JB (1986) L'œsophagite par reflux et ses complications: ulcère, sténose, endobrachy-œsophage. Encycl Med Chir (Paris, France) ORL 20822 A10, 10–(16 p)
13. Vane DW, Harmel RP, King DR, Boles ET (1985) The effectiveness of Nissen fundoplication in neurologically impaired children with gastroesophageal reflux. Surgery 98: 662–667

Surgical indication in stenosis

H. Richelme, and *B. Limouse* (Nice)

The treatment of peptic esophageal strictures has been the subject of many studies since the report of Chalnot and Richard [5] at the 70th Surgical Congress in 1968. Some degree of improvement in the difficult management of these benign polymorphous lesions has emerged. Thus endoscopy and surgery are not in conflict but are used in combination to make excisional surgery exceptional and to yield good results with conservative methods.

Peptic esophagitis is the outcome of gastroesophageal reflux and peptic stricture represents the most severe stage of evolution (grade 4) of this esophagitis. The anatomic features of the peptic stricture lesion are at issue: the site, extent and severity of the narrowing; the existence of brachyesophagus or endobrachyesophagus; whether the stricture is fibrosed and fixed or retains a degree of flexibility; the assuredness of its benign nature. All these are questions that must be answered definitely before making any therapeutic decision.

This underlines the importance of endoscopy with biopsies, a major factor in definition of the lesion in unequivocal terms and in appropriate treatment. Such definition rests on four criteria: clinical, i.e. dysphagia; radiologic, i.e. constant reduction of esophageal caliber; endoscopic, the impossibility of traversing the stricture with the fiber-gastroscope; and histologic, the absence of evidence of malignancy. It must always be added that our understanding of the physiopathology of gastroesophageal reflux and peptic esophagitis [41] still rests on the manometric and pH measurement data, even obtained peri-operatively.

Thus the treatment of peptic stenosis is based on many factors, but all are indispensable if failures of medical or surgical treatment are to be avoided. We are concerned here in specifying the time for surgical treatment and thus its place in relation to medical treatment. We shall consider the different surgical concepts before defining the surgical indications.

Surgical Procedures

• *A. The surgery of reflux*

The aim is to deal with a benign disorder with a benign procedure. The methods are based on the physiopathology of the peptic disorder. One must distinguish the classical "direct" methods aimed at reestablishing an effective and continent inferior esophageal sphincter and the "indirect" methods aimed at "denaturing" the composition of the reflux fluid and also at "deviating" it.

Anti-reflux procedures

Since Hayward in 1961 [13] maintained for the first time that a certain number of strictures regress when protected by an antireflux procedure, a great many techniques have been studied [14, 20, 24, 28, 49, 50]. All have in common the combination with a pre or postoperative dilatation maneuver. Several papers affirm the better efficacy of the Nissen-Rossetti complete type of fundoplication [2, 34, 39] although the long-term disadvantages or failures are beginning to be stressed [29]. However it also appears that the need for a topographic reconstruction has been discussed by some workers, hence the performance of different procedures without bringing down the cardia:
- Nissen's intrathoracic procedure [20, 26, 38].
- tubulation of the lesser curvature combined with fundoplication [30, 31, 32, 38, 43].
- construction of a sleeve on a gastric cone [25].

Total duodenal diversion

The experimental and clinical proofs of the harmfulness of alkaline and mixed forms of reflux have been given by Wangensteen and Levin as far back as 1913 [46], Lambert in 1962 [21], Gillisson in 1972 [11], Pellegrini, and DeMeester and Skinner in 1978 [33]. In 1961, Holt and Large [19] reported for the first time cures of peptic stricture after Billroth type 2 gastrectomy obtained by total duodenal diversion.

Since then, the literature has provided over a hundred published cases in two etiologic conditions of peptic stricture: 1) most often, for severe esophagitis after gastrectomy (usually of the upper pole) or for failed anti-reflux operation for brachyesophagus or complicated gastroesophageal reflux [7, 10, 15, 17, 18, 36, 44, 45]. 2) more rarely, as the treatment of first intention for a "primary" peptic stricture [9, 42, 46, 47].

• *B. Excisional surgery*

Two procedures find a place here; colopasties of the Belsey type and gastroplasties of the Santy-Lewis type.

Coloplasty retains its value not only because historically it remains attached to the name of R. Belsey but also because it is a method that radically attacks the reflux and its stricture while respecting the gastric reservoir. The major series of Belsey [3] and Reboud [12] witness that it should not be qualified as very serious surgery as was done in the report of Chalnot and Richard [5].

On the other hand, the Santy-Lewis type of operation performed by a double abdominal and thoracic approach certainly sacrifices the gastric reservoir but benefits from low operative risk.

Indications for surgery

These are determined by three important points:

1. precise anatomic, histologic and physiopathologic assessment of the peptic stricture.
2. long-term assessment of the results of endoscopic treatment by instrumental dilatation [2, 4, 7, 8, 22, 23, 40, 49, 50]
3. the risks and results of surgical operations.

For schematic purposes we shall contrast simple and complicated strictures and discuss the intermediate cases which are always more difficult to place within a therapeutic framework. Finally we shall deal with the particular case of patients already operated on. In every case our discussion and proposals relate to operable patients.

Simple strictures

These are strictures that are not very tight (> 10 mm), short (< 2 cm), localized to the lower third of the esophagus and readily dilatable. The real problem here is whether or not to combine dilatation with surgery to correct the gastroesophageal reflux and the answer is provided by complete investigation of esophageal function performed after instrumental dilatation [17,41].

If the tests show positive massive and prolonged reflux the question of a surgical antireflux procedure must be raised. In our view this means performing a Nissen-Rossetti complete type of fundoplication.

Complicated strictures

These strictures are very tight (< 5 mm) or high or extensive (> 6 cm) and irregular, difficult to dilate or reforming rapidly. They are also suspicious at the histologic level. They are currently much fewer in number. In our view they should be dealt with by excision. Since the operative mortality risk is low (less than 10%) and the results of good quality, a Santy-Lewis type of gastroplasty is preferable to a coloplasty.

Complex cases

These are strictures that are moderately tight (between 5 and 10 mm) and moderately extensive (between 2 and 6 cm), above a hiatus hernia of long and capricious symptomatic duration despite medical treatment. Here the operative indication after instrumental dilatation is clear and imperative. The findings of the functional esophageal assessment taken together with those obtained during operation itself will lead to adoption of the best choice of technique.

Three aspects should lead to rejection of a Nissen type of antireflux procedure: the first has to do with function, the existence of disorders of esophageal motor function which lead to functional failures as stressed by Skinner [41].

The second is anatomic, the existence of a cardia that cannot be brought down and leads to the effective performance of an intrathoracic Nissen procedure, which is unacceptable. Indeed in this case the extent of early and late postoperative complications, particularly gastric fistulae (nearly 20%) with a considerable mortality rate (around 10%) has been stressed in the literature [11, 39].

The third is taken from the randomized study of Washey, Royston and Spencer [47] who showed that total duodenal diversion gave the best 5 year results (91% of good results) and further emphasized the absence of mortality in 22 diversions compared to 2 deaths in 22 Nissen operations. For these various reasons, total duodenal diversion should be proposed in these complex cases.

Peptic strictures in already operated patients.

These patients have already undergone an antireflux procedure for hiatus hernia or brachyesophagus, or a polar gastrectomy for ulcer. Here total duodenal diversion has an undeniable place though the stricture must be certainly assessed as dilatable and benign beforehand. The technical difficulties of the essential truncal vagotomy due to the previous surgical procedure can be usefully evaded by a short left thoracic approach [9].

References

1. Baulieux J, Gianello P, Peix JL, Goudin JL, Caillot JL, Pouyet M, (1984) Les fistules œsophagiennes après cure de hernie hiatale Lyon Chir 180–183
2. Behar J, Sheahan DG, Biancani P, Spiro HM, Storer EH (1975) Medical and surgical management of reflux oesophagitis, a 38 month report on a prospective clinical trial N Eng J Med 293: 263–268
3. Belsey R (1969) Traitement chirurgical des sténoses bénignes fibreuses de l'œsophage. Lyon Chirurgical 65: 832–841
4. Bigard MA, Champigneule B, Gaucher P, Dollet JM, Schmit JL, Aussedat Ph (1985) Peut-on proposer les dilatations oesophagiennes comme seul traitement des sténoses peptiques oesophagiennes. Endoscopie digestive 8: 11–16
5. Chalnot P, Richard CA (1968) Les œsophagites peptiques. 70ème Congrés Français de Chirurgie Paris. Presses Universitaires de France Edit Paris
6. Dupin B, Castro R, Dumon JP, Meric B (1984) Notre expérience de la dilatation œsophagienne. A propos de 1138 dilatations. Ann de Gastro-entérologie et d'hépatologie, 20–5: 299

7. Elias D, Lasser Ph, Leclercq B, Nitenberg G (1983) La diversion duodénale modifiée dans le traitement des œsophagites par reflux biliaire compliquant une gastrectomie polaire supérieure. J Chir 120: 651–653
8. Evreux M, van Niewenhuyx A, Tete R, Trepo C, Brette R (1983) Traitement des sténoses peptiques de l'œsophage par dilatations endoscopiques à l'appareil d'Eder-Puestow isolées ou couplées à la chirurgie conservatrice. Journal de Medecine de Lyon 64: 357–361
9. Fekete F (1985) Total duodenal diversion in DeMeester TR, Skinner DB: Esophageal disorders pathophysiology and therapy. New-York, Raven press
10. Fekete F (1983) Œsophagites peptiques graves. Traitement par diversion duodénale totale NPM, 12, 36: 2239–2242
11. Gillison EW, De Castro VAM, Nyhus LM, Kusakari K, Bombeck CT (1972) The significance of bile in reflux esophagitis. Surg Gynecol Obst 134: 419–424
12. Giudicelli R, Fuentes P, Dumon JF, Riera P, Reboud E (1983) Traitement des sténoses peptiques de l'œsophage. A propos de cent cas. Ann Chir 37: 627–628
13. Hayward (1961) The treatment of fibrous strictures of oesophagus associated with hiatal hernia, Thorax 16: 36–45
14. Henderson RD, Manyatt RM (1983) Total fundoplication gastroplasty long term follow-up in 500 patients. J Thorac-Cardiovasc Surg 85: 81–87
15. Herrington JL, Mody B (1976) Total duodenal diversion for treatment of reflux esophagitis uncontrolled by repeated antireflux procedures. Ann Surg 183: 636–44
16. Hill L, Asplund C, Roberts P (1984) Intraoperative manometry: adjunct to surgery for esophageal motility disorders. Am H of Surg 147: 171–174
17. Hivet M, Mahoux P (1974) Œsophagite grave après œsogastrectomie polaire superieure. Deux cas traités par gastrectomie inférieure complémentaire. Ann Chir 28: 989–994
18. Hollender LF, Meyer Ch, Marric A, Keller D, Zeyler B, Goldschmidt P (1981) La place de la fundo-jejunostomie sur anse exclue en Y dans les échecs therapeutiques chirurgicaux du reflux gastro-oesophagien. Chirurgie 107: 139–145
19. Holt CJ, Large AM (1961) Surgical management of reflux esophagitis. Ann Surg 153: 555–562
20. Keenan SJ, Hamilton JRL, Gibbous FRCS, Stevenson HM (1984) Surgery for benign oesophageal stricture. J Thorac Cardiovasc Surg 88: 182–188
21. Lambert R (1962) Relative importance of biliary and pancreatic secretions in the genesis of esophagitis in rats. Am I Dig Dis 7: 1025–1033
22. Lequerler Y, Le Guillou M, Vallot Th, Robaszkiewicz M, Gouerou H (1985) Sténoses peptiques dilatées par la méthode d'Eder-Puestow. Devenir à moyen et long terme. Endoscopie Digestive 8: 3–9
23. Leichtmann GA, Novis BA, Samara M (1984) Dilatation instrumentale des sténoses œsophagiennes à l'aide du catheter de Gruntzig et du dilatateur de Celestin. Résultats préliminaires. Gastro entérol Clin Biol 8: 616–620
24. Loygue J, Parc R, Letoublon C, Cugnenc H (1980) Traitement des sténoses peptiques de l'oesophage. A propos de 40 cas Chirurgie 106: 636–643
25. Maillet P, Cazagoux JF, Baulieux J (1980) La voie abdominale dans le traitement conservateur des sténoses peptiques de l'œsophage. Ann Chir 34: 380–381
26. Maher JW, Hocking MP, Woodward ER (1984) Supradiaphragmatic fundoplication. Long term follow-up and analysis of complications. Am I Surg 147: 181–186
27. DeMeester TR, Johnson LF, Kent AH (1974) Evaluation of current operations for prevention of gastroesophageal reflux. Ann Surg 180: 511–525
28. Moghissi K (1980) Sténoses hautes de l'œsophage thoracique et leur traitement chirurgical. Chirurgie 106: 711–718
29. Nègre JP (1984) La fundoplicature de Nissen: échecs et inconvenients à long terme. Ann Chir 38: 275–280
30. Orringer MB (1983) The combined Collis-Nissen operation. Early assessment of reflux control. Ann Chir 37: 633
31. Paris F, Benages A, Ridocci MT, Tarazoua V, Molina R, Mora F, Pastor J, Lloret D, Garrida G (1977) Allongement œsophagien avec le stapler et valvulo-plastie comme opération antireflux. Ann Chir 16: 335–341
32. Pearson JG, Henderson RD (1976) Long term follow-up of peptic strictures managed by dilatation modified Collis-gastroplasty and Belsey hiatus hernia repair. Surgery 80: 396–404

33. Pellegrini CA, DeMeester TR, Werly JA, Johnson LF, Skinner DB (1978) Alkaline gastroesophageal reflux Am I Surg 135: 177–783
34. Polk HC (1976) Fundoplication for reflux esophagitis: misadventures with the operation of choice. Ann Surg 183: 645–652
35. Richieri JP, Mathieu B, Pin G, Touchene B, Remacle JP, Blachere P, Mouges H (1980) Sténoses peptiques de l'oesophage. Traitement par le dilatateur d'Eder-Puestow. NPM 9, 13: 955–958
36. Royston CMS, Dowling BL, Spencer J (1975) Antrectomy with Roux en Y anastomosis in the treatment of peptic oesophagitis with stricture. Br I Surg 62: 605-607
37. Salo JA, Lampinen H, Kivilaakso (1985) Partial gastrectomy with Roux en Y reconstruction of persistent or recurrent oesophagitis after Nissen fundoplication. Br I Surg 72: 623–625
38. Saubier EC, Gouillat C (1983) Traitement des sténoses peptiques de l'oesophage par fundoplicature intrathoracique avec dilatation per operatoire de la sténose. Chirurgie 109: 494–500
39. Saubier EC, Gouillat C, Teboul F (1986) Traitement du reflux gastro-œsophagien par fundoplicature complète de Nissen. Résultats de 112 observations. Chirurgie 112: 123–131
40. Stoddard CJ, Simons JM (1984) Dilatation of benign oesophageal strictures in the out patient departement Br I Surg 71: 752–753
41. Skinner DB (1985) Pathophysiology of gastroesophageal reflux. Ann Surg 202, 5: 546–556
42. Tanner NC, Westerholm P (1968) Partial gastrectomy in the treatment of esophageal stricture after hiatal hernia Am J Surg 115: 449–453
43. Vankemmel M, Rwamasirabo E, Binot D (1983) Traitement du reflux gastro-oesophagien par cardioplastie Ann Chir 37: 634–635
44. Viard H, Favre JP, Sala JJ, Sicard C, Hillon P, Cougard P (1985) La diversion duodenale totale dans le traitement des oesophagites peptiques. Lyon Chir 81: 3–6
45. Viard H, Favre JP, Cayot M, Trigalou D, Chevilotte P (1978) Le traitement chirurgical de l'oesophagite peptique après oeso-gastrectomie polaire supérieure. Plaidoyer en faveur de l'antrectomie suivie de gastro-jéjunostomie en Y Ann Chir 17: 217–221
46. Wangensteen OH, Levin NL (1949) Gastric resection for oesophagitis and stricture of acid peptic origin. Surg gynecol obstet 88: 560–570
47. Washer GF, Gear MWL, Dowling BL, Gillison EW, CMS Royston, Spencer I (1984) Randomized prospective Roux en Y duodenal diversion versus fundoplication for severe reflux oesophagitis. Br I Surg 71: 181–184
48. Weaver AW, Large AM, Walt AJ (1961) Surgical management of reflux oesophagitis Ann Surg 119: 15–20
49. Réunion internationale sur la pathologie oesophagienne Marseille 1982. Ann Chir 37, 8: 582–636
50. Le traitement conservateur des sténoses peptiques de l'oesophage de l'adulte Table ronde. Journées Chirurgicales de Normandie. Ann Chir 1980, 34, 5: 376–383

When a peptic esophageal lesion is healed, is maintenance therapy nevertheless indicated?

R. Colin, and *E. Lerebours* (Rouen)

The posing of this question calls for a preliminary remark before attempting a reply. The concept of healing usually applies to the complete repair of the macroscopic lesions (most often as seen at endoscopy) whether these be ulcerations or erosions; but is has been shown that there is a poor correlation between this macroscopic "healing" and that of the histologic or functional disturbances [5]. This fact explains certain divergences during the selection of patients in controlled studies. A precise reply, firmly suited to the question, cannot be given; nevertheless, it is possible, on the basis of published studies, to assemble a certain number of arguments that may help in the decision.

Maintenance treatment after the healing of the lesions of esophagitis may aim at diverse objectives.

The prevention of relapse of symptoms

It has been shown that the prevention of symptomatic relapse is possible provided powerful maintenance treatment is used identical with that of acknowledged efficacy in the acute treatment of esophagitis: ranitidine 300 mg/day in the study of McCallum et al. [3], cimetidine 1.6 g/day together with antacids in the study of Wesdorp et al. [8]. On the other hand, treatment with reduced doses of anti-H_2 agents such as ranitidine 150 mg at night [3] or by antacids is ineffective.

The prevention of recurrences of esophagitis after healing

A recent study [2] reveals that maintenance treatment with ranitidine in a dose of 150 mg at night, the efficacy of which has been demonstrated in preventing relapses of gastroduodenal ulceration, did not prevent relapses of esophagitis, which occurred at 6 months in 14 out of 33 cases on ranitidine and in 10 out of 28 cases on placebo. Conversely two studies using 1.6 g/day of cimetidine alone [7] or together with antacids [8] show a preventive effect on the reappearance of the progressive lesions of esophagitis.

Improvement of the natural history of severe peptic esophagitis

The studies of Ferguson et al. [1] and of Starlinger et al. [7], though employing the same therapeutic schedule (cimetidine 1.6 g/day long-term) in the maintenance treatment of esophagitis with stricture, gave conflicting results. The first study found no preventive effect on recurrence as assessed by the anatomic findings and the need for dilatation whereas for Starlinger et al, this same treatment continued for 6 years in some patients prevented recurrence and the redevelopment of stricture.

Modification of the natural history of endobrachyesophagus

The combination of cimetidine 1.6 g/day and antacids though effective against the symptoms and lesions of esophagitis produced no regression of the endobrachyesophagus after continuous treatment for 2 years [8]. There have even been reports of the development of a complication in the shape of stricture of an endobrachyesophagus despite continuous treatment with H_2 antagonists [4]. Finally, no medical treatment has shown any efficacy in preventing the development of cancer in endobrachyesophagus [6].

These differing reports suggest the following conclusions:

- prophylactic medical treatments of symptomatic and structural relapses must, if they are to be effective, comprise drugs and dosages similar to those proved necessary for the initial treatment of esophagitis.
- as the natural history of reflux esophagitis is still not fully understood and is probably marked by stages of acute exacerbation, the utility of routine prophylactic treatment for recurrence of esophagitis has not been demonstrated
- it may be suggested that, though there may exist a subgroup of patients justifying prophylactic medical treatment, it is probably opportune to discuss the alternative of surgical treatment with these patients.

References

1. Ferguson R, Dronfield MW, Atkinson M (1979) Cimetidine of reflux oesophagitis with peptic stricture. Br Med J 2: 472–474
2. Koelz HR, Birchler R, Bretholz A et al (1986) Healing and relapse of reflux esophagitis during treatment with Ranitidine. Gastroenterology 91: 1198–1205
3. McCallum RW, Sontag SJ, Vlahcevic ZR et al (1985) Ranitidine versus placebo in long term treatment of gastroesophageal reflux (abstract)/Am J Gastroenterol 80: 864
4. Salzman M, Barwick K, McCallum RW (1982) Progression of Cimetidine-treated reflux esophagitis to a Barrett's stricture. Dig Dis Sci 27: 181–186.
5. Sonnenberg A, Lepsien G, Muller-Lissner SA et al (1982) When is esophagitis healed? Esophageal endoscopy, histology and function before and after Cimetidine treatment. Dig Dis Sci 27: 297–302
6. Spechler SJ, Goyal RK (1986) Barrett's esophagus. N Engl J Med 315: 362–371
7. Starlinger M, Appell WH, Schemper M, Schiessel R (1985) Long-term treatment of peptic esophageal stenosis with dilatation and Cimetidine: factors influencing clinical result. Eur Surg Res 17: 207–214
8. Wesdorp ICE, Bartelsman J, Schipper MEI, Tytgat GN (1981) Effect of long-term treatment with Cimetidine and antacids in Barrett oesophagus. Gut 22: 724–727

Is it necessary to consider standardizing the methods of evaluation in order to compare the different treatments?

S. Bonfils (Paris)

Standardization of the different methods of assessment for different treatments of esophagitis is eminently desirable. However, while this is an essential in terms of trials designed for comparative evaluation of various drugs the problem takes another aspect when it is matter of studying of "drugs against surgery", and still more so in considering a series of individual cases. In the last instance the therapeutic benefit may be based on different features, according to the patients.

Two further preliminaries of the greatest importance must be mentioned:

1. the dissociation frequently noted between functional symptoms and anatomic lesions in the lower esophagus
2. the fact that among the special techniques of examination (endoscopy, pH measurement, manometry) some refer to a structural lesion and others to physiopathology.

Now the correction of a physiopathologic disorder may itself create new disorders (such as an over-tight Nissen procedure) or may end by substituting one pathogenic factor for another (total correction of acid hypersecretion being replaced by biliary reflux).

In view of these considerations, the possible methods of assessment may be listed in the following manner:

- clinical:
  disappearance of pyrosis, disappearance of postural syndrome, disappearance of all alimentary sensitivity,
- endoscopic:
  disappearance of endoscopic lesions,
- physiopathologic:
  improvement of results of esophageal pH measurement, controlled reduction of acid secretion, acceleration of gastric emptying, control of the state of inferior esophageal sphincter(?)

It is generally agreed that esophageal biopsies are not considered of the first interest, as macroscopic restitution ad integrum should suffice as the endoscopic criterion of cure.

For my part I consider that if the absolute criterion of therapeutic efficacy is the disappearance of all functional disorder, lesions or anomalies, simultaneous normalization of the three aspects is virtually never obtained medically. Which of these should be accorded the most importance? For any given patient the percentage of functional and structural improvement in relation to the initial state is always an absolutely valid criterion.

In other words in patients with great discomfort or with esophageal ulceration the control of minor functional disorders or of esophagitis is itself a success. Is this satisfactory, can this benefit be compared with the absolute disappearance of symptoms in a patient with little distress?

J. P. Galmiche (Nantes)

It seems desirable to distinguish between the assessment of a therapy by a controlled trial (based on groups of patients) and the interpretation of the result, whether a success or (especially) a failure, obtained in an individual patient submitted to antireflux treatment.

In the case of the controlled trial (against placebo or a reference treatment) certain methodologic recommendations deserve mention. The "preferred" assessment criterion should be exactly defined before the trial and it is desirable to avoid multiplication of assessment criteria. One also must ensure that the trial is authoritative enough for a reply to the question raised, notably by including an adequate number of patients. As regards reflux and peptic esophagitis, these rules, elementary as they are, have usually been little respected, and the published trials generally relate to small series (less than 50 in each group). As for the assessment criteria themselves, evaluation may be based on functional symptoms (possibly grouped in a single symptomatic score) and/or on the macroscopic endoscopic lesions (in practice, on the epithelial "defects").

While the organization of a trial comparing medical and surgical treatment raises problems of organizational practice undeniably more complex than the comparison of two forms of medical treatment, the methods and criteria of assessment nevertheless remain the same and are in my view essentially clinical; in fact apart from very severe lesions of esophagitis (ulcer, stricture, extensive endobrachyesophagus), functional symptomatology seems to me as important as the endoscopic findings. Indeed the risk of long-term development of an erosive esophagitis towards a severe strictured esophagitis is undoubtedly very small, if not nil, and this is even more true for catarrhal esophagitis.

The only problem is the inclusion in a trial of patients with atypical symptoms, which may be desirable if one wishes to deal with a population more representative of the disease than one composed only of patients with characteristic pyrosis and postural syndrome. In this case, especially if the endoscopy is normal, positive pH measurment may constitute an indispensable criterion for inclusion.

In general terms pH measurement, manometry and functional studies are not essential to the conduct of a controlled therapeutic trial, though they may assist in interpreting certain results, notably after surgical intervention.

Thus, a good clinical result is not always correlated with a good result in terms of pH measurement; failures in terms of pH measurement doubtless explain the long-term deterioration in clinical results after posterior hemi-fundoplication, and are themselves explained by inadequate restoration of the cardiac continence. Conversely, it would be incorrect to consider a good pH result as a therapeutic success in a patient with major undesirable effects of medication (e.g. metolopramide) or with sequelae of surgical treatment (dysphagia, gas-bloat syndrome after a Nissen procedure).

In principle, the clinical state still constitutes the preferred assessment criterion in a therapeutic trial; other methods are useful for objective and/or quantitative evaluation, but they are not, in the strict sense, essential to the demonstration of therapeutic success.

The problem is a little different in the care of an individual patient, as interpretation of the therapeutic result can no longer be expressed in statistical terms. If medical or surgical treatment appears to fail the clinical status is not enough. Esophageal pH measurement will be required to confirm the diagnosis if the symptoms are not characteristic, and for repetition during treatment to ensure the efficacy or non-efficacy of the latter (short of being able to certainly predict its *utility*!). In this case, pH measurement may also help in adjusting the dosage of an antisecretory agent or the optimal partitioning of combined treatment, e.g. the combination of antisecretory and prokinetic medication.

A "multifactorial" and physiopathologic approach then seems to me rational and desirable. Such an approach may call also for evaluation of cardiac continence and esophageal peristalsis (by manometry) and gastric secretion and emptying, for lack of the ability at present to investigate the resistance of the esophageal mucosa by simple means.

Finally, standardization of the assessment criteria is desirable, but the same criteria should not be applied routinely to all therapeutic situations, whether clinical or experimental.

Conclusion

J. F. Rey (St. Laurent du Var)

Medical treatment of gastro-esophageal reflux

The gastro-esophageal reflux is a common disease which has benefited from physiopathological knowledge and development of new techniques such as 24 hour pHmonitoring. The frequency of this trouble and its development are uncertain and in most cases, appropriate dietetic measures relieved symptomatic disorders.

If the reflux leads to mild esophagitis the treatment could be based on two kinds of drugs: drug increasing esophageal motility and antacids.

a) Metoclopramide and domperidone have about the same efficacy on the esophageal motility. Early trials on cisapride are extremely promising in cases of esophagitis.
b) antacids and alginates are a logical prescription for basic treatment. Sucralfate seems more accurate in case of esophagitis.

In case of moderate or severe esophagitis diagnosed by endoscopy, blockers of H_2 receptors were an important step in the management of the patients. Ranitidine and cimetidine relieved symtomatic pain. These two H_2-blockers act directly on esophageal sensitivity and in reducing gastric acidity. Moderate esophagitis is cured in 75% of cases. Prescription should be given twice or even three times a day; at 300 mg per 24 hrs for ranitidine, or 800 mg per 24 hrs for cimetidine. Marked increases of this regimen do not affect the clinical results.

Initial treatment should for be at least 3 months, but these two H_2-blockers do not prevent relapse. There is no significant correlation between evolution of clinical symptoms and histologic or endoscopic patterns during treatment.

If we look to new molecules, two have been extensively tried: prostaglandins and omeprazole. Clinical effects of prostaglandins in esophagitis seem disappointing. Efficiency of omeprazole has been clearly shown but its routine use is impaired by potential side-effects. Side-effects related to H_2-blockers appear minor if we compare a world-wide 10 years prescription, and they remain a logical prescription in cases of esophagitis.

Surgical treatment of peptic esophagitis

President: *Mark B. Orringer* (Ann Arbor)

Free Commentators: *Y. Chapuis* (Paris)
Ph. E. Donahue (Chicago)
P. Hautefeuille (Paris)
R. Parc (Paris)
R. Stoppa (Amiens)
K. Thor (Stockholm)

What are the factors contributing to the continence of the cardia? Increase of the LES

P. E. Donahue, C. T. Bombeck, and *L. M. Nyhus*
(Chicago)

The absolute strength of the squeeze pressure exerted by the Lower Esophageal Sphincter (LES) has long been recognized as an important factor in maintaining the competence of the gastroesophageal junction. However, to the dismay of both physicians and surgeons, the absolute LES sphincter pressures have not proven to be the absolute discriminant factor capable of distinguishing a population of "refluxers" from the rest of the population. Therefore, measurements of esophageal pressure have become a curiosity to be obtained or not obtained, depending on the bias of the individual. Even the enthusiasts for these measurements must admit that the information obtained has only been of incidental value, and of primary use in reference to the investigation of patients after anti-reflux surgery.

DeMeester et al. have emphasized the fact that competence of the cardia is a multifactorial process including both the length, the position and the strength of the sphincter [1]. The current status of this concept has been expanded by the recent work of Bombeck et al. showing that the important factors include those mentioned plus factors relating to the symmetry of the sphincter, and the presence of "weak spots" in the longitudinal array of contractile elements.

At the beginning of this presentation it is appropriate to mention the seminal work of several investigators working in the laboratories at the University of Illinois Hospital; the studies referred to initiated our investigation of the multivariate nature of reflux based upon a comparison of the standard measures of LES pressure, the concept of LES Opening Pressure (LESOP) and the analysis of the symmetry of the component parts of the antireflux mechanism [2, 3].

The concept of LESOP has a special place in this story since it was the beginning of our insight into functional aspects of the sling fibers of the cardia, and because it allowed some insight into the contribution of the sling fibers of the proximal stomach to the antireflux mechanism. Parenthetically, we had previously recognized a paradoxical situation that excision of the lower esophageal segment only in some of our experimental animals did *not* produce clinical evidence of reflux. When Pettersson et al. investigated LESOP in the laboratory they showed that elements of gastric distention and tension in the gastric wall might be playing a role in the normal function of the anti-reflux mechanism [4]. They also suggested the congruence of this concept with the elegant anatomic studies of Liebermann-Meffert et al. which had shown anatomic equivalents of a sphincter in the collar of Helvetius and the "clasp-like" arrangement of the discrete muscular components of the cardia [5].

Returning to the central theme of LES pressure as part of the anti-reflux mechanism, then, there are two types of evidence which must be considered in constructing the answer to the question. First, the clinical laboratory has shown many times that the efficacy of anti-reflux operations is *not* determined absolutely by the changes or lack thereof in measured postoperative LES pressures. On the contrary, when a postoperative pressure is extremely high, there is a good chance that a "supercompetent" valve has been created and that the patient will have traded symptoms of pathologic reflux for those due to a valve which will not allow normal gastroesophageal reflux [6]. This has been true whether the pressures have been measured as single values, or when they have been compared as part of a computerized axial manometry system which considered the absolute pressures in conjunction with spatial organization of contractile pressures along the axis of the distal esophagus and proximal stomach. In both cases, the absolute value of the sphincter is only part of the answer to the question, and must be considered only in conjunction with other values which relate to the competency of the cardia [7].

References

1. O'Sullivan GC, DeMeester TR, Joelsson BE, Smith RB, Blough RR, Johnson LF, Skinner DB (1982) Interaction of lower esophageal sphincter pressure and length of sphincter in the abdomen as determinants of gastroesophageal competence. Am J Surg 143: 40–48
2. Samelson SL, Abuabara SF, Bombeck CT (1982) The failing lower esophageal sphincter: a multivariate analysis. Gastroenterol 82: 1169
3. Petterson GB, Bombeck CT, Nyhus LM (1980) The Lower Esophageal Sphincter. Mechanisms of Opening and Closure. Surgery 88: 307–313
4. Pettersson GB, Bombeck CT, Nyhus LM (1980) The Dynamics of the Lower Esophageal Function. Current Surgery 37: 143–145
5. Liebermann-Meffert D, Allgower M, Schmid P, Blum AL (1979) Muscular equivalents of the lower esophageal sphincter. Gastroenterology 76: 31–42
6. Donahue PE, Samelson S, Nyhus LM, Bombeck CT (1985) The Floppy Nissen Fundoplication – Effective long-term control of pathologic reflux. Arch Surg 120: 721–730
7. Bombeck CT, Vaz O, DeSalvo J, Donahue PE, Nyhus LM (1987) Computerized axial manometry of the esophagus: a new method for the assessment of anti-reflux operations. Presented at the American Surgical Association Meeting, April

How does the length of the abdominal esophagus contribute to the continence of the cardia?

T. R. DeMeester (Omaha)

The function of the lower esophageal sphincter is to protect the esophageal mucosa from excessive exposure to gastric juice. This function depends upon the resistance the sphincter imposes to the flow of gastric juice from an environment above atmospheric pressure, the stomach, into an environment below atmospheric pressure, the esophagus. This resistance is due to the integrated mechanical effect of sphincter pressure, the length of sphincter exposed to the positive environmental pressure of the abdomen and the overall sphincter length. The most common mechanical cause of incompetency is an inadequate distal esophageal sphincter pressure, but the efficiency of a sphincter with normal pressures can be nullified by an inadequate abdominal length or an abnormally short overall length. The grounds for this statement are as follows.

A relationship between sphincter pressure and its abdominal length can be demonstrated in an in vitro model designed to simulate the forces acting on the distal esophageal sphincter. Fig. 1 shows that the competency of the sphincter to challenges of intra-abdominal pressure is related to the length of sphincter exposed to the positive pressure environment of the abdomen, and the shorter the length exposed, the greater the sphincter pressure necessary to maintain competency. A minimum length of 1 cm of sphincter is required to protect against challenges of increases in intra-abdominal pressure since the amplitude of pressure necessary to achieve competency with less than this amount becomes infinite [1].

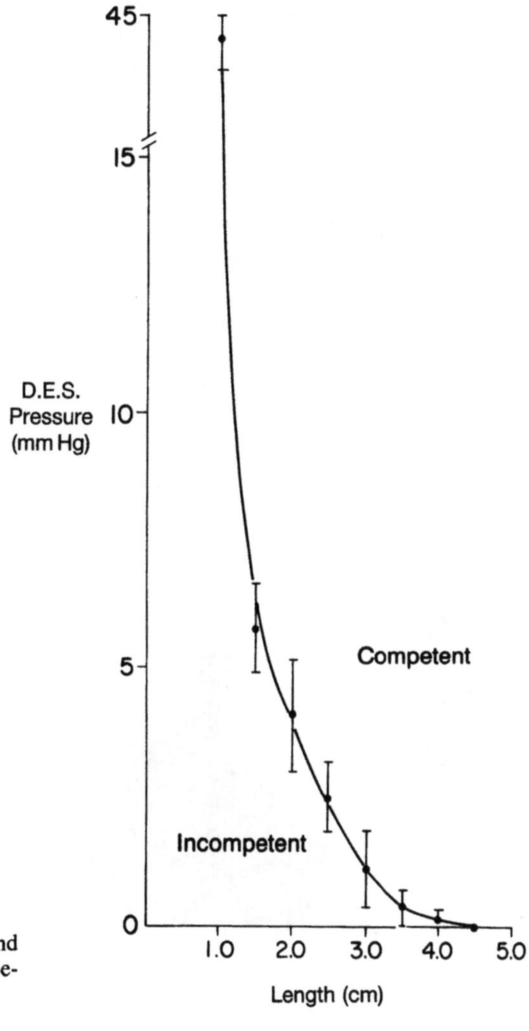

Fig. 1. Relationship of DES pressure and length of abdominal esophagus to competency of the cardia

Table 1

Maneuver	Thoracic Esophagus	Distal esophageal sphincter Thor. part (DES-T)	Abdom. part (DES-A)	Gastric Fundus
Valsalva	30.2 (±3.6)	24.9 (±4.6)$^{\times}$	30.7 (±2.3)$^{\times}$	36.4 (±1.3)
Leg Raising	0.38 (±0.1)	3.7 (±3.5)*	16.3 (±2.8)	17.2 (±3.3)
Muller	> −22 mm Hg	14.9 (±3.8)	16.1 (±4.7)	7.3 (±1.9)

All Measurements differ significantly from resting pressure ($p < .05$) except for *. Comparison between thoracic and abdominal portions of DES are all significant ($p < .05$) except for $^{\times}$

Table 1 shows that the sphincter in man reflects changes in its environmental pressure induced by various maneuvers. Each portion of the sphincter, abdominal or thoracic, is independently affected by changes in its environmental pressure. An increase in abdominal pressure causes an increase in the abdominal portion of the sphincter and stomach, while the thoracic portion and esophagus remain unaffected and vice versa. The study further showed that at least 1 cm of the sphincter must be exposed to the positive pressure of the abdomen in order for this response to occur. Lesser amounts places the sphincter at a mechanical disadvantage [2].

Fig. 2 shows the distribution of the abdominal sphincter length measured in 50 healthy volunteers Fig. 3 shows these normal values stratified according to percentiles. Ninety-five percent of normal subjects have an abdominal sphincter length longer than 1 cm; that is, greater than the critical value predicted by the former two studies [3].

Fig. 4 shows the distribution of the abdominal length of the lower esophageal sphincter in 622 patients who had the competency of their sphincter assessed by 24-hour esophageal pH monitoring. Eighty percent of patients with an abdominal length less than 1 cm (shaded area), that is, below the 5th percentile of normal, had an abnormal esophageal exposure to acid gastric juice [3].

Fig. 5 shows the specific manometric abnormalities in 196 patients with reflux and abnormal sphincter manometries. The most common isolated abnormality was a low

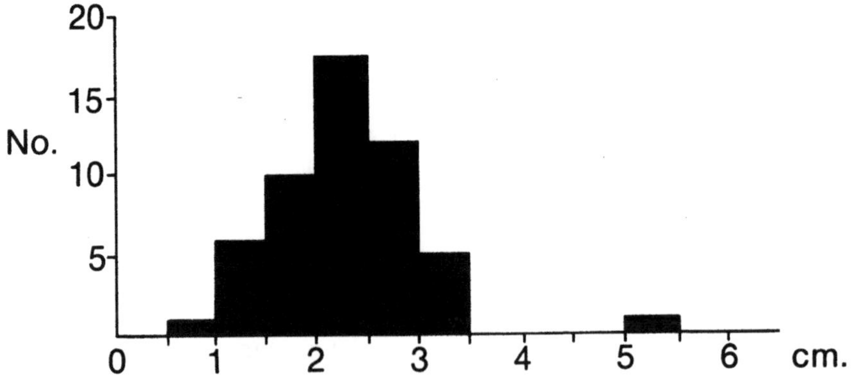

Fig. 2. Distribution of abdominal sphincter length in 50 healthy volunteers

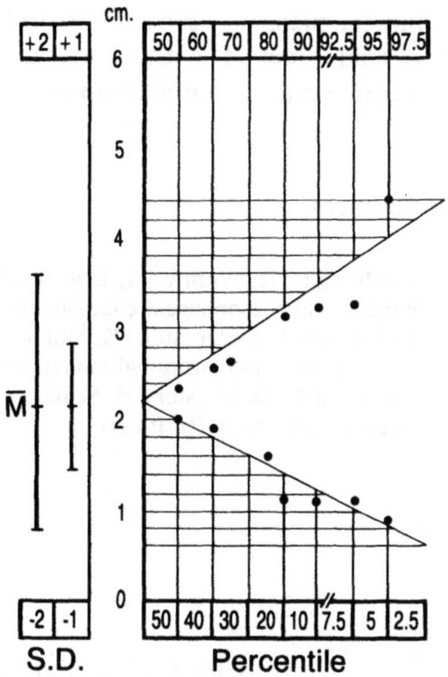

Fig. 3. Sphincter abdominal length

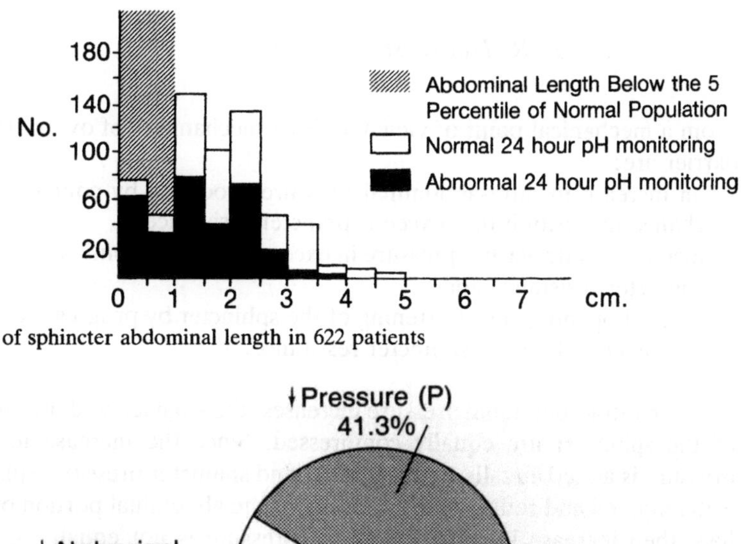

Fig. 4. Distribution of sphincter abdominal length in 622 patients

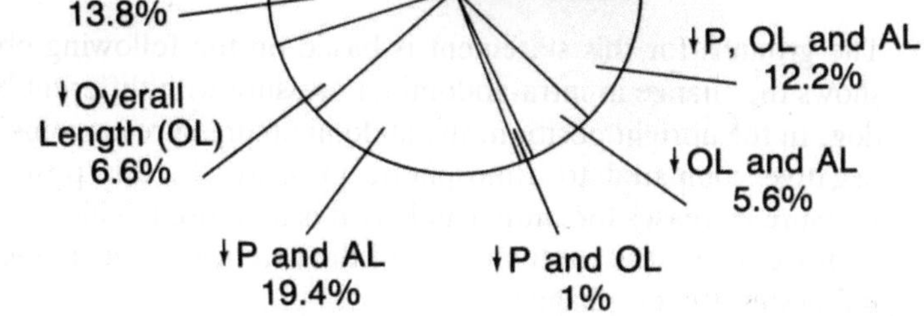

Fig. 5. Specific manometric abnormalities in 196 patients with reflux and abnormal sphincter manometrics

sphincter pressure (≦6 mm Hg). The second, was an abdominal sphincter length less than 1 cm. The third was an overall sphincter length less than 2 cm. The remainder was a combination of the three [3].

References

1. DeMeester TR, Wernly JA, Bryant GH, et al (1979) Clinical and in vitro analysis of determinants of gastroesophageal competence. Am J Surg 137: 39–46
2. Pellegrini CA, DeMeester TR, Skinner DB (1976) Response of the Distal Esophageal Sphincter to respiratory and positional maneuvers in humans. Surg Forum 27: 380-382
3. Zaninotto G, DeMeester TR, Schwizer W, et al: The Lower Esophageal Sphincter in health and disease. Am J Surg (In Press)

How does intra-abdominal pressure contribute to the continence of the cardia?

T. R. DeMeester (Omaha)

From a mechanical point of view the three mechanisms of overriding the antireflux barrier are:
- an increase in intra-abdominal pressure produced by coughing, straining, or a change in position that exceed sphincter resistance;
- increase in intragastric pressure in excess of intra-abdominal pressure that exceed sphincter resistance and;
- gradual opening and shortening of the sphincter by progressive gastric dilatation with eventual loss of sphincter resistance.

When intra-abdominal pressure increases, the stomach and the abdominal portion of the sphincter are equally compressed. Since the increase in intra-abdominal pressure is added equally to intragastric and sphincter pressure, sphincter resistance is maintained and reflux does not occur. If the abdominal portion of the sphincter is lost, then increase in intra-abdominal pressure is not equally applied and reflux occurs.

1. The grounds for this statement is based on the following observation: Table 1 shows the change in intra-abdominal pressure with different body position in the dog. In the upright position, the abdominal pressure surrounding the sphincter is negative compared to atmospheric pressure. In this position, the abdominal pressure increases the more caudally it is measured. This pressure gradient tends to move the gastric contents toward the cardia and encourages the occurrence of reflux into the esophagus.

Table 1. Intra-abdominal pressure, CM. of water under diaphragm

Position of animal	on inspiration	on expiration	in lower part of abdomen
Supine	3.0	3.5	5.5
Erect	−3.5	−3.0	10.0
Head down	11.0	16.0	0.5
Head up (45 degrees)	−2.5	−2.0	8.0
Head down (45 degrees)	6.0	5.5	2.0
Supine (second reading)	3.0	3.5	5.5

In contrast, in the supine position, the pressure gradient diminishes, and the abdominal hydrostatic pressure under the diaphragm increases [1].

2. The grounds for this statement is based on the following observation: Fig. 1 shows that sphincter pressure in normal subjects is significantly higher in the supine position than in the upright position. This reflects the apposition of the hydrostatic pressure of the abdomen to the abdominal portion of the sphincter when supine [2].
3. The grounds for this statement is based on the following observation: Fig. 2 shows the effects of progressively increasing abdominal pressure in cats when the sphincter is in its normal position and after it has been surgically placed in the chest. In the normal position, stepwise increases in abdominal pressure caused an identical stepwise increases in sphincter pressure without changing the amounts of gastric pressure necessary to overcome sphincter competency. When the sphincter was in the chest, stepwise increases in abdominal pressure did not result

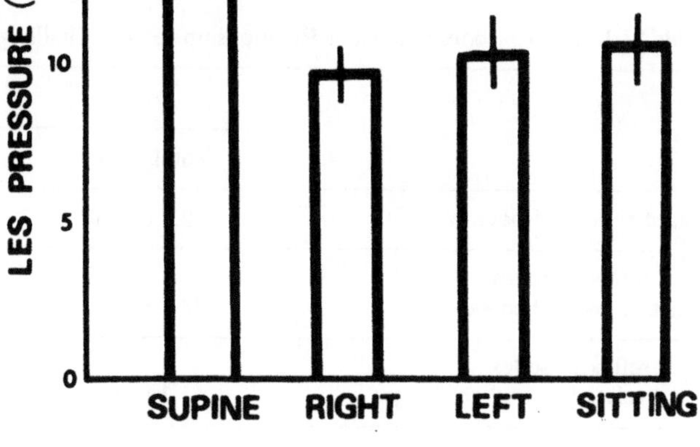

Fig. 1. Mean resting lower esophageal sphincter (LES) pressure in 20 normal subjects in the supine, right decubitus, left decubitus, and sitting positions. Vertical lines indicate ± SE of the mean

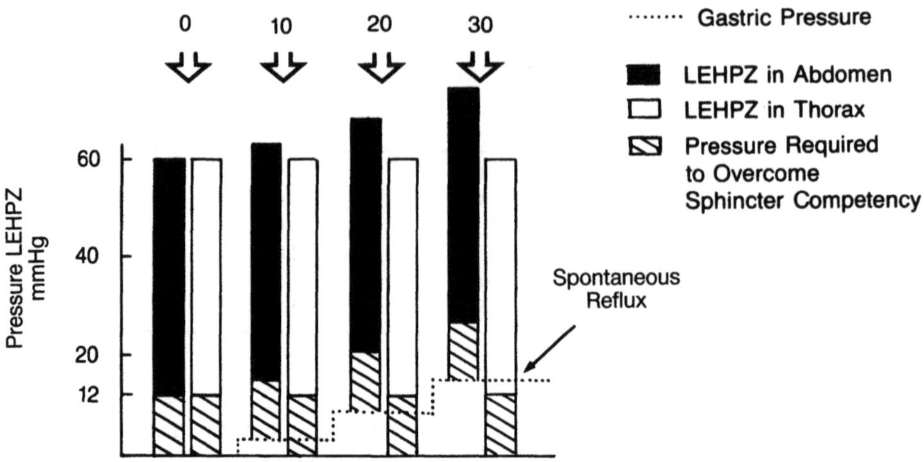

Fig. 2. Abdominal Compression (mmHg)

in stepwise increases in sphincter pressure and reflux occurred spontaneously when abdominal pressure reached the level necessary to overcome sphincter resistence.

4. The grounds for this statement is based on the following observation: The relationship between the magnitude of the abdominal pressure challenge and the efficiency of the intra-abdominal esophagus to respond to the challenge can be demonstrated in an in vitro model designed to simulate the forces acting on the distal esophageal sphincter. The minimal length of abdominal esophagus necessary for competency decreased as the magnitude of the intra-abdominal pressure challenge increased. Alternatively, the higher the intra-abdominal pressure challenge the shorter the length of abdominal sphincter necessary to maintain competency [3].
5. The grounds for this statement is based on the following observation: Table 2 shows the results of simultaneous 24-hour monitoring of esophageal pH and intra-abdominal pressure in 19 patients with gastroesophageal reflux. Increases in intra-abdominal pressure accounted for 38% of the reflux episodes recorded. The sphincter was challenged by frequent episodes of increases intra-abdominal

Table 2. Reflux Episodes and Their Relationship to IAP Challenges

	Period		
	Total 24-hr	Upright	Supine
No. of reflux episodes/hr	2.7± 1.5	3.1± 1.7	2.1± 1.9
% of reflux episodes caused by IAP challenges	38.7±18	38.7±20.2	34.7±21.8
% of reflux episodes not related to IAP challenges	61.3±18	61.3±20.2	65.3±21

pressure but only eight percent resulted in a reflux episode. This indicates that even in patients with symptomatic reflux, the sphincter is able to resist the majority of episodes of increased intra-abdominal pressure [4].

6. The grounds for this statement is based on the following observation: Fig. 3 shows the relationship of sphincter pressure and abdominal length to the percent

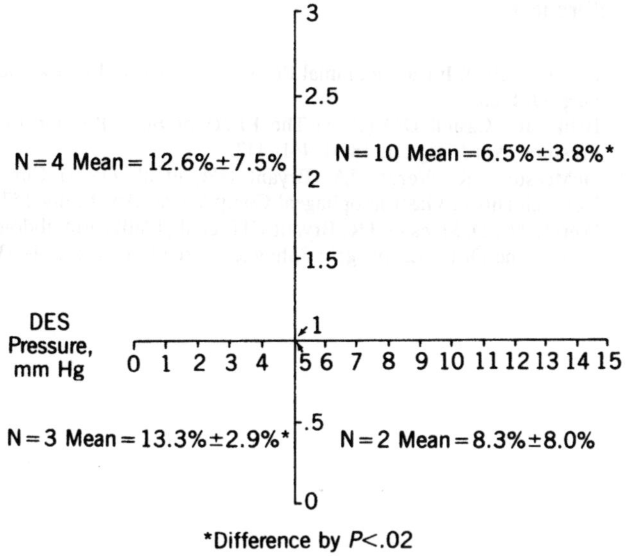

Fig. 3. Length of Abdominal Esophagus, cm

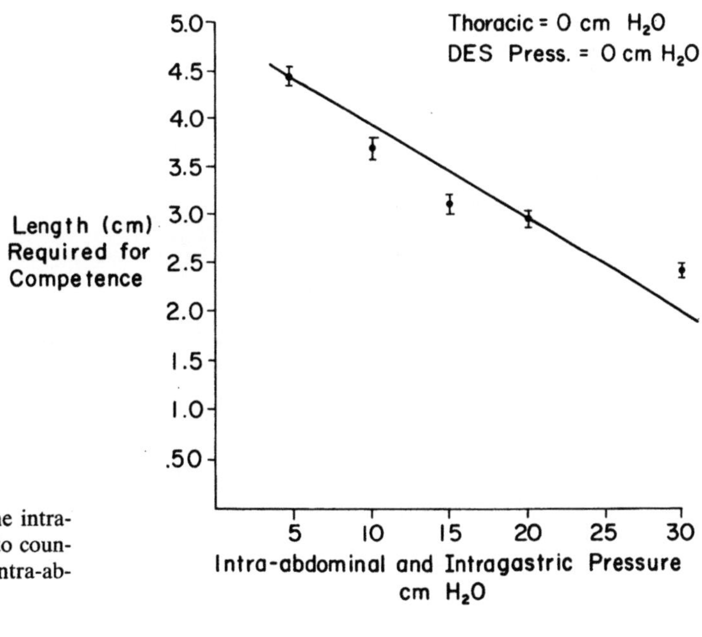

Fig. 4. Efficiency of the intra-abdominal Esophagus to counteract challenges of intra-abdominal Pressure

of intra-abdominal pressure challenges resulting in a reflux episode in the 19 patients referred to in point 5. Patients with a low sphincter pressure and short abdominal length are more able to resist challenges of increased intra-abdominal pressure if the abdominal length is long [4] (Fig. 4).

References

1. Lam CR (1939) Intra-abdominal Pressure: A Critical Review and an Experimental Study. Arch Surg 39: 1006
2. Babka JC, Castell DO (1973) The Effect of Body Position on Lower Esophageal Sphincter Pressure. Am J Dig Dis 18(5): 441–442
3. DeMeester TR, Wernly JA, Bryant GH, et al: (1979) Clinical and In Vitro Analysis of Determinants of Gastroesophageal Competence. Am J Surg 137: 39–46
4. Wernly JA, DeMeester TR, Bryant GH, et al (1980) Intra-abdominal Pressure and Manometric Data of the Distal Esophageal Sphincter. Arch Surg 115: 534–539

Conservative surgical procedures (1)

Anatomical procedures

F. Kümmerle (Mainz)

Anatomical reconstruction procedures intend to restore or at least imitate normal anatomy and the function of the esophageal-gastric sphincter.

Many mechanisms are suggested to control esophageal reflux and to prevent reflux disease: Angle of His, diaphragm, elastic occlusion by unipolar muscular structure, fluttervalve, ligamentum phrenicoesophageale, abdominal pressure, peristaltic waves. The most acceptable hypothesis is the manometrically defined digestive sphincter (Fig. 1).

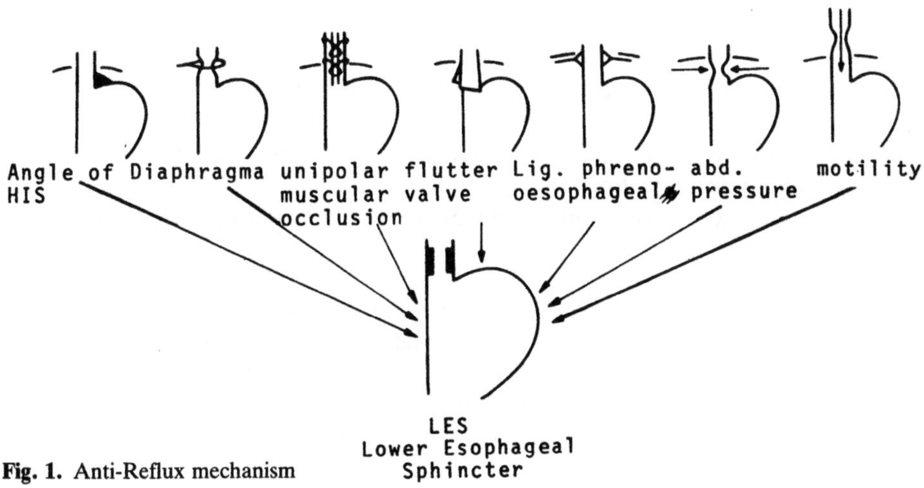

Fig. 1. Anti-Reflux mechanism

According to the mechanism involved in lower esophageal sphincter function, surgical techniques used in the therapy of reflux disease vary, and is a sure sign that no approach is clearly superior.

The many modifications can be classified in two general principles: anatomical reconstructions and valvuloplasties (Table 1).

- *Hiatoplasties* have lost importance since they have no proven anti-reflux effect.
- *Gastropexia* according to Nissen, attaching the anterior gastric wall to the anterior abdominal wall, is restricted to paraesophageal hernias. It is contraindicated in reflux disease and hiatal hernia.
- The *anti-reflux operations* for anatomical reconstruction have a proven effect on the distal esophageal sphincter demonstrated by manometry as well as by clinical follow-up examinations.

Table 1. Anti-reflux surgery, principles

1. Anatomical reconstructions
   1. Hiatoplasty (Allison)
   2. Gastropexia (Nissen)
   3. Anti-Reflux procedures
      A) Esophagofundopexia (Lortat-Jacob)
      B) Fundophrenicopexia (Kümmerle)

2. Valvuloplasties
   1. Fundoplication (Nissen-Rossetti)
   2. Belsey Mark 4
   3. Gastropexia posterior (Hill)

- Esophagofundopexia (Lortat-Jacob) is performed by narrowing the hiatus posteriorly and then fixing the fundus to the esophagus.

- Our own anatomical anti-reflux procedure is called: Fundophrenicopexia (Fig. 2).

  It is an effective but more simple procedure:
- The sphincter region is replaced into the abdomen. Circular mobilization of the esophagus is not necessary.
- The hiatal ring is loosely closed by narrowing the crura by 2 – 3 sutures (silk), controlled by the index finger (Fig. 2 a + b).
- The fundus is fixed to the diaphragm with 4–5 sutures, starting very close (0.5 to 1 cm) to the cardia (Fig. 2 c + d).

Fundophrenicopexia has several technical advantages: simple procedure, no mobilization of the esophagus, no sutures in the esophagus, no compression of the cardiac-region and less dangerous reoperation, but we must emphasize that none of these reconstructive anatomical procedures have been subjected to controlled study to prove their therapeutic effect conclusively.

Our opinion on the question anatomical reconstruction or valvuloplasty is documented by the distribution of our operations. In the last 20 years 413 anti-reflux operations have been performed: in almost 80% of cases, fundophrenicopexia, was preferred to Nissen fundoplication (Table 2).

Table 2. Surgical procedures in reconstruction of gastro-esophageal junction

	N	%
Fundophrenicopexia	326	78.9
Fundoplication	87	21.1
Summary	413	

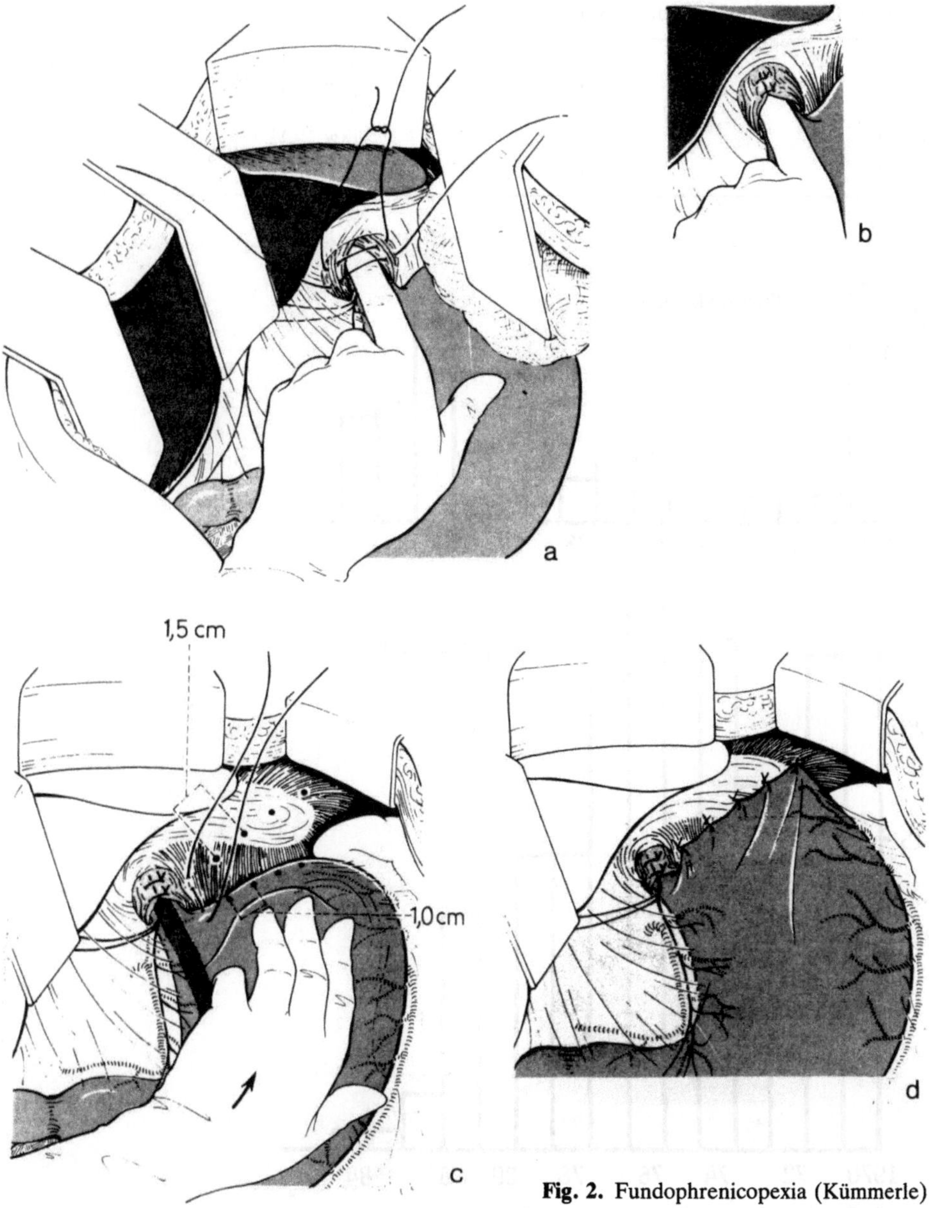

Fig. 2. Fundophrenicopexia (Kümmerle)

In summary the clinical results of fundophrenicopexia are similar to those of Nissen fundoplication, but postoperative side effects and specific syndromes occur less frequently. However, postoperative reflux-episodes are more frequent (Table 3).

H_2-receptor antagonists caused a remarkable decline in anti-reflux surgery. In our department, the both number of patients admitted due to reflux disease and the number of operations have decreased (Fig. 3).

Table 3. Clinical fundophrenicopexia (n=326)

Visick	1	68%	80%
Visick	2	12%	
Visick	3	14%	20%
Visick	4	6%	

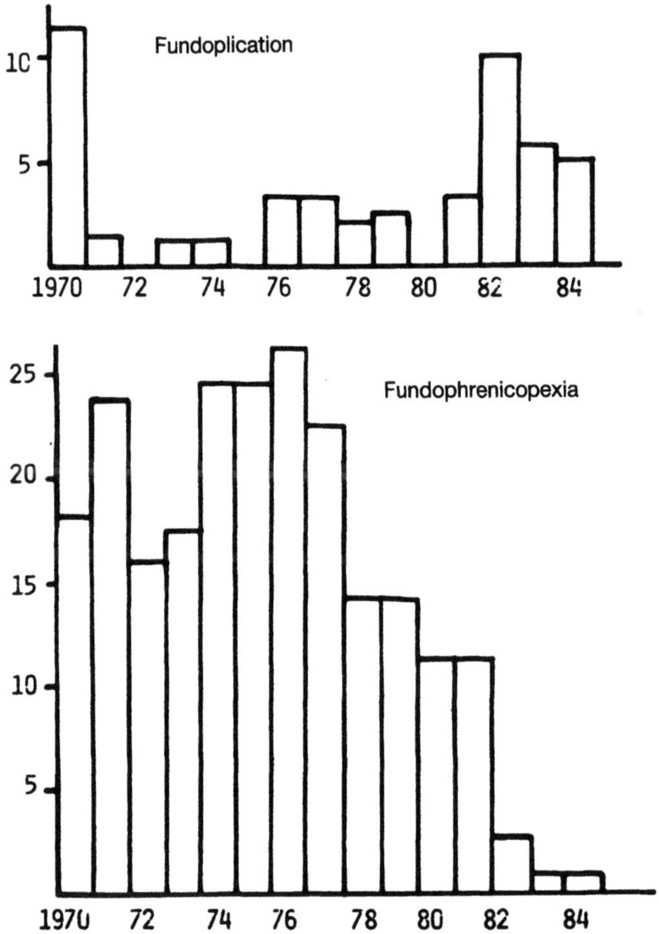

Fig. 3. Decline of surgical treatment in reflux-disease

The choice of operative procedure has also changed: since grades 1–3 are treated medically, anatomical reconstructions (such as fundophrenicopexia) have lost their importance. In advanced therapy-resistant stages of reflux disease, valvuloplasty (fundoplication) is indicated primarily.

Trends in anti-reflux treatment tend to prolonged medical management and less surgery. However, the problems are evident:

- Life-long medical therapy?
- Side effects of H_2-receptor-antagonists?
- Compliance?

Finally I think there will always be patients who are resistant to conservative therapy, have complications of the reflux disease, and will require surgical treatment.

The Lortat-Jacob procedure

J. L. Lortat-Jacob (Paris)

Some authors have compared the hiatal region to the pelvic corridor of the levator ani. This compares the pelvic muscular support system to the diaphragmatic loop, and the defective suspension of the female genital apparatus by collagen tissue to the defective fixation of the esophago-cardio-gastric region by the peritoneum, while the role of pelvic gravity is analogous to descending traction on the cardia by the longitudinal contractions of the esophagus. Without exactly sharing this interpretation of the pathogenesis of the disorders engendered by hiatus hernia, I nevertheless devised in 1948 a procedure somewhat evocative of the treatment of genital prolapse. The principles of this technique are as follows:

Except in very stout persons, this is done through a median supra-umbilical abdominal incision, with insertion of a subxiphoid retractor.

- Freeing of the abdominal esophagus, the cardia, the fundus and their more or less loose or even abnormal peritoneal attachments, and exposure of the right and left crura of the diaphragm, respecting the 2 vagus nerves, the left in front, the right behind and more remote.
- Maximum bringing down of the abdominal esophagus
- Approximation of the crura of the diaphragm behind the esophagus, leaving a hiatal opening only a finger's-breadth wider than the esophagus
- Reattachment of the fundus to the subdiaphragmatic peritoneum
- Construction of an anti-reflux valve by reconstruction of the cardio-fundal angle of His supporting the intragastric valve of Gubarov, while fixing the right margin of the fundus to the left margin of the esophagus by a line of interrupted sutures.

With major reflux, this line can be reinforced by a second line 2 cm distant, or by a gastric pleat attached to the right crus of the diaphragm either in front of the abdominal esophagus or behind it (according to Dor or Toupet).

Dr Goutallier from Orléans, will provide you with useful details on this procedure, whose the clinical and radiologic results (Figs. 1 and 2) are excellent in over 90% of cases.

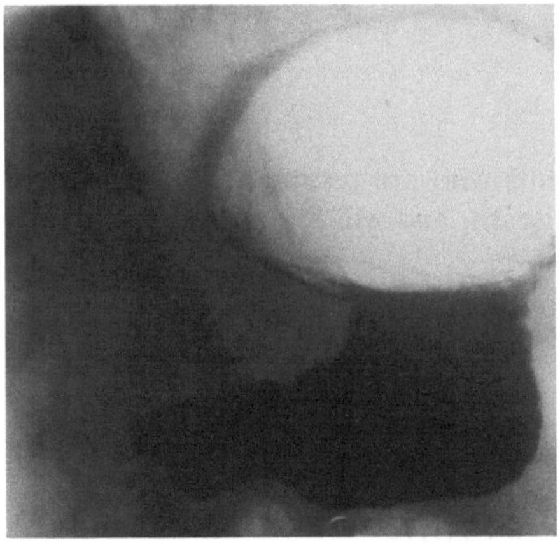

Fig. 1. Gastric air-pocket

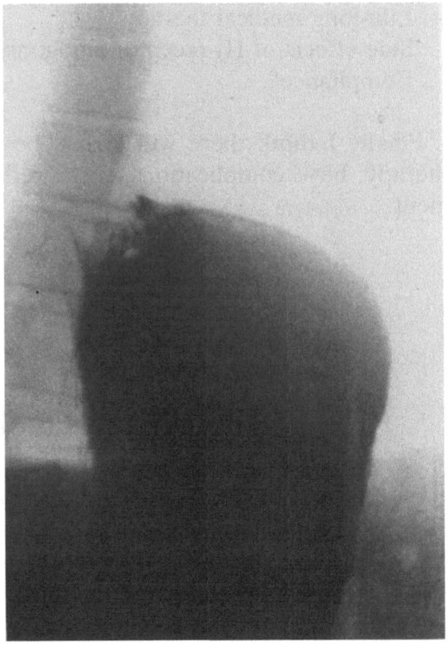

Fig. 2. Appearance in procubitus with compression

Ph. Goutallier (Orléans)

The initial description of the clinical syndrome associated with hiatus hernia was founded on anatomic considerations. These are, briefly, as follows:

- the esophageal hiatus constituted by the interlacing of two muscle bands arising from the right crus of the diaphragm;
- the length of the abdominal esophagus (4–5 cm);
- the attachments: the Bertelli-Laimer membrane; the mesoesophagus, abnormal elongation of which could cause cardio-fundal malpositions.

To these anatomical bases are added factors acting on cardiac continence and therefore resisting gastroesophageal reflux (GER):

- the right crus of the diaphragm surrounding the abdominal esophagus acts as an external sphincter
- the angle of His formed by the convergence at an acute angle of the lower esophagus and the right margin of the fundus
- the valve of Gubarov, the mucosal endogastric counterpart of the angle of His, acting as a valve opposing reflux of acid gastric fluid towards the unprotected esophageal mucosa during excess intragastric pressure.

Based on the deterioration of these various elements, J. L. Lortat-Jacob produced one of the first surgical procedures aimed at repairing the anatomic disorders accompanying hiatus hernia and eliminating their physiologic consequences. Thus the Lortat-Jacob operation acts on 3 anatomic factors to produce narrowing of the hiatal orifice, elongation of the abdominal esophagus and reconstitution of the angle of His.

Technique (Fig. 1)

The value of this technique lies in its performance by the abdominal route. True, it may be made difficult by the patient's physique (obesity, narrow sternocostal angle). For this reason a bi-subcostal approach may be preferable to a midline supra-umbilical approach in some cases. Use of a block will give the best exposure of the subdiaphragmatic region. The costal overhang is retracted and it is usually necessary to mobilize the left lobe of the liver by section of the left triangular ligament, avoiding damage to the subdiaphragmatic vein.

Peritoneal section is begun by incision of the pars condensa of the lesser omentum, avascular or easy to secure hemostasis, followed by incision of the pre-esophageal peritoneum without concern for a possible sac. The aim is to achieve perfect exposure of the lateral crura and of the anterior arc of the hiatus. If correctly exposed, the crura nearly always appear adequate in quality to allow their subsequent final approximation.

In most of the recurrences that we have to reoperate we frequently note inadequacy or even absence of this crural dissection, indicating that it is their peritoneal covering and not the actual fleshy crus that has been used.

The meso-esophagus is ruptured with a finger round the esophagus, isolated from its crura. A stout blunt clamp then makes it possible to surround the esophagus itself and to load it into a noose, taking care that the right vagus accompanies the esophagus. The stomach, which has ascended more or less through the hiatus, is

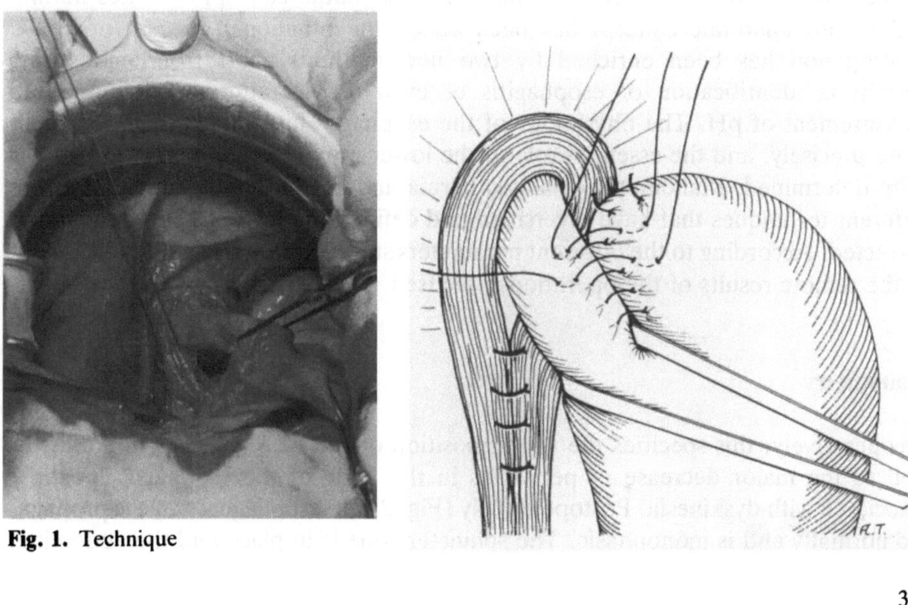

Fig. 1. Technique

then restored to its subdiaphragmatic position. The noose marks the theoretic position of the angle of His. The hiatal region and the abdominal esophagus now appear exposed in an absolutely anatomic fashion, allowing subsequent stages of the operation to be performed with complete efficiency.

Approximation of the crura is effected by means of 2 or 3 stout nonabsorbable stitches, either by drawing the esophagus to the left (which allows approximation entirely to the right of the esophagus) or by drawing the esophagus first to the right to catch the left crus and then to the left to catch the right crus, the needle and the free end of the stitch being taken over to the right behind the esophagus between the two stages. Once the hiatal orifice is so narrowed, it will admit a finger alongside the esophagus with only mild friction.

After approximation of the crura to narrow the hiatus, the second main stage of the technique is reconstruction of the angle of His. This is performed by a row of stitches (of less stout thread but also nonabsorbable) joining the right margin of the fundus and the left margin of the abdominal esophagus. It seems desirable for each stitch to catch the stomach twice, the uppermost stitch also including the left crus of the diaphragm. At the same time as the fixed reconstitution of the angle of His, this series of sutures ensures restoration of a correct length (about 5 cm) of the abdominal esophagus.

Parietal closure is made without drainage.

Minor postoperative dysphagia, disappearing in 4 to 6 weeks, constitutes the only complication ever encountered.

The advantages of this technique are based on

- its ease of execution by the abdominal route (though we have seen that its performance must be scrupulous, in particular with perfect exposure of the muscular crura and bringing the cardia well down)
- the good quality of the results in over 90% of operated cases.

The last 25 years have seen confirmation of the initial concept of hiatus hernia, and to this anatomic concept has been added the functional concept of GER. Investigation has been enriched by two new methods apart from endoscopy, permitting identification of esophagitis or even of ulceration: manometry and measurement of pH. The physiology of the esophagus has thus been investigated more precisely, and the essential role of the lower esophageal sphincter (LES) has been determined. Manometry of hiatus hernia and pH measurement in GER are different techniques that have diversified and defined the factors to be treated and corrected. According to the different parameters studied, they also allow assessment of the remote results of the operations practised.

Manometry

Preoperatively, this specifies the wrong position of the LES and its hypotonus, as well as the major decrease of peristalsis in the body of the esophagus, possibly associated with dyskinesia. Postoperatively (Fig. 2) the esophageal wave is propagated normally and is monophasic. The sphincter zone is in place and the abdominal

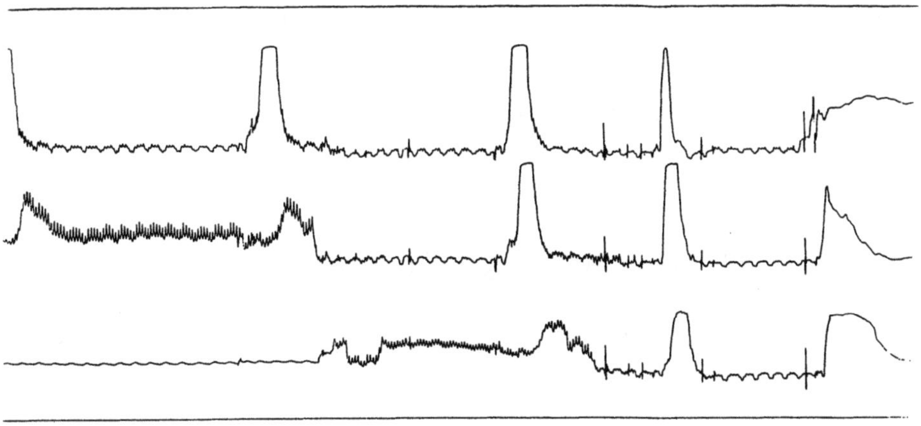

Fig. 2. Postoperative manometry

esophagus measures 4.8 cm. Sphincter tone is normal (17 cm of water). Relaxation obviates only 50% of preexisting sphincter tone.

pH measurement

Measured over 3 hours, this confirms the absence of GER. Made at different levels, it shows normal pH values of 1.5 in the stomach and 6.15 to 7.2 in the esophagus. Over a 3 hour study period the global score confirming the absence of GER is close to 0.

The manometric and pH data have arrived, late in the day, to confirm the sound foundation of a technique based initially on anatomic principles. Certain basic principles have been reinforced:

- to secure an adequate length of abdominal esophagus (4 cm seems the desirable minimum
- to establish close relations between the abdominal esophagus and the gastric fundus
- to secure intra-abdominal fixation of the arrangement.

The Lortat-Jacob operation satisfies these 3 great principles. Subsequent discussion will elicit that the majority of the other techniques, while supplying variable modifications, retain the essential points of this technique.

Long-term results

The assessment of these has demonstrated some deterioration of the results of the Lortat-Jacob operation. But one must insist on the absence of parallelism between the functional results and the results of the different para-clinical investigations. In any case, any treatment of hiatus hernia and its consequences is marked by some deterioration of the long-term results. Precise and meticulous performance of the different stages we have described remains the best guarantee of continued cure. This is why it seemed important to recall the Lortat-Jacob operation at the start of this session on the surgical treatment of hiatus hernia.

The Belsey Mark IV procedure

R. Belsey (Chicago)

Principle

Restoration and maintenance of a 4 cm and 5 cm segment of lower esophagus in the high pressure infradiaphragmatic position. Effective if:

a) Principle strictly observed.

b) No technical modifications.

Indications

1. Routine ARP in many centres.
2. Applicable in cases of functional dysmotility, following myotomy.
3. Applicable to infants and children.
4. Avoids postoperative gas-bloat, dysphagia.
5. No late catastrophic complications; only recurrent reflux.
6. Laboratory confirmation of the principle.
7. Evidence available on long term results.
8. Final procedure when all other techniques have failed.

Contraindications

1. Chronic ulcerative esophagitis with acquired shortening sufficient to prohibit the principle.
2. Inadequate training in technique. More demanding.
3. Gross pulmonary insufficiency may contraindicate thoracotomy.

Technique

The technique has been adequately recorded elsewhere. Basic principles;
1. Adequate exposure.
2. Extensive mobilization of lower esophagus and cardia.

3. Removal of anterior fat pad.
4. Mobilization of vagi in continuity to a posterior position for protection.
5. A 240° anterior fundoplication to retain the LES below the diaphragm.
6. Manual reduction of the hernia.
7. Creation of a posterior buttress for counterpressure.
8. Repair of the thoracotomy.

Common errors:
1. Inadequate exposure.
2. Inadequate mobilization of esophagus and cardia.
3. Faulty placement of fundoplication sutures.
4. Too aggressive suturing when performing the fundoplication.
5. Excessive narrowing of the hiatus.
6. Incorrect indications.
7. Faulty thoracotomy technique.

Advantages of the Mark IV technique

1. Satisfies the criteria demanded of any antireflux procedure.
2. Long term results have been adequately documented.
3. 89% long term success rate in centres dedicated to a resident training program.
4. Avoids mechanical obstruction in presence of dyskinesia.
5. Avoids early postoperative complications.
6. Only late complication recorded has been recurrent reflux when the procedure has been incorrectly performed, or on the wrong indications.
7. No modifications have been necessary in 35 years.

Cardiopexy with umbilical ligament

J. B. Flament, H. Plet, J. P. Palot, J. F. Delattre,
and *J. Rives* (Reims)

Treatment of gastroesophageal reflux had been associated for a long time with hiatal hernia repair, but we cannot take this association into account any longer for surgical indications: on the one hand, the frequency of hiatal hernia increases with age and an operation can be contemplated only if the reflux is complicated by esophagitis. On the other hand routine endoscopic examinations showed that reflux esophagitis could exist without evidence of hiatal hernia.

Appreciation of the role of the lower esophageal sphincter (LES) in prevention of the acid reflux led to the creation of procedures designed to reinforce the LES and restore its normal competence. The numerous articles devoted to this problem emphasized the importance of creating an artificial valve at the G.E. junction – preferably behind the esophagus – lengthening the subdiaphragmatic esophagus, and necessarily maintaining the sphincter mechanism into the positive pressure environment of the abdominal cavity. The narrowing of the hiatus itself is no longer considered essential, even if it can be a useful additional procedure. These principles should bring about an improvement of our results through a reduced rate of the fair and poor results, rated at about 15% in the surgical literature until recently. This figure approximately represents the results we obtained with the excellent procedure of J. L. Lortat-Jacob which already met the goals of modern treatment. We used this procedure for a long time with satisfactory results: failures were rare and incomplete and were never as severe as those we occasionally observed with Nissen's fundoplication.

The present report describes our experience of 76 operations in which we combined the Lortat-Jacob procedure with a cardiopexy using the ligamentum teres. This technique was inspired by the publications of Pedinielli [8] and Rampal [9, 10] and corresponds to the procedure used by G. Marchal for many years, with the good results recently reported in the thesis of his assistant D. Bories-Azeau [2].

Material and methods

Population studied

Over a five year period, from January 1982 to December 1986, 107 consecutive patients were operated on for gastroesophageal reflux. Out of these, 76 underwent an operation derived from the Rampal-Marchal procedure including the slinging of the G.E. junction with the ligamentum teres and the creation of a posterior semifundoplication. There were 32 female and 44 male patients. The mean age was slightly higher in female (56.6 years with a range of 33 to 81) than in male (47.9 with a range of 25 to 85).

4 patients were operated on for recurrent reflux esophagitis (2 and 6 years after a prior operation). The other 72 had a primary repair: 35 were suffering from an isolated G.E. reflux uncontrolled by medical therapy; in 41 patients the G.E. reflux was associated with another digestive disease (27 gallstones, 13 duodenal ulcers and 1 colonic cancer). Reflux was the main complaint in 13 of these 41 patients and it was not in the other 28, but in all cases G.E. reflux was clinically evident and was documented by endoscopic and/or manometric studies (we have never effected preventive repair of a hiatal hernia non complicated with reflux or esophagitis in the course of a supramesocolic operation).

Pre-operative evaluation

Nearly all the patients were evaluated with fiberoptic endoscopy (73/76=96%). Esophagitis was scored in 4 grades according to DeMeester's scale [4]: grade 0: no esophagitis (18 patients), grade 1: erythematous mucosa (9 patients), grade 2: presence of erosions and pseudomembranous mucosa (25 patients), grade 3: ulceration or stenosis (21 patients). Thus a high proportion of the patients were scored in grades 2 and 3 (46/76=63%).

Upper GI Xray examination was carried out in 44 patients.

Manometric study was performed in 40 patients and post-prandial 3 hour pH monitoring in 29 patients.

Operative technique (Fig. 1)

Our procedure includes three major steps:
1 – approximation of the crura of the diaphragm
2 – cardiopexy with the ligamentum teres
3 – porterior semifundoplication

All operations were performed transabdominally, 51 through an upper midline incision, 25 through an upper transverse incision, depending on the morphology of the patient.

The first step is to dissect and to free the ligamentum teres from its umbilical insertion up to the bottom of the fissure for the ligamentum teres on the inferior surface of the liver.

The second step is the exposure of the hiatus. We use a self retaining Olivier's retractor to elevate the thoracic wall; the left triangular ligament is divided and the left lobe of the liver retracted. The vestibule of the lesser sac is then divided and the anterior and posterior nerves of Latarget are retracted medially along side the lesser curvature of the stomach. They must be carefully protected. Division of the upper part of the gastrohepatic ligament provides excellent exposure of the right crus of the diaphragm. The esophagus is then mobilized after division of the peritoneal reflection and the phrenoesophageal membrane. Distal esophagus is dissected until a long intra abdominal segment is obtained which has always proved possible but necessitated a bilateral truncal vagotomy on 14 cases (18.4%). The esophagus and the anterior vagus nerve are encircled with a tape and the posterior vagus nerve is usually left posteriorly off the tape. Finally dissection of the gastrophrenic ligament and division of 1 or 2 short gastric vessels provide a wide exposure of the left crus.

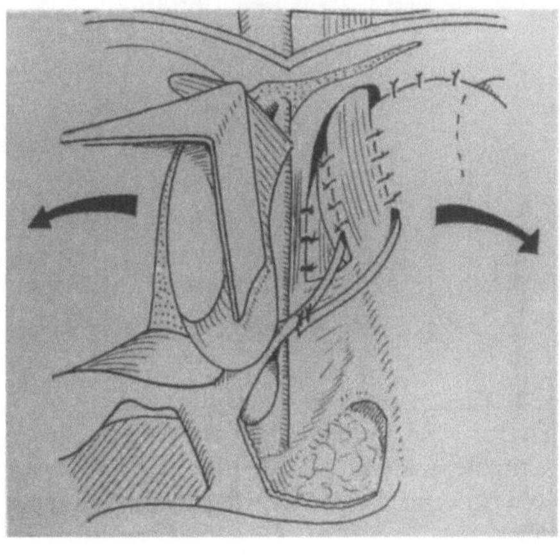

Fig. 1. *Cardiopexy with the ligamentum teres.* The cardiopexy is associated with approximation of the crura, posterior semifundoplication and gastropexy to the diaphragm

The third step is the approximation of the crura of the diaphragm posteriorly to the esophagus with 3 or 4 heavy non absorbable sutures. These sutures must be tied with a tension that causes tissue approximation but avoids any laceration of the muscles. The esophageal hiatus thus narrowed is displaced forewards and upwards and must accept the insertion of the surgeon's index finger alongside the esophagus.

The fourth step is the mooring of the G. E. junction. The ligamentum teres is pulled behind and around the esophagus from the right to the left and then fixed to itself by 2 ou 3 non absorbable stitches in order to form a loop. This must not be too tight and must accept a fingertip alongside the esophagus but the ligament may be fairly taut (Fig. 2).

The last step of the procedure is the creation of a semifundoplication including an anterior and a posterior fundic fold. The fundus is pulled behind the esophagus with a Duval clamp and then sutured on its right border with a vertical row of 5 or 6 non absorbable stitches. An anterior valve is obtained similarly and fixed by a second row of stitches placed either right or left of the anterior vagus nerve.

This description corresponds to our standard procedure which we effected in most cases (Fig. 3). In some cases variations were introduced: too short a ligament was reinforced by a skin strip in 6 cases, there was no hiatus closure in 15 patients, and finally the ligamentum teres was fixed to the anterior abdominal wall in 15 patients at the beginning of our experience.

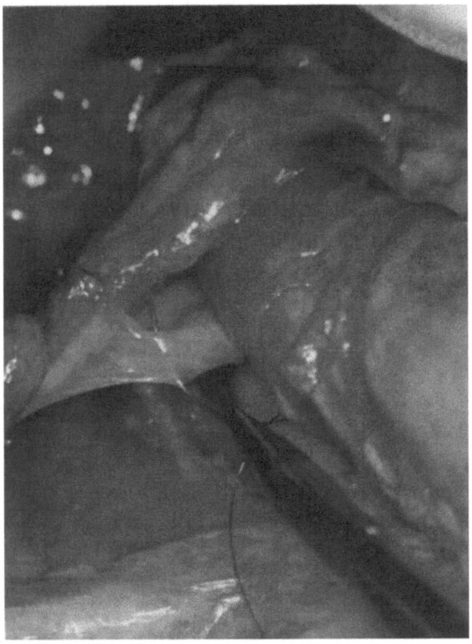

Fig. 2. *Cardiopexy with the ligamentum teres:* operative view. Suture is performed with non absorbable material. Note that stitches are placed superficially in order to preserve blood supply

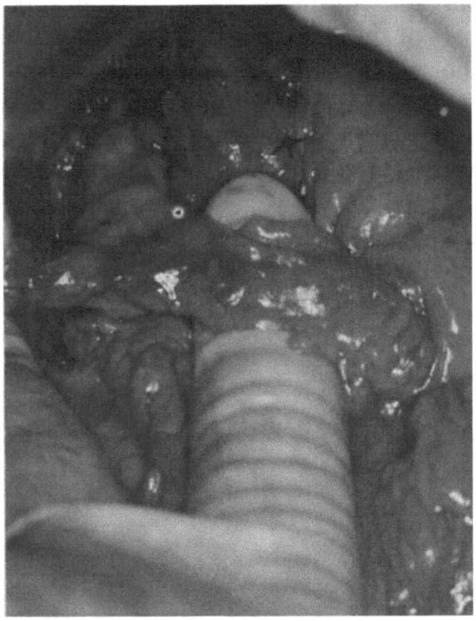

Fig. 3. *Operative view of the cardiopexy.* The loop accepts the surgeon's index finger alongside the esophagus

Other procedures were associated in 41 patients: operation on biliary tract in 27 cases, treatment of duodenal ulcer in 13 cases (11 parietal cell vagotomies and 2 bilateral truncal vagotomies) and right hemicolectomy for cancer in 1 case.

Post-operative evaluation

Clinical evaluation was effected after 3 weeks, 6 months then annually. Immediate post-operative controls also included 58 upper gastro-intestinal Xray examinations, 35 fiberoptic endoscopies and 32 manometric studies associated with 3 hour pH monitoring.

Results

Mortality

There was one post-operative death (1/76=1.3%): a 70 year old patient dies suddenly after an operation that included cholecystectomy and external biliary drainage for angiocholitis. A pulmonary embolus was confirmed at autopsy.

Morbidity

There were ten minor splenic tears without consequence. 5 splenic injuries required subsequent splenectomy (6.5%), one of the patients whose subphrenic space had not been drained developed a subphrenic abcess.

In two patients dissection of the esophagus produced an esophageal tear simply closed and buttressed by the fundoplication without consequence.

11 wound infections (14.6%) were responsible for 1 immediate post-operative evisceration (successfully treated with an absorbable prosthesis) and for two delayed incisional hernias.

Early post-operative results

- symptoms of G.E. reflux immediately disappeared in all cases. 14 patients (18.6%) suffered from a transient dysphagia relieved in all cases within 3 weeks to 6 months. Only 1 patient reported painful belching which disappeared after 8 months.
- endoscopic examination was performed in 35 patients: 12 out of the 21 grade 3 and 12 out of the 20 grade 2 patients were examined post-operatively: the mucosa of the esophagus was normal in all cases.
- Xray examination was performed in 58 patients with satisfactory results in 48 cases (Fig. 4). An esophageal dilation was present in 10 patients but only five suffered from dysphagia.

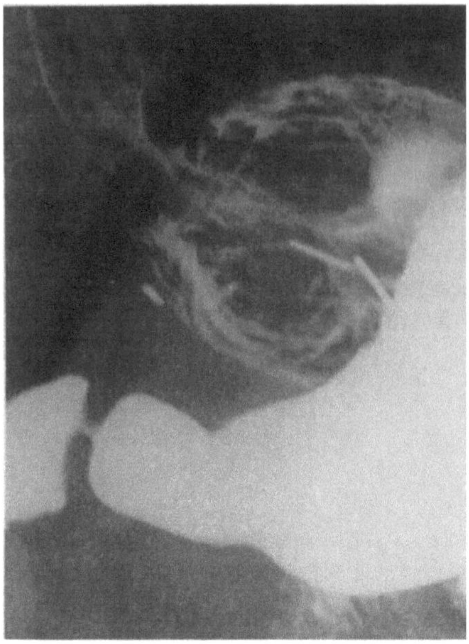

Fig. 4. *Post-operative radiologic study.* Note the lengthening of distal esophagus

- functional study by manometry was carried out in 31 patients and gave evidence of the restoration of a competent LES in all cases: the average lower esophageal sphincter pressure (LES) was indeed 13.45 cms H20 before and 24.3 cms H20 after operation. This difference his highly significant ($p. < 0.001$).

In 20 patients manometric studies showed motility disorders in distal esophagus whose interpretation is unclear but were accompanied in 6 cases with transient dysphagia.

Finally, pH monitoring verified the absence of reflux in the 31 patients examined post-operatively.

Long term results

One patient died 3 months after surgery from intercurrent disease. The other 74 patients were all submitted to post-operative clinical evaluation (follow up: 100%). The follow up period ranged from 6 months to 5 years.

On subjective clinical evaluation 72 out 74 patients (97%) are quite satisfied with the results of the operation. Recurrent symptoms are present in 2 patients: a 60 year old woman whose reflux is well controlled by medical therapy, and a 45 year old woman operated on for recurrent reflux presenting intermittent regurgitations but normal endoscopic findings.

Asymptomatic reflux was evidenced by upper GI Xray examination in only one female patient, with whom endoscopic and manometric controls were normal.

In 2 cases a persistant reflux was demonstrated by pH monitoring in the absence of any clinical symptom.

Discussion

In 1958 L. Pedinielli [8] was the first to propose a procedure of cardiopexy slinging the G.E. junction and called it "technique du collet". For this purpose he used a strip of skin cut from the abdominal wall at the beginning of the operation. He slung it around the distal esophagus and sutured it to itself. Then he attached it fairly tensely to the anterior abdominal wall. This principle was attractive and the first results published were satisfactory. Yet questions remained concerning the evolution of the cutaneous strip in the absence of any blood supply.

This explains why M. Rampal, P. Perillat and R. Rouzaud [9] proposed in 1964 to resort to the ligamentum teres to perform a cardiopexy whose principle was directly inspired from Pedinielli's "snare". The advantages were the following:

1. blood supply for the ligamentum teres is provided by a little artery branching from the hepatic artery, thus preventing long term resorption.
2. the ligament moors the G.E. function to the left lobe of the liver which acts as a "floating anchor" through its movements accompanying respiration.
3. the system thus obtained is most likely to maintain the angle of His as it pulls the G.E. junction forward, dowward and toward the right.

But the author considered that this procedure could not prevent reflux in itself and had to be associated with closure of the hiatus and anterior gastropexy.

In 1967, G. Marchal [6] adopted Rampal's technique with a few modifications, insisting on the restoration of the angle of His by creating a close anatomic contact between the fundus and distal esophagus. His results were published recently in thesis of D. Bories Azeau. We reached the same conclusions and confirmed the interest of gastropexy with the ligamentum teres.

The very good results of this procedure are due to its respecting a number of theoretical criteria: sliding hiatal hernia is an acquired disease linked with the failure of the posterior attaches of the G.E. junction and preceded by shortening of the abdominal portion esophagus. The hernia is accompanied in most cases by pathologic reflux due to deterioration of gastroesophageal sphincter competence. The goal of surgery is to reduce the hernia and to prevent the reflux. Thus, ideal treatment should be conducted along two different concepts, and the operation include two main steps:

1. a "plastic" step corresponding to the creation of an artificial valve. The simplest procedure is to restore the angle of His by suturing the fundus to the distal esophagus. J. L. Lortat-Jacob demonstrated its importance [5]. Creation of a zone of hyperpressure by partial (Toupet) or total (Nissen) wrapping of the distal esophagus with the gastric fundus is probably the best way to prevent reflux: indeed variations of intragastric or intra-abdominal pressure are immediatly transmitted to the distal esophageal sphincter, then preventing reflux. Adlay [1] showed that a 270° semi fundoplication was sufficient and avoided the side effects of Nissen's fundoplication.

   Such a high pressure zone does exist in normal subjects and corresponds to the diaphragmatic canal limited by the two muscular bundles of the hiatus (A. Delmas). Its role in improving the LES has been clearly demonstrated by J. F. Delattre [3].

2. a "pexic" step aiming at anchoring the G.E. junction inside the abdominal cavity. This step ensures a lengthening of the subdiaphragmatic esophagus that favors the transmission of the variations of intra-abdominal pressure. Fixation of the valve to the posterior parietal structures, either the median arcuate ligament as advocated by Hill or the crura of the diaphragm as recommended by Toupet, seems in our view a fairly rigid system.

On the other hand, the attachment of the G.E. junction by the ligamentum teres provides a flexible system, concomitantly mobile with the liver. It can even be considered that this represents a self-adapting and self-regulating system. Indeed, contractions of the diaphragm that increase intraabdominal pressure and provoke reflux when the esophageal hiatus is enlayed, pull the liver and subsequently the insertion of the ligamentum teres downwards: the more powerful the contraction of the diaphragm, the more powerful the traction on the ligament.

This procedure reproduces the normal anatomic and physiologic conditions of cardiac competence as they were summarized by H. Monges and J. Gambarelli [7].

Conclusion

Over the past five years we have been using a procedure combining hiatus closure, cardiopexy with the ligamentum teres and a 270° semifundoplication. We consider this procedure easy to perform, benign, and reliable. In our view the results obtained with this technique are slightly superior to those obtained in other series. Post prandial pH monitoring shows the absence of post-operative reflux in all cases. Healing of reflux esophagitis can be verified by endoscopy in 100% of cases. Finally manometric measurements indicate effective restoration of LESP. These results remain stable with time and there are no uncomfortable side effects.

This procedure seems to be interesting and should be developed further.

References

1. Adlay ES, Goldsmith HS (1973) Efficacity of fundoplication in preventing gastric reflux. Am J Surg 126: 322–324
2. Bories-Azeau D (1982) Etude critique du traitement chirurgical de la hernie hiatale. Place de la cardiopexie par le ligament rond. Thèse Montpellier
3. Delattre JF (1984) Les piliers du diaphragme et la traversée diaphragmatique de l'œsophage. Application au reflux gastro-œsophagien et à son traitement chirurgical. Mémoire Laboratoire d'Anatomie de Paris
4. DeMeester TR, Johnson LF (1975) Evaluation of the Nissen antireflux procedure by esophageal manometry and twenty-four hour pH monitoring. AM J Surg 129: 94–100
5. Lortat-Jacob JL, Dromer M, Lebas P, Maillard JN, Richard CL (1962) A propos de 221 interventions pour hernie par l'hiatus œsophagien chez l'adulte. Etude d'une statistique hospitalière intégrale. Ann Chir 16: 985–990
6. Marchal G, Balmes M, Bousquet M, Olivier G, Dayan L (1967) Traitement des hernies hiatales par la technique de Rampal. Montpellier Chir 479–482
7. Monges H, Gambarelli J, Jouve-Fournier P (1956) Sur le mécanisme de la continence gastro-œsophagienne et la physio-pathologie du reflux gastro-œsophagien. Marseille Med 8: 655–678

8. Pedinielli L (1964) Traitement chirurgical de la hernie hiatale par la "technique du collet". Ann Chir 18: 1461–1474
9. Rampal M, Perillat P, Rouzaud R (1964) Notes préliminaires sur une nouvelle technique de cure chirurgicale des hernies hiatales: la cardiopexie par le ligament rond. Marseille Chir 16: 488
10. Rampal M, Perillat P, Figarella J, Julie R, Bonnet J (1967) Traitement des hernies hiatales et du reflux oesophagien par la cardiopexie avec le ligament rond du foie. Presse Med 75: 615–620

What is the real function of a gastro-esophageal valve?

K. B. Å. Thor, and *L. D. Hill* (Stockholm and Seattle)

The gastroesophageal (GE) junction maintains a pressure gradient between the esophagus and the stomach and allows the ingestion of food and liquid without gross reflux. The nature of this closing mechanism has been a matter of dispute since the eighteenth century. Several factors have been suggested to explain this "cardiac sphincter" and include the lower esophageal sphincter (LES), the intraabdominal location of the GE junction, the diaphragm, the phrenoesophageal membrane and the flap valve created by the acute angle of His. The concept of a flap valve mechanism at the GE junction is more than 100 years old but the physiological importance of a flap valve mechanism has however been minimized despite several previous studies indicating such a mechanism [1–4].

The flap valve consists of the oblique entrance of the esophagus into the stomach with a sharp angle between the left wall of the abdominal esophagus and the right side of the gastric fundus. In order to establish whether there is a flap valve mechanism present at the GE junction and to determine its importance a study in cadavers has been carried out [5]. In a cadaver with no active muscle function left, the importance of the LES should be negligible. Other mechanisms must therefore be responsible for the observation that postmortem the stomach can be filled with water without eliciting GE reflux.

Cadavers were investigated with open manometry catheters in the esophagus and stomach without mobilization of the aorta, esophagus, stomach or the diaphragm. The experimental setting is shown in Fig. 1. Stepwise (50 ml) filling of the stomach demonstrated a GE pressure gradient of 4.6±1.6 cm H_2O. This gradient could be significantly increased to 12.5±3.1 cm H_2O ($p < 0.05$) by performing a valvuloplasty procedure through a gastrotomy through the anterior part of the stomach (Fig. 2). The flap valve was grasped with Babcock forceps and lengthened by traction caudally. Three stiches were then placed in the anterior and posterior aspects of the valve, carrying the sutures cephalad through the GE junction, thereby accentuating it (valvuloplasty) (Fig. 3). The stomach was then closed with running suture.

By depressing the fundus of the stomach, the angle of His was made more obtuse and the flap valve component eliminated (Fig. 4). This maneuver resulted in reflux

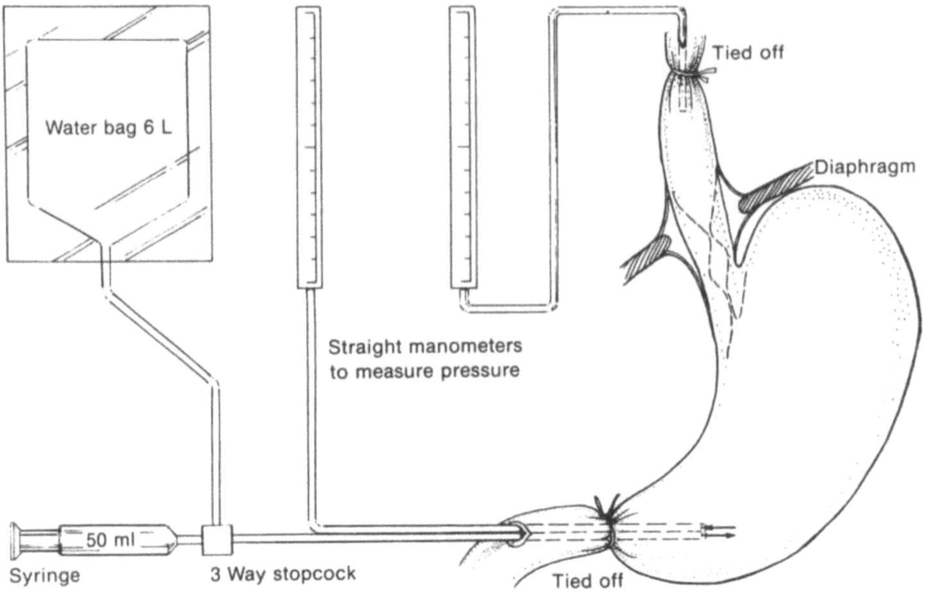

Fig. 1. The diagrammatic plan of the experiments

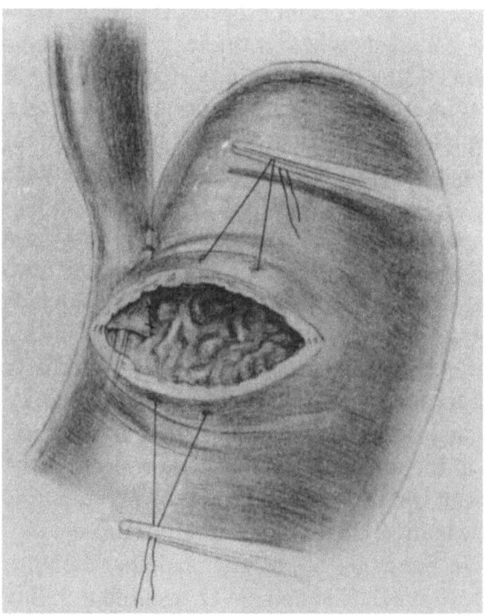

Fig. 2. The site of the gastrotomy and the appearance of the flap valve after valvuloplasty

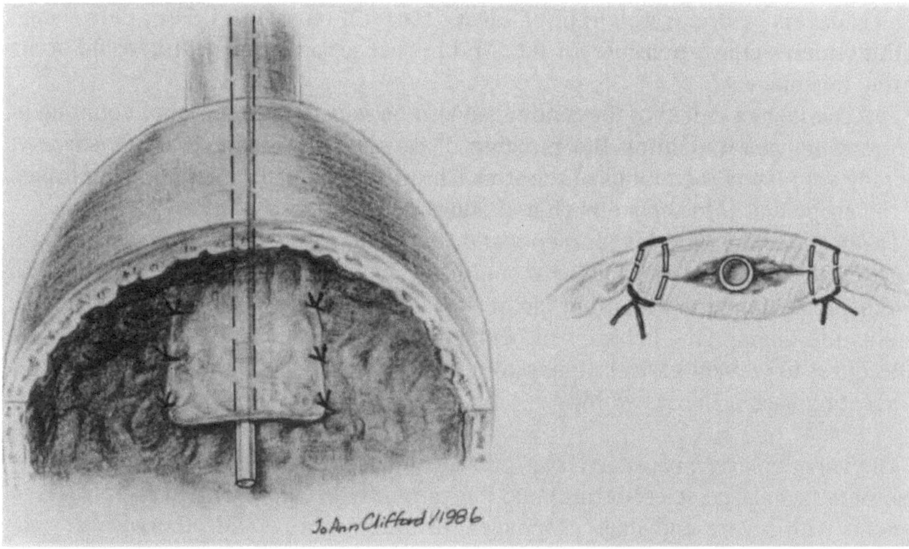

Fig. 3. The appearance of the valvuloplasty seen from the greater curvature and in cross-section. (The tube inserted for clarification)

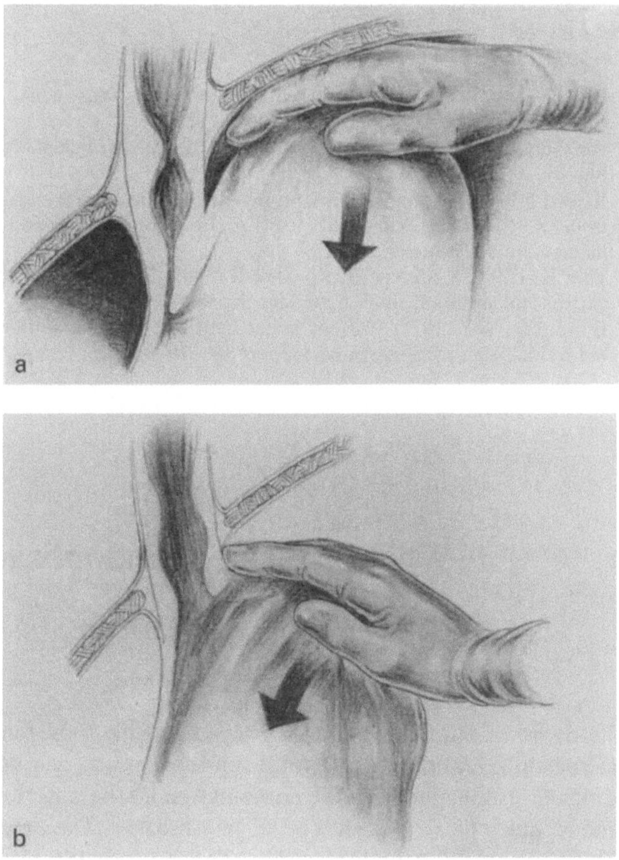

Fig. 4. The hand is placed on top of the fundus of the stomach **(a)**. Caudal movement of the hand increases the angle between the esophagus and the stomach, the valve is eliminated, whereupon the free reflux occurs **(b)**

in all cadavers before as well as after valvuloplasty: if only the LES or "narrowing" at this region were responsible for the GE pressure gradient, no reflux would occur during this maneuver.

This caudal movement of the fundus can also be seen during the act of vomiting in the retching phase. During the retching phase the diaphragm descends sharply, thereby depressing the fundus of the stomach which eliminates the oblique entrance of the esophagus into the stomach and allows free reflux to occur.

Taken together, these experiments and observations together with our valvuloplasty procedure indicate that there is a flap valve mechanism at the GE junction working in conjunction with other factors like LES and intraabdominal esophagus as well as the diaphragm. It has even been suggested that the most commonly used procedures to prevent gastroesophageal reflux (Hill, Nissen, Belsey) actually do this by creating such a flap valve [6].

The valvuloplasty procedure is at present under study in patients with motility disorders (achalasia, scleroderma) and has presently been performed in 23 cases in patients with severe end-stage esophageal disorders who would otherwise be candidates for esophageal resections.

References

1. Braune W (1878) Topographisch-anatomischer Atlas nach Durchschnitten an gefrorene Cadavern. Kleine Ausgabe. Leipzig 113–114
2. von Gubaroff A (1886) Über den Verschluß des menschlichen Magens an der Cardia. Arch Anat Physiol 395
3. Barrett NR (1954) Hiatus hernia: a review of some controversial points. Br J Surg 42: 231–244
4. Collis JL, Kelly TD, Wiley AM (1954) Anatomy of the crura of the diaphragm and the surgery of hiatus hernia. Thorax 9: 175–189
5. Thor K, Hill LD, Mercer D, Kozarek R (1987) Reappraisal of the flap valve mechanism in the gastroesophageal junction. Acta Chir Scand 153: 25–28
6. Butterfield WC (1971) Current hiatal hernia repairs: similarities, mechanisms, and extended indications – an autopsy study. Surgery 69: 910–916

What is a Nissen fundoplication?

G. Beauchamp, and *A. Duranceau* (Montreal)

The name of Rudolf Nissen is associated with total fundoplication for control of gastroesophageal reflux. By total fundoplication, one understand the wrapping of the lower esophagus with the combination of the anterior and posterior wall of the fundus, much like a Witzel type of gastrostomy. The anterior wall alone can also be used to complete a fundoplication. The anterior fundus is then slipped around the esophagus without cutting the short gastric vessels. After the fundoplication, the crurae are closed. My understanding is that Rudolf Nissen has described at least two variations of fundoplication [1, 2].

Now, what is the misunderstanding about the Nissen fundoplication [3]? Well, it is only the number of additions, modifications and variations to the original 5 to 6 cm fundoplication done on large gastric tube: among the variations are the use of more or less fundus, of a long or short wrap, of a tight or very loose (floppy), wrap [4]. Some have added a truncular vagotomy or a supraselective vagotomy [5, 6] or have excluded the posterior vagus from the wrap [7]. Others have felt the necessity to anchor the fundoplication to the arcuate ligament [8]. Others have left the fundoplication in the chest without closing the crurae [9, 10, 11]. The very last variation appears to be the use of Teflon pledget in the making of the fundoplication [12].

The many variations are symptomatic of a problem: patients and surgeons are not completely satisfied with the original Nissen operation. Why is this? The reason is that the patients, after a total fundoplication, present with too many side effects from the surgery [13, 14].

From 1980 to 1985, I have performed more than 200 antireflux procedures. One hundred twenty have been Nissen procedure using the anterior fundus and cutting the short gastric vessels: I have observed during the follow-up that all the patients operated for a Nissen procedure have developed a post-fundoplication syndrome. For some patients, the symptoms are mild. For the others, the symptoms have been embarrassing and they are not completely satisfied with the operation. Only a minority of patients have needed reoperation.

The syndrome is more complex than the early description of the gas bloat syndrome [15]. The post-fundoplication syndrome involves esophageal, gastric, small and large bowel symptoms. It may also manifest itself with cardiologic and neurologic symptoms.

The symptoms are secondary to the utilization of the fundus, which has another physiologic role than simply serving as a valvular mechanism. The fundus is normally used for the stocking of food and air. The fundus also plays an important role in gastric emptying. During digestion, input from excitatory nerves causes a sustained increase in fundus tone and increases the intragastric pressure, which forces intragastric content from oral to caudal stomach.

The post-fundoplication syndrome can happen because the surgical technique is not appropriate or because the selection of the patients is not appropriate for this type of surgery [16]. I strongly believe that it is because using the fundus is not anatomically or physiologically sound. That is the reason why all the patients develop a post-fundoplication syndrome. The severity of the syndrome depends on how much fundus is used and how easy belching is for the patient (tightness of fundoplication). Patients personal eating habits also affect the results.

The type of fundoplication and its modifications may affect the results and, there is a need for every surgeon who performs a total fundoplication and publishes on it to describe his operation, and the variations from the original operation. But more than that, we need to better understand the mechanism of the fundoplication. Thus, we might be able to design a more precise and predictable operation.

References

1. Nissen R (1961) Gastropexy and "fundoplication" in surgical treatment of hiatal hernia. Am J Dig Dis 6(10): 954–961
2. Nissen R (1970) Reminiscences – Reflux esophagitis and hiatal hernia. Rev Surg 27: 307–314
3. Jamieson GG, Duranceau A (1984) What is a Nissen fundoplication? Surg Gynecol Obstet 159: 591–593
4. Donahue PE, Samelson S, Nyhus LM, Bombeck T (1985) The floppy Nissen fundoplication. Arch Surg 120: 663–668
5. Bahadorzadeh K, Jordan PH (1975) Evaluation of the Nissen fundoplication for treatment of hiatal hernia: Use of parietal cell vagotomy without drainage as an adjunctive procedure. Ann Surg 181: 402–408
6. Jordan PH (1978) Parietal cell vagotomy facilitates fundoplication in the treatment of reflux esophagitis. Surg Gynecol Obstet 147: 593–595
7. Herrington JL, Meacham PW, Hunter RM (1982) Gastric ulceration after fundic wrapping. Vagal nerve entrapment, a possible causative factor. Ann Surg 195: 574–581
8. Kaminski DL, Codd JE, Sigmund CJ (1977) Evaluation of the use of the median arcuate ligament in fundoplication for reflux esophagitis. Am J Surg 134: 724–729
9. Safaie-Shirazi S, Zike WL, Anuras S, Condon RE, DenBesten L (1974) Nissen fundoplication without crural repair. A cure for reflux esophagitis. Arch Surg 108: 424–427
10. Maher JW, Hocking MP, Woodward ER (1984) Supradiaphragmatic fundoplication. Long-term follow-up and analysis of complications. Am J Surg 147: 181–186
11. Richardson JD, Larson GM, Polk HC (1982) Intrathoracic fundoplication for shortened esophagus. Treacherous solution to a challenging problem. Am J Surg 143: 29–35
12. DeMeester TR, Bonavina L, Albertucci M (1986) Nissen fundoplication for gastroesophageal reflux disease. Ann Surg 204: 9–20
13. Menguy R (1978) A modified fundoplication which preserves the ability to belch. Surgery 84: 301–307
14. Negre JB, Markkula HT, Keyrilainen O, Matikainen M (1983) Nissen fundoplication. Results at 10 year follow-up. Am J Surg 146: 635–638
15. Bushkin FL, Neustein CL, Parker TH, Woodward ER (1977) Nissen fundoplication for reflux peptic esophagitis. Ann Surg 185: 672–676
16. Ellis FH, Crozier RE (1984) Reflux control by fundoplication: a clinical and manometric assessment of the Nissen operation. Ann Thorac Surg 38: 387–392

P. E. Donahue, and *C. T. Bombeck* (Chicago)

Introduction

Following its first description 1956 the Nissen fundoplication has been widely recognized as the most effective of several alternative operative procedures for pathologic gastroesophageal reflux. However, there are still many local variations in the manner in which this operative procedure is performed, and a corresponding difference in the clinical results obtained after operation. In attempting to rationalize the different operative approaches, it seems obvious that the goal of minimizing postoperative symptoms is almost as important as control of the primary complaint; since the patients have a benign disease to begin with, they are intolerant of any abnormality postoperatively. Memory is sometimes short with regard to the reasons for having correction of reflux symptoms, so that a patient who is forced to live with one of the moderate discomfort syndromes characteristic of some variations on the fundoplication theme may ultimately wish that the operation had never been performed.

Therefore, it is worthwhile to restate the objectives of antireflux therapy and to reiterate the concept of the "Floppy Fundoplication", a technique which maximizes the opportunity for control of pathologic reflux and minimizes the chance for unpleasant sequellae.

Discussion

The mechanism by which fundoplication prevents pathologic reflux is by enhancing the antireflux mechanism at the lower end of the esophagus and the proximal end of the stomach. While several experimental studies have suggested that there is a physiologic component to the antireflux barrier created by fundoplication [1, 2], several recent studies suggest that the mechanical buttress provided by the fundoplication causes changes in the physiological function of the cardia which are indistinguishable from those cause by insertion of an inert material such as the Angelchik prosthesis [3, 4]. Furthermore, the increasing awareness of separate anatomic and functional components of the antireflux mechanism provides other insights into the way which pathologic reflux events occur [5, 6]. However, while the investigation of precise mechanisms by which the antireflux operations achieve their goal is important, other valid questions relating to technical creation of a fundoplication also deserve an answer, and can be addressed at this time.

"What is a fundoplication?" This question has several components, including the method of construction, the suture material employed, the treatment of the vagus nerves, and the precise treatment of the esophageal hiatus. Also, the postoperative measurement of esophageal physiology can provide insights into the mode of action of fundoplication, and part of the answer to related concerns regarding the effects of Nissen fundoplication. These include the question of whether effective operations must create a supercompetent valve, and whether it is ever possible to make a fundoplication "too-loose".

When we first described the technique of the Floppy Nissen Fundoplication (FNF) we were concerned about the possibility of gas-bloat as a consequence of effective operation. At that time we began a series of experiments to demonstrate the comparison of several varieties of fundic wrap, and found that the FNF provided an effective reflux barrier.

The details of this procedure are illustrated below (Fig. 1–2); what must be stated at the outset, however, is the fact that it was impossible to make a wrap so loose that it would not function as an effective anti-reflux barrier. Indeed, the way of performing the wrap which became the standard in the West Side Medical Center in Chicago was the FNF made as patulous as possible. Another corollary of this experience has been the realization that in patients in whom the physical dimensions of the esophagogastric junction preclude a standard FNF, such as patients of small stature, the surgeon must only employ a fundic wrap which is as loose as possible for that particular patient.

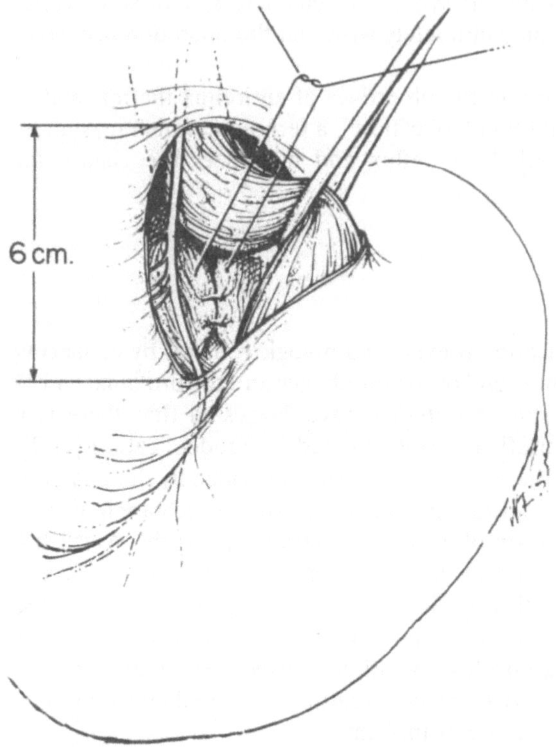

Fig. 1. The lower six cm of the esophagus have been cleared, maintaining the plane of dissection in the periesophageal space. The vagus nerves are identified and pushed to the patient's right side prior to closing the crura of the diaphragm. The diaphragmatic sutures are not tied until after checking the degree of "tightness" of the hiatus with respect to the distended esophagus

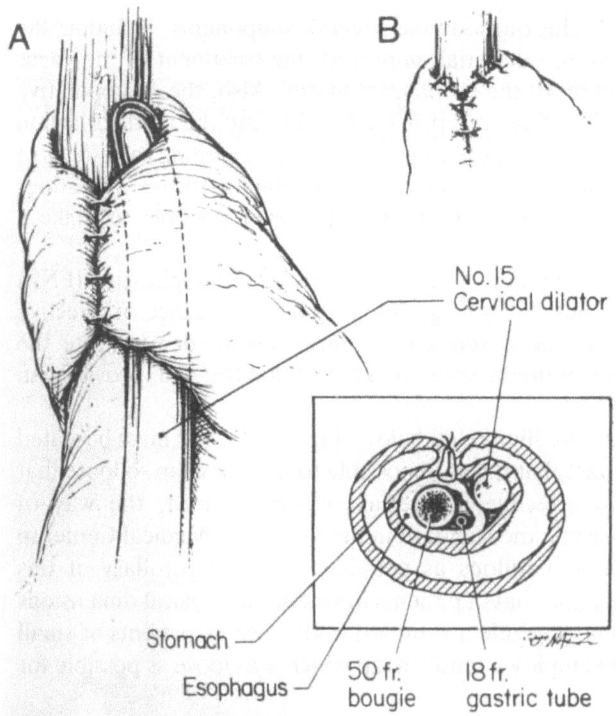

Fig. 2. The Floppy Nissen Fundoplication is made as "loose" as possible by using both the anterior and posterior walls of the stomach. All sutures are of 2–0 nylon material, and care is taken to maintain the position of the greater curvature of the wrap "in-line" with the greater curve of the stomach. The "collar" stitches also prevent slipping of the wrap

The most important part of the operation from this point of view is that the anterior as well as the posterior portions of the fundus must be included in the construction of the wrap. If the plicated fundus consists predominantly of the anterior wall, and mobilization of the posterior wall is avoided, then it is physically impossible to make the wrap "floppy". This technical point deserves emphasis in light of methods of fundoplication which are performed by pushing the anterior wall of the stomach behind the esophagus, toward the patient's right side, and are completed by sutures between the remnant of the anterior wall remaining to the left of the esophago-gastric junction.

The importance of using a loose wrap is widely recognized at this time, and may help explain the excellent results obtained with this method [7]. The length of the fundoplication is variable in most clinics, but we support the concept that a wrap must be 2–3 cm long; from a practical point of view, this is achieved by 3–4 sutures placed as shown in the illustration. As shown by the theoretical work from the Bombeck laboratory, the explanation for a successful anti-reflux procedure may reside in the lowest or "offloading" suture instead of the length of the fundoplication per se [8].

For many years the suture material employed was 2–0 silk. At that time we did not appreciate the potential for silk sutures to fragment and disintegrate after many years in situ. Since then, we have adopted the practice of using 2–0 nylon sutures for the fundic wrap as well as for repair of the crura of the diaphragm. Parenthetically, the disintegration of silk sutures could explain some of the late failures after fundoplication. In this regard, late failure is one of the unanswered questions after fundoplication, with several clinics reporting recurrent disease in more than 20% of their patients. Therefore, the tendency to employ non-absorbable suture materials is increasingly recognized and supported [8].

The repair of the esophageal hiatus is another technical aspect of fundoplication which deserves critical appraisal. When fundoplication was first performed, there was some debate about the necessity of reconstructing the esophageal hiatus, especially in those patients without antecedent hiatus hernia. The proponents of non-repair could point to the efficacy of intrathoracic fundoplications in preventing reflux, and from this point of view the repair of the diaphragm seemed superfluous. However, when patients with fundoplication were followed for long periods of time it became apparent that gradual migration of the fundoplication into the thorax resulted in complications similar to those observed with incarcerated para-esophageal hernia. That is, ulcerations of the stomach, perforation of an incarcerated stomach, or recurrent reflux due to distention of a trapped fundic pouch were recognized [9, 10]. The evolution of this type of complication can be very gradual, and the eventual crisis may be the first untoward postoperative event reported by the patient.

However, it is not too surprising that this problem would occur, (especially in retrospect), since the performance of effective fundoplication requires destruction of anterior and posterior phrenoesophageal supports (ligaments?) as well as the division of the structural integrity of the gastropancreatic fold and hepatogastric ligaments which provide additional resistance to migration of the cardia and fundus in the postoperative period.

Therefore, reconstruction of the esophageal hiatus has been recognized as an important feature of the operation in patients of all ages [11]. The problem which remains is, "how tight?" In my view, the esophagus should be distended with a bougie prior to tightening any of the sutures inserted into the crura of the diaphragm. The ultimate goal is to leave an opening in the diaphragm which allows a No. 15. Hegar dilator to enter the esophageal hiatus alongside the distended esophagus. The danger is that one might narrow the esophagus too-much, resulting in postoperative dysphagia. Also, the repair is ideally performed with nylon sutures, since the silk sutures might fragment over a period of many years.

The treatment of the vagus nerves is left to the preference of the operating surgeon; the choices are to perform a fundic wrap with the vagus nerves included within the wrap. The other alternative is to develop a plane of dissection in the periesophageal space, toward the goal of specifically isolating and protecting these nerves.

At times the posterior vagus is so closely applied to the posterior aspect of the cardia that inadvertent damage can occur unless the nerve is dissected clear of the site of plication; on the other hand, proponents of "inclusion" of vagus nerves within the wrap might rightly maintain that the nerves are more likely to be protected by not disturbing their anatomic position. Obviously, this is a technical point which is left to the discretion of the operator; however, I believe that the exposure provided by identification of the periesophageal space affords several discrete advantages to the surgeon [12]. The advantages include the possibility of a more precise and therefore safer isolation of the esophagus, the chance to place the "collar" sutures of the fundic wrap more precisely, and the potential benefit a wrap performed in the absence of interposed fat and connective tissue has less potential for disruption or migration. The last point, of course, is conjectural, since the major factor in preventing the slippage of a fundoplication is the insertion of sutures between the apex of the wrap and the esophagus. With respect to the suture material uniting the apex of the fundic wrap and the esophagus, it sems advisable to use nylon suture material in this location as well. The individual sutures are placed at one cm intervals between the apex of the fundus and the esophagus, and are designed to prevent "telescoping" of the fundoplication.

When the above considerations are performed faithfully, there is an outstanding possibility that the patient's preoperative difficulties will be relieved, and a corresponding likelihood that postoperative complications will not occur.

Finally, when evaluating patients who have some digestive or retrosternal complaints in the postoperative period, it is important that someone with experience and judgement regarding surgical procedures be involved in the evaluation process. In the past we have described the endoscopic appearance of the Nissen fundoplication (Fig. 3), and believe that one should be very cautious about interpreting ascribing complaints to recurrent reflux disease if the "nipple" is characteristic. On the other hand, a partial nipple is often associated with pathologic reflux, and a non-surgical physician may not discern the differences of the endoscopic appearances of some of the common antireflux operations. This fact reinforces our view that surgeons must continue to be involved with the practice of endoscopy, and that the surgeon has an important role as a consultant as well as a technical expert [13] reconstructions.

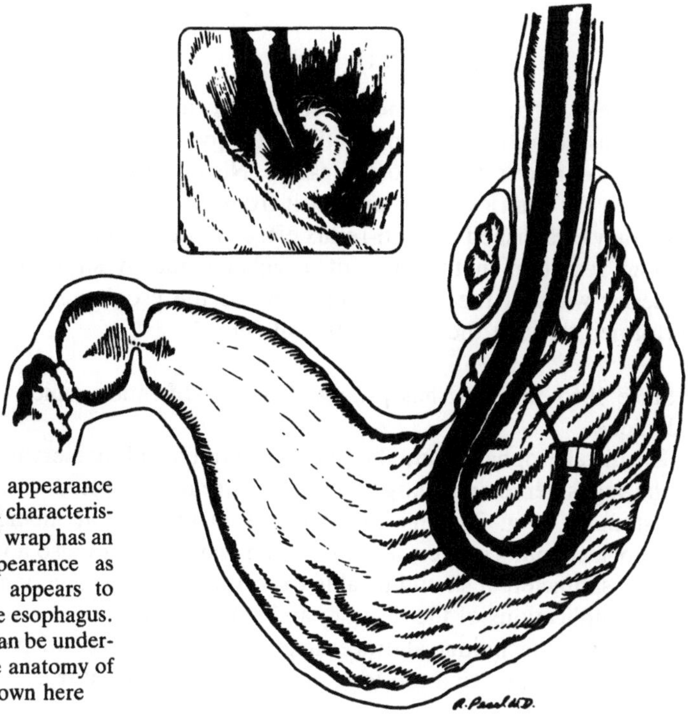

Fig. 3. The endoscopic appearance of a fundoplication has a characteristic appearance. The 360° wrap has an almost paradoxical appearance as seen endoscopically: it appears to surround only 270° of the esophagus. This apparent paradox can be understood by considering the anatomy of the fundoplication as shown here

References

1. Siewert R, Jenneawern HM, Waldeck F (1974) Experimentelle und klinische Untersuchungen zum Wirkungsmechanismus der Fundoplikatien. Helv Chir Acta 41: 39–41
2. Donahue PE, Bombeck CT (1977) The modified Nissen fundoplication – reflux prevention without gas bloat. Chir Gastroent 11: 15–27
3. Angelchik J-P, Cohen R (1979) A new surgical procedure for the treatment of gastroesophageal reflux and hiatal hernia. Surg Gynecol Obstet 148: 246–248
4. Samelson S, Bombeck CT, Siewert R, Weiser HF, Ludkte FE, Holscher AH, Abuabara SF, Nyhus LM (1983) A new concept in the surgical treatment of gastroesophageal reflux. Ann Surg 197: 254–257
5. Pettersson GB, Bombeck CT, Nyhus LM (1976) The lower esophageal sphincter: Mechanisms of opening and closure. Surgery 88: 307–314
6. Liebermann-Meffert D, Allgower M, Schmid F et al (1979) Muscular equivalent of the lower esophageal sphincter. Gastroenterology 76: 31–38
7. Siewert R (1978) Operative Behandlung der Refluxkrankheit. Chirurg 49: 137–145
8. Donahue PE, Samelson S, Nyhus LM, Bombeck CT (1985) The Floppy Nissen Fundoplication: effective; pmg-term control of pathologic reflux. Arch Surg 120: 663–668
9. Richardson JD, Larson GM, Polk HC Jr (1982) Intrathoracic fundoplication for shortened esophagus. Treachersous solution to a challenging problem. Am J Surg 143: 29–35
10. Maher JW, Hocking MP, Woodward ER (1984) Supradiaphragmatic fundoplication. Long-term follow-up and analysis of complications. Am J Surg 147: 181–186
11. Dedinsky GK, Vane DW, Black CT, Turner MK, West KW, Grosfeld JL (1987) Complications and reoperation after Nissen fundoplication in childhood. Am J Surg 153: 177–183
12. Donahue PE, Nyhus LM (1981) Exposure of the periesophageal space. Surg Gynecol Obstet 152: 218–220
13. Donahue PE, Yoshida J, Bombeck CT, Nyhus LM (1986) Endoscopic Skills – an imperative for surgeons. Digestive Surgery 3: 1–3

M. Rossetti (Liestal)

In the year 1955, Nissen and Rossetti performed the first fundoplication history, which was an antireflux construction, derived from the principle of the continent anastomosis after resection of the cardia (Nissen 1937) and where the esophagus was buried in the gastric wall to protect it from the reflux.

As they established the anti-reflux effect of the technique, they decided to apply it without resection in the form of a jacket made by suturing the anterior to the posterior walls of the fundus anteriorly to the esophagus. 2 of the sutures were performed through the esophagus wall (Fig. 1).

Since 1965, Rossetti has proposed the modification which is now the standard technique.

The distal esophagus and the fundus are freed with preservation of both branches of the vagus nerve and a large loose plicature is performed with the anterior wall of the stomach (Fig. 2). This procedure is in anatomical, manometrical and pharmacological points of view not only a one-way valve but also a true substitute of the inferior sphincter. It should be able to correct the reflux, its symptoms and the long-term complications of the disease, and stop its course.

The current technique allows eructation and vomiting and avoids the so-called gas bloat stomach, due to a too long or a too narrow plicature.

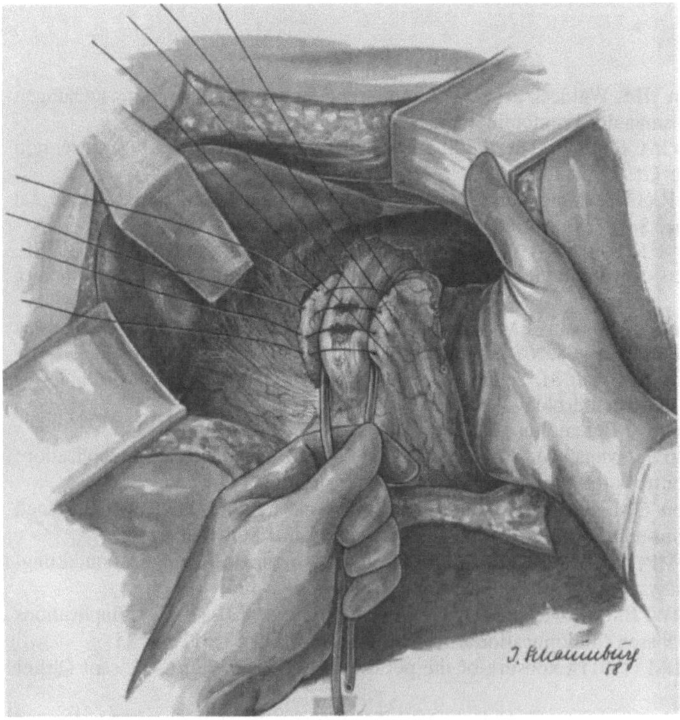

Fig. 1. Former technique (anterior and posterior wall)

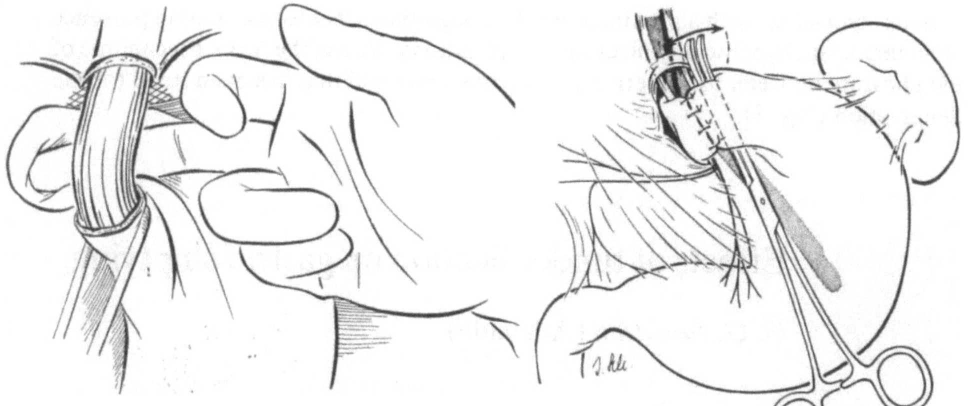

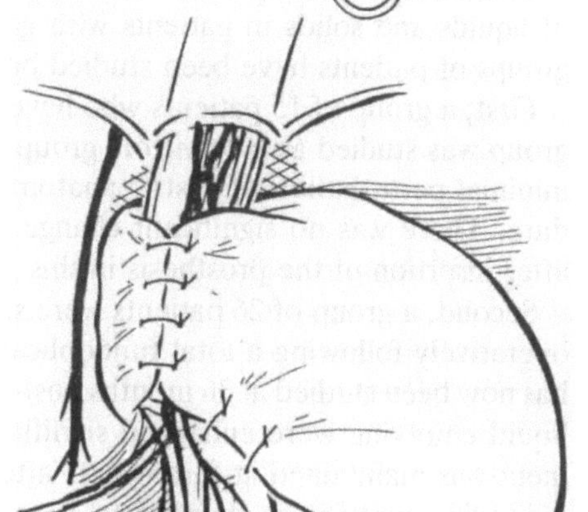

Fig. 2. Present standard technique (anterior wall)

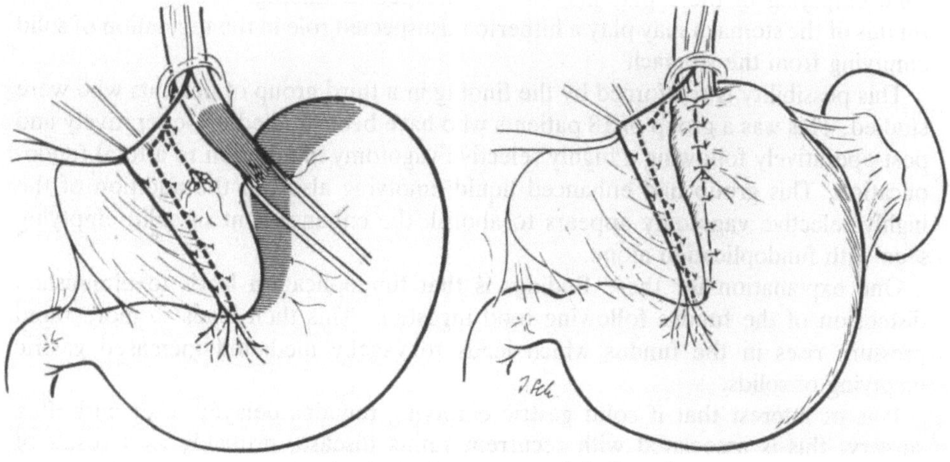

Fig. 3. Technique used when proximal selective vagotomy is indicated

In its association with a proximal selective vagotomy (that is indicated in presence of an important hyperacidity ulcerous complications) we use the former technique of the plicature between the anterior and the posterior wall that has been freed for the denervation (Fig. 3).

Effects of fundoplication on gastric emptying

G. G. Jamieson (Adelaide)

A dual isotope technique has been used to study simultaneously the gastric emptying of liquids and solids in patients with gastro-esophageal reflux disease [1]. Several groups of patients have been studied both before and after antireflux surgery.

First, a group of 15 patients who have had an Angelchik prosthesis inserted. This group was studied as a "control" group. It was reasoned that the operation caused minimal perturbation of gastric anatomy and yet still acted as an antireflux procedure. There was no significant change in the gastric emptying of solids or liquids after insertion of the prosthesis in this group.

Second, a group of 26 patients were studied preoperatively and at 6 months post-operatively following a total fundoplication. A further 17 of this group of patients has now been studied at 36 months post-operatively. It was found that both solid and liquid emptying were enhanced significantly by fundoplication, and this enhancement was maintained at three years after antireflux surgery.

Liquid emptying is thought to be controlled by fundic tone [2] and thus the decreased fundal capacity in these patients provides a ready explanation for the acceleration in liquid emptying. However solid emptying is thought to be controlled by antral function, and the fundus of the stomach is not usually regard as playing a significant role in the gastric emptying of solids [2]. Therefore the enhancement of solid emptying in these patients was an unexpected finding. It suggests that the fundus of the stomach may play a hitherto unsuspected role in the regulation of solid emptying from the stomach.

This possibility is reinforced by the finding in a third group of patients who were studied. This was a group of 18 patients who have been studied pre-operatively and post-operatively following a highly selective vagotomy in addition to a total fundoplication. This group had enhanced liquid emptying also but the addition of the highly selective vagotomy appears to abolish the enhancement of solid emptying seen with fundoplication alone.

One explanation for these findings is that fundoplication leads to diminished distension of the fundus following food ingestion. This then leads to more rapid pressure rises in the fundus which leads to vagally mediated increased gastric emptying of solids.

It is of interest that if solid gastric emptying remains delayed after antireflux surgery, this is associated with recurrent reflux disease, probably as a result of breakdown of the repair. We have studied a group of 38 patients who have had failure of antireflux surgery, and when studied at a median of 40 (6–180) months after their antireflux repair, we found that solid emptying was significantly delayed compared with both the 6 and 36 months follow-up in the patients who have had their gastric emptying assessed prospectively before and after antireflux surgery.

References

1. Maddern GJ, Chatterton BE, Collins PJ, Horowitz M, Shearman DJC, Jamieson GG (1985) Solid and gastric emptying in patients with gastro-oesophageal reflux. Br J Surg 72: 344–347
2. Kelly KA (1980) Gastric emptying of liquids and solids: roles of proximal and distal stomach. Editorial review. Am J Physiol G71–76

Results of the Nissen procedure

F. H. Ellis (Boston)

There is ample experimental [1] and clinical [2] evidence that the Nissen total 360 degree fundoplication is the best antireflux operation available. However, the operation has been criticized as being subject to a number of potential postoperative complications particularly dysphagia and the "gas bloat" syndrome. My personal experience with the use of this operation, which I will briefly summarize, suggests that if properly performed, these sequalae are uncommon. This view is shared by other esophageal surgeons and the recent report by DeMeester and associates [3] is a representative example. Analysis of a consecutive series of 100 patients treated over a 10 year period disclosed a 91% success rate.

Surgical Technique

The surgical technique which I employ has been detailed elsewhere [4]. An abdominal approach through an upper midline incision is preferred, a thoracic approach being used only when esophageal shortening is suspected or a previous thoracotomy has been done. The left lobe of the liver is mobilized and the gastric fundus is completely freed by division of the short gastric and posterior gastric vessels. A segment of abdominal esophagus is mobilized to provide an adequate length for the wrap, care being taken to preserve the vagus nerves. With traction on an encircling penrose drain, the freed gastric fundus is passed behind the esophagus, grasped with a Babcock clamp and the adjacent margins of anterior and posterior gastric fundus are loosely approximated around the freed esophagus using heavy non-absorbable sutures. I currently prefer a short wrap, of 2 to 3 cm long, loosely fashioned with a 42 F Maloney dilator acting as intraluminal stent. The esophageal hiatus is narrowed posteriorly to prevent cephalad migration of the wrap into the mediastinum.

Case Material and Results

Between January 1970 and January 1987, 241 fundoplication procedures were performed at the Lahey Clinic of which 157 were of the Nissen type. There were 48 Collis-Nissen procedure, 20 Collis-Belsey operations, 13 Belsey Mark 4 antireflux procedures and 3 Hill posterior gastroplasties. Of the 157 Nissen procedures, 36 are not included in this evaluation for they were either reoperations for symptoms other than reflux after antireflux surgery performed elsewhere, or the wrap was placed around a fibrotic stricture or left in the chest, procedures that I now consider contraindicated. Thus there remain 121 Nissen fundoplications which were done for gastroesophageal reflux without stricture with the wrap placed within the abdomen. 91 of these were primary procedures, the remaining 30 being reoperations most of which were secondary procedures but 4 patients had actually had three previous operations and were undergoing their fourth procedure. In all of these patients reflux was the result of hypotension of the lower esophageal sphincter (LES) associated with a diaphragmatic hernia in 79 patients, while in 5 patients a previous destructive operative procedure on the esophagogastric junction had led to a hypotensive LES. In 37 patients there was no obvious anatomic defect nor disease entity responsible for the hypotensive LES.

The surgical approach was a transabdominal one in 100 of these patients, while in the remaining 21, a thoracotomy was employed. Additional procedures were required in 29 patients. Six patients underwent a splenectomy. Five had an associated paraesophageal hiatus hernia treated with a Collis repair. There were five operative procedures on the billiary tract, 3 pyloromyotomies, 2 vagotomies and pyloroplasties and 2 patients who had undergone previous gastrectomy required fashioning of a Lawrence jejunal pouch while 2 patients had concomitant parietal cell vagotomy. Postoperative complications developed in 13 patients, an incidence of 10.7%. Four patients developed a postoperative ileus. There were four wound infections, two urinary tract infections, one dehiscence, one postoperative paraesophageal hernia requiring repair and one case of thrombophlebitis. There were no postoperative deaths.

Results

The results in some of these patients have been reported previously [5], in a follow-up study averaging 5¾ years in duration. The operation was a success in permanently controlling the symptoms of reflux in 90.2% of patients. One of the criticisms of the operation concerns the ability to belch postoperatively which was evaluated in most patients and 80% of those questioned could do so. In evaluating the overall result of the operation both its success is preventing reflux and the patient's overall condition were considered. The success rate was slightly lower than if only the effect of the operation on gastroesophageal reflux had been considered. For those undergoing operation for the first time, the overall success rate was 84.5% whereas it was only 75% in those patients undergoing reoperation. When the poor results were analyzed, persistent and/or recurrent gastroesophageal reflux was the most common cause occurring in 8 patients, 3 of whom were reoperated on with good results as was one patient with the "gas bloat" syndrome and one patient with a postoperative paraesophageal hernia. Of the remaining 5 patients with poor results, one had severe diarrhea, another had dysphagia requiring dilations and the remaining 3 complained of multiple seemingly unrelated symptoms that defyed analysis. Because of the high incidence of recurrent gastroesophageal reflux in the early cases, a larger stent has been used for the past 10 years with no examples of recurrent reflux. Current evaluation of the patients operated on since our earlier report, reveals a success rate in relieving reflux symptoms of 93% with an overall improvement rate of 83%. As in our earlier report the results of primary procedures was better than that following reoperations, three of the five poor results occurring in patients having secondary procedures.

Summary

The Nissen 360 degree fundoplication is an extremely successful antireflux procedure. If performed loosely over a short length of intra-abdominal esophagus, post operative complications are rare and the risk of recurrent reflux, dysphagia or "gas bloat" is negligible.

References

1. Leonardi HK, Lee ME, El-Kurd MF, Ellis FH Jr (1977) An experimental study of the effectiveness of various antireflux operations. Ann Thorac Surg 24: 215
2. DeMeester TR, Johnson LF, Kent AH (1974) Evaluation of current operations for the prevention of gastroesophageal reflux. Ann Surg 180: 511
3. DeMeester TR, Bonavina L, Albertucci M (1986) Nissen fundoplication for gastroesophageal reflux disease, evaluation of primary repair in 100 consecutive patients. Ann Surg 204: 9–20
4. Ellis FH Jr, Gibb SP (1974) Fundoplication for hypotensive lower esophageal sphincter. Hosp Pract 9: 80
5. Ellis FH Jr, Crozier RE (1984) Reflux control by fundoplication: a clinical and manometric assessment of the Nissen operation. Ann Thorac Surg 38: 387–392

S. Seineldin (Rosario)

One hundred and ninety-six patients were operated on with the Nissen technique at the Hospital Provincial de Rosario (Argentina), from 1962 to 1980.

We conducted a restrospective study in 1982 in order to evaluate the influence of the short esophagus on the hiatal hernia repair.

Seventy-eight patients were included in the study and further assigned to one of the following groups, according to clinical, radiological, endoscopic and surgical criteria:
Group 1: Patients with an apparently normal esophagus (55 patients)
Group 11: Patients with evidence of short esophagus (23 patients)

Table 1

AGE (Years)	N° of patients	GROUP I	GROUP II
0–10	7	2	5
11–30	1	0	1
31–50	12	10	2
51–70	36	31	5
71–82	22	12	10
TOTAL	78	55	23

Table 2

FOLLOW UP	GROUP I		GROUP II	
	N°	%	N°	%
20<15	4	7.3	–	–
15<10	10	18.2	2	8.7
10< 5	18	32.7	7	30.4
5< 2	23	41.8	14	60.9
TOTAL	55	100	23	100
	$\bar{x}$=7.4		$\bar{x}$=5.5	

There were 40 women and 38 men, aged 4 months to 82 years (mean age 39,3 years, (Table 1)). The follow up is shown in table 2.

Regarding previous history of gastroesophageal reflux symptoms, 43.6% of cases in Group I had been symptomatic for less than one year: on the other hand, 43.4% of patients in Group 2 had reflux symptoms for more than 10 years (Table 3).

Sliding hiatal hernia was found in 83.6% of Group 1 and 91.3% of Group 2 cases. The presence of gastroesophageal reflux by radiology was routinely investigated in Group 1. Spontaneous reflux was found in 30.9% of cases, while another 45.4% had evidence of induced reflux. Gastroesophageal reflux could not be properly evaluated in Group 2 patients due to the high incidence of stricture of the esophageal lumen.

From the endoscopic standpoint, 65% of patients in Group I had no evidence of lesions, while 91.3% in Group 2 presented lesions classified as "severe" by the endoscopist (Table 4).

Manometric esophageal studies were performed in a low number of cases by that time, so we cannot draw any conclusion.

We observed a suggestive high incidence of associated conditions in Group 1, particularly regarding ulcer and cholecystopathy; on the contrary, Group 2 showed mainly complications of the acid-peptic reflux (Table 5).

Table 3

Duration of reflux symptoms (years)	GROUP 1		GROUP 2	
	N°	%	N°	%
<1	24	43.6	1	4.3
1–2	19	34.5	3	13.0
3–4	12	21.8	2	8.7
5–10	–		7	30.4
>10	–		10	43.4
TOTAL	55	100	23	100

Table 4

ESOPHAGOSCOPY	GROUP 1		GROUP 2	
	N°	%	N°	%
Normal	36	65.4	–	
Esophagitis 1	9	16.3	–	
Esophagitis 2	6	11.0	2	8.6
Esophagitis 3	4	7.2	5	21.7
Stricture	–		16	69.5
TOTAL	55	100	23	100

Table 5

ASOCIATED DISEASES	GROUP 1	GROUP 2
Cholecystopathy	21	1
Duodenal Ulcer	9	–
Umbilical hernia and cholecystopathy	7	–
Pharyngoesophageal diverticula	1	–
Megaesophagus	–	1
Inguinal hernia	1	–

This latter observation is valid, since in 67.2% of patients in Group I the surgical procedure was decided according to the presence and evolution of the associated condition, as opposed to that in Group 2, surgery was exclusively prescribed taking into account the severity of the esophageal lesions.

Symptoms developed after fundoplication in 14.5% of patients with normal esophagus and 39.1% with short esophagus (Table 6). Swallowing discomfort, inability to belch and vomit and persistent dysphagia were the most frequent complaints: late recurrence of reflux symptoms was referred by 21.7% of Group 2 patients, compared with 7.2% of Group 1.

Table 6

POST-FUNDOPLICATION SYMPTOMS	GROUP 1		GROUP 2	
	N°	%	N°	%
Swallowing disconfort	6	10.9	3	13.0
Inability to belch	3	5.4	5	21.7
Inability to vomit	5	9.0	4	17.3
Persistent disphagia	3	5.4	7	30.4
Upper abdominal pain	2	3.6	4	17.3
Recurrence G.E.R. symptoms	4	7.2	5	21.7
Abdominal meteorism	4	7.2	2	8.6
Diarrhea	2	3.6	–	–
N° PATIENTS	8	14.5	9	39.1

Table 7

RADIOLOGY	GROUP 1		GROUP 2	
	N°	%	N°	%
Recidivant hernia	2	3.6	–	
Displacement of hernia repair	2	3.6	5***	21.7
Disruptid of fundoplication	1	1.8	5**	21.7
Intussusception	–		2*	8.6
TOTAL	5	9.0	12	52.2

* Number of reoperations

Radiological abnormalities of the cardio-hiatal region (Table 7) were documented in both Group 1 and 2, with an incidence of 9 and 52.2%, respectively; Group 2 disclosed more severe complications, like thoracic displacement of the repair (21.7% of cases), disruption of fundoplication (21.7%) and intussusception (8.6%), that required a high number of reoperations (26.0%).

Conclusions

An effective antireflux procedure should achieve control of the acid-peptic manifestations and good post-operative quality of life.

The Nissen technique is probably the most efficient procedure for the surgical treatment of gastroesophageal reflux. However, a number of complications has limited its use.

Based on our unfavourable results, we do not advise the performance of this technique in cases of long history of reflux symptoms, peptic stenosis, severe ulcerative esophagitis, obesity, recurring hiatal hernia, chronic lung disease and tissue friability of the cardio-hiatal region.

However, in such cases, good short term results can be obtained with few postoperative complaints by careful selection of patients and providing great attention to the technical details of the operation.

M. Rossetti (Liestal)

Around 2000 publications deal with this subject in the five continents (and their number increases every month). The results of the studies are hard to compare because of the different methods of evaluation that are used and we shall thus avoid giving a pseudo-scientific or mathematic aspect to statistics that concern a biological and human matter with computerized percentages that could not be taken seriously.

The Table 1 gives a synthesis of the results that concern our 30 years of experience, and those of many other authors:

It is understandable that the tissue degradation and the technical mistakes are both responsible for failures and long-term recurrences.

The Table 2 summarizes our newest statistics:

Table 1. Global Results of the Fundoplication

90% of mid-term clinical healing (2 years)
75% of long-term clinical healing (2–20 years)

Table 2. Liestal Clinic. 1975–1983

Fundoplications		377	(14 surgeons)
Results			
	good	326	86%
	modest	41	11%
	bad	10	3%
Recurrence	with reflux		
	in 2 years	14	4%
	6 years	28	8%
	without reflux	9	3%
Operative mortality		2	

Conservative surgical procedures (2)

President: *Mitsuo Endo* (Tokyo)

Free Commentators: *J. H. Alexandre* (Paris)
P. Carabalona (Montpellier)
R. J. Earlam (London)
F. H. Ellis (Boston)
S. Mantonakis (Athens)
J. L. Ribardière (Paris)
P. Barron (Tokyo)

Partial fundoplication

R. D. Henderson (Toronto)

Partial fundoplication procedures are commonly used as a method of management of gastroesophageal reflux. Although not as effective as total fundoplication in reflux control each method has its advantages and disadvantages.

My experience using partial fundoplication is with the standard Belsey repair and with the partial fundoplication gastroplasty (TFG: Belsey gastroplasty). Other partial fundoplications which have been extensively reported include the Hill and Allison repairs.

With partial fundoplication the HPZ is reduced below the diaphgram and some form of partial fundoplication added. The extent of fundoplication varies from 30–270° of wrap. This procedure is less effective than total fundoplication as a method of reflux control. With total fundoplication, increases in gastric pressures are circumferentially applied to the HPZ and distal esophagus. This method of pressure transmission will prevent reflux when the junction is in either chest or abdomen. Pressure transmission is obviously less effective with partial fundoplication. Once a partial fundoplication is in the chest it becomes ineffective in reflux control.

There is serious question as to whether a partial fundoplication is important in prevent reflux or whether its sole purpose is to anatomically fix the HPZ below the diaphragm. If the wrap does not add to reflux control then the effectiveness of the procedure would depend upon HPZ tone and its reduction and fixation within the abdomen (Fig. 1)

There is no doubt that partial fundoplications are effective in many patients. Ample longterm studies are available indicating 85% excellent results 10 years after surgery; despite this quality of result, there are reports indicating radiologic or pH

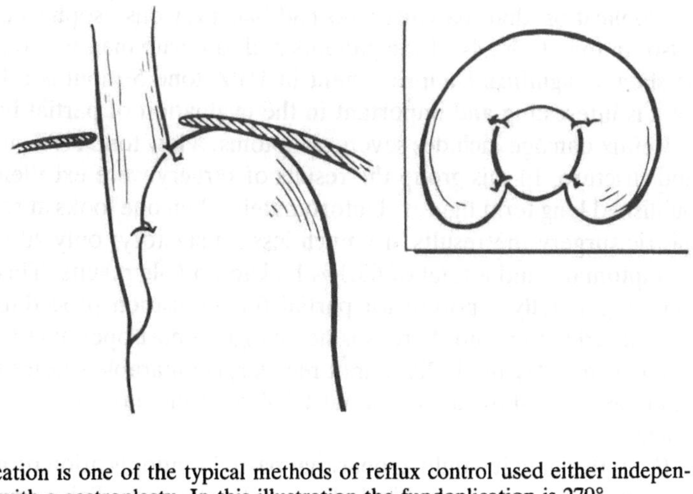

Fig. 1. Partial fundoplication is one of the typical methods of reflux control used either independently or in association with a gastroplasty. In this illustration the fundoplication is 270°

reflux occurring in 44 to 56% of patients studied. Clearly reflux alone is not the sole criteria of success. Perhaps, although reflux is present, the amount of reflux has been reduced to a level where symptoms can improve.

Having established that partial fundoplications are effective in the majority of patients it would be helpful to evaluate the success of the procedure under varying pathologic conditions. In my own experience using partial fundoplication gastroplasty in 125 patients the results after 10 years of followup have been evaluated as follows:

a) Asymptomatic and eating normally
b) Improved but with some persistent symptoms
d) Failure of surgical management

Table 1. Results of partial fundoplication Gastroplasty

	Total Group 125 Patients	Reflux Pathology Only 60 Patients	Recurrent Surgery 65 Patients
A	63.2%	88.3%	40%
B	17.5%	11.7%	23.1%
C	19.2%	0%	36.9%

Analysing the total group (Table 1) 63.2% were asymptomatic, 17.5% had some persistent symptoms and 19.2% were failure of surgical management.

Sixty of the 125 patients had reflux pathology only. In this group of 60 patients 88.3% were asymptomatic, 11.7% had some persistent symptoms and none were failures.

Sixty-five patients had recurrent hiatal hernias or previous gastric surgery: forty percent of these were asymptomatic, 23.1% had residual symptoms and 36.9% were considered failure of surgical management.

In this study patients with reflux injury only responded much better to partial fundoplication than patients who had had previous esophageal or gastric surgery. Also, in this study, 44 of the patients had followup manometric studies which failed to show a significant improvement in HPZ tone 5 months following surgery; this data is interesting and important in the evaluation of partial fundoplication.

Reflux damage includes severe symptoms, a low tone HPZ, ulcerative esophagitis and stricture. In this group the results of surgery were excellent and equal to most published long term figures. Unfortunately when one looks at revision esophageal or gastric surgery the results are much less satisfactory: only 40% of this group were asymptomatic and a total of 63.1% had acceptable results. This data is much worse than is generally reported for partial fundoplication procedures. Furthermore, in manometric follow-up there was no change in post-operative HPZ tone, suggesting that in some way the HPZ cannot recover; comparable studies in patients with total fundoplication show a substantial HPZ tone increase with a return to the normal range.

From this data it would appear that partial fundoplication procedures are effective for reflux injury up to and including peptic stricture. This same operation is clearly not suited for management of anatomic recurrence, and much better results have been reported with the management of recurrence using total fundoplication.

Since pre-operative pathology is not reported in most follow-up studies of hernia repair, this key information is not generally recognized. Obviously, the reported results of hernia repair will vary with the patient mix and the pre-operative findings.

In summary, partial fundoplication procedures have been extensively used in surgical reflux control. These various operations have been reported as showing excellent results, however some of their problems should be recognized and these are outlined as follows:

- Partial fundoplication is ineffective once the esophagogastric junction is in the chest.
- Partial fundoplication is less effective than total in reflux control.
- Partial fundoplication is less likely to produce overcompetence than total fundoplication.
- The operation is effective in the management of primary reflux injury.
- In patients requiring revision surgery after hernia repair or gastric surgery, partial fundoplication is much less effective than total fundoplication and should be avoided.

References

1. Collis JL (1961) Gastroplasty. Thorax 16: 197
2. Pearson FG, Langer B, Henderson RD (1971) Gastroplasty and Belsey hiatus hernia repair; an operation for the management of peptic stricture with acquired short esophagus. J Thorac Cardiovasc Surg 61: 50
3. Henderson RD, Marryatt GV (1985) Total fundoplication gastroplasty (Nissen gastroplasty): Five-year review. Ann Thoracic Surg 39: 74–79

What is the value of an intrathoracic fundoplication?

J. Baulieux, and *P. Maillet* (Lyons)

In 1977, we reported details on our experience on the treatment of peptic stenosis concerning 139 cases (Table 1) [5]. The conservative procedure without resection was the method chosen most often. Only 13 intrathoracic fundoplications were performed (Table 2).

There was a postoperative fatal outcome with 2 patients. 1 patient was lost to follow up. The follow up assessment of surviving patients between 1 and 7 years showed 7 excellent results and 3 poor results.

1 patient required further surgery for hemorrhagic gastric ulcer. Since this period, 53 peptic stenosis were operated on; only 3 thoracic Nissen fundoplications were performed. Since 1980, no thoracic fundoplication has been performed.

Table 1. Peptic stenosis – treatment

Non conservative	48	Esogastrectomies Interpositions		34 14
Conservative	82	Abdominal Approach =46	Fundoplications other types	33 13
		Thoracic Approach =36	ITFP Mark 4 Esogastrostomies	13 18 5
Medical treatment	9			
Total	139			

Table 2. 13 intrathoracic fundoplications

• Post-operative mortality	2
• Unknown	1
• Late results (1 year → 7 years)	
– excellent =	7
– poor =	3

Discussion

Many authors [7, 8, 10] have reported their experience with this procedure.

Woodward et al. [10], and Moghissi [8] stated that, in their hands, the transthoracic Nissen fundoplication with the left supradiaphragmatic repair has provided excellent results, without incident. Many authors emphasized accidents with this procedure [6].

Gastric ulcers, early and late, are often reported (Table 3 = 20%). Saubier [8] has seen 2 early gastric fistulas and 4 late-onset fistulas with an experience of 29 cases. Bremner [2] thought alkaline reflux was responsible. Bushkin [4] considered the

Table 3. Complications

Gastric ulcers	early late onset fistulae
Saubier – Bremner – Bushkin – Scobie – Mansour	
Causes	• Alkakine reflux, • Gastrin hypersecretion, • Ischemia, • Mechanical factors.

cause to be gastrin hypersecretion secondary to gaseous distension. Scobie [9] postulated that mechanical factors related to diaphragmatic trauma may be relevant. Mansour [6] emphasized the possibility of recurrence after suture of the gastric ulcer, with bronchial fistulas. We have treated one patient, with bronchial fistula, with total gastrectomy, left inferior lung lobectomy and coloplasty.

Diaphragmatic hernias are another late complication (Saubier [8]: 4 cases, Balison [1]: 5 cases). Late intrathoracic migration of abdominal organs can be prevented by a careful closing of the diaphragm. It is a severe complication which needs reoperation.

Functional sequellae are not exceptional. Typical functional sequellae of the Nissen procedure are well-known. (dysphagia – "gas bloat syndrome"). We have confirmed limitation of the vital capacity (25%) by gaseous distension of the intrathoracic stomach.

Conclusion

The intrathoracic Nissen fundoplication gives good functional results, but it is evident from this review that intrathoracic Nissen wrap is subject to potentially lethal complications. These complications suggest that the indications should be limited [6] and the conservative methods by abdominal route are preferable.

References

1. Balison JR, MacGregor A, Woodward ER (1973) Post-opérative diaphragmatic herniation following trans-thoracic fundoplication. Arch Surg 106: 164–166
2. Bremner CG (1977) Gastric-ulcer after the Nissen fundoplication. S Afr Med J 1: 791
3. Burnett HF, Read RC, Morris WD, Campbell GS (1977) Management of complications of fundoplication and Barrett's oesophagus. Surgery 82: 521–530
4. Bushkin FL, Woodward ER, O'Leary JP (1972) Occurrence of gastric ulcer after Nissen fundoplication. Am Surg 42: 821
5. Maillet P, Baulieux J, Boulez J, Dumurgier CL (1977) Valeur des méthodes conservatrices dans le traitement chirurgical des sténoses peptiques de l'œsophage chez l'adulte. J Chir 114: 443–450
6. Mansour KA, Burton HG, Miller J, Hatcher CR (1981) Complications of intra-thoracic Nissen fundoplication. Ann Thorac Surg 32: 173– 178
7. Moghissi K (1983) Intra-thoracic fundoplication for reflux stricture associated with short esophagus Thorax 36–40
8. Saubier E, Gouillat EC (1983) Traitement des sténoses peptiques de l'œsophage par fundoplicature intrathoracique avec dilatation per-opératoire de la sténose. Etude critique de 29 observations. Chirurgie 109: 494–500
9. Scobie BA (1979) High gastric ulcer after Nissen fundoplication Med J Aust 1: 409
10. Woodward ER, Thomas HF, McAlhany JC (1971) Comparison of crural repair and Nissen fundoplication in the treatment of esophagus hiatus hernia with peptic esophagitis. Ann Surg 173: 782–792

L. A. Praderi, and O. Balboa (Montevideo)

Nissen's fundoplication is currently considered to be the most effective technique for gastroesophageal reflux and therefore for esophagitis. [5, 9, 10, 18]. However, there is intense controversy over fundoplication placed in the thorax, which is considered either reliable or high-risk by some surgeons, [12, 18] while it is supported, for some particular cases, by others. [11, 15]. We have consistently used Nissen-Rossetti's fundoplication since 1965 (179 patients), [16, 17, 19] and we have had to place it in the thorax in only 5 cases (2.8%). In our very limited experience, we have seen that intrathoraxic Nissen is very well tolerated by some patients, while it is poorly tolerated by others, causing severe and multiple symptoms!

Cases

L.A.R. age 5: Operated at age 3 for diaphragmatic hernia and esophageal stricture. An Alisson technique was utilized and failed. The patient was reoperated on at age 5. The cardioesophageal junction could not be reduced so an intrathoracic Nissen repair was left. Gastric dilation ensued (Fig. 1) and an erosive gastritis which was relieved by medical treatment. At age 20 she is symptom-free and tolerating well the procedure.

P.R. de V. age 32: Asthma since childhood. Treated for pulmonary tuberculosis 1½ years ago. Currently receiving steroids. She had recurrent asthmatic attacks. Severe gastroesophageal reflux, hiatal hernia and esophagitis were found. In june 1978 a Nissen procedure was performed and a good clinical response was observed with subsidence of asthma. Two years after, hiatal hernia recurred with intrathoracic Nissen without reflux, associated with gastric ulcer (Fig. 2). She was reoperated on and a subtotal gastrectomy was performed. She is now symptom-free.

This different response to apparently similar situations resembles the inconsistent behavior of hiatal hernia and reflux, which can be the origin of severe disturbances or quite asymptomatic and just be diagnosed as a radiologic finding.

In order to explain these clinical facts we must search for physiopathologic interpretations. The cardioesophageal junction is placed in the middle of the thoraco-abdominal coelomic cavity where the esophagus slides up and down through the esophageal hiatus of the diaphragm. At this particular level where negative intrathoracic pressure meets positive intraabdominal pressure, the esophagus is tethered to the musculo-aponeurotic hiatus. We must also bear in mind the fact that negative thoracic and positive abdominal pressures can change a great deal due to many causes. Thus abdominal pressure increases considerably towards the pelvis (related to voiding functions) while standing up, and decreases down to almost zero at the gastric fundus close to the diaphragm. This explains the evolution and migration of many pathologic processes (subphrenic abscess, etc.)

Since 1977, we have studied the relationship between reflux and respiratory disease. We have recorded a series of 570 patients with both disturbances [14, 17, 19].

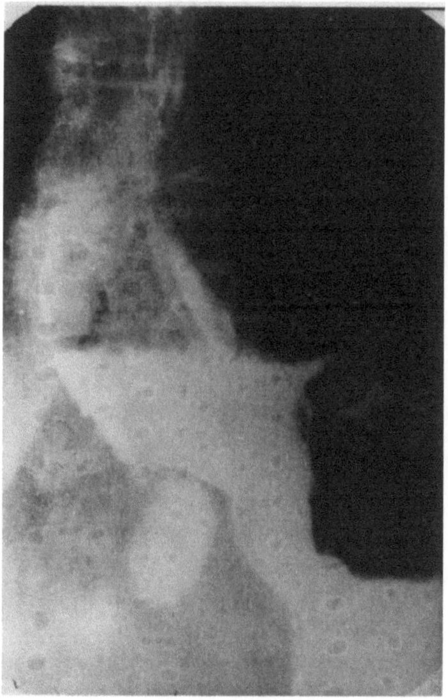

Fig. 1. Intrathoracic Nissen tolerating

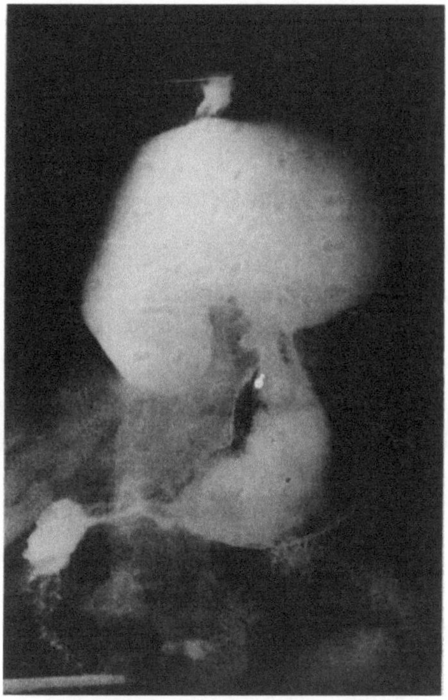

Fig. 2. Hiatal hernia recurred with intrathoracic Nissen. Associated with gastric ulcer

According to our own manometric studies, intrapleural pressure can become so low as to overcome the high pressure zone (HPZ) and cause reflux. We have found cases of reflux with normal lower esophageal sphincter pressure [2, 3], which can be caused therefore by the dominance of negative intrapleural pressure as a suction force (Fig. 3, 4).

Fundoplication immediately supresses reflux. This can be easily corroborated after surgery [16–17], due to the fact that either fundoplication substitutes for the incompetent esophageal sphincter or because it generates better conditions for the recovery of normal sphincteric function [6, 4, 8].

The first hypothesis would explain the efficacy against reflux of Nissen's procedure surrounding Collis' gastroplasty, where there is no esophageal sphincter [13].

When placed within the thorax, fundoplication can overcome negative pressure and prevent reflux. This would explain the absence of reflux in intrathoracic Nissen repairs. Much lower intrapleural negative pressures cause the failure of this procedure and favor stasis and dilation of the gastric cavity [18].

*

In our series of 232 patients operated on for esophageal cancer utilizing Ivor Lewis' technique, the stomach within the thorax dilated only in one case (gastric hypotonus) two years after the operation, in spite of a pyloroplasty. We do not know

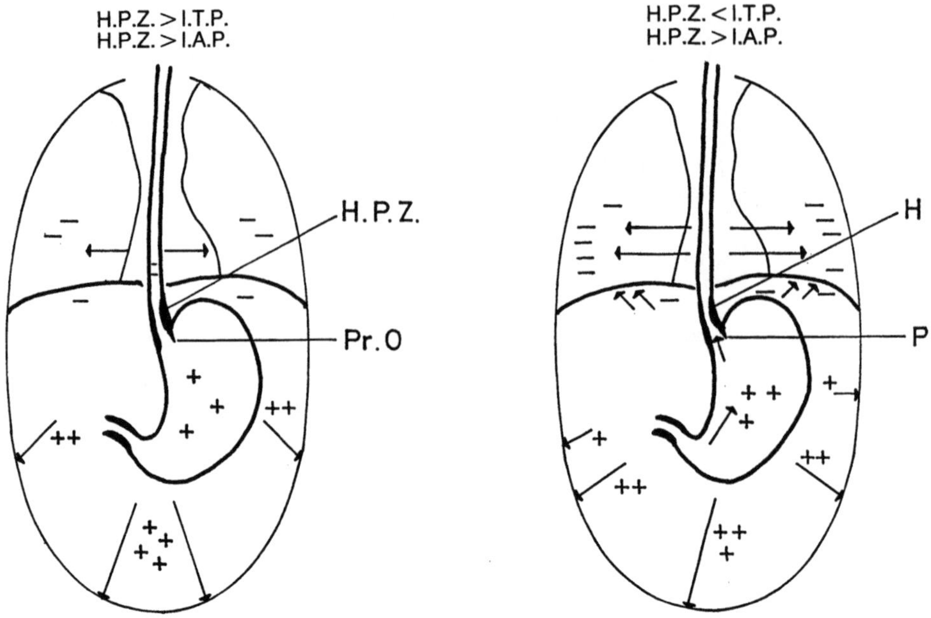

Fig. 3 NORMAL C.O.L.D.

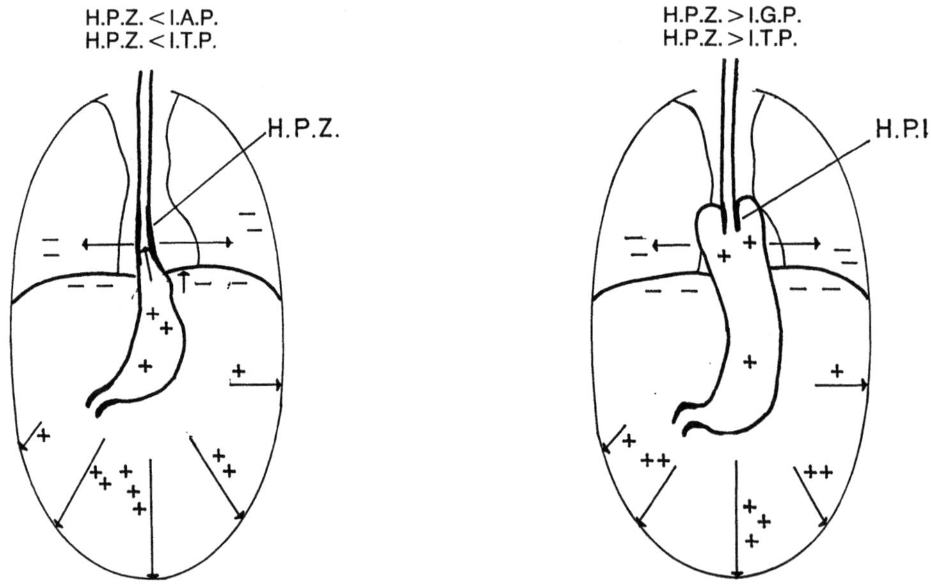

Fig. 4 GASTROESOPHAGEAL REFLUX INTRATHORACIC FUNDOPLICATION

Fig. 3–4. Schematic drawing of the dynamic pressure of the thoraco – abdominal coelomic cavity. H.P.Z. = High pressure zone; I.T. P. = Intrathoracic pressure; I.A.P. = Intraabdominal pressure; C.O.L.D. = Chronic obstructive lung disease; I.G.P. = Intragastric pressure the cause, but we must point out that this was a patient with a chronic obstructive lung disease (C.O.L.D.) and increased pleural pressure [18].

Cardioesophageal surgery must be performed by surgeons trained in abdominal and thoracic surgery. The lack of experience to deal with unfamiliar ground across the diaphragm has led to incomplete solutions. Therefore complicated esophagites must be operated on by experienced surgeons, with wide knowledge of esophageal pathology.

In our practice, it's unusual to be unable to reduce cardioesophageal junction into the abdomen (2.8%). The main goals are to suppress reflux, choosing a safe and simple procedure according to a benign condition.

As a review of publications shows, the search for an appropriate technique goes on. We think it has not been found yet and this is the source of current difficulties.

We have given up esophagogastric anastomoses because they are justified only when it is not possible to rule out a neoplastic disease, and we have currently other choices. Although attractive for their ingenuity, many of them have been shown to create complications and are not considered worthwhile. Such is the case of the Collis-Belsey procedure. Others, such as jejunal interposition (Merendino) or left colonic interposition ("Short" Belsey) are complex procedures, demanding the opening of viscera. Postoperative severe risk or even lethal complications should not happen at all when performing a functional and reconstructive procedure. For all these reasons we believe that intrathoracic Nissen repair is still warranted for unusual situations, due to the fact that it is executed rapidly and simply and provides a remarkably competent valve that can usually resist the suction from negative intrapleural pressure. According to the physiopathologic concepts that we have mentioned above, fundoplication would not be indicated in patients with chronic obstructive lung diseases, because of negative intrapleural pressure.

*

As a primary condition for the success of this procedure, an impeccable technique is mandatory, as for an intraabdominal Nissen.

- Floppy fundoplication (not tight) [7, 17]
- Diaphragmatic closure must not constrict the fundoplication at the hiatus. The stomach must not be sutured to the diaphragm, according to our experience with surgery for cancer of the esophagus where we do not do this. We have never had colonic hernia.
- Pyloroplasty (whether instrumental or digital), if a vagotomy has been needed to free the mediastinal esophagus.

  Complications of thoracic and abdominal fundoplicature are in most cases derived from surgical technique failures [17]. We have never seen bleeding from veinous hypertension, or gastric perforation, mediastinitis, etc. [1, 13, 18].

In summary: We believe that the Nissen repair must remain below the diaphragm, so we fix the stomach according to Cordano (Fig. 5). A Nissen repair sliding into the thorax is a complication that is difficult to treat and must be prevented.

The intrathoracic Nissen repair is the procedure of choice for unusual situations. One should try to obviate it by placing the cardioesophageal junction in the abdomen by means of an appropriate surgical technique.

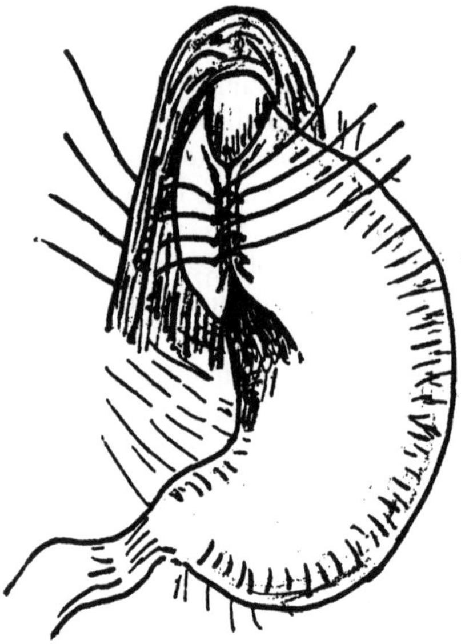

Fig. 5. Nissen repair with sutures passed through the right crus of the diaphragm to prevent upward displacement

References

1. Asole F, Clemente G, Colosimo C, Puglionisi (1983) Le complicanze della fundoplicatio di Nissen e la loro complicazione. Chir Gastroent 17: 3
2. Balboa O, Delgado F, Voeiker R (1979) Incompetencia del esfínter esofágico inferior normotenso-Su relación con las variantes de presión intraabdominal e intratorácica. Cir del Uruguay 49: 559
3. Balboa O (1982) El esfínter esofágico inferior. Tesis de docencia. Montevideo
4. Bonavina L, Evander A, DeMeester TR, Walther B, Cheng SCH, Palazoo L, Concannon J (1986) Length of the Distal Esophageal Spincter and Competency of the Cardia. The Am J of Surg 151: 25
5. DeMeester TR, Johnson L, Kent A (1974) Evaluation of current operations for the prevention of gastroesophageal reflux. Ann Surg 180: 511
6. DeMeester TR, Weruly JA, Bryant GG, Little AG, Skinner DB (1979) Clinical and in vitro Analysis of determinants of gastroesophageal competence. The Am J Of Surg 137: 39
7. Donahue P, Bombeck C (1977) The modified Nissen Fundoplication reflux prevention without gas bloat. Chir Gastroenterolog 11: 15
8. Ellis FH, El Kurd MFA, Gibb SP (1976) The effect of fundoplication on the lower esophageal sphincter. SGO 143: 1
9. Ferraris V, Sube J (1981) Retrospective study of the surgical management of reflux esophagitis. SGO 152: 17–21
10. Guarner V, Martinez M, Gavino J (1980) Ten Years evaluation fundoplasty in the treatment of Gastroesophageal reflux: long term and comparative study in 135 patients. Am J Surg 139: 200
11. Hollenbeck JL, Woodward ER (1985) Treatment of peptic esophageal stricture with combined fundic patch fundoplication. Am Surg 182: 472–478
12. Mansour KA, Burton HG, Miller JL Jr, Hatcher CR Jr (1981) Complications on intrathoracic Nissen fundoplication. Ann Thorac Surg 32: 173–178
13. Orringer MB, Sloan H (1977) Complications and failing of the combined Collis/Belsey operation. The Journ of Th and Cardiov Surg 74: 726
14. Overholt R, Vorhees R (1966) Esophageal reflux as a "Trigger" in asthma. Dis Chest 49: 464–466

15. Pennell TC (1981) Supradiaphragmatic correction of esophageal reflux strictures. Ann Surg 193: 655–665
16. Praderi LA La funduplicatura de Nissen en la hernia hiatal por deslizamiento. Indicaciones, Técnica, Resultados. Rev Cir Uruguay 37: 53–62
17. Praderi LA, Balboa O (1984) Esofagitis por reflujo no complicada. Cir del Uruguay 54: 248–257
18. Richardson JD, Larson GM, Polk HC (1982) Intrathoracic Fundoplication for shortened esophagus. The Am J of Surg 143: 29
19. Tomalino D, Praderi LA, Romano D, Balboa O, Fugasot LE, Gutierrez H, Touya E, Ricciardi N, Colamonici O (1982) Patología Respiratoria y reflujo gastroesofágico. La Prensa Médica Uruguaya 5: 1

The fixed retroesophageal valve

G. Champault, B. Baranger, and *Ph. Boutelier* (Paris)

In the long controversy over the choice of technique in the surgical treatment of gastroesophageal reflux (GER) certain aspects are now accepted, thanks to the development of investigations of gastroesophageal function, particularly manometry and pH measurement [15] and to the early results of controlled studies [8, 12, 14, 17] evaluating the efficacy of the more commonly employed techniques in the short- and mid-term.

Facts and arguments

The inferior esophageal sphincter (LES), a manometric entity [15], has a normal tonus of 25±10 cm H_2), which is appreciably higher than the gastric pressure at rest. The LES is situated over the last 4–5 cm of the esophagus. Under the control of a great many hormonal and nervous factors, it is the chief element in maintaining cardiac continence [3].

In GER, the tonus of the LES is very frequently, and variably, reduced [15]. Its length, too, is sometimes decreased. The object of surgical treatment is the restoration of permanent tonus adequate to prevent the gastric contents from attacking the esophagus.

The aggressive nature of the GER is assessed by endoscopy and by pH measurement [13] over 3–24 hours [15], and should be specified before operation to provide a criterion for postoperative comparisons in the short- and mid-term.

The essential stage in the surgical cure of GER is the restoration of an abdominal esophagus of adequate length (4 cm) [1]. When GER is associated with low sphincteric tonus, this mere reposition of the sphincter significantly increases the pressure [11], the gain habitually exceeding the passive transmission due to the increase in abdominal pressure [1]. This effect is due to the tightening of the fibers of the LES when the cardia is reduced into the abdomen [18]. On the other hand, the length of the zone of high pressure seems to remain unchanged [11, 13].

Csendes [5] has shown that patients with a pathologic GER have a cardiac perimeter significantly greater than that of healthy subjects. Stretching of the esophagus may, in itself, reduce the cardiac diameter. Certain procedures act directly (Hill) or by using the gastric fundus as a wrapping [7].

Partial or complete wrapping of the esophagus with the gastric fundus [10, 19] increases the tone of the LES [7] and is considered by some [13] as the main factor in continence. All studies are agreed [2, 8, 13] that, the more complete the fundoplication, the greater the increase in LES pressure. Peroperative recording of the pressure [9] gives perfect correlation of LES tone and the degree of fundoplication.

For want of fixation, the intra-abdominal repositon of the esophagus is subjected to the double strain of abdominal pressure [3] and the retractile power of the esophagus. Good continence is maintained by retaining the LES, ie. the esophagus, within the abdomen, whether this be by direct fixation of the cardia to the arcuate ligament (Hill) or to the crura of the diaphragm (Toupet) [19] (Boutelier) [1]. Objective analysis by manometry and pH measurement in the short-or mid-term of the chief technical procedures currently employed [4, 12, 14, 16, 17, 18] shows that none is really superior to the others and that deterioration in the results occurs between 3 and 6 months later in 10 to 25% of cases.

The study of unsatisfactory manometric or pH findings confirms that the postoperative tonus of the LES appears to be the factor determining the success or failure of the operation, as against the acid secretory response [13] or the quality of gastric emptying as studied by the technique of double dilution of a colored indicator for the emptying of fluids and of radio-opaque markers for solids [13]. All authors [14, 27] have noted the frequent inconsistency between the clinical results (good in 90% of cases) and the manometric and pH findings (early deterioration).

Finally, while there is as yet no objective long-term follow-up as regards antireflux procedures, the experience of some workers [1, 4, 10, 19] provides an excellent idea of the mortality (1–3%) and morbidity of these operations.

Choice of method

This must satisfy the following requirements: reconstitution of an abdominal esophagus of sufficient length [5, 11]; reinforcement of the tonus of the LES by fundoplication [7]; intra-abdominal fixation [3]; the least possible morbidity [4]; no reduction of gastric acidity [18]; an associated emptying maneuver [18].

Apart from Hill's operation, which otherwise satisfies most of these criteria, the problem is essentially to decide between the posterior fundoplication of Toupet [19], which corresponds to sheathing of 180° of the esophagus by the mobilized fundus, fixed to the crura behind and the esophageal margins in front, and Nissen's complete (360°) wrapping of the esophagus [10]. These two operations, the most widely used, have been studied in numerous publications whose main importance is the acknowledgment of a very low mortality (0 to 1%), and of a moderate morbidity that is nevertheless rather higher (5%) for Nissen's operation than for posterior fundoplication (dysphagia, gas-bloat syndrome, etc). They are used for reference in most current controlled studies and in the objective assessment of their short- and mid-term results [8, 13, 14, 17]. There is agreement on the following points:

a) the mortality is almost nil (but the series are short); morbidity is higher after the Nissen procedure.
b) at 3 and 6 months, clinical efficacy as regards signs of reflux (pyrosis) is excellent (92.96%) and comparable. Dysphagia persists in a third of the cases in both groups [12] but disappears more rapidly in posterior fundoplication. Manometry and pH measurement gives comparable results [12], although Galmiche [8] reports a 25% incidence of gastro-esophageal reflux after posterior fundoplication.
c) at 24 months, Ottignon [14] reports a 34% incidence of pyrosis after posterior valve construction as against 8% after Nissen's operation, confirmed by manometry and pH measurements.

Segol [17] reports the results of a controlled trial comparing the Nissen, Toupet and Lortat-Jacob procedures. At 2 years, 87% of the operated patients were symptom-free and the symptomatic 13% included no Nissen procedures, 10% Toupet and 26% Lortat-Jacob operations. The difference between the Nissen and Lortat-Jacob techniques was at the limits of significance. At pH measurement performed in 46 patients, 63% had a good result and 37% an abnormal pH value with a Minaire score of 4 or higher: Nissen 21%, Toupet 45% and Lortat-Jacob 60%. The difference in the Minaire score was significant (p 0.05) only between the Nissen and Lortat-Jacob procedures (Table 1).

Finally, at manometry performed in 43 patients the sphincter had normal tonus in 77% of the Nissen, 44% of the Toupet and 29% of the Lortat-Jacob procedures, again with a significant difference (p 0.05) between the Lortat-Jacob and Nissen operations. Thus, the efficacy of the posterior valve, identical with that of the Nissen procedure in the immediate postoperative period, seems of deteriorate with time (30% at two years, though without any clinically evident differences) [17].

Fixed retroesophageal fundoplication raises several problems. The technical variants are numerous, which makes their evaluation difficult, and relate essentially to the level of the procedure, the mode of fundoplication and its type of fixation (or nonfixation). We opted for a level of around 4 cm and complete mobilization of the fundus, either by total liberation of its posterior surface or by section of the short

Table 1. Results of a controlled trial comparing the Nissen, Toupet and Lortat-Jacob procedures

		Nissen	HFP	Lortat-Jacob	
Clinic	O. 87%				
	+ 13%	0	10%	26%	
pH	N. 63%				
	Path. 37%	21%	45%	60%	S
Manometry	LES N	77%	44%	29%	

Segol (AURC) – 24 months

gastric vessels, which permits the creation of a supple fundoplication and good fixation to the crura of the diaphragm. As for the degree of sheathing of the esophagus, this varies according to the preoperative manometric figure; it should be at least 180 to 200°, reaches 360° where the LES is destroyed (endobrachyesophagus, tight peptic stricture) and involves only ¾ of the circumference in intermediate cases.

Thus, the choice between the Toupet and Nissen procedures involves a range of variants in terms of the extent of the fundoplication required to suit the preoperative tone of the LES. This "modulated" attitude seems best suited to an essentially functional type of surgery, the quality of whose results largely depends on adaptation of the set-up to each individual case.

Conclusion

In our present ignorance of the ideal procedure for the surgical treatment of GER, and while awaiting the long-term results of procedures in current use, the choice must be oriented between the known efficacy of the methods and their drawbacks and therefore to navigate between Toupet and Nissen, with preoperative manometry as the best guide [9].

References

1. Boutelier Ph (1973) Les hernies hiatales de l'adulte et leur traitement chirurgical Masson Edit Paris
2. Boutelier Ph, Jonsell G (1982) An alternative fundoplicative maneuver for gastro-esophageal reflux Am J Surg 143: 260–264
3. Boutelier Ph (1983) Critique des différentes méthodes chirurgicales du reflux gastro-oesophagien Actualités Digestives 7: 309–310
4. Breil Ph (1983) Etude critique des résultats de la chirurgie des reflux gastro-œsophagiens. Actualités Digestives, 7: 315–317
5. Csendes A, Larrain A (1972) Effect of posterior gastropexie on gastro-esophageal sphincter pressure and symptomatic reflux in patients with hiatal hernia Gastroenterology, 63: 19–24
6. DeMeester TR, Johnson LF Evaluation of the Nissen anti-reflux procedure by esophageal manometry and 24 hours pHmonitoring
7. Ellis FH Jr, El Kurd NFA (1976) The effect of fundoplication on the lower esophageal sphincter Surgery Gynecol Obstet 143: 1–4
8. Galmiche JP, Téniere P, Ducrotte P, Denis P, Colin R, Testart J (1983) Traitement du reflux gastro (œsophagien acide par hémifundoplicature postérieure. Résultats cliniques et pHmétriques. Gastro Entérologique Clin et Biol 7: 385–391
9. Jonsell G, Boutelier Ph (1979) Gastro-esophageal reflux. Evaluation of two fundoplicature methods by intra-operative esophageal manometry Acta Chir Scand 493 (suppl): 47
10. Nissen R (1961) Gastropexie and fundoplication in surgical treatment of hiatus hernia. Am J Dig Dis 6: 654–658
11. O'Sullivan GC, DeMeester TR, Joelson BE (1982) Interaction of lower esophageal sphincter pressure and length of sphincter in the abdomen as determinants of gastroesophageal competence. Am J Surg 143: 40–47
12. Ottignon Y, Mantion G, Sava P, Clement C, Birgen C, Carayon P, Pelissier E, Gillet M (1984) Evaluation clinique, pHmétrique et manométrique de la fundoplicature complète de Nissen et de l'hémifundoplicature postérieure de Toupet chez 41 malades souffrant de reflux gastro-œsophagien (résultats préliminaires). Actualités Digestives 1: 17–20

13. Ottignon Y, Ampelas M, Voigt J, Chassigneul J, Pascal JP (1984) Comparaison de trois méthodes d'enregistrement du pH œsophagien dans le diagnostic du reflux gastro-œsophagien acide. Gastro-entérol. Clin Biol 8: 609–615
14. Ottignon Y, Mantion G, Pelissier E, Birgen C, Deschamps JP, Carayon P, Gillet M (1987) Evaluation à court et moyen terme de la fundoplicature complète de Nissen et de l'hémifundoplicature postérieure de Toupet chez 64 malades souffrant de reflux gastro-œsophagien. J Chir à paraître (abstract 88e Congrès Français de Chirurgie)
15. Le reflux gastro-œsophagien (1983) 2e colloque de gastro-entérologie de l'hôpital Beaujon (4 juin 1983) Actualités Digestives, 5, 7: p 271
16. Segol P, Baptiste P, L'hirondel C, Marchand P, Gignoux M (1982) Effets de la fundoplicature sur le sphincter inférieur de l'œsophage: étude manométrique pré et post-opératoire. Gastroentérol Clin Biol 6: 222–228
17. Segol Ph (26/4/1986) Le traitement chirurgical du reflux gastro-œsophagien, Nissen, Toupet ou Lortat-Jacob 2èmes journées de l'Aurc (Abstract)
18. Touchais JY, Lerebours E, Sauger F, Testart J, Teniere P, Ducrotte P, Guillard JF, Paley D, Galmiche JP, Denis P, Colin R (1985) Analyse des différents facteurs conditionnant les résultats du traitement chirurgical du reflux gastro-œsophagien Gastroentérolog. Clin Biol 9: 712–718
19. Toupet A (1963) Technique d'œsophago-gastroplastie avec phéno-gastropexie appliquée à la cure radicale des hernies hiatales et comme complément de l'opération de Heller dans les cardiospasmes Mem Acad Chir 89: 394–501
20. Vansant JH, Baker JW (1976) Complications of vagotomy in the treatment of hiatal hernia Ann Surg 183: 629–635

The degradation of posterior fundoplication

J. P. Galmiche, P. Denis, P. Tenière, P. Ducrotte, J. Y. Touchais, P. A. Lehur, and *J. Testart*
(Nantes and Rouen)

Questions about surgery in gastroesophageal reflux (GER) are the following [1]:

a) Are currently used surgical repairs effective in preventing reflux?
b) For how long are surgical manipulations effective? Indeed Brand et al. [2] reported late deterioration of clinical, manometric, histological and pHmetric results 5 to 8 years after surgery.
c) What are the causes of failures and/or late clinical deterioration after surgical repair?

These questions prompted us to use esophageal pH measurement to evaluate the effects of current operations performed for treatment of GER. The method of esophageal pH measurement we used for this purpose has been described previously [3]. Three hour post-prandial recording of esophageal pH was performed after a standard test meal. As described by Kaye, results were expressed using a scoring index system. The so called Kaye score takes into account both the time spent at a low pH level and the magnitude of each pH drop. The maximal normal value, defined as mean plus 2 standard deviations is 90. In patients with typical symptoms of heartburn and regurgitations its sensitivity was 0.81 for a specificity of 1.00.

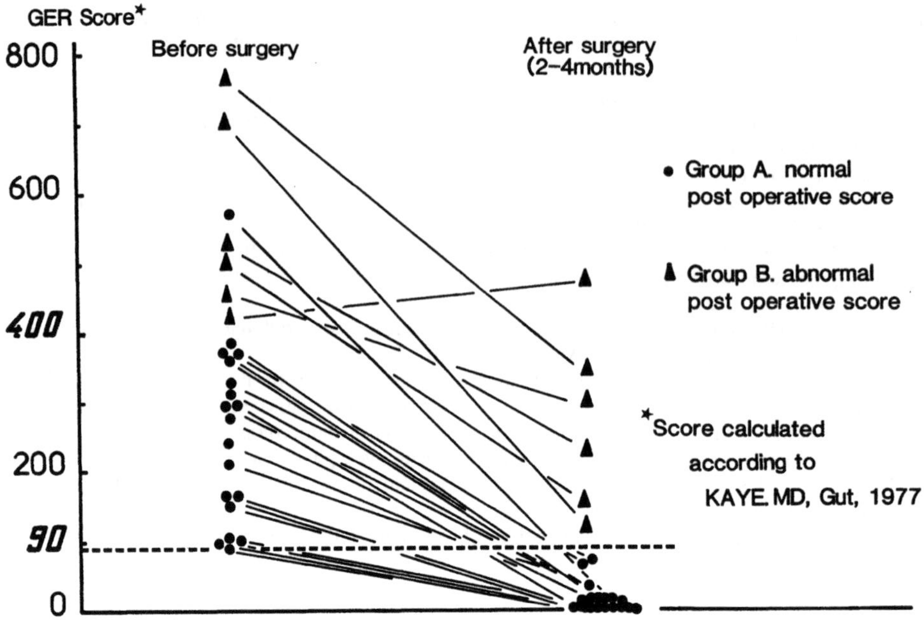

Fig. 1. Changes in esophageal pHscore after posterior hemifundoplication (from reference 4)

Results

First study [4]

Fig. 1 shows changes in esophageal pH score after posterior hemifundoplication (called Toupet's operation in France). This prospective study [4] included 25 patients with reflux symptoms and/or endoscopic esophagitis resistant to medical treatment. All patients were operated on by the same surgical team and evaluated by a clinical interview and a 3-hour pH test 2 to 4 months after surgery. At this time all patients except one were very satisfied, being nearly symptom free. Indeed when compared to preoperative values, after surgery pH score was decreased in 24 patients. However pH score returned to normal values in only 19 patients called group "A". In the 6 remaining patients refered to as group "B", pH score was clearly above the physiological range, although they were clinically asymptomatic.

We had the opportunity to conduct a follow up study in 23 of them who were interviewed about 2 years later; symptom relapse occurred more frequently in group B than in group A. The difference of relapse rate was not statistically significant, mainly because numbers of patients were low in each subgroup. However recurrence of reflux was documented in 3 out of 4 cases in group B whereas pH score was normal in 5 of the 6 group A patients who alleged clinical deterioration (Table 1).

Table 1. Follow up after posterior hemifundoplication. Late post-operative interview (median=21 mo)

	No relapse	Symptom relapse
Group A (n=17)	11	6 (a)
Group B (n=6)	2	4 (b)

a) mild and rare symptoms in 3 cases; pH score normal in 5 cases and abnormal in 1 case
b) GER confirmed by 3-h pH test in 3 cases

Second study [5]

We have compared the esophageal pH changes after different types of surgical repair, including a fundic wrap or not (Fig. 2); we also tried to correlate these changes with several factors considered as potential determinants in the pathogenesis of reflux, such as the lower esophageal sphincter (LES) tone, gastric acidity and emptying.

Patients included were sent to our laboratory for esophageal and gastric function tests prior to surgery and 2 to 4 months later. They underwent 4 different surgical procedures according to possibilities and choices made by the surgeons (Fig. 2).

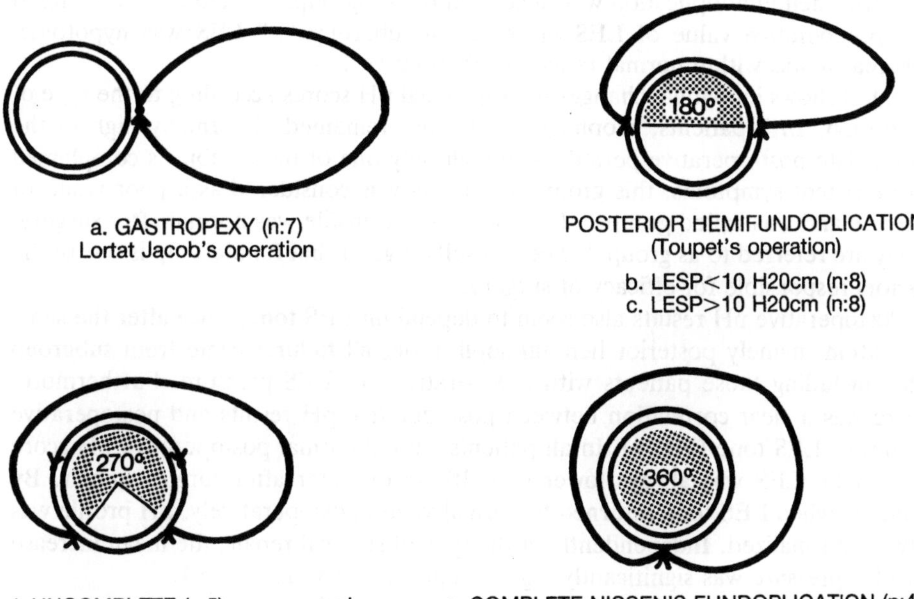

a. GASTROPEXY (n:7)
Lortat Jacob's operation

POSTERIOR HEMIFUNDOPLICATION
(Toupet's operation)
b. LESP<10 H20cm (n:8)
c. LESP>10 H20cm (n:8)

d. UNCOMPLETE (n:5) and e. COMPLETE NISSEN'S FUNDOPLICATION (n:4)

Fig. 2. Esophageal pH test after different operations for gastroesophageal surgery (GER) (from reference 5)

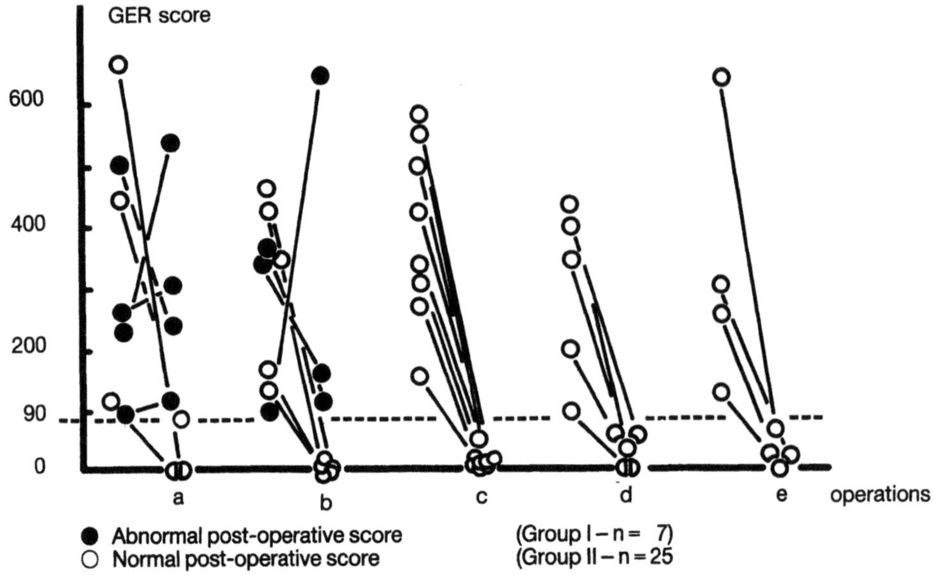

Fig. 3 Changes in esophageal pHscores after various types of GER surgery (study 2) (from reference 5) – see figure 2 for operations

Seven patients had a simple anatomical repair without a fundic wrap. Fundoplication was performed in 25 patients with different degrees of wrap around the distal esophagus. For the purpose of analysis, the group of 16 patients who underwent posterior hemifundoplication was divided into 2 subgroups, "b and c", according to the preoperative value of LES pressure. In subgroup "b" LES was hypotonic, whereas it was within normal range in subgroup "c".

Fig. 3 shows individual changes in esophageal pH scores according to the type of operation. In 7 patients, esophageal pH score remained abnormally high in the immediate post-operative period. Although only one of these subjects complained of persistent symptoms, this group of patients was considered as a poor result of surgery and was called group 1. In 5 patients pH profile was normal after surgery. They are referred to as group 2. These results suggest that fundic wrap is one of the factors responsible for efficacy of surgery.

Postoperative pH results also seem to depend on LES tone, since after the same operation, namely posterior hemifundoplication, all failures came from subgroup "b", including those patients with preoperative low LES pressure. Furthermore, there was a clear correlation between postoperative pH results and postoperative values of LES tone (Fig. 4). In all patients with abnormal postoperative pH score (group 1), LES was always lower than 10 cm of water after surgical repair. By contrast when LES tone returned to normal values postoperatively, pH profile was always normalized. Independently of the type of surgical repair, the mean increase in LES pressure was significantly higher in group 2 than in group 1.

Maximal gastric acid secretion in response to a liquid protein meal was measured in all patients before surgery, using the intragastric titration method with bicarbonate. Patients with abnormal postoperative pH score were not different from those

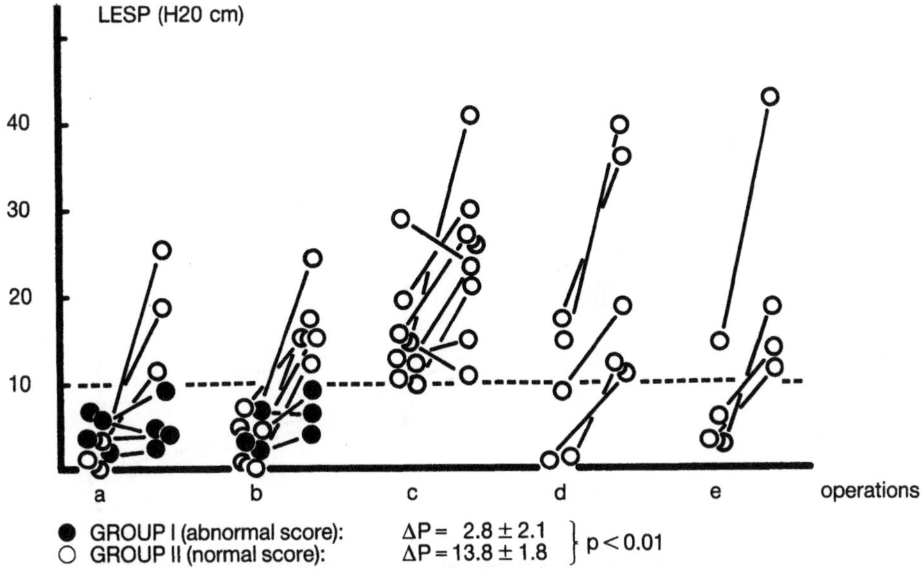

Fig. 4. Correlations between surgical results (pHscores) and changes in lower esophageal sphincter tone (from reference 5)

Table 2. Maximal gastric acid secretion (MAO mmol/h)* and results of GER surgery

Healthy subjects (n=23)	24.0±6.6
Group 1 (n=7)	24.4±3.2
Group 2 (n=25)	23.6±2.0

* acid response to a liquid protein meal (Gastric titration)
Group 1: postoperative esophageal pH score >90
Group 2: postoperative esophageal pH score <90

of group 2. Acid outputs of reflux patients were within the normal range of our laboratory values (Table 2).

Finally, we also studied gastric emptying of indigestible solids. One hundred solid radio-opaque markers were given with a French standard test meal. Using plain abdominal film, the markers found in the stomach area were counted at different times after the test meal. Although there was a slight tendency to delayed gastric emptying in patients of group 1, that is with abnormal postoperative pH profiles, the differences with patients of group 2 and with healthy controls were not statistically significant (Fig. 5).

Conclusions

1. Esophageal pH measurement is a simple and useful tool for objective assessment of results after GER surgery.

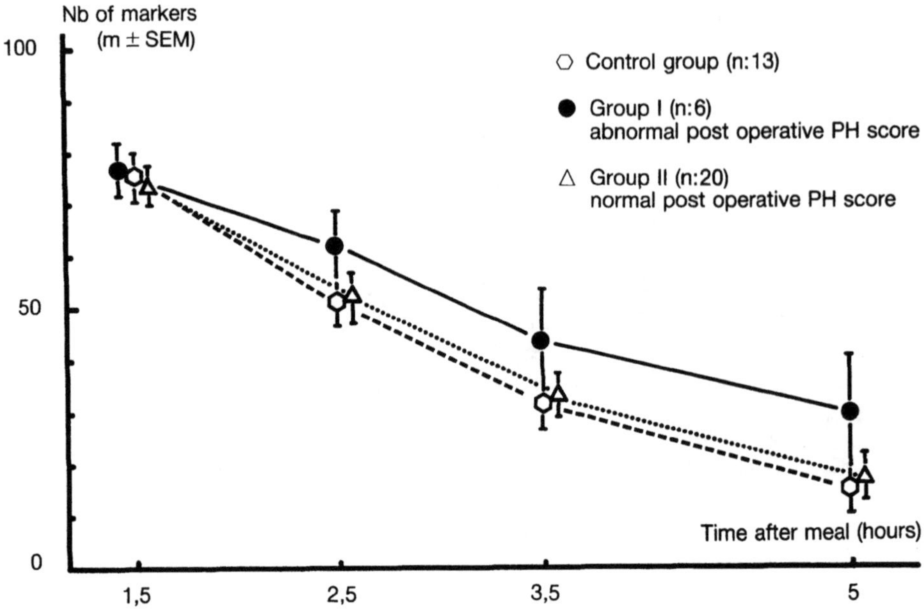

Fig. 5. Gastric emptying of solid radio-opaque markers after GER surgery and in control subjects

2. After GER surgery, an abnormal pH profile may persist in asymptomatic patients and seems to carry an increased risk of late deterioration.
3. Poor pHmetric results after GER surgery are mainly associated with incomplete restoration of LES tone (whereas gastric acid secretion and emptying of solids do not seem to play a major role).

References

1. Behar J (1979) Surgical treatment of reflux esophagitis: how well does it work? Gastroenterology 77: 183–191
2. Brand DL, Eastwood IR, Martin D, Carter WB, Pope CE (1979) Esophageal symptoms, manometry, and histology before and after antireflux surgery. Gastroenterology 76: 1193–1401
3. Galmiche JP, Guillard JF, Denis P, Boussakr K, Lefrançois R, Colin R (1980) Etude du pH œsophagien en période post-prandiale chez le sujet normal et au cours du syndrome de reflux gastro-œsophagien. Intéret d'un score de reflux acide; Gastroenterol Clin Biol 5: 531–539
4. Galmiche JP, Teniere P, Ducrotte P, Denis P, Colin R, Testart J (1983) Traitement du reflux gastro-œsophagien acide par hémifundoplicature postérieure. Résultats cliniques et pHmétriques. Gastrenterol Clin Biol 7: 385–391
5. Touchais JY, Lerebours E, Sauger F et al (1985) Analyse des différents facteurs conditionnant les résultats du traitement chirurgical du reflux gastro-œsophagien. Gastroenterol Clin Biol 9: 712–718

The Hill procedure

K. B. Å. Thor, and *L. D. Hill* (Stockholm and Seattle)

Technique

Gastroesophageal restoration (Hill operation) is accomplished through an upper midline abdominal incision. The abdomen is explored. The pylorus is examined carefully for any evidence of pyloric stenosis that might impede gastric emptying. The triangular ligament of the left lobe of the liver is divided and the liver retracted to the patient's right. The upper hand retractor is placed to facilitate exposure. The phrenoesophageal membrane is divided on the diaphragm removing as much of the fibroareolar tissue as possible (Fig. 1).

These bundles will be used in the repair.

The lesser omentum is divided and the esophageal hiatus is exposed. The esophagus is gently diverted to the patient's right and the attachment of the cardia to the diaphragm is divided. As few short gastric arteries as possible are divided. This dissection must be done with care so as not to tear the spleen. Division of the phrenogastric and superior portion of the gastrosplenic ligament mobilizes the upper part of the gastric fundus.

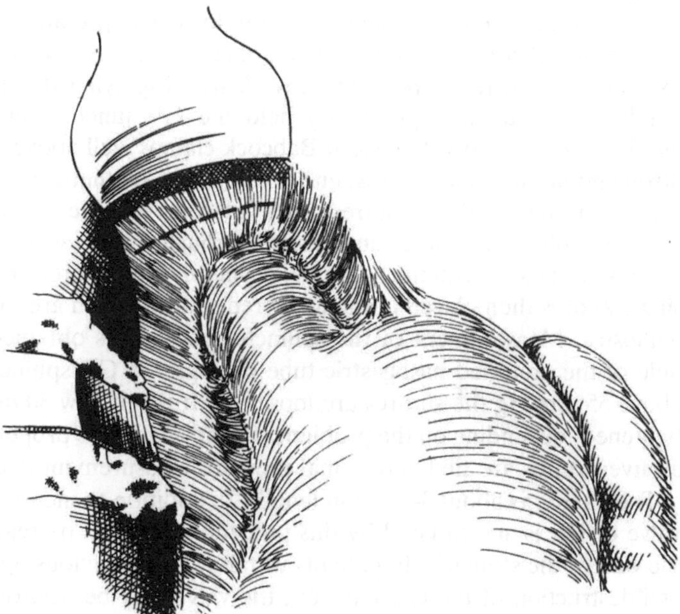

Fig. 1. The dotted line in the illustration is the line at which the dissection of the fibroareolar tissue from the diaphragm is begun in order to obtain as much tissue of the phrenoesophageal bundles as possible. These bundles are used in fixing the GE junction to the preaortic fascia

The fundus can then be rotated so that the posterior part of the stomach can be visualized. This allows the GE junction to be retracted down and the hernia is reduced.

By retracting the anterior and posterior phrenoesophageal bundles an intraabdominal segment of esophagus becomes visible. The anterior and posterior vagus nerves are visualized and kept in view so as not to be damaged. Retracting the stomach to the patient's left exposes the preaortic fascia. The median arcuate ligament lies immediately above the celiac trunk. It can be exposed by careful blunt dissection at the midpoint of the aorta. The celiac artery usually arises cephalad to the median arcuate ligament.

Dissection of the celiac axis has been a deterrent to performing this operation in many hands. If it is difficult to locate the ligament or if the surgeon is not familiar with vascular surgery and is uncomfortable in dissecting out the celiac axis, a safer alternative procedure is recommended. By retracting the esophagus to the patient's left, the surgeon can expose the esophageal hiatus. The fibroareolar tissue overlying the aorta and the esophageal hiatus can be simply divided by sharp dissection, thereby exposing the aorta. A finger is then passed gently beneath the preaortic fascia, down the celiac artery, and the preaortic fascia is lifted off the aorta. This can then be grasped with the Babcock clamp and the sutures simply placed through the fascia. Care must be taken not to damage short branches that pass from the aorta to the crura. By staying in the midline, these branches are avoided. If a branch of the celiac or the aorta is avulsed, brisk bleeding may occur. This may be dealt with simply by gentle pressure with a finger, exposure of the branch, and ligation with a vascular suture.

The crura of the esophageal hiatus are loosely approximated behind the esophagus with nonabsorbable sutures. The stomach is then rotated in a clockwise direction to expose its posterior part, thereby clearly displaying the anterior and posterior bundles of tissue that previously held the GE junction in the diaphragm. The bundles are grasped with special Babcock clamps well above the left gastric artery. Strong nonabsorbable sutures, either 0-silk or 0-synthetic material, are used for the repair. Usually five sutures are placed in the anterior and posterior phrenoesophageal bundles and carried through the preaortic fascia (Fig. 2). These sutures are placed with the vagus nerves in full view in order not to damage them. A single knot is then placed in the top three sutures which are then clamped with long hemostas. Measurement of the sphincter pressure is obtained by passing the side hole of the modified nasogastric tube through the GE sphincter. If the pressure is above 55 mm Hg the sutures are loosened. If it is below 30 mm Hg the sutures are tightened, depending on the problem at hand. After the proper pressure is obtained, all five sutures are tied and a final pressure measurement is taken (Fig. 3).

The barrier is about 3–4 cm in length. In addition to measuring the sphincter, the valve of His is accentuated by this procedure and can be readily palpated through the wall of the stomach. In patients who have had previous operations with scarring and destruction of the GE junction, the valve may be destroyed or inadequate. In these cases, a gastrotomy is performed and the valve is secured with sutures in the anterior and posterior edges of the valve, thereby lengthening the valve to 3–4 cm.

Attempts to calibrate the cardia with a bougie are unsatisfactory. It is difficult to determine whether the wrap around the bougie is tight or loose.

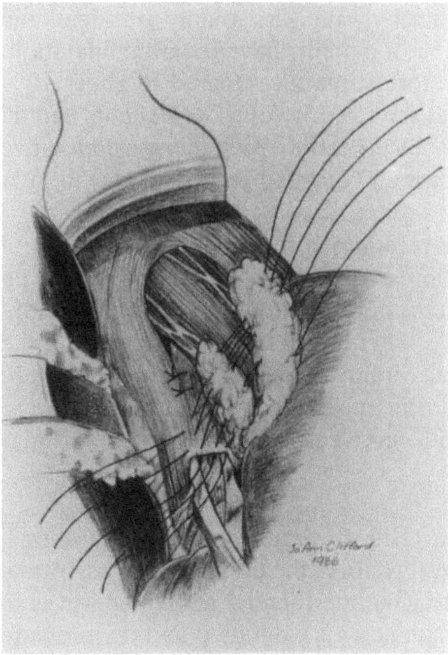

Fig. 2. The anterior and posterior phrenoesophageal bundles have been demonstrated and heavy, nonabsorbable, sutures are passed through the bundles and the preaortic fascia and median arcuate ligament

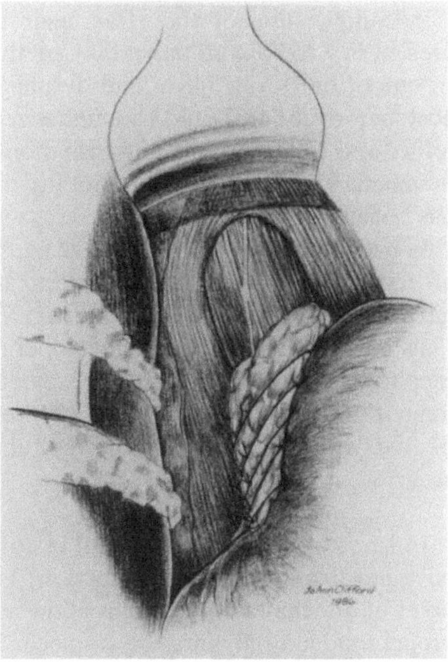

Fig. 3. The final appearance of the repair. The phrenoesophageal bundles are anchored securely to the preaortic fascia and the median arcuate ligament. The GE valve has been accentuated with tension on the collarsling musculature. The vagus nerves have been preserved

Results

The most important criterion of success of patients is patient satisfaction: if a patient is free of heartburn, can eat a full meal, can resume normal activity including bending over in the garden and indulging in strenous exercise without reflux or heartburn, then the operation should be considered a success. On the other hand, we have been particularly meticulous in our follow-up using pH and pressure studies two to three months after surgery whenever possible. In those patients who refuse pH and pressure studies, we obtain a GE tract x-ray series of scintiscan to test the effectiveness of the operation designed to curtain reflux.

Three major retrospective studies of the long-term effect of surgical treatment with the Hill repair have been performed by us in more than 1.300 patients out of 1.640 patients operated upon over a 24 year period.

The results are summarized as follows: excellent or good results have been obtained in over 95%, with a failure and recurrence rate of 1.5–5%. The complication and mortality rates have been very low, (0.2%), with one death in the last 500 operations for primary repairs. In 114 reoperations (mainly failed Nissen repairs) the mortality rate has been 1.7% and for strictures 0.5%.

A complication of the Hill repair has been dysphagia, usually transient and present in 5 to 20% of patients. Less than 5% of patients have required dilatation. In one of our series, 48% had dysphagia before surgery compared to about 20% postoperatively; it should be emphasized that the majority of those patients had no reflux and tolerated this new situation without dilatation. Whether postoperative dysphagia is due to persistent motility disorders and counted preoperatively in 41% has not yet been evaluated.

In over 1.600 operations we have had brisk bleeding from branches from the aorta or celiac artery in only 8 instances. Ligation of these vessels has produced no discernible complications. In one series 28% of our patients had pulmonary symptoms before surgery and 6% postoperatively. There have been 4 fistulas from the esophagus. Two of these were treated with drainage and expired. These were treated early in our experience before Celestin tubes were available. Two were treated with insertion of Celestin tube and survived. Only one of the fistulas occurred in a primary repair.

In summary, gastroesophageal restoration (Hill procedure) restores the normal posterior fixation of the GE junction. This also restores the esophagus to its normal point of attachment or fulcrum allowing it to generate forceful peristaltic waves to propel food aborally into the stomach. The sphincter is calibrated and the pressure measured so that a range of pressure is created that is high enough to prevent reflux but not so high as to create dysphagia. The acute angle of His is accentuated by stress on the collarsling musculature which restores the GE valve. The mortality and morbidity are low and the operation is reproducible in other hands with good results.

The Toupet procedure

J. Y. Barbin, J. G. Barbin, and *Ph. Chaillou* (Nantes)

In 1963, A. Toupet presented to the Academie de Chirurgie his technique of "esophagogastroplasty with phrenogastropexy employed in the radical cure of hiatus hernia and as an adjunct to Heller's operation in cardiospasm". He took the opportunity to review the anatomic basis of his technique in 1968 during a symposium on the treatment of hiatus hernia [12, 13].

Toupet's original technique [12] consisted of three stages:

- a first stage of freeing of the abdominal esophagus
- a second stage of freeing of the posterior aspect of the gastric fundus
- a third stage of esophago-gastroplasty with phreno-gastropexy.

After liberation of the abdominal esophagus, the second stage of Toupet's original technique consisted of freeing of the posterior surface of the gastric fundus. In this technique, the freeing was done from above downwards hugging the posterior surface of the stomach and directed downwards and inwards below the left gastropancreatic fold (sheath of the left gastric artery). Because of the danger of this to the spleen, which can be torn during this maneuver, and in particular to the superior polar vessels and the short gastric vessels, the author practices "almost routinely, section of the left gastric artery".

This stage, considered as of major importance, must be completed by section of the areolar-fatty tissue still attaching the upper part of the lesser curvature to the posterior abdominal wall, thus permitting very wide freeing of the posterior surface of the gastric fundus to right and left, and displaying well its posterior wall. After identification of the vagus nerves, which must in never be included in the sutures, the third stage consists of fixation of the gastric fundus to the right margin of the esophagus, followed by fixation of the fundus to the right pillar of the hiatus by 4 or 5 sutures, the upper stitch catching esophagus, fundus and pillar, and one stitch catching the fibrous portion of the aortic hiatus. It is then necessary to fix the fundus to the left crus of the diaphragm by separate sutures, beginning with the lowermost suture, then to fix the fundus to the left margin of the esophagus, and finally to fix the upper part of the esophagogastroplasty to the pre-esophageal peritoneum. If the esophageal hiatus is too wide, the pillars may be sutured together by one or two stitches in front of the esophagus (Figs. 1, 2).

This very attractive technique for treatment of uncomplicated hiatus hernia, thanks to its posterior half-valve, makes it unnecessary to attack the other fixation elements of the "abdominal esophagus" and the cardio-fundal region, often very defective, and to avoid the drawbacks of the fundoplication procedure described by Nissen and Rossetti. The importance of these methods of fixation has been described repeatedly and at length in the literature. Our concern is not to repeat this study, but to specify some very particular embryologic and anatomic points.

*

The organization of the esophago-fundal region and its relations with the diaphragm is very complex, resulting from the development of the esophagus and diaphragm, and from the modifications produced by the intra-embryonal celom.

As regards the esophagus [6], on the 32nd day (5 mm stage) the esophagus is a short narrow, tube, which will lengthen rapidly because of the development of the heart and thorax. At the 39th day (12 mm stage) the esophagus is pressed ventrally and to the left by the aorta. At the 18 mm stage the abdominal esophagus is well differentiated and clearly visible, but will regress progressively in the course of fetal life. The esophagus, as the embryonal digestive tube, is fixed to the posterior wall by a mesentery which is crossed at the level of the primitive posterior mesogastrium by two branches given from the celiac axis: cranially the left gastric artery, caudally the common hepatic artery.

The diaphragm is composed of elements of different embryonic origin [1]. It is identifiable very early, as from the 3rd week there develops a thick transverse mesodermal layer separating the vitelline stalk and the primordial cardiac and pericardiac structures. During the 4th week it forms an incomplete septum between the pericardial and peritoneal cavities. Its development continues dorsally with the periesophageal mesoderm, and thus with the primitive posterior mesoesophagus.

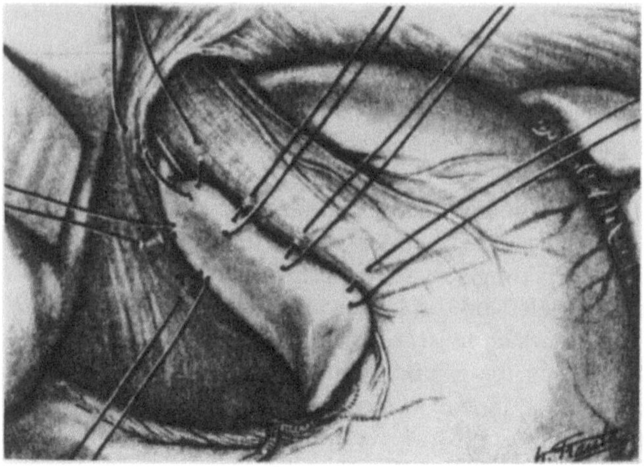

Fig. 1

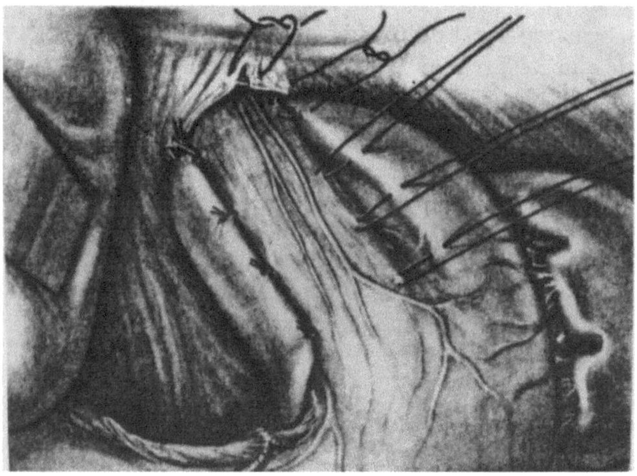

Fig. 2

Fig. 1, 2. Esophago-gastroplasty with phreno-gastropexy

From the 32nd day, the intraembryonic coelom is divided by the development of the transverse septum into a cranial pleuro-pericardial cavity and a caudal peritoneal cavity. It is very important to stress that in the median sagittal plane the septum transversum extends as far as the digestive tube, thus separating these two cavities along the median plane, which communicate laterally by the pericardio-peritoneal canal [6].

From the 34th day (7 mm stage) the pleuroperitoneal membranes appear, differentiating at the level of the septum transversum. All these elements are in place very early, even before the development of the lungs and the elongation of the esophagus, at a stage when this region corresponds to the 3rd, 4th and 5th cervical somites. A little later the development of the lungs and thorax displaces the pleuro-peritoneal membrane towards the caudal region. This membrane extends progressively, and closes completely around the 48th day (20 mm stage). The pleural and peritoneal cavities are then completely separated and it is only later that the peripheral part of the diaphragm progressively extends [6].

Thus, the ontogenesis led the classical authors to regard the definitive diaphragm as composed of the following components:

- an unpaired anterior portion derived from the septum transversum which will become the central tendon
- a second unpaired posterior portion originating the crura of the diaphragm, therefore derived from the periesophageal mesodermal tissue
- two paired dorsal portions derived from the pleuroperitoneal membranes which, during normal ontogenesis, become continuous with the dorsal and lateral part of the central tendon
- a peripheral portion arising from the progressive expansion of the pleuroperitoneal membrane and dependent on the somites.

Thus, there a continuous mesodermal layer of very early origin seems to exist, constituted by the septum transversum, which is extended into the periesophageal tissue dorsally, and laterally by the pleuroperitoneal layers. The early appearance of this transverse septum locates it opposite the cervical comites C3-C4-C5. It is from this period that the anterior motor branch of C4, and secondarily of C3 and C5, comes to join the homolateral septum, which explains the innervation of the diaphragm by the phrenic nerve.

Delattre and Hureau [6] even consider that there is a single muscular layer divided by the median sagittal plane into a right hemilamina, innervated by the right anterior primary branches of the spinal nerves C3-C4-C5 constituting the right phrenic nerve, and a left hemilamina likewise innervated by the left phrenic nerve. It is possible to consider the lumbar (prevertebral) portion of the diaphragm as an unpaired rudiment derived, as we have seen, from the periesophageal mesodermal tissue. Delattre and Hureau [6] find this difficult, since two fibromuscular components exist in the adult, one situated to the right of the esophagus and innervated by the right phrenic nerve, and the other on the left, innervated by the left phrenic nerve.

As shown by Boutelier [4], this embryologic element, known as the posterior mesentery of the esophagus, plays a special part in fixation of the esophagus around the esophageal hiatus. Let us note that Delattre and Hureau [6] consider that this cellulo-fibrous layer, containing no vessels between the aorta and the terminal portion of the esophagus, should no longer be given this name. In fact, as already noted, it constitutes the prolongation of the mediastinal mesoesophagus, displaced somewhat to the right due to gastric rotation, which produces slight rotation of the lower part of the esophagus. This posterior mesoesophagus cannot be isolated from the cellulofibrous tissue that is continuous on the right with the lesser omentum in its most cranial portion (pars condensa); a defect in this means of fixation, whether due to embryologic causes or ageing, in certain morphotypes and in certain forms of respiration, would explain the creation of this intramediastinal gastric "prolapse", as Toupet has suggested [13]. This would seem to exclude the possibility of looking to these structures to refix the esophageal-cardiac-fundal region.

This periesophageal tissue extends downwards in the retroperitoneal region as far as the left gastro-pancreatic ligaments, the cranial limit of the entry into the caudal recess of the omental bursa (epiploic foramen). We have seen that certain authors (Nissen, Toupet) [10, 12] advise section of this ligament, yet its the anatomic arrangement does not seem to confirm the hypothesis that it constitutes an important means of fixation of the esophageal-cardiac-fundal region. Indeed, its concave orientation downwards does not seem capable of resisting ascent of the cardia. Further, during surgical treatment of hiatus hernia, it seems that there has been an elongation of the left gastric vascular elements. It therefore seems unnecessary to sacrifice this artery.

Again, during the freeing of the lower part of the esophagus it soon becomes apparent that the structures fixing the region of the cardia are constituted much more by the nervous structures of the posterior and anterior vagus than by vascular elements. It is their placing under tension that limits the bringing down of the cardia.

This periesophageal tissue is extended to the left by the gastrophrenic ligament. This more or less developed ligament is continuous to the left with the pancreato-splenic and gastro-splenic ligaments. The short gastric vessels travel within this ligament, and this often necessitates their section between two ligatures.

At its upper part, the gastric fundus rests directly on the diaphragm and is closely applied to this in the gap between the two sheets of the gastro-phrenic ligament, by means of fibrous tissue (the former suspensory ligament of the stomach of Gregoire). Laterally, the two peritoneal layers of the gastro-phrenic ligament are applied to each other and are continuous with the two layers of the phrenicosplenic ligament. Medially, the inferior layer of the gastro-phrenic ligament is continuous with the left layer of the left gastropancreatic ligament, and the superior layer with the left layer of the "mesoesophagus".

In addition, we have shown [2] that the crura of the diaphragm are normally powerful muscular structures, as witnessed by the depth of their attachments to the dorsolumbar spine, much more marked on the right than the left. The lesser importance of the left crus results from the lateralization of the aorta to the left, but nonetheless it is functionally important. The esophageal hiatus constitutes the diaphragmatic canal and, like Delmas [7] and Delattre and Hureau [6], we believe there is no abdominal esophagus but certainly a diaphragmatic esophagus, the abdominal esophagus only being created during dissection by rupture of the periesophageal cellulo-fibrous structures. The abdominal esophagus sems to us to be an artefact of dissection.

We have also shown [2] that at the moment of deep inspiration, the contraction of the crura fixes the entire central zone of the diaphragm, immobilized between the two domes. It is their action that ensures the amplitude of respiratory movements, but the central portion of the diaphragm on which the heart rests, and which is traversed by the inferior vena cava in its foramen obviously cannot follow the movement of the domes. The inferior vena cava traverses an inflexible fibrous canal, which is functionally explicable. The periesophageal diaphragmatic structures allow the esophagus a certain degree of freedom and maintain an anatomic and functional equilibrium in this conflicting zone, which resists reflux while allowing esophageal movement.

Thus, during contraction of the crura of the diaphragm in the course of deep inspiration there is an undeniable "lasso" effect; the cardia is drawn downward and

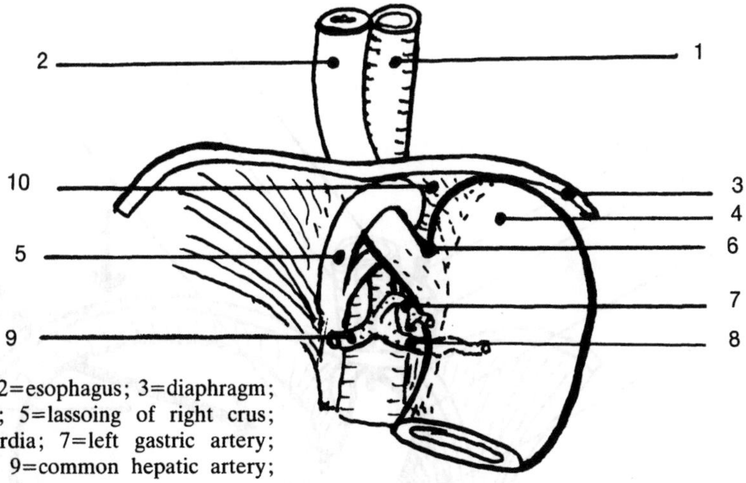

Fig. 3. 1=aorta; 2=esophagus; 3=diaphragm; 4=gastric fundus; 5=lassoing of right crus; 6=incision of cardia; 7=left gastric artery; 8=splenic artery; 9=common hepatic artery; 10=left crus of diaphragm

backward, whatever the variability of anatomic constitution of the lasso. Contraction of this pillar by its pre- and retroesophageal elements would risk considerable reduction of the esophageal lumen if the synchronous contraction of the left crus, whose fibers are attached to the left component of the right crus did not exert an adjustment permitting persistent equilibrium in this region (Fig. 3).

In the functional study of the diaphragm [2] we showed that because of the fixation of the central part of the muscle and the play of the domes of the diaphragm, the gastric fundus attached to the dome by the phrenogastric ligament and lodged under the dome was subject to the lowering of the dome in deep inspiration. In this movement the gastric fundus is lowered and must be displaced downward and to the right, i.e. it must close the cardiac incisura (angle of His) (Fig. 4). This has been confirmed by Delattre [6]. Thus, during deep inspiration, added to contraction of the diaphragmatic lasso and the balancing of this contraction by the left crus there is a gliding movement of the gastric fundus to the right, accentuating or restoring the normality of the cardio-esophageal angle.

*

We may conclude from this brief ontogenic and anatomic review:

- that there is anatomo-embryologic unity between the crura of the diaphragm and the other so-called means of fixation of the esophageal-cardiac-fundal region
- that fixation of the central median sagittal part of the diaphragm by contraction of the crura allows normal play of the domes
- that the harmonious contraction of the two crura straightens the esophagus sagitally in its lower portion
- that normally no anatomic abdominal esophagus exists. This abdominal portion of the esophagus can come into existence only through failure of the constituent elements of the diaphragmatic canal, consisting of the esophageal hiatus and the surrounding cellulo-fibrous structures, or through the artifice of dissection.

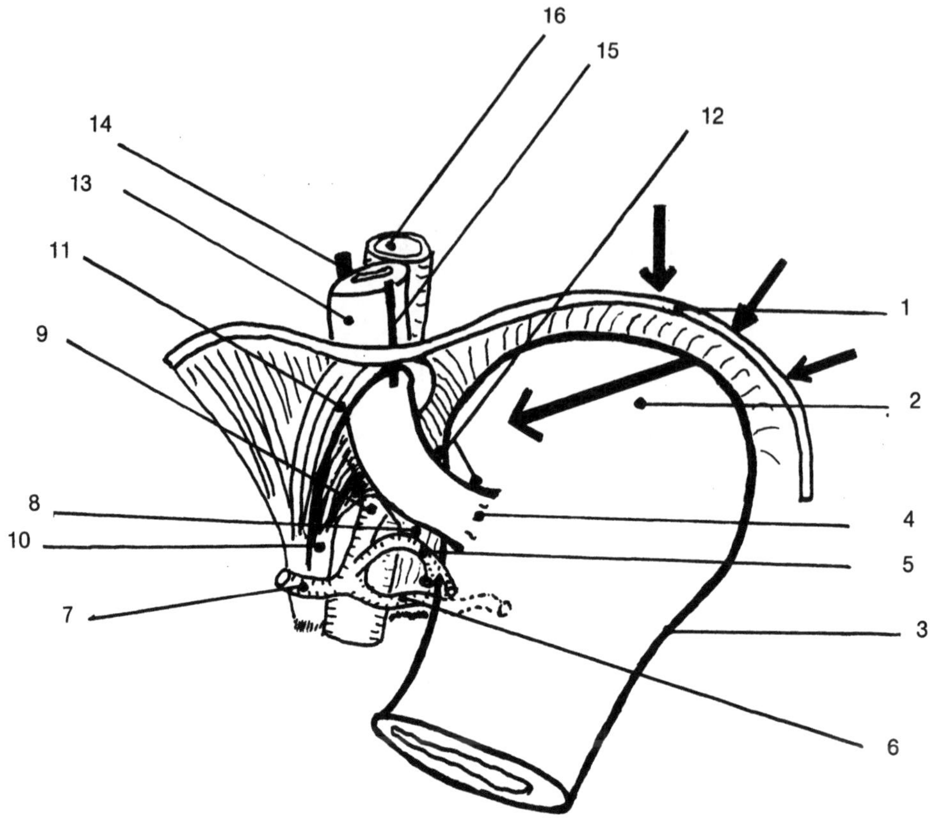

Fig. 4. 1=left dome of diaphragm; 2=gastric fundus; 3=greater curvature; 4=cardia 5=left gastric artery; 6=splenic artery; 7=common hepatic artery; 8=left crus of diaphragm; 9=celiac trunk; 10=right crus of diaphragm; 11=lasso; 12=cardiac notch; 13=esophagus; 14=right vagus nerve; 15=left vagus nerve; 16=aorta

- that the antireflux system also consists of a movement of the fundus towards the esophagus during inspiration, reconstituting the cardio-esophageal angle (of His) to prevent gastroesophageal reflux, while recognizing the existence of a zone of high pressure in the distal part of the esophagus due to the complex ensemble of intrinsic and extrinsic factors (respiration, quality of the crura of the diaphragm) [2].

Restoration of the cardio-esophageal angle has been proposed by many authors, particularly by Lortat-Jacob, taking into account the normal gliding movement of the fundus towards the left margin of the lower esophagus, whose abnormal mobility due to failure of the "continent" system may be made good, where this is possible, by repair of the crura of the diaphragm behind the esophagus. The techniques described by different authors (Boerema, Pedinielli) address this reconstruction of the cardio-esophageal angle.

These procedures may be supplemented by a gastrophrenopexy restoring the anatomic relations between the gastric fundus and left dome of the diaphragm.

When the lower esophagus has been dissected to create an abdominal esophagus, and if there is no wish to deal with the so-called fixational structures of the esophagus, then the cardio-esophageal angle must be restored by accentuating the movement of the gastric fundus from left to right to a greater degree than Lortat-Jacob's technique provides. It is the importance of this gliding movement of the fundus towards the esophagus that gave rise to the techniques of fundoplication (Nissen and Rossetti, Dor, Toupet) [10, 12]. Toupet's procedure has inspired other workers (Vayre, Hureau, Roux, Boutelier) [14, 15, 16, 4]. These techniques have in common the "taming" of this movement of the fundus in more or less ample fashion to allow permanent contact between the fundus and the dissected abdominal esophagus, which generally makes it unnecessary to touch the other structures of the esophageal-cardiac-fundal region.

Thus, in order to slip the gastric fundus behind the esophagus over a depth sufficient for permanent contact between the two organs, the esophagus must be afforded a certain length. It is essential to dissect it from the inframediastinal space to the subperitoneal abdominal region after incision of the peritoneum, as specified by Barraya and Carles [3]. In this way an abdominal esophagus created or lengthened. Whether this fundoplication is total (Nissen and Rossetti) [10], anterior (Dor) or a posterior half-valve (Toupet) [12], its success requires dissection of the lower esophagus.

The originality of Toupet's procedure lies in that it combines the gliding of the fundus from left to right with substitution of the support structures, since it fixes the fundus to the crura of the diaphragm. Vayre and Hureau fix the fundus to the crura with repair of the cardio-esophageal angle in a single common plane, which is the simplest procedure, but the fixation may just as well be made to the right crus when this appears to be the more valid structure.

It is possible to secure fixation to the crura, with repair of the cardio-esophageal angle in two separate planes by suturing the right posterior part of the fundus, usually to the right crus if this is of good quality.

The construction of a valve by slipping the fundus from left to right behind the esophagus requires section of the gastrophrenic ligament, which is of varying extent, as we have seen.

However, it should be noted that in the technique described by Nissen and Rossetti [10], after dissection of the esophagus, the noose passed round it produces a fold on the anterior aspect of the fundus, which is brought upwards behind the esophagus and which must provide the material necessary to surround it through 360°. If this maneuver is impossible, Nissen and Rossetti [10] advise opening the upper part of the omental bursa to expose the posterior aspect of the stomach, but it is then necessary to divide the upper part of the gastrohepatic ligament (pars condensa of the lesser omentum) between two ligatures.

These authors state that division of vessels must extend as far as the left gastric artery, whose chief branches must be respected. Then, by sliding a hand over the posterior aspect of the fundus, a gastric fold must be created behind the cardia to make the fundoplication.

Toupet's technique [12] likewise requires vascular freeing of the fundus and cardiac region descending down the lesser curvature as far as the left gastric artery inclusive. This also applies to the procedures derived from that of Toupet.

To avoid the problems created by maneuvers executed so close to the spleen and avoid ligature of the short gastric vessels, one of us (J. G. Barbin) has suggested passing via the inferior omental recess to reach the omental bursa. Access to this is easy below the arterial circle of the greater curvature. The incision of the gastrocolic ligament must be wide enough to admit the hand.

*

The technique we employ is as follows:

The approach is bisubcostal, giving an excellent exposure of the subdiaphragmatic region to be operated on after retraction of the costal margin. The patient is tilted head downwards. The left triangular ligament of the liver is divided. The esophagus is dissected in the classical manner, but the posterior vagus is left on the medial aspect of the right crus of the diaphragm where it lies. Once the esophagus is on a noose, the gastrohepatic ligament must be incised in its upper part (pars condensa of the lesser omentum) as far as, but respecting, the left gastric artery. This permits better dissection of the crura and freeing of the esophagus from the cellulo-fibrous tissue that surrounds it, the residue of the posterior mesoesophagus that tethers it more or less loosely laterally and behind.

The second stage consists of opening the inferior omental recess below the vascular circle of the greater curvature. The avascular adhesions joining the posterior stomach wall to the posterior parietal peritoneum in the omental bursa are freed. These ties are avascular; if not, one is in the transverse mesocolon. One thus arrives from below upward at the right part of the gastrophrenic ligament. This ligament is not attached to the upper border of the fundus but to its posterior aspect, due to embryologic peritoneal fusion obliterating the summit of the omental bursa. Section of the right part of the gastrophrenic ligament communicates the omental bursa with the zone of cardio-esophageal freeing. It is then sufficient to use the right hand to displace the posterior aspect of the stomach from below upwards, and slightly from left to right (Fig. 5).

A great deal of stomach substance is then available without any attention to the spleen or short gastric vessels. The spreading of the posterior surface of the stomach behind the fundus permits the latter to come to lie very largely behind the esophagus and cardia and to the right of the esophagus. This gastric "bursa" is sutured to the right crus of the diaphragm according to the technique of Toupet. It then becomes evident that the amount of gastric substance so carried upwards widely overlaps the esophagus, both to the right and to the left, and comes spontaneously, extensively and without any traction in contact with the gastric "bursa" situated to the right of the esophagus (Fig. 6).

It only remains to join the two gastric bursae by catching the right margin of the esophagus between them. The right vagus is left on the medial aspect of the right crus; the left vagus, on the anterior left face of the esophagus, is not involved in this suture. If so desired, a gastrophrenopexy can be made subsequently. Toupet, in his report to the Académie de Chirurgie [12], compared sliding hiatus hernia to genital prolapse, and his suggested treatment for this condition to a "pexy obliteration of

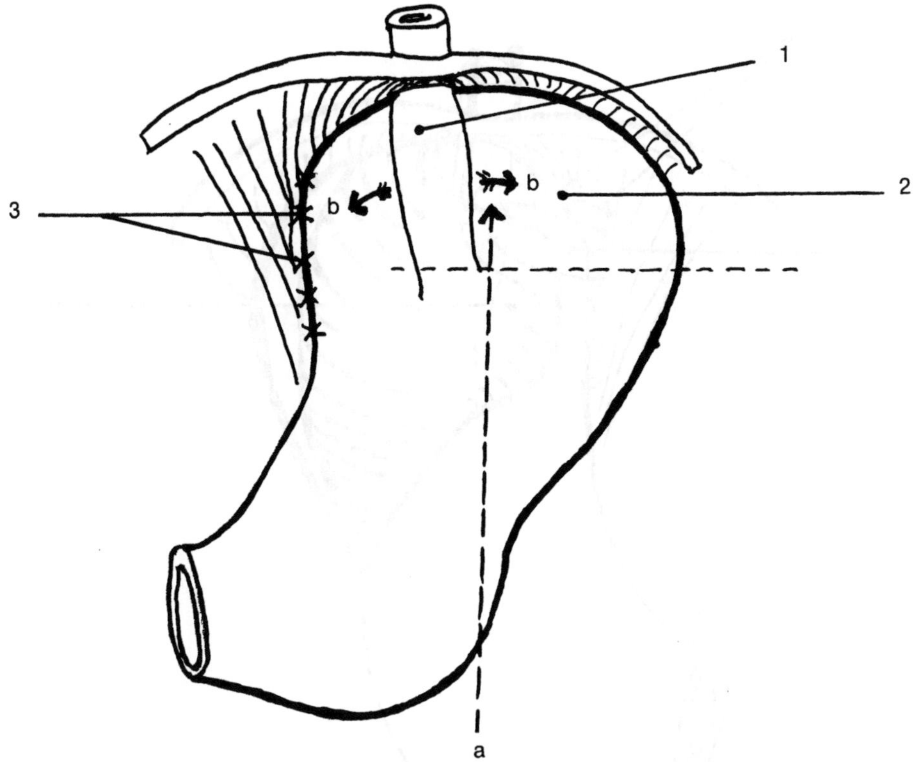

Fig. 5. Upward displacement of the gastric fundus by unfolding of the posterior aspect of the stomach. 1=esophagus; 2=gastric fundus; 3=suture of "right gastric bursa" to right crus of diaphragm
The arrow a) represents the action of the right hand passed into the omental bursa to unfold the posterior face of the stomach. This extends widely to right and left of the esophagus: arrows b)

the cul de sac, and freshening of the deperitonealized surfaces", the suture of the esophageal orifice being secondary.

The aim of our method is to deal with this very real "fundal prolapse" by a kind of columnization (identical with that proposed by Muller and Savariaud for genital prolapse), thus fixing the esophageal cardiac fundal region. As Toupet had recommended, this technique comprises of:

- freeing the abdominal esophagus, leaving the right vagus on the right crus of the diaphragm
- a stage of freeing the posterior aspect of the stomach, but effected here by freeing the entire posterior surface of the body of the stomach, approached by opening the gastrocolic ligament at the inferior border of the greater curvature, so allowing access to the inferior omental recess and the omental bursa.

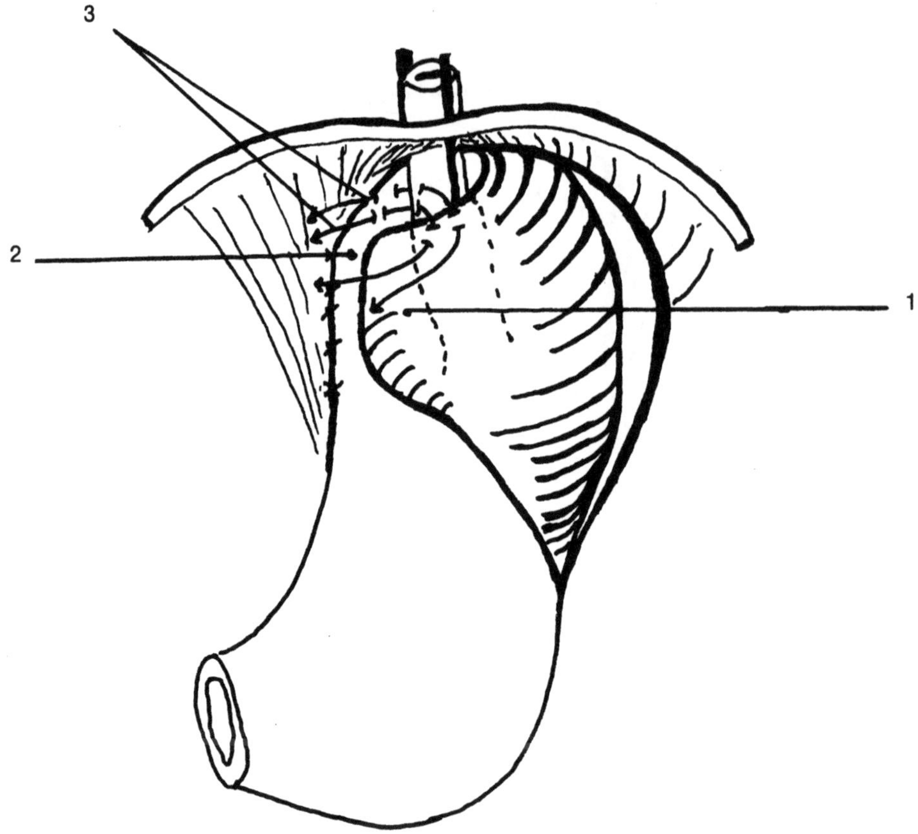

Fig. 6. Construction of the gastroesophagopexy and of the gastrophrenopexy. 1=Left gastric bursa brought in front of the esophagus and sutured to the right gastric bursa; 2=right gastric bursa sutured to right crus of diaphragm; 3=sutures catching the left and anterior bursa, the right margin of the esophagus and the right and posterior bursa

This stage of freeing the posterior aspect of the stomach and fundus is made from below upwards, and no longer from above downwards, and vertically and not from left to right – a stage of esophagogastroplasty, joining the two pre- and retroesophageal gastric bursas with the right margin of the esophagus, and a phrenogastropexy that attaches the fundus only to the right crus of the diaphragm. Thus, the cardioesophageal angle (of His) is perfectly reconstructed.

Thus, attracted by the considerable advantages of the procedure described by Toupet, but at grips with certain stout and deep patients, "poorly welcomed" by the left hypochondrium (Jourdan), we have sought an easier approach to the fundus. The direct approach to the inferior omental recess via the gastrocolic ligament and the very bringing upward of the posterior aspect of the stomach has greatly helped us in constructing the posterior valve called for by Toupet. But this route of approach has allowed us to state that an anterior valve places itself spontaneously in position, so that we only need to make use of the facility offered by the anatomy.

*

Thus, this method combines the procedure of a posterior valve fixed to the right crus of the diaphragm with a Nissen type of fundoplication; this makes it possible to attach the two half-valves together and to join them with the right margin of the esophagus, without worrying about the vagi and without the problems raised by Nissen's technique.

We have found this method easy to perform and the immediate results very favorable; but we need much more perspective to assess the late results, as is the case for all the procedures attacking the problem of hiatus hernia.

This is why we readily conclude, with Rudler, that "it is enough to have experienced the history of the surgery of hiatus hernia from its outset, that is, to have witnessed the birth and disappearance of numerous operative procedures, to be persuaded that we shall see still new ones appear that will be abandoned in their turn. It may be that we shall never find a satisfactory technique for every case".

References

1. Barbin JY, Barbin JG, Collin C, Armstrong O (1985) Embryologie du diaphragme. 7e réunion du Groupe de recherches et d'études de la paroi abdominale. Juin
2. Barbin JY, Barbin JG, Collin C, Armstrong O (1985) Essai d'anatomie fonctionnelle du diaphragme. Société anatomique de Paris. Juillet
3. Barraya L, Carles R Hernie diaphragmatique de l'adulte. Encycl Méd Chir Paris. Techniques chirurgicales appareil digestif 4, 3.03, fasc 40–250, 25–42
4. Boutelier Ph, Lefort R (1970) Etude anatomique du "méso-oesophage abdominal". Déductions chirurgicales. J Chir 100, 5: 371–384
5. Carey JM, Hollineshead WH (1955) Anatomy of the oesophageal hiatus related to repair of hiatle hernia. Proceedings of the staff meetings of the Mayo Clinic, 30, 11: 223–226
6. Delattre JF (1984) Les piliers du diaphragme et la traversée diaphragmatique de l'œsophage. Application au reflux gastro-œsophagien et à son traitement chirurgical Mémoire pour le D.E.R.B.H. Laboratoire d'anatomie d'U.E.R. Bio-médicale des Saint Pères (Professeur Hureau J) Paris
7. Delmas A, Roux J (1938) Les gaines de l'œsophage diaphragmatique. Ann D'an path 15, 6: 635–640
8. Hill LD, Tobias J, Morgan EH (1966) Newer 37 Concepts of the Pathophysiology of hiatal hernia and oesophagitis. Am the Journ surg 111: 70–79
9. Marchand E (1959) Anatomy of oesophageal hiatus of the diaphragm and pathogenesis of hiatus herniation. J thoracic surg 37, 1: 81–92
10. Nissen R, Rossetti M (1965) Surgery of hiatal and other diaphragmatic hernias. J of the international Coll of surg 43, 6: 663–674
11. Schwarz GS (1967) Historical aspect of the anatomy of the cardia with special references to hiatus hernia. Bull NY Acad Méd 43, 2: 112–125
12. Toupet A (1963) Technique d'œsophago-gastroplastie avec phréno-gastropexie appliquée dans la cure radicale des hernies hiatales et comme complément de l'opération de Heller dans les cardiospasmes. Mém Acad Chir n° 11–12–13: 374–399
13. Toupet A (1968) Les hernies hiatales non compliquées. Anatomie chirurgicale Méd et Hyg (Genève), 26, 26: 831, 786–787, Méd Prati novembre 1968, 24: 344–347
14. Vayre P, Hureau J (1968) Cure chirurgicale des hernies hiatales dites par glissement chez l'adulte. Presse Méd 76, 19: 925–927

15. Vayre P, Hureau J, Roux M (1969) La cure chirurgicale des hernies hiatales de l'adulte. Faits anatomiques et pathologiques. Déductions thérapeutiques à propos de 212 cas opérés. Arch Franc Mal appar dig 58, 3: 184–185
16. Vayre P, Hureau J (1975) La cardio-gastro-phrénopexie par voie abdominale. Méd Chir dig 4: 175–179

What is the effect of an antireflux procedure on esophageal dyskinesis?

P. Denis, J. Y. Touchais, F. Michot, and *P. Ténière* (Rouen)

The problem posed is the risk of postoperative dyskinesia when the operation includes the risk of contributing an additional obstacle to the progression of the alimentary bolus. This question is often raised, since the probability of dyskinesia increases with the degree of esophagitis [1], progression towards a peptic stenosis is more frequent in cases of esophageal motor disorders [2]. In addition to the dyskinesia related to the actual reflux, indications for antireflux surgery may occur in patients with a motility disorder, e.g. scleroderma or peripheral nervous disorder, or when the antireflux action is combined with cardiomyotomy. Finally, it is important to bear in mind that 25% of subjects oder than 60 with no digestive symptoms present esophageal peristalsis anomalies [3].

When the dyskinesia results from reflux, it is tempting to think that the disappearance of the reflux after surgery will correct the motility disorders. The amplitude and duration of manometric contraction can thus be rendered normal by a fundoplication [4], although the propagation velocity remains abnormal (Table 1) [4]. In addition, the aperistaltic esophagus remains in that state after surgery and the

Table 1. Postoperative frequency of dysphagia, not correlated with anomalies of the main esophagus

	Nissen fundoplication	
Esophageal contractions	Gill. Gastroenterology 1986	Eckardt Gastroenterology 1977
Amplitude	↗	→
Duration	↗	→
Velocity of propagation	→	→
Preoperative absence of peristalsis, unimproved after operation		

esophagus of some patients becomes aperistaltic after the operation [4]. Although no correlation with the persistence of a dysphagia has been observed [4], it appeared necessary to attract attention to the non confirmation of those results by others [5], and to the possibility of the occurrence of radiological megaesophagus with peristaltism and severe dysphagia in five personal cases after Nissen's operation (Fig. 1).

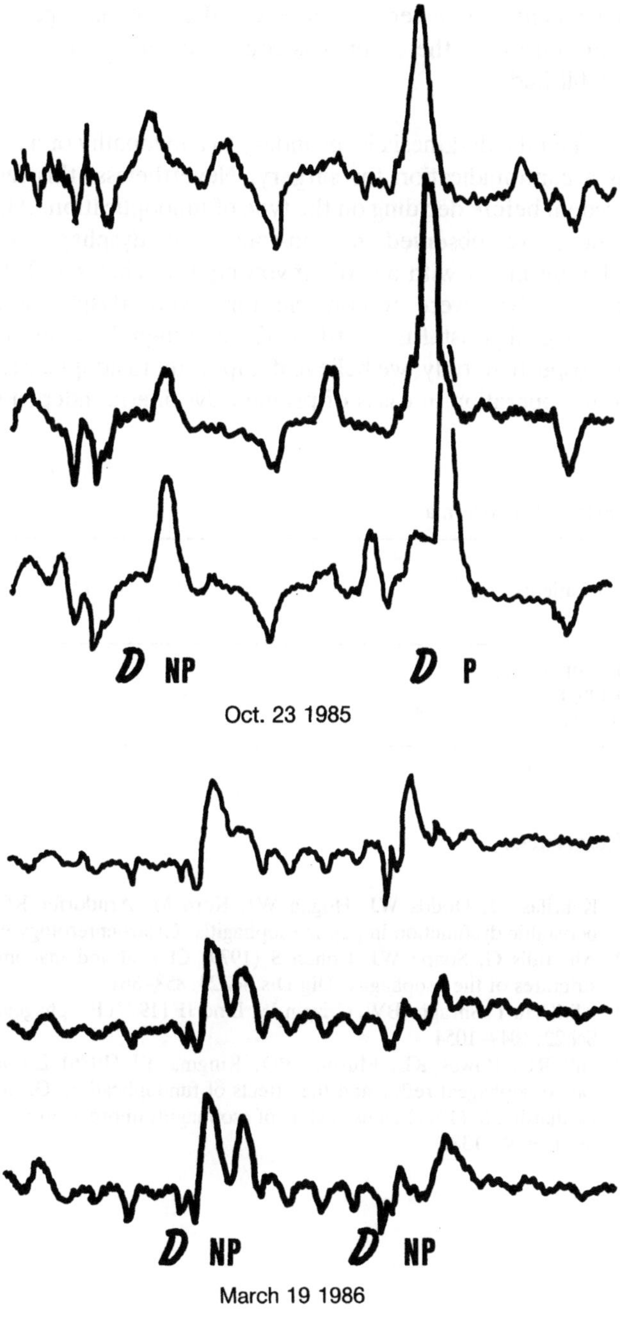

Fig. 1. Preoperative curve from a patient showing by way of example on the right a propagated response to swallowing (P) and on the left a non propagated response of low amplitude (NP)
After a Nissen operation, all the responses to swallowing are of low amplitude and non propagated, coinciding with the development of megaesophagus as shown radiologically

Preoperative manometry in these cases had shown the existence of repetitive or simultaneous contractions, or of motor coordination disorders. This type of preoperative anomaly currently does not lead to the prediction of an unambiguous occurrence of complications, since they may be related to the reflux itself and thus corrected by the operation. In the context of a gastroesophageal reflux today, it is very difficult to affirm if this type of anomaly is a motility disorder which is dependent or independent of acid reflux. The exaggeration of these anomalies by acid infusion of the esophagus could have a predictive value, which remains to be established.

When the dyskinesia is secondary to a myopathy or a neuropathy, it was not taken as a contraindication for surgery. Nevertheless, this factor should be taken into account before deciding on the type of fundoplication. After Toupet's hemifundoplication, we observed no postoperative dysphagia in patients afflicted with scleroderma or with a cardiomyotomy for achalasia (Table 2). On the other hand, larger valves were responsible for severe dysphagia in the elderly presenting esophageal peristalsis disorders. Even though these observations are clinical and not a prospective study, we believe it important to adopt a cautious attitude in the choice of the operation in cases of primary dyskinesia independent of reflux.

Table 2. Scleroderma

• 7 Patients:	HFP 180°: n=6	
	HFP 270°: n=1	
post-operatory	HFP: 180°	HFP: 270°
pH metry	N	N
Dysphagia	Abs.	Severe

References

1. Kahrilas PJ, Dodds WJ, Hogan WJ, Kern M, Arndorfer RC, Reece A (1986) Esophageal peristaltic dysfunction in peptic esophagitis. Gastroenterology 91: 897–904
2. Ahtaridis G, Snape WJ, Cohen S (1979) Clinical and manometric findings in benign peptic strictures of the esophagus. Dig Dis Sci 24: 858–861
3. Ali Khan T, Shragge BW, Crispin JS, Lind JF (1977) Esophageal motility in the elderly. Dig Dis Sci 22: 1049–1054
4. Gill RC, Bowes KL, Murphy PD, Kingma YJ (1986) Esophageal motor abnormalities in gastroesophageal reflux and the effects of fundoplication. Gastroenterology 91: 364–369
5. Eckhardt US, (1977) Does healing of esophagitis improve esophageal motor function? Gastroenterology 92: 1380

When is it appropriate to add vagotomy to an antireflux procedure?

J. H. Alexandre, and *J. L. Bouillot* (Paris)

Despite the numerous techniques put forward, it is still difficult to obtain more than 85% of good results after the surgical treatment of peptic esophagitis due to gastroesophageal reflux [19, 1]. The failures of treatment are associated with technical imperfections responsible for recurrence or with residual hyperacidity.

Choice of best valvular system

Two main procedures for the treatment of gastroesophageal reflux by the abdominal route have been proposed: esophago-cardio-fundal fixation as illustrated by Hill's procedure and the so-called "valvular" techniques. These latter create a zone of high pressure at the level of the abdominal esophagus, so re-establishing the correct functional conditions for the inferior esophageal sphincter and resisting gastroesophageal reflux. This increase in the pressure of the inferior sphincter of the esophagus (LES) has been demonstrated in numerous studies [4, 20]. Two valvular procedures are currently in use, that of Nissen and that of Toupet.

Nissen's operation, proposed in 1956 and modified by Rossetti in 1966, employs a fundal valve entirely surrounding the esophagus. It is credited with 85% of good results and with less than 5% of late recurrences, but the postoperative complications are high (30%) with a reoperation rate of 2 to 8% [5, 8]. Late functional disorders are serious. In a series of 226 patients Negre found 46% with changed bowel habits, 38% with abdominal meteorism, 31% with inability to vomit, 9% unable to eructate and 12% with epigastric pain, the overall symptomatology being a nuisance in 26% of cases and disabling in 10% of patients [15].

The functional sequelae of this operation seem to be linked to several factors:

1. a valve system that is too tight around the esophagus, despite shortness of the valve (a valve of over 4 cm is responsible for even more frequent dysphagia)
2. traumatic lesions of the vagus nerves. True gastric ulcers occurring after Nissen's operation have been reported, due either to direct injuries of the vagus nerves or to a preexistent pyloric lesion [7, 9, 14]
3. disorders of esophageal motility not recognized at the time of operation and appearing subsequently [8].

Critical analysis of Toupet's operation shows that it produces a disguised selective vagotomy by extensive freeing of the lesser gastric curvature and ligature of the left gastric pedicle [24]. Dissection of the hernial funnel and of the periesophageal sleeve inevitably necessitates incision of the "pars condensa", producing contusion, displacement or section of a certain number of nerve fibers. These are fibers of the right vagus going to the esophagus and the lesser curvature or fibers of the left vagis going to the liver, gallbladder and duodenum. In many cases this results in a blind partial vagotomy, which may even amount to pure and simple section of the nerve of

Latarjet. Toupet's operation includes a complementary pyloroplasty. The sequelae of this pyloroplasty seem to us to proscribe this maneuver, but we retain from the original technique the freeing of a very large gastric valve without dissection of the fundus, a posterior valve which is sutured to the right crus of the diaphragm.

Arguments for associated hyperselective vagotomy

Studies dealing with vagotomies associated with the cure of gastroesophageal reflux are rare [11, 16, 18, 21, 25, 26]. The great majority of authors mention its importance only in cases of postoperative recurrence. The efficacy of hyperselective vagotomy in the control of gastric acidity no longer needs demonstrating, and antiulcer drugs (cimetidine, ranitidine) are prescribed in over a half of the patients with esophagitis.

Hyperselective vagotomy does not alter the functioning of the LES, as many studies show [20, 23]. The only risk of this combined maneuver is of producing serious devascularization of the lesser curvature which could bring about its necrosis [13, 21]. The effectiveness of such vagotomy in the control of reflux has been proved retrospectively by the work of Csendes et al., who found symptomatology of reflux in almost 40% of patients needing operation for peptic ulcer, and in whom the esophageal symptoms regressed after vagotomy [3].

This vagotomy does not involve the pylorus, so avoiding the alkaline reflux responsible for some forms of severe esophagitis and for some bad results of truncal vagotomy associated with the cure of hiatus hernia [17, 25]. However, the long-term consequences of digestive anacidity are still not well-known.

Finally, the performance of highly selective vagotomy facilitates the technical construction of the posterior valve, which is to ensheath the esophagus over 270 to 330° [12]. In practice, faced with gastroesophageal reflux responsible for esophagitis and not regressing under medical treatment, we investigate the reflux by fiberoscopy with biopsies, a barium study to check reflux, esophago-gastric scintigraphy to provide information on possible disorder of esophageal motility, quantifying the degree of reflux and the speed of gastric emptying, and finally measurement of pH over 24 hours is required particularly when alkaline reflux esophagitis is suspected [6].

Technique employed

Midline supra-umbilical incision. After freeing the left triangular ligament, the stomach – elevated on a Faucher's tube – is drawn downwards as a whole. The highly selective vagotomy is begun at the level of the pes anserinus, as for duodenal ulcer, and then one ascends along the lesser curvature to free this completely in two or three planes. The dissection is taken up to the right margin of the esophagus, which is isolated and placed on a noose. Some peritoneal folds and adhesions are freed and sectioned at the fundus. After identification of the crura, these are sutured with a few nonabsorbable stitches. The posterior valve is then constructed by traction on the posterior aspect of the fundus and sutured to the right crus by four nonabsorbable stitches. The set-up is always well vascularized, without retroesophageal stricture, the valve measuring 6 to 7 cm. Its anterior portion is then fixed to the antero-right border of the esophagus. A third series of stitches joins the upper part of the fundus to the upper part of the left crus of the diaphragm and to the adjacent esophagus, performing envelopment of the left margin of the esophagus. The Faucher tube is removed and replaced by a stomach tube to ensure, by a routine methylene-blue test, that no tear of the esophagus should pass unnoticed. The lesser curvature is peritonized and the abdomen closed without drainage. The set-up is checked routinely by barium study and scintigraphy at the 8th postoperative day.

Using this technique, we have operated on 26 patients of average age 49.2 years during the last 3 years. All had preoperative fiberoscopy and scintigraphy. In more recent cases, measurement of pH has been routinely requested. There has been no postoperative mortality and no major complications have ensued. All patients were subjected to postoperative radiologic and scintigraphic monitoring.

At the functional level, all the patients have been improved, even though postoperative exploration showed persistence of reflux (though of less severity) in 5 cases. One patient had a poor result, as assessed by fiberoscopy, radiography and scintigraphy. This failure may be explained by a major postoperative gastric paresis, possibly connected with truncal section of the vagi.

References

1. Belsey RHR (1980) Gastroesophageal reflux. Am J Surg 139: 775–781
2. Braasch JW, Sala LE, Ellis HF Jr et al (1980) Parietal cell vagotomy. Its effect on lower oesophageal sphincter function. Arch Surg 115: 699–701
3. Csendes A, Oster M, Moller JT et al (1978) Gastroesophageal reflux in duodenal ulcer patients before and after vagotomy. Ann Surg 188: 804–808
4. DeMeester TR, Wang CL, Vernly JA et al (1980) Technique, indications and clinical use of 24 hour esophageal pH monitoring. J Thorac Cardiovasc Surg 79: 656–670
5. Festen C (1981) Paraesophageal hernia: a major complication of Nissen's fundoplication. J Oed Surg 16: 496–499
6. Galmiche JP, Denis P, Desechalliers JP (1981) Valeur des examens complémentaires au cours du reflux gastro-oesophagien de l'adulte. Gastroentérol Clin Biol 5: 1014–1025
7. Gay RJ, Tuner LJ, Doubek LJ (1978) Gastric ulceration after fundoplication for gastroesophageal reflux. Langenbecks Arch Chir 347: 311–315
8. Gelfand MD (1981) Irreversible esophageal motor dysfunction in postvagotomy dysphagia. Am J Gastroenterol 76: 347–350
9. Herrington JL, Meacham PW, Hunter R (1970) Gastric ulceration after fundic wrapping. Ann Surg 172: 638–651
10. Hocking MP, Maher JW, Woodward ER (1982) Definitive surgical therapy for incapaciting "gas bloat" syndrome. Am Surgeon 48: 131–133
11. Jones NAG, Anders CJA (1979) A new approach to the surgical treatment of reflux oesophagitis. Ann R Coll Surg Engl 61: 48–50
12. Jordan PH Jr (1978) Parietal cell vagotomy facilitates fundoplication in the treatment of reflux esophagitis. Surg Gynecol Obste 147: 593–595
13. Kennedy T, Magill P, Johnston GW, Parks TG (1979) Proximal gastric vagotomy fundoplication and lesser-curve necrosis. Br Med J 1: 1455–1456
14. Maher JW, Cerda JJ (1982) The role of gastric stasis in the genesis of gastric ulceration following fundoplication. World J Surg 6: 794–799

15. Negre JB (1983) Post fundoplication symptoms. Do they restrict the success of Nissen fundoplication. Ann Surg 198: 698–700
16. Oster MJ, Csendes A, Funch-Jensen P et al (1982) Parietal cell vagotomy and modified Hill procedure as surgical treatment of reflux esophagitis. World J Surg 6: 412–417
17. Papazian A, Nguyen-Phuoc BK (1982) Le reflux duodéno-gastrique: mise en évidence, affections associées, conséquences, traitement. Gastroentérol Clin Biol 6: 1020–1028
18. Pearson FG, Stone RM, Parris RM et al (1969) Role of vagotomy and pyloroplasty in the therapy of symptomatic hiatus hernia. Am J Surg 117: 130–137
19. Russel COH, Hill MD (1983) Gastroesophageal reflux. Curr Probl Surg 20: 211–278
20. Segol P, Baptiste P, L'Hirondel C, Marchand P, Gignoux M (1982) Effets de la fundoplicature sur le sphinter inférieur de l'œsophage: étude manométrique pré et post-opératoire. Gastroentérol Clin Biol 6: 222–228
21. Stoppa R, Adamski C, Verhaeghe P et al (1982) A propos de la vagotomie suprasélective associée à la fundoplicature. J Chir 119: 668
22. Temple JG, McFarland J (1975) Gastroesophageal reflux complicating highly selective vagotomy. Br Med J 2: 168–169
23. Temple JG, Goodall RJR, Hay DJ et al (1981) Effect highly selective vagotomy upon the lower esophageal sphincter. Gut 22: 368–370
24. Toupet A (1963) Technique d'œsophagoplastie avec phrénogastropexie appliquée dans la cure radicale des hernies hiatales et comme complément de l'opération de Heller dans les cardiospasmes. Mém Acad Chir 89: 394–399
25. Vansant JH, Baker JW Jr (1976) Complications of vagotomy in the treatment of hiatal hernia. Ann Surg 183: 629–635
26. Vayre P, Hureau J, Roux M (1970) La cure des hernies hiatales de l'adulte. Facteurs anatomiques et pathologiques. Déduction thérapeutique à propos de 230 cas opérés. Ann Chir 24: 627–636

F. Gayral, and *H. Larrieu* (Paris)

Introduction

The initial object of combining vagotomy with an anti-reflux procedure was reduction of gastric acidity. The early operations, in the form of truncal or selective vagotomy, reduced gastric acidity and sometimes promoted duodeno-gastric reflux through the drainage procedure required, such drainage being customarily a pyloroplasty. The technique of selective vagotomy led to dissection of the esophagus, respecting the trunk of the right vagus; this limited this vagotomy to the stomach and avoided a more complete vagotomy such as may be done accidentally during the conduct of separate anti-reflux procedures.

The subsequent employment of highly selective vagotomy combined these different objectives for the better. It reduces gastric acidity without requiring a drainage procedure; the wide dissection of the gastroesophageal junction allows easy performance of the anti-reflux procedure and preserves antral innervation and the trunk of the right vagus, whose distribution goes beyond the stomach. Thus, it is legitimate to claim to avoid the postoperative disorders attributed to anti-reflux procedures alone, such as difficulties of gastric emptying the "gas bloat syndrome" and other alimentary disorders such as diarrhea and dumping, which are very likely due to accidental vagotomy and may be explained by injury to the vagal trunks during closure of the crura of the diaphragm, construction of the half-valve or fundoplication, or fixation to the arcuate ligament of the diaphragm.

Material and methods

From 1972 to 1986 a vagotomy was combined with an anti-reflux procedure in 73 patients, 50 men and 23 women, with a mean age of 51 years (25–77 years). In 37 cases the indication was symptomatology of gastroesophageal reflux resistant to treatment and/or lesions of moderate esophagitis (erythema-ulceration, grades 1–II; in 36 cases there was severe esophagitis, with ulceration and/or stricture in 6 cases (grades 3–4).

The duration of symptoms before operation was 5.6 years. The associated lesions were: ulcerative bulbitis 5 times, gallbladder stones 6 times, leiomyoblastoma of the gastric antrum 1 case. In 4 cases endobrachyesophagus was recognized.

During the early years, truncal (TV) or selective (SV) vagotomies were performed in combination with a pyloroplasty (P). Later, preference was given to highly selective vagotomy (HSV). The anti-reflux procedure (AR) usually consisted of a Nissen fundoplication, except in 4 cases where a posterior half-valve was made and in 3 cases of repair of the cardioesophageal angle and suture of the crura of the diaphragm (Table 1).

Table 1. Operations performed:

TV/SV – P: 16	TV + P: 6 + Nissen	
	SV + P: 10	8 Nissen
		2 cardioesophageal angle + crura
HSV: 57	52 Nissen	
	4 posterior half-valves	
	1 cardioesophageal angle + crura	

Results

- Immediate results: one woman patient, an asthmatic treated with corticoids, died from cardiovascular complications on the 2nd postoperative day. Other nonfatal complications were 1 pulmonary embolism, 1 pneumopathy, and 1 transient ulnar nerve paralysis.
- Early functional results: the assessment sought to judge the functional disorders specifically linked to the surgical treatment and their outcome one year after the operation. (Table 2): diarrhea was rarer after HSV+AR than after TV/SV+AR ($p < 0.05$) and always transient. 2 patients exhibited diarrhea persisting beyond a year after TV+AR; dumping syndrome and "gas bloat" were equally short-lasting. The dysphagia observed in 32% of cases after HSV+AR usually regressed in the first postoperative weeks except for 2 cases, where intermittent moderate episodes of dysphagia without stricture were noted after 1 year.

Table 2

	Diarrhea	Dumping syndrome	Gas-bloat	Dysphagia	
At 1 month					
TV/SV + AR: 14	5	3	4	3	
	$p < 0.05$				NS
HSV + AR: 56	5	3	15	18	
At 1 year					
TV/SV + AR: 10	2	1	2	2	
HSV + AR: 42	0	0	1	2	

- Remote results: the mean period of surveillance for the entire group of patients (except 2 early lost from sight) was 43.2 months (3–138 months). The results were assessed in patients with a follow-up of at least 1 year, allowing for early failures in the first year with inadequate follow-up. Thus 56 cases were analysed. In the only patients presenting persistent disorders, clinical investigations were carried out (esophageal manometry, pH measurement, barium, transit). These results were assessed by Visick's classification. The TV/SV+AR group is too limited and nonuniform to allow specific commentary. Details of results are given for the HSV+AR group (Table 3).

Table 3

Results Visick's classification	Excellent or good 1–2	Mediocre 3	Poor-Failed 4
TV/SV + AR: 14	10	2	2
HSV + AR: 42	29	7	6

The excellent or good results (Visick 1–II) correspond to total absence of symptoms, or very minor symptoms producing no lasting handicap and not requiring treatment. They were observed in 67.6% of cases after HSV+AR. The mediocre results (Visick 3) showed moderate handicap, transient gastroesophageal reflux and/or an esophagitis of grade II or less responding favorably to medical treatment. In 3 out of 7 cases after HSV+AR, the inadequacy of the AR procedure seemed attributable in 2 cases to disruption of the operative set-up, once because of violent abdominal exertion and once due to use of absorable sutures. In these 7 mediocre results, the addition of HSV to the AR procedure may have prevented a more severe form of recurrence.

The failures or poor results (Visick 4) relate to patients presenting recurrence or persistence of esophagitis requiring continued medical treatment or reoperation. These appeared linked to immediate inadequacy of the AR procedure or its poor performance, notably by excessive tightening of the lower part of the cuff, isolating a gastric pouch above, that permanently floods the lower esophagus. Technical faults seem to be due to the heterogeneity of the operators and lack of initial experience among some. Among the 6 failures observed after HSV+AR, 1 exhibited an ulcerated esophagitis and was lost sight of 30 months after operation. The other 5 patients were reoperated by total duodenal diversion 4 times and repair of the AR+vagotomy procedure in 1 case. One patient, having undergone duodenal diversion, still showed symptomatology of troublesome reflux. The other 4 reoperations had a favorable effect.

Discussion

The indication for combining vagotomy with an anti-reflux procedure was one of principle and there was no randomized study to confirm its value. The propriety of this combination involves discussion of the risk of harmful effects, secondary to the different types of vagotomy.

Use of a truncal vagotomy risks disorders of gastric emptying and specific complications such as the dumping syndrome and diarrhea; we observed 3 such complications more than a year after operation. In a comparative non-randomized series, Vansant observed, after the combination of a truncal vagotomy with an anti-reflux procedure, twice as much diarrhea and vomiting and one dumping in the single group of vagotomized patients [17]. Other authors had previously reported these harmful effects [in 1]. At the physiologic level, the length of the inferior esophageal sphincter appears decreased after truncal vagotomy for duodenal ulcer and the pressure locally decreases in the first postoperative months, though regaining a normal level at 6 to 12 months after the operation [16]. As for the preventive effect, in Vansant's series truncal vagotomy did not protect against recurrences of gastroesophageal reflux [17]. For all these reasons, the addition of truncal vagotomy to an anti-reflux procedure is no longer recommended. Selective vagotomy has rarely been associated with anti-reflux procedures and our series is too limited to afford any conclusions.

That performance of a highly selective vagotomy facilitates that of the anti-reflux procedure is widely acknowledged [1, 5, 8, 12, 14, 15]. The criteria for monitoring the efficacy of the anti-reflux procedure in these circumstances and the absence of a comparative series are not such as to confirm its value, which must be left to the judgment of the surgeon. This value can be justified only in the absence of effects of HSV on esophageal motility, and in particular on the pressure of the inferior esophageal sphincter and gastric emptying. In practice, highly selective vagotomy does not alter the sphincter pressure [3, 11, 13] and, by itself, does not increase the gastro-esophageal reflex [6]. It is probable, therefore, that its addition does not increase the risk of recurrence of gastroesophageal reflux when combined with an anti-reflux procedure.

As regards gastric emptying, disturbance of which may favor recurrence of GER [10] or other symptoms, globally HSV, produces little or no disturbance of motility; it accelerates the early gastric emptying of fluids and slows down, but only moderately, the emptying of solids [2, 7, 4]. This is consistent with the customary absence of specific disorders associated with HSV in the surgery of duodenal ulcer and with the improvement in functional results long after the operation.

Mention should be made of the risk of necrosis of the lesser curvature of the stomach after HSV, reported in 3 out of 33 operations by Kennedy [9]. This risk has not been noted by other workers. In our series, an ulceration of the lesser curvature raised the question of ischemic etiology, but it was asymptomatic, it was found 2 years after operation and healed under medical treatment.

Though it is common to observe dysphagia transiently after HSV, its addition to an anti-reflux procedure does not seem to add to this risk and no severe dysphagia was permanent. Long after the operation, certain well-tolerated recurrences of reflux may indicate the probable value of vagotomy, which has produced the equivalent of an antisecretory treatment. However, some recurrences have been severe despite vagotomy; a mechanical factor in performance of anti-reflux procedures may develop in these cases in the form of tightness of the fundoplication or excessive tightness of its lower part.

Because of the quality of surgical exposure it provides, HSV should allow prevention or reduction in future of the technical failures due to lack of uniformity in the conduct of the anti-reflux procedure itself.

References

1. Bahadorzadem H, Jordan PH (1975) Evaluation of the Nissen fundoplication for treatment of hiatal hernia: use of parietal cell vagotomy without drainage as an adjunctive procedure. Ann Surg 181: 402–408
2. Berger T, Ceder L, Hamfelt A et al (1981) Effect of highly selective vagotomy on gastric emptying. Scand J Gastroenterol 80: 922–927
3. Braasch JW, Sala LE, Ellis FH et al (1980) Parietal cell vagotomy – Its effect on lower esophageal sphincter function. Arch Surg 115: 699–701
4. Faxen A, Alpstein M, Cederblad A et al (1978) The effect of parietal cell vagotomy and selective vagotomy with pyloroplasty on gastric emptying of a solid meal. A prospective randomized study. Scand J Gastroenterol 13: 545–550
5. Hancock DM, Sankar MY, Old JM et al (1978) The combination of proximal vagotomy with a rotational posterior gastropexy for duodenal ulcer. Br J Surg 65: 706–711
6. Hook III VH, Williams NS, Johnson D et al (1986) Gastroesophageal reflux is not increased by highly selective vagotomy. Surg Gynecol Obstet 163: 547–551
7. Jian R, Kilian D, Grall Y et al (1985) Effets de la vagotomie fundique sur la vidange gastrique des solides et des liquides d'un repas chez des patients avec et sans récidive ulcéreuse duodénale post-opératoire. Gastroenterol Clin Biol 9: 486–490
8. Jordan PH (1978) Parietal cell vagotomy facilitates fundoplication in the treatment of reflux esophagitis. Surg Gynecol Obstet 147: 593–595
9. Kennedy T, Magill P, Johnson GW et al (1979) Proximal gastric vagotomy, fundoplication and lesser-curve necrosis. Br Med J 1: 1455–1456
10. Maddern GJ, Jamieson GG, Chatterton BE et al (1985) Is there an association between failed antireflux procedures and delayed gastric emptying? Ann Surg 202: 162–165
11. Mazur JM, Skinner DB, Jones EL et al (1973) Effect of transabdominal vagotomy on the human gastroesophageal high-pressure zone. Surgery 73: 818–822
12. Mouiel J (1980) Le traitement des hernies hiatales avec reflux gastro-oesophagien. Manchonnage de l'œsophage abdominal par plicature de la petite courbure après vagotomie ultra sélective. Nouv Presse Med 9: 2915–2917

13. Ogilvie AL, Atkinson M (1984) Influence of the vagus nerve upon the reflex control of the lower esophageal sphincter. Gut 25: 253–258
14. Oster MJ, Csendes A, Funch-Jensen P et al (1982) PCV and modified Hill procedure as surgical treatment of reflux esophagitis. Results in 108 patients. World J Surg 6: 412–417
15. Samama G, Mercier V, Mouvier S (1986) Traitement du reflux gastro-œsophagien. Intérêt de la vagotomie acidofundique associée à la fundoplicature de Nissen. Presse Med 15: 255–256
16. Thomas PA, Earlam RJ (1973) The gastro esophageal junction before and after operations for duodenal ulcer. Br J Surg 60: 717–719
17. Vansant JH, Baker JW (1976) Complications of vagotomy in the treatment of hiatal hernia. Ann Surg 183: 629–633

Methods nonetheless conservative

Migration of the cardia and the posterior aspect of the stomach in large irreducible hiatal hernias

L. Couraud, J. F. Velly, Ph. Clerc, and *P. Lefebvre*
(Bordeaux)

The irreducibility of hiatal hernia and impossibility of putting the cardia, the fundus and their valvular device back into the abdomen can result from two types of lesions:

1. a congenital or acquired short esophagus. In this case the problem of reflux to be solved necessitates either a lengthening of the esophagus by a Collis type procedure or a Niessen intrathoracic valvuloplasty;
2. acquired fibrous adhesions of the stomach into the endothoracic hernial sac. In this case difficulties occur in reducing herniated viscera through an abdominal route. Nevertheless the ability to reducing the cardia, the fundus and a new antireflux valve in the abdomen remains through an appropriate approach: the thoracic route.

This case of irreducibility and its technical implications will be studied through a series of 19 cases of extremely voluminous hiatal hernias.

Frequency

Fibrous adhesions of the fundus and cardia into the thoracic sac are unusual in common hiatal hernia cases. Still, their frequency is high if related to extensively developed hernias where the stomach has wholly migrated into the thorax: in our series they were registered in 15 cases out of 19 and judged to be very tightened in 10.

Mechanism

The fixed parts of the cardio-tuberosity area are the cardia by the Bartelli-Laimer membrane and the meso-esophagus, the upper part of the lesser curvature fixed by its vessels and the posterior side of the fundus fixed by the phreno-gastric ligament.

In irreducible voluminous hiatal hernia one can find the following anatomic dispositions, which result in irreducibility (Fig. 1):

- an extensive distension of the hiatal passage, often linked to an atrophic left pillar or with a common aortoesophageal hiatus.
- a variable ascension of the cardia in 13 out of 15 cases causing both rolling and sliding hernia. Only two patients had their cardia in the right place and a plain rolling hernia.
- a sliding movement of the posterior side of the fundus into the endothoracic sac: in this ascension the upper pole of the stomach keeps its parietal attachment by the phrenogastric ligament subject to the same movement. Thus the upper pole

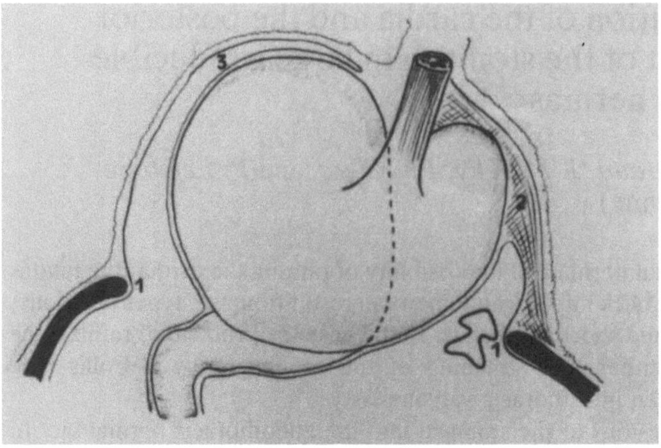

Fig. 1. Sliding of the phrenogastric ligament in the intrathoracic sac in voluminous hiatal hernia

of the stomach become fixed in an intrathoracic position by close posterior attachments which have to be cut before the stomach can be reintegrated into the abdomen.

The intrathoracic volvulus of the anterior side of the stomach and the antrum does not lead to the same effects because these parts are not fixed, so they are easily reducible by traction.

Nevertheless, through a completely different mechanism, a large volvulus that has suffered from ischemia during sub-occlusive episodes can acquire inflammatory adhesions to the hernial sac and the diaphragmatic passage, which can make the mobilization of the stomach and its laying back to the abdomen difficult.

In short the sliding shift of the phrenogastric ligament into the thorax and possible acquired post-ischemic adhesions constitute the mechanisms which make a number of voluminous hiatal hernia non-reducible.

Treatments and results

Because straightforward tractions do not permit lowering the stomach, a careful division of the thoracic attachments is needed, under sight control.

Laparotomy is an inappropriate approach to this aim. Sometimes the extensive dilatation of the hiatus and the thinness of some patients do allow completion of the operation, which in these privileged cases became a kind of transhiatal thoracic surgical approach. But a safe control of dividing thoracic attachments needs a left thoracic route.

Among the 15 voluminous hernias with endothoracic adhesions, 8 were treated through a laparotomy and 7 through a left thoracotomy. Final succes was obtained in all cases. Nevertheless the extremely good evolution does not give evidence of the technical difficulties encountered through laparotomy in some cases: in one case, the total impossibility of dividing intrathoracic attachments led to proceeding to an additional left thoracotomy. In another, a patient suffering from serious metabolic acidosis, a double surgical route was estimated to be an intolerable procedure and sectioning of thoracic adhesions was achieved under incontrolled and dangerous maneuvers which have to be avoided.

On the other hand, after freeing the upper pole of the stomach, the reintegration of the cardia in the abdomen and an antireflux valvuloplasty were possible in all cases.

Comments and conclusions

Unless a supporter of a systematic left thoracic approach for surgical repair of hiatal hernia, these intrathoracic adhesions have to be foreseen in voluminous hernias, because from our point of view, among others they are specific indication for the thoracic route.

This anticipation is supported by the following signs:

- the volume of the hernia, which was always of prime importance in our observations, and should be the first mark to hold attention even though it is not synonymous with irreducibleness.
- the intrathoracic sliding of the posterior side of the fundus and to a lesser degree the intra-thoracic migration of the cardia. The systematic evidence of such a phenomenon is revealed by barium roentgenogram of the upper pole of the stomach, and should be studied in lateral and oblique views.
- Moreover, repeated and serious subocclusive attacks with metabolic acidosis revealing ischemia, that can result in acquired inflammatory adhesions.

For the supporters of elective indications for the surgical route, these signs are to be considered as specific indications for a left thoracic approach.

How can a conservative procedure be considered in view of a stenosis on an irreducible cardia?

R. D. Henderson (Toronto)

In the situation where the esophagus is severely damaged by reflux there are strong advocates for both resective and conservative reconstructive surgery. The choice of surgical management depends on more than just stenosis and shortening. Three major factors should be considered before the surgical method is decided.

1. Previous esophageal or gastric surgery: the type and number of procedures
2. Reflux induced esophageal shortening
3. Peptic stenosis: its length and dilatability

Previous esophageal or gastric surgery is of great importance. The difficulty of surgical repair is increased with each operation and is particularly complex following previous gastric surgery. As the number of previous operations increases, so does the difficulty of repair. Inappropriate or inadvertent esophageal myotomy further compounds the problem.

Esophageal shortening is a separate problem. This is produced by reflux, and is associated with ulceration and scar formation. At this stage there is no absolute preoperative test of esophageal length. However, several investigations are helpful. In general shortening is found in patients with a giant or radiologically irreducible hernia, as well as patients with severe ulceration and stenosis.

An esophageal stricture is easily identifiable as being associated with shortening. However, minor web strictures are likely to be a problem and true shortening is almost always associated with severe active ulceration and long strictures.

These various factors must be considered carefully in all patients with advanced esophageal reflux pathology before considering resection or reconstruction [1, 2]. As part of this process one must also develop a method of deciding whether or not the esophagus is shortened and what surgical options are available (Fig. 1) Surprisingly very little is written regarding the differentiation and recognition of esophageal scar shortening. Using a transthoracic surgical approach, true esophageal shortening is difficult to judge. When a thoracoabdominal or abdominal incision is used, it is possible to judge the length of esophagus below the diaphragm. In the normal subject there is a 2.5 cm segment of intra-abdominal esophagus. When the esophagus is mobilized this segment is increased to 4 cm. If anesthetic relaxation wears off in the operating room the 4 cm intra-abdominal length reduces to the normal 2 to 2.5 cm (Fig. 2).

Under most of the previously described pathologic circumstances shortening is moderate. The esophageal wall is palpably thickened and the esophagus when fully

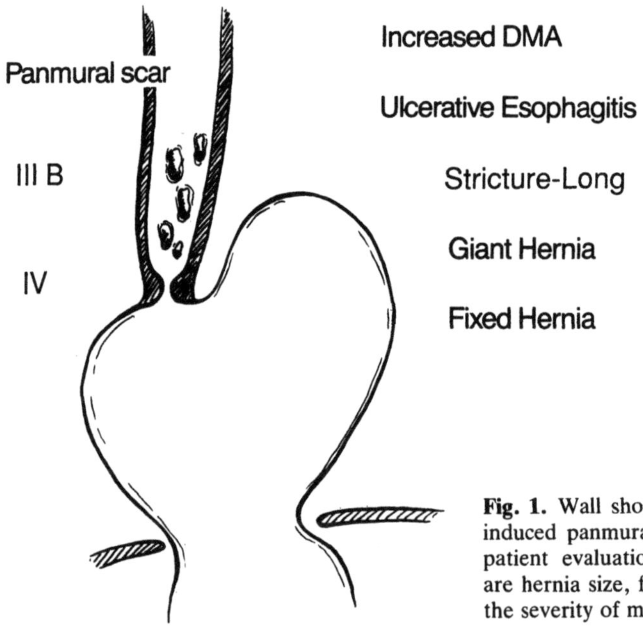

Fig. 1. Wall shortening is secondary to reflux induced panmural esophagitis and scar. From patient evaluation the demonstrable changes are hernia size, fixity, ulceration, stricture and the severity of motor change

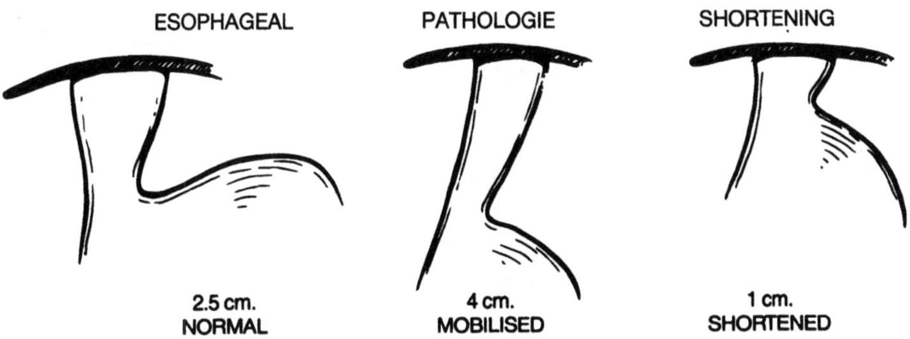

Fig. 2. Normal intra-abdominal esophageal (I.A.E) length is 2.5 cm and increased to 4 cm following surgical mobilization. If anesthetic relaxation disappears, the esophagus shortens by 1–2 cm. When panmural esophagitis is present the wall is palpably thickened and the I.A.E. is short

mobilized will lie 2 cm below the diaphragm rather than the 4 cm previously noted. Only in extreme circumstances will esophageal shortening absolutely prevent HPZ reduction below the diaphgram. The type of surgery must be tailored to esophageal length.

In the situation where a stricture is present, if the esophagus is palpably normal and intra-abdominal reduction is normal, then a standard hernia repair of a Belsey Hill or Nissen variety is possible. Such stricture would almost always be short webs with minor ulceration. For these standard operations to be effective an intra-abdominal length of 3–4 cm is necessary to achieve an appropriate length of fundoplication below the diaphragm.

When shortening is present and 2 cm or less of esophagus can be reduced below the diaphragm after full mobilization, then an intrathoracic Nissen or gastroplasty would be appropriate. It is in this situation that major controversy exists: clearly, a standard repair under tension is at risk of anatomic recurrence and many surgeons, rather than using a gastroplasty, would prefer resection and bowel interposition.

In my personal experience a total fundoplication gastroplasty (T.F.G.) can be used for the surgical correction of reflux in the majority of patients with an esophageal stricture and demonstrable shortening. This opinion is based on the surgical management of 100 consecutive patients with a peptic stricture out of a total experience of 1040 patients requiring T.F.G. for reflux control.

In this group of 100 stricture patients 13 had scleroderma and 4 previous esophageal caustic injury complicated by reflux. The remaining 83 were pure reflux injury. Within this group 35% had extensive ulceration, 38% had had previous esophageal surgery, and 10% had a Barrett's esophagus. Less severe ulcerative esophagitis was present in 62% of patients.

From our analysis of this data all had strictures and more than half had a significantly shortened esophagus. Ninety eight of these patients were treated by T.F.G. and only 2 required resection and interposition. In followup of the 98 treated by T.F.G., 87 are asymptomatic, 6 have minor residual symptoms and 4 moderate residual symptoms. Only one patient has required further surgery.

Table 1

	No.	Asymptomatic	Mild Residual	Mod Residual	Revision Surgery
Esophageal Stricture only	46	97.8%	0	2.2%	0
Plus 1 factor	35	91.4%	5.7%	2.9%	0
Plus 2 factors	15	66.6%	26.7%	6.7%	0
Plus 3 factors	2	0	0	50%	50%

Added factors: severe ulceration; scleroderma; revision surgery

More detailed analysis of preoperative pathology identified three major risk factors in surgical management. These risk factors were pancreas, esophageal or gastric surgery, scleroderma or severe ulcerative esophagitis. The results achieved surgically were clearly affected by these risk factors.

In the patients with a peptic stricture as the only factor high quality results were obtained in 97.8%. When one risk factor was present the optimal result was achieved in 91.4% With two risk factors this was further reduced to 66.6% and with all three risk factors in two patients there were no good results (Table 1).

Both patients treated by surgical resection had had previous surgery and both has severe ulcerative esophagitis and a severe stricture.

The decision to resect was based on factors other than esophageal shortening.

The information presented clearly demonstrates a conservative approach using T.F.G. is effective in the management of esophageal strictures and shortening. Using this approach all but the most severe pathology can be managed with results only slightly worse than those achieved in the management of uncomplicated reflux pathology.

Reflux induced shortening is not by itself a reason for esophageal resection.

Resection and interposition has a place in the management of reflux, however this should be confined to the management of very advanced pathology complicated by previous esophageal or gastric surgery.

References

1. Henderson, RD (1980) The Esophagus: reflux and primary motor disorders. Williams and Wilkins, Baltimore/London
2. Henderson RD, Pearson FG (1976) Preoperative assessment of esophageal pathology. J Thoracic & Cardiovasc Surg 72: 512

D. Rignault (Paris)

This operation consists of stapling with a TA 55 clip, parallel to the lesser curvature of the stomach. This stapling, performed by an abdominal approach, creates a "neo-esophagus" flanked by an augmented angle of His, on which the intragastric pressure is exerted. The effect of this is to approximate the walls of this "neo-esophagus" (and of the subjacent "neo-cardia"), making it continent by an internal valve action.

The most useful aspect of this antireflux mechanism is that it can be obtained even if reduction of the anatomic cardia is impossible, in other words in cases of irreducible brachyesophagus.

Our first operation of this nature was in 1976; it was described and reported in 1978 [1]. 90 such operations were performed between 1976 and 1985. In these 90 patients, 12 had a cardia partly reducible as far as the hiatus. In 9, the cardia was frankly intrathoracic and absolutely irreducible. 6 of these 21 patients also suffered from esophageal stricture, and in these bougie dilatation was combined with the continent tubulation. Postoperatively, immediate disappearance of reflux was constant, including the cases of brachyesophagus. Our operated patients were monitored at three levels: clinical, radiologic and fiberoscopic, some also by manometry and pH measurement. In 90% of cases the successful result persisted in the long term (average follow-up 5 years), but in the middle and long term the risk of unsealing was not entirely theoretic and was noted in 2 out of the 90 cases.

This led us to modify the original technique, using a fundoplication to surround the "neo-esophagus", so augmenting the antireflux action of the tubulation but especially perpetuating this neo-esophagus even in the event of partial unsealing. This variation is similar in principle to the technique described by Maillet under the name of "conisation".

Reference

Rignault D (1978) A new antireflux technique that can be performed by a purely abdominal route. Chirurgie 104, 99: 942–945

The Collis-Nissen procedure

G. Beauchamp (Montreal)

The gastroplasty, as described by Collis [1, 2, 3], is a tube made of the lesser curvature of the stomach to lengthen the esophagus. Although the tube has no valvular mechanism, it can reduce gastroesophageal reflux. However, some surgeons felt that the tube was not enough for controlling gastroesophageal reflux.

They have combined the gastroplasty to a valvular mechanism such as a Belsey [1] procedure.

The Collis-Belsey was introduced by FG Pearson and RD Henderson with good results in handling peptic stenosis [4, 5, 6]. After a few years, RD Henderson felt the partial fundoplication was not effective enough to give a complete and lasting control of gastroesophageal reflux. He then associated the gastroplasty to a Nissen procedure [2, 7, 8].

Orringer has followed the same route [9, 10, 11, 12, 13]. However, the results were not that good because the Nissen fundoplication has to be reduced to a smaller length [1½ cm) and done on a large bougie to reduce postoperative dysphagia [14].

During the first years of experience, the gastroplasty and antireflux have been used for more difficult cases (redoo, peptic stenosis, short esophagus). After a few years, it has become the operation of choice for the first repair in order to reduce anatomical recurrence of hiatal hernia. The procedure was first designed to be executed through the chest. Now, the gastroplasty tube can also be constructed from the abdomen [15]. The technique has been modified (uncut gastroplasty) since it first description and used by different other authors with good results [16, 17, 18, 19, 20, 21, 22].

We have performed a Collis gastroplasty and short Nissen fundoplication through the chest in 53 patients and through the abdomen in 5 patients that we followed for 1 to 5 years and evaluated with radiology, endoscopy and manometry; and each patient was examined at each visit (i.e. each 3 months for 2 years and after every 6 months).

Among these patients, we found 17 patients relatively obese, and 16 patients with a severe stenosis associated or not to a Barrett. Of the 16 patients, 5 had previous antireflux surgery. Seven patients sustained a gastroplasty and Nissen for persistent reflux and esophagitis after a first or second antireflux. Eighteen patients could have been done with a transabdominal Nissen procedure, but were elected for a transthoracic gastroplasty and Nissen.

Three mortalities are found in the follow-up, one related to the surgery and 2 unrelated (all were redoo). 2 patients had major complications i.e. gastroplasty tube fistula, of which one died. There were no other major immediate complications.

Fifty-six patients are available for the follow-up: the follow-up with a questionnaire of wellbeing showed 31 patients with excellent result, no reflux, and very slight post-fundoplication syndrome. Sixteen patients had a good result with complete control of gastroesophageal reflux, but with side effects of the fundoplication affecting then wellbeing. Two patients had severe post-fundoplication syndrome but with good control of gastroesophageal reflux.

Six patients had a bad result because control of reflux was not effective (2), or because of post-fundoplication syndrome, chest pain after the thoracotomy (2), or recurrence of hernia (2).

Gastroplasty and Nissen can be done through the chest or abdomen and is a very effective operation for the control of gastroesophageal reflux [23, 24]. It is especially useful for obese patient, recurrent stenosis and severe esophagitis. Recurrence of postoperative hiatal hernia or paraesophageal hernia is rare although always possible [25]. Gastroplasty and Nissen carries the risk of a post-fundoplication syndrome. The gastroplasty tube and Nissen was not always effective in the recurrences. These patients should probably have had a resection.

Gastroplasty and Nissen is now chosen for obese patient and redo surgery. It can be done very effectively through the abdomen with the proper instrumentation, and avoid post-thoracic pain.

Control of reflux has been generally excellent except in those patients with second and third redoo. However, patients are at risk of developing a postfundoplication syndrome as well as chest pain.

The gastroesophageal reflux is present in different types of patients with different degrees of complication. The surgeon must then choose the ideal operation for the patient. The Belsey should be used for patients with motility problems such as achalasia or scleroderma. In contradiction to Orringer, we disagree with the use of Collis-Nissen gastroplasty in scleroderma [26].

The transabdominal Nissen fundoplication is used as a routine operation for the management of primary surgical reflux. Gastroplasty and Nissen fundoplication is used for obese patients, short esophagus as well as redoo or severe stricture.

References

1. Collis JL (1961) Gastroplasty. Thorax 16: 197–206
2. Collis JL (1976) Surgical control of reflux in hiatal hernia. Clin Gastroenterol 5: 187–204
3. Collis JL (1957) An operation for hiatus hernia with short esophagus. Thorax 12: 181–188
4. Pearson FG (1973) Henderson RD Experimental and clinical studies of gastroplasty in the management of acquired short esophagus. Surg Gynecol Obstet 136: 737–744
5. Pearson FG, Henderson RD (1976) Long-term follow-up of peptic strictures managed by dilatation, modified Collis gastroplasty and Belsey hiatus hernia repair. Surgery 80: 396–404
6. Pearson FG (1977) Surgical management of acquired short esophagus with dilatable peptic stricture. World J Surg 1: 463–473
7. Henderson RD (1977) Reflux control following gastroplasty. Ann Thorac Surg 24: 206–214
8. Henderson RD (1979) Nissen hiatal hernia repair: problems of recurrence and continued symptoms. Ann Thorac Surg 28: 587–593
9. Orringer MB, Sloan H (1974) An improved technique for the combined Collis-Belsey approach to dilatable esophageal structures. J Thorac Cardiovasc Surg 68: 298–302
10. Orringer MB, Sloan H (1976) Collis-Belsey reconstruction of the esophagogastric junction. Indications, physiology and technical considerations. J Thorac Cardiovasc Surg 71: 295–303.
11. Orringer MB, Sloan H (1977) Complications and failings of the combined Collis-Belsey operation. J Thorac Cardiovasc Surg 74: 726–735
12. Orringer MB, Sloan H (1978) Combined Collis-Nissen reconstruction of the esophagogastric junction. Ann Thorac Surg 25: 16–21
13. Orringer MB, Orringer JS (1982) The combined Collis-Nissen operation: Early assessment of reflux control. Ann Thorac Surg 33: 534–539
14. Henderson RD, Marryatt GV (1985) Total fundoplication gastroplasty (Nissen gastroplasty): Five-year review. Ann Thorac Surg 39: 74–79
15. Henderson RD, Marryatt G (1981) Recurrent hiatal hernia: Management by thoracoabdominal total fundoplication gastroplasty. Can J Surg 24: 151–157
16. Bingham JAW (1974) Evolution and early results of constructing an antireflux valve in the stomach. Proc Roy Soc Med 67: 4–8
17. Bingham JAW (1977) Hiatus hernia repair combined with the construction of an anti-reflux valve in the stomach. Br J Surg 64: 460–465
18. Demos NJ (1976) A simplified, improved technique for the Collis gastroplasty for dilatable esophageal strictures. Surg Gynecol Obstet 142: 591–592

19. Demos NJ, Smith N, Williams D (1975) A gastroplasty for short esophagus and reflux esophagitis: experimental and clinical studies. Ann Surg 181: 178–180
20. Piehler JM, Payne WS, Cameron AJ, Pairolero PC (1984) The uncut Collis-Nissen procedure for esophageal hiatal hernia and its complications. Probl Gen Surg 1: 1–14
21. Vankemmel M (1982) Etude comparée schématique de quatre procédés de correction du reflux gastro-oesophagien par voie abdominale. J Chir (Paris) 119: 295–301
22. Rignault D (1978) Une technique anti-reflux simple et efficace réalisable par voie abdominale pure. Chirurgie 104: 942–945
23. Thomas-Ridocci M, Paris F, Carbonell-Antoli C and al (1985) Total fundoplication with or without gastroplasty for gastroesophageal reflux. Comparative study. Ann Thorac Surg 39: 508–511
24. Henderson RD, Marryatt G (1983) Total fundoplication gastroplasty: Longterm follow-up in 500 patients. J Thorac Cardiovasc Surg 85: 81–87
25. Henderson RD (1986) Surgical management of the failed gastroplasty. J Thorac Cardiovasc Surg 91: 46–52
26. Orringer MB, Orringer JS, Dabich L, Zarafonetis CJD (1981) Combined Collis gastroplasty -fundoplication operations for scleroderma reflux esophagitis. Surgery 90: 624–630

The advantage of Collis-Nissen procedure via an abdominal or thoracic approach

S. Sancho-Fornos, C. R. Magallon, A. P. Carrillo, J. Orbis, C. Marquez, and *C. Gil* (Valencia)

The Collis gastroplasty, with the creation of a neoesophagus, made at the expense of the smaller gastric curvature, is the most suitable antireflux technique, when the cardioesophageal junction cannot be reduced in the abdomen without tension.

In some idiopatic circumstances, the so called "short esophagus" occurs, and more frequently, in cases of peptic stenosis, reproduced hiatal hernia, and in old and voluminous ones. In all these cases the cardia remains in the thorax, fixed by the inflammatory adhesions created by the surrounding structures.

Twenty-five years ago, Leigh Collis solved this problem, with his esophageal lengthening technique, and achieved very good results.

Despite that, the procedure was not generalised, probably because of technical difficulties and the special ability that was required.

In recent years, with the appearance of the mechanical autosuture devices, which makes the critical point of the procedure easier; it was reintroduced by some authors (Pearson, Orringer, Henderson). All of them add some type of funduplication, which gives even better results. The apparatus used was the GHIA, and the approach, transthoracic.

However, we think that the use of the thoracic route can again prevent diffusion of this optimal method. We think it interesting to present our experience with the use of the abdominal approach, more familiar to many surgeons, and which allows us to deal with associated abdominal pathologies, if present.

We have employed the abdominal approach, using the TA 55 auto-suture device, and systematically add a Nissen vavuloplasty since 1976. In this period we have operated on 404 with hiatal hernia, and 180 (44.5%) with associated pathologies. Gastroplasty has been performed in 77 patients (19.05%) with Nissen funduplication in 67 cases.

Controlled by a protocolized procedure, including endoscopic, manometric and pH metric evaluation, we present, in this paper only, our experience with a follow up between 3 and 10 years.

Material and Methods

Patients

46 cases, 25 females. Average age, 39 years (range 12–75), with a 3 year minimum follow up, with complete instrumental control.

The cardial irreductibility was due to four causes:

- Peptic Stenosis: 19 cases

Half of them were classified as severe (10/19 not counting infantile gastroscope not allowed) and the rest as moderate (gastroscopy accomplished with the infantile apparatus, but not with the adult one).

The locations of the strictures were: 4 middle third
2 upper third
10 lower third
3 double third

All of them were treated with pre, intra and post-operative dilatations with Maloney's bougie, the post-operative ones for two or twenty-one months after surgery.

- Giant and old hernias: 12 cases

With nine females, nearly one third had no reflux clinically or at pHmetric evaluation prior to the operation; this subgroup continued with chronic bleeding.

All had adherent sacs to the pleura and diaphragm. Eight had very tiny crura and in five approximation was impossible.

- Recurrent hernias: 9 cases

The previous procedures were: teres cardiopexia (2), Lortat-Jacob (4), Nissen 360 (3).

- Short "idiopatic" esophagus: 6 cases

None had periesophageal, inflamatory evidence. Four had Barret epitelium, one with esophageal ulcer.

Methods

Instrumentation

- Adults and children, gastroscopes (Olympus, internaldiameter 15 and 10 millimeters respectively)
- 7754B HP polygraph; syringes, Harvard type infusion pump (before 1982) and hydropneumocapilar, low compliance pump since 1982, for manometry (Winam-Harris technique).

- Silver pre-electrodes with ClK bridge and recently with solid bridge, for pHmetric evaluations (34% Sart method, 2 hour monitoring, the rest).

Complete clinical and instrumental protocol follow-up at three months, and at one, three, five, eight and ten years after surgery. In this study we present only the cases with more than three years after surgery, because the peptic stricture group submitted to dilatation needs an important lapse before being catalogued.

Results

Mortality: none

Complications:

pleural suffusion	3 cases	6%
spleen injury	2 cases	4%
peritoneal abscess	1 case	2%
myocardial infarct	1 case	2%
wound infection	3 cases	6%
mechanic ileus	1 case	2%

Antireflux clinical Evaluation

Based on a protocolized questionnaire modified from DeMeester.

We found "gas bloat" in 18% of the cases, but when asked for spontaneous complaints about this sequela, only 9% appeared.

The postoperative dysphagia is detected in the same way in 15%, but it is troublesome (not counting cases with peptic strictures) in only 4%. None has needed dilatation.

- pHmetric Control

Effected on 92 occasions, 27 of them with the 24 hour monitoring test. We have one positive test at the 5 year control.

The statistic calculations indicate that we can expect a recurrence rate of 4% at post-operative period 5 year.

- *Manometric findings*

The characteristic feature after this operation is an enlarged HPZ (4–6 cm) abdominally placed in more than the 75%, with an average pressure of 13 mmHg (sd 5.3). This pressure, mainly due to the Nissen valvuloplasty, as documented by some authors, decreased with time.

The change between the results of one and five years is not statistically significant (13×.4.6 SD and ×=11, SD=5.8 respectively) but reaches a T of 0.01 if compared with the eight year results (×=8.5, SD=3.4).

The descent enters the maximum and significant range in the latest period (T=0.5 between 5 and 8 years results).

One interesting fact, not previously reported, is that with time, the length of intraabdominal ZAP also changes, decreasing in favour of the thoracic extent (88% to 50%).

*

Among the anti-reflux surgical techniques, the Collis gastroplasty is the unique alternative against esophageal resection procedures, when the cardioesophageal junction cannot be made to descend to the abdomen.

This happens in some idiopatic circumstances, the so-called "short esophagus", and more frequently in cases of peptic stenosis reproduced hiatal hernia, and in the old and voluminous ones.

In all these circumstances, the esophagus cannot be reduced in the abdomen without tension because of adhesions with the surrounding strictures.

The esophagogastric junction appears absolutely fixed in a thoracic position with a frequency between 10 and 25% of the cases surgically treated. The incidence in special centres attracts the worse cases, like the surgical recurrences, or peptic strictures.

The possibilities for surgical management, to restore the stomach to its normal abdominal position are two: resection with intestinal interposition, or esophageal enlargement techniques.

The Collis gastroplasty is characteristic of the second group. It allows normal abdominal positioning of the gastroesophageal function, with internal dilatation of strictures if necessary. Collis did not add other antireflux mechanisms, and had excellent results. Probably, the existence of a tube, like the neo-esophagus, in the abdomen, is in itself a factor of continence.

In this sense, there is a great amount of experimental, theoretic and clinical evidence. The experimental design, repeated with some variants, is the most important: it consists in the excision of the distal esophagus, including the LES, in different mammalians, and resuturing with the stomach. The critical fact, determining the appearance of reflux esophagitis is the length of esophagus positioned below the diaphragm: if this segment is at least 4 cm, esophagitis does not occur. If, on the contrary, the esophagus is placed above the diaphragm in all its length, pathologic reflux is the rule.

DeMeester gave the human correlation with these experiences. With 24 hour esophageal pH monitoring, he found an inverse correlation between the length of the abdominal esophagus and the positiveness of the test. The strength of the LES was also measured manometrically: the pressure needed for preventing reflux was very low, 5 mmHg, if the abdominal esophagus measured manometrically is of 3 cm, and none, if the viscus placed below the diaphragm is of 5 cm or more. On the other hand, if the length of the abdominal esophagus is about one centimeter, only cases with an LESP of more than 15 mmHg do not present reflux. When all the esophagus is placed above the diaphragm, reflux appears, no matter how powerful the LES are. The theoretical explanation that best correlates the facts is the Laplace law. According to this, resistance to collapsing in hollow and elastic strictures, against externally applied pressure, is directly related to the radius. The application of this implies that as result of abdominal pressure, the esophagus collapses in its infradiaphragmatic extension, the stomach remaining unaffected.

DeMeester also demonstrated that the LES only acts if the part of the esophagus where the pHmeter is placed, receives direct abdominal pressure.

The occurrence of reflux relapses after gastroplasty has been attributed to the fact that sometimes the average enlargement obtained is insufficient: in very few instances, a sliding hernia, even minimal, can be demonstrated. But, manometrically, the existence of an aperistaltic segment of more than 3 cm proximal at the PIP, suggesting that the neoesophagus has been displaced above the diaphragm, is the rule.

After Collis all authors add as a rule of caution some kind of valvuloplasty. The Belsey procedure was used in the first place, but was soon abandoned for two main reasons. First, despite the immediate good results, as time passed they were not very different from those obtained with gastroplasty alone, according to Collis's publications. Second, the Nissen procedure was at the time giving better antireflux results.

So this was the elective valvuloplasty added to Collis enlargement. For us there is another strong reason for the use of Nissen fundoplication: it can be easily done through the abdominal approach, that is our standard route, and the Belsey type cannot.

- We have seven cases of Collis-Belsey, all of them with more than five year post-op. period, and four of them repeatedly explored: in four there is not yet an esophageal abdominal segment, of one or more cm, another four had LESPS of neglectable value, below 3 mmHg, and one between 3 and 5. The cases in the last group are failures of the Belsey technique: all of them had values above 11 mmHg in previous determinations.

Fortunately only 2 patients had pathologic pH reflux (SART and pH-24 h). In both, abnormal facts are present: atonic LES, and thoracic displacement of the neoesophagus.

- Among our Collis-Nissen results, we found 5 cases with LESP below 5 mmHg, and 3 with all the LES length positioned in the thoracic cavity. Another four have more than 50% of the LES above the PIP. The one patient who has pathological reflux presents a LESP of 2 to 3 mmHg, 75% of the high pressure zone above the PIP. We have detected another patient with both findings; but he does not reflux at present.

In the group of hypotonic sphincters, the critical decrease, below 5 mmHg appeared in 3 in the 3 year control, and in two others in the 5th year. Taking into account the percentages of corresponding calculations, we can expect 12% of cases to have a LESP below 5 mmHg at five years. The lapse between operation and valvuloplasty failure cannot be reported more accurately.

In patients controlled at 3 months, 1, 3, 5, 8 and 10 years after surgery, the loosening of the fundic wrap appeared between 1 to 5 years, and the facts are that 7 cases had pressures above 10 mmHg in the 3 month and 1 year controls.

The decrease is not linear: four patients had pressure controls, with previous values above 10 mmHg, and do not develop more decreases in subsequent manometric evaluation.

The post-operative shortening of the neo-esophagus increases with time but does not affect all the cases. The process appears in 25% of the patients, with an increase in thoracic extent of the LES of 50% or more.

In order to do more precise studies which could detect less important changes, we are going to change our system of manometric procedure. In the cases reported here the extraction of the probe has been done by the stationary pull-through system retiring 1 cm in each instance. This cannot allow the detection of changes of less than one cm and that represents 25% of the total sphincter length. Now we are using a system of low continous extraction, with a mechanical device.

The actuarial and statistic calculations give a result of 5.3% of bad instrumental results. At the 5 year follow-up, this implies the simultaneous presentation of a weakened Nissen wrap and an intrathoracic high pressure zone.

This number, the best that can be expected among the antireflux procedures, is inferior to our own clinical results expressed in the Visick table.

This is because there are some cases without reflux but with dysphagia, and basically, gas bloat: in this field, the method gives very good results again. The dysphagia, clinically checked, appears in 8%, and gas-bloat, which is detected with the same intensity in 27% of our 360° Nissen cases (with more than 5 year follow-up), is reported in only 13% in the Collis-Nissen group.

We conclude that this method, despite being employed in the worst situations, gives better results, without increasing immediate complications of less aggressive reflux, in which we expect to improve results and reduce sequelae.

R. D. Henderson (Toronto)

The Collis-Nissen operation requires careful definition. In 1961 Collis described the original gastroplasty as a tubed portion of stomach with fundus sutured to its lateral wall. By 1971 the fundoplication was increased to 270° and by 1978 to 360°. Since neither Belsey nor Nissen were involved in the operative design the terms partial (270°) and total fundoplication (360°) gastroplasty are more appropriate. Using this terminology the questions posed will be analysed from observations made on a group of 351 transthoracic total fundoplication gastroplasties (T.F.G.) followed for 5–10 years, and 250 transabdominal gastroplasties followed for 1–4 years.

In my original experience with T.F.G., first reported in 1978, my preference was to use a transthoracic approach for primary hernia repairs and a thoracoabdominal approach for recurrent hernias. During the past four years the approach has been modified to a transabdominal incision in selected patients as follows:

- The thoracoabdominal approach is optimal for the management of a recurrent hernia as this allows direct vision dissection of both the intrathoracic esophagus and the esophagogastric fundus. Also a pyloromyotomy can be added for gastric drainage.
- In patients without previous surgery who are not excessively obese, the choice of incision depends upon esophageal length. As a general rule the esophagus lies 2.5 cm below the diaphragm in the normal subject. When the esophagus is mobilized

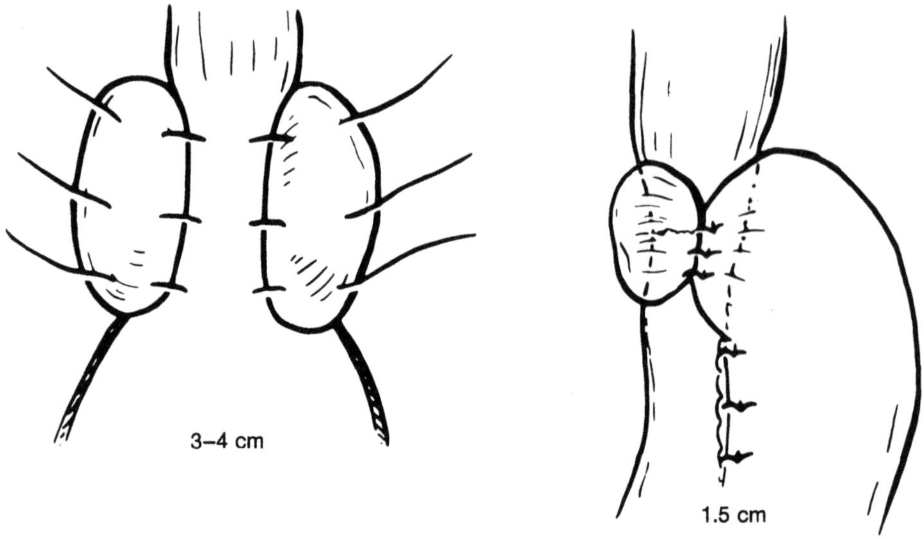

Fig. 1. With a standard Nissen suturing placed in a gastro-esophago-gastric fashion. By using this technique the intra-abdominal length is the same as the fundoplication length. Using a total fundoplication gastroplasty the fundoplication is tailored and the completed fundoplication reduced to 1.5 cm

surgically 4 cm will lie below the diaphragm. When the anesthetic relaxation wears off the esophagus will shorten to its normal length. In my view a standard Nissen or Belsey requires 3–4 cm for fundoplication while a gastroplasty requires only 1.5 cm (Fig. 1). This accounts for the effectiveness of gastroplasty in the management of a shortened esophagus. Under exceptional circumstances a hernia repair is possible by gastroplasty with no intraabdominal esophagus.

Length of esophagus is critical to the choice of operative approach. With minor shortening of up to 2 cm, the abdominal route can be used in a non-obese patient. Esophageal length can be predicted from preoperative evaluation. Shortening is present in patients with a giant fixed hernia, severe esophageal secondary motor disorders, a long stricture or severe ulcerative esophagitis.

Having described the method of incision selection, one can evaluate the relative merits of each approach. With a transthoracic approach the major problem is incisional pain. This prolongs convalescence, is occasionally a major physical restriction and is commonly a longterm nagging problem. With the transabdominal approach incisional pain is eliminated. The major problems related to the abdominal approach in 250 patients was splenectomy in 2 (0.8%); wound evisceration in 1 (0.4%) and ventral hernias in 8 (3.2%). Eliminating significant wound pain by using an abdominal incision has proved to be a major advantage.

Using any one of these operative approaches the operative design is identical. The esophagogastric junction is fully mobilized and the esophagogastric fat pad removed. Posterior crural sutures are placed and tied at the completion of the operation.

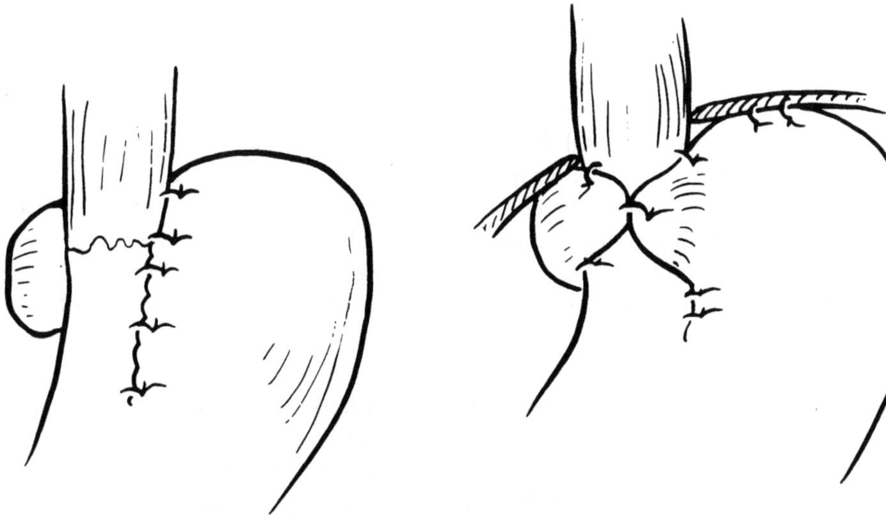

Fig. 2. The total fundoplication gastroplasty creates a 5 cm gastroplasty tube plus 1.5 cm of LES for a total of 6.5 cm intra-abdominal length. The completion fundoplication is 1.5 cm

The gastroplasty tube is from the lesser curvature of stomach over a # 60 Fr. Maloney bougie and the tube closed in two layers with 00 Dexon and invaginating continuous 000 silk (Fig. 2a). The fundus is now rotated around the gastroplasty tube and distal 1.5 cm of esophagus and the fundus approximated with interrupted 00 mattress silk sutures (Fig. 2b). This first suture line creates a 6.5 cm intraabdominal segment and creates operative stability.

Following this, the completion of fundoplication is approximated over a distance of 1.5 cm using 3 interrupted 00 mattress silks. The completed fundoplication is responsible for reflux control. Too long a completed fundoplication produces overcompetence and too short a fundoplication produces reflux.

Having reviewed the operative design and the surgical approach, the ultimate question is: are the results comparable for a transthoracic, a thoracoabdominal and a transabdominal approach? The answer unfortunately is complex. In my own experience with 351 patients using a transthoracic approach, 335 have adequate evaluation: there was no operative mortality. An anatomic recurrence rate of 1.2% has occurred. The incidence of significant dysphagia was 3%, however in recent years this has decreased to 1% by reducing the length of the completed fundoplication. At this stage 93.1% eat normally without heartburn; 3.9% have either persistent or recurrent significant symtoms.

Within this group of patients are many who would now be treated transabdominally. Also within this group 40% have had previous esophageal or gastric surgery and would have been treated by a thoracoabdominal incision, T.F.G. and pyloromyotomy. These patients have been followed 5–10 years while the 250 with an abdominal incision are all primary repairs, there is no major esophageal shortening and follow-up is only 1–4 years.

It can be shown that the quality of result produced by T.F.G. is dependent on the severity of the preoperative pathology. In general the important factors which affect the quality of result are stricture, severe ulceration, previous esophageal or gastric surgery or scleroderma. The number of complicating factors is also important.

Since the patients for a transabdominal T.F.G. have limited major preoperative pathology one would expect a better quality of result. At this stage, allowing for the preoperative pathology and for the shorter follow-up the results are identical regardless of the incision used. Since identical results can be achieved in selected patients using transabdominal T.F.G. this would appear to be the route of choice as the operation is well tolerated, and there is no residual intercostal pneumonitis.

*

Total fundoplication gastroplasty (T.F.G.) is an operative design which has been shown to be effective in long term follow-up. Properly constructed, the operation has a very low mortality, a 1.2% anatomic recurrence rate and over 90% high quality results. In selected patients the transabdominal approach is optimal, however a thoracoabdominal incision is an important approach for recurrent hernias.

References

1. Henderson RD (1977) Reflux control following gastroplasty. Ann Thoracic Surg 24: 206–214
2. Henderson RD, Marryatt GV (1985) Total fundoplication gastroplasty (Nissen gastroplasty): Five-year review. Ann Thoracic Surg 39: 74–79
3. Henderson RD, Marryatt GV (1985) Transabdominal total fundoplication gastroplasty to control reflux: A preliminary report. Can J Surg 28: 127
4. Orringer MB, Sloan J (1978) Combined Collis-Nissen reconstruction of the esophagogastric junction. Ann Thoracic Surg 25:16

Results of Collis-Nissen operation

M. B. Orringer (Ann Arbor)

Since 1976, we have performed the combined Collis gastroplasty-Nissen fundoplication operation in 320 patients. The operation is performed transthoracically, and after mobilization of the esophagogastric junction and dilation of any stricture that is present, a 5 cm long gastroplasty tube is constructed using the GIA surgical stapler. The elongated gastric fundus resulting from construction of the gastroplasty tube is then passed posteriorly around the tube and is positioned for construction of the fundoplication. Seromuscular sutures are then placed between gastric fundus, gastroplasty tube, and then gastric fundus again. Four such sutures 1 cm apart are placed so that the total length of the fundoplication is 3 cm. The fundoplication is then reduced back through the diaphragmatic hiatus and into the abdominal cavity, and the posterior crural sutures previously placed are tied.

Table 1. Indications – Collis-Nissen operation – 320 pts

	No.	%
Reflux esophagitis (peptic stricture)	161 (59)	50% (18%)
Obesity	117	37%
Type 3 hiatal hernia – short esophagus	43	13%
Esophagomyotomy for spasm	24	8%

We have performed the Collis-Nissen operation not only in patients with reflux strictures and esophageal shortening, but also in those with factors which we believe predispose them to recurrence after any of the standard operations. These factors include recurrent reflux requiring reoperation, a history of a prior distal esophageal operation which interferes with accurate placement of lower esophageal sutures, marked obesity, and a history of one or more abdominal wall hernias, either incisional or inguinal, which implies an inherent tissue weakness in these individuals.

Of our 320 patients, 154 were woman and 166 men, and their average age was 51 years (Table 1). The indications for operation included the presence of reflux esophagitis in 50% of these patients, 18% having peptic strictures. Thirty-seven per cent of our patients were markedly obese, 13% had large combined sliding and paraesophageal hiatal hernias with associated esophageal shortening, and 8% required an esophagomyotomy for esophageal spasm, and the Collis-Nissen operation was used in hopes that the gastroplasty tube would provide a better distal esophagus around which to perform the fundoplication. Twenty-three per cent of our patients had undergone one or more prior distal esophageal or periesophageal operations including thoracic or abdominal hiatal hernia repairs and vagotomy (Table 2). Four patients in this series died postoperatively for a mortality of 1.3%. Causes of death included an unrecognized leak from an esophagomyotomy with secondary mediastinitis and sepsis, bowel obstruction, aspiration pneumonia, and a pulmonary embolus. Twenty-eight patients experienced significant complications.

Table 2. Indications – Collis-Nissen operation – 320 pts

	No.		%
Periesophagitis from prior operations	75		23
thoracic hiatal hernia repair		34	
abdominal hiatal hernia repair		37	
vagotomy		17	
repair of perforation		3	
esophagomyotomy, diverticulum resection		3	
repair-esophageal atresia		1	

Table 3. Collis-Nissen complications – 320 pts

	No.
Gastroplasty tube leak	2 (0.6%)
Perforated stricture	2
Perforated diverticulum site	1
Perforation-repeat – myotomy	1
Perforation-distal esoph (RE-DO)	1
Splenic injury	3 (0.9%)
Hemorrhage	4 (1.3%)

Table 4. Collis-Nissen complications – 320 pts

	No.
Gastric atony	2 (0.6%)
Crural repair dehiscence	2
Small bowel obstruction	2
Wound infection	5 (1.6%)
Pulmonary embolus	2
Chylothorax	1

These complications included (Table 3) leaks from the distal esophagus or gastroplasty tube, intraoperative splenic injury requiring splenectomy, postoperative bleeding requiring reexploration, and various miscellaneous complications (Table 4) including gastric atony, bowel obstruction, and wound infection. The majority of these complications were not related to the specific operative technique of the Collis-Nissen operation.

This procedure was undertaken with a firm commitment to long-term follow-up of these patients not only with personal interview, but also with objective esophageal function studies including manometric assessment of the lower esophageal sphincter pressures and reflux control as documented with the intraesophageal pH electrode. Among our 320 patients, 76% have been followed at least six months, and the average follow-up for these 242 patients is 41 months (Table 5). Postoperative

Table 5. Collis-Nissen follow-up – 320 pts

242 (76%) – followed at least 6 mos. (avg. 41 mos.) Post-operative esophageal function tests
118 (49%) – 6 months
183 (76%) – 12 months
129 (53%) – 24 months
84 (35%) – 36 months
58 (24%) – 48 months
44 (18%) – 60 months

esophageal function tests have been performed in 49% of our patients at six months, in 76% at 12 months, in 53% at 24 months, in 35% at 36 months, in 24% at 48 months, and in 18% at 60 months (Table 6a). At the time of their most recent evaluation, 85% of these patients have no reflux symptoms whatsoever. Five per cent have mild symptoms (rare heartburn in the supine position relieved with occasional antacids) and remain extremely satisfied with the results of operation. Five per cent of these patients have moderate reflux symptoms, which have required resumption of a strict antireflux medical regimen for control, and 4% have had severe recurrent reflux uncontrolled with medical therapy and frequently requiring reoperation. Post thoracotomy incisional pain, early satiety (gas bloats), and post vagotomy diarrhea have been experienced by a minority of these patients (Table 6b).

Virtually every antireflux operation is associated with some degree of postoperative dysphagia. Our patients have been carefully questioned about the presence of *any* degree of difficulty swallowing after operation (Table 6c). Fifty-four per cent of these patients deny any dysphagia whatsoever. Twenty per cent admit to occasional slow emptying of the esophagus for some solid foods and bread which has required no treatment and is not regarded as a major problem for them. Twenty-six per cent have had moderate or severe dysphagia requiring either periodic or regular esophageal dilations.

Table 6a. Collis-Nissen – Subjective results – 242 pts

	No.	%
Reflux		
none	206	85
mild	13	5
moderate	13	5
severe	10	4

Table 6b. Subjective results (Cont. 1)

	No.	%
Thoracotomy pain	21	9
Early satiety ("Bloats")	9	4
Post-vagotomy diarrhea	3	1

Table 6c. Subjective results (Cont. 2)

	No.	%
Dysphagia		
none	130	54
mild	49	20
moderate	46	19
severe	17	7

Table 7. Dysphagia after Collis-Nissen repair. 112/242 pts (46%)

Esophageal pathology	No.	Dysphagia mild-occasional	Dysphagia requiring dilation
Uncomplicated			
Hernia or GER	135	27 (20%)	24 (17%)
Stricture	53	6 (11%)	25 (47%)
Type 3 HH	33	12 (36%)	3 (9%)
Spasm	21	4 (19%)	11 (52%)
Total	242	49 (20%)	63 (26%)

The degree of dysphagia after a Collis-Nissen repair can be related to the underlying esophageal pathology (Table 7). Nearly half of the patients with esophageal strictures will require postoperative esophageal dilations. Because half of our patients with esophageal spasm who underwent an esophagomyotomy with a concomitant Collis-Nissen repair developed postoperative dysphagia that necessitated dilation, we have abandoned this operative approach in the patient with spasm. In fact, our long-term results with relief of pain and dysphagia in the patient with esophageal spasm is so poor, that we now rarely operate upon these patients whose disease is primarily psychological. Objective postoperative esophageal function tests (Table 8) have shown that the lower esophageal high pressure zone pressures and length substantially increase over preoperative levels, and these increases remain fairly constant in long-term follow-up. While 92% of these patients demonstrated abnormal gastroesophageal reflux with the intraesophageal pH electrode preoperatively, approximately 11% have demonstrated abnormal reflux in long-term follow-up postoperatively.

In summary (Table 9), of our 242 patients who have undergone Collis-Nissen operations and have been followed for an average of 41 months, subjective reflux control has been good or excellent in 90%, while recurrent reflux symptoms have appeared in 9%. Objectively, 11% have demonstrated abnormal reflux with the pH

Table 8. Collis-Nissen esophageal function tests

	No pts.	HPZ pressure (mmHg)	HPZ length (cm)	moderate-severe reflux (%)
Pre-op	289	4.4	1.6	92%
Post-op				
6 mos.	116	12.0	4.4	4 (3%)
12	177	11.6	4.3	10 (6%)
24	119	11.0	4.4	13 (11%)
36	77	10.8	4.2	7 (9%)
48	52	10.3	4.5	9 (17%)
60	40	11.1	4.0	5 (12%)

Table 9. Overall results – Collis-Nissen repair – 242 pts

Subjective:	no reflux	– 206 (85%)
	mild reflux	– 13 (5%)
	mod-severe reflux	– 23 (9%)
Objective (pH probe):		
	poor control – 27 (11%)	
	no symptoms – 10 (37%)	
	mild symptoms – 6 (22%)	
	reoperation – 11 (41%)	
	good control – 215 (89%)	

electrode: of this latter group of 27 patients, 37% have no symptoms of reflux, 22% have very mild reflux symptoms which require no regular therapy, and 41%, or 11 patients, have required reoperation for reflux control. Good control of reflux as documented with the intraesophageal pH electrode has been achieved in 89% of our patients.

These results substantiate excellent reflux control with the Collis-Nissen procedure and justify its continued use in appropriately selected patients with gastroesophageal reflux and its complications.

References

1. Orringer MB, Sloan H (1974) An improved technique for the combined Collis-Belsey approach to dilatable esophageal strictures. J Thorac Cardiovasc Surg 68: 298
2. Orringer MB, Sloan H (1977) Complications and failings of the combined Collis-Belsey operation. J Thorac Cardiovasc Surg 74: 726
3. Orringer MB, Sloan H (1978) Combined Collis-Nissen reconstruction of the esophagogastric junction. Ann Thorac Surg 25: 16
4. Orringer MB, Orringer JS (1981) The combined Collis-Nissen operation: early assessment of reflux control. Ann Thorac Surg 33: 534

The Collis-Belsey procedure

F. G. Pearson (Toronto)

We reported initial experience with this operation in 1971 [1]. Collis' technique of gastroplasty was somewhat modified, and a long partial fundoplication was added rather than a Collis' repair. Our modification uses a transthoracic approach through the left sixth intercostal space. Several technical features warrant emphasis:

1. Exposure and mobilization of the esophagus, cardia and proximal stomach is identical to that used for a Belsey Mark 4 repair.

2. The addition of gastroplasty requires a more extensive removal of the esophagogastric fat pad than the Mark 4 repair.
3. The length and luminal diameter of the gastric tube are considered important features of the anti-reflux mechanism. The tube is fashioned snugly over a No. 48 French bougie, is of uniform diameter from top to bottom, and is usually about 5 cms. in length.
4. A 270 degree partial fundoplication is created over a length of 4 to 5 cms. The length of fundoplication is longer than that used for a standard Belsey repair, – and is created using three rather than two tiers of fundoplicating sutures.

Material

Since 1964 we have used this operation in almost 500 patients with selected complications of reflux esophagitis. The indication for adding gastroplasty was due to one or more of the following findings.

1. Short esophagus and stricture – 304 cases
2. Short esophagus without significant stricture – 113 cases
3. Redo cases – 118 cases
4. Massive herniation – 54 cases
5. Associated primary motor disorder – 37 cases

Follow-up was conducted by annual interview with completion of a specific questionnaire and barium studies at one, five and 10 years. Only patients with recurrent symptoms were routinely submitted to follow-up endoscopy, manometry and pH studies.

Four hundred and thirty patients have been followed between two and 20 years. Two hundred and fifty of these cases have been followed for more than five years and 101 patients for more than 10.

Results

Morbidity and mortality are listed in Table 1.

The complications observed in this series are similar in severity and frequency to those anticipated following any of the standard hiatus hernia repairs. There were six esophageal fistulae, none were fatal, and three of the six occurred in patients undergoing redo surgery.

Table 1

Complications	424 Patients
Atelectasis, pneumonia	18
Wound infection	12
Esophageal fistula	6
Prolonged incisional pain	17
Other	30

Functional results are classified as follows: Good – asymptomatic, or with inconsequential symptoms requiring no therapy. Fair – improved, but with symptoms and/or endoscopic findings requiring intermittent therapy (anti-reflux medication or dilatation). Poor–unimproved or worse. Table 2 is a tabulation of results which have been subdivided into four categories for purposes of this review.

Table 2. Results by category

	No. cases	Results		
		Good	Fair	Poor
Short esophagus – stricture (138) esophagitis (77) (excluding redo cases and motor disorders)	215	93% (199)	4% (10)	3% (6)
"Redo cases" – 1 or more prior unsuccessful antireflux operations	118	80% (93)	12% (15)	8% (10)
Peptic stricture [25], or esophagitis [12], associated with a primary motor disorder	37	54% (19)	24% (9)	22% (8)
Intrathoracic stomach	54	91% (49)	9% (5)	0% (0)

In this series of patients with acquired short esophagus due to esophagitis and dilatable peptic stricture, good results were obtained in 93% of patients who did not have an underlying primary motor disorder or a history of previous anti-reflux surgery. Re-operation following unsuccessful prior anti-reflux surgery yielded significantly fewer good results – 80%. The most challenging and difficult problems have been patients presenting with ulcerative reflux esophagitis and peptic strictures associated with underlying primary motor disorder (Table 3). Only about half of these patients have had good results sustained over the long period of follow-up. Furthermore, results have tended to deteriorate with the passage of further time.

Among these motor disorders, achalasia is the most difficult. When ulcerative reflux esophagitis and stenosis develop after esophagomyotomy for achalasia, there appears to be no conservative operation which controls both reflux and dysphagia,

Table 3

Primary motor disorders:	No. Cases	Results		
		Good	Fair	Poor
Scleroderma	16	9(57%)	4	3
Achalasia	14	6(43%)	4	4
Diffuse spasm	7	5(71%)	1	1

and good results were sustained in only six of our 14 patients. Three of the four patients with poor results have since undergone resection of the thoracic esophagus and gastric replacement. We currently recommend serious consideration of resection in any patient with achalasia who has endoscopic confirmation of gross ulcerative peptic esophagitis or peptic stricture.

Subsequent Adenocarcinoma

Adenocarcinoma developed in the distal esophagus in five patients. All five cases had some degree of acquired columnarlined esophagus and three of the five had peptic strictures. The diagnosis of carcinoma was established between three months and seven years after operation. In two patients, the adenocarcinoma was identified at three and nine months following repair, and was probably present as an occult tumor at the time of repair. In the remaining three patients, the tumor was identified at two and one-half, three and seven years after repair. One of these latter three patients had poor reflux control.

Comparison of Collis-Nissen and Collis-Belsey procedures

F. París, M. T. Ridocci, F. Mora, and *A. Benages*
(Valencia)

Reflux structure of the esophagus represents the end of a pathologic spectrum that begins as a simple esophagitis. From February 1973 to May 1986, we have operated on 47 patients sufferring from esophageal peptic strictures. Our most preferred policy today is the dilatation of the stricture associated with an antireflux procedure (A.R.P.).

Our series is composed of forty one Collis gastroplasties associated with partial plication in ten patients (Fig. 1) and total plication in 31 patients (Fig. 2, 3).

Thirty three patients were followed more than five years and an other five more than three years. Six secondary resection substitutions were performed (Fig. 4). In total, fifty five operations were carried out, including eight resection-substitutions "per primam". From 1979 only two patients required resection, as primary operation, because the esophageal stricture was perforated during intraoperative dilatation.

In patients with esophageal reflux stricture, we prefer the thoracic approach for several reasons:

1. It allows the choice between a Collis gastroplasty or a resection-reconstruction;

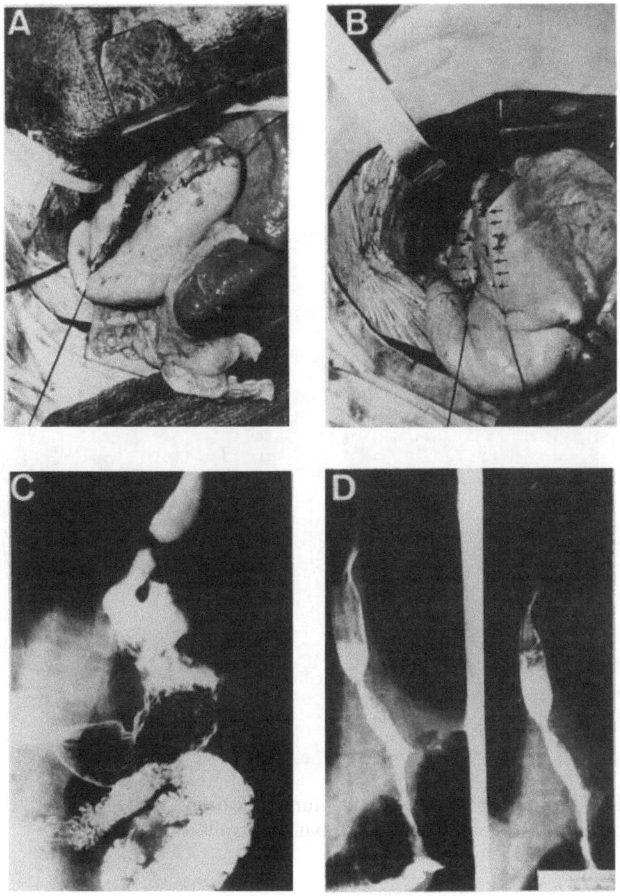

Fig. 1. Gastroplasty with partial fundoplication: (Collis-Nissen) **a)** Gastroplasty tube; **b)** Partial wrapping (the arrows are at the sutures from gastric fundus to the tube); **c)** and **d)** Preoperative and postoperative barium swallows

2. We can identify the severity of the esophageal panmural fibrosis and the exposure is better than that obtained through the abdominal route;
3. It helps esophageal dilatation (perorally and/or retrograde) of the stricture, at the operation;
4. It is the only surgical approach able to meet the diagnosis of an esophageal perforation during intraoperative dilatation.

Concerning the antireflux procedure, in 1976 we have abandoned the Collis-Belsey in favour of the Collis-Nissen operation, because 4/10 recurrences reappeared when partial plication was used: These four patients, after having had early good results, needed a new operation because of recurrence of heartburn and reflux to the throat, and recurrence of esophageal stricture. They were treated by resection substitution (2 patients) and total plication (2 patients).

The results of the 31 cases submitted to the Collis-Nissen procedure were: 25 good (81%), one bad, one death and four patients needing secondary esophageal resection-substitution (12%). These last four patients did not complain of reflux symp-

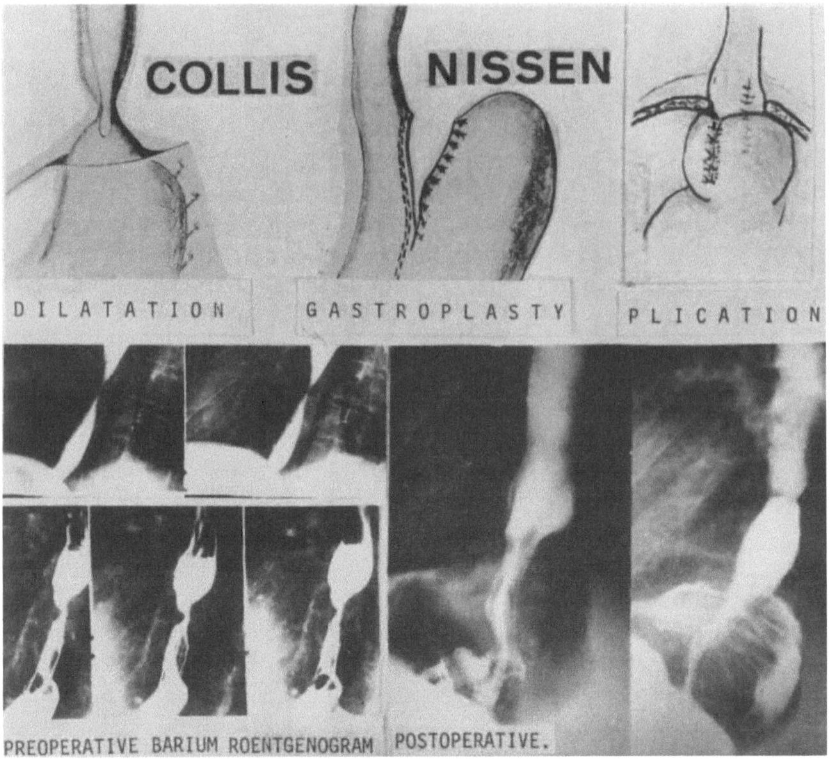

Fig. 2. Gastroplasty with total fundoplication. Above operative steps of the procedure; below preoperative and postoperative barium swallows

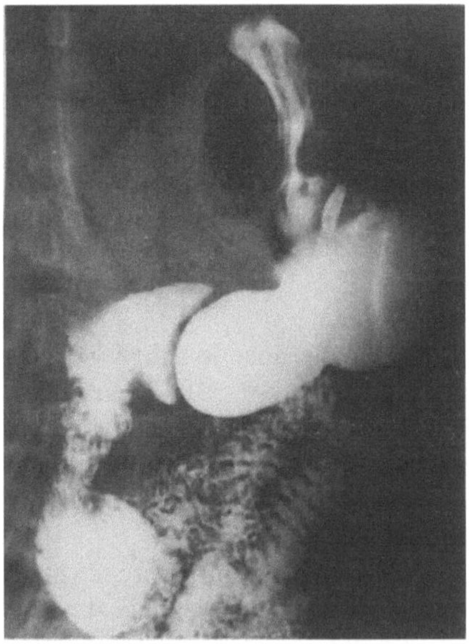

Fig. 3. Barium swallow examination in a patient after Collis-Nissen operation. The Collis neo-tube is surrounded by the adjacent gastric fundus

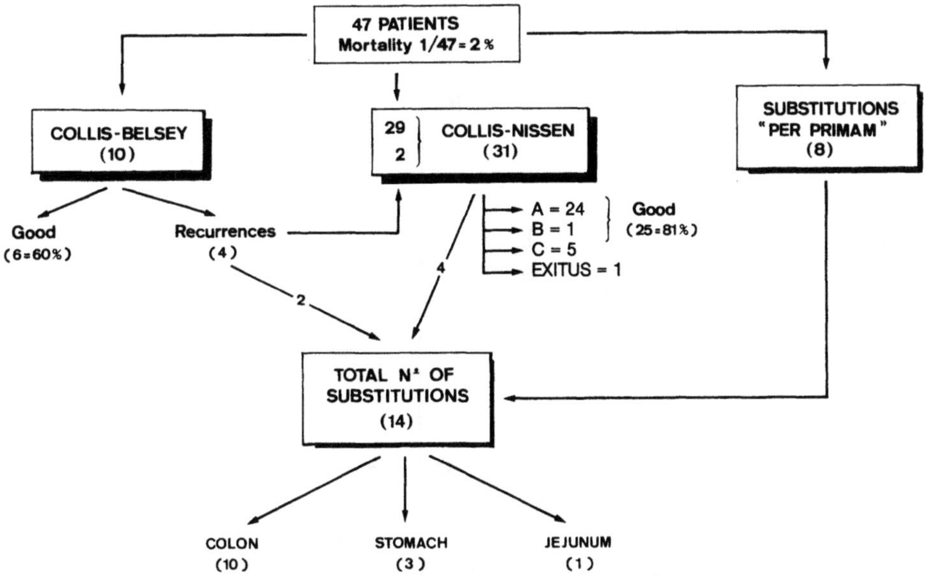

Fig. 4. Clinical evolution in our series of patients with reflux esophageal strictures

toms after the primary A.R.P. In our opinion, the stricture recurrences presented in this group should be related to the previous panmural fibrosis.

The differences between the results achieved by the Collis-Belsey and Collis-Nissen procedures had an easy explanation. When a lengthening of the esophagus is performed, the gastroesophageal competence is achieved, principally by the collapses of the neoesophagus by high abdominal pressure and wrapping of the fundus. Many authors [1, 2, 3] have demonstrated the superiority of the total wrapping in increasing the preoperative LESP (Fig. 5).

Our studies [4] showed that when a Collis-Belsey procedure is performed (Fig. 6) the mean esophageal high pressure zone, which is increased in early postoperative studies (2–3 months), decreased in later studies (12–24 months). The mean preoperative LESP of 11.2±8.2 mmHg, increased after the operation to 17.3±7.2 mmHg, but decreased in the second studies to 13.7±7.2 mmHg. The difference between preoperative and early postoperative studies was significant ($p. < 0.01$, paired t test), but was not significant between the preoperative and second postoperative studies. In the second studies, the manometric common cavity test and the short pH reflux tests were positive in 28% and 23% respectively (Fig. 7 and 8).

When a Collis-Nissen procedure was performed [4] the preoperative high pressure zone of 9.3±4.8 mmHg (Fig. 6) increased after the surgical procedure to 17.7±7.5 mmHg, did not decrease in the second postoperative studies, 16.4±8 mmHg. The percentage of positive tests were null in the first postoperative control and only 3% in the second postoperative studies.

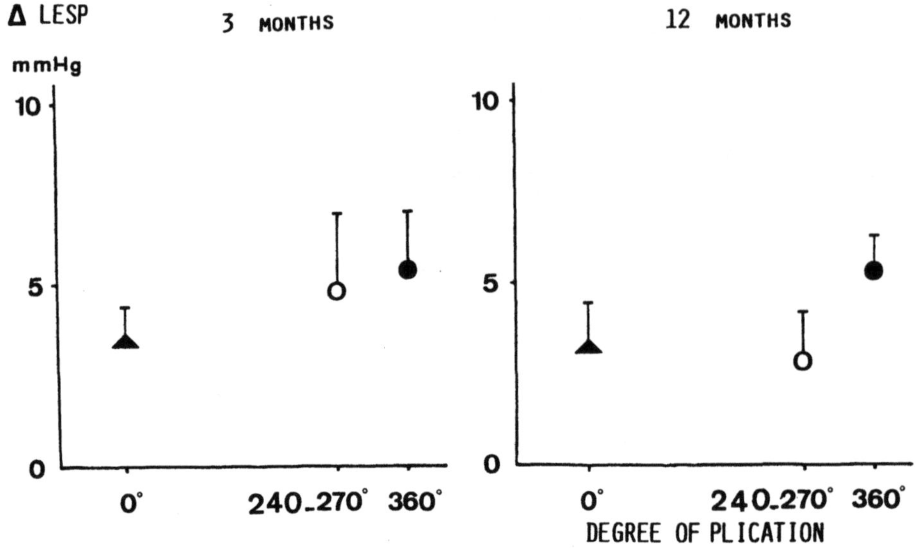

Fig. 5. Mean postoperative increasing of the LESP (mmHg) after the operation (left) and 12 months later (right)
0°=anatomical reconstruction
240–270°=partial fundoplication
360°=total fundoplication

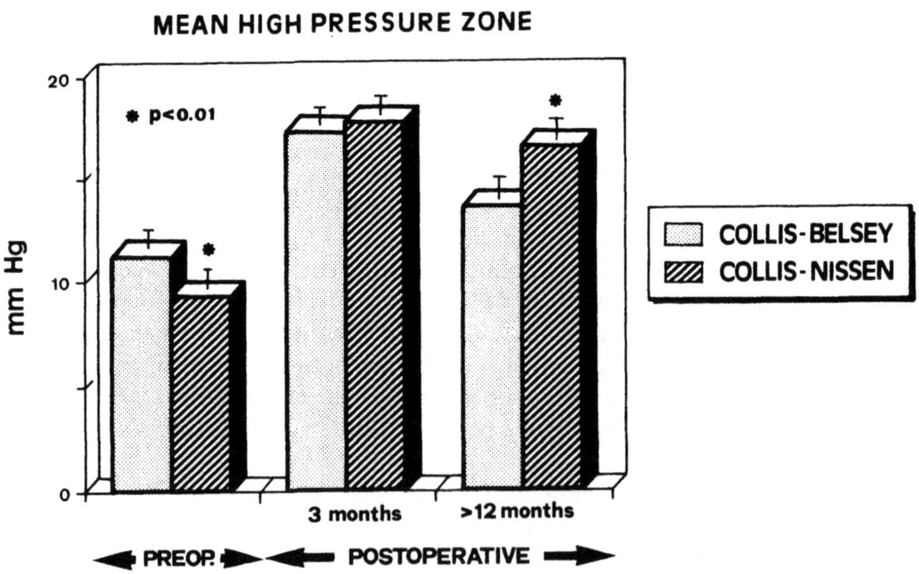

Fig. 6. Pre and postoperative mean high pressure zone in patients submitted to the Collis-Belsey and Collis-Nissen procedures

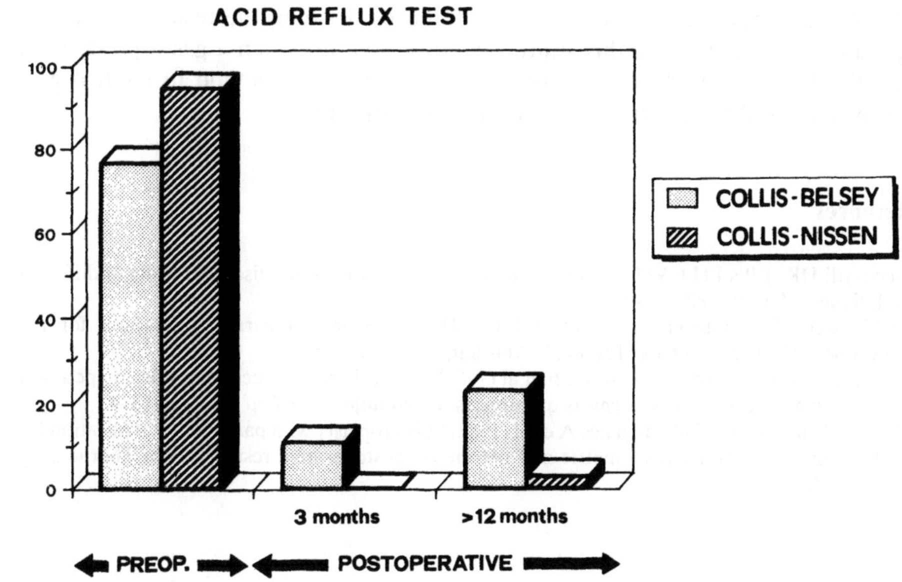

Fig. 7. Pre and postoperative short acid reflux tests

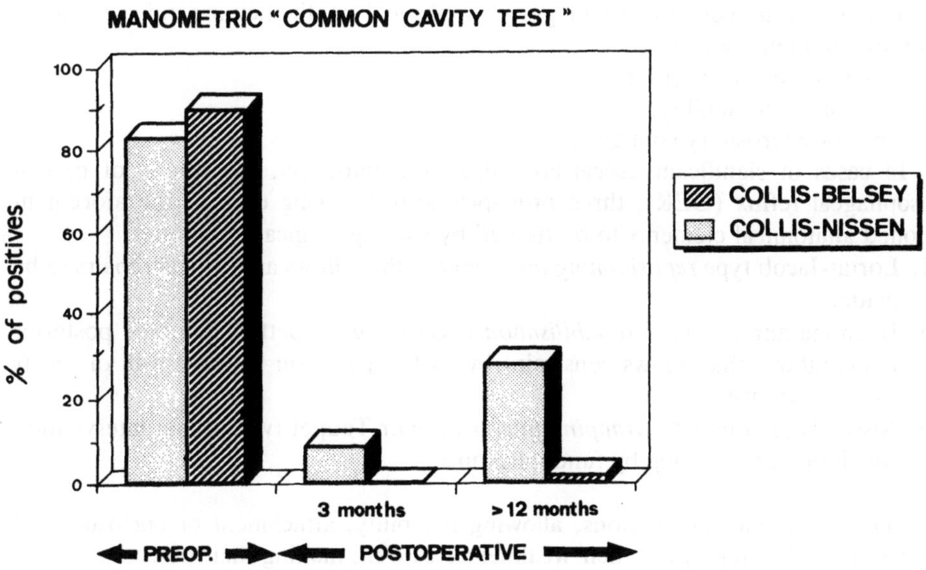

Fig. 8. Pre and postoperative manometric "Common cavity test"

We should emphasize the significant differences between the results of the two surgical procedures used in this study. They were better when a gastroplasty with total plication was employed, offering the most effective method to control gastroesophageal reflux in patients with esophageal stricture.

References

1. Leonardi HK, Ellis FH (1977) "Experimental fundoplication: comparison of results of different techniques". Surgery 82: 514–520
2. DeMeester TR, Johnson LE, Kent AH (1974) "Evaluation of current operations for the prevention of gastroesophageal reflux". Ann Surg 180: 511–525
3. Tomás Ridocci M, Benages A, Mora F et al (1986) "Analisis de los mecanismos de competencia gastroesofágica tras diversas técnicas quirúrgicas antirreflujo". Cir Esp 40: 1308–1314
4. París F, Tomás Ridocci M, Benages A et al (1982) "Gastroplasty with partial or total plication for gastroesophageal reflux: manometric and pH-metric postoperative results". Ann Thorac Surg 33: 540–548

Are there still indications for cardioplasty?

M. Vankemmel, C. Goachet, and *M. F. Brandt* (Lille)

General Principles

The anatomical requirements of gastroesophageal continency are ruled by three interrelated imperatives:
- a harmonious disposition,
- a satisfactory stability,
- an eso-tuberositary contiguity.

In cases of significant esocardiophrenic destabilisation, the source of gastroesophageal reflux (GER), three principles arise allowing each of the aforementioned anatomical elements to be treated by varying surgical techniques:
1. Lortat-Jacob type *repositioning intervention*, that allows anatomical repairs to be made.
2. Boerema anterior type *restabilisation intervention* or better, Hill type posterior intervention, that allows constraint by gastric pexy, on its front wall or on its small curvature.
3. Nissen type complete *wrapping intervention* or Toupet type partial intervention which permits clasping by fundoplicature.

These different interventions, allowing flexibility, attachment or enclosure; all have their advantages, but their weaknesses as well, making their objective partial and limited.

To bring together all three anatomical principles in a single intervention appears to be a presumptuous objective:

1. In the case of a malpositioned cardia, the difficulties of performing a good anatomical repositioning force us to perform transpositioning of the cardia by cardioplasty.
2. In the case of increasing instability of the esocardial junction, the difficulties of stabilization of the orifice force us to attach the valve, created in advance, by valvulopexy near its base.
3. In the case of non-contiguity caused by esotuberositary stretching, the difficulties of utilizing the virtual posterior space (retro-esophageal) force us to recover the front wall of abdominal esophagus, by the large tuberosity, the only available side which thus preserves its function of a vast air pocket.

This original "cardioplasty-valvulopexy-backup" or "cardioplasty-pexy" (CP-pexy) seems to us to renew both the anatomic and physiologic essentials of esophagogastric dynamics and gastroesophageal continence in a free way, without stiffness or constraint. This freedom is conditioned by suppression of lower esophageal widening, with reestablishment of a narrow esophageal junction, implanted no longer on the gastric dome, but on the lesser curvature. This gives the reshaped lower esophagus the appearance of a flute mouthpiece, whose vibratory and valvular membrane ensures the harmonious and unidirectional functioning of the arrangement, and is only forced open when necessary (Fig. 1).

Patients and Methods

From January 1980 until March 1987, we performed 243 esocardiophrenic restabilisations, following this technique (cardioplasty-pexy) by retensioning of the esophageal gap each time it appeared weakened. In addition to the 23 CP-pexies to correct a regional destabilization, along with other interventions (vagotomy, Heller, gastrectomy...) and of 88 surgical cures by opportunity of average severity GER treated during another abdominal intervention, 32 patients were sent to us for treatment of a particularly debilitating GER. All these patients benefited from a CP-pexy; among them, 10 suffered from a peptic stenosis, complicating a severe esophagitis.

These 10 patients – 6 men and 4 women – are between 30 and 59 years old (average age: 49.4 years). All these patients had a cardio-tuberositary malposition (n=4) or a hiatus hernia (by sliding: n=5 or mixed: n=1) complicated by an old pyrosis, by difficulties in swallowing, that in 2 cases corresponded to a recent and permanent dysphagia. There were bronchopulmonary signs in two patients (post-eating or nocturnal cough), and food rejection or vomiting blood in 2 others. Two patients had already benefited (before being brought to us) from a treatment of their GER (a woman, ten years earlier, by the thoracic route, and a man nine months earlier, by a Toupet intervention.

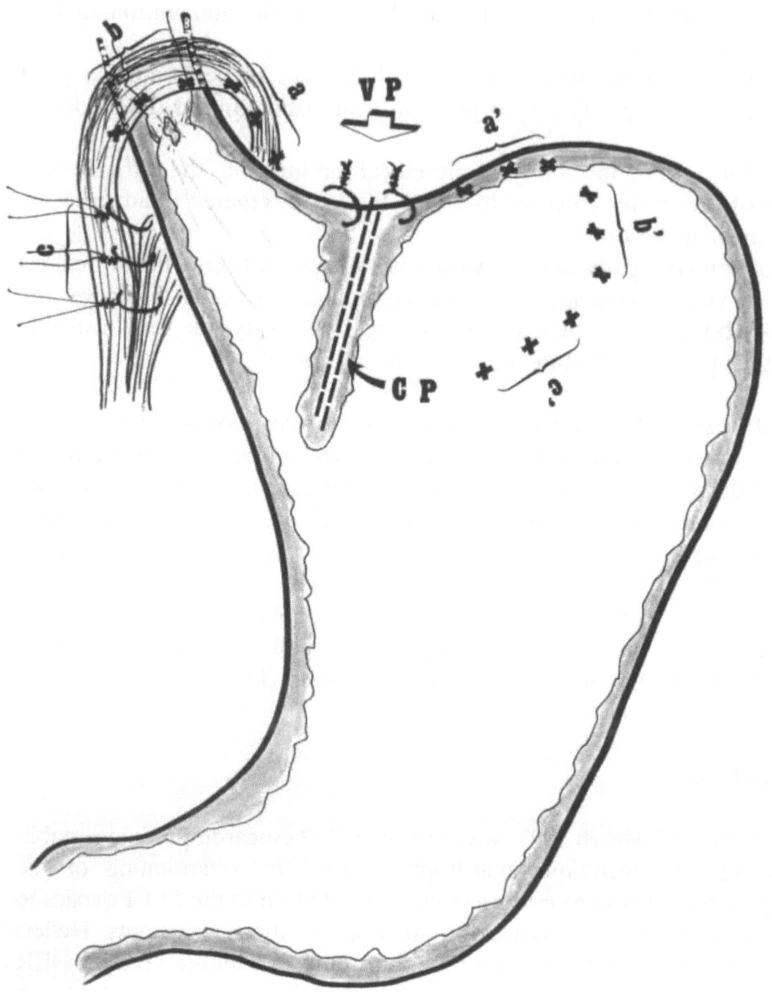

Fig. 1. Sliding hiatus hernia, complicated by an ulcerated and narrowing esophagitis: after esophageal dilatation with a Savary tube, surgical treatment by posterior myorraphy and "cardioplasty-pexy" (cardioplasty.CP–valvuloplasty.VP and anterior back-up of the tuberosity – abc –). It results the formation of a conic abdominal neo esophagus, like a flute-tip juxtaposed and recovered by a large gastric air pocket

The lesions of stenosis and esophagitis were confirmed

- by upper gastro-intestinal opacity: 8 slight narrowings on the lower esophagus, and 2 more important stenoses, the first one short and curved at the junction of middle 1/3 and upper 1/3 of the esophagus, and the second, severe and extensive, on about 10 cm of the lower 1/3 of the esophagus,
- by endoscopic exploration: for the 2 severe stenosis cited above, the esophagus below the stenosis could only be explored by a pediatric fibroscope (1 case) or after dilatation. The observed lesions of esophagitis were ulcerated in 4 cases

(Stadium 2a: 2 cases; Stadium 2b: 2 cases) frequently associated with aspects of gastric heterotopy, with 4 endobrachyesophagus, and once to an ulcer of the hernial collar. Biopsies were performed in 8 cases and it has been possible to confirm inflammatory alteration of the mucous wall of the esophagus with gastric metaplasia (n=3) and areas of intermediate dysplasia (n=2).

The intervention consisted of approximating the pillars of the esophageal hiatus (in all the cases except one) by posterior myorraphy associated with CP-pexy which combines cardioplexy-valvuloplasty and anterior tuberosity recovery:

- the cardioplasty has been and must be done with the Russian stapler YO 60, provided with loaders and staples of 5.5 length (the different TA 55 staplers – U.S.S.C. model – or SL 60 – Ethicon model – with staples 4.8 mm must be rejected for this. The pressing of these staples used without the guide wire is flawed. Besides, the 4.8 mm staples are too short for the thickness of the tissues for suturing near the gastric small curvature. The oblique orientation of the cardioplasty line (from the esocardiotuberositary angle of His to the gastric little curvature), and the calibration of the neocardia are assured by momentary insertion of the Savary tube (11 mm in diameter) into the stomach. So we obtain a conic neo-esophagus uni-directional, shaped like a flute-tip.
- the valvulopexy consists of the bond of the "hinges" of the valvular door, neoformed by suture of the top of the angle of His to the pre-aortic curvated ligament.
- the tuberositary recovery on the anterior wall of the abdominal esophagus and then on the neo-esophagus, is assured by a suture fastening the large tuberosity on the left, upper, and right edges of the hiatal opening without tension.

Results

There was no post-operative mortality

After surgery, only the patient already operated on by the abdominal approach according to Toupet needed an urgent reoperation, seven days after the first, for localized peritonitis caused by a perforation of the large tuberosity; this was cured by simple suture. This perforation corresponded to a very localized necrosis caused by the extraction of a big metallic clip which was found on the large tuberosity and whose extraction seemed to us to be necessary to complete the cardioplasty and anterior tuberosity recovery.

The average duration of hospitalization was 13.4 days with extremes from 7 to 40 days. Only three patients remained slightly dysphagic for thick fragments staying 3 to 5 weeks and only one had to be treated up to 30 days with dilatations using a Savary tube.

X-rays during the third month enabled us to see an elongation of the abdominal esophagus with lowering of the neocardia, compared to the archeocardia, and disappearance of signs of esophageal stenosis. As the same time endoscopy enabled us to see a healing of evolutive and ulcerated lesions of the esophageal mucous membrane. However, in the patient with a stenosis of middle 1/3 of the esophagus (totally regressive) it must be said that healing of all mucous lesions, with the exception of a small residual ulceration observed for the 3rd time during the 5th month that corresponded to a suspended zone of severe dysplasia, with carcinomatous transformation. This lesion justified surgical removal, with a gastric transplant (subtotal esophagectomy; the results remain excellent after 7 years). pH measurements of the esophagus were performed on 5 patients during the 6th and 12th months, and confirmed the favorable clinical results.

Only one patient (cardioplasty-pexy after Toupet, and operated on again seven days after surgery), after the 15th post-operative month, after complete disappearance of the symptomatology of his mucous lesions, associated with weight increase of 26 kgs, suffers from intermittent dysphagia with sometimes a complete food stoppage, without any obstruction. These different disturbance disappear systematically after inserting a Savary tube Nr. 12.8 into the esophagus. With this patient, endoscopy enabled us to confirm the persistence of the integrity of the esophageal mucous wall. Esophageal pressure measurements found a spastic aspect of the antireflux system. Esophageal measurements of pH showed only a slight gastroesophageal reflux of basic nature. At present, four years after the cardioplasty-pexy, clinical examination shows a hepatosplenomegaly with a collateral abdominothoracic circulation, caused by an old and relevant alcoholism.

Comments

The original technique [1, 2, 3], adopted in 243 patients for treatment of their GER [4] and applied to ten of them who suffered from a peptic stenosis, enables us to correct the deficiencies of the three essential antireflux systems that are classically accepted:

- orificial: correction of the hiatal gab by a posterior myorraphy;
- valvular: strengthening of the deficient valve of Gubaroff by cardioplasty and valvulopexy.
- tensional: new contiguity between the esophagus and the large tuberosity by reconstitution of a large air pocket, backed against a narrow and cylindroconic esophageal duct. So, it's possible to regularize the tension of the classical lower esophageal sphincter (anatomicaly, it corresponds to a real high pressure sieve depending on tensional variations, chiefly transmitted by the large tuberosity).

Moreover this cardioplasty-pexy, performed by the abdominal approach, can be used for an important inflammation around the esophagus, when the cardia can't be lowered because of the presence of a narrowing and retractile periesophageal sclerosis. This intervention needs neither a large dissection nor an important traction. With simple cardioplasty, by suture and without section, it is possible to perform the elongation of the abdominal esophagus and the abdominal transposition of the cardia together.

In an important esophageal narrowing, the dilatation must be and has been performed before surgery, with the Savary tube, to obtain passage of tube number 11 at least. Whenever the peptic stenosis can be enlarged this way, conservative surgical treatment appears to be possible and desirable, if there isn't any important dysplasia or any sulfomucines in the biopsic esophageal samples.

The cardioplasty-pexy is a logical complement to this technique, because it needs a Savary tube number 11 in the esophagus to give the calibre of the neo-esophagus and the neo-cardia. After five years, the good and very good results in 95% of the cases from this simple and physiological technique are strenghtened by the results of this short series of ten peptic stenoses. The radiologic and chiefly endoscopic follow-up associated with biopsy samples must be maintained a long time after the surgery to confirm disappearance of the stenosis and especially of the mucous lesions. Such a follow-up enabled us to detect the evolution of a small permanent esophageal ulceration in a carcinoma during the 6th month after surgery. It's interesting to notice that neither the esophagetomy nor the gastric tubulization was disturbed by the cardioplasty-pexy. Moreover, the excellent results have remained for seven years. The quality of the results achieved allows us to give the CP-pexy a good position in the therapeutic techniques for peptic esophagitis, even if they have a narrowing evolution.

References

1. Vankemmel M (1982) Etude comparée schématique de 4 procédés de correction du reflux gastro-oesophagien, par voie abdominale. J Chir 119: 295–301
2. Vankemmel M, Francke-Mauroy B (1982) Cardioplastie anti-reflux par suture mécanique: Bases physio-pathologiques et résultats (46 cas). Ann Chir 36: 459–467
3. Vankemmel M, Rwamasirabo E, Binot D (1983) Traitement du reflux gastro-oesophagien par cardioplastie. Ann Chir 37: 634–635
4. Vankemmel M, Goachet C, Leblance E, Bertaux D, Martin F (1987) La cardioplastie-pexie: indications et résultats (243 cas) Chirurgie 113 (sous presse)

Total duodenal diversion

H. Viard, J. P. Favre, A. Bernard, and *O. Haas* (Dijon)

Introduction

Total duodenal diversion (TDD) associating antrectomy and truncal vagotomy (TV) or distal gastrectomy (DG), to prevent acid reflux, with Roux en Y gastrojejunostomy, to eliminate biliary-pancreatic reflux, is a treatment in peptic esophagitis. The good results in our previous experience [5, 6] allowed extension of the indication.

The results on 23 patients operated on between 1970 and 1986 let us specify indications and their future.

Material and Methods

23 TDD for peptic esophagitis performed between 1970 and 1986 are analysed.

There are 17 men and 6 women, the mean age in 58 years (28 to 82).

In 8 cases, peptic esophagitis followed upper partial gastrectomy (UPG) performed for 6 cardia adenocarcinomas and 2 benign lesions. Gastroesophageal reflux caused severe discomfort with early appearance in all cases. After a 14 months delay on average, TDD couldn't be avoided. Esophagitis has associated digestive bleeding (2 cases) and peptic stenosis (3 cases) that have been treated by endoscopic dilatations.

In 5 cases peptic esophagitis followed a hiatal hernia recurrence (1 Hill and 4 Nissen, one of them on gastric cone). Esophagitis has associated digestive bleeding (1 case) and peptic stenosis (3 cases) without dilatation. TDD was performed 38 months later on average.

In 3 cases peptic esophagitis followed gastroesophageal reflux after Heller's procedure for achalasia. This reflux was late (8, 6 years later on average); all cases have associated stenosis treated by endoscopic dilatations (2 cases) and inferior esophagectomy and short coloplasty by left thoracotomy (1 case). TDD was performed, on average after 23 years, with Heller's procedure.

In 3 cases, peptic esophagitis has associated ulcer recurrence treated by distal gastrectomy with Finsterer's gastrojejunostomy (2 cases) and by TV with gastroenteroanastomosis (GEA) and anti-reflux procedure (1 case). The delay between TDD and previous gastric surgery was 18 years on average.

In 1 case peptic esophagitis followed a gastroesophageal reflux on a gastric catheter revealed 30 days later in a postoperative period. Finally, in 3 cases, peptic esophagitis was primitive, with unknown gastroesophageal reflux.

Operative procedure varies according to previous surgery.

In 10 cases, TV was performed previously (8 UPG, 1 esophagectomy, 1 TV with GEA for duodenal ulcerous stenosis), TDD was an antrectomy in 8 cases and in 2 cases duodenal exclusion without resection, with Roux en Y gastrojejunostomy.

In 13 cases, TV had not been performed. In 4 cases, the hiatus was accessible (3 primitive oesophagitis, 1 postoperative stenosis), TDD was antrectomy with TV and Roux en Y gastrojejunostomy. In 7 cases the hiatus was inaccessible (5 hiatal hernia recurrence) or dangerous (2 Heller procedure); TDD was distal gastrectomy in 5 cases, antrectomy with simultaneous thoracic TV in 1 case, and isolated antrectomy in 1 case with Roux en Y gastrojejunostomy. In the 2 cases with previous distal gastrectomy (duodenal ulcer) TDD was TV with Roux en Y gastrojejunostomy and antireflux procedure.

Indications, operative procedure, results and follow up are summarized in Table 1.

Results

The postoperative death rate is 2/23 cases: 1 catheter induced septicemia, 1 diabetic coma.

Table 1

Esophagitis reason	Delay before TDD	TDD procedure	Results	Follow up
UPG: 8 cases	14 months	7 A + Y 1 Dε + Y	1 death (septicemia) 7 good results	1 to 9 years
Hiatal hernia recurrence: 5 cases (1 Hill, 4 Nissen)	38 months	3 D.G. + Y 1 A+ thoracic TV + Y 2 isolated A + Y	4 good results 1 peptic ulcer	1 to 36 months
Heller procedure: 2 cases Heller esophagocoloplasty after: 1 case	23 years	2 D.G. + Y 1 A + Y	1 digestive draining trouble 2 good results	3 to 48 months
Ulcer after DG + F: 2 cases TV + GEA + ARP: 1 case	18 years	2 TV + Y + ARP 1 Dε + Y	3 good results	2 to 10 months
Primitive stenosis: 3 cases Postoperative: 1 case		2 A + TV + Y + ARP 1 A + TV + Y 1 A + TV + Y	3 good results 1 death (diabetic coma)	2 to 15 months

UPG: upper partial gastrectomy; TDD: total duodenal diversion; D: duodenal exclusion; A: antrectomy; DG: distal gastrectomy; TV: truncal vagotomy; Y: Roux en Y gastrojejunostomy; GEA: gastro entero anastomosis; ARP: anti-reflux procedure; F: Finsterer's gastrojejunostomy

Postoperative morbidity was 2 gastroplegia, 1 subphrenic abcess, 1 intestinal occlusion and 1 eventration. But no gastric necrosis was observed.

In the other patients, post operative follow up has been 35 months.

We obtained 19 good results: 18 directly, 1 after gastrojejunostomy refection 4 months later.

The 2 bad results are: 1 gastrojejunal draining trouble persisting 48 months later (distal gastrectomy for reflux after Heller); endoscopy doesn't reveal esophagitis but a good gastrojejunostomy permeability; 1 peptic ulcer 2 months after TDD (distal gastrectomy for reflux recurrence after Nissen's procedure that have migrated into the thorax) with a successful medical treatment.

Discussion

TDD in peptic esophagitis treatment gives good results (19/21 cases in our series) in agreement with others [1]. The 2 postoperative deaths are independent of surgical procedure (1 septicemia, 1 diabetic coma). With Fekete [1], we have observed gastroplegia (2 cases). The 2 bad results are reliable to procedure error: 1 peptic gastrojejunal ulcer after insufficient gastrectomy actually medically treated, 1 gastrojejunal draining persisting trouble. No dumping syndrome [3], and no gastric necrosis [2] were observed.

Peptic esophagitis after hiatal surgery is the best indication (17/23 cases). After UPG (8 cases) no gastric necrosis was observed; the 9 months delay between the 2 gastric resections allowed a neovascularisation development of the untouched gastric segment; Hivet describes 1 case of gastric necrosis but only endoscopically [2]. In hiatal hernia, surgery (5 cases) resection must be distal gastrectomy or antrectomy with thoracic TV to avoid peptic ulcer: 1 case in our series; gastric resection importance was overestimated because the Nissen was intrathoracic. In peptic esophagitis after Heller (3 cases), we have 2 good results and in one of them TDD was performed after an inferior esophagectomy with short coloplasty, confirming Popovici's results [4]. Esophagitis after TV for duodenal ulcer (1 case) is also a good indication.

These TDD good results induced us to use this procedure in esophagitis after distal gastrectomy for ulcer (2 cases), in primitive peptic esophagitis (3 cases really primitive, 1 case after gastric catheter). In these 2 indications an antireflux procedure must be associated with TDD.

Washer, in a randomized study, showed TDD to be better than Nissen for gastroesophageal reflux primary treatment [7], and TDD should certainly be weight against Collis-Nissen procedure in severe peptic esophagitis with unlowerable cardia.

References

1. Fekete F, Hugentobler GL, Breil Ph (1983) Place de la diversion duodénale totale dans le traitement de l'œsophagite peptique: à propos de 15 observations. Actualités Chirurgicales 82–89, Masson, Edit Paris
2. Hivet M, Mahoux P (1974) Œsophagite grave après œsogastrectomie polaire supérieure: 2 cas traités par gastrectomie inférieure complémentaire. Ann Chir 28: 989–994
3. Hollender LF, Meyer Ch, Marrie A, Keller D, Zeyber B, Goldschmidt P (1981) La place de la fundo-jéjunostomie sur anse exclue en Y dans les échecs thérapeutiques chirurgicaux du reflux gastro-œsophagien. Chirurgie 107: 139–145
4. Popovici Z (1986) La diversion duodénale totale dans l'œsophagite du reflux après l'œsophagoplastie colique. J Chir (Paris) 123: 500–503
5. Viard H, Favre JP, Cayot M, Trigalou D, Chevillotte P (1978) Le traitement chirurgical de l'œsophagite peptique après œsogastrectomie polaire supérieure. Plaidoyer en faveur de l'antrectomie suivie de gastro-jéjunostomie en Y. A propos de 5 observations. Ann Chir: Chir Thorac Cardiovasc 17: 217–221
6. Viard H, Favre JP, Sala JJ, Sicard C, Hillon P, Cougard P (1985) La diversion duodénale totale dans le traitement des œsophagites peptiques. Lyon Chir 81: 3–6
7. Washer GF, Gear HLW, Dowling BL, Gillisson ZW, Royston CMS, Spencer J (1984) Randomized prospective trial of Roux en Y duodenal diversion versus fundoplication for severe reflux oesophagitis. Br J Surg 71: 181–184

Must duodenal diversion be reserved for alkaline reflux?

H. Viard (Dijon)

In answering this question, it is important to note that two populations may be opposed in our series: those of esophagitis after UPG (Uppen Polar Gastrectomy) (8 cases), where the result of duodenal diversion is regularly good and long-lasting, and those of esophagitis after recurrence of hiatus hernia (5 cases) or after Heller's operation (3 cases), which include the 2 poor results. This contrast is probably linked to the nature of the reflux. In UPG the reflux is alkaline, since there has been a TV (Truneal Vagotony) and an extensive gastric resection; the esophagitis is then early and severe. In recurrences after hiatus hernia or Heller operations the reflux is acid and the esophagitis develops later. But when there is no anatomic explanation to arouse suspicion of alkaline reflux, its diagnosis may encounter technical difficulties. In fact, endoscopy and scintigraphy with technetium-99 can diagnose duodeno-gastric reflux [3] but pH measurement cannot prove alkaline esophageal reflux since the esophageal pH is normally elevated and the recording is disturbed by the alkaline saliva [4].

This accounts for the uneven quality of the results of duodenal diversion in postoperative biliary gastritis [1, 2, 3] and makes it impossible to predict the success of duodenal diversion in peptic esophagitis.

References

1. Jebira A, Benamor N, Ayachi K, Ben Younes MA, Gargouri M, Fourati M (1986) La diversion duodénale totale: à propos de 4 cas. Me Chir Dig 15: 559–562
2. Malagelada JR, Phillips S, Shorter RG, Higgins JA, Magrina C, Van Heerden JA, Adson MA (1985) Post-operative reflux gastritis: pathophysiology and long term outcome after Roux en Y diversion. Ann Intern Med 103: 178–183
3. Ritchie WP Jr (1986) Alkaline reflux gastritis: late results on a controlled trial of Diagnosis and treatment. Ann Surg 203: 537–544
4. Schlesinger PK, Donahue PE, Schmid B, Layden TJ (1985) Limitations of 24-hour intra-oesophageal pH-Monitoring in the hospital setting. Gastroenterology 80: 797–804

From the clinical point of view, do peptidic hormones have an effect on LES?

T. Chevalier, and *S. Bonfils* (Paris)

A large number of peptidic hormones exert a pharmacologic action on the LES. The chief of these are gastrin and motilin, which produce contraction, and the pancreozymin cholecystokinin (CCK) and secretin, which produce relaxation of the LES. Should it therefore be concluded that a hormonal regulation of sphincteric tonus under physiologic or certain pathologic conditions exists? There is no definite answer to this question, even though it is now accepted that the LES is essentially under the control of the autonomic nervous system.

The peptidic hormones could have a modulating role, in view of the close interrelation of nervous and hormonal regulation at various levels of the alimentary tract. Certain peptidic hormones are present in both the nerve fibers and the endocrine cells and have an action of endocrine and/or paracrine nature. The hormonal action may be exerted via the nerve-endings or directly on the smooth muscle.

The demonstration of a physiologic hormonal effect is based on a group of arguments:

1. correlation between the levels of circulating hormones and the corresponding LES pressure in the postprandial period or during trials of gastric acidification or alkalinization
2. modification of LES pressure after injection of specific antibodies (antigastrin, antisecretin) in animals
3. modification of LES pressure in response to prolonged perfusion of hormones at levels reproducing physiologic plasma variations.

These studies are subject to certain limitations. They usually involve plasma variations of a single hormone, which are not necessarily representative of tissue concentrations, and the data obtained do not allow integration of the complex problem of hormonal and neurohormonal interactions. This may explain the contradictory results of numerous studies seeking to demonstrate a regulatory role of gastrin on the LES under physiologic conditions [2].

This role might be more obvious in certain pathologic conditions of hormonal hypersecretion. This is the case in the Zollinger-Ellison syndrome (ZES), characterized by an abnormal secretion of gastrin of tumoral origin and in which an increased LES pressure correlated with plasma gastrin levels has been reported [3].

These sphincteric changes might reduce the risks of esophagitis associated with acid gastric hypersecretion by reinforcing the “anti-reflux barrier”.

The fact thus far admitted has not been confirmed in a recent study, where it appears that esophagitis is common in ZES [4]. Again, several studies have shown no increase of LES pressure in patients affected by the ZES, despite very high average levels of plasma gastrin, thus casting doubt on the action of gastrin on the LES [1].

References

1. Roze C (1980) Régulation de la motricité oesophagienne et gastrique; aspects physiologiques et pharmacologiques récents. Gastroenterol Clin Biol 4: 486–496
2. Meyer GW, Castell DO (1982) Physiology of the esophagus. Clin Gastroenterol 11: 439–451
3. Isenberg J (1971) Resting and paentagastrin stimulated gastro-esophageal sphincter pressure in patients with Zollinger-Ellison syndrome. Gastroenterology 61: 655–658

4. Ollyo JB (1986) L'oesophagite par reflux au cours du syndrome de Zollinger-Ellison; à propos de 33 cas. Mémoire pour le titre d'assistant étranger; Université de Paris 7, Faculté de médecine Xavier Bichat

J. W. Maher (Iowa City)

The answer to this question is not entirely clear at this juncture. Evidence from canine studies indicates that pancreatic polypeptide release, secondary to vagal stimulation, the presence of protein in the duodenum, or both are responsible for the postprandial increase in lower esophageal sphincter pressure [1–5]. If one experimentally excludes the duodenum of dogs from contact with gastric chyme, this normal postprandial increase in sphincter pressure is eliminated and pancreatic polypeptide release is attenuated [1, 2].

Perfusion of the excluded duodenum with peptone solution is associated with increases in both lower esophageal sphincter pressure and pancreatic polypeptide levels [6]. Additionally, suppression of enteral hormone release by somatostatin infusion eliminates both the postprandial increase in sphincter pressure and the increase seen in response to duodenal peptone infusion [6]. Finally, administration of pancreatic polypeptide in doses that produce plasma levels similar to those seen postprandially, result in increased LESP, similar to that which is observed postprandially [7].

There is also evidence that this phenomenon may occur in man. Recently, Funch-Jensen et al. have reported that in patients with an "abnormal duodenal loop" (e.g. Billroth II), there is a paradoxical decrease in postprandial lower esophageal sphincter pressure [8].

Nonetheless, it is impossible, at present, to say what contribution the postprandial increase in sphincter pressure makes to overall gastroesophageal competence. Postprandial gastroesophageal reflux is common in controls; however, Baldi et al. have found increased postprandial reflux in esophagitis patients [9].

Further experiments to estimate the importance of the postprandial increase in sphincter pressure are essential: if this increase in sphincter pressure is found to be an important defense mechanism, it might become necessary to reconsider the physiologic rationale for duodenal diversion in treating patients with esophagitis. Nevertheless, the excellent results reported with duodenal diversion in reoperations for esophagitis continue to make this procedure a viable therapeutic option at this point [10].

References

1. Maher JW, Olinde AJ, McGuigan JE (1982) The effects of duodenal exclusion on postprandial lower esophageal sphincter pressure. Surgical Forum 33: 139
2. Maher JW, Olinde AJ, McGuigan JE (1984) Suppression of postprandial lower esophageal sphincter pressure and pancreatic polypeptide by duodenal exclusion. J Surg Res 37: 467–471

3. Coltharp WH, Maher MS, Maher JW, Koury AM, McGuigan JE (1985) The effect of vagotomy on lower esophageal sphincter pressure response to pancreatic polypeptide. Surg Forum 36: 119–121
4. Olinde AJ, Maher MS, Maher JW, McGuigan JE (1986) The effect of varying levels of vagotomy on postprandial lower esophageal sphincter pressure and pancreatic polypeptide. W J Surg 10: 809–813
5. Maher JW The etiology of the postprandial increase in lower esophageal sphincter pressure: Evidence for control by pancreatic polypeptide and vagal influences. In Proceedings of International Esophageal Week. Springer Verlag (in press)
6. Maher JW, Olinde AJ, Coltharp WC, McGuigan JE (1984) The role of the duodenum in regulation of postprandial lower esophageal sphincter pressure (abstract). Gastroenterology 86: 1171
7. Coltharp WH, Maher MS, Maher JW, Koury AM, McGuigan JE (1985) Effect of vagotomy on lower esophageal sphincter pressure response to pancreatic polypeptide. Surg Forum 36: 119–121
8. Funch-Jensen P, Oster MJ, Thommesen P (1981) Food-stimulated gastroesophageal sphincter pressure in patients with abnormal duodenal loop compared with controls. Scand J Gastroent 16: 527–530
9. Baldi F, Ferrarini F, Balestra R (1984) Diurnal pattern of esophageal motility and acid reflux in normal subjects and in patients with esophagitis. Gastroenterol (abstract) 86: 1018
10. Fekete F (1985) Total duodenal diversion. In Esophageal Disorders: Pathophysiology and Therapy. DeMeester TR and Skinner DB (Ed) Raven Press, New York

Surgical resection

Evaluation of surgical results

President: *Robert D. Henderson* (Toronto)

Free Commentators: *H. Charleux* (Paris)
R. E. Condon (Milwaukee)
C. A. Hiebert (Portland)
F. G. Pearson (Toronto)
M. Rossetti, B. Meyrat (Liestal)
P. Vayre (Paris)

Introduction

H. Charleux, and *J. P. Marmuse* (Paris)

From February 1984 to February 1987, 12 patients (7 men and 5 women) with a mean age of 61 years (range 28–84 years) benefited from esophageal resection for peptic structure. Eleven were operated electively because of an extensive undilatable stricture. One was operated on urgently for perforation during a dilatation session. All had been treated medically for several years with repeated sessions of dilatation in addition. 5 had already been operated for hiatus hernia (1 Nissen and 4 Toupet procedures), 1 was followed up for a ZE syndrome, and 1 has had a gastrectomy. Apart from the patient operated as an emergency, the indication for operation was the failure of dilatation sessions and the impermeable nature of the stricture.

Operation

Excision was always performed by the trans-hiatal route. No esophageal restoration was done for the patient operated urgently and the operation ended with a cervical esophagostomy and a gastrostomy. This patient is now in excellent condition and restoration will be done in a month. In the other 11 patients, restoration will be done as follows: 2 by left coloplasty (the patient with the ZE syndrome and the patient with previous gastrectomy); 9 by tubulated gastroplasty using the lesser curvature, vascularization being assured by the pyloric and right gastro-epiploic vessels.

Pyloroplasty was done routinely. All the plasties were placed in the posterior mediastinum; the anastomosis was performed by continuous vicryl suture in all patients. There were no peroperative complications. The postoperative course was straightforward. 1 patient had a left subphrenic abscess, reoperated and cured. There was no fistula, no pneumopathy and the duration of stay in intensive care was always less than a week. All patients were discharged less than 3 weeks after operation, nourished normally by mouth (solid diet, bread, etc). The late results are excellent. There was no recurrent paralysis and no reflux; one stricture of the cervical anastomosis was cured by two sessions of dilatation.

Discussion

This procedure has several advantages. It permits excision of the stenosis, but also of the proximal esophagus, often the site of motor disorders. The risk of mediastinal fistula is nil, which is important for an benign type of lesion since these fistulae still have a mortality that is very high (over 50%). There is no reflux, probably due to the intrathoracic position of all the residual stomach. The functional results of gastroplasty are excellent, those of coloplasty less so. Mortality nil.

Gastric replacement

P. Fuentes, P. Thomas, R. Giudicelli, B. Dupin, V. Fulachier, and *E. Reboud* (Marseilles)

In the past, it was not uncommon to perform esophageal resection for peptic esophagitis. Today, however, thanks not only to widespread use of modern dilatation techniques but also to surgical procedures such as duodenal diversion and gastroplasty fundoplication, the indications for esophagectomy are much less frequent [1, 3, 5, 8, 13]. The rate of esophageal resection for peptic esophagitis is currently about 10% (Table 1). Esophageal resection for peptic esophagitis accounts for around 25% of all esophagectomies performed for benign lesions of the esophagus (Table 2) [3, 8]. It is important to say that in the present study patients undergoing a retrosternal by-pass without esophagectomy are not considered. This procedure should in fact not be used since it leaves in place the diseased esophagus which is still exposed to gastroesophageal reflux (G.E.R.) and inaccessible to endoscopic surveillance.

Table 1. Rate of esophagectomy for peptic esophagitis

Neville	1962	10/27	=37%
Belsey	1967	229/270	=85%
Williamson	1971	12/83	=14.4%
Gatzinski	1976	12/57	=21%
Keenam	1977	27/94	=28.7%
Reboud	1986	14/115	=12.2%

Table 2. Esophagectomy for benign disease

	Benign lesions	Peptic esophagitis
Hankins – 1982 –	23	6=26%
Orringer – 1985 –	65	15=24%

From a perusal of the literature (Table 3), it is possible to define a certain number of situations in which esophagectomy is indicated for peptic esophagitis. They are as follows:

1. Failure of forceful dilatation. With the advent of the Savary system, dilatation is feasible in almost all cases except perhaps those involving very extensive lesions. In some cases even though dilatation may be initially successful, recurrence is rapid despite appropriate drug therapy.
2. Anatomic difficulties preventing the cardia from being lowered into the abdomen [11]. Although its existence has been disputed, all authors have at some point in their experience encountered the problem of a short esophagus (brachyesopha-

Table 3. Peptic esophagitis – resection – esophageal reconstruction

	Resection	Gastro plasty	Colonic interposition	Jejunal interposition
Neville 1962	10	2	8	
Belsey 1967	229	41	188	
Payne 1970	6	6		
Williamson 1971	12	9	1	2
Gatzinski 1976	12	12		
Keenam 1977	27		17	10
Orringer 1985	15	10	4	
Reboud 1985	14	6	8	

gus). In such cases, esophagectomy is, however, not the only surgical option available and conservative procedures such as duodenal diversion [2, 12]. Nissen intrathoracic fundoplication and Collis-Nissen fundoplication may still be possible [7–10].

3. Inability to rule out malignancy in spite of multiple biopsy samples. Histologically speaking Barrett's esophagus associated with moderate or severe dysplasia has a great potential for malignant transformation. In our opinion esophagectomy is an appropriate therapy for long term survival in these cases [11].
4. Unfeasibility of repeated antireflux surgery. Antireflux surgery may be unavailable as a result of previous surgery or because of associated esophageal disease (achalasia, scleroderma, ...). Again in this case esophagectomy is not the only alternative, but it may be the best in terms of long term results [1, 6].

Of these four situations, the last two most frequently motivate esophagectomy for high grade peptic esophagitis. That is to say when malignancy cannot be ruled out or when antireflux surgery can no longer be performed with a reasonable hope of success.

Gastroplasty is one means used to reestablish digestive patency after esophagectomy. Several gastroplasty procedures have been described:

1. After partial esophagectomy and mobilization of the stomach, gastroplasty can be performed with an intrathoracic anastomosis. Several insertion techniques or valve mechanisms have been proposed to protect this type of anastomosis from recurrence of GER, but none have been very successful. Thus this procedure is generally not advocated by the various authors.
2. Total esophagectomy (with or without thoracotomy) or subtotal esophagectomy with a gastroesophageal anastomosis by thoracotomy at the top of the thorax are the most widely recommended resection procedures. Under these conditions, the stomach is a very versatile esophageal substitute [8] that can be used in its entirety, or according to the technique of Akiyama, or by tubularization of the greater curvature. In our department we prefer the latter method because it always provides a sufficiently long graft with a guaranteed blood supply. Other forms of gastroplasty that may be suitable in some cases are the Celerier and the Gavriliu procedures. The esogastric anastomosis is made either by thoracotomy at the top of the thorax or by left cervicotomy.

The series reported in the literature are too small and too diverse and in most cases the follow-up is too short to allow statistical comparison of these various procedures [1, 5, 8]. Better results with regard to operative mortality and morbidity as well as in terms of function do however appear to be gained by following a few simple guidelines:
- perform total or subtotal esophagectomy;
- position the gastric substitute in the bed of the resected esophagus. This facilitates swallowing;
- make the esogastric anastomosis as high as possible. This should preclude the risks of recurrent esophagitis upstream.

Peptic esophagitis is not a malignant disease. Unlike cancer, the long term prognosis after esophagectomy is good. Thus the operation must be a riskfree as possible and provide functional results compatible with a long life. Esophagectomy can be carried out with or without thoracotomy and followed by gastroplasty either in the same operation or in a separate stage. This depends on individual factors such as age, overall status, and especially on previous surgical history and the condition of the esophagus.

In some patients who have undergone previous antireflux procedures, the stomach cannot be used as an esophageal substitute. It is thus important to recall that prior to 1975 colonic interposition according to Belsey was a widely used technique of esophageal reconstruction [13]. Since then this type of procedure has fallen into disuse the stomach being more and more frequently preferred as a substitute in cases of esophageal cancer. The experience garnered in the treatment of malignant esophageal disease was transfered to esophageal replacement after esophagectomy for peptic esophagitis. At the present time, however, valid statistical studies comparing these two esophageal substitutes are unavailable since the series are too small. While the colon is a very reliable esophageal substitute, the stomach, when usable, may be a better alternative since the operation is simpler and mortality lower. Moreover functional results can be excellent if the anastomosis is performed very high.

References

1. Fuentes P, Giudicelli R, Riera P, Dumon JF, Dupin B, Reboud E (1985) Treatment of Esophageal Peptic Strictures Esophageal Disorders: pathophysiology and therapy, DeMeester and Skinner Ed. Raven Press 253–256
2. Hesselink EJ, Sloof MJH, Bleichrodt RP, Jansen W, Edens EJ (1986) B2 Gastrectomy and Roux en Y duodenal diversion as treatment for severe esophagitis International Esophageal Week, Munich
3. Hankins JR, Cole FN, McLaughlin JS (1984) Colon interposition for benign esophageal disease: experience with 23 patients. The Annals of Thoracic Surgery 37: 192
4. Mansour KA, Hansen HA, Hersh T, Miller JI Jr, Hatcher CR Jr (1981) Colon interposition for advanced non malignant esophageal stricture: Experience with 40 patients. The Annals of Thoracic Surgery 32: 584
5. Keenan JM, Hamilton JRL, Gibbons J, Stevenson HM (1984) Surgery for benign Esophageal Stricture J Thorac Cardiovasc Surg 88: 182–188

6. Mercer CD, Hill LD (1986) Surgical management of peptic esophageal stricture Twenty year experience. J Thorac Cardiovasc Surg 91: 371–378
7. Orringer MB (1986) Combinend Collis Gastroplasty – Nissen Fundoplication operation for esophageal reflux strictures. International Esophageal Week, Munich
8. Orringer MB (1986) Tranhiatal esophagectomy for benign disease. J Thorac Cardiovasc Surg 90: 649–655
9. Pearson FG, Pizza D, Cooper JD, Patterson GA, Todd TR, Waters PF (1986) Gastroplasty and partial fundoplication in patients with peptic esophagitis and acquired shortening: results in long term follow-up International Esophageal Week, Munich
10. Pearson FG (1985) Collis-Belsey procedure for peptic strictures: Five to 15 year follow-up Esophageal Disorders, Pathology and Therapy. DeMeester-Skinner Ed. Raven Press 257–260
11. Skinner DB, Walther BC, Little AG (1985) Surgical treatment of Barrett's esophagus Barrett's esophagus: pathophysiology, diagnosis and management – Spechler S, Goyal RAJ-K – Elsevier 211–222
12. Washer GF, Gear MWL, Dowling BL, Gillison EW, Royston CMS, Spencer J (1984) Randomized prospective trial of Roux-en-Y duodenal diversion versus fundoplication for severe reflux esophagitis Br J Surg 71: 181–184
13. Belsey R (1965) Reconstruction of the esophagus with left colon. J Thorac Cardiovasc Surg 49: 33–55

P. F. Waters, F. G. Pearson, T. Todd, G. A. Patterson, M. Goldberg, R. J. Ginsberg, J. D. Cooper, J. Ramirez, and *L. Miller* (Toronto)

It has been pointed out by many authors that, in neuromuscular disorders of the esophagus, the best chance of a successful outcome will be present at the patient's first surgical procedure. For this result a careful diagnosis, using all available techniques including manometry, radiology and endoscopy is important. Furthermore, a well planned and appropriate procedure by a surgeon experienced in such disorders is crucial. Once the initial procedure has failed then the likelihood of further reconstructive surgery of revisional surgery in the lower esophageal area being successful diminishes.

In a patient with a motor disorder characterized by aperistalsis, either iatrogenic or as the primary disorder, the development of a peptic stricture is the final nail in the coffin of unsatisfactory swallowing. Any attempt at revision will be difficult to accomplish. One must balance the obstruction caused by an anti-reflux procedure and the subsequent dysphagia made worse by the aperistalsis against the problem of recurrent reflux and ongoing peptic esophagitis and stricture. It is virtually impossible to achieve this balance in exactly the correct way.

We have felt, therefore that patients with motor disorders who present with peptic stricture, and in particular this refers to the group of patients with achalasia, revisional surgery on the lower esophagus is ill-advised. We recommend at that time an esophageal resection.

Similarly, patients with complex reflux disorders which have resulted in peptic stricture and in whom several previous attempts have unsuccessfully controlled reflux have again been recommended for resection rather than repeat anti-reflux surgery. This of course is providing that the anti-reflux surgery previously performed has been satisfactorily carried out.

Other motor disorders including spasm have also come to resection. In this group of patients the myotomy has been performed and aperistalsis is iatrogenic. Once again when reflux occurs as a post-operative complication in these patients the development of a stricture makes this situation almost impossible to salvage without resectional surgery. The final group of patients to be mentioned are those having suffered multiple complications following trauma or instrumental perforation.

We have had the opportunity to review our experience with resectional surgery for complex benign disease. In a ten year period between 1976 and 1986 we collected a group of twenty-one such patients who were treated with total thoracic esophagectomy and replacement with stomach. Simultaneously, close to five hundred patients were seen and treated surgically for benign esophageal disorders so that this group of patients represents a small number in our total practice.

Of these twenty-one patients, all had previous operations designed to relieve symptoms of benign esophageal disorders. All patients had at least one and some had up to four previous procedures performed. Sixteen of the twenty-one patients had primary motor disorders. Nine patients had the diagnosis of achalasia and were treated with Heller myotomy. These patients presented with aperistalsis and peptic stricture secondary to esophagitis and gastroesophageal reflux. In seven patients, esophageal spasm had been treated by esophageal myotomy with dysphagia and reflux causing an unsatisfactory result. There were eleven patients who had multiple operations for gastroesophageal reflux and peptic esophagitis. These patients remained severely symptomatic usually with severe reflux and/or dysphagia.

We elected to perform total thoracic esophagectomy in all twenty-one cases favouring this approach over the intrathoracic anastomosis because of the much decreased incidence of reflux related problems using the anastomosis in the neck. The resection was carried out via a right thoracotomy, laparotomy and neck incision in five patients and in sixteen patients the operation was performed transhiatally without thoracotomy.

There were no serious intra-operative complications. There was one perioperative death which occurred from massive aspiration resulting in respiratory failure and death following transhiatal esophagectomy for a failed Heller myotomy. Other complications included an anastomotic leak in three. All were treated conservatively and resolved spontaneously. In one patient a tracheoesophageal fistula followed an anastomotic leak, again managed conservatively and eventually responding to this treatment. There was one recurrent nerve palsy which required treatment. In two patients hoarseness was transient.

We have been able to record good to excellent functional results in twelve patients, fair results in seven and poor results in one. It is felt that this outcome in this very difficult patient group is quite acceptable and respresents a better result than could be expected from further local revisional surgery. We therefore recommend esophageal resection for benign disease in the situations as described; the patient with failed multiple operations who have neuromuscular disorders of the esophagus and the patient who has had multiple procedures for gastroesophageal reflux may benefit from resection rather than further attempts at local surgery.

We feel that total thoracic esophagectomy with the use of stomach as replacement organ is by far the more straight forward and easily performed procedure. We recommend its use whenever possible; and also favour the esophagogastric anastomosis in the neck as opposed to intrathoracic anastomosis for the reasons we have mentioned. We once again urge that the initial procedure for such motor disorders be carefully planned and performed by an experienced surgeon in order to lessen the likelihood that a failed procedure will result in eventual resection.

References

1. Orringer MB, Orringer JS (1982) Esophagectomy: Definitive treatment for esophageal neuromotor dysfunction. Ann Thor Surg 34 (3): 237
2. Mullen DC, Young WG Jr, (Sealy WC (1968) Results of twenty years experience with esophageal replacement for benign disorders. Ann Thor Surg 5: 481
3. Belsey RHR (1965) Reconstruction of the esophagus with left colon. J Thorac Cardiovasc Surg 49: 33
4. Orringer MB, Kirsh MM, Sloan H (1977) New trends in esophageal replacement for benign disease. Ann Thor Surg 23: 409

Colon interposition

R. Belsey (Chicago)

The advantages of left colon for replacement:

1. Adequate length of viscus to replace the entire esophagus up to the pharynx.
2. Reliable, anatomically constant blood supply from left colic artery.
3. Smaller caliber than right colon; trained to propel a solid bolus.
4. Applicable to children.
5. Long term functional results satisfactory in 85% of cases.
6. Available for bypass as well as replacement.
7. Operative mortality can be no higher than 5%.
8. Functional results improve progressively in time.
9. Late complications are rare.

Contraindications

1. Intrinsic colonic disease.
2. Mesenteric arteritis.
3. Previous colonic surgery; debatable.
4. Previous abdominal surgery may have interfered with the blood supply.
5. Sluggish colon in 15% of cases.

Technique

1. Extended left thoracotomy, 6th interspace.
2. Inspection of left colic artery and branches.
3. Mobilization of colon segment. Pyloromyotomy.
4. Colocolic anastomosis. Single layer interrupted steel wire technique.
5. Cologastric anastomosis, low posterior.
6. Selection of route for transplant; mediastinal, transpleural, substernal in that order of preference.
7. Esophagocolic anastomosis, thoracic or cervical. Cervical for preference.
8. Correction of any redundancy. Fixation to hiatus.
9. Review of blood supply. Venous drainage, is as important as arterial in flow.
10. Repair of thoracotomy.
11. Postoperative care. Normal alimentation can be started in 48 hours if steel wire anastomotic technique is employed.

Complications

1. Loss of transplant; interference with arterial inflow. Kinking, torsion. Obstruction of venous drainage.
2. Progressive fibrosis at proximal end; chronic venous obstruction.
3. Intrathoracic redundancy. Preventable.
4. Anastomotic strictures. Steel wire technique. End-to-end anastomoses.
5. Gastrocolic reflux. Preventable; low posterior cologastric anastomosis.
6. Functional inadequacy. Sluggish, atonic, colon. Preoperative investigation.
7. Transient diarrhea.
8. Antiperistaltic transplants.

Common technical errors

1. Inadequate exposure.
2. Excessive handling of mesocolon and nutrient vessels.
3. Kinking the left colic vascular pedicle round the lesser curve when attempting an anterior cologastric anastomosis.
4. A cologastric anastomosis at the cardia or apex of the fundus. The low posterior anastomosis creates an effective antireflux mechanism.
5. The transmediastinal or transpleural route is the most direct and least likely to embarrass the arterial supply and venous drainage.
6. The retrosternal route is more tortuous and accompanied by a higher incidence of complications at the esophagocolic anastomosis.
7. Multilayer anastomotic techniques. The single layer end to end steel wire technique has proven the most effective.
8. Failure to anchor the transplant to the margin of the hiatus may permit intrathoracic prolapse and redundancy.
9. Antiperistaltic transplants must be avoided. The results are functionally inadequate or lethal.

D. B. Skinner (Chicago)

There are many options for esophageal replacement including left and transverse colon, right and transverse colon, jejunum, whole stomach, partial stomach, gastric tube, free intestinal grafts, skin tubes, or extracorporeal tubes. Among these the procedure of choice in our clinic is isoperistaltic left and transverse colon interposition.

Factors which influence the choice for esophageal replacement include the presence of other diseases such as ulcer disease making the stomach undesirable, or colonic disease precluding the use of colon interposition. Pancreatitis or portal hypertension may cause problems in managing the mesentery. Prior surgery involving the colon, stomach, or small intestine obviously influences the choice.

The nature of the disease requiring esophagectomy may influence the decision. A palliative operation for malignant disease is best concluded as rapidly as possible, and this usually means advancing the stomach as the simplest replacement. However, the acid secretion of the stomach has the potential for causing severe esophagitis in long-term survivors. When the prognosis is excellent or the operation is done for benign disease, the problems of esophagitis make the use of stomach less desirable. Whenever an intestinal segment is used, it should be used in an isoperistaltic direction, as there is good evidence that the colon or jejunal segments function actively. The long-term results from antiperistaltic colon interposition are not as good as for isoperistaltic colon interpositions as documented by Fujimaki and others [1].

Advantages of the isoperistaltic left colon include its location in the left upper quadrant where it sits immediately adjacent to the proximal stomach and distal esophagus. It is readily accessible through a left thoracotomy as well as abdominal incisions. The left colon usually has a reliable blood supply based on the ascending branch of the left colic artery. Often the left branch of the midcolic artery may also be preserved to provide a double arcade. In only 5% of our cases has the blood supply prevented use of this bowel segment. The diameter of the transverse and descending colon is closer to that of the esophagus than is the right colon. If an anastomotic leak occurs, the absence of digestive secretions leads to a higher probability of secondary healing. Contraindications to the use of the colon segment include diverticulosis, colitis, polyps, obesity, hypertension, atherosclerosis, or portal hypertension.

Key technical considerations include exposure: by separating the diaphragm around its periphery and retracting it upwards into the chest, the splenic flexure is readily visualized. It is quite possible to mobilize the descending colon down to the level of the sigmoid and across to the hepatic flexure through a left thoracotomy incision without a thoracoabdominal extension or a separate laparotomy.

The omentum is completely removed from the colon and mesocolon by dissecting in the avascular fusion plane between omentum and the mesocolon.

The colon should be mobilized down to the sigmoid level to provide ample slack for the colonic anastomosis. The blood supply is inspected during the operation by application of vascular clamps at the points of proposed transsection with verification of the persistant pulsations. Preoperative angiography is unnecessary. The colon is tunnelled posteriorly to the stomach and usually placed in the posterior mediastinum. For substernal interpositions the pedicle is still placed behind the stomach to protect it from injury during subsequent laparotomies. The site for the cologastric anastomosis is important and should be placed high on the greater curvature. A segment of colon is left intraabdominally to permit abdominal pressure compression of the segment. The fundus of the stomach is partially wrapped around the colon segment by anchoring the fundus to the undersurface of the diaphragm around the hiatus in a horseshoe fashion. The colon segment should be fixed carefully to the hiatus to prevent an upward migration of the colon causing intrathoracic stasis, or herniation of other bowel through the hiatus.

In an earlier report from Frenchay Hospital, follow-up of reconstructions following esophagectomy for stricture demonstrated that the recurrent esophagitis rate was 17% after gastric reconstruction and 0% after colonic interposition. Postoperative mortality was also higher in the gastric reconstruction group related to a higher incidence of serious anastomotic leaks and aspiration [2].

In a more recent personal series of esophageal reconstructions from 1969 to 1986, 60 reconstructions were done following esophagectomy for benign disease: isoperistaltic left and transverse colon was employed in 42 of these cases, 29 for peptic strictures, 6 for motor disorders, 5 (1 death) for perforation, and 2 (1 death) for lye or radiation stricture. In this series, the anastomotic leakage rate was 3, or 6%. In 2 cases vascular problems led to removal of the colon segment, and there were two incidences of late colonic perforation from diverticulosis and from vasculitis.

Long-term follow-up has been carried out for 53 colon interpostions for benign disease at the University of Chicago from 1974 to 1986 [3]. Two patients (3.8%) (same as above) died, and postoperative esophagitis occurred in 26%. Based on patient satisfaction interviews, 75% of the patients regard the outcome to be good or excellent. Based on objective analyses of organ function, 72% of colon interpositions are performing well, with a mean follow-up of 5 years. These results are comparable or better to those obtained from other types of esophageal replacement, and speak to the merit of this method for esophageal replacement.

References

1. Fujimaki, et al. In press. In *Diseases of Esophagus*. Siewert JR, Holscher AH, eds Berlin: Springer
2. Skinner DB, Belsey RHR (1967). Surgical management of esophageal reflux and hiatus hernia: long-term results with 1030 patients. *J Thorac Cardiovasc Surg* 53: 33-57
3. Curet-Scott MJ, Ferguson MK, Little AG, Skinner DB. In press. Colon interposition for benign esophageal disease. Presented at the 44th Annual Meeting of the Central Surgical Association, Louisville, Kentucky, March 5, 1987. Accepted for publication in *Surgery*

Can a jejunal loop offer more resistance to acidity?

A. Sicular (New York)

When loss of anti-reflux function between the esophagus and the stomach occurs from destruction of the distal esophagus by ulceration, fibrosis or perforation, the ability to construct a competent valve surgically (Nissen, Hill or Belsey), is lost. In these cases, interposition reproduces a structure that prevents reflux acid burn of the distal esophagus. Human colon and jejunal segments are available. In my opinion, based on the literature and my own experience, the jejunal loop will offer a uniquely better resistance to esophageal acidity if properly interposed between the esophagus and the stomach. The basis for this rests on anatomic, radiographic and physiologic phenomena.

Firstly, if a loop longer than twelve inches is interposed, the data of multiple series (Merendino, Polk, Sicular [1, 3] demonstrates that reflux does not occur under normal physiologic conditions into the distal esophagus from the stomach.

Secondly, aboral gastrostomy barium refluxes only 8 cm.

Thirdly, all pH measurements proximal to a functioning esophagojejunal interposition made in a 17 patients, 10 to 17 year follow-up, were alkaline [2]. The physiologic basis for anti-reflux action for all substances is the maintenance of an isoperistaltic segment which responds to distension by propulsion. Careful canine model studies [4] with isoperistalsis demonstrated integrated isoperistalsis when two sequential mesenteric neurovascular pedicles are preserved to the interposed loop.

Employing this principle, I preserved isoperistalsis in my patients. In the 15 patients whom I have followed (three or more years), none complain anymore of heartburn. Furthermore, in those patients in whom post-operative X-ray studies have been done years later (Moylan [2] and Merendino [1] Polk [3], not a single patient has antiperistaltic action or evidence of esophagojejunal reflux when the loop is more than 15 cm long. In a single patient of Garlock's followed 20 years (SW), re-X-rayed by Marshak in 1983 following a 1965 interposition where the segment was only 12 cm long, supine asymptomatic reflux was observed.

Several corollaries of the use of this loop exist:

Firstly, because of its length, X-rays show these loops to be S-shaped or curved in situ. This appearance in no way prevents peristalsis from carrying substances from the esophagus to the stomach and does not interfere with the physiologic passage of food.

Secondly, the question has been raised as to the possibility of marginal ulceration occurring in the jejunal gastric connection distal to the interposition. As a clinical fact, these ulcers rarely occur. Only one or two patients of the fifty followed developed distal marginal jejunal ulcers. In one explored by me and one by Dr. Polk, acute cholecystitis was the indication for re-exploration. Therefore, innervated gastric remnants may be maintained, precluding gastric emptying problems. However, in cases in which vagotomy is necessary, a pyloroplasty has been done by me in all cases.

Thirdly, to avoid an outlet obstruction problem to the stomach, it is very important, as both Dr. Polk and I have indicated in our personal series, not to take the jejunal loop for interposition any closer than nine inches from the ligament of Treitz. Several patients where I have made a more proximal interposition have developed duodenojejunal obstruction due to the band-like action of the neurovascular pedicle upon the remaining duodenum or jejunum and a severe retrograde obstruction can occur; one aspirated and died in my series. Two patients required gastrojejunostomy and gastrostomy or chronic pharmacologic stimulation and antibiotics for "retained loop syndrome".

Jejunum may be preferable to colon because colon peristalsis is intermittent and may be bi-directional even though the colon loop is isoperistaltic [6]. Interposed colon, of course, contracts promptly to acid reflux stimulation [5] and is a reasonably and technically simpler alternative for high insertions because of its long neurovascular pedicle [7].

In conclusion, however, I think that the properly selected jejunal loop provides the best substitution for the impaired or destroyed anti-reflux mechanism of the esophagogastric junction.

References

1. Merendino KA, Dillard DH (1955) The concept of sphincter substitution by an interposed jejunal segment for anatomic physiologic abnormalities at the esophagogastric junction. Ann Surg 142:486
2. Moylan JP, Bell JW, Cantrell JR, Merendino KA (1971) The jejunal interposition operation: A follow-up on seventeen patients followed 10 to 17 Years. Ann Surg 172:205
3. Polk HC (1980) Jejunal interposition for reflux esophagitis and esophageal stricture unresponsive to valvuloplasty. World J Surg 4:731-736
4. Burrows L, Frankel A (oral permission)
5. Jones EL, Skinner DB, DeMeester TR, Elkins RC, Zuidema GD (1973) Response of the interposed human colonic segment to an acid challenge. Ann Surg 177:75
6. Wilkins EW Jr (1980) Long-segment colon substitution for the esophagus. Ann Surg, Vol 192, #6, pp 722–24
7. Belsey R (1965) Reconstruction of esophagus with left colon. J Thorac Cardiovasc Surg 49:33

M. Mignon, and *F. Ratineau* (Paris)

Since its original description by Roux (1907), several works have tested the comparative qualities of jejunal interposition between stomach and esophagus as a reconstructive procedure after esophageal resection for benign peptic stricture.

These qualities were tested in terms of:

a) mechanical characteristics, i.e. adequate peristaltis.
b) resistance to gastro-esophageal reflux whatever the nature of the refluxed material, i.e. acid, bilious or both.
c) operative difficulty greater than after colonic transplant.

Informative experimental [1–2] and clinical data [3–4] are available as far as question b is concerned.

Sirak et al., notably, have shown in the dog that jejunal as well as colonic transplants resisted well to unstimulated gastric secretion. In contrast, however, after maximal histamine stimulation both segments became eroded (colonic more than jejunal) although the sub-jacent esophagus was protected. Additional studies by Dillard and Merendino [2] have confirmed the previous findings.

Clinical observations in man have also clearly indicated that jejunal interposition is exposed to alteration from refluxed material as well as colonic transplant.

Thus, whether it is interposed between the esophagus and the stomach or used as a drainage procedure after gastric surgery for peptic ulcer, the jejunum is greatly exposed to peptic ulceration. In both situations, thus, it is necessary to perform some kind of gastric acid secretion reducing procedure, usually vagotomy (plus drainage).

References

1. Sirak HD, Clatworthy HW, Elliot DW (1954) An evaluation of jejunal and colic transplants in experimental esophagitis. Surgery 36: 399–410
2. Dillard DH, Merendino KA (1956) New studies in the dog supporting the concept of equal resistance of various levels of the intestinal tract to acid peptic digestion. J Surg Gynec Obstet 103: 289
3. Ferrer JM, Bruck HM (1969) Jejunal and colonic interposition for non-malignant disease of the oesophagus. Ann Surg 169: 533–543
4. Pasch AR, Putnam T (1985) Jejunal interposition for recurrent gastro-oesophageal reflux in children. Am J Surg 150: 246–251
5. Mignon M, De Mestier Ph, Zielinski B (1984) The problem of remaining gastric acidity. In Cancer of the Esophagus in 1984. OESO international Congress. Maloine Publ p 280–281

The Thal procedure, combined with that of Nissen

J. W. Maher (Iowa City)

Optimum therapy of strictures of the esophagus requires of the operating surgeon a wide repertoire of procedures suited to the individual circumstance. Strictures can ordinarily be classified as either annular or longitudinal: the annular stricture is characterized by an area of submucosal fibrosis covered with intact mucosa. The longitudinal stricture is associated with transmural fibrosis which infiltrates the full-thickness of the esophageal wall from an ulcerated mucosa. The inflammation and scarring is accompanied by scar contraction in all three dimensions. This produces a lesion that is characterized by esophageal shortening as well as stenosis.

Annular strictures may be treated satisfactorily by esophageal dilatation combined with an antireflux procedure with a high success rate. However, dilatation of the truly transmural stricture produces hemorrhage, formation of granulation tissue, fibroblast proliferation, collagen deposition, and finally recurrent stenosis due to the cross-linking and contraction of collagen. This basic biologic phenomenon cannot be altered by an antireflux procedure.

The combined Thal fundic patch-fundoplication procedure should be used in the patient with a longitudinal transmural stricture which cannot be easily dilated. When used in this setting, it widens the distal esophagus with a patch of pliable well-vascularized fundus lined by a skin graft and provides effective protection against gastroesophageal reflux. The skin graft prevents reepithelialization of the esophageal wall by granulation tissue and thus minimizes contraction of the lumen when compared with an unsurfaced patch [1].

Maher and coworkers reported 68 patients who underwent combined Thal-Nissen procedures for longitudinal peptic strictures [2] (Table 1). The mean stricture length was 4 cm (range 2.5–11 cm). Operative mortality was 4%. The average length of follow-up was over five years: fifty-seven of 68 patients had an acceptable result (84%). Four per cent had an early recurrence of their strictures, while an additional 4% had late recurrence of their stricture after an initially good response period of from two to 11 years (Table 2) four of the six patients with poor results had motility disorders preoperatively (either: achalasia with stricture following myotomy, scleroderma, or diffuse esophageal spasm).

The combined Thal-Nissen procedure represents optimum therapy for the patient with an undilatable transmural stricture of the esophagus. When used in this setting, satisfactory results will be achieved in a large majority of patients with a low operative mortality. Colonic or jejunal interposition should be reserved for those patients who either fail to respond to a combined Thal-Nissen procedure or who demonstrate sufficiently disordered peristalsis to render the esophagus an unsatisfactory conduit for the passage of food.

Table 1. Thal-Nissen (68 Patients)

Mortality	4%
Average Follow-up	68 months
Average Stricture Length	4 cm (2–11 cm)
Good Results	85%

Table 2. Thal-Nissen poor results

Early Recurrence	3 Patients	(1-achalasia following Heller)
Late Recurrence	3 Patients	(1-scleroderma – 2 years) (1-achalasia – 6 years) (1-DES – 11 years)

References

1. Tsukamoto M, Thal AP (1966) Correction of experimental esophageal stricture with the use of the skin-lined fundic patch. J Thorac Cardiovasc Surg 52: 682–689
2. Maher JW, Hocking MP, Woodward ER (1981) Long-term follow-up of the combined fundic patch fundoplication for treatment of longitudinal peptic strictures of the esophagus. Ann Surg 194: 64–69

L. Couraud, S. Mériot, P. Clerc, and *P. Lefebvre* (Bordeaux)

Introduction

The surgeon is sometimes confronted with situations where lower esophagus preservative surgery has become impossible or unsatisfactory and where esophagus resection is judged too dangerous or too mutilating.

This situation can result from the pre-operative examination, but it often arises during an operation when the surgical approach does not allow cardio-esophageal resection without an additional surgical route, and when this additional approach is considerated to be too stressing for a patient in poor condition.

The Thal operation seemed therefore to offer an alternative to the resection anastomosis of the lower esophagus and the cardia for 13 stenosis cases. With a follow up of 6 and 20 years later, we are able to show their results.

Patients

The operation was performed on 13 patients aged 32 to 76 years (average 58 years old). Most of them were very weak having suffered from a dysphagiant pathology for a long period. Five of them had already undergone surgery on the lower esophagus and mostly for achalasia.

The first stenosis pathogenia is not always clearly established but the lesions recorded at the time of the operation were:

- primary peptic esophagitis — 5 cases
- esophagitis on previously operated achalasia — 5 cases
- esophagus perforation — 3 cases
  (After endoscopic dilatation of a caustic stenosis (1 case) or during a surgical procedure for a pathology linking spasm and esophagitis (2 cases))

Methods

- Longitudinal broadening esophagotomy was done over a length of 3 to 8 centimeters, depending upon the position and extension of the stenosis.

- The gastric patch stitched to the edges of the opening of the esophagus is only effective in the treatment of stenosis. It was therefore felt that another technique should be added to deal with physiopathologic requirements of this region or to correct the complex physiological manifestations of the original disease.
- A valvuloplasty wrapping 3/4 of the esophagus circumference inside the fundus of the stomach (3/4 of Niessen fundoplication) and overshooting the upper end of the esophagus opening 3 to 5 centimeters was always associated with the broadening patch. When the valvula was lifted into thoracic position (8 cases out of 13) a wider phrenotomy was made to avoid the strangulation of the stomach in a narrow diaphragmatic passage. The stomach was carefully fixed to the edges of the phrenotomy but as we shall see it did not always prevent secondary hernia in the area of the incision.

An esophagitis caused by reflux was either evident or possible, that is why we have almost always took additional precautions which consisted in guarding against possible excessive gastric acidity or in draining the stomach:

- vagotomy: 9 cases out of 13 (of the nerve trunk or supra-selective)
- pyloroplasty: 9 cases

In most cases the surgical approach was thoracic (7 cases) or both thoracic and abdominal (1 case), sometimes only abdominal (5 cases) to treat lower stenosis (in these cases valvulas were situated in the abdomen).

Results

The early results after surgery were good in all cases, there was neither mortality nor morbidity.

After a long period of 3 to 16 years (average period 7.3 years) six old patients died from natural causes not linked in anyway with their esophagus stenosis (average age 74 years old); seven are still alive (average age 63 years old) having been under medical supervision for 9 to 18 years).

Secondary morbidity was as follows:

Paravalvular diaphragmatic hernia: 3 cases

It is a common complication, all the more as it only happened in the 8 cases where the patients had had a phrenotomy and an endothoracic valve in spite of the care taken in closing the diaphragmatic opening. The weakness of the gastric and epiploic purchase explains this high frequency. They have been successfully reoperated on and there has been no further recurrence.

Failure and esophagitis recurrence: 1 case

This is the only serious failure of the group. An extensive distension of the esophagus that couldn't be satisfactorily wrapped in a restricted fundus rendered the valve inadequate. An early esophagitis with anemia and then a serious hemorrhagic ulcer led us to an emergency resection anastomosis 8 years later. Today five years later the result is good.

Persistent reflux: 2 cases

Two patients after 9 and 13 years suffer respectively from regurgitation and burning sensations necessitating antacid treatment periodically but repeatedly: the endoscopy reveals neither esophagitis not stenosis. pHmetry confirms that there is a reflux and the manometry reveals the absence of the lower esophagus sphincter. In both cases, given the patients psychosocio professional context, the importance of the clinical disorder may be regarded as uncertain but there is no doubt about the reality of the reflux even if thanks to the anti-acidic treatment it does not lead to any endoesophageal lesion.

The anatomic and functional results may be judged valid in 10 cases after medical supervision for an average of 11 years in spite of some considerable deviations from the recommended diet: the reflux is absent or mild and very intermittent. Some dysphagia sensations in swallowing large pieces of meat were reported by some patients. One patient was found to have a very narrow lower oesophagus, he underwent a dilatation which was beneficial. Others had a normal diameter of the esophagus and it was esteemed that they suffered from a functional disorder resulting from a loss of the peristalsis over a substantial part of the lower esophagus. This phenomenon is however unfrequent and patients lead a normal life without treatment or special diet.

Comments

The Thal operation in association with valvuloplasty and procedure reducing excessive gastric acidity is far from ideal operation since out of 13 cases, it produced 1 failure and 2 fair or poor results. Moreover, 3 diaphragmatic hernias had to be subsequently reoperated.

This is not a perfectly workable corrective operation and it should not be compared with isolated valvuloplasties or with simple esophageal dilatations followed by valvuloplasty.

Technically speaking it is however a safe operation procedure (no death – no fistula) and the long term adverse effects are mild in comparison with these of the resection-anastomosis procedures which, in our experience are the only alternative to the Thal operation and therefore the only point for comparison.

In addition, the results are lasting: our bad results showed themselves within a year and the favourable results remained steady whatever the period of medical supervision and have lasted for the length of time the patients lived afterwards.

For all these reasons, the Thal operation with valvuloplasty still has an undeniable place in the lower esophagus surgery. But it should be used in selected cases. The irregular performance of the valve, the occasional poor functionning of the lower esophagus (probably caused by the opening of the esophagus and the loss of the lower esophageal sphincter) make this operation unsatisfactory in the treatment of extensive primitive stenosing peptic esophagitis.

On the other hand, it does seem to treat satisfactorily short stenosis of the lower esophagus. Thus in the case of sclerosed and inflammatory stenosis of the old megaesophagus where myotomy was not possible and after occasional failures of the Heller operation with terminal esophagitis, we had good results. The fact that the valvula could be reintegrated in the abdomen led to fewer complications and more favourable results.

The perforations of the lower esophagus: either endoscopic or peroperative during myotomy on sclerosed tissues proved to be a safe and useful indication on three occasions. In the case of such operations on frail people, the Thal operation is surely far less traumatic than an esophageal resection and the results can be expected to be just as good. But to be successful, the broadening patch should not be considered as the only goal of this surgery but should be completed by an anti-reflux operation and a reduction of the acidopeptic flow of the stomach.

In those indications, and when part of the techniques dealing with the physiopathology of the gastroesophageal reflux, this preservative operation therefore seems to deserve its role as a sometimes preferable alternative to the resection of the lower esophagus.

Evaluation of surgical results

Why have so many antireflux procedures been devised? Can specific factors be defined in order to properly choose the procedure to offer?

W. S. Payne (Rochester)

Antireflux operations are like fine wines in that some travel well and some do not. Few techniques upon general application have lived up to the expectations suggested by initial reports. Lack of skill? Difficult to teach? The master's touch? Possibly a bit of each of the above! More obvious is that all are effective [5, 6, 7, 9, 10, 11], but not for all patients or all circumstances [12, 13]. We are only just beginning to understand some of the essential features of antireflux procedures and why they usually work but sometimes fail.

The goal of surgical treatment for gastroesophageal reflux is not only restoration of competence but also elimination of associated subjective and objective complications of reflux (Table 1) without superimposing new morbidity related to the repair itself.

In an earlier review [1], the author alluded to a study of over 400 Mayo Clinic patients undergoing repairs of the types described by Nissen, Belsey and Hill, as well as those designated as Collis gastroplasty with Belsey or Nissen type fundoplications: it was found that all were relatively safe and all provided restoration of competence with relief of symptoms, but not universally free of morbidity, mortality or frank failure to obtain competence. Of special note was the observation that only the Nissen repair provided reliable competence, provided the anatomic integrity of the Nissen repair was maintained. Unwrapping of the 360° fundoplication, or more commonly, telescoping of the esophagogastric junction cephalad out of an intact wrap, proved disastrous. The other observation of note was that patients managed by Collis gastroplasty rarely experienced any type of anatomic recurrence. The cut gastroplasty proved to be unnecessary unless there was significant esophageal shortening. It was replaced by an uncut Collis gastroplasty.

Table 1. Complications of gastroesophageal reflux

Intractable subjective distress
Esophagitis
Bleeding
Stenosis of esophagus
Reversible
Irreversible
Shortening of esophagus
Reversible
Irreversible
Esophageal-ulcer penetration or perforation
Columnar epithelial-lined lower esophagus (Barrett's esophagus)
Motility disturbances of esophagus
Contraction ring of lower esophagus (Schatzki's ring)
Respiratory aspiration

We and others have come to appreciate that the major complications of the Nissen relate to anatomic reduction under tension, with failure of stitches between the stomach and esophagus to maintain reduction (leading to telescoping). We believe this to be eliminated by the frenulum effect of the uncut gastroplasty. Further, a short length (1–2 cm) and looseness of the wrap (floppy short Nissen) have proved important in preventing esophageal obstruction (dysphagia), even in patients with absent peristalsis; if the fundus is inadequate for a truly loose 360° wrap, then a 270° Belsey type partial fundoplication will prevent obstruction in the absence of peristalsis. Not all patients present with an adequate fundus, especially those with a shortened esophagus or those reoperated on following a failed previous antireflux procedure. Under the latter circumstances a cut Collis with Nissen [2] is a potential alternative.

In the author's experience, none of the antireflux procedures are applicable to achalasia patients with gross mega-esophagus since a gastric fundus of the largest size would be dwarfed by the huge, often tortously angulated amotile esophagus. The techniques of the author's current methods of effecting an uncut Collis Nissen have recently been published [2, 3]. Our group experience to date with over 300 patients [4] has shown the procedure to be safe (1 death) and to date, symptomati-

Table 2. Conclusions

1. Keep Nissen short and floppy
2. Avoid linear tension (and telescoping) by uncut gastroplasty
3. Reduce entire stomach and fundoplication below diaphragm
4. Avoid intrathoracic Nissen
5. Repair crura behind esophagus
6. Obturate esophagus with 50 French mandril during gastroplasty fundoplication and crural repair to prevent obstruction
7. Avoid injury to vagal trunks
8. Select alternatives to classical Nissen fundoplication if peristalsis absent, fundus deficient in size or esophagus shortened
9. Avoid splenectomy (left transthoracic transhiatal approach?)
10. Avoid operations in patients with uncorrectable downstream gastrointestinal motility or stasis problems

Table 3. Goals

Applicable to the obese patient
Competence at cardia
Unobstructed swallowing
Retain belch and emesis capacity
Avoid "gas-bloat" syndrome
Avoid splenectomy
Low morbidity-mortality as possible
Short hospitalization
Short period of post-surgical disability
Long-term effectiveness
Reproducible results (easily taught)

cally effective (90%) with no incidental splenectomies and a brief hospitalization (8 days).

Table 2 lists this author's considered conclusions regarding his interpretation of those factors which contribute to a successful antireflux operation and ultimate goal of therapy (Table 3).

References

1. Piehler JM, Payne WS, Cameron AJ, et al (1984) The uncut Collis-Nissen procedure for esophageal hiatal hernia and its complications. Probl Gen Surg 1: 1–14
2. Payne WS (1986) Reflux Esophagitis with Stricture: Alternative Methods of Management. In Dudley H, Carter DC, Jackson JW, Cooper DKC (eds): Rob & Smith's Operative Surgery, 4th edition. London: Butterworths, pp 314–235
3. Payne WS (1985) The esophagus and esophagogastric junction. In Remine WH, Payne WS, and van Heerden JA: Manual of upper gastrointestinal surgery. Edited by Egdahl RM. New York: Springer-Verlag, pp 1–60
4. Payne WS, Pairolero PC and Trastek VF: Unpublished data
5. Henderson RD and Marryatt G (1983) Total fundoplication gastroplasty: long-term follow-up in 500 patients. J Thorac cardiovasc Surg 85: 81–87
6. DeMeester TR, Johnson LF and Kent AH (1974) Evaluation of current operations for the prevention of gastroesophageal reflux. Ann Surg 180: 511–525
7. Donahue PE and Bombeck CT (1977) The modified Nissen fundoplication – reflux prevention without gas-bloat. Chir Gastroenterol 11: 15–21
8. Henderson RD (1983) Diffuse esophageal spasm. Surg Clin North Amer 63: 951
9. Richardson JD, Larson GM and Polk HC Jr (1982) Intrathoracic fundoplication for shortened esophagus: treacherous solution to a challenging problem. Amer J Surg 143: 29–35
10. Leonardi HK, Lee ME, El-Kurd MF, et al (1977) An experimental study of the effectiveness of various antireflux operations. Ann Thorac Surg 24: 215–222
11. Wald H, Polk HC Jr (1983) Anatomical variations in hiatal and upper gastric areas and their relationship to difficulties experienced in operations for reflux esophagitis. Ann Surg 197: 389–392
12. Leonardi HK, Crozier RE and Ellis FH Jr (1981) Reoperation for complications of the Nissen fundoplication. J Thorac Cardiovasc Surg 81: 50
13. Polk HC Jr (1976) Fundoplication for reflux esophagitis: misadventures with the operation of choice. Ann Surg 183: 645

Is intra-operative manometry useful?

D. E. Low, and *L. D. Hill* (Seattle and Stockholm)

Background and Technique

Intraoperative manometrics has been used in several centers as an objective measurement of the lower esophageal sphincter pressure during various types of esophageal surgery [1–4]. These reports cite its utilization and success with the

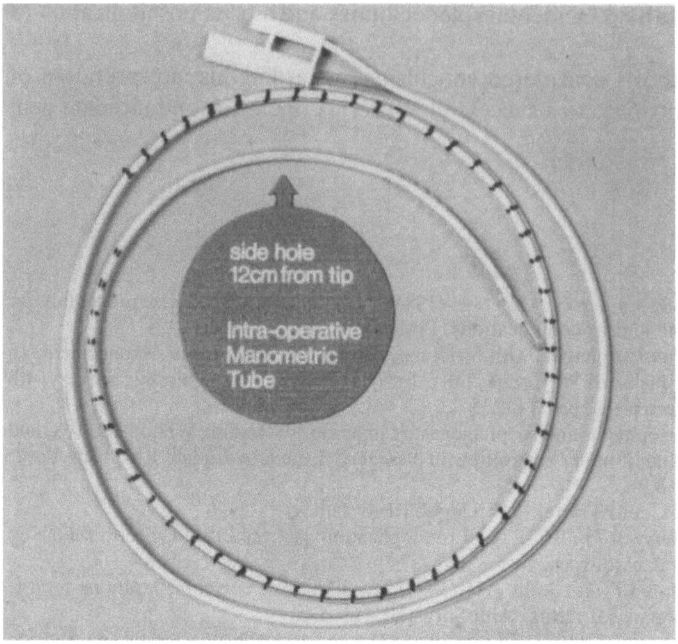

Fig. 1. Hill manometric tube: polyvinyl pressure tube with side hole located 12 cm from the tip of an attached 16 French nasogastric tube

Nissen, Belsey and Hill antireflux operations and in both the pediatric and adult populations.

We have utilized this technique to improve results in the operative management of gastroesophageal reflux (Hill procedure) and in surgery for various esophageal motility disorders. In association with antireflux surgery, it provides an impression at the time of operation of whether the repair has augmented the lower esophageal sphincter pressure (LESP) sufficiently or conversely if the repair has been constructed too tightly.

LESP measurement is obtained using a repeated, slow pullthrough technique with modified nasogastric tube (Physio Control Corp) with a side opening 12 cm from the tip (Fig. 1). The pressure tube is attached to a Harvard pump and perfused with sterile water at a rate of 0.7 ml/min. Recordings are made on the manometer (Fig. 2) which produces a digital readout and a recording (Physio Control Corp). An alternative to the specially constructed manometric machine is simply connecting the Hill pressure tubing to an arterial pressure line setup. We have found this is an easy and inexpensive mechanism for providing ongoing pressure readouts and a taped recording when desired.

The average time required for taking the three necessary pressure measurements is approximately 10 minutes once operating room support personnel are familiar with the technique.

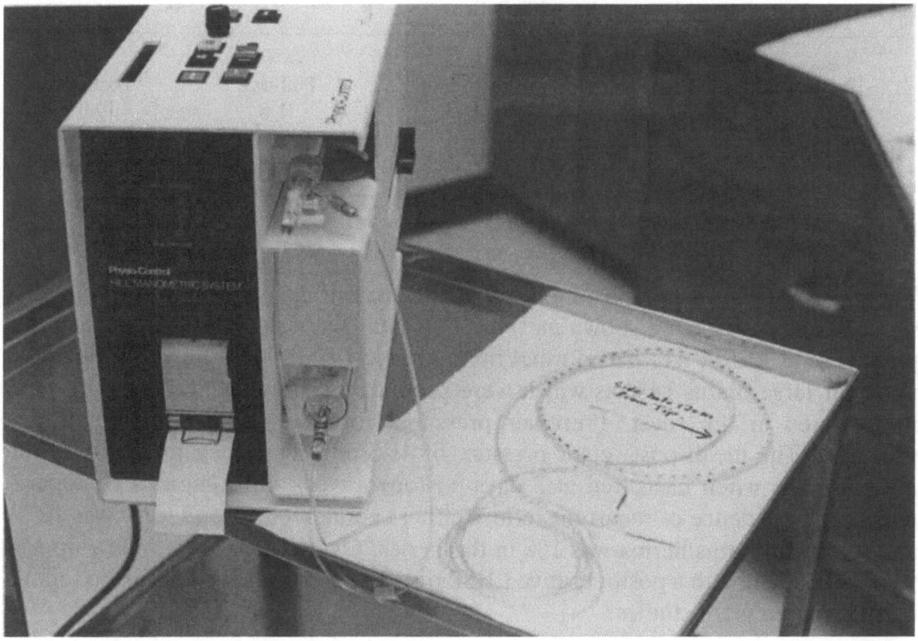

Fig. 2. Hill manometric recorder: provides readout of ongoing and peak pressure on digital display and manometric recording tape

Our initial study examined 200 patients undergoing either primary or secondary antireflux surgery with the Hill posterior gastropexy (Table 1). All patients had failed a trial of medical management for their reflux and had undergone preoperative pH and pressure studies and endoscopy.

At operation, before the dissection is begun, an initial LESP measurement is taken with the Hill manometric tube prior to the construction of the Hill posterior gastropexy. Before the repair sutures are permanently tied down to the median arcute ligament, the first two are snugged down with a one throw tie and clamped. A repeat pressure measurement is done to give an immediate indication of the adequacy of the repair. At this point, depending on the pressure, the sutures can be loosened or tightened appropriately.

Initially we accepted a pressure range of 45 to 57 mm Hg. However, over the past 10 years, pressures between 40 and 50 mm Hg have given good postoperative pressures while at the same time further decreased the incidence of postoperative dysphagia. If this initial pressure is within the acceptable range, all sutures are tied down to the median arcuate ligament and final pullthroughs are sequentially done, an average of which provides a final post-repair LESP. In patients with scleroderma or achalasia (post myotomy) undergoing antireflux surgery, the intraoperative pressure is reduced to approximately 40 mm Hg in an attempt to minimize postoperative dysphagia in these patients with aperistaltic or hypomotile esophagus.

Table 1. Intraoperative Manometrics – 200 Patients

	Intraoperative			
Preop	Pre-repair	Post-repair	Pull-out	Post-op
5.5	5.0	41.5	21.8	19.0

Results

The mean pre, intra and postoperative LESP measurements achieved in our first series of 200 patients are shown in Table 1. Ninety-six per cent of patients had low preoperative LESP, 4% had normal preoperative LESP but were being operated upon for large hiatus hernias which were producing symptoms because they were incarcerated in the chest. Prerepair pressures correlate well with preoperative pressures. The mean post repair pressure of 41.5 mm Hg is seen to drop into the normal range when measured at 3 days postoperatively and 3 months postoperatively. The incidence of recurrent reflux (either spontaneous or induced) was 1.5% and recurrent hiatus hernia was 1% in this series. Overall long-term follow-up was 93%: no patient with a postoperative LESP of > 15 mm Hg showed reflux on follow-up pH and pressure studies.

In a more recent series completed in 1984, 196 patients were reviewed: the relationship between intraoperative, post repair (mean 47.5 mm Hg) and three month post repair LESP measurements (mean 17.6 mm Hg) was once again seen. In addition, a significant rise ($p > 0.001$) was seen between preoperative (mean 8.6 mm Hg) and postoperative LESP measurements (mean 17.6 mm Hg). Overall, 95% were considered to be excellent or good results.

In addition to using intraoperative manometrics in cases of primary antireflux procedures, its role in recurrent repairs may be even more important. In these cases, the tissue is destroyed or attenuated and there is a higher risk of constructing an inadequate repair. Having objective intraoperative data in these difficult cases has produced satisfactory results in our most recent review of 116 patients undergoing reoperation following failed Nissen fundoplication: postoperative results demonstrated excellent or good outcomes in 86% and fair results, i.e., improvement but requiring antacid therapy or dilations, in 9%.

We also utilize intraoperative manometrics as an adjunct to surgery in patients with esophageal motility disorders, i.e., achalasia and diffuse esophageal spasm. In achalasia we have utilized intraoperative pressure measurements to help us determine the amount of muscle to divide to relieve dysphagia but at the same time avoid initiating uncontrollable reflux [5]. By reducing the overall length of the LES to approximately 1–2 cm, the patients get relief from dysphagia with minimal reflux sequelae (Table 2).

In the 19 patients undergoing the Heller procedure for achalasia in our reported series, LES pressures were reduced to normal or high normal levels and the length of the LES was decreased to approximately 2 cm. Intraoperative pressure measurements were especially valuable in our series of patients operated upon for failed esophagomyotomy for achalasia. In these difficult patients it was a useful

Table 2. Average manometric results after various surgical procedures

Surgical procedure	Premyotomy Pressure (mm Hg)	Premyotomy Length (cm)	Postmyotomy Pressure (mm Hg)	Postmyotomy Length (cm)	Follow-up (mo)	Results
Primary repair for achalasia (n=15)	42	5.5	20	2.1	34 (5–56)	7 excellent, 7 good, 1 unchanged
Reoperation for achalasia (n=4)	28	3.5	16	2	36 (17–64)	2 good, 1 unchanged, 1 poor
Myotomy for diffuse esophageal spasm (n=6)	41	13	22	2	29 (3–51)	5 excellent, 1 poor

adjunct not only to ensure that an adequate secondary procedure was done, but it often helped identify the reason for failure of the original procedure.

In diffuse esophageal spasm we have used intraoperative manometrics as a guide to demonstrate the extent or length of the myotomy required in each patient.

*

Summary

We have found intraoperative manometrics to be an invaluable adjunct in many facets of surgery of the esophagus. If surgeons believe that low preoperative LESP is one criteria for operation and a normal postoperative LESP is an indication of success, then it follows that intraoperative adjustment of the LESP during construction of the antireflux repair is prudent and ultimately will improve results. To simply measure postoperative LESP at which time nothing can be done to modify the measurement, provides follow-up only. Intraoperative manometrics is a safe and relatively easy technique by which on-the-spot objective data can be used to improve results.

References

1. Hill LD (1978) Intraoperative measurement of lower esophageal sphincter pressure. J Thorac Cardivasc Surg 75: 378–81
2. Cooper JD, Gill SS, Nelems JM, Pearson FG (1977) Intraoperative and postoperative esophageal manometric findings with Collis gastroplasty and Belsey hiatal hernia repair for gastroesophageal reflux. J Thorac Cardiovasc Surg 74: 744–51
3. Puglionisi A, Asole F, Clemente G, Villani A (1984) Effectiveness of intraoperative LES pressure measurement during the Nissen-Rossetti fundoplication. Ital J Surg Sc 14(2): 91–6
4. Noble HG, Christie DL, Cahill FL (1982) Follow-up studies on patients undergoing Nissen fundoplication utilizing intraoperative manometry. J Pediatr Surg 17(5): 490–493
5. Hill LD, Asplund CM, Roberts PN (1984) Intraoperative manometry: adjunct to surgery for esophageal motility disorders. Am J Surg 147: 171–174
6. Mercer CD, Hill LD (1986) Reoperation after failed esophagomyotomy for achalasia. Can J Surg 29: 177–180

M. B. Orringer (Ann Arbor)

Intraoperative measurement of lower esophageal sphincter pressure was first proposed by Doctor Lucius Hill [2] as a means of insuring adequate control of gastroesophageal reflux at the time of an antireflux procedure. This is an appealing concept for it suggests that in the operating room, the surgeon may calibrate the distal esophageal high pressure zone to a specific desirable pressure that will correlate with subsequent postoperative manometric values that have been associated with successful reflux control.

Unfortunately, early reports about intraoperative esophageal manometry contained no statistical analysis of the data obtained. We therefore undertook a study to determine the effects of general anesthesia and operative manipulation of the esophagus on intraoperative HPZ determinations and the statistical relationship between intraoperative and postoperative HPZ values.

Forty-five adult patients undergoing a transthoracic combined Collis gastroplasty-Nissen fundoplication procedure for control of gastroesophageal reflux were included in this study (Table 1). Twelve had ulcerative esophagitis, and eight had reflux strictures. Eight had undergone prior antireflux operations, nine had scleroderma, and eight had diffuse esophageal spasm. At the time of the Collis-Nissen procedure, eight patients underwent intraoperative dilation of strictures and eight underwent esophagomyotomy for spasm.

Table 1. Intraoperative esophageal manometry Collis-Nissen operation 45 patients

Esophagitis without stricture	12
Stricture	8
Diffuse spasm	8
Scleroderma	9
Prior operation	8

The combined Collis-Nissen operation [3] was performed through a left posterolateral thoracotomy, dilating strictures when present intraoperatively, constructing the gastroplasty tube over a 54 to 56 French dilator with the GIA stapler, and then passing the gastric fundus posterior to the gastroplasty tube prior to a 360° fundoplication which is finally reduced below the diaphragm. HPZ pressures and length were determined preoperatively with pullback measurements (Table 2) using triple lumen perfused catheters. The same equipment and technique were used for intraoperative HPZ measurements made with the patient under general anesthesia

1. prior to opening the chest in the right lateral decubitus position (38 patients),
2. after mobilizing the distal esophagus and cardia prior to beginning the gastroplasty (38 patients),
3. after completion of the gastroplasty, with the gastric fundus reduced below the diaphragm (29 patients), and

Table 2. HPZ Determinations – 45 pts

Pre-operative	43
Intraoperative	
chest closed	38
cardia mobilized	38
gastroplasty complete	29
repair complete	45
Postoperative	
6 months	35
12 months	21

4. following the fundoplication, with reduction below the diaphragm and the posterior crural sutures tied with the chest open (45 patients).

Two sequential pullback tracings were made for each determination, and the six HPZ values obtained were averaged to give a single HPZ pressure and length. The intraoperative HPZ values were compared with postoperative HPZ determinations and acid reflux tests performed without sedation or anesthesia after one to three weeks (44 patients), six months (35 patients), and twelve months (21 patients).

Results

Fig. 1 shows the *mean* HPZ pressures for the entire group at various intervals before, during, and after operation plotted graphically: the average intraoperative HPZ pressure obtained at the conclusion of the Collis-Nissen repair was 21 mm Hg. This decreased to 15 mm Hg at 1–3 weeks and 11–12 mm Hg at 6 and 12 months postoperatively. These data are similar to those reported by others indicating that

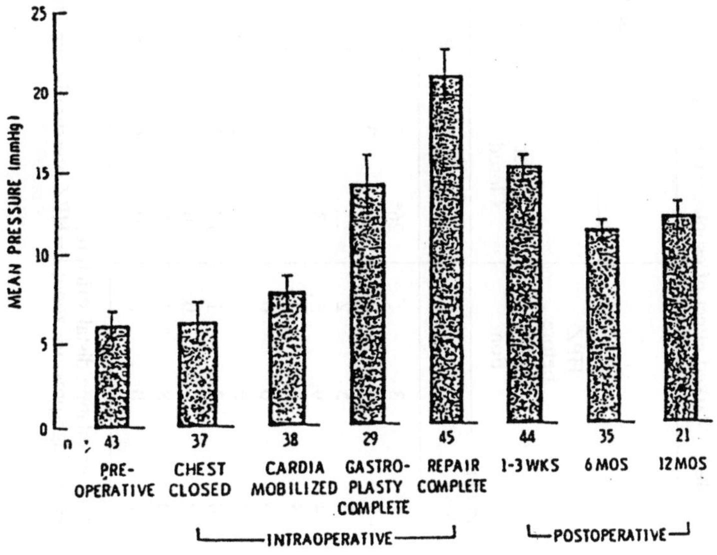

Fig. 1

Table 3. Marked effect of esophageal manipulation on High-Pressure-Zone values in 11 patients

Patient	HPZ before Operation		HPZ under general anesthesia: Chest Closed		Cardia Mobilized		Gastroplasty Complete		Repair Complete		HPZ after operation: 1 to 3 Wk		6 Mo		12 Mo	
No.	P	L	P	L	P	L	P	L	P	L	P	L	P	L	P	L
1	3	1	26[a]	2	25	5	...	...	34	6	13	6	15	6	12	6
2	0	0	28[a]	3	29	4	34	5	59	7	18	6	12	4	10	3
3	5	2	...	...	10	3	...	...	14	4	12	4	...	...	...	...
4	9	3	3	2	12	6	15	6	14	6	23	4	15	5	9	4
5	9	3	...	...	13	3	32	4	22	6	16	4	10	4	10	3
6	0	0	...	...	13	2	18	4	23	9	28	7	16	6	21	8
7	6	5	8	3	14	6	16	5	17	5	12	6	6	5	6	7
8	3	1	10	2	15	4	15	5	18	6	13	5	...	...	...	...
9	0	0	0	0	7	4	9	4	15	5	9	5	6	3	...	...
10	8	4	5	4	7	5	8	5	13	6	12	5	8	5	...	...
11	0	0	0	0	6	5	0	0	12	7	10	5	7	4	...	...

[a] After dilating distal stricture.
HPZ=high-pressure zone; P=HPZ pressure in mm Hg; L=HPZ length in centimeters

the *mean* intraoperative pressures obtained for the entire group at the completion of an anti-reflux procedure are approximately twice as high as subsequent mean recordings obtained 6 and 12 months after operation. Unfortunately, a more detailed evaluation of the data and statistical analysis demonstrate the errors inherent in relying on intraoperative determinations: for example, in these 11 patients or 24% of the group (Table 3), dilation of peptic strictures or manipulation of the esophagus required for mobilization of the cardia, prior to even beginning the repair, produced these increases in HPZ tone to levels 50% or more of the final HPZ value obtained at the conclusion of the gastroplasty and fundoplication. In two patients, dilating distal strictures alone produced HPZ determinations of 26 and 28 mm Hg, respectively.

Further, although these *mean* values obtained during operation at each successive stage of the repair and postoperatively at 6–12 months are statistically significantly different (p. < 0.1), if the intraoperative and subsequent postoperative pressures obtained in *individuals* are compared statistically, *no significant correlation* is found. Irrespective of the final intraoperative HPZ value, *no* patient undergoing acid reflux testing with the pH probe at 6–12 months after operation had any gastroesophageal reflux.

In conclusion, intraoperative esophageal manometry [4] adds a minimum of 30–45 minutes to the operation, and the information gained is of little practical or statistical significance. Based upon our data, we question the rationale for altering the technique of an operation simply to obtain an "ideal" intraoperative HPZ value. We do not believe that intraoperative esophageal manometry is a valid scientific concept.

References

1. Cooper JD, Gill SS, Nelems JM, et al (1977) Intraoperative and postoperative esophageal manometric findings with Collis gastroplasty and Belsey hiatal hernia repair for gastroesophageal reflux. J Thorac Cardiovasc Surg 74: 744
2. Hill LD (1978) Intraoperative measurement of lower esophageal sphincter pressure. J Thorac Cardiovasc Surg 75: 378
3. Orringer MB, Sloan H (1978) Combined Collis-Nissen reconstruction of the esophagogastric junction. Ann Thorac Surg 25: 16
4. Orringer MB, Schneider R, Williams GW, Sloan H (1979) Intraoperative esophageal manometry: is it valid? Ann Thorac Surg 30: 13

F. G. Pearson (Toronto)

There is little reported experience on the application of intraoperative pressure studies in esophageal surgery. Manometry can be used intraoperatively to quantify or calibrate the pressure created in the distal esophagus by an anti-reflux reconstruction. It may also be used to define pressure changes resulting after esophagomyotomy for achalasia or diffuse spasm.

Intraoperative Manometry for anti-reflux Surgery

Hill routinely uses a simple technique of intraoperative manometry to calibrate the pressure generated at the cardia by his repair [1]. Using his technique for pressure measurement, he has demonstrated that the data is reproducible on repeated pullthrough studies and can be used to define the adequacy of repair at the time of operation. He has found that an intraoperative pressure in the lower esophageal sphincter area between 45 and 55 mmHg is consistent with good reflux control and avoidance of dysphagia. If the pressure in the repair is below this range intraoperatively, – reflux may be inadequately controlled. Dysphagia frequently complicates a repair which generates pressures above this range. Hill notes that the postoperative pressure falls to about half the level observed intraoperatively.

We have conducted intraoperative manometry in a series of 61 patients with acquired short esophagus managed by gastroplasty and partial fundoplication [2]. The following conclusions were derived from this study:

1. The lower esophageal high pressure zone (HPZ) can be measured with the patient under general anesthesia, and the pressure so recorded correlates well with preoperative measurements.
2. The gastric cardia in man, when fashioned into a tube of esophageal diameter, functions like the lower esophageal sphincter in that it is hormonally sensitive and relaxes with swallowing.
3. The pressure recorded in the gastroplasty tube at the time of operation is the same whether the tube lies in the chest or in the abdomen, – tone is intrinsic and not related to abdominal compression.
4. A zone of elevated pressure is generated throughout the full length of the gastroplasty tube. The narrower the diameter of the tube, the higher the level of pressure created.
5. Addition of a fundoplication enhances the tone in the gastroplasty segment.
6. Within a few weeks to one month of operation, – the level of pressure in the gastroplasty and fundoplication falls to about half of the recorded intraoperative value. It appears to remain stable thereafter.

At the present time, we do not believe that intraoperative manometry offers us a practical guide at the time of operation for either a Belsey Mark IV repair, or for gastroplasty and fundoplication. I believe, however, that the technique is practical and very useful for the Hill operation.

*

Intraoperative Evaluation of Motor Disorders

Intraoperative manometry (IOM) can be used to determine the completeness of esophagomyotomy in patients with achalasia or diffuse spasm. In our experience, a conventional esophagomyotomy for achalasia does not completely ablate the distal sphincter pressure. Matteoli and colleagues [3] in Bologna have shown that the pressure in the cardia is only abolished if the myotomy is carried for at least three or four centimeters beyond the EG junction and onto the front of the stomach. They content that complete ablation of the pressure through extension of the gastric end of the myotomy results in better esophageal emptying than that achieved by conventional myotomy.

We have found IOM to be most useful in patients requiring re-operation after previous esophagomyotomy. The anatomy of the previous myotomy and definition of the esophagogastric junction are sometimes obscured in these redo cases, and intraoperative pressure evaluation will insure that a subsequent myotomy is adequate.

References

1. Hill LD (1978) Intraoperative measurement of lower esophageal sphincter pressure. J Thorac Cardiovasc Surg 75: 378–382
2. Cooper JD, Gill SS, Nelems JM, Pearson FG (1977) Intraoperative and postoperative esophageal manometric findings with Collis gastroplasty and Belsey hiatal hernia repair for gastroesophageal reflux. J Thorac Cardiovasc Surg 74: 744–751
3. Matteoli S, Gozetti G, Pilotti V, Spangaro M (1986) Intra-operative manometry for achalasia. International esophageal week (Münich), in press

What are the criteria for evaluation of the results of an operation for peptic esophagitis?

P. E. Donahue, C. T. Bombeck, and *L. M. Nyhus* (Chicago)

The results of any operation for peptic esophagitis are to be considered in light of the efficacy of the operation for the primary problem and the sum total of postoperative complications related to the operative procedure. Almost all of the senior surgeons practicing today have been witness to a fascinating evolution of operative therapy for the problem of peptic esophagitis. In retrospect the question of assessing the results of operations seems more clear than it was in prospect; indeed, the rich store of information regarding operations for reflux must be viewed as a "treasure house" of data obtained by those individuals whose interest in the problem led them to apply modern technology to a difficult question.

When Allison began this story many years ago, modern gastrointestinal physiology was still in its infancy compared to the present: esophagoscopy was still a technique which had limited application, was difficult to employ, and had inherent complications which limited its use. The Barium meal was still the most important part of the diagnostic equation, and the relationship between hiatus hernia and pathologic reflux was not understood. Esophageal manometric examinations were in their infancy, and the functional relationships of the lower esophageal sphincter and cardia were largely unknown.

What a different situation exists today! The modern gastrointestinal surgeon has precise knowledge of the mucosal reaction to reflux via the insight provided by flexible fiberoptic endoscopy. The relationship between motility disorders of the esophagus and symptoms of pathologic reflux is becoming more clear. The availability of 24 hr pH monitoring has revolutionized the evaluation of patients with atypical symptoms of gastroesophageal reflux, and the recent description of computerized analyses of the components of the anti-reflux mechanism promise to add further to our knowledge of this common problem. Furthermore, the combination of these diagnostic modalities has made it more clear than ever that we can investigate those patients with failure after primary surgical treatment and categorize them into groups with primary failure of the operation ("bad" operations), those with specific complications related to the operation, and those with an unrelated disease complex [1].

What, then, is the problem about assessing the results of operations for pathologic reflux? With all of these techniques, why is it that everyone is not completely satisfied after having an operative procedure? The answer is that the surgical community in some ways has not been able to keep pace with the discoveries of the last twenty years. We have seen descriptions of the ways in which operations can be standardized, but still find that every clinic seems to use a different procedure. There is still no "gold standard" for evaluating the problems after reflux surgery. There are still surgeons who have not found out about the need for careful reconstruction of the cardia. There are still individuals who have not adopted the flexible endoscopic insights as the keystone of their investigation of patients with problems.

To evaluate the patient who has had surgical therapy for peptic esophagitis we need to know the answer to the four questions:

1. Are the symptoms improved?
2. Are there any persistent problems postoperatively?
3. Has the operation been seen to become less effective with time? (This is especially important since so many reports indicate a late failure rate after operation.)
4. Has the surgeon attempted to stay informed about his or her patients after operation, or has postoperative assessment been relegated to non-surgical colleagues who do not appreciate all of the problems which may supervene? Have endoscopic examinations in the postoperative clinic been performed with the guidance of the surgeon's view, and have the objective means of evaluating results been employed? [2]

While the answers to these questions will aid in the management of most of the problems which are observed after surgery, there are still biological questions relating to several of the "great questions" in peptic esophagitis. What is the ultimate fate of the columnar lined esophagus? What is the role of resection for peptic stricture? What, if any, risk of cancer exists in those patients with severe reflux following corrective surgery?

Several of these questions are being addressed in this symposium, but it seems clear that there will be a continuing need for experienced clinicians to remain involved with their patients and study the results of their efforts. No doubt, there will be many additional modifications to the armementarium of the antireflux practitioner, and I predict that these will be made by surgeons who have an interest in this problem, and who continue the outstanding research efforts which have been described in this symposium.

References

1. Donahue PE, Yoshida J, Bombeck CT, Nyhus LM (1986) Endoscopic Skills – an imperative for surgeons. Digestive Surgery 3: 1–3.1
2. Donahue PE, Samelson S, Nyhus LM, Bombeck CT (1985) The Floppy Nissen Fundoplication: effective long-term control of pathologic reflux. Arch Surg 120: 663–668

The effects of the different procedures on the opening pressures of the LES

P. E. Donahue, C. T. Bombeck, and *L. M. Nyhus* (Chicago)

The concept of a lower esophageal sphincter opening pressure (LESOP) has direct relevance to the questions of gastroesophageal competence. The LESOP is a means of looking at the reflux episode from the gastric side, and is a helpful way of investigating the mechanical effects of the various antireflux procedures; unfortunately, it is almost impossible to obtain valid material relating to this parameter in the human laboratory. In an in vitro canine model designed to investigate the effect of hiatus hernia, the elements of sphincter failure were related to four factors: LES resting pressure, the point of insertion of the phrenoesophageal membrane, the elasticity of the hernia sac (if present), and the size of the hiatus hernia. The LESOP was found to give additional information about the effects of anatomic variables listed above in the genesis of a reflux episode when the LES was held constant [1].

The LESOP has also proven useful in the definition of the role of the gastric sling fibers as part of the anti-reflux mechanism: Samelson et al. measured LESOP and % Time pH <4 in dogs before and after excision of the LES, excision of the sling fibers, and after excision of the LES-sling muscle complex. The LESOP and the pH study independently revealed that reflux episodes were progressively more severe depending upon the status of the sling fibers, and worst when both LES and sling fibers were absent [2]. The data are of interest in relation to other operative procedures used for pathologic reflux, including the Angelchik procedure, the Narbona sling technique, and all of the common valvuloplasty procedures. What all of these techniques have in common is the creation of a reinforcement for the sling fibers, analogous to the artificial (circular string ligature) used as an "unloading" device in the study of artificial hiatus hernia. The most important part of an anti-reflux procedure, therefore, is not the absolute level of the LES pressure, but rather the way in which that pressure coexists in relation to the remainder of the anti-reflux mechanisms at the cardia.

The LESOP is only one of several means of measuring the tendency for mechanical failure of the LES-complex. Recently we have described a comparison of the LESOP with the Timed-pH measurement in the esophagus in a pharmacologic model of gastroesophageal reflux: the pH test was at least as sensitive as the LESOP, with the advantage that no invasive operative procedures such as gastrostomy are required [3].

References

1. Pettersson GB, Bombeck CT, Nyhus LM (1976) The lower esophageal sphincer: mechanisms of opening and closure. Surgery 88: 307–314
2. Samelson S, Bombeck CT, Siewert R, Weiser HF, Ludkte FE, Holscher AH, Abuabara SF, Nyhus LM (1983) A new concept in the surgical treatment of gastroesophageal reflux. Ann Surg 197: 254–257
3. DeSalvo J, Bombeck CT, Vaz OP, Donahue PE, Nyhus LM (1987) A new canine model of gastroesophageal reflux. Submitted to Surgical Forum, March

A comparison of manometric and pH measurements in different continence procedures

J. Baulieux (Lyons)

Fortunately, this complex procedure is not systematically used for all patients. However, it becomes classical to use this objective method in comparing the surgical procedures for continence restitution.

The aim of pH-metry and manometry in the post-operative phase

The method is interesting in 3 situations:

1. When a patient has some *functional postoperative symptoms* that are difficult to analyze, this examination is useful to understand these symptoms. This is the case in *postoperative dysphagia*. This method can differentiate a "too tight" procedure on a minor achalasia, that was unknown in the preoperative phase, and that was increased by the surgical technique. Sometimes it is possible to detect a scleroderma by finding a dyskinetic esophagus which is the first symptom of the thickness.

2. In case of suspicion of recurrence before performing surgical therapy, the pH and manometric study are absolutely imperative. A reoperation cannot be only indicated by functional and clinical symptoms. Gatzinsky [6] has clearly underlined the sensibility of pHmetry, which is superior to the X-Ray examination. A question is the outcome of the examined patients in the early postoperative phase, with a pathologic pHmetry, but without any clinical symptoms. An attentive follow-up is likely justified in these cases. Indeed Brand and Pope [2] have emphasized the positivity of early pHmetry in forecasting a later true recurrence.
3. *The comparison of surgical techniques by this method* is naturaly very tempting and a lot of authors (who cannot be all mentioned) have done this type of research.

   We will mention *4 retrospective studies*:
   - Woodward [8] compared 259 cases, the usual crural repair that gives 54% of pH-metric recurrence and the Nissen procedure that gives 39% of recurrences.
   - Dilling [4] compared the "Belsey Mark 4" (47% reccurence) and Nissen (9%).
   - Sillin [7] obtained the same results, on a series of 89 fundoplications and 46 Hill procedures.
   - In France, Galmiche [5] did this kind of study after posterior hemiwrap ("Toupet" type). They found 25% of pH metric recurrences in the short term.

Prospective studies are less frequent:

The DeMeester's publication [3] is classical: it concerns 15 Nissen, 15 Hill and 15 Belsey Mark 4. It uses 24-Hour esophageal pH monitoring, at a mean of 154 days following the surgical repair. He concluded that the Nissen procedure was the procedure of choice.

We did this kind of evaluation in the Aubry's [1] thesis. It concerns 81 patients operated between 1979 and 1980 and who were all submitted to a complete exploration between the 2nd and the 3rd postoperative month. For some of them, a second evaluation was performed at approximately the 30th postoperative month. The surgical techniques used were 30 Nissen, 29 Hill and 22 posterior hemiwrap: the early results have quickly shown us the superiority of Nissen and Hill's procedures, and led us at the same time to abandon the practise of the posterior hemiwrap before the end of this study. The late pHmetric results are more serious than the clinical results and have confirmed the early ones. Among the evaluated patients, 2 Nissen of 8 showed a pHmetric reccurence, 3 Hill of 10, and 5 posterior hemiwrap of 10.

Conclusions

On the basis of this study, it is concluded that all procedures with an hemiwrap repair, whether anterior or posterior, are not completely certain. It is the same for the Belsey Mark 4.

The most effective technics are Nissen and Hill and, on the sole basis of reflux correction (without considering other criteria), the Nissen procedure is probably the most efficient.

References

1. Aubry C (1985) Résultats tardifs du traitement des hernies hiatales. Comparaison de la fundoplicature, de la cardiopexie postérieure et de l'hémivalve postérieure. Thèse Lyon
2. Brand DL, Eastwood IR, Martin D, Carter WB, Pope CE (1974) Esophageal symptoms, manometry and histology before and after anti-reflux surgery. A long term follow-up study. Gastroenterology 76: 1393–1401
3. DeMeester TR, Johnson LF, Kent AH (1974) Evaluation of current operations for the prevention of gastroesophageal reflux. Ann Surg 180: 571–581
4. Dilling EW, Peyton MD, Cannon JP, Kanaly PJ, Elkins RC (1977) Comparison of Nissen fundoplication and Belsey Mark IV in the management of gastroesophageal reflux. Am J Surg 134: 730–733
5. Galmiche JP, Teniere P, Ducrotte P, Denis Ph, Colin R, Testart J (1983) Traitement du R.G.O. acide par hémifundoplicature postérieure. Résultats cliniques et pH-métriques. Gastroentérol Clin Biol 7: 385–391
6. Gatzinsky P, Sandberg N, Sihlbom H (1979) Gastroesophageal reflux after surgical treatment of hiatal hernia with and without severe reflux complications. Acta Chir Scand 145: 45–53
7. Sillin L, Condon R, Wilson J, Worhan L (1979) Effective surgical therapy of oesophagitis. Experience with Belsey, Hill and Nissen operations. Arch Surg 114: 536–541
8. Woodward ER, Thomas HF Alhany MC (1971) Comparison of crural repair and Nissen fundoplication in the treatment of esophageal hiatus hernia with peptic-esophagitis. Ann Surg 173: 782–792

G. Mantion, Y. Ottignon, E. Pelissier, and *M. Gillet* (Besançon)

The Nissen fundoplication is generally considered to be an effective surgical procedure, recommended for gastroesophageal reflux, although it has yet to be evaluated on a long-term basis. Moreover, this procedure causes certain definite side effects. It is for these reasons that some surgeons prefer the Toupet posterior hemifundoplication, despite the fact that only one long-term study has been conducted on this procedure.

The purpose of this study was:

1. to compare the efficacy of the two surgical techniques in the short term (3 to 6 months);
2. to detect possible deterioration of the antireflux repair (24 months postsurgery);
3. and to seek possible correlations between the parameters investigated and the development of complications or failures.

Material and Methods

64 patients with gastroesophageal reflux disease secondary to a hiatus hernia or to cardio-tuberositary malposition underwent surgery performed by two surgical teams. The first team performed surgery on 38 patients using the Nissen procedure, and the second team used the Toupet posterior hemifundoplication technique on 26 patients. The two groups of patients were made up in terms of the recruitment of the two surgical teams.

- Criteria for patient selection were as follows:
  - evidence of an abnormal pattern of esophageal acid exposure shown on esophageal pH monitoring (for more than 10% of the recording time);
  - the clinical presence of one of the following symptoms:
    - typical symptoms:
      - ascending retrosternal heartburn,
      - regurgitations,
      - postural syndrom,
    - atypical symptoms:
      - painful dysphagia,
      - retroxyphoid pain,
      - vomiting,
    - Dysphagia
- Criteria for patient exclusion were the following:
  - alkaline reflux,
  - presence of a gastric or duodenal ulcer or systemic disease,
  - evidence of esophageal ulceration or stricture on endoscopy,
  - association with another esophageal disease such as diverticula, achalasia, myomatosis, and spasmodic disease,
  - any patient having a visceral defect or psychiatric disorders or for whom a 2-year follow-up evaluation could not be conducted,
  - associated surgical act other than cholecystectomy,
  - special surgical difficulties such as cardia resistance (brachyesophagus).

The mean age of the patients in this study is 51 years in both groups, and the average weight is 71.5 kilograms. The distribution according to sex, however, is somewhat different:

- 25 men, 13 women for the Nissen procedure
- 10 men, 16 women for the Toupet operative technique

A clinical evaluation of the patients was carried out three times during this study by an outside medical team: presurgery, from 3 to 6 months postsurgery, and then, 24 months postsurgery. This pre- and postoperative evaluation included a direct interview with the patient, 3-hour post prandial esophageal pH monitoring, and esophageal manometry according to the perfused catheter technique. Twelve patients did not grant permission for all or part of the short or mean term follow-up examinations (6 Nissen, 6 Toupet).

The patient filled in the clinical questionnaire himself, classifying the intensity of his symptoms on a 4-stage scale of increasing gravity ranging from 0 to 3.

Results

Initially, the typical signs almost completely disappeared. After 24 months, however, a recurrence of these signs was observed in 8% of the cases (Nissen repair) and in 36% of the other cases (Toupet repair) (Fig. 1).

Early postoperative follow-up showed that the atypical signs were affected to a lesser degree by the surgery and returned to their initial level after 24 months (Nissen procedure) (Fig. 2).

The incidence of dysphagia after the Nissen repair remained high whereas the Toupet procedure resulted in a significant decrease after 24 months (Fig. 3).

In the short term, the Nissen procedure brought about outstanding improvement, as shown on esophageal pH monitoring: all the values returned to normal, the mean value decreasing from 54% to 0.34% (Fig. 4). The results following the Toupet repair (Fig. 4) are quite comparable with the exception of two asymptomatic pH monitoring failures and a mean value decreasing from 51% to 2.9% (Fig. 5).

At 24 months postsurgery, follow-up evaluations were carried out on the first 12 patients who had undergone the Nissen operation. The results remain unchanged except for one patient. The first 11 patients having received Toupet repairs were also examined. A clear deterioration was observed since 6 patients (Fig. 6) showed abnormal or borderline values. This result, however, is not statistically significant (Fig. 7).

Esophageal manometry revealed an overall increase in LES pressure (N between 10 and 40 cm H_2O) in both operative procedures and in the short term. The mean pressure increased from 11 to 22, 5 cm H_2O following the Nissen repairs (Fig. 8), and from 13.8 to 24.4 after the Toupet repairs (Fig. 9). Subsequent measurements

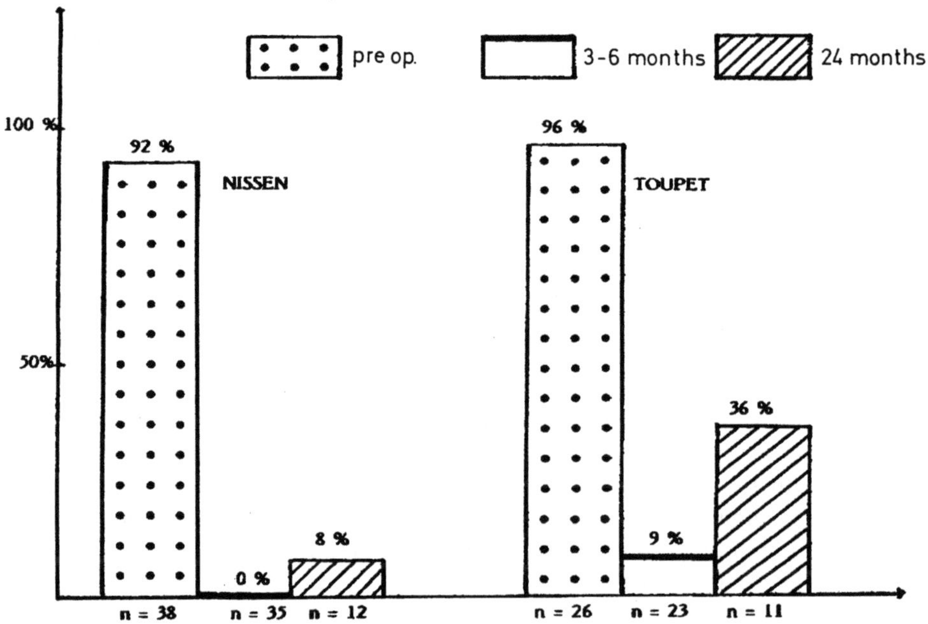

Fig. 1. Frequency of typical features

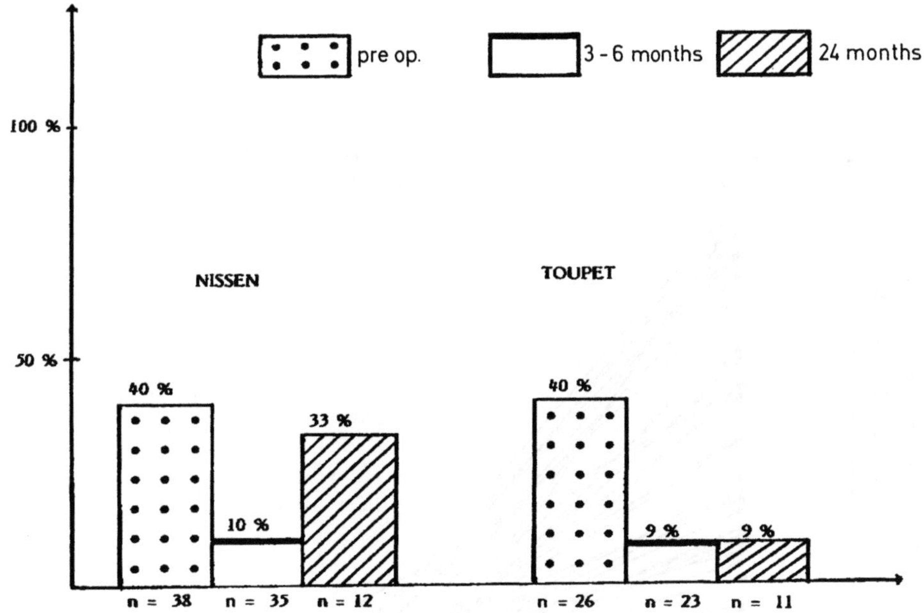

Fig. 2. Frequency of atypical features

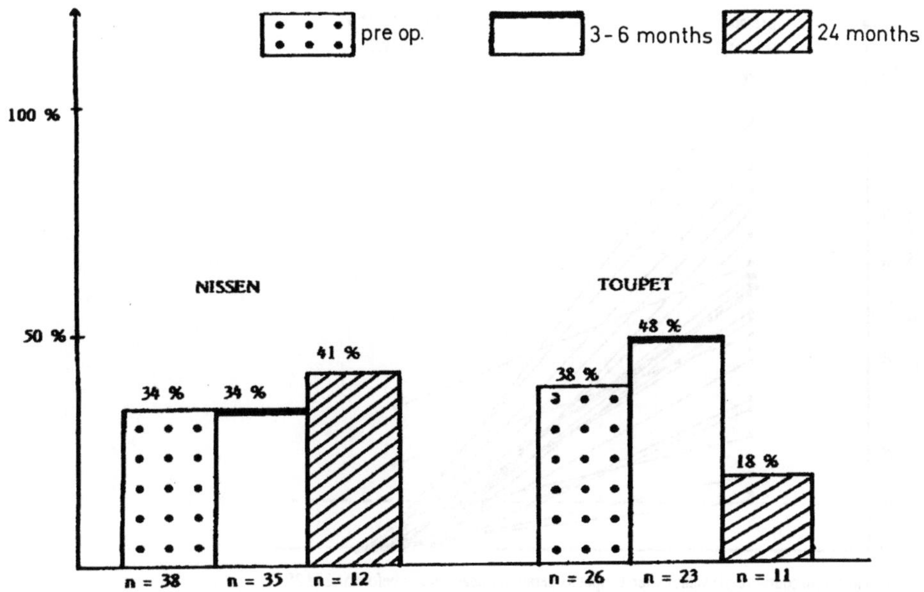

Fig. 3. Incidence of dysphagia

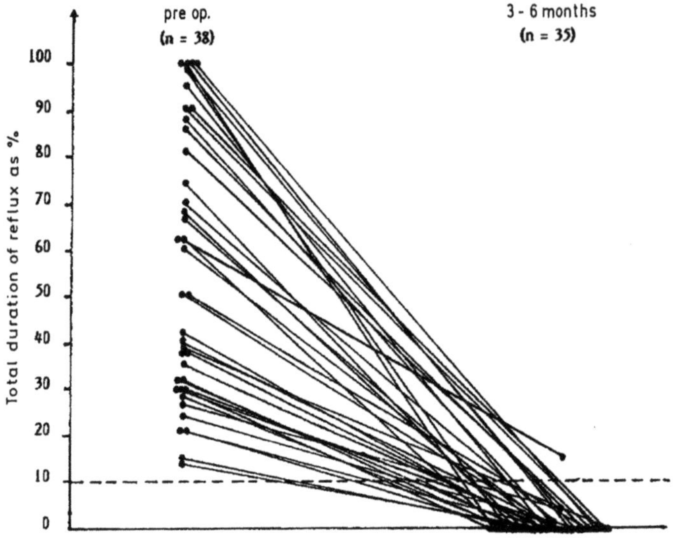

Fig. 4. Short-term course of pH values after Nissen's operation (mean values: before 54±27; after 0.34±0.75) ($p < 0.0001$)

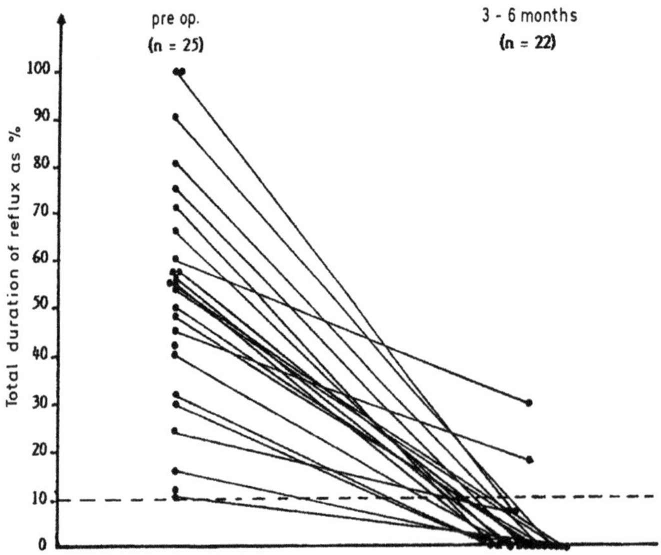

Fig. 5. Short-term course of pH values after Toupet's operation (mean values: before 51.37±25.43; After 2.9±6.9) ($p < 0.0001$)

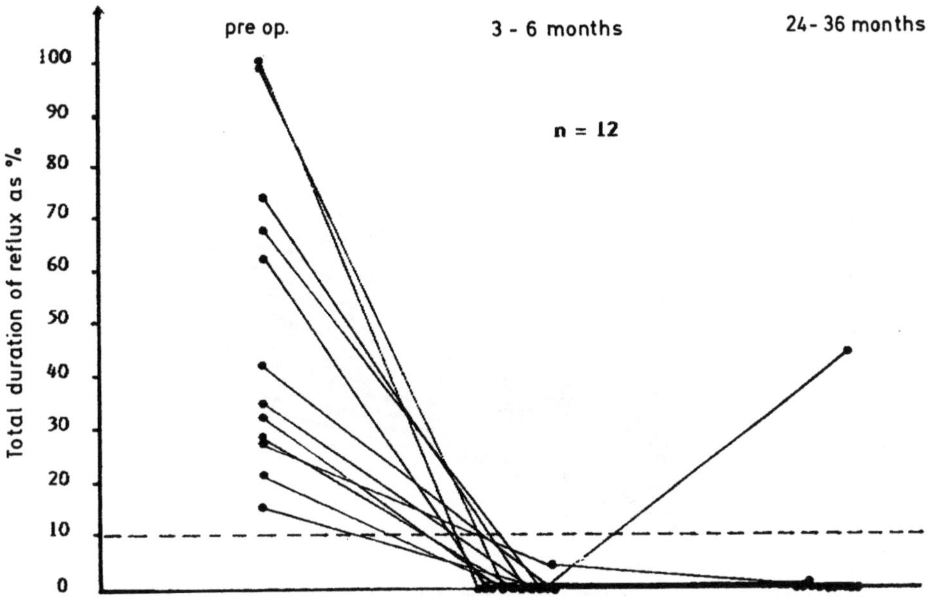

Fig. 6. Long-term chances in pH values after Nissen's operation (mean value at 24 months: 5.08±11.79) (NS)

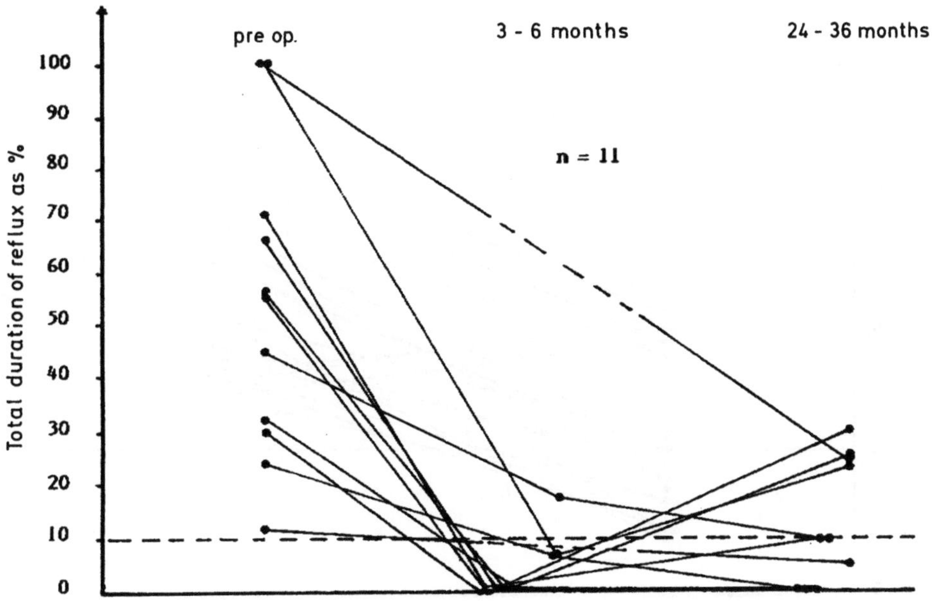

Fig. 7. Long-term chances in pH values after Toupet's operation (mean value at 24 months: 12.70±11.14) (NS)

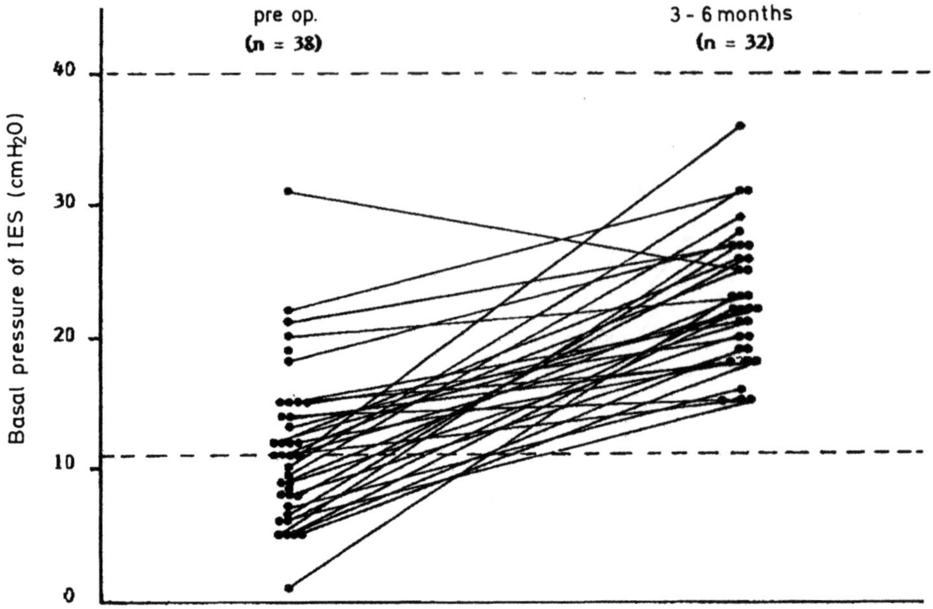

Fig. 8. Short-term changes in basal pressure of LES after Nissen's operation (mean values: before 11±5.11; after 22.5±5.13) ($p<0.0001$)

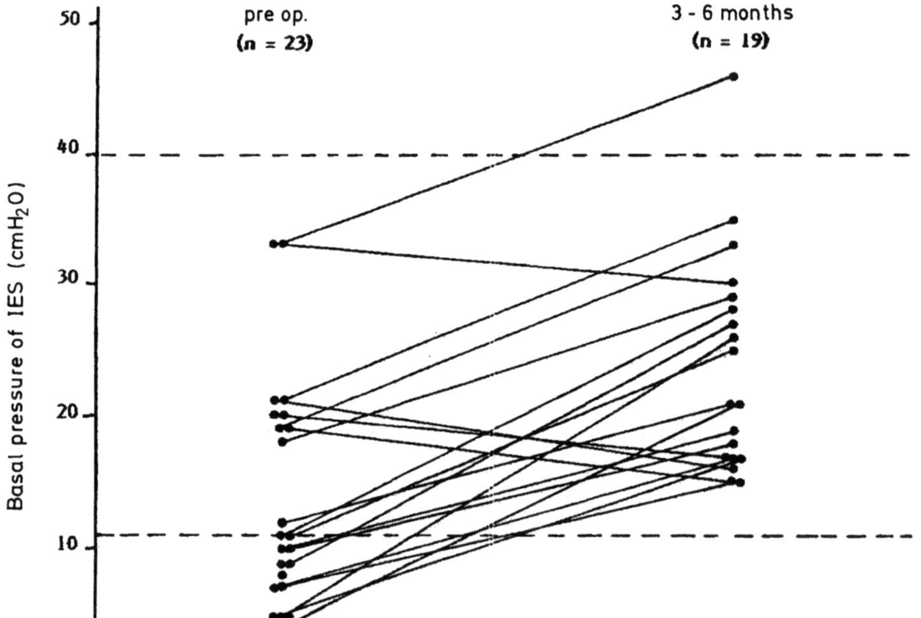

Fig. 9. Short-term changes in basal pressure of LES after Toupet's operation (mean values: before 3.8±8.55; after 24.4±7.33) ($p<0.0001$)

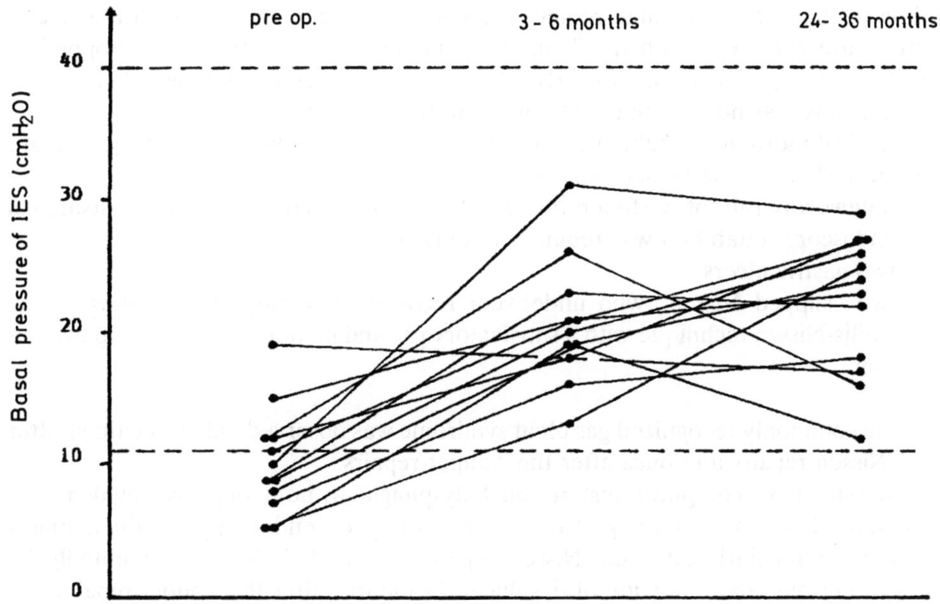

Fig. 10. Long-term changes in basal pressure of LES after Nissen's operation (mean value at 24 months: 22.2±4.48) (NS)

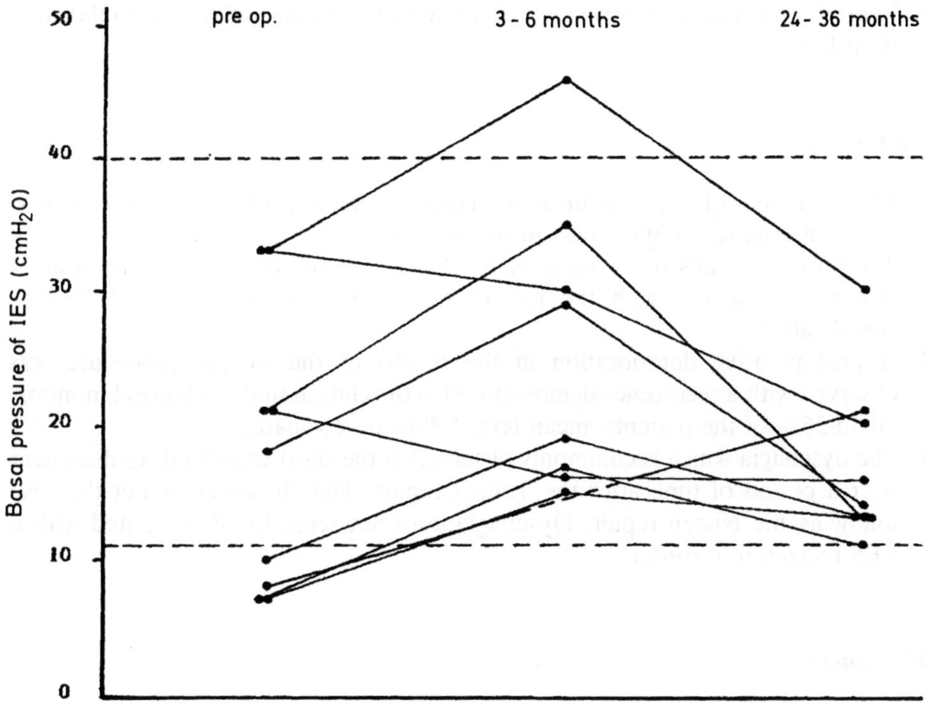

Fig. 11. Long-term changes in basal pressure of LES after Toupet's operation (mean value at 4 months: 16.5±5.85) ($p<0.05$)

showed that the mean value remained unchanged at 22.2 cm H_2O with the Nissen procedure (Fig. 10). With the Toupet technique, however, the value dropped to 16.5, revealing a decrease in nearly all the individual values (9 patients) (Fig. 11).

Mortality was non-existent (0%) in each of the groups.

Surgical morbidity resulting from both operative procedures appears quite high, particularly after the Nissen repairs:

- noteworthy rate of postoperative dysphagia though not disturbing. Postsurgical endoscopic dilatation was required in only one case.
- two gastric ulcers
- two "slipped Nissen" who underwent reconstructive surgery according to the Collis-Nissen technique with a satisfactory pH and manometric follow-up evaluation.

The commonly recognized gas bloat syndrome was observed only three times after the Nissen repairs and once after the Toupet repairs.

Among these complications, residual dysphagia without objective evidence of stricture demonstrated on gastro-intestinal study or endoscopy is still a major concern praticularly after the Nissen repairs. A parallel should undoubtedly be drawn between the reduction of dysphagia 24 months after the Toupet repairs and the deterioration of clinical, esophageal pH monitoring, and manometric results.

A comparative study of dysphagia and LES relaxation suggests that (Fig. 12, 13):

1. There is no correlation between pre- and postoperative dysphagia.
2. In a certain number of cases, the fundoplication causes LES relaxation disorders.
3. There is no correlation between postoperative dysphagia and the LES relaxation disorders.

Conclusion

1. The two operative procedures are equally effective in the control of gastroesophageal reflux symptoms in the short term.
2. The positive results observed after the Nissen repairs remain unchanged at 24 months postsurgery with the risk of the occurrence of a "slipped Nissen" complication.
3. A postoperative deterioration in the results of the Toupet procedure was observed with a recurrence demonstrated in the clinical findings and pH monitoring in 36% of the patients' mean term follow-up evaluations.
4. The dysphagia which is commonly observed in the short term tends to disappear over a period of time after the Toupet repair. This, however, is not the case following the Nissen repair. Dysphagia does not seem to be associated with a LES relaxation disorder.

References

1. DeMeester TR, Johnson LF, Kent AH (1974) Evaluation of current operations for the prevention of gastroesophageal reflux. Ann Surg 180: 511–525

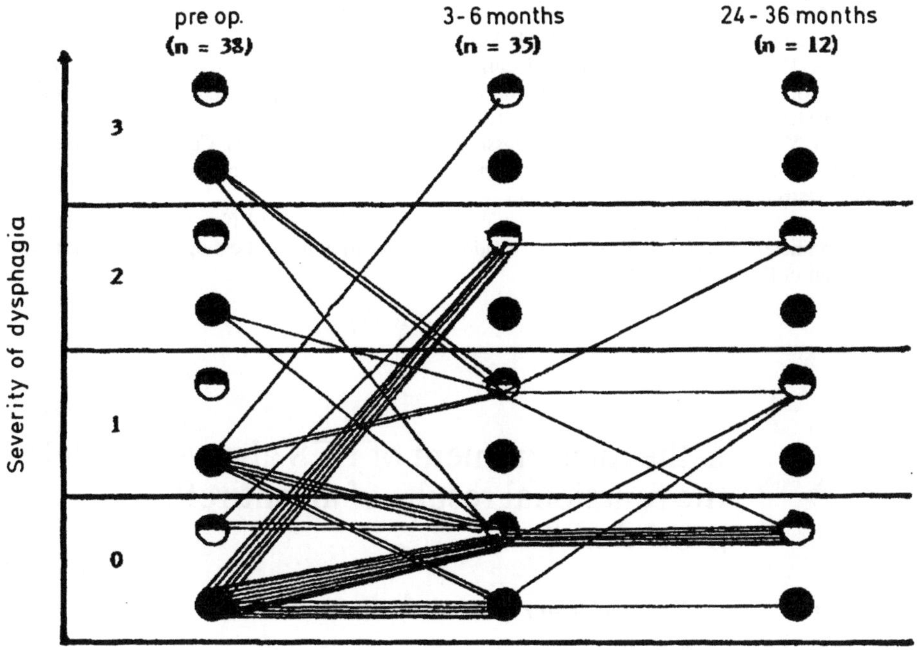

Fig. 12. Course of dysphagia and relaxation of LES after Nissen's operation. ●=complete relaxation of LES; ◓=incomplete or no relaxation of LES

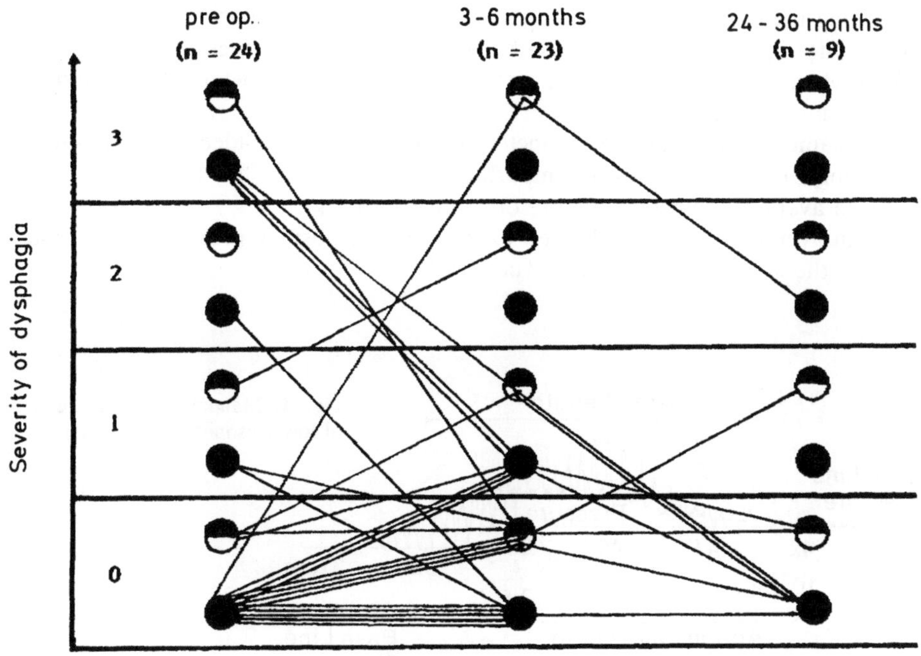

Fig. 13. Course of dysphagia and relaxation of LES after Toupet's operation. ●=complete relaxation of LES; ◓=incomplete or no relaxation of LES

2. Fink SM, McCallum RW (1984) The role of prolonged esophageal pHmonitoring in the diagnosis of gastroesophageal reflux. Jama 252: 1160–1164
3. Galmiche JP, Teniere P, Ducrotte P, Denis P, Colin R, Testar J (1983) Traitement du reflux gastro-œsophagien acide par hémifundoplicature postérieure. Résultats cliniques et pHmétriques. Gastroentérol Clin et Biol 7: 385–391
4. Ottignon Y, Ampelas M, Voigt JJ, Gassigneul J, Pascal JP (1984) Comparaison de trois méthodes d'enregistrement du pH œsophagien dans le diagnostic du reflux gastro-œsophagien acide. Gastroentérol Clin Biol 8: 609–615
5. Segol P, Baptiste P, L'Hirondel C, Marchand P, Gignoux M (1982) Effets de la fundoplicature sur le sphincter inférieur de l'œsophage: étude manométrique pré et post-opératoire. Gastroentérol Clin et Biol 6: 222–228

Is the measurement of LES always parallel to the functional results of an antireflux procedure?

T. R. DeMeester (Omaha)

Increased esophageal exposure to gastric juice can be caused by esophageal, sphincter or gastric abnormalities. An antireflux procedure is a mechanical therapeutic approach to the problem of increased esophageal acid exposure by improving the competency of the sphincter. It will reduce esophageal exposure to gastric juice regardless of the cause but is less likely to produce troublesome side effects when used to correct a manometrically defective sphincter. The grounds for this statement are as follows:

1. Mechanical failure of the sphincter is recognized by inadequate manometric findings. Fig. 1 illustrates the important measurements. They are:
   a) an average sphincter pressure of 6 mm Hg or less;
   b) an average length of sphincter exposed to the positive pressure environment of the abdomen of less than 1 cm; and/or

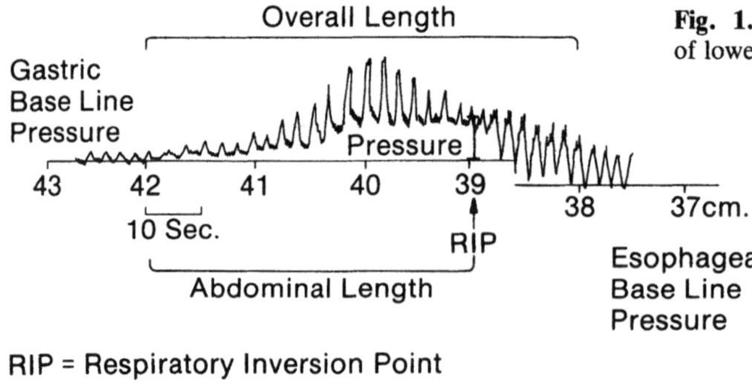

Fig. 1. Manometric measurements of lower esophageal sphincter

c) a sphincter with an average overall length of less than 2 cm. The key factor in the competency of the cardia is at the distal esophageal sphincter pressure, but the efficiency of the pressure can be nullified by inadequate abdominal length or an abnormally short overall sphincter length.

2. Figs. 2, 3, 4 and 5 show that the Nissen fundoplication can correct these manometric abnormalities without causing deterioration or augmentation of esophageal contractility. The correction is associated with a reduction of esophageal acid exposure to normal base on both symptomatic improvement and objective measurement of esophageal pH [1].

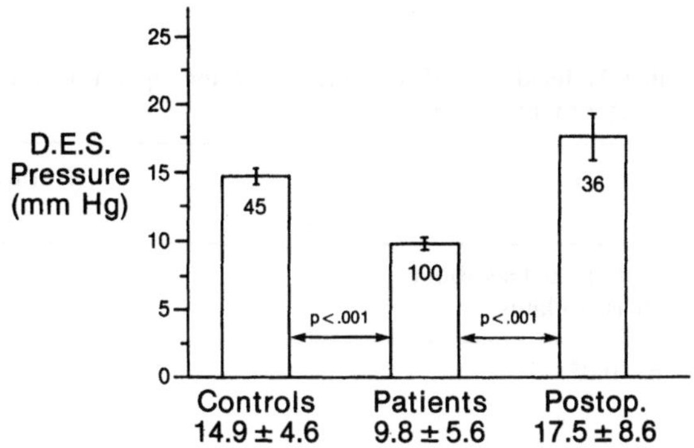

Fig. 2. Comparison of the mean distal, esophageal sphincter pressure measured in control subjects, and in patients before and after surgery

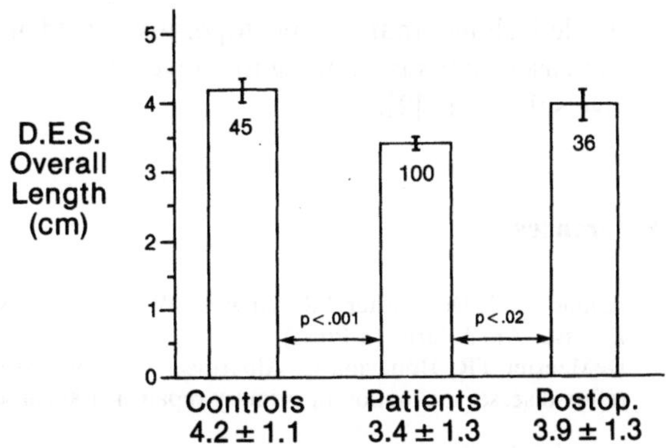

Fig. 3. Comparison of the mean overall length of the distal esophageal sphincter measured in control subjects, and in patients before and after surgery

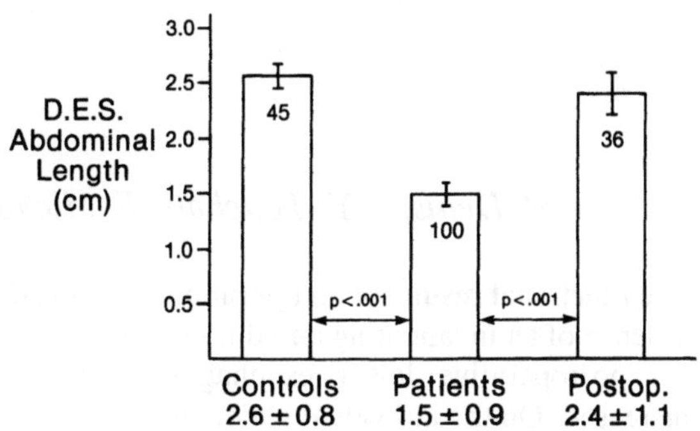

Fig. 4. Comparison of the mean abdominal length of the distal esophageal sphincter measured in control subjects and in patients before and after surgery

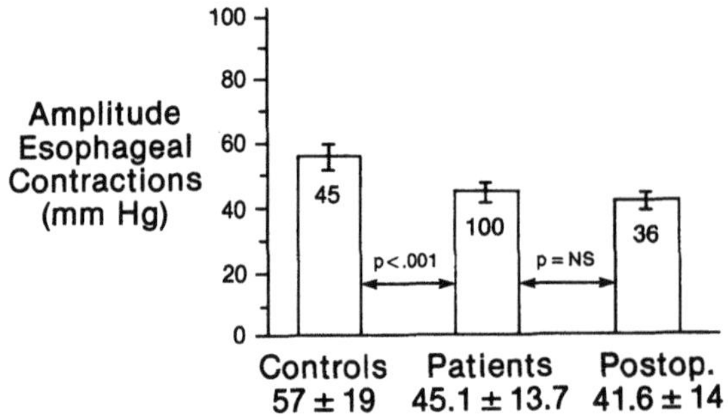

Fig. 5. Comparison of the mean amplitude of esophageal contractions measured in control subjects, and in patients before and after surgery

Table 1. Incidence of side effects of the operation related to preoperative distal esophageal sphincter manometrics

	Normal L.E.S. (n=43)	Defective L.E.S. (n=57)
Symptomatic Gas Bloat	44%	23%*
Increased Flatus	75%	48%*

* $p < 0.05$

3. Table 1 shows that the postoperative incidence of symptomatic gas bloat and increased flatus is significantly lower in patients who had manometrically defective sphincters [2].

References

1. Zaninotto G, DeMeester TR, Schwizer W et al The Lower Esophageal Sphincter in Health and Disease. Am J Surg (In Press)
2. DeMeester TR, Bonavina L, Albertucci M (1986) Nissen fundoplication for gastroesophageal reflux disease: evaluation of primary repair in 100 consecutive patients. Ann Surg 204(1): 9–20

P. Denis, J. Y. Touchais, F. Michot, and *P. Ténière* (Rouen)

The functional results of an operation are judged by the correction of reflux and the absence of an invalidating and durable dysphagia. When patient groups are studied, the postoperative lower esophageal sphincter (LES) pressure is significantly increased. On the individual scale, the reflux correction is observed in the absence of an increase in the postoperative LES pressure in comparison to the preoperative value [1]. But reflux occasionally persists in spite of a clearcut improvement in the postoperative pressure [1]. In these conditions, it must be admitted that pressure measurement does not always affirm the effectiveness of the operation (this effectiveness can only be judged by a pHmetry study). When discordance exists between the LES pressure and the pHmetry results, other factors are invoked: abnormal esophageal clearance, decreased gastric emptying rate, gastric hypersecretion of acid or of other elements of the cardia continence. Insufficient correction of the elastic properties of the LES after surgery is a seductive theoretical explanation, but one which not been extensively studied (Fig. 1) [2]. The length of the postoperative abdominal esophageal segment is not correlated with the effectiveness of the operation [3–4–5]. Transitory relaxations of the LES cause reflux when the residual LES pressure during the relaxations is very low. As a result of the increased postoperative resting LES pressure, the residual pressure during transitory relaxations is sufficient to prevent reflux (Fig. 2) [6].

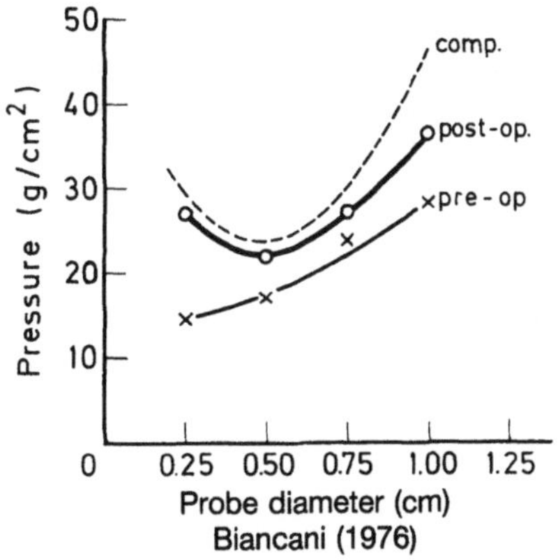

Fig. 1. Values of inferior esophageal sphincter pressures for dilatation with bougies of increasing diameter – the preoperative pressure curve is normalized by operation

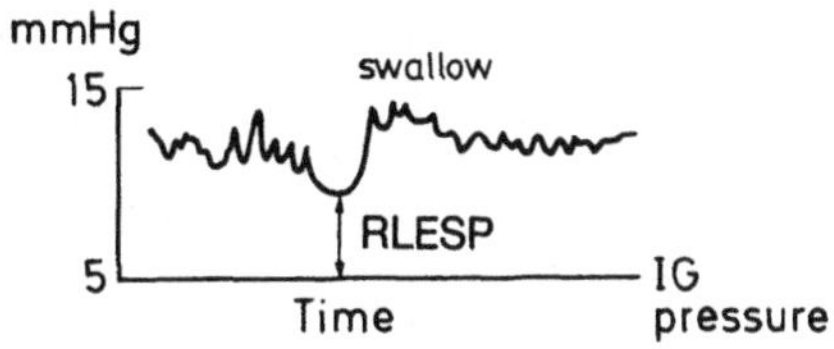

Fig. 2. Swallowing produces incomplete relaxation of the inferior esophageal sphincter, leaving a residual pressure (RLESP) of 5 mm of mercury Kiroff (1984)

Personal work (Fig. 3) [3] had shown that reflux never occurred when postoperative pressure was greater than 10 cm H_2O. In addition, we never observed postoperative dysphagia in the absence of LES hypertonia, confirming prior data [7]. In these conditions, it appears that in the absence of a perfect parallelism between the postoperative LES parameters and the results of reflux correction, only pHmetry results can judge the effectiveness of the operation. The return to normal of the LES pressure appears to us to be the primary aim to correct reflux.

This is the reason for our undertaking a prospective study where a 270° fundoplication was done in cases of preoperative hypotonia of the LES, and 180° in cases of normal postoperative tone. The postoperative LES pressure was always higher than 10 cm H_2O in the first 12 patients and none retained pathological postprandial reflux or suffered from a durable dysphagia (Table 1). These results suggest that the criterion of effectiveness remains the pHmetry results and that LES pressure could guide the choice of the operation.

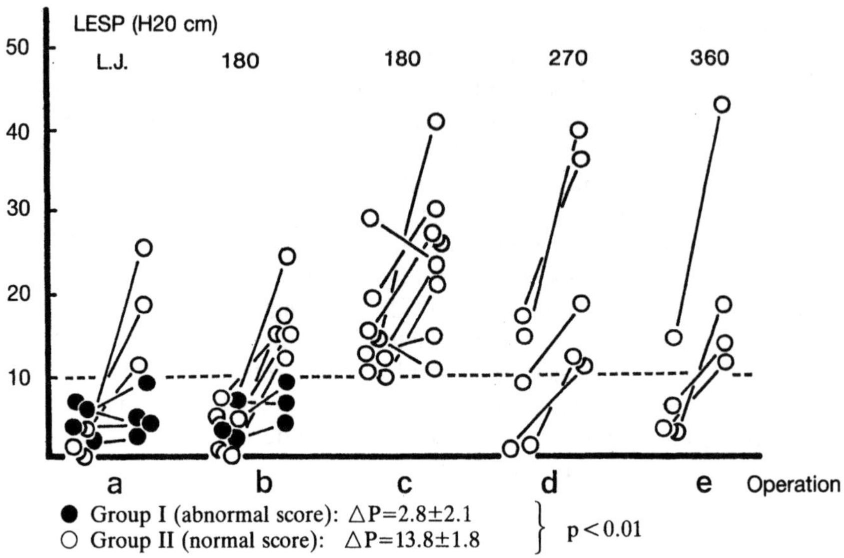

Fig. 3. Preoperative (left) and postoperative (right) inferior esophageal sphincter pressure in patients having undergone a Lortat-Jacob operation (a), a 360° fundoplication (e), a 270° fundoplication (d), and a 180° fundoplication with a reduced (b) or normal (c) preoperative LES pressure

Table 1. Prospective study

Preliminary results
12 patients with reflux demonstrable by pH measurement
Hemifundoplication of: – 180° if LES pressure exceeds 10 cm H_2O preoperatively – 270° if LES pressure is below 10 cm H_2O preoperatively
3 months postoperatively: – no reflux – no dysphagia

References

1. DeMeester TR, Bonavina L, Albertucci M (1986) Nissen fundoplication for gastroesophageal reflux disease. Evaluation of primary repair in 100 consecutive patients. Am Surg 204: 9–20
2. Biancani P, Zabinski MP, Behar J (1976) Pressure, tension, and force of closure of the human lower esophageal sphincter and esophagus. J Clin Invest 56: 476–483
3. Touchais JY, Lerebours E, Sauger F, Testart J, Teniere P, Ducrotte P, Guillard JF, Paley D, Galmiche JP, Denis P, Colin R (1985) Analyse des différents facteurs conditionnant les résultats du traitement chirurgical du reflux gastroesophagien. Gastroenterol Clin Biol 9: 712–718
4. Bancewicz J, Mughal M, Marples M (1987) The lower esophageal sphincter after floppy Nissen fundoplication. Br J Surg 74: 162–164
5. O'Sullivan GC, DeMeester TR, Joelsson BE, Smith RB, Blough RR, Johnson LF, Skinner DB (1982) Interaction of lower esophageal sphincter pressure and length of sphincter in the abdomen as determinants of gastroesophageal competence. Am J Surg 143: 40–47
6. Kiroff GK, Maddern GJ, Jamieson GG (1984) A study of factors responsible for the efficacy of fundoplication in the treatment of gastroesophageal reflux. Aust N Z J Surg 54: 109–112
7. Segol P, Baptiste P, L'Hirondel C, Marchand P, Gignoux M (1982) Effets de la fundoplicature sur le sphincter inférieur de l'œsophage: étude manométrique pré et post-opératoire. Gastroenterol Clin Biol 6: 222–228

The role of incomplete LES relaxation in postoperative dysphagia

P. Verhaeghe, and *R. Stoppa* (Amiens)

The frequency of postoperative dysphagia is variously assessed by authors and differs with different surgical techniques. After excluding early postoperative dysphagia, which is common and resolves in a few weeks in the great majority of cases, incomplete relaxation of the inferior esophageal sphincter may be proposed for some 20% of those operated. This last hypothesis can only be discussed after having excluded the hypotheses of secondary peptic stricture, slipping of the valve, and even aperistalsis (scleroderma, intermittent esophageal spasm, etc.).

Demonstration of disturbed relaxation

A manometric study can in itself demonstrate disordered relaxation of the LES and also makes it possible to measure the severity of this defect in relaxation. Gastroesophageal fiberoscopy and esophageal pH measurement [9] are required to define the condition of the esophageal mucosa and reveal a persistent or recurrent reflux [15]. The absence of parallelism between the lesions of the esophageal mucosa and the clinical symptomatology adds to the difficulties of interpretation [5].

Mechanism of relaxation disturbance

Interpretation of the mechanism(s) of disorders of relaxation is far from being unanimous: lack of flexibility of the periesophageal scar [4, 5]; the role of the vagus nerve [19, 14]; though the cure of hiatus hernia may correct disturbed motility induced by reflux [12], this surgical maneuver will be ineffective for "primary" anomalies of the inferior sphincter [3]; elevated pressure of the LES [7], which constitutes an effective barrier against reflux [1, 6], may hinder the expression of other physiologic potentials of this sphincter [10, 11]; also, why is the dysphagia often not in evidence until the 7th postoperative day [4]?

Causal link between disordered relaxation and dysphagia. This link is often difficult to demonstrate [2]. Ideally, it would call for routine preoperative manometry, something rarely carried out by surgical units since such preoperative manometry does not supply a decisive factor in the choice of surgical technique. In the absence of this decisive element we are confined to analysing the disjointed results of published series [13, 16, 17, 18].

Dysphagia is observed with the same frequency after medical or surgical treatment. Disturbance of relaxation, once demonstrated, proves variable in time in one and the same patient. Does this phenomenon explain why some authors have not observed disorders of relaxation [8]? Measurement of disordered relaxation lacks precision, while disturbed relaxation may be observed in operated individuals without dysphagia. Different surgical techniques give different rates of disturbed relaxation, as might be expected; but the same technique (the Nissen-Rossetti type of procedure) in the hands of different surgeons gives different incidences of disturbed relaxation. This is explicable partly by the impossibility of strict reproducibility of these techniques.

In conclusion, the way in which sufferers from hiatus hernia are investigated preoperatively often renders differentiation of pre- and postoperative disorders of motility very difficult. Disturbance of relaxation of the LES may account for some postoperative dysphagia, but what is the exact role and frequency of this incomplete relaxation?

Operations of the Nissen type (a 360° valve) are certainly the most effective in preventing recurrence of reflux, but they do not restore a normal sphincter; they create an effective cuff without the adaptability of the physiologic sphincter. The ideal procedure remains to be discovered.

References

1. Behar J, Biancani P, Spiro HM, Storer EH (1974) Effect of an anterior fundoplication on lower esophageal sphincter competence. Gastroenterology 67 (2): 209–215
2. Bonavina L, Evander A, DeMeester TR, Walther B, Cheng SC, Palazzo L, Concannon (1986) Length of the distal sphincter and competency of the cardia. The American Journal of Surgery 151: 25–34
3. Brand DL, Eastwood IR, Martin D, Carter WB, Pope CE (1979) Esophageal symptoms, manometry and histology before and after antireflux surgery. A long term follow up study. Gastroenterology 76: 1393–1401
4. Edwards DAW (1970) Post-vagotomy dysphagia. The Lancet 7663: 90–92
5. Edwards DAW (1982) The antireflux mechanism, its disorder and their consequences. Clinics in Gastroenterology 11 (3): 479–496
6. Fisher RS, Malmud LS, Roberts GS, Lobis IF (1977) The lower esophageal sphincter as a barrier to gastrophageal reflux. Gastroenterology 72: 19–22
7. Goodall RJR, Temple JG (1980) Effect of Nissen fundoplication on competence of the gastroesophageal junction. Gut 21: 607–613
8. Higgs RH, Castell DO, Farrell RL (1975) Evaluation of the effect of fundoplication on the incompetent lower esophageal sphincter. Surgery Gynecology and Obstetrics 141 (4): 571–575
9. Hollender LF, Meyer CH, Calderoli H, Blanchot P, Starlinger M (1976) Apports de la manométrie cardio-œsophagienne dans l'étude pré et post-opératoire des hernies hiatales. Chirurgie 102: 804–814
10. Leonardi HK, Lee ME, El-Kurd MF, Ellis FH (1977) An experimental study of the effectiveness of various antireflux operations. The Annals of Thoracic Surgery 24 (3): 215–222
11. Leonardi HK, Ellis FH (1983) Complications of the Nissen fundoplication. Surgical clinics of North America 63 (6): 1155–1165
12. Lind JF, Burns CM, MacDougall JT (1965) "Physiological" repair for hiatus hernia – manometric study. Archives of Surgery, 91 (2): 233–237
13. Negre JB (1983) Nissen fundoplication: Results at 10 year follow up. The American Journal of Surgery 146: 635–638
14. Olinde AJ, Maher JW, Mac Guigan JE (1986) The effect of varying levels of vagotomy on postprandial lower esophageal sphincter pressure and pancreatic polypeptide. World Journal of Surgery 10: 809–813
15. Richter JE, Castell DO (1982) Gastroesophageal reflux: pathogenesis and therapy. Annals of Internal Medicine 97: 93–103
16. Segol P, Baptiste P, L'Hirondel C, Marchand P, Gignoux M (1982) Effets de la fundoplicature sur le sphincter inférieur de l'œsophage: étude manométrique pré et post-opératoire. Gastroentérologie clinique et biologique 6: 222–228

17. Siewert R, Weiser F, Jennewein HM, Waldeck F (1974) Clinical and manometric investigations of the lower esophageal sphincter and its reactivity to pentagastrin in patients with hiatus hernia. Digestion 10: 287–297
18. Touchais JY, Lerebours E, Sauger F, Testart J, Teniere P, Ducrotte P, Guillard JF, Paley D, Galmiche JP, Denis P, Colin R (1985) Analyse des différents facteurs conditionnant les résultats du traitement chirurgical du reflux gastro-œsophagien. Gastroentérologie Clinique et Biologique 9: 712–718
19. Vansant JH, Baker JW (1976) Complications of vagotomy in the treatment of hiatal hernia. Annals of Surgery 183 (6): 629–635

Is it possible to quantify dysphagia to enable comparison between patients?

R. D. Henderson, and *A. H. Zalev* (Toronto)

Perfect quantitation of dysphagia is not possible, however there are some useful methods of investigation which allow fair comparison. There are two types of dysphagia, mechanical stricture related dysphagia and motor dysphagia. Each of these must be considered separately.

When a mechanical stricture is present, the major variables in dysphagia are the diameter and length of the stricture, the proximal peristaltic thrusts of the esophagus and the consistency of the food bolus. In evaluating the dysphagia each of these variables must be considered.

The end point of calibration is the patient's recognition of what can and cannot be swallowed. Variation depends on the food consistency, diligence in chewing and the consistency and fragmentation of the particles. Clearly, the patient recognizes what will go down and mechanical strictures produce a bolus size specific obstruction (Fig. 1).

Esophageal stricture [1] diameter produces appropriate dysphagias; as the length of the stricture increases the dysphagia becomes worse. Peristaltic power is an important factor. In the presence of an adynamic sclerodermatous esophagus, even a minor stricture will produce major dysphagia.

Having examined the factors affecting mechanical dysphagia, how can one investigate and categorize the problems. Several methods are possible:

1. Radiologic quantification.
2. Isotope studies.
3. Manometric evaluation.
4. Symptom analysis.

Radiologically, with mechanic obstruction a retention air fluid level will indicate major or total obstruction. With mechanical obstruction solid bolus dysphagia is more important and can be documented by recording the progress of a barium sandwich or barium impregnated marshmallow. The quality of radiologic evaluation

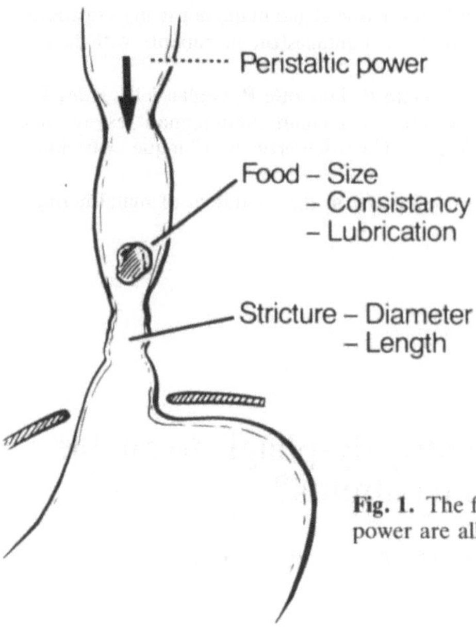

Fig. 1. The food size, lumen size, food consistency and motor power are all important

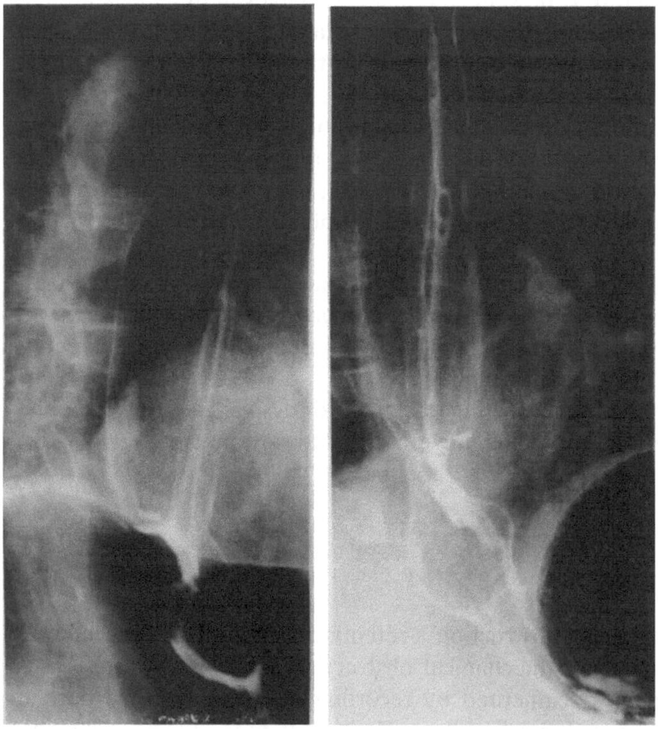

Fig. 2. Using the tube air insufflation, esophagogram demonstrates clearly the stricture width and length. These dimensions can be related to the severity of dysphagia

of stricture diameter and length can be greatly improved by using an air insufflation tube esophagus (Fig. 2).

For mechanical obstruction, radioactive solids can be swallowed and recorded. There is no advantage in this method over standard radiology.

Manometry is of more diagnostic value and does not quantify, but secondary disordered motor activity is increased in the presence of chronic obstruction. Of more importance manometry quantifies motor power in the presence of scleroderma (Fig. 3).

The endpoint is symptom analysis. In obtaining a history, it is important to record the presence or absence of dysphagia, its duration, whether it occurs with liquids, solids or both, its frequency, and the occurrence of regurgitation.

With a carefully taken history, radiologic evaluation of stricture and length, and manometric evaluation of motor power, it is possible to grade mechanical dysphagia

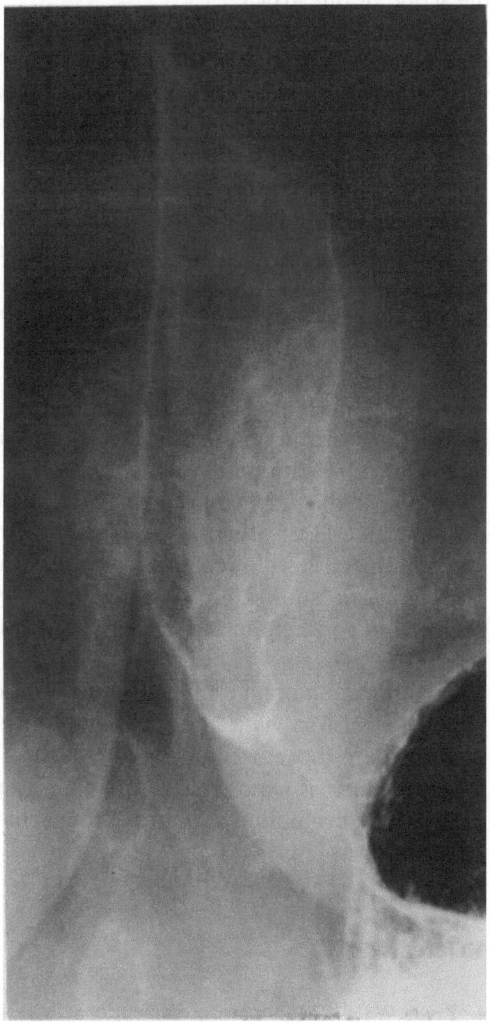

Fig. 3. In this patient there is a mild stricture illustrated by air insufflation tube esophagogram. This patient has an adynamic sclerodermatous esophagus and disproportionate dysphagia

at least to the level of mild, moderate, severe and very severe. In my own system I use the following symptomatic classification:

1. Mild dysphagia – less than once per week with normal food.
2. Moderate – daily with normal food, but easily corrected by chewing and reasonable selection.
3. Severe – all foods unless pureed.
4. Very severe – all liquids and occasionally even saliva.

*

While mechanical obstruction is difficult to quantify, motor obstruction [2] is even less accurate. There are several types of motor obstruction including achalasia, diffuse esophageal spasm (D.E.S.), reflux, scleroderma and surgically induced over-competence. Motor problems also exist at the cricopharyngeal level, but are beyond the scope of this article.

Obstruction in achalasia is secondary to the absence of HPZ relaxation and proximal esophageal dilatation. With untreated achalasia, some obstruction occurs with all meals, however this is often not recognized by the patient.

Diffuse spasm produces severe motor spasm with obstruction. Dysphagia with scleroderma is usually secondary to an esophageal stricture; the lack of esophageal peristalsis with scleroderma [3] makes dysphagia more severe.

The commonest cause of dysphagia is gastroesophageal reflux. In my experience, 80% of patients with reflux have dysphagia, 70% are motor and only 10% are secondary to a peptic stricture. One other group of motor dysphagias are those produced by surgical hernia repair. This problem is particularly prevalent in patients with an over-competent total fundoplication.

Radiologic studies may be normal with motor dysphagia as the dysphagia is usually intermittent. Solid food particles are often necessary to demonstrate the obstruction. In the absence of mechanical stricture, the radiologist must evaluate motor function with particular care.

Isotope studies can be used to quantitate dysphagia as they will show prolonged holdup at the level of motor obstruction. Isotope studies are of particular value in assessing hiatal hernia repair and demonstrating esophageal emptying times.

Manometric studies are essential for a specific diagnosis of the type of motor obstruction and help in evaluating and quantifying the degree of dysphagia.

Quantification of an esophageal motor disorder is difficult; with care it is possible to use the history as a guide to symptom severity and the investigative methods described are those used as a guide to the exact diagnosis.

In summary, it is possible to quantify dysphagia: the methods lack accuracy and need careful evaluation to improve the technique. Quantification by history gives an effective overview.

References

1. Payne WS, (1970) Surgical treatment of reflux esophagitis and stricture associated with permanent incompetence of the cardia. Mayo Clin Proc 45: 553

2. Henderson RD (1980) The Esophagus: Reflux and Primary Motor Disorders. Williams and Wilkins, Baltimore and London
3. Perdue GD, Morris AJ (1962) Surgical manifestations of scleroderma. Surg Gynecol Obstet 115: 745

Can the pharmacological improvement of gastric emptying improve the results of certain procedures?

R. W. McCallum (Charlottesville)

Although delayed gastric emptying of liquids or solids may be one of the mechanisms that increases the volume of gastric contents available for reflux into the esophagus, investigations of this possible relationship have yielded conflicting results.

Studies using scintigraphy [1] and the double sampling method [2] both demonstrated that patients with reflux esophagitis emptied liquids in a normal fashion. However, antral contractility and cumulative antral activity were observed to be decreased in the presence of gastroesophageal reflux [1]. On the other hand, another scintigraphic study showed delayed gastric emptying of liquids in reflux esophagitis patients [2]. Two additional studies [3, 4] using radiolabelled solid-liquid meals disclosed that gastroesophageal reflux was associated with significant delay in emptying, although these meals did not allow precise discrimination between solid and liquid emptying.

Investigators using a gastroduodenal intubative method found that patients with gastroesophageal reflux and normal controls had similar amounts of acid secretion and duodenogastric reflux, as well as similar solid and liquid gastric emptying rates [5].

However, dual isotope scintigraphic studies demonstrated that, as a group, gastroesophageal reflux patients had significant solid-food retention [6]: 57% had delayed gastric emptying of solids, indicative of a disturbance in antral motility; reflux patients with abnormal solid emptying were shown to have normal emptying of liquids (that is normal fundic motility). Interestingly, only 25% of reflux patients with delayed gastric emptying had symptoms, such as nausea and vomiting, which are usually associated with gastric stasis [3].

Whether delayed solid emptying in the presence of gastroesophageal reflux is a primary or secondary phenomenon remains to be determined.

Nevertheless, these studies illustrate the heterogeneity of gastric solid retention and their results have important therapeutic implications. It must also be noted that infants with severe gastroesophageal reflux who fail to thrive or have pulmonary aspiration exhibited marked gastric retention of a liquid meal [7, 8]. Gastroesophageal reflux of infancy appears to be a pathogenetically distinct entity, possibly involving fundic dysmotility.

An antireflux operation, especially fundoplication, is often successful in patients with reflux esophagitis. When gastric emptying studies are performed, surgical failures appear to correlate with slower solid emptying [9], while there was more increased liquid emptying probably attributable to surgically induced impaired receptive relaxation related to damage and/or entrapment of the vagus nerve. I have also made the observation that a population of post-fundoplication patients presenting with increasing symptoms of gastroesophageal reflux, and therefore termed relative failures or absolute failures, have an accompanying delay in gastric emptying.

The cause of the delayed gastric emptying in this failed operative group may reflect that the patient had the delay in gastric emptying from the onset, as has been summarized above, and there would be no reason to believe that a fundoplication would really improve the rate of gastric emptying of solids. It is interesting that the literature would indicate that symptoms tend to recur over a period of 3 to 5 years, such that by five years there is significant documentation of reflux by esophageal pH studies. It may be indicative that the continued delay in gastric emptying slowly impairs the efficacy of the antireflux procedure: obviously one possible mechanism would be the continual gastric distention related to delayed gastric emptying placing stress on the antireflux construction, leading to its gradual weakening with time. Another proposal would be that the delay in gastric emptying produces gastric distention, which in turn promotes more transient relaxations of the lower esophageal sphincter, as has been reported, and this would contribute significantly to postprandial reflux and undermine the role of the surgery [10].

McCallum et al. have reported [11] that the slow gastric emptying of solids in the population of GER patients can be correlated with the degree and severity of antral gastritis. The more severe grades of gastritis; some including small intestinal

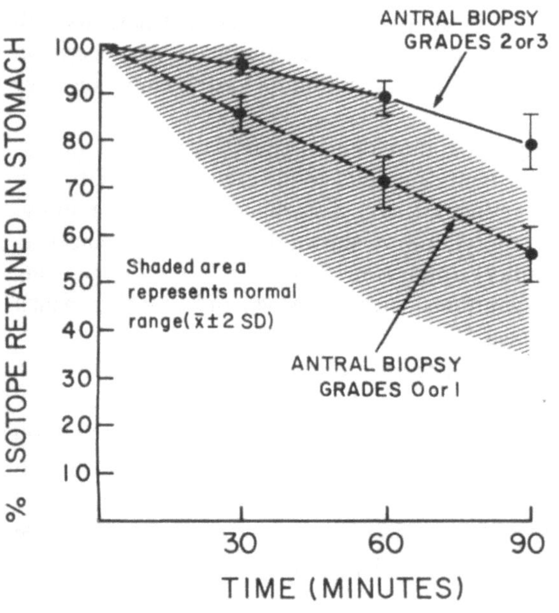

Fig. 1. Relationship of histologic antral gastritis and gastric emptying in gastroesophageal reflux patients. Patients with grades 2 or 3 (severe) gastritis retained significantly more isotope (mean ±S.E.M.) at 30 ($p<0.05$), 60 ($p<0.01$), and 90 ($p<0.01$) minutes after the test meal, compared to patients with grades 0 or 1 gastritis, and also compared ($p<0.01$) to the rate of gastric emptying for normal subjects (shaded area)

metaplasia, were associated with the slowest gastric emptying (Fig. 1). Presumably this antral gastritis continues after surgery. The etiology of the gastritis is not clear: could gastric stasis itself lead to gastritis or could gastritis induce a smooth muscle impairment? The etiology for the latter gastritis could be bile reflux (some comparisons with the gastritis of gastric ulcer), and raises questions of the competence of the pylorus and the status of duodenal motility in GER disease.

Another possibility is that at the time of fundoplication, there is vagal damage in the form of an accidental vagotomy or perhaps entrapment of the vagus nerve in the fundoplication wrap. There are estimates which could imply that accidental vagotomies and/or vagal nerve damage could occur in as many as 30% of patients undergoing fundoplication and particularly in the setting of a second antireflux operation. Such vagal damage would certainly explain the more rapid gastric emptying of liquids found in the post-operative setting [9], and at the same time this could result in impaired antral innervation and delayed gastric emptying of solids.

How does one approach this therapeutically and/or how does this alter the surgical approach in the future? It would be my concept that medical management of a recurrence of gastroesophageal reflux symptoms in the post-fundoplication state would or should be treated with a prokinetic agent such as Metoclopramide (primperan) or Domperidone (motilium). This would promote gastric emptying and decrease distention and minimize the transient lower esophageal sphincter relaxations and the potential weakening of the fundoplication procedure; I have not seen any indication at the present time to consider the role of more extensive surgery such as an antrectomy and drainage procedure at the time of surgery.

I believe the potential for bile reflux into a slowly emptying or atonic stomach results in more post-operative complications than would be acceptable; in patients in whom a very high acid secretion rate has been documented, as well as gastroesophageal reflux disease (less than 5% of the reflux population) [11], there could be rationale for a selective parietal cell vagotomy to decrease acid secretion and also accelerate gastric emptying of liquids. Such an operation may also be useful in the treatment of Barrett's esophagus in order to guarantee minimal acid exposure to the metaplastic esophageal mucosa.

More prospective studies are required to understand the pre and post-operative gastric emptying status of patients, and the correlation of gastric stasis with recurrence and severity of GER symptoms.

References

1. Behar J, Ramsby G (1978) Gastric emptying and antral motility in reflux esophagitis. Gastroenterology 74:253–256
2. Csendes A, Henriquez A (1978) Gastric emptying in patients with reflux esophagitis or benign strictures of the esophagus secondary to reflux compared to controls. Scand J Gastroenterol 13:205–207
3. Baldi F, Corinaldesi R, Ferrarini F (1981) Gastric secretion and emptying of liquids in reflux esophagitis. Dig Dis Sci 26:886–889
4. McCallum RW, Berkowitz DM, Lerner E (1981) Gastric emptying in patients with gastroesophageal reflux. Gastroenterology 80:285–291

5. Donovan IA, Harding LK, Keighley MRB, et al. (1977) Abnormalities of gastric emptying and pyloric reflux in uncomplicated hiatus hernia. Br J Surg 64: 847–848
6. Coleman SC, Rees WDW, Malagelada JR (1979) Normal gastric function in reflux esophagitis (abstr). Gastroenterology 76: 1115
7. McCallum RW, Mensh R, Lange R (1981) Definition of the gastric emptying abnormality present in gastroesophageal reflux patients (abstr). Gastroenterology 80: 1226
8. Hillemeier AC, Lange R, McCallum RW, et al (1981) Delayed gastric emptying in infants with gastroesophageal reflux. J Pediatr 98: 190–193
9. Maddern MB, Jamieson GG, Chatterton BE, Collins PJ (1985) Is there an association between failed antireflux procedures and delayed gastric emptying. Ann Surg 202: 162–165
10. Holloway RH, Hongo M, McCallum RW (1985) Gastric distention. A mechanism for postprandial gastroesophageal reflux. Gastroenterology 89: 779–784
11. Fink SM, Barwick K, DeLuca V, Sanders FJ, Kandathil M, McCallum RW (1984) The association of histologic gastritis with gastroesophageal reflux and delayed gastric emptying. J Clin Gastroenterol 6: 301–309

R. Jian, F. Ducrot, and *M. Lehmann* (Paris)

Important advances have been achieved in recent years in the treatment of gastric emptying disorders (GED), especially in gastric stasis. Indications of such medical treatment for improvement of results of the surgical correction of gastroesophageal reflux (GER) are linked to the existence and the physiopathologic importance of gastric stasis in such patients.

Impairments of gastric emptying in patients who underwent surgical treatment of a GER

Such impairments can be present before surgery, revealed by surgery or induced by surgery.

1. studies assessing gastric stasis in GER patients are contradictory [1]. However, 9 of the 13 studies analysed concerning more than 350 adult patients conclude that gastric stasis is a feature of GER; most of them use scintigraphic measurement of gastric emptying; 29% evidence a selective stasis of emptying of solids. 14% a stasis of the liquid fraction, and 29% a delay of gastric evacuation of both phases of the meal. Interpretation of pediatric studies is even more misleading.

   Even when a GED is found, it only concerns a sub-group of GER patients (approx. 50%). Finally, even if gastric stasis is a common feature of GER patients, its interpretation has still to be defined: coincidence of two frequent disorders or physiopathologic relation between gastric stasis and GER? Gastric stasis should be detected and its role discussed before surgical management of GER patients.
2. gastric stases induced or revealed by GER surgery are often caused by previous treatment.
   - Some of them are the consequence of an accidental vagotomy occurring during the anti-reflux procedure. Although the incidence of such accidents cannot be appreciated, they are in our experience the most frequent cause of

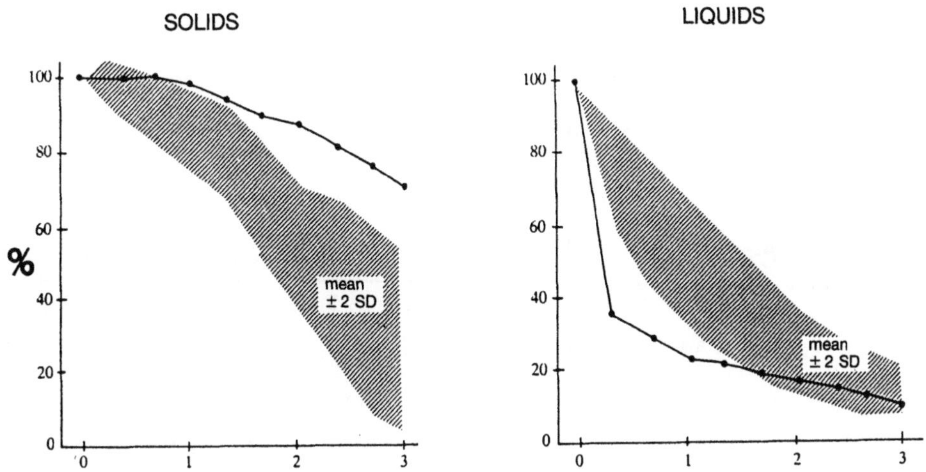

Fig. 1. Gastric stasis following accidental vagotomy during fundoplication

post-operative gastric stasis. It is well documented that although troncular vagotomy/pyloroplasty and proximal vagotomy have hardly no influence on gastric emptying [2], troncular vagotomy induces an antral hypomotility and a gastric stasis. Its usual scintigraphic pattern is a delay of solid emptying and acceleration of liquid emptying (Fig. 1), but it can also result in stasis of both phases of the meal. In that case only a Hollander test can authenticate the origin of the disorder.

- Symptoms of gastric stasis and antral hypomotility have been found after fundoplicature in patients whose Hollander test attested the absence of accidental vagotomy [3]. Symptoms were not influenced by medical treatment, and in 3 of the 6 patients, were severe enough to need antrectomy. It remains to be established whether these disorders were induced by the surgical procedure or only revealed by it.

Medical treatment of gastric stasis

Several drugs have proven their efficacy on gastric stasis and symptoms of dyspepsia. Most of these studies however did not specifically study gastric stasis occurring after GER surgery.

Nevertheless, the efficacy of metoclopramide (Primperan R), domperidone (Motilium R) and cholinergic drugs on gastric stasis of miscellaneous origin as well as secondary to vagotomy is proven [4, 5, 6].

We have assessed the effect of cisapride on gastric emptying. This new drug stimulates digestive motility by enhancing post-ganglionic secretion of acetylcholine. Its potency and specificity seem important, and it does not have any of the usual side effects of cholinomimentic drugs. In a first study [7], we assessed the acute effect of this drug (4 injection of 8 mg of cisapride or placebo in a double blind randomized study) on gastroparesia of diverse etiology, including post-vagotomy

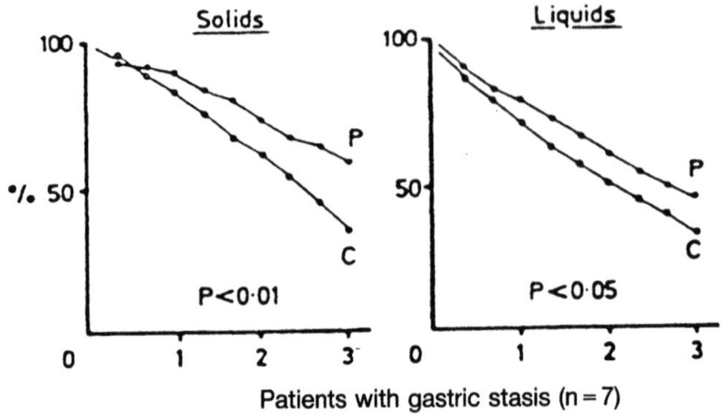

Fig. 2. Acute effect of Cisapride Vs placebo on patients with gastric stasis

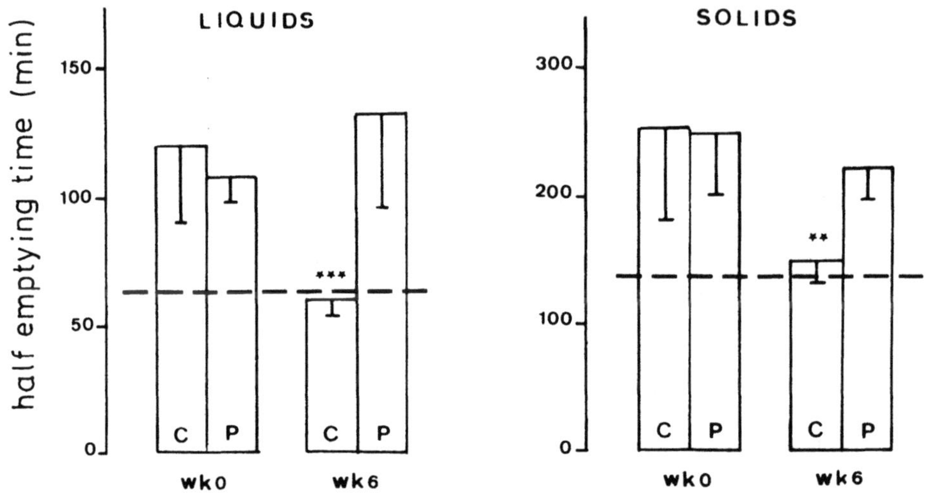

Fig. 3. Effect of chronic administration of Cisapride Vs placebo with idiopathic dyspepsia
c=Cisapride (3 mg/day) P=placebo
---normal gastric emptying (mean of control group)

patients: a significant acceleration of gastric emptying was evidenced for both the solid and the liquid phases of the meal, and increased with the degree of initial gastric stasis (Fig. 2).

In a second work [8] we studied the effect of chronic administration of cisapride (10 mg tid vs placebo in a double-blind study design); gastric emptying was measured before and after a six week treatment period. While placebo had no effect on gastric stasis, cisapride normalized gastric emptying rates of solids and liquids in nearly all the patients with a previous stasis (Fig. 3) and improved their symptoms. Although that study only concerned patients with idiopathic dyspepsia, it seems reasonable to assume that a similar study with secondary dyspepsia patients would have yielded similar results.

Conclusion

Gastroparesia can therefore sometimes be evidenced in patients who underwent surgical management of GER. This anomaly can be responsible for sometimes very disturbing dyspetic symptoms. Furthermore, gastric stasis could contribute to failure of surgical procedure, for mechanical reasons (by increasing intra-gastric post-prandial pressure) or more complex ones (such as promoting the occurrence of spontaneous relaxation of the lower esophageal sphincter). The clinician now has several potent drugs that specifically enhance gastric motility. It is therefore likely that pharmacologic stimulation of gastric emptying could improve the results of some anti-reflux surgical procedures, or at least of some of their failures.

References

1. Jian R (1986) Reflux gastro-œsophagien et motricité gastrique. Gastroenterol Clin Biol 10: 319–321
2. Jian R, Kilian D, Grall Y, Ducrot F, Valleur P, Hautefeuille P, Bernier JJ (1985) Effet de la vagotomie fundique sur la vidange gastrique des solides et des liquides d'un repas chez des patients avec et sans récidive ulcéreuse duodénale post-opératoire. Gastroentérol Clin Biol 9: 486–490
3. Stanghellini V, Malagelada JR (1983) Gastric manometric abnormalities in patients with dyspeptic symptoms after fundoplication. Gut 24: 790–797
4. Brogden RN, Carmine AA, Hoel RC, Speight TM, Avery GS (1982) Domperidone. A review of its pharmacolocical activity, pharmacokinetics and therapeutic efficacy in the symptomatic treatment of chronic dyspepsia as an antiemetic. Drugs 24: 360–400
5. Harrington RA, Hamilton CW, Brogden RN, Linkenwich JA, Romankiewicz JA, Heel RC (1983) Metoclopramide. An updated review of its pharmacological properties and clinical use. Drugs 25: 451–494
6. Malagelada JR (1982) Gastric emptying disorders. Clinical significance and treatment. Drugs 86: 1592–1610
7. Jian R, Ducrot F, Piedeloup C, Mary JY, Najean Y, Bernier JJ. Measurement of gastric emptying in dyspeptic patients: effect of a new gastrokinetic agent (cisapride). Gut 26: 352–358
8. Jian R, Ruskone A, Ducrot F, Chaussade S, Rambaud JC, Bernier JJ (1986) Radionuclide and therapeutic assessment of chronic idiopathic dyspepsia (CID). Gastroenterology 90: 1477

Longterm evaluation of surgery

President: *W. Spencer Payne* (Rochester)

Free Commentators: *G. Beauchamp* (Montreal)
D. Gardiol (Lausanne)
J. A. Gruwez (Leuven)
J. Moreaux (Paris)
D. Rignault (Paris)
S. J. Spechler (Boston)

Can we specify the differences existing between endoscopic healing and histologic healing?

J. R. Siewert (Munich)

From the point of view of the clinician two important hints are at hand to indicate that an endoscopic healing of esophagitis is not always necessarily accompanied by microscopic healing.

1. In a study using cimetidine performed in 1978, we could demonstrate that the disturbance of the motility in the tubular esophagus persisted in spite of an endoscopic-macroscopic healing of esophagitis: acid clearance, the Bernstein test, and motility remained in pathologic ranges also after healing of esophagitis under cimetidine therapy. A microscopic persistance of the inflammation could explain these findings.
2. The high recurrence rate of esophagitis after medical longterm maintenance therapy could be another indication: this recurrence rate amounts to 30% in 6 months under ranitidine (Fig. 1) in a study by Koelz, and in one of our own studies under cimetidine (Fig. 2), we found a recurrence rate of 20% in the same time period. Persistent inflammation in microscopical ranges could also serve as explanation.

Therefore, in a study including 240 patients, we have checked the correlation between endoscopic-macroscopic and microscopic-histologic findings.

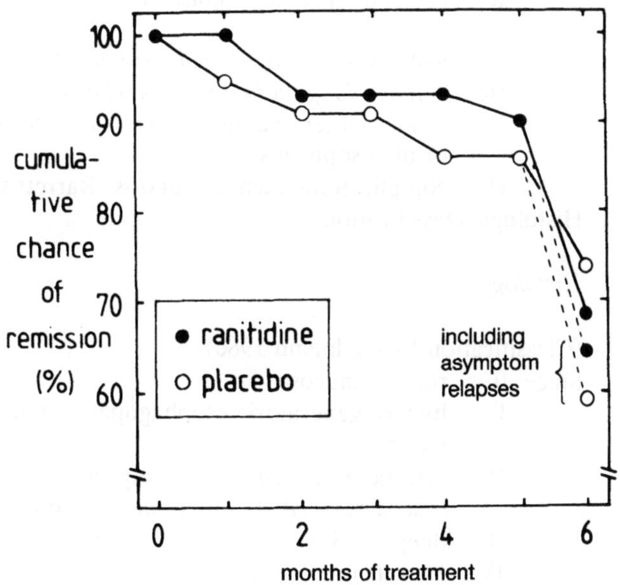

Fig. 1. Relapse of esophagitis

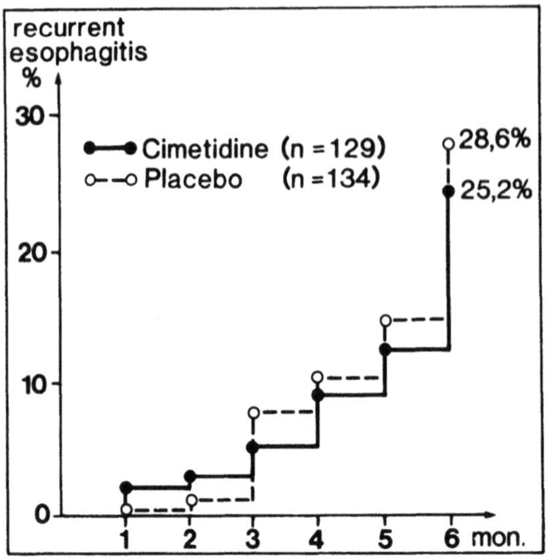

Fig. 2. Reflux esophagitis-longterm maintenance treatment

We have used the following classifications:

1. Macroscopic classification:

Endoscopy

(Classification by Savary and Miller, modified by Ottenjann/Siewert 1986)

Stage	0	regular mucosa
	Ia	isolated red *maculate* lesions *without* white fibrinous coat
	Ib	isolated *maculate* lesions *with* white fibrinous coat
	IIa	isolated red *longitudinal* lesions *without* white fibrinous coat
	IIb	isolated *longitudinal* lesions *with* white fibrinous coat
	III	lesions larger than in stages I or II, covering the whole circumference of the esophagus
	IV	complications such as stenosis, Barrett ulceration, etc.

2. Histologic classification:

Histology

(Classification by Heilmann 1986)

Stage	0	regular mucosa
	I	hyperregeneratoric esophagopathy, papillary ectasia, intraepithelial leucocytes
	II	infiltrates of leucocytes, superficial erosions (polymorphonuclear leucocytes > 10 + superficial erosions)
	III	deep erosions
	IV	Barrett mucosa, ulcers.

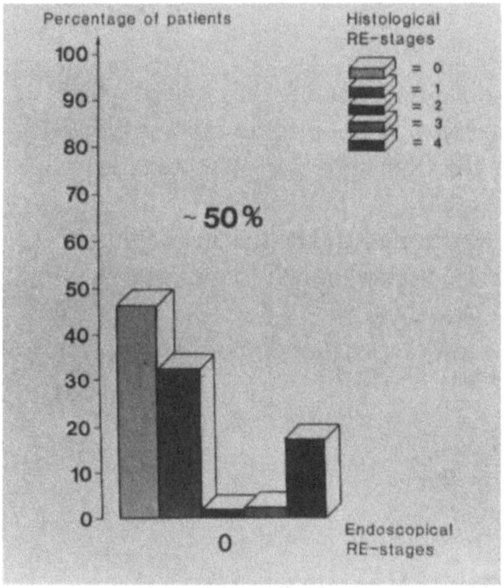

Fig. 3. Correlation between endoscopical and histological RE-stages

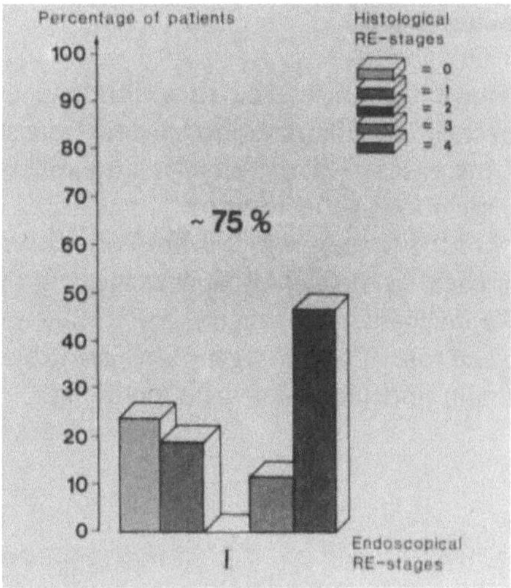

Fig. 4. Correlation between endoscopical and histological RE-stages

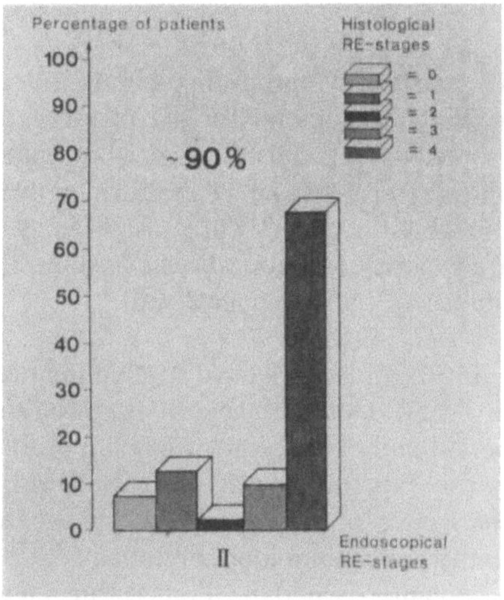

Fig. 5. Correlation between endoscopical and histological RE-stages

The results are shown in Fig. 3, 4 and 5.

- In endoscopic stage 0, that is after healing of esophagitis, in only 50% of the cases can a microscopic healing also be found. On the other hand it has to be considered whether the so-called hyperregeneratoric esophagopathy is really to be seen as a pathologic finding, although histologic examination of the biopsies in some 25% of the patients serious pathologic signs of inflammation were found.
- In endoscopic stage 1 and by selective sampling, the correlation of macroscopic and microscopic findings was better.

In conclusion

It must be considered that although an endoscopic healing has taken place, a microscopic inflammation can still persist in at least 25% up to a maximum of 50% of the cases. This possibly is an explanation for the high rate of recurrence after medical long-term therapy.

For the time being, it is not yet quite clear how long it takes for an esophagitis to also heal in the microscopic range, but obviously, it takes much longer than healing of a macroscopic change.

The role of persisting motility disturbances – as demonstrated in our study – has to remain undecided for the time being.

Healing of esophagitis and intraparietal esophageal collagen

H. J. Mud (Rotterdam)

The relief of symptoms in patients undergoing treatment for reflux esophagitis is not a reliable parameter for the reversal of histologic and motor abnormalities in the esophagus [1]. Histological abnormalities in severe reflux esophagitis include mucosal erosions or ulcerations, polymorphonuclear infiltration of the wall and probably the onset of fibrosis: stricture formation and shortening of the esophagus are two major complications of reflux esophagitis of long duration and are related to fibrosis of the esophageal wall.

In Rotterdam we have studied the problem of mural fibrosis in reflux esophagitis in a rat model, with special attention to the influence of the duration of the reflux period and of subsequent healing of the esophagitis [2].

The experiment was conducted with male Wistar rats. Reflux was induced by transection of the intraabdominal esophagus and end to side esophagojejunostomy to the first jejunal loop, optionally combined with total gastrectomy (Fig. 1). Reflux esophagitis ensued in all rats within a few days and looked macroscopically as shown on Fig. 2. Microscopically (Fig. 3) mucosal erosions or ulcerations where seen together with a dense panmural inflammatory reaction.

Acknowledging collagen as the main constituent of fibrous tissue we measured intraparietal collagen after 7, 14, 28 and 42 days of reflux and compared it to control values obtained from normal rats:

The data show a gradual rise in collagen content of the esophageal wall already demonstrable after 7 days of reflux. The difference with control values reaches statistical significance after 42 days of reflux.

After the assigned period of reflux rats were subjected to a reflux abolishing operation, a Roux en Y deviation (Fig. 4).

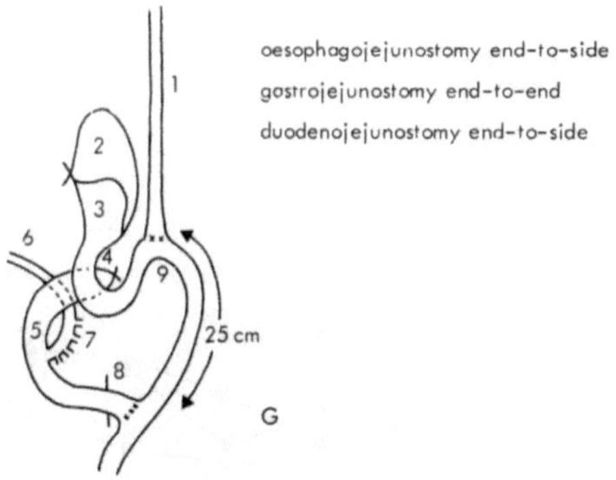

Fig. 1. Surgical design of the experiment

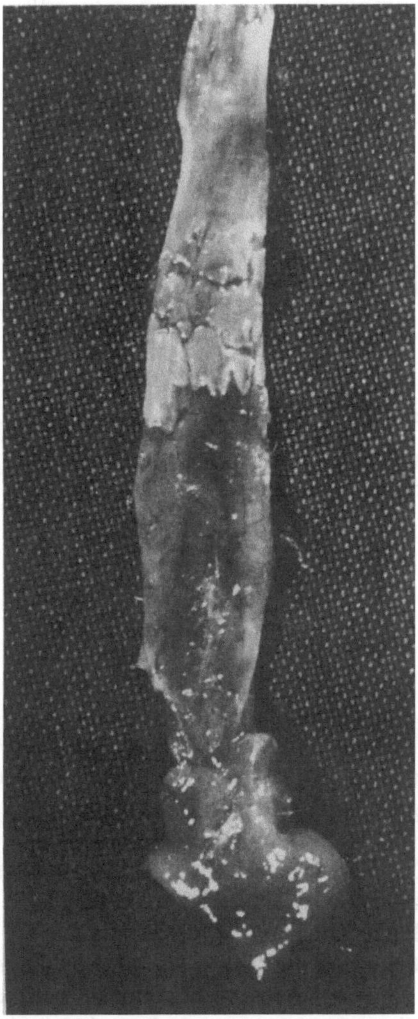

Fig. 2. Macroscopic appearance of rat esophagitis

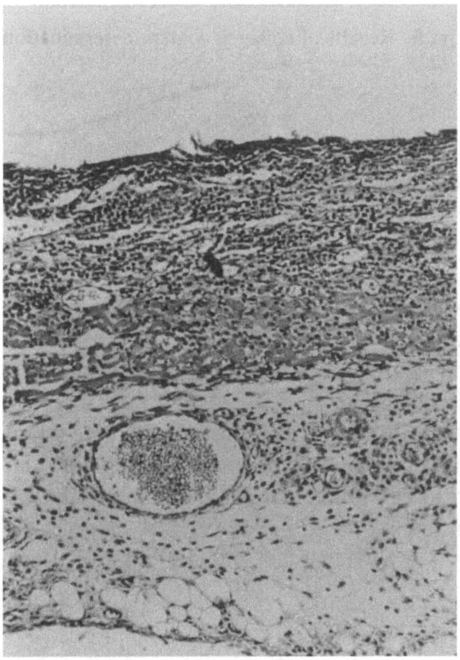

Fig. 3. Microscopic appearance of rat esophagitis

The effects of this operation were studied after 2, 4 and 6 weeks: The epithelial defects all healed within 2 weeks, though often there was a marked hyperkeratosis present.

After 6 weeks, the esophageal wall looked normal again on microscopic examination, but the collagen content determinations showed a different picture.

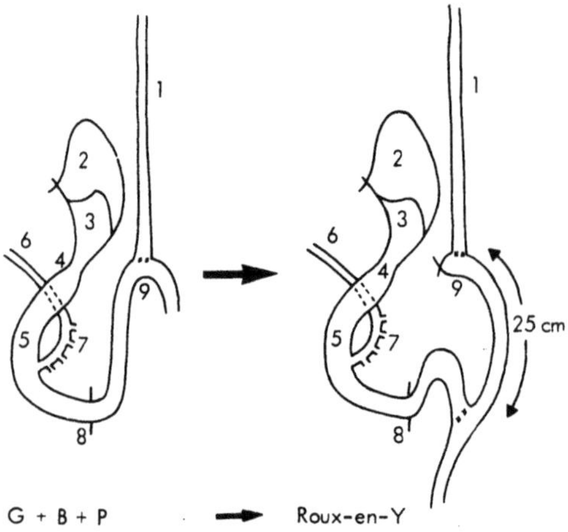

Fig. 4. Surgical design of the reflux abolishing operation

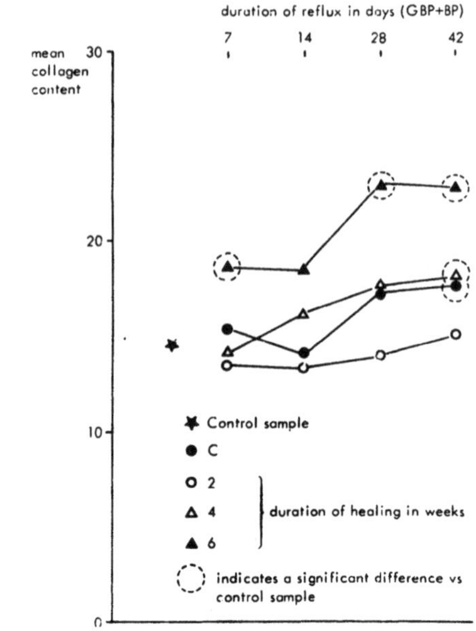

Fig. 5. Results of collagen content determination

Values continued rising and at evaluation 6 weeks after the reflux inducing operation reached a significant difference with control values in 3 out of 4 reflux groups (Fig. 5).

These finding show that already after a short period of severe esophagitis there is a considerable build up of collagen. Secondly, the amount of collagen increases with longer duration of reflux and thirdly, when healing is already nearing completion, the amount of intraparietal collagen is still rising.

Of course results of animal experimentation should be interpreted with care when discussing human pathology, but perhaps it is permissible to speculate that residual increased intraparietal collagen after a period of esophagitis could contribute to the persistence of demonstrable motor defects.

References

1. Sonnenberg A, Lepsien G, Muller-Lissner SA, Koelz HR, Siewert JR, Blum AL (1982) When is esophagitis healed? Dig Dis Sci 27: 297–302
2. Mud HJ, Kranendonk SE, van Houten H, Westbroek DL (1985) Mural collagen in experimental reflux esophagitis in rats. J Surg Res 38: 97–104

Recurrences and technical pseudo-recurrences

M. Rossetti (Liestal)

Between 1965 and 1986 (Table 1) we had the disputable privilege to deal with 78 cases operated because of reflux diseases in Europe. Only a few of them had been operated in our Clinic, and necessitated a new operation after the most diverse operative procedures.

Table 1. 78 reoperations after antireflux procedures

39	after actual or attempted fundoplication
11	after simple gastropexy – which cannot control reflux!
9	after Dor procedure
6	after Belsey procedure
13	after indeterminate procedures: most patients for reoperation come from a distance, often without records!

The technical recurrence is generally an early one as opposed to the biological recurrence, which is mostly a late one and accompanied by tissue degradation. We use the term "pseudorecurrence" when the operation was not able to control the disease or aggravated the symptoms without an interval of improvement (Table 2).

The post-surgical pathology is very diverse and we found the most difficult situations in the consequences of a non-successful fundoplication, or after an attempt at fundoplication.

Table 2. Reoperations for recurrence or pseudorecurrence

1. Transabdominal esophagogastrolysis, refundoplication with vagotomy.
2. Dilatation of a stenosis.
3. Distal (2/3) gastric resection with antrectomy and vagotomy and Roux-en-Y anastomosis

To simplify, we shall mention the telescope phenomenon, where the wrap loosens and slides upward, the development of paraesophageal diverticula, anemias, ulcer

Table 3. Operations in recurrence or pseudorecurrence. 1965–1986

78	Reoperations
49	transabdominal procedures
29	transthoracic procedures
37	gastric rections with Roux-en-Y anastomosis.
	Results of a study in 1981
27	operated patients between 1970–1977
21	improved or with minor symptomatology.

complications and the reflux disease that continues in a maltreated esophagus, with or without secondary peptic stenosis and always with a serious perifocal fibrosis.

The surgical attitude (Table 2) should always be a careful one and attempted only when all the other medical treatments have been exhausted (Table 3).

The reoperation should be done by an expert surgeon because of the risks it involves.

Table 2 summarizes our general policy in such cases; Table 3 shows corresponding figures.

What follow-up period is required to assess the results of surgical treatment?

A. Moraldi, C. Iascone, M. Zerilli, P. Chieco Addario M. Accordino, and *S. Stipa* (Rome)

From 1972 to 1977 we have observed 140 patients with symptoms of gastroesophageal reflux (GER); 30 pts, 21.4% were submitted to surgery after failure of medical treatment.

In the period between January 1978 and December 1986, 486 patients with symptoms of GER were studied and reflux was proved to be abnormal in 173 (35.6%). 93 out of these 173 patients were our patients and 36% underwent surgery, while 64% were treated by medical therapy; the remaining 80 patients were referred to us to have a complete esophageal study and 54% underwent medical treatment while 46% were operated upon elsewhere.

Altogether, (Table 1) 100 patients, out of 626 observed with symptoms of GER, were submitted to surgery (15.9 %).

Table 1. Gastroesophageal reflux (1978–86)

Our patients	93	33 (36%) surgical treatment
		60 (64%) medical treatment
Pts. referred to us	80	37 (46%) surgical treatment
		43 (54%) medical treatment

100/626 (15.9%) pts. underwent surgery

In our Department, we have operated on 63 patients, 31 male and 32 female, with a mean age of 49 years.

The Belsey Mark IV antireflux procedure has been our operation of choice, by a left thoracic approach. We lost two patients due to respiratory problems in the immediate post-op. period. Five patients were lost to follow-up and six died during the follow-up period, between 36 and 90 months after the operation (Table 2).

Table 2. Gastroesophageal reflux: Follow-up 63 pts

Operative mortality	2
Pts. lost at follow-up	5
* unrelated mortality	6

* Pts. dead from 36 to 90 mths. after surgery

The follow-up consists of a personal interview and X-ray examination for all patients; endoscopy and 24 hour pH-monitoring of distal esophagus were performed in those complaining of heartburn and/or dysphagia. Results were considered as excellent if patients were completely asymptomatic, good if one symptom (pyrosis, regurgitation or dysphagia) was present occasionally, fair if one or more symptoms were present frequently and failure when there was no improvement after the operation, with persistence of symptoms and esophagitis. The mean follow-up was 92 months, median 95 months, ranging from 3 to 180 months.

Results were excellent (30 pts) or good (12 pts) in 75% of patients and fair in 5 pts (9%). We have had 9 failures, or 16% (Table 3). It is interesting to note that in patients where the Belsey Mark IV was the first operation (44) or the second procedure (13), excellent or good results were almost similar: 77% vs 70%, whereas the rate failure was 13.6% (6/44 pts) vs 23% (3/13 pts) respectively.

Table 3. Gastroesophageal reflux results (56 pts.)

Excellent	30 pts.	(75%)
good	12 pts.	
Fair	5 pts.	(9%)
failure	9 pts.	(16%)

As far as recurrences are concerned we have observed 3 failures within the first year, 2 between the first and second year, one after the fourth, 2 after the sixth and one, nine years post-op (Table 4).

Table 4. Gastroesophageal reflux. Recurrences after surgery

Pts.	3	2	1	2	1
Year	1st	2nd	4th	6th	9th

Scleroderma (3 patients), reoperation (3 patients), stenoses (2 patients), obesity (2 patients) and Barrett's esophagus (1 patient) were considered as factors contributing to recurrence in six patients.

As far as treatment of failures is concerned, we performed one reoperation successfully, and one underwent surgery elsewere unsuccessfully, 3 underwent medical therapy plus dilatation with two good results, and 4 are under medical treatment (3 of them are currently free of symptoms).

Orringer, Skinner and Belsey [5] in their well-known study on long-term results of the Belsey Mark IV operation, report an overall recurrence rate of 11%; the recurrence rate in patients followed from 3 to 10 years was 12%, and 14.7% in patients followed more than 10 years. Most recurrences occurred within 5 years of the initial operation.

Brand et al. [1] studied 25 pts with reflux preoperatively, 8 months after surgery and 13 of them 69 months postoperatively. At the late follow-up, only 2 out of 13 had return of heartburn, but 4 of 9 with no early postoperative reflux had positive tests; 5 out of 8 whose biopsies had become normal were again abnormal, and the mean lower esophageal sphincter pressure decreased significantly from 14.8 to 10.9 mmHg. The authors conclude that it is reasonable to expect 5–6 years of relief from heartburn after antireflux surgery, but late postoperative deterioration is possible, and suggests that further refinement of surgical technique may be necessary.

Henderson and Marryatt [3] agree on the length of the follow-up period, that should be at least five years; their results from total fundoplication gastroplasty performed on 335 patients are excellent in 93% of the cases after an average follow-up of 6.5 years (range 5 to 85 years).

Hill reported 0.8% early recurrence rate with posterior gastropexy, but a later study demonstrated that at 5 years 18% of the patients had clinically significant reflux [4]. DeMeester et al. [2] studied 100 consecutive patients who underwent a Nissen fundoplication for gastro-esophageal reflux; they report three symptomatic recurrences occurring 6 months, 2 years and 7 years after operation. 36 pts underwent 24-hour pH-test within one year from the operation and 9 volunteered for a second postoperative study. All nine patients were normal on their first postoperative 24-hour pH-test: on the second study, performed 3 to 9 years after the operation, four of them remained normal and five had become abnormal.

In conclusion, in our opinion, patients submitted to surgery for gastroesophageal reflux must have a minimum five-year period of follow-up, because although the majority of recurrences will present within 3 years, it is also true that many patients become symptomatic with recurrent reflux and esophagitis ten years and more after the operation.

References

1. Brand DL, Eastwood IR, Martin D, Carter WB, Pope II CE (1979) Esophageal symptoms, manometry and histology before and after antireflux surgery. A long-term follow-up study. Gastroenterology 76: 1393
2. DeMeester TR, Bonavina L, Albertucci M (1986) Nissen fundoplication for gastro-esophageal reflux disease. Evaluation of primary repair in 100 consecutive patients. Ann Surg 204: 9
3. Henderson RD, Marryatt GV (1985) Total fundoplication gastroplasty (Nissen gastroplasty): five-year review. Ann Thorac Surg 39: 74
4. Hill LD (1977) Progress in the surgical management of hiatus hernia. World J Surg 1: 425
5. Orringer MB, Skinner DB, Belsey RHR (1972) Long-term results of the Mark IV operation for hiatal hernia and analyses of the recurrences and their treatment. J Thorac Cardiovasc Surg 63: 25

Should the reported failure of a method be linked to its popularity?

R. Belsey (Chicago)

Failure can be defined in the context of the surgical management of peptic esophagitis as the need for further surgery to control symptoms or complications unresponsive to medical treatment, and is the criterion adopted here.

The incidence of failure can be stated as a percentage of the total number of procedures performed, or as the number of failures referred back, or to other centres, for correction. The increasing incidence in the second category suggests that the published evidence on relative percentage failure is often misleading. The definition of success is a subjective assessment restrained by no generally accepted criteria. The significant late results are directly related to the duration of the postoperative follow-up, if any. No follow-up; no failures!

The popularity of any technique is influenced by various factors:

1. Technical ease. In the case of antireflux surgery the abdominal approach will be preferred.
2. Propaganda. The more a technique is discussed, the greater the incentive to give it a trial.
3. Low incidence of early postoperative morbidity and mortality. Most malpractice suits are motivated by early complications rather than late failures.
4. Published "success" rates; frequently at variance from the incidence of failures referred back for surgical correction, but nevertheless powerful advertisements for any technique and its advocate.
5. Too few centres pursue an adequate long term follow-up program. Failures may gravitate to other centres and are "lost" to the surgeon responsible for the initial treatment.
6. No universally recognized indications for surgical intervention. Popularity may be influenced by considerations that are not strictly medical. Frivolous surgery distorts genuine popularity and increases the incidence of failures by not relating to the cause of the patients symptoms.

The solution lies in greater reticence in premature publication, more concern with the objective assessment of late results, and peer review. In centres where a second opinion is deemed mandatory before any surgical intervention, the number of interventions has fallen dramatically. And presumably the number of subsequent failures.

So, the answer to the opening question appears to be a qualified "yes". The qualification stems from the infrequency with which surgical failures are ever published.

Recurrences with different techniques

P. Fuentes, E. Ragni, R. Giudicelli, B. Dupin, A. Barthelemy, and *E. Reboud* (Marseilles)

Assessing the rate of recurrence of gastroesophageal reflux (GER) after surgical treatment as a function of the technique used is difficult for various reasons [6, 9]. Preoperative and postoperative investigative techniques differ widely from one group to another. Variants of the same technique are often designated by the same name. The definition of recurrence is not standardized. Most studies are retrospective and the longest follow-up is 3 years.

The present study was undertaken in an effort to critically analyze data reported in the largest series.

The Nissen procedure [1, 7, 16] is a very widely used antireflux technique (Table 1).

It effectively prevents GER no matter what methods are used to evaluate results (clinical examination, X-ray imaging, manometry, or 24h pH monitoring). Moreover long term results are very stable.

The Hill procedure [1, 2, 14] (Table 2) brings good results from a clinical standpoint. However a prospective study using 24h pH monitoring (DeMeester) showed the recurrence rate to be 34% at one year.

Table 1. Recurrence after a Nissen procedure

	Patients	Investigative Technique	Rate of Recurrence	Follow-up
Ellis (1985)	86	Clinical Manometry	10%	
Rossetti (1973)	1700	Clinical X-ray	3–4%	3 years
DeMeester (1974)	15	24h pH monitoring	0%	2 years

Table 2. Recurrence after a Hill procedure

	Patients	Investigative Technique	Rate of Recurrence	Follow-up
Hill (1967)	149	Clinical	3%	
Hemreck (1980)	53	Clinical Manometry	15%	3 years
DeMeester (1974)	15	24h pH monitoring	34%	1 year

Table 3. Recurrence after a Belsey procedure

	Patients	Investigative Technique	Rate of Recurrence	Follow-up
Belsey-Skinner Orringer (1972)	632	Clinical	7%	5 years
DeMeester (1974)	15	24h pH monitoring	70%	2 years

In a retrospective study involving a very large series of Belsey procedures [1, 3] (Table 3), the recurrence rate was found to be 15% with a follow-up of 10 years. In his prospective study using 24h pH monitoring before and after Belsey surgery, DeMeester reported that the recurrence rate at 2 years was 70%.

After a Toupet procedure [4, 5, 15, 17] (Table 4), clinical and X-ray findings are generally good. Only two prospective studies have been published and both have short follow-ups. In one of these reports, the author. Galmiche stated that the rate of recurrence at 18 months was 25%. However, in this study, the duration of pH monitoring was 3 hours and only 10 patients were thoroughly investigated. In the second study made in our department, all patients were investigated by means of a personal interview, X-ray imaging, manometry, 24h pH monitoring, and esophageal scintigraphy. These examinations were carried out postoperatively at 3, 9, and 12 months and then yearly. The follow-up is now 18 months and the recurrence rate is 9%.

Table 4. Recurrence after a Toupet procedure

	Patients	Investigative Technique	Rate of Recurrence	Follow-up
Boutelier (1982)	110	Clinical Manometry	0%	
Guarner (1980)	135	Clinical X-ray	5%	5 years
Galmiche (1983)	25	3h pH monitoring	25%	20 months
Reboud (1986)	50	24h pH	9%	18 months

With regard to placement of Angelchik prosthesis [10, 11, 13] (Table 5), though good clinical results have been reported by its inventor, other studies, based on sounder investigative techniques and in particular on pH monitoring, show a recurrence rate of 20 to 25 % at one year.

Table 5. Recurrence after placement of an Angelchik prosthesis

	Patients	Investigative Technique	Rate of Recurrence	Follow-up
Angelchik (1977)	122	Clinical	8%	7 years
Durrans (1985)	41	Clinical pH monitoring X-ray	25%	2 years
Wale (1985)	50	pH monitoring	20%	1 year

Finally, a recent development in the field of antireflux surgery is a technique combining the lengthening of the esophagus by means of a plasty fashioned from the lesser curvature of the stomach (Collis) with fundoplication (Table 6). Orringer [8, 12] has published two prospective studies regarding this type of procedure. Though pH monitoring lasted only 3 hours, it is noteworthy that, in association with Collis gastroplasty, the Nissen procedure appears to give much better results than does the Besley procedure.

Table 6. Recurrence after gastroplasty – fundoplication

	Patients	Investigative Technique	Rate of Recurrence	Follow-up
Collis-Belsey (Orringer) (1977)	83	pH monitoring Manometry	34%	3 years
Collis-Nissen (Orringer) (1985)	161	pH monitoring Manometry	7%	2 years

Study of the different series brings out the determinant role of certain factors in recurrence:

- All authors stress the importance of obesity and chronic bronchopulmonary disease in precipitating relapse.
- It is obvious that the rate of recurrence after antireflux surgery is higher for patients with peptic stenosis and/or a previous history of surgery responsible for periesophagitis and/or hyperacid reflux.

On the basis of these observations, it is possible to class patients according to the number of risk factors that they present. For low risk patients, fundoplication procedures (Nissen or Toupet) can bring excellent results. For high risk patients the combined Collis gastroplasty/Nissen fundoplication procedure may be required.

Thus it appears that Nissen procedure is the most effective antireflux procedure in terms of immediate and long term results. It is important to note that for the same surgical technique, the more precise the preoperative and postoperative investigations are, the higher the recurrence rate is. Simply interviewing the patient is not a satisfactory method of evaluation since fully one third of all recurrences detected by pH monitoring are asymptomatic. Manometric study [9] should not be limited to the lower esophageal sphincter but rather extended to the whole thoracic esophagus. Some symptoms that persist in spite of a technically successful antireflux procedure are caused by esophageal motility disorders existing prior to surgery. pH monitoring must be carried out for 24 hours both preoperatively and postoperatively; this method is the only means to assess acid and alkaline reflux physiologically. Finally five-year prospective studies should be started with yearly investigations.

References

1. DeMeester TR, Lawrence LTC, Johnson F, Col. MC, Alfred H, Kent MC (1974) Evaluation of current operations for the prevention of gastro esophageal reflux. Ann Surg 180: (511–525)
2. Hermreck A, Coates NR (1980) Results of the Hill antireflux operation. Am J Surg 140: 764–767
3. Orringer MB, Skinner DB, Belsey RHR, (1972) Long term results of the mark IV operation for hiatal hernia and analyses of recurrences and their treatment. J Thoracic-Cardiovasc Surg 63: 1
4. Guarner V, Nelson Martinez, JF Gavino C (1980) Ten year evaluation of posterior fundoplasty in the treatment of gastro esophageal reflux. Am J Surg 139: 200–204
5. Galmiche JP, Teniere P, Ducrotte P, Denis P, Colin R, Testart J (1983) Traitement du reflux gastro-œsophagien acide par hémi-fundoplicature postérieure. Résultats cliniques et pH métriques. Gastroentérol Clin Biol 7: 385–391
6. Little G, Fergusson MK, Skinner DB (1986) Reoperations for failed antireflux operations. J Thorac Cardiovasc Surg 91: 4, 511–517
7. Ellis FH – Nissen Fundoplication (1985) A clinical and mannometric assessment of results. Esophageal disorders. DeMeester TR –Skinner DB – Raven Press (p. 197–201)
8. Orringer MB (1985) The Combined Collis-Nissen fundoplication for Gastroesophageal reflux. Esophageal Disorders. DeMeester TR, Skinner DB Raven Press (p. 203)
9. Skinner DB, Little G, DeMeester TR, Belsey RH (1985) Assessment of failed antireflux repairs. Esophageal Disorders. DeMeester TR, Skinner DB, Raven Press (p. 303–313)
10. Wale RJ, Royston LMS, Benet JR, Buckton GK (1985) Prospective Study of the Angelchik anti-reflux prothesis. Br J Surg 72: 520–524
11. Durrans, Armstrong CP, Taylor TV (1985) The Angelchik anti-reflux Prothesis – Some Reservations. Br J Surg 72: 525–527
12. Orringer MB, Sloan H (1977) Complications and failings of the combined Collis-Belsey operation. J Thorac Cardiovasc Surg 74: 5
13. Angelchik JP, Cohen R (1979) A new surgical procedure for the treatent of gastroesophageal reflux and hiatal hernia. Surg Gynecol Obstet 148: 246–248
14. Hill LD (1967) An effective operation for hiatal hernia: an eight year appraisal. Ann Surg 166: 681–692
15. Boutelier Ph, Jonsell G (1982) An alternative fundoplication maneuver for gastro esophageal reflux. Am J Surg 143: 260
16. Rossetti M (1973) Fundoplication for Treatment of Hiatal Hernia. Progress in Surgery 12
17. Fuentes P, Dupin B, Giudicelli R, Reboud E (1986) Posterior fundoplication for gastro esophageal reflux. International Esophageal Week – Munich

F. G. Pearson (Toronto)

Recurrence or failure has been analyzed in 424 patients with complex reflux problems managed by gastroplasty and partial fundoplication since 1964. Results are analyzed in three categories 54 patients who had gastroplasty and fundoplication for the management of massive hiatal hernia (intra-thoracic stomach) are excluded from detailed analysis. Over all complications are shown in Table 1.

Table 1

Complications	424 Patients
Atelectasis, Pneumonia	18
Wound infection	12
Esophageal fistula	6
Prolonged incisional pain	17
Other	30

"Uncomplicated" Short Esophagus (215 patients)

Stricture and esophagitis without previous repair, no primary motor disorder: There were 17 unsatisfactory results in this group (8%). Eleven results were categorized as fair because of dysphagia in eight cases, reflux in one and both reflux and dysphagia in one. All of the six poor results were due to dysphagia, although some reflux symptoms may have been present: three of the six patients with poor results were re-operated because of persistent ulcerative esophagitis and re-stenosis, and in each case the partial fundoplication was taken down and then reconstructed using a 360 degree Nissen-type wrap.

Two additional patients in this group (both with good reflux control) required re-operation for complications of subsequent duodenal ulcer: One required an antrectomy for pyloric stenosis, and the other an emergency omental patch for a perforated duodenal ulcer.

Re-operation for failed anti-reflux repair (118 patients)

This group of patients had undergone one or more prior, unsuccessful anti-reflux operations. There were 149 prior operations in 118 cases. Twenty-two patients had had two or more previous procedures. Thirty-eight of these 118 patients had a persistent or recurrent peptic stricture. The types of prior repair were: transabdominal Nissen : 65, transthoracic Belsey Mark IV : 31, transabdominal Hill : 9, transthoracic Thal procedure : 3, gastroplasty and fundoplication : 1, and unidentifiable repair : 9.

Unsatisfactory results occurred in 25 of these patients on longterm follow-up (20%). In 15 patients, the result was classified as fair because of both symptomatic reflux and dysphagia in 10 cases, and dysphagia alone in 5. A poor result observed in 10 patients (8%) was due to reflux and dysphagia in six cases, dysphagia alone in three, and reflux alone in one. Three of the 10 patients with poor results were re-operated on and all were managed by revision with complete fundoplication.

Associated Primary Motor Disorder

There were 37 patients with an underlying primary motor disorder: Scleroderma -16, achalasia -14, and diffuse spasm -7. All 37 patients in this group had gross endoscopic ulcerative peptic esophagitis, and there was some degree of peptic stricture in 25 of the 37 cases.

In patients with achalasia, reflux esophagitis is only seen as a complication which follows esophagomyotomy. All 14 patients with achalasia had had a prior myotomy, and six of the 14 had an additional anti-reflux operation in an attempt to control the subsequent reflux.
Results are summarized in Table 2.

Table 2

Primary motor disorders:		Results		
	No. cases	good	fair	poor
Scleroderma	16	9 (57%)	4	3
Achalasia	14	6 (43%)	4	4
Diffuse spasm	7	5 (71%)	1	1

Good results were sustained in only 54% of these patients. The worst results were observed in cases of achalasia, and three of these patients developed unmanageable progressive dysphagia due to continued reflux, – and were submitted to thoracic esophagectomy and cervical esophagogastrostomy.

Mortality of reoperations

J. W. Maher (Iowa City)

The answer to this question varies from author to author. Hill, in 1971 reported 63 patients with recurrent hiatal hernia managed secondarily by posterior gastropexy; mortality was 3.3% [1]. Ellis and Crozier recently documented a series of 29 patients undergoing reoperation utilizing fundoplication with 75% satisfactory result and no mortality [2]. Polk has utilized jejunal interposition with excellent success and a four per cent mortality [3]; however, other authors have reported up to a 15% mortality with the same approach [4, 5].

Maher et al. recently documented a series of nearly 60 reoperations of varying types, predominantly transthoracic fundoplications and combined fundic patch-fundoplications with a four per cent mortality and 80% good results on long-term followup [6]. In contrast, Zucker et al. have detailed 17 patients who suffered an 18% mortality and a disturbing 29% incidence of esophageal leaks [7].

These procedures can be extraordinarily difficult to perform. The author prefers a transthoracic approach in most candidates if there is no overriding reason to favor a transabdominal repair. The transthoracic approach allows the surgeon to sidestep the "footprints" of the previous operator. Avoiding the tedious and sometimes hazardous dissection of the stomach from the left upper quadrant minimizes iatrogenic holes in the stomach and permits a more precise anatomic reconstruction. Additionally, should there be any acquired shortening, the esophagus may be mobilized to the aortic arch, which may allow the fundoplication to be replaced into the abdomen. If the wrap cannot be reduced, it may be left in the chest without any detrimental effects [8, 9].

The author now chooses the transabdominal approach for reconstruction only in patients where abdominal pathology dictates this route, or when the surgeon feels that posterior gastropexy is the procedure of choice.

Reoperations for reflux following unsuccessful antireflux procedures constitute an effective means of controlling recurrent esophagitis and compare similarly with primary operations in both mortality and success rate.

References

1. Hill LD (1971) Management of recurrent hiatal hernia. Arch Surg 102: 296–302
2. Ellis FH, Crozier R (1985) The Nissen fundoplication: a clinical and manometric assessment of results, in *Esophageal Disorders: pathophysiology and management.* DeMeester TR, Skinner DB (Ed) Raven Press, New York
3. Polk HC (1980) Jejunal interposition for reflux esophagitis and esophageal stricture unresponsive to valvuloplasty. World J Surg 4: 731–736
4. Ferrer JM, Bruck HM (1967) Jejunal and colonic interposition for non-malignant disease of the esophagus. Ann Surg 169: 533–543
5. Merendino KA, Dillard DH (1955) The concept of sphincter substitution by an interposed jejunal segment for anatomic and physiologic abnormalities at the esophagogastric junction. With special reference to reflux esophagitis and cardiospasm and esophageal varices. Ann Surg 142: 486–509
6. Maher JW, Hocking MP, Woodward ER (1985) Reoperations for esophagitis following a failed antireflux procedure. Ann Surg 201: 723–727
7. Zucker K, Peskin GW, Saik RP (1982) Recurrent hiatal hernia repair. Arch Surg 117: 413–414
8. Jones EL, Booth DJ, Cameron JL et al (1971) Functional evaluation of esophageal reconstructions. Ann Thorac Surg 12: 331–346
9. Maher JW, Hocking MP, Woodward ER (1984) Supradiaphragmatic fundoplication: long term follow-up and analysis of complications. Am J Surg 147: 181–186

H. F. Weiser (Munich)

In contrast to primary fundoplication, it is not the anti-reflux operation that gives rise to problems in re-fundoplication, but undoing the situation created by the previous operation, which is the most difficult step and at the same time leads to complications. According to the literature mortality is up to 18% [1, 2, 3].

In our own hospital re- or corrective operations have increased and transabdominal re-fundoplication has become the technique of choice, irrespective of the type of primary operation. The results of this technique will be compared with a collective of primary fundoplications performed during the same period of time.

From 1.7.82 till 31.3.87 (Fig. 1), 52 patients (25 male, 27 female), mean age 51.7 ± 15.8 years were operated at the Department of Surgery, Technical University Munich. In all cases the indication for anti-reflux surgery was severe reflux disease, resistant to conservative treatment.

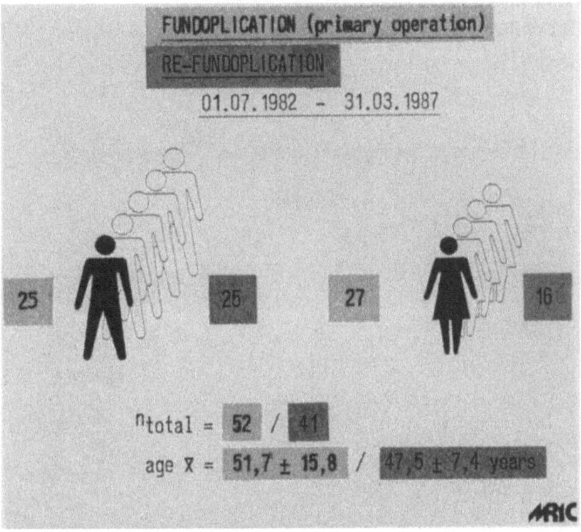

Fig. 1

At the same time 41 patients (25 male, 16 female), mean age 47.5 ± 7.4 years, had a refundoplication: in 21 cases there was recurrent reflux due to an open fundoplication; in 15 cases recurrent reflux was combined with severe therapy-resistent dysphagia due to a telescope phenomenon and 5 patients complained of dysphagia caused by a too narrow fundoplication (Table 1).

Table 1. Indications for Re-Fundoplication

– recurrent reflux opening of the cuff		n=21
– recurrent reflux + dysphagia telescope phenomenon		=15
– dysphagia narrowed cuff		n= 5
	total	=41

Despite the fact that in all cases primary fundoplication was performed transabdominally, two postoperative pulmonary complications occurred. Two patients showed delayed wound healing. One patient had to undergo splenectomy. There were no deaths.

Postoperative complications were markedly increased in refundoplication: in six cases splenectomy had to be performed. 2 patients developed pulmonary complications and there were two cases of delayed wound healing. One patient with postoperative pancreatitis could be treated conservatively. There was one death due to necrosis of the fundus, which leads to a mortality rate of 2.4% (Fig. 2).

Postoperative complaints following re-fundoplication were surprisingly few (Fig. 3). Only one of 33 patients followed up after re-fundoplication showed severe dysphagia which was so strong, that this patient must be classified as Visick grade 3.

In both groups preexistent esophagitis had healed completely on gastroscopic control. The resting pressure at the LES reached normal values following primary as well as secondary fundoplication (13.2 ± 2.7 mmHg). Gastro-esophageal reflux was overcorrected in both groups; in other words preoperative pathological GER was decreased to values clearly below normal physiological values (pH < 7%/measuring period).

POSTOPERATIVE COURSE :	PRIMARY FUNDOPLICATION	RE-FUNDOPLICATION
	n = 52	41
hospitalisation :	13,6 ± 6,8	16,4 ± 14 days
morbidity : pleural exsudate / pneumonia	n = 2	2
disturbed wound healing	n = 2	2
splenectomie	n = 1	6
postop. pancreatitis	n = 0	1
necrosis of fundus	n = 0	1 (+)
mortality :	n = 0	1

ARIC

Fig. 2

FUNCTIONAL RESULTS :		PRIM. FUNDOPLICATION	RE-FUNDOPLICATION
Visick I + II		n = 44	32
Visick III + IV		n = 0	1
Endoscopy	esophagitis	ø	ø
Manometry	LESP mmHg	15	12
24-H-pH-Metry	- empty stomach phase %/h	0	2,7
	- postprandial phase %/h	0	0
	- sleeping phase %/h	0	0

ARIC

Fig. 3

Conclusions

1. Refundoplication showes a markedly increased morbidity and mortality for transthoracic as well as transabdominal approach compared to primary fundoplication. Our mortality rate of 2.4% seems rather satisfactory, but since we are dealing with a benign disease, it is still extremely high.
2. In view of the excellent functional results, refundoplication has a promising prognosis even after unsatisfactory results of the primary operation.
3. Since the underlying pathology is situated almost exclusively intraabdominally, a transabdominal approach should be chosen, that can be extended into the thorax if necessary.

References

1. Maher JW, Hocking MP, Woodward ER (1984) Subdiaphragmative fundoplication: Long-term follow-up and analysis of complication Am J Surg 147: 181–186
2. Siewert JR, Weiser HF (1984) Reinterventionen nach Antirefluxoperationen. Chirurg 55: 373–380
3. Zucker K, Peskin GW, Saik RP (1982) Recurrent hiatal hernia repair. Arch Surg 117: 413–414

Does the persistence of histologic signs suggest that other factors than acidity could occur?

Ch. Fontolliet, D. Gardiol, Ph. Monnier, J. B. Ollyo, and *M. Savary* (Lausanne)

Various histologic features have been described in connection with reflux esophagitis. In particular, these include hyperplasia of the basal layer, elongation of the vascular connective tissue papillae, infiltration of the lamina propria by lymphoplasmocytes [3] or by neutrophil and/or eosinophil granulocytes [8, 9, 12] and vascular changes [1, 4].

There is no unanimity about any of these criteria, since some authors have found a similar incidence of these changes in healthy subjects [5, 8] or have shown that their presence largely depends on the type and site of samples and the method used to obtain them [10, 11].

The cellular and vascular inflammatory features described above are nearly always associated with losses of substance which do not normally transgress the muscularis mucosae [2].

In our own experience [6, 7] reflux esophagitis in its early stages constitutes a localized disorder; biopsies made at the same level as the peptic erosion, in a mucous membrane that is macroscopically healthy, reveal a perfectly normal epithelium and lamina propria.

Apart from peptic erosion or ulceration, we therefore do not consider that histologic features specific to reflux exist. In consequence, we are unable to supply an answer to the question.

References

1. Geboes K, Desmet V, Vantrappen G, Mebis J (1980) Vascular changes in the esophageal mucosa. An early histologic sign of esophagitis. Gastrointest Endosc 26:29–32
2. Hendrix TR, Varoley JH (1976) Consequences of gastroesophageal reflux. Clin Gastroenterol 5:156–174
3. Ismail-Beigi F, Horton PF, Pope CE (1970) Histological consequences of gastroesophageal reflux in man. Gastroenterology 58:163–174
4. Kobayashi S, Kasugai T (1974) Endoscopic and biopsy criteria for the diagnosis of esophagitis with a fibreoptic esophagoscope. Dig Dis 19:345–352
5. Meier RF, Sieber R, Bauerfeind P, Blum AL (1986) Endoscopy as final arbiter in controlled clinical trials in peptic disorders. Clin Gastroenterol 15:377–391
6. Monnier P, Savary M (1984) Contribution of endoscopy to gastroesophageal reflux disease. Scand J gastroenterol 19: Suppl 106:28–45
7. Savary M, Monnier P (1980) Le reflux gastro-oesophagien: l'apport de l'endoscopie dans l'indication opératoire et les contrôles postopératoires. Helv Chir Acta 47:693–706
8. Seefeld U, Krejs GI, Siebenmann RE, Blum AM (1977) Esophageal histology in gastroesophageal reflux. Morphometrics findings in succion biopsies. Am J Dig Dis 22:956–964
9. Sonnenberg A, Lepsien G, Muller-Lissner SA, Koelz HR, Siewert JR, Blum AL (1982) When is esophagitis healed? Esophageal endoscopy, histology and function before and after cimetidine treatment. Dig Dis Sci 27:297–302
10. Tumala V, Barwick KW, Sontag SJ, Vlahcevic RB, McCallum RW (1987) The significance of intraepithelial eosinophils in the histologic diagnosis of gastroesophageal reflux. Am J Clin Pathol 87:43–48
11. Weinstein WM, Bogoch ER, Bowes KL (1975) The normal human esophageal mucosa: a histological reappraisal. Gastroenterology 68:40–44
12. Winter HS, Madara JL, Stafford RJ (1982) Intraepithelial eosinophilis: a new diagnostic criterion for reflux esophagitis. Gastroenterology 83:818–823

What is the incidence of gastric epithelium lying below a treated peptic stenosis?

J. B. Ollyo, D. Gardiol, M. Savary, J. Wellinger, Ph. Monnier, J. J. Gonvers, and *Ch. Fontolliet* (Lausanne)

The esophageal columnar epithelium associated with peptic stricture may be circumferential or more rarely in the form of "tongues" [7, 8]. The majority of strictures associated with circumferential columnar epithelium are located at the top of this epithelium, 85% [101/119] in our series. The rare benign strictures located within the columnar epithelium that we saw, 15% [18/119], were either ulcerations that were too severe to succeed the metaplastic healing or ulcers developing on

Table 1. Prevalence of endobrachyesophagus (CLE) in patients with esophageal peptic stenosis (EPS)

		Patients with EPS	EPS + CLE
Baldi F. et al	(1)	224	26 (10.6%)
Borrie J. et al	(2)	45	45 (100%)
Davidson J. S.	(3)	202	46 (22.7%)
Mercer et al	(5)	160	37 (23.1%)
Savary M. et al	(*)	345	149 (43.2%)
Siewert R. et al	(9)	118	89 (75.4%)
Total		1114	392 (35.2%)

* Non-published data. (Chuv, Lausanne, Suisse: 01. 01. 1963–31. 12. 1986)

residual epidermoid epithelium [4, 8]. The "tongue" forms of columnar epithelium are rarer, 30 cases in our series, and are always located proximally to the stricture.

It is difficult to estimate the true prevalence of Barrett's esophagus in patients with a peptic stenosis since, in the majority of retrospective series it ranges from 10.6% to 100% (Table 1). This discrepancy may be explained by differences in patient selection in the various medical centers. Also biopsies were not always routinely performed proximal and distal to the stricture at the initial endoscopy. Without routine biopsies even an experienced endoscopist may often miss Barrett's epithelium [6].

For Spechler et al. [10] the incidence of columnar epithelium in patients with peptic stenosis treated by dilatations is 44%, whereas in our series the majority of patients are treated by antireflux surgery and the incidence is 17.5%. This difference may for a large part be explained by the difference in treatments (Table 2). A functioning antireflux operation heals reflux esophagitis and prevents appearance or progression of columnar epithelium. Dilatations may increase the gastroesophageal reflux and favour progression of Barrett's epithelium.

In conclusion, the exact prevalence and incidence of columnar epithelium in patients with peptic stricture is not known. If the treatment does not correct the gastroesophageal reflux (dilatations alone or antireflux operation not functioning) the incidence of columnar epithelium may be very high [10].

Table 2. Incidence of endobrachyesophagus in patients with peptic stenosis

	Nb of patients	mean follow-up	Type of treatment	Incidence of CLE
Spechler S. J. et al (10)	25	50.5 months	Bougienage 20/25	11/25 (44%)
Savary M. et al (*)	63	61 months	Nissen (n=41) Bougienage (n=22)	4/41 (9.7%) 7/22 (31.8%)

* Non-published data (Chuv, Lausanne, Suisse: 01. 01. 1963–31. 12. 1986)

References

1. Baldi F, Ferrarini F, Morselli Labate AM, Barbara L (1985) Prevalence of esophagitis in patients undergoing routine upper endoscopy: a multicenter survey in Italy. Esophageal Disorders. Pathophysiology and Therapy. Edited by DeMeester TR, Skinner DB. Raven Press, New York 213–219
2. Borrie J, Goldwater L (1976) Columnar cell-lined esophagus: Assessment of etiology and treatment. J Thorac Cardiovasc Surg 71: 825–834
3. Davidson JS (1976) High peptic stricture of the oesophagus. Thorax 31: 1–14
4. Lackey Ch, Rankin RA, Welsh JD (1984) Stricture location in Barrett's esophagus. Gastrointest Endosc 30: 331–333
5. Mercer CD, Hill LD (1986) Surgical management of peptic esophageal stricture. J Thorac Cardiovasc Surg 91: 371–378
6. Sarr MG, Hamilton SR, Marrone GC, Cameron JL (1985) Barrett's esophagus: Its prevalence and association with adenocarcinoma in patients with symptoms of gastroesophageal reflux. Am J Surg 149: 187–193
7. Savary M, Miller G (1977) L'œsophage. Manuel et atlas d'endoscopie. Gassmann SA, édit, Soleure
8. Savary M, Monnier P (1985) Diagnosis, pathophysiology, and adenocarcinogenesis of Barrett's esophagus. Esophageal disorders: pathophysiology and therapy. Edited by: DeMeester TR, Skinner DB. Raven Press, New York 101–108
9. Siewert R, Lepsien G, Schattenmann G, Weiser HF (1980) Chirurgie peptischer Oesophagusstenosen. Langenbecks Archiv Chir 352–600
10. Spechler SJ, Sperber H, Doos WG, Schimmel EM (1983) The prevalence of Barrett's esophagus in patients with chronic peptic esophageal strictures. Dig Dis Sci 769–774

What value should be attributed to the persistence of radiological signs of reflux or persistent acid pH without clinical signs following anti-reflux surgery?

P. Kohek, P. Rehak, F. M. Jüttner, and *G. Friehs* (Graz)

The variety of diagnostic procedures detecting gastroesophageal reflux (GER) has given us a deeper insight into the gastroesophageal junction. The more we know about the pathogenesis of GER the less operative procedures are in use. Conservative treatment based on endoscopic-, manometric- and pH-monitoring findings has established as the preferred therapeutic approach in nearly 90% of the cases. Nowadays less than 10% of GER patients underwent surgical anti-reflux treatment, according to the literature.

For the documentation of the therapeutic efficacy of antireflux surgery the same criteria should be used as in the pretherapeutic evaluation. Clinical symptoms (acc. to DeMeester's HRD score) manometry, pH monitoring and endoscopy with biopsy can give an objective assessment about anti-reflux surgery achievment. According to Leisner et al. (1978) esophageal radiography shows low sensitivity, and does not allow any essential statements about the reflux (clearance, LES pressure, day and night reflux episodes).

Continuous 24 hr pH monitoring of the esophagus has brought an enormous advantage into the diagnosis and therapeutic approach to GER. Different investigators classify reflux by different standards, 24 hr long term pH monitoring helps us to differ between physiological and pathological reflux. Registration of the acid clearing time and documentation of day and night reflux episodes with or without clinical symptoms are also possible.

Evaluation Schedule

To document and evaluate the efficacy of antireflux surgery, we use the following scheme 12 weeks after the operation: clinical symptoms are classified by the HRD score of DeMeester; 24 hr pH monitoring allows essential statements about esophageal clearance and reflux episodes under almost physiological conditions. The LES resting pressure and the LES motility is documented by esophageal manometry; endoscopy and biopsy demonstrate any structural damage or inflammation of the esophagus. Not one of the diagnostic procedures mentioned has enough diagnostic value to lead to any therapeutic consequences.

If radiological signs of reflux are shown by X rays, or persistent pH is pointed out by pH monitoring without any clinical symptoms, manometry and endoscopy are indicated to establish adequate therapy; if reflux is pointed out only by radiography in the absence of clinical symptoms, we would suggest no therapy due to the lack of value of this diagnostic procedure.

Persistent acid pH without clinical symptoms is however a matter of defining the standards suggesting pathology. We have compared the standards of Aggestrup and DeMeester with histologically verified reflux esophagitis: the DeMeester standards showed high specificity. On the other hand high sensitivity was pointed out in Aggestrup's published parameters (Fig. 1).

For selection of appropriate therapeutic procedures, esophageal clearance, LES pressure and/or endoscopic findings have to be considered.

Results

In our study, we have investigated 134 patients suffering from GER from 1984–1986: In only 9 patients (7%) conservative treatment did not improve GER. These patients underwent antireflux surgery according to Nissen Rossetti's fundoplication. In the 12 weeks postoperative follow-up, none of them was suffering from typical GER symptoms, one patient showed dysphagia, which was treated by bougienage. Esophagitis was reported after biopsy in 3 cases. The average resting LES pressure was 11.2 mm Hg. The Clearance Index (C.I.)*, which considers the reflux time between pH5 and pH4 and pays attention to the slope of the pH after an episode, was more than 7 minutes in two cases we consider 7 minutes to be the borderline between sufficient and insufficient clearance.

---

* C.I. = pH5–pH4 in minutes divided by the number of reflux episodes

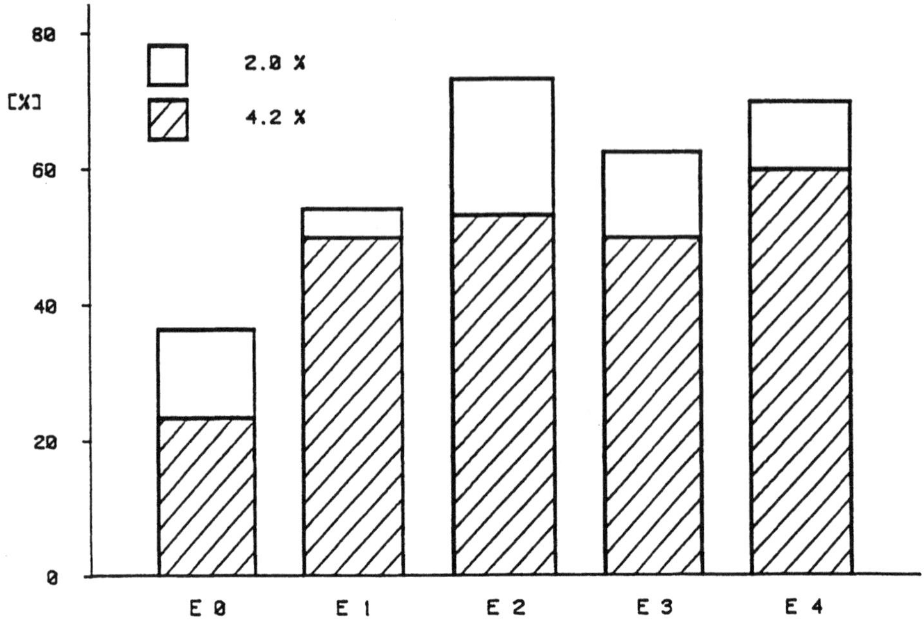

Fig. 1. Long-term pH-monitoring (pH < 4) > Limit vs. Esophagitis-SM-stage

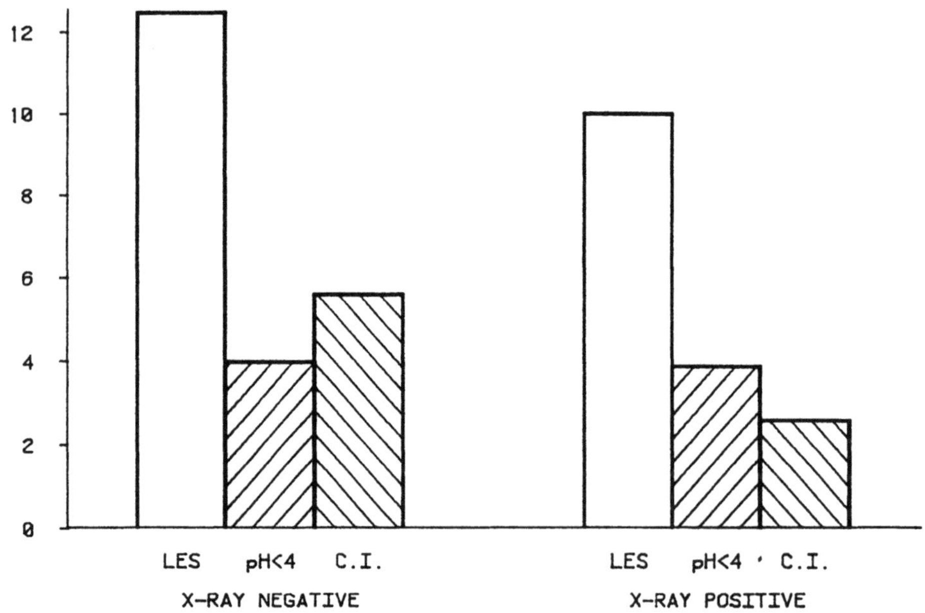

Fig. 2. Reflux diagnosis. Fundoplication (n=9 patients=7%)

Radiologic signs of GER were documented in 5 cases (2 with esophagitis, 3 without esophagitis) (Fig. 2).

In cases with esophagitis, H2 antagonists combined with metoclopramide according to LES pressure and C.I. were given to support the antireflux surgery for another 12 weeks; in the other cases without esophagitis, we felt fundoplication should be sufficient without any supplementary conservative therapeutic procedure.

K. Jeyasingham (Bristol)

The isolated finding of radiologic or acid reflux on pH testing without symptoms of reflux is often indicative of the small degree of such reflux and the efficacy of the esophageal clearance.

These are not infrequent in patients who have undergone antireflux surgery, but have recently developed an increase in the adipose tissue in the abdomen. A further factor in the finding of radiologic reflux is the enthusiasm with which the radiologist employs various manoeuvres to induce reflux; some of these manoeuvres are entirely unphysiological, e.g. the water siphon test, or the Mueller manoeuvre, and even the Trendelenburg position with pressure to the abdomen. Not many middle aged post repair patients go through these manoeuvres in their daily existence, and the significance attached to such findings are often limited.

The appearance of a small pouch of stomach behind the esophagus with contrast regurgitating into this pouch is an occasional finding after a 270° partial fundoplication. This is totally asymptomatic, and in itself is not a significant cause for concern.

If, however prolonged pH testing with an indwelling probe shows a high score for the various pH levels, then one has to pay attention to the result, and ensure by endoscopy that there is no reflux esophagitis and by histological examination of the lower esophageal mucosa to exclude inflammation. These patients will require close follow-up with, if necessary, conservative measures to minimize the reflux.

Do radioactive methods enable a better approach to reflux by evaluating the esophageal clearance?

C. G. Bremner (Johannesburg)

In 1976 Fisher et al. [1] applied scintiscanning techniques to detect and quantitate gastroesophageal reflux. A dose of ^{99m} Tc-sulphur colloid was instilled into the stomach either via a nasogastric tube or by swallowing and a scintiscan detected reflux. Menin et al. [2] used scintiscanning to assess the severity of reflux and correlated the results with endoscopic esophagitis.

Modification of the technique allowed transit to be quantitated [3, 4]. The method of assessing esophageal transit (or clearance) introduced an alternative method to the previous method of using a bolus of 15ml of 0.1N HCl introduced via a catheter, and detecting pH changes [5].

Several investigators have used the radioactive methods to compare conventional methods of detecting reflux, esophageal transit and motility disorders. We need to evaluate the evidence supporting the accuracy of radionuclide tests to detect these abnormalities.

Is scintigraphy an accurate method of assessing gastroesophageal reflux

It is generally accepted that radiology is an inaccurate method of assessing GE reflux. Scintiscanning detects and quantitates reflux in much the same way as radiology detects the passage of barium into the esophagus, but it has the advantage of quantifying the results. It is a noninvasive tubeless test, and the many reports attest to its value in detecting reflux, especially in children.

Kaul et al. [6] detected reflux in 86% of 101 symptomatic patients, whereas endoscopy and biopsy were only positive in 68% and 58% respectively. Fisher et al. [1] also reported on a 90% positive result as compared to 40% on endoscopy and 46.7 on biopsy. Fung et al. [7] found GE scintigraphy of little value in the diagnosis of GE reflux.

From the number of reports, the test is used widely. Most tests compare results with conventional methods of detecting reflux and have not used ambulatory pH recording to substantiate the accuracy of the method.

In 1983 the author [8] used radioactive scintiscanning and transit tests to quantitate and measure transit time in 37 patients with symptoms of GER. The results were compared with manometric evaluation of esophageal function, pH pull-through tests, and the SART. A positive reflux index was found in 11 patients, and a prolonged transit time (>15 secs, Fig. 1) in 11 patients. There was no correlation between symptoms, LESP, hypomotility, pH reflux tests, and either the reflux index or RT time (table).

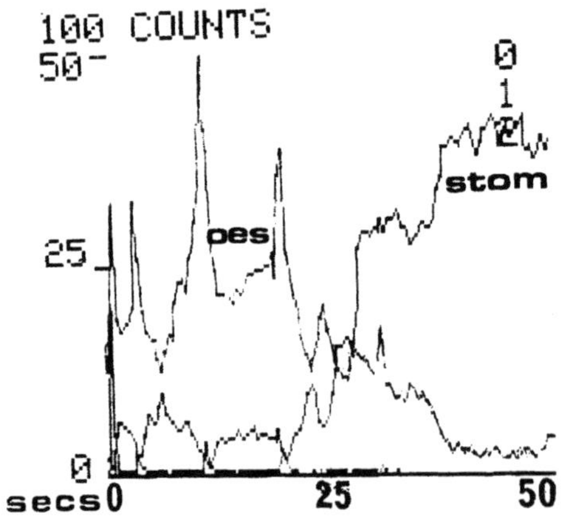

Fig. 1. Study on a patient who has delayed transit

Transit time and motility disorders

Esophageal transit measurement has been reported to be a useful test for patients suspected of having an esophageal motility disorder. The sensitivity of RT in detecting dysmotility has been shown in one study to be 75% as compared to 83% sensitivity when manometry was used [9].

The concordance between the two tests was 71%, and there was a disparity of 29% in which RT detected 18 patients with abnormalities (normal motility) and motility detected 26 abnormalities (normal RT). Motility disorders associated with gastroesophageal reflux was diagnosed in 27 of 150 patients with symptoms.

The major areas of disagreement between the 2 test were in nutcracker esophagus, the hypertensive lower esophageal sphincter and diffuse esophageal spasm [10]. Radionuclide transit is unable to detect high pressure areas. Richter et al. [10] using RT and manometry testing, found that RT time was independant of the amplitude and duration of peristalsis of the lower esophageal sphincter pressure. Mughal et al. [11] found that RT had a sensitivity of only 44% when compared to 99% sensitivity of esophageal motility.

Transit time and reflux

Using 3 areas of interest [3] the transit time of a bolus of radioisotope can be measured from the pharynx to the stomach. A delay in transit implies either a dysmotility or the compounded result of reflux and transit. If the acid clearing of the esophagus is complete, and is followed by subsequent peaks in the radioisotope measurement in the esophagus, reflux is diagnosed. These peaks coincide with a decrease in gastric radioactivity [4].

How accurate is this test, and will it replace more direct methods of measuring reflux such as ambulatory pH recording?

Styles et al. [12] found that the sensitivity of reflux scintigraphy to detect GE reflux as determined by esophageal histology was 70%, and its specificity 87%. There was no relationship between the magnitude of the symptoms and the volume of the reflux. Seibert et al. [13] performed simultaneous pH monitoring and gastroesophageal scintigraphy in 49 infants and children, forty-seven of these patients being later monitored by a 24hr pH probe. The sensitivity of the gastroesophageal scintigraphy when compared to the 24hr probe as a standard, was 79%, and its specificity was 93%.

As stated above (Table), the results of our comparative study, made in 37 symptomatic patients, of radionuclide transit in relation to symptoms, manometric evaluation, pH pull-through and SART did nod show correlation between symptoms, LES pressure, pH reflux tests and transit time.

Conclusion

Gastrointestinal scintigraphy is a safe noninvasive method of assessing esophageal motility disorders, and the combination of scintigraphy and motility has given a high

Table 1

	No	Reflux index	Transit time > 15 secs	ph test + ive
Heartburn (HB)	23	9	6	14
No heartburn	14	5	2	7
HB + dysphagia	11	4	1	7
Poor LESP	32	8	10	17
Hypomotile body	18	6	7	13
Reflux (Tuttle) + ive	7	5	2	
Reflux (provocative) + ive	15	3	7	
Reflux (radiological) + ive	10	4	2	7

accuracy rate in some studies. Scintigraphy is also an accurate way in which to measure transit time, but it is not as sensitive a method of detecting reflux as is the 24hr pH probe. Scintigraphy does enable a better approach to reflux because it will alert the clinician and surgeon to motility abnormalities which may modify treatment. As yet however, it does not replace either manometry or 24hr pH testing.

References

1. Fisher RS, Malmud LS, Roberts GS, Lobis IF (1976) Gastroesophageal (GE) Scintiscanning to detect and quantitate GE reflux. Gastroenterology 70(3): 301–307
2. Menin RA, Malmud LS, Petersen RP, Maier WP, Fisher RS (1980) Gastroesophageal scintigraphy to assess the severity of gastroesophageal reflux disease. Ann Surg 191(1): 66–71
3. Tolin RD, Malmud RS, Reilly J, Fisher JS (1979) Esophageal scintigraphy to quantitate esophageal transit. Gastroenterol 76: 1402–1408
4. Russell COH, Pope CE, Gannan RM, Allen RD, Velasco N, Hill LD (1981) Does surgery correct esophageal motor dysfunction in Gastroesophageal Reflux. Ann Surg 194(3): 290–296
5. Skinner DB, Booth DJ (1970) Assessment of distal esophageal function in patients with hiatal hernia and/or gastroesophageal reflux. Ann Surg 172: 627
6. Kaul B, Halvorsen T, Petersen H, Grette K, Myrvold HE (1986) Gastroesophageal reflux disease. Scintigraphic, endoscopic and histologic considerations. Scand J Gastroenterol 21(2): 134–138
7. Fung WP, van der Schaaf A, Grieve JC (1985) Gastroesophageal scintigraphy and endoscopy in the diagnosis of esophageal reflux and esophagitis. Am J Gastroenterol 80(4): 245–247
8. Bremner CG, Bremner CH, Powers M (1983) Gastroesophageal scintiscanning and radionuclide transit measurement to detect and quantitate reflux and oesophageal motor function. S Afr J Surg 21(3): 139–140
9. De Caestecker JS, Blackwell JN, Adam RD, Hannan WJ, Brown J, Heading RC (1986) Clinical value of radionuclide esophageal transit measurement. Gut 27(6): 659–666
10. Richter JE, Blackwell JN, Wu WL, Cowan JT, Johns DM, Castell DO (1983) Assessment of liquid bolus transit by simultaneous radionuclide transit and esophageal manometry. Gastroenterol 84: 1285
11. Mughal MM, Marples M, Bancewicz J (1986) Scintigraphic assessment of esophageal motility: what does it show and how reliable is it? Gut 27(8): 946–953
12. Styles CB, Holt S, Bowes KL, Jewell L, Hooper HR (1984) Gastroesophageal reflux and transit scintigraphy: a comparison with esophageal biopsy in patients with heartburn. J Can Assoc Radiol 35(2): 124–127
13. Seibert JJ, Byrne WJ, Euler AR, Latture T, Leach M, Campbell M (1983) Gastroesophageal reflux – the acid test: scintigraphy or the pH probe? AJR 140(6): 1087–1090

J. Domergue (Montpellier)

Radioactive techniques supply precise information in the evaluation of gastroesophageal reflux (GER). Two methods are available to display the ascent of a radioactive agent into the esophagus. Esophageal scintigraphy (ES) is performed in a fasting patient after absorption of 1 mCi of ammonium sulphide or colloidal antimony labeled with $technetium_{99}$. Gastric filling is completed with 300 ml of water, which allows esophageal washout. The examination is conducted in the sitting position, and then in Trendelenburg position to facilitate the development of reflux. The recording is made over 45 minutes, by means of 90 images at 30 second intervals of the stomach and esophagus.

Biliary scintigraphy with HIDA is used to visualize duodeno-gastric biliary reflux that may enter the lower esophagus. Recording is made over one hour, beginning 30 minutes after injection of the radioactive agent.

The combination of these methods with long-term measurement of pH allows assessment of their respective sensitivity.

Such comparison indicates that ES is less efficient than pH measurement because

1. it does not specify the nature of the fluid refluxing into the esophagus (acid, basic or neutral),
2. in the absence of precise quantification of the parameters recorded, it does not allow discrimination between physiologic and pathologic reflux, and
3. it gives information that is too immediate in time and would benefit by techniques such as pH measurement sensitive to changes produced by meals.

ES does not constitute a better approach to GER, but represents a supplementary method of quite some value in particular situations, such as assessment of GER after cardioesophageal surgery or in the analysis of the physiopathology of angina or asthma.

Are the disorders of esophageal motility corrected by anti-reflux surgery?

C. G. Bremner (Johannesburg)

For more than 20 years, motor disturbances associated with esophagitis have been recognized. Motility studies have documented a weak lower esophageal sphincter, incoordination, hypomotility, non-peristaltic contractions and even complete motor failure in patients with esophagitis. Olsen and Schlegel [1] found that the degree of disturbance was, in general, proportional to the severity of the esophagitis. The fact that these abnormalities are associated with reflux esophagitis does not imply that reflux was responsible for the damage. In the experimental baboon model however, acid perfusion results in a steady decrease in the lower esophageal sphincter pressure (LESP) and of the amplitude in swallow contractions in the body of the esophagus [2]. Should antireflux surgery result in a return to normal motility patterns, the pathogenesis of the abnormalities would be more easy to understand. Failure to correct the disorders would suggest that the damage was permanent or otherwise unrelated to reflux. Studies of the motility changes after antireflux surgery have examined these changes in the LES and responses in the body of the esophagus and the crico-pharyngeal sphincter.

Lower esophageal sphincter pressure, length and responses

Most reports show that antireflux surgery results in a significant increase in LESP, and this increase results in the majority of cases with competence of the LES (Table 1) [3–7]. The increases in LESP vary between 50–400%. An increase in the length of the LES has also been reported by DeMeester et al. [3] (1.5–2.4 cm). Surprisingly, a return of the sphincter responses (relaxation and contraction) has also been reported [8], and it has been suggested that fundic muscle has the same properties of relaxation and contraction as the LES.

Table 1. Improvement in LESP after anti-reflux surgery

Author and Date			Operation	Pre-op LESP mmHg	Post-op LESP mmHg
Bremner	[2]	1974	Nissen	1.7 (±1.9)	11.4 (±4.5)
Dimarino	[4]	1975	Hill	4.4 (±0.4)	13.9 (±0.5)
Bowes	[5]	1975	Nissen	12.6 (±2.0) cm H_2O	16.5 (±1.5) cm H_2O
Fisher	[6]	1975	Nissen	8.2 (±1.3)	12.0 (±1.5)
Ellis	[7]	1984	Nissen	7.2 (±0.5)	15.6 (±1.5)
DeMeester	[3]	1986	Nissen	9.8 (±5.6)	17.6 (±8.6)

Responses in the body of the esophagus

Recent evidence suggests that the abnormalities of esophageal motility may not be due to reflux, but could have antedated reflux. Esophageal spasm, hypomotility and incoordinate peristaltic waves have been described in esophagitis. It is also possible that these abnormalities could occur in stages of severity of gastroesophageal reflux [9], and that they are irreversible.

There are relatively few reports on studies of esophageal motility which describe the changes after surgery in the body of the esophagus. Two studies found no correction of abnormalities after surgery: Arana et al. [10] studied 14 children with symptomatic reflux before and after a Nissen fundoplication that had corrected the reflux. A high percentage of tertiary non-propulsive esophageal waves remained high several months postoperatively. Russel et al. [11] used radionuclide transit studies in 29 patients and found that the motility abnormalities in 52% of the patients persisted 3 months after a Hill posterior gastropexy repair. Katz et al. [12] studied 13 patients with gastroesophageal reflux disease while in remission on medical treatment, and found that there was no improvement in LES pressure or peristaltic pressure in the body of the esophagus.

These persistent abnormalities could be related to impairment of vagal function as supported by Ogilvie et al. [13]. In our own study [2] we measured the height of contractions following wet swallows before and after fundoplication in 10 patients and found a significant decrease in responses after the operation.

Esophageal emptying

Maddern et al. [14] studied esophageal emptying in patients with gastro-esophageal reflux by using a radionuclide technique. Emptying was delayed in patients with GER, and following fundoplication there was no significant difference in the emptying pattern.

Cricopharyngeal resting pressure and swallow responses

In our studies before and after fundoplication in 10 patients, there was no change in the resting tone of the cricopharyngeal muscle, but there was a decrease in the contraction responses after swallowing [2]. Henderson et al. [15] noted pharyngoesophageal dysphagia in 51.3% of 1000 consecutive patients with gastroesophageal reflux. Cricopharyngeal incoordination was demonstrated by high speed manometry in 20 of 52 patients studied. Antireflux surgery corrected the symptoms in most patients. Cricopharyngeal myotomy corrected the dysphagia in those patients with persistent symptoms after reflux had been corrected. Ekberg and Lindgren [16] found a positive radiologic correlation between dysfunction of the cricopharyngeus muscle and gastroesophageal reflux.

The cricopharyngeus muscle is difficult to evaluate by conventional manometrical equipment, and there is little data to substantiate changes after antireflux surgery.

Conclusions

Following antireflux surgery, there is an increase in the tone and swallowing responses in the lower esophageal sphincter. The abnormalities in esophageal motor function have been found to persist in the few studies on this subject. Surprisingly, symptoms improved despite the fact that the motility defects were not corrected. This suggests that symptoms are due to the acid reflux and not due to the motility abnormalities.

Clinical and radiologic evaluation of cricopharyngeal sphincter abnormalities suggests an improvement in most patients after antireflux surgery, but because of the difficulties in upper-esophageal manometry, there is a paucity of conclusive evidence.

References

1. Olsen AM, Schlegel JF (1965) Motility disturbances caused by esophagitis. J Thorac Cardovasc Surg 50(5): 607–612
2. Bremner CG (1974) Manometric Assessment of Oesophageal Function after the Nissen Fundoplication. S Afr J Surg 12(2): 73
3. DeMeester TR, Bonavina L, Albertucci M (1986) Nissen Fundoplication for Gastroesophageal Reflux Disease. Ann Surg 204(1): 9–20
4. Dimarino AJ, Rosato E, Rosate F, Cohen S (1975) Improvement in lower esophageal sphincter pressure following surgery for complicated gastroesophageal reflux. Ann Surg 181(2): 239–242
5. Bowes KL, Sarna SK (1975) Effect of fundoplication on the lower esophageal sphincter. Can J Surg 18(4): 328–333
6. Fisher RS, Malmud LS, Lobis IF, Maier WP (1975) Antireflux surgery for symptomatic gastroesophageal reflux. Ann Surg 181(2): 239–242
7. Ellis FH Jr, Crozier RE (1984) Reflux control by fundoplication: A clinical and manometric assessment of the Nissen operation. Ann Thorac Surg 38(4): 387–392
8. Higgs RH, Castell DO, Farrell RL (1975) Evaluation of the effect of fundoplication on the incompetent lower esophageal sphincter. Surg Gynecol Obstet 141(4): 571–575
9. Bremner CG (1982) Benign strictures of the esophagus. Current problems in Surgery. Year Book Medical Publishers
10. Arana J, Tovar JA, Garay J (1986) Abnormal preoperative and postoperative esophageal peristalsis in gastroesophageal reflux. J Pediatr Surg 21(8): 711–714
11. Russel COH, Pope CE II, Gannan RM, Allen FD, Velasco N, Hill LD (1981) Does surgery correct esophageal motor dysfunction in gastroesophageal disease? Ann Surg 194(3): 290–296
12. Katz PO, Knuff TE, Benjamin SB, Castell DO (1986) Abnormal esophageal pressure in reflux esophagitis: cause or effect? Am J Gastroenterol 81(9): 744–746
13. Ogilvie AL, James PD, Atkinson M (1985) Impairment of vagal function in reflux esophagitis. Q J Med 54(213): 61–74
14. Maddern GJ, Jamieson GG (1986) Oesophageal emptying in patients with gastroesophageal reflux. Br J Surg 73(8): 615–617
15. Henderson RD, Woolf C, Marryatt G (1976) Pharyngoesophageal dysphagia and gastroesophageal reflux. Laryngoscope 86(10): 1531–1539
16. Ekberg D, Lindgren S (1986) Gastroesophageal reflux and pharyngeal function. Acta Radiol 27(4): 421–423

N. Kockel, B. Ulrich, W. Berges, and *K. Kremer* (Düsseldorf)

In the course of reflux disease there is the accumulated dysfunction of esophageal motility [1, 2, 3]. This is itself proven by cineradiography and also by manometric demonstration. A valid manometric sign of dysfunction is shown as a continuous peristaltic wave, visible in multipoint manometry, as far as the contraction amplitude.

We have investigated whether swallowing function is restored following the teresplasty operation. Teresplasty is a dynamic pexis-method [4], as shown in Fig. 1.

Since 1977, teresplasty was performed in 52 patients with severe peptic esophagitis. The follow-up includes 29 patients who were operated on more than 3 years ago, with regard to their motility functions pre- and post-operatively: the catamnesis, the clinical investigations, the endoscopies with histologic examinations

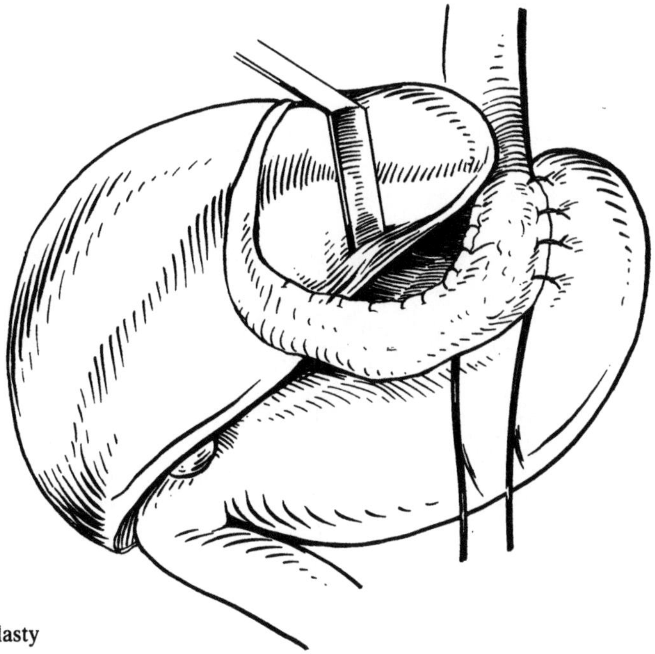

Fig. 1. Scheme of the teresplasty

and pH-measurements showed that 28 of these 29 patients with pre-operative complaints were without symptoms [5]. The singular exception here was due to a technical error during the operation, as the herniated stomach was thought to be the distal esophagus.

Cineradiography showed esophageal motor disfunction in 25 of 29 patients pre-operatively and only in 3 patients post-operatively. The improvement in motility caused by the operation was statistically proven ($p < 0.0001$; X^2-test).

In 22 patients manometric findings were compared pre and post-operatively. The average pressure of the LES increased significantly from 8.27 mm Hg to 16,41 mm Hg post-operatively ($p < 0.0001$; student-test). In 3 patients, the preoperative disorders of LES relaxation was found to be corrected following the operation.

Functional disturbance in the tubular esophagus was found by manometry in 19 of 22 patients preoperatively, post-operatively however only in 2 cases. Comparable cineradiographic findings also demonstrated an improvement motility by the operation ($p < 0.0001$; X^2-test).

Figs. 2 and 3 present typical multi-point manometry passing-through-curves in these patients. Three distinct differences are obvious:

1. A regular peristaltic wave is only visible in the post-operative period.
2. The pressure of the lower esophagus sphincter (LES) increases from 8 mm Hg to 14 mm Hg postoperatively.

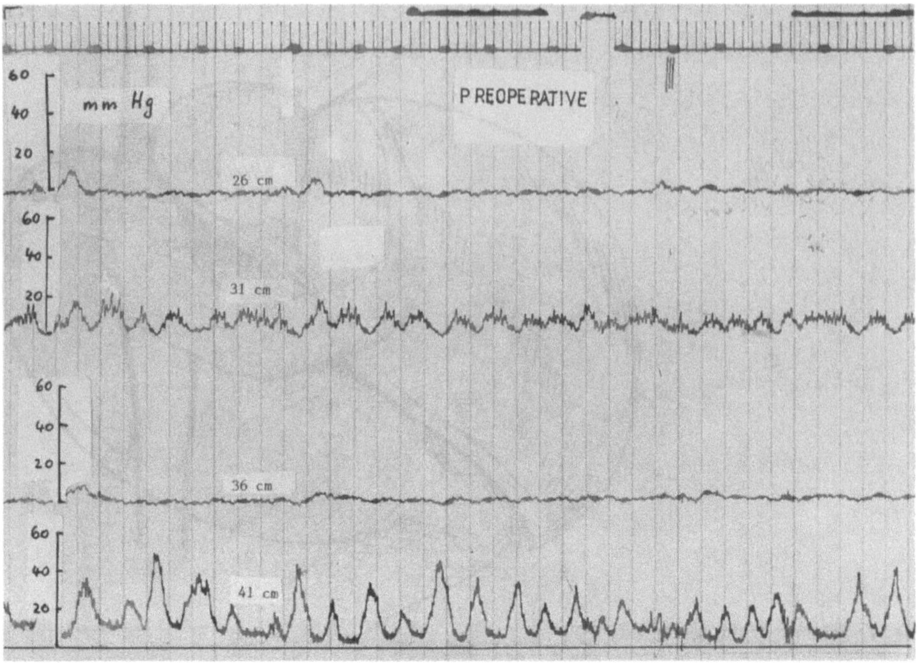

Fig. 2. Multipoint manometry in a patient with reflux esophagitis

3. The maximal amplitude of contraction rises from 30 mm Hg pre-operatively to 80 mm Hg post-operatively.

Summary

Our follow-up examinations show that by the use of Teresplasty, more than 95% of patients with peptic esophagitis could be cured. Both cineradiography and manometry support that most preoperative disorders of esophageal motility could be corrected by the Teresplasty operation.

References

1. Kahrilas PJ, Dodds WJ, Hogan WJ, Kern M, Arndorfer RC, Reece A (1986) Esophageal Peristaltic dysfunction in peptic esophagitis. Gastroenterology 91: 897–904
2. Burns TW, Venturatos SG (1985) Esophageal motor function and response to acid perfusion in patients with symptomatic reflux esophagitis. Digestive Disease and Sciences 30: 529–535
3. Dodds WJ, Dent J, Hogan WJ et al (1982) Mechanisms of gastroesophageal reflux in patients with reflux esophagitis. N Engl J Med 307: 1547–1552
4. Mahmud H, Ulrich B, Kremer K (1979) Die Teres-Plastik. Chirurg 50: 322
5. Ulrich B, Kremer K (1986) Die dynamische Pexie (Teresplastik) zur Behandlung der Reflux-ösophagitis. Zent bl Chir 111: 853–861

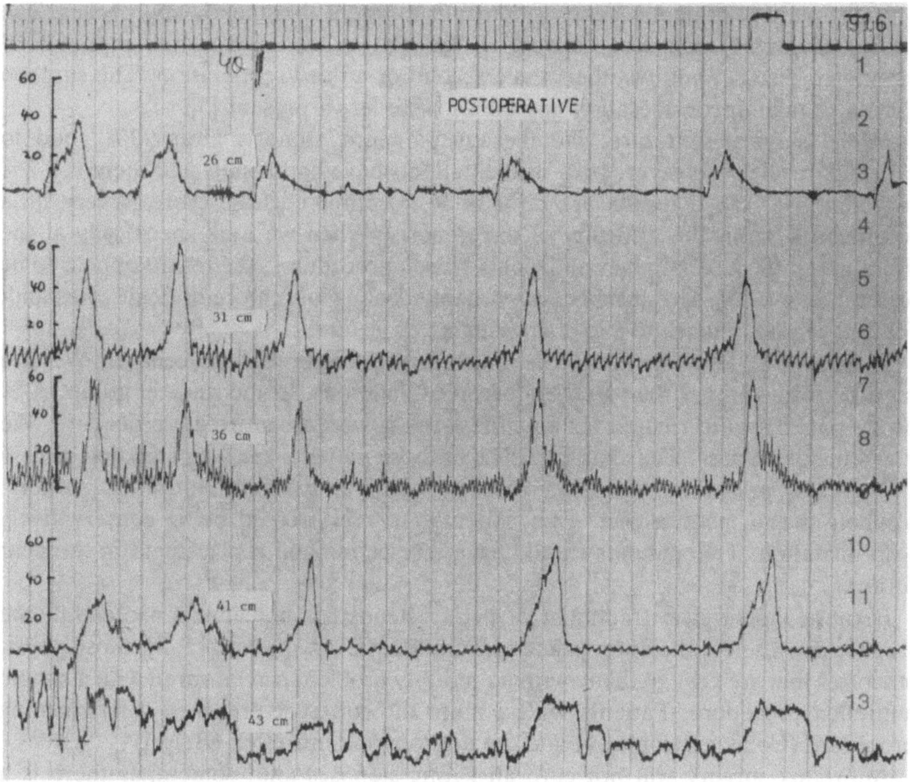

Fig. 3. Multipoint manometry in the same patient (see Fig. 2) postoperatively

How does one interpret peptic stenosis occurring after antireflux surgery?

G. Beauchamp, and *G. Jobin* (Montreal)

The benefit of a fundoplication on the healing of esophagitis has been described [1]. However, very little data is found in the literature about the healing of peptic stenosis after an antireflux procedure. The literature is scant on the subject because many strictures arise in old patients who are not operated [2]. The other reason is that the peptic stenosis that come to surgery vary greatly [3]. Peptic stenosis can be symetrical or asymetrical, long or short, high or low, associated or not with a motility disorder such as achalasia or scleroderma. It can be associated with a Barrett's esophagus [4] or not.

Such a variety of peptic stenoses demands different therapeutic approaches. The choice of surgery will also depend on the age of the patient, the presence of associated disease, and whether it is a second or a third reoperation. The surgeon must also take in consideration any motor disorder, if present [5].

In the surgical literature, the therapy of peptic stenosis gives 90% good to excellent results. However, 10% of the patients have bad results and there is a 2% mortality [6]. These results are difficult to interpret because there is very little information about the difficulty of the stenosis. When we look specifically at the literature of the Collis-Belsey and Collis-Nissen procedures, the results appear to be less impressive [6]. The authors are probably dealing with more difficult cases and, for that reason, choose to use a lengthening procedure.

From 1980 to 1985, we have done more than 200 antireflux procedures. We also have performed more than 1000 endoscopic dilatations. In the surgical group, 30% of the patients were treated for a peptic stenosis with an antireflux procedure. We had 4 major failures. The characteristics of those patients are long standing disease >10 years, presence of Barrett disease, multiple previous antireflux surgery, alcoholism and malnutrition. Two patients are now treated being conservatively with dilatation. Two patients should have a resection and replacement in the near future.

Because the surgical treatment of peptic stenosis is not always successful, the surgeon must select the appropriate technique for every patient [7, 8]: those peptic strictures that are easy to dilate with no motility problem can be cured with a simple antireflux procedure. Patients with a more difficult stricture need a lengthening procedure (Collis gastroplasty) and the appropriate antireflux (Belsey vs Nissen).

Antireflux surgery will not cure all peptic stenoses and, sometimes there is a tendency to recurrence [9]. After multiple failures, there is no other alternative than the resection, and replacement of the esophagus with colon or stomach [10].

References

1. Richardson JD, Kuhns JG, Richardson RL, Polk HC (1983) Properly conducted fundoplication reverses histologic evidence of esophagitis. Ann Surg 197: 763–770
2. Wesdorp ICE, Bartelsman JFWM, Den Hartog Jager FCA, Huibregtse K, Tytgat GN (1982) Results of conservative treatment of benign esophageal strictures: A follow-up study in 100 patients. Gastroenterology 82: 487–493
3. Sandry RJ (1972) Pathology of reflux esophagitis. In Skinner DB, Belsey RHR, Hendrix TR et al (eds): Gastroesophageal reflux and hiatal hernia. Boston, Little Brown & Co
4. Savary M, Miller G (1978) The esophagus. Handbook and Atlas of Endoscopy. Edition Gassman Ag Solothurn Switzerland
5. Bremner CG (1982) Benign strictures of the esophagus. Curr Probl Surg XIX: 406–489
6. Siewert R (1981) Surgical therapy of peptic stenoses. In Medical and Surgical Problems of the Esophagus. Serono Symposia, Vol 43. Edited by Stipa S, Belsey RHR and Moraldi A. Academic Press, London and New York: 146–153
7. Payne WS (1984) Surgical management of reflux – induced oesophageal stenoses: results in 101 patients. Br J Surg 71: 971–973
8. Keenan DJM, Hamilton JRL, Gibbons J, Stevenson HM (1984) Surgery for benign esophageal stricture. J Thorac Cardiovasc Surg 88: 182–188
9. Brand DL, Eastwood IR, Martin D, Carter WB, Pope CE (1979) Esophageal symptoms, manometry, and histology before and after antireflux surgery. A long-term follow-up study. Gastroenterology 76: 1393–1401
10. Little AG, Ferguson MK, Skinner DB (1986) Reoperation for failed antireflux operations. J Thorac Cardiovasc Surg 91: 511–517

Is the progression of the stenosis controlled permanently after treatment?

H. J. Mud (Rotterdam)

There are two, possibly three factors which determine the obstruction caused by reflux-induced stenosis, inflammatory reaction, fibrosis and possibly spasm [1]. Progression of the stenosis can be monitored by assessment of the severity of dysphagia. In most reports the severity of dysphagia is expressed in the need for repeated dilatations of the stricture.

Progression of the stenosis can also be measured directly with standardized barium contrast studies of the esophagus.

What treatment are we talking about? There is a fair amount of unanimity among authors writing about strictures that reflux may be implemented as the cause of the severe esophagitis from which strictures result [2, 3, 4]. Not surprisingly, for most authors the control of reflux is a major goal of therapy [5, 6].

Internists rely on pharmacological control of reflux, combined with postural treatment and life rules concerning body weight and eating habits [7]. In case of stricture they add bougienage and several reports show that in time the number of dilatations decreases [8, 9, 10]. Another author does not add antireflux therapy to bougienage and reports a very large number of dilatations per patient [11], and finally a better compliance with antireflux therapy is associated with better control of dysphagia [12].

Surgeons either remove the stricture and replace the esophagus or perform an antireflux operation combined with dilatations, and spontaneous regression of strictures following adequate antireflux surgery without dilatation has been reported [13].

Surgical operations that effectively control reflux may relieve the patient's dysphagia after a single dilatation [15, 16], but operations designed to remove the stricture without proper control of reflux are doomed to failure [14].

As for the factors that cause the obstruction in strictures of the esophagus and their fate once reflux has been controlled, spasm and inflammatory reaction, consisting of edema an polymorphonuclear infiltration of the esophageal wall, are likely to subside, and spontaneous resolution of the stricture may occur. It is unlikely that fibrotic changes will also disappear, in fact they have been shown to persist. However, they do not progress provided control of reflux is adequate. The control of progression of stenosis depends on the control of reflux, and one may speculate that the number of dilatations required is higher with medical therapy because surgery controls reflux more effectively.

Notwithstanding my own experimental work, in which I showed that in rats the amount of collagen in the esophageal wall increases even after cessation of reflux [17], in man there seems to be little evidence that stricture formation continues after reflux has been controlled effectively. Whether that is a permanent situation remains to be answered.

References

1. Schildberg FW, Witte J, Stücker FJ (1978) Refluxbedingte Oesophagusstenose Chirurg 49: 146–154
2. Wagensteen OH, Logan Leven N (1949) Gastric resection for esophagitis and stricture of acid-peptic origin. Surg Gynec Obst 88: 560–570
3. Brunnen PL, Karmody AM, Needham CD (1969) Severe peptic oesophagitis Gut 10: 831–837
4. Payne WS (1970) Surgical treatment of reflux esophagitis and stricture associated with permanent incompetence of the cardia. Mayo Clin Proc 45: 553–562
5. Skinner DB (1977) Benign esophageal strictures. Adv in Surgery 10: 177–197
6. Lanza FL (1978) Conservative management of esophageal stricture using dilatation and antireflux therapy. South Med J 71 suppl (1): 8–9
7. Cooper JD, Jeejeebhoy KN (1981) Gastroesophageal reflux: medical and surgical management Ann Thor Surg 31: 577–593
8. Lanza FL, Graham DY (1978) Bouginage is effective therapy for most benign esophageal strictures JAMA, 240: 844–847
9. Ferguson R, Dronfield MW, Atkinson M (1979) Cimetidine in treatment of reflux oesophagitis with peptic stricture. Brit Med J (2): 472–474
10. Wesdorp ICE, Bartelsman JFWM, den Hartog Jager FCA, Huibregtse K, Tytgat GN (1982) Results of conservative treatment of benign esophageal strictures: A follow-up study in 100 patients. Gastroenterology 82: 487–493
11. Glick ME (1982) Clinical course of esophageal stricture managed by bouginage. Dig Dis Sci 27: 884–888
12. Starlinger M, Appel WH, Schemper M, Schiessel R (1985) Long-term treatment of peptic esophageal stenosis with dilatation and cimetidine: factors influencing clinical results. Eur Surg Res 17: 207–214
13. Larrain A, Csendes A, Pope CE II (1975) Surgical correction of reflux. Gastroenterology 69: 578–583
14. Gatzinsky P, Bergh NP, Löf BA (1979) Hiatal hernia complicated by oesophageal stricture. Acta Chir Scand 145: 149–158
15. Watson A (1984) The role of antireflux surgery combined with fiberoptic endoscopic dilatation in peptic esophageal stricture Am J Surg 148: 346–349
16. Mercer CD, Hill JD (1986) Surgical management of peptic esophageal stricture. J Thorac Cardiovasc Surg 91: 371–378
17. Mud HJ, Kranendonk SE, van Houten H, Westbroek DL (1985) Mural collagen in experimental reflux esophagitis in rats. J Surg Res 38: 97–104

Do the classifications of peptic stenosis allow a definition of the risk of degeneration?

J. B. Ollyo, M. Savary, Ph. Monnier, J. Wellinger, J. J. Gonvers, and *F. Levi* (Lausanne)

Four different classifications of peptic strictures of the esophagus have been described [5, 7, 9].

Classification according to extent

A "long" and a "short" form have been described. In the majority of cases, peptic strictures are short and localized. The long tubular image seen in contrast radiography is only an artefact due to insufficient filling of the esophagus distal to the stenosis.

Classification according to site

Peptic stricture is usually localized to the middle and distal thirds of the thoracic esophagus. It is usually adjacent to squamous epithelium, at the top of a hiatus hernia or a Barrett's esophagus (Table 1, Fig. 2).

Table 1. Peptic strictures: classification by extent and site

Extent (at esophagoscopy)		Site in thoracic cavity	
"Short" stricture (< 2 cm)	: 270 (78%)	Upper 1/3	: 6 (1.7%)
"Long" stricture (> 2 cm)	: 34 (10%)	Middle 1/3	: 114 (33 %)
Length not reported	: 41 (12%)	Lower 1/3	: 206 (59.7%)
Min. and max. lengths (cm)	: 1–10	Not reported	: 19 (5.5%)

Classification according to degree of stricture

An absolute stricture can only be differentiated from a relative stricture by comparison of the diameters observed during maximum inspiration and endoscopic air inflation. On inspiration, the absolute stricture shows a diameter which is narrower

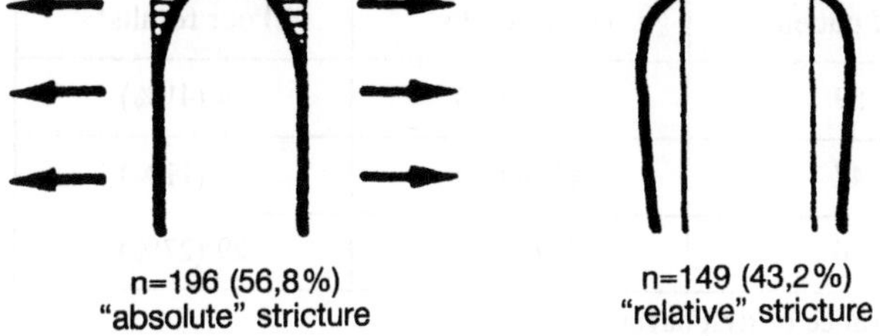

Fig. 1. Classification according to degree of stricture

than that of the adjacent parts of the esophagus. The relative stricture shows, on inspiration, a diameter which is the same as that of the rest of the esophagus. It may be recognized only by powerful inflation of air (Fig. 1).

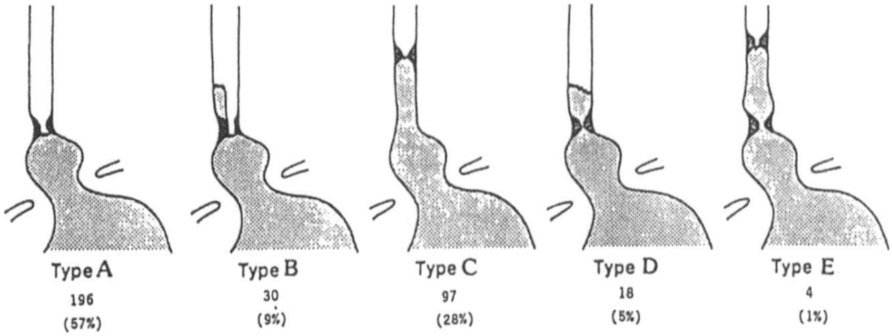

Fig. 2. Peptic stenosis and Barrett's epithelium: after Savary

Classification according to the associated epithelium

In our series, 43% of peptic strictures were associated with columnar epithelium which was localized or circumferential (Barrett's esophagus). This columnar epithelium was usually in the segment distal to the stricture (Fig. 2).

In our experience, the long-term outcome of peptic stricture depends only on the degree of stricture and the presence of columnar epithelium whereas the length and site of the stenosis are of little importance. Likewise the results of antireflux surgery depend on the degree of stricture (Table 2), [6]. Barrett's esophagus is clearly a precancerous condition. These patients have a 40 times greater probability of developing a carcinoma at any site (adenocarcinoma or epidermoid carcinoma) and are at 300 to 1200 times greater risk of esophageal adenocarcinoma than an individual without columnar epithelium [10, 3]. The few epidermoid carcinomas associated with Barrett's esophagus are usually located either within residual squamous epithelium surrounded by columnar epithelium (type II Barrett's esophagus of the Savary classification) [9] or at the proximal edge of the columnar epithelium [1, 2, 4, 8, 11].

Table 2. Long-term results (90 months) of conservative surgical treatment (Nissen) of peptic strictures

Type of stricture	No. of patients	Good results*	Poor results*
"Absolute"	59	35 (59%)	24 (41%)
"Relative"	47	42 (89%)	5 (11%)
Total	106	77 (73%)	29 (27%)

* Good results: complete disappearance of dysphagia
* Poor results: persistence or early recurrence of dysphagia

References

1. Allan NK, Weitzner S, Scott L, Khalil KG (1986) Adenocarcinoma arising in Barrett's esophagus with synchronous squamous cell carcinoma of the esophagus. South Med J 79: 1036–1039
2. Banner BF, Memoli VA, Warren WH, Gould VE (1983) Carcinoma with multidirectional differentiation arising in Barrett's esophagus. Ultrastruct Pathol 4: 205–217
3. Bell RCW (1987) Barrett's esophagus. N Engl J Med 316: 277
4. Burke EL, Sturm J, Williamson D (1978) The diagnosis of microscopic carcinoma of the esophagus. Dig Dis Sci 23: 148–151
5. Davidson JS (1976) High peptic stricture of the esophagus. Thorax 31: 1–14
6. Moghissi K (1979) Conservative surgery in reflux stricture of the esophagus associated with hiatal hernia. Br J Surg 66: 221–225
7. Paulson DL (1967) Benign stricture of the esophagus secondary to gastroesophageal reflux. Ann Surg 165: 765–779
8. Resano CH, Cabrera N, Gonzalez Cueto D, Sanchez Basso AE, Rubio HH (1985) Double early epidermoid carcinoma of the esophagus in columnar epithelium. Endoscopy 17: 73–75
9. Savary M, Miller G (1977) L'œsophage. Manuel et Atlas d'endoscopie. Gassmann SA., édit Soleure
10. Spechler SJ, Robbins AH, Bloomfield Rubins H et al (1984) Adenocarcinoma and Barrett's esophagus. An overrated risk? Gastroenterology 87: 927–933
11. Tamura H, Schulman SA (1971) Barrett-Type esophagus associated with squamous carcinoma. Chest 59: 330–333

What is the respective incidence of peptic stenosis and columnar epithelium lined lower esophagus (Barrett's esophagus)?

C. G. Bremner (Johannesburg)

This question will be dealt with in 3 sections:

What percentage of patients with reflux esophagitis will develop peptic stenosis?

Quoted figures are difficult to interpret, because detail is often lacking. Palmer [1] stated that less than 5% of patients with reflux esophagitis will present with an established stricture. Of approximately 1600 patients with reflux symptoms referred to us for motility tests, 304 had a stricture (19%).

What percentage of patients with reflux esophagitis present with Barrett's epithelium?

Naef et al [2] investigated 1225 patients with reflux esophagitis and diagnosed a columnar lined esophagus (CLE) in 140 (11,4%) and Sarr et al [3] found that 8.2% of 1020 patients had a CLE. Dahms et al [4] found 13 cases of CLE in 103 children with gastroesophageal reflux (12.6%) and Roberts et al [5] found 7 of 23 developmentally disabled children with upper-gastrointestinal symptoms had a Barrett's esophagus. Forty (9.1%) of the patients in Starnes et al [6] series were also found to have a CLE. We have had 95 cases of CLE in our own series of 1600 patients (5.9%).

What percentage of strictures resulting from reflux esophagitis are associated with a CLE?

Allison and Johnstone [7] found 11 cases of CLE in a series of 104 strictures (9.5%). Spechler [8] diagnosed a CLE in 11 of 14 strictures (44%) and we have had 55 patients with CLE in our 304 strictures (18%).

Why reflux esophagitis should result in fewer cases of Barrett's stricture than peptic stricture is speculative. Possibly a severer degree of reflux and poorer acid clearing are responsible.

Conclusion

A wide variation of results has been reported. Of 100 cases of reflux esophagitis 5–19% will have a stricture, 9–12% a Barrett's esophagus and 3% a Barrett's stricture.

References

1. Palmer ED (1968) The hiatus-hernia-esophagitis-esophageal stricture complex. Am J Med 44:566–579
2. Naef AP, Savary M, Ozzello L, Pearson FF (1975) Columnar-lined lower esophagus. Surgery 70: 826–834
3. Sarr MG, Hamilton SR, Marrone GC, Cameron JL (1985) Barrett's esophagus: Its prevalence and association with adenocarcinoma in patients with symptoms of gastroesophageal reflux. Am J Surg 149(1):187–193
4. Dahms BB and Rothstein FC (1984) Barrett's esophagus in children: a consequence of chronic gastroesophageal reflux. Gastroenterology 86(2):318–323
5. Roberts IM, Curtis RL, Madara JL (1986) Gastroesophageal reflux and Barrett's esophagus in developmentally disabled patients. Am J Gastroenterol 81(7):519–523
6. Starnes VA, Adkins RB, Ballinger JF, Sawyers JL (1984) Barrett's esophagus: A surgical entity. Arch Surg 119(5):563–567
7. Allison PR, Johnstone AS (1953) The esophagus lined with gastric mucous membrane. Thorax 8:87–100
8. Spechler SJ, Sperber H, Doos WG, Schimmel EM (1983) The prevalence of Barrett's esophagus in patients with chronic peptic esophageal strictures. Digestive diseases and Sciences 28:769

D. B. Skinner (Chicago)

The incidence of peptic stenosis from reflux depends upon the definition of a stricture: If the definition is radiographic narrowing, the incidence is higher than if it is based on endoscopic criteria. The radiographic appearance includes some cases of spasm through which an endoscope can be passed. The better criteria for defining peptic stenosis is ability or inability to pass a particular size endoscope, and the visualization that the cause of the stenosis is indeed reflux esophagitis, with ulceration and fibrosis.

The incidence of stenosis also depends on the total pool of patients under investigation. In my personal practice at the University of Chicago from 1972 to 1986, a total of 406 patients have been evaluated and treated for reflux esophagitis and its complications. Among these 119 or 29% had a reflux-induced narrowing or stricture confirmed endoscopically. Among 78 patients requiring reoperations for previously failed antireflux surgery, 22 or 28% had definite reflux-induced strictures, indicating that the prevalence of strictures is similar among patients who present initially for treatment of reflux esophagitis as well as in the group in which previous surgery has failed.

The likelihood of stricture in patients with Barrett's esophagus is higher, as over 50% of patients with benign Barrett's esophagus whom we have treated present with a developed stricture from esophagitis [1].

The prevalence of Barrett's esophagus among patients referred for treatment of symptomatic reflux esophagitis is high. In some published series, the incidence of Barrett's esophagus identified during upper-GI endoscopy is stated to be approximately 10%. Savary, et al state that over 60% of patients with grade 4 esophagitis have Barrett's epithelium [2]. In a review of patients evaluated in my unit from 1975 to 1986, 58 (16%) of 357 patients referred for possible surgical treatment of reflux esophagitis were found to have definite evidence of Barrett's esophagus defined as gastric-type epithelium extending at least 3cm above the junction of the tubular esophagus with a gastric pouch.

It appears that the likelihood of identifying Barrett's esophagus among patients with symptomatic gastroesophageal reflux is in the range of 10–15%. This incidence has only been appreciated in recent years and is not noted in reports from earlier studies. Whether this reflects the improved optics of modern endoscopy or a true change in the epidemiology of Barrett's esophagus remains uncertain.

References

1. Skinner DB, Walther BC, Little AG (1985) Surgical treatment of Barrett's esophagus. In Barrett's Esophagus: Pathophysiology, Diagnosis, and Management. S.J. Spechler, R. Goyal, eds New York: Elsevier Science Publishing Co
2. Savary M, Monnier Ph, Miller G (1983) Diagnosis and pathophysiology of Barrett's oesophagus. In Pathological Gastro-Oesophageal Reflux. Proc Workshop Diagnosis and Treatment Pathological Gastro-Oesophageal Reflux. H. A. van Heukelem, H. G. Gooszen, J. L. Terprstra, R. H. R. Belsey, eds. Leiden, Netherlands: Noordwijk

Barrett's esophagus (1)

President: *Sergio Stipa* (Rome)

Free Commentators: *B. Husemann* (Erlangen)
G. G. Jamieson (Adelaide)
E. Lira (Santiago)
H. Nahum (Paris)
F. Potet (Paris)
P. Schlag (Heidelberg)

What is the definition of Barrett's esophagus?

J. L. Lortat-Jacob (Paris)

This word "endobrachyesophagus", which I believe I created, applies to the esophagus whose external morphology is normal or appreciably normal with preservation of an abdominal esophagus and its relations with the gastric fundus, while internally the malpighian mucosa does not occupy the entire length of the esophagus (Fig. 1). A certain length of the lower esophagus may be clothed on its inner aspect with a gastric mucosa of fundal type or a metaplastic, even intestinal, mucosa.

My teacher, Paul Lecène, an eminent surgical professor of the 1920s, who died at the age of 50 in 1929 when I was a first year intern in his unit, uttered this thought that Robert Giuli has reproduced in the tables set out here:

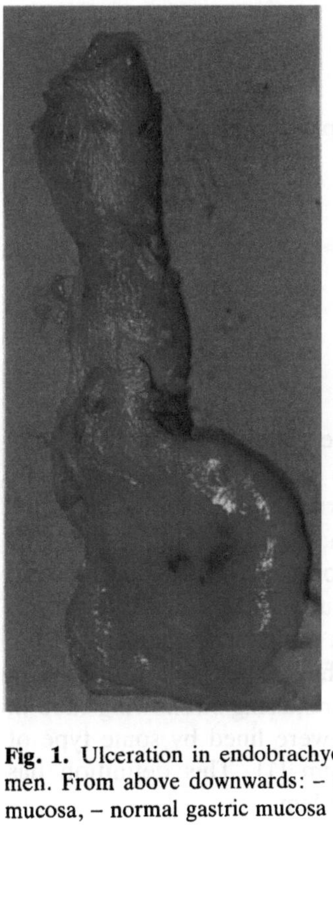

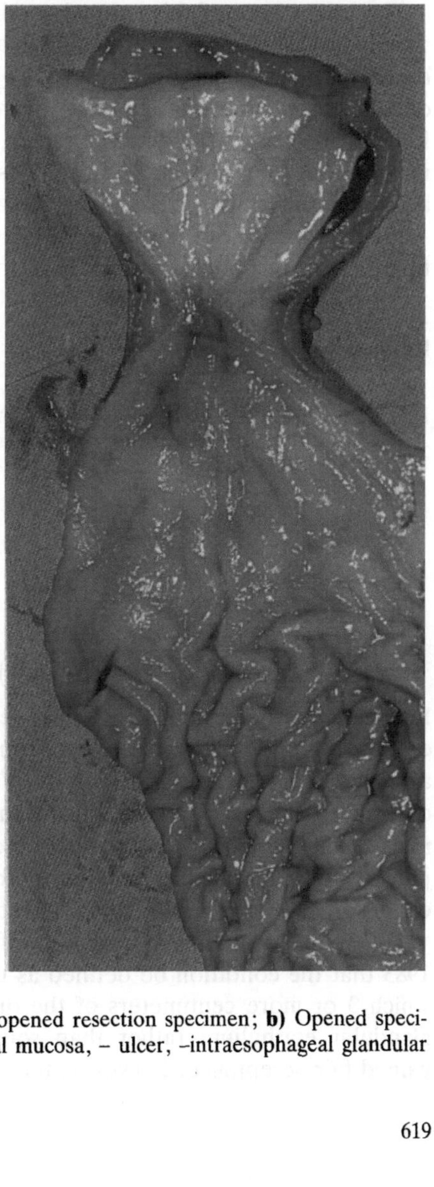

Fig. 1. Ulceration in endobrachyesophagus. **a)** Unopened resection specimen; **b)** Opened specimen. From above downwards: – normal esophageal mucosa, – ulcer, –intraesophageal glandular mucosa, – normal gastric mucosa

When men who are sincere and, at the same time, qualified, have totally different opinions on a precise point, that means that, either they are not speaking about the same thing, or that the question is of no importance.

Fortunately, this aphorism does not apply to Barrett and myself. It was at much the same time [1, 2] that Barrett and I described in somewhat different terms "the lower esophagus lined by columnar epithelium" or "lined by gastric mucosa". Evidently I prefer "endobrachyesophagus" to "Barrett's esophagus". My definition is strictly anatomic, making the essential distinction between brachyesophagus, involving the entire organ, and endobrachyesophagus, involving only the inner lining. It is fundamental that this makes no assumptions about the nature of the mucosal lining existing in the part of the esophagus intermediate between the malpighian mucosa and the mucosa of the stomach, whereas Barrett's esophagus envisages only columnar epithelium.

The importance of this anomaly and its nosologic implications lies in facilitating radiologic diagnosis. My original idea about its origin was a congenital metaplasia, based on the existence in the rest of the esophagus in certain cases of islets of mucosa of diverse appearance proximal to the malpighian limit of the endobrachyesophagus. Later, it became clear that very often this mucosal anomaly resulted from a very imperfect healing process of a reflux esophagitis, a cardio-fundal malposition often being associated with this endoesophageal anomaly.

Indeed, despite our few differences, the smile that Barrett and I exchange on the first page of this book is evidence of the accord of our points of view.

References

1. Barrett NR (1957) The lower esophagus lined by columnar epithelium Surgery, 41: 881
2. Lortat-Jacob JL (1957) L'Endo braeky esophage. Semauce des Hôpitaes, Annales de Chir 11: 17, 18, 1247–1255

D. B. Skinner (Chicago)

For advances to be made in the understanding of the glandular-lined (Barrett's) esophagus, widespread agreement on the definition of the condition must be achieved. This is complicated by the fact that the normal distal esophagus, when defined as the muscular peristalsing tube, has columnar-type epithelium lining its most distal 1–2 cm; when the gastroesophageal junction is defined as the mucosal junction rather than the junction of the swallowing tube with a digestive pouch, confusion as to the incidence of Barrett's esophagus is rampant.

To establish a stringent diagnosis of Barrett's esophagus, we have proposed in 1983 that the condition be defined as the muscular peristalsing swallowing tube in which 3 or more centimeters of the distal esophagus were lined by some type of glandular epithelium rather than squamous epithelium [1]. This definition has gained fair acceptance. However, there remains a problem.

The glandular lining of the normal distal 1–2 cm of esophagus is simple columnar epithelium. When such epithelium extends 5 or 6 centimeters up into the peristalsing esophagus, there is general agreement that this represents a Barrett's esophagus. However, a pathological hallmark of Barrett's esophagus is metaplastic epithelium including distinctive goblet cells, this lining being not normally present at the cardia. When such metaplastic epithelium is found by biopsy within the distal 3 centimeters of esophagus, the argument can be made that this also should be included as a case of Barrett's esophagus.

Accordingly we now modify the definition of Barrett's esophagus to include all cases in which the metaplastic goblet cell-type of epithelium is found within the esophageal lumen at any level provided it is in continuity with gastric epithelium distally, as well as including all cases in which any type of glandular epithelium is found extending more than 3 cm cephalad in the muscular peristalsing esophagus.

This definition must be based on endoscopic findings and proven by biopsies. Because of the mobility of the esophagus, especially in cases of hiatal hernia, the measurements of 3 cm or more of gastric-type epithelium should be made both during the downward passage and withdrawal of the endoscope. The actual level of the biopsies may vary during scope withdrawal or insertion because of the sliding nature of the hiatal hernia usually present; however, the relationship of the bottom of the narrow swallowing tube to the gastric pouch compared to the level of the squamo-columnar junction should be relatively constant during both scope insertion and withdrawal, and hence confirm the presence of the Barrett's esophagus.

An antireflux operation typically relocates the distal esophagus to an intraabdominal location and lengthens the overall esophagus. This has the effect of causing a downward placement of the squamo-columnar junction. When discussion is made of possible regression of Barrett's esophagus, it must be based upon a comparison of the early post-operative endoscopic findings to subsequent follow-up rather than an assessment of the preoperative location of the squamo-columnar junction compared to the follow-up evaluations.

Reference

1. Skinner DB, Walther BC, Riddell RH, Schmidt H, Iascone C, DeMeester TR (1983) Barrett's esophagus: comparison of benign and malignant cases. Ann Surg. 198: 554–565

The various degrees of differentiation toward gastric or intestinal epithelium seem to predispose to dysplasia and cancer

H. D. Appelmann (Ann Arbor)

For Barrett's esophagus, what are the various degrees of differentiation toward gastric or intestinal epithelium which seem to predispose to dysplasia and cancer?

It has become clear that there are three basic types of mucosa which occur in Barrett's esophagus, and not all of them occur in every case.

First, there is a mucosa which resembles gastric cardia, and this has been termed "junctional". It contains pits and glands of about equal depth. There tend to be fewer glands and more lamina propria than in normal cardiac mucosa.

The second type, also a gastric type mucosa, is a modified fundic or body mucosa in which the pits and glands are also of roughly equal depth, but the glands contain the usual body constituents of parietal cells and chief cells in addition to mucus cells.

The third type of mucosa seems to be quite unique to Barrett's esophagus, and it has been designated as the "specialized" type. This is an expanded mucosa which seems to be composed of gastric style pits which, toward the lumen, expand so as to produce a villiform surface configuration. The epithelium lining these pits and villi is composed of a mixture of gastric surface type cells with apical mucus droplets and scattered intestinal type goblet cells. This epithelial alteration has been designated as incomplete intestinal metaplasia.

When these mucosal types were first defined, it was felt that the specialized or intestinalized type was more likely to be most proximal, with the modified fundic type the most distal, and the modified cardiac or junctional type in between. We have recognized that although these patterns of distribution tend to occur in general, actually the mucosae are mosaics with mixtures of these types, especially of the specialized and junctional types.

If we define dysplasias as epithelial alterations which are truly neoplastic and, on occasions, which may be invasive, then we recognize dysplasias as occurring in both the intestinalized mucosa and the non-intestinalized. Furthermore, there is considerable evidence that the intestinalized mucosa which is associated with dysplasia is that form of incomplete intestinal metaplasia in which the gastric type surface cells between the globet cells often contain sulfated acid mucopolysaccharide.

In general, it appears that dysplasia is more likely to occur in the specialized type of Barrett's mucosa. However, in some dysplastic Barrett's mucosa, the dysplastic epithelium has completely obliterated the underlying mucosa from which it arose, so it is impossible to tell where such dysplasia evolved.

Is the initial anomaly definitely congenital in certain cases?

C. G. Bremner (Johannesburg)

Certain aspects of the columnar-lined esophagus have suggested that some cases may be congenital in origin. The following arguments have been put forward in favour of a congenital original.

1. The fetal esophagus is lined by a simple columnar epithelium that gradually changes to a stratified squamous type and matures by the sixth month. Persistence of this fetal columnar epithelium would account for a congenital columnar lining. However, a columnar lined esophagus has not been reported in any neonate autopsy study.

2. Islands of heterotopic gastric mucosa have been described in all esophageal segments, including the postcricoid area. Weingart et al. [1] described such islands in 125 patients.
   By definition, a columnar lined esophagus is one in which a segment of the organ is totally lined by columnar epithelium in continuity with the stomach. Such islands do not constitute a Barrett esophagus.
3. Borrie and Goldwater [2] suggested that there may be a congenital and an acquired type because of the bimodal age range in their series (0–10 and 48–80 years). However, Dahms and Rothstein [3] described a CLE in 13 children who had gastroesophageal reflux, and Hassal et al. [4] reported on 11 children (6–14 years) with a CLE all of whom had longstanding reflux. In order to explain these cases on a congenital theory, one would also have to postulate a congenital incompetence of the lower esophageal sphincter (LES); it is highly likely that the LES has failed to develop or is weak in these cases, allowing reflux to occur from an early age. It is not the columnar lining which is congenital, but the incompetence of the lower sphincter.
4. Variations in the squamo-columnar junction suggest two different types. The flame-shaped junction, according to Stadelman et al. [5] is the acquired type, and the type with a clear-cut demarkation is the congenital variety.
5. Familial Barrett's has been described in two sisters aged 66 years [6], both of whom had hiatal hernias and a poor LES on manometry. Again, there is more evidence for a reflux history to explain the CLE. Hague [7] described a single case of total esophageal columnar lining in a patient with a long history of reflux.

*

The evidence for the congenital origin of a Barrett's esophagus is virtually non-existent. There is evidence, however, for a congenital absence or incompetence of the lower esophageal sphincter, which in turn could lead to a columnar-lined esophagus in some cases.

References

1. Weingart J, Seib HJ, Elster K, Ottenjann R (1984) Gastric mucosa heterotopies in the upper gastrointestinal tract. Leber Magen Derm 14(4): 155–160
2. Borrie J, Goldwater L (1976) Columnar cell-lined esophagus. Assessment of etiology and treatment. J Cardiovasc Thor Surg 71: 825–834
3. Dahms BB, Rothstein FC (1984) Barrett's esophagus in children: a consequence of chronic gastroesophageal reflux. Gastroenterol 86(2): 318–323
4. Hassall E, Weinstein WM, Ament ME (1985) Barrett's esophagus in children. Gastroenterol 89(6): 1331–1337
5. Stadelman O, Elster K, Kühn HA (1981) Columnar-lined esophagus (Barrett's syndrome) – congenital or acquired? Endoscopy 13(4): 140–147
6. Prior A, Whorwell PJ (1986) Familial Barrett's esophagus. Hepatogastroenterol 33(2): 86–87
7. Haque AK, Merkel M (1981) Total columnar-lined esophagus: a case for congenital origin. Arch Pathol Lab Med 105(10): 546–548

Y. Kawaura (Kanazawa)

There has been divided opinion about whether the abnormally located columnar epithelium, so called Barrett's esophagus [1] is a congenital anomaly or is acquired heterotopia caused by injury of the squamous epithelium.

The author experienced 824 cases of esophagitis (without post-operative esophagitis) and 35 cases of Barrett's esophagus between 1960 and 1982. Among them, 685 cases have reflux esophagitis which accompanied 28 cases of Barrett's epithelium. The other 139 cases were non-reflux esophagitis accompanying 7 cases of Barrett's epithelium. Definite diagnosis of the Barrett's esophagus and reflux esophagitis was made by endoscopy.

Among Barrett's esophagus, ulcer was seen in 8 cases. As regards lesions associated with Barrett's esophagus, hiatal hernia was seen in 7 cases of Barrett's ulcer and in 5 cases of Barrett's epithelium. Regarding mucosal findings, 85.7% of Barrett's ulcer and 71.4% of Barrett's esophagus accompanied inflammation, 15 biopsied cases showed a high incidence of gastric or intestinal metaplasia. The Barrett's epithelium was seen mainly in older patients (mean 54.8 years old) (Table 1).

It is difficult to decide whether the Barrett's esophagus is a congenital or acquired anomaly in certain cases.

The author tried to divide the Barrett's esophagus into 3 categories (Table 2).

Allison and Johnstone [2] published the congenital theory of Barrett's esophagus.

Islets of ciliated columnar epithelium have been noted in post-mortem examination of esophagus from premature and newborn infants.

Recent observations, documenting the ascent up the esophagus of the squamous-columnar junction, support the concept of an acquired dynamic epithelium within the sheet of columnar epithelium and could be interpreted as the more resistant remmants of squamous epithelium that survived the erosive action of digestive secretions. This phenomenon is less easily explained by the congenital theory.

To find a hiatal hernia in the cases with gastroesophageal reflux is common, and the refluxing gastric sections would appear to be responsible for the acquired heterotopic columnar epithelium. These findings favoring the congenital theory point only to the patients having columnar epithelium in the esophagus without a

Table 1. Total number of cases

Age (mean)	54.8 years
Number of Esophagitis	824 cases
Reflux Esophagitis	685 cases
Non-Reflux Esophagitis	139 cases
Barrett's Esophagus	35 cases
Diffuse Barrett's Esophagus	7 cases
with Ulcer	8 cases
with Hiatal Hernia	12 cases
with Metaplasia	15 cases

Table 2. Classification of Barrett's Esophagus

	distinctly congenital	probably congenital	acquired
Age	neonatal	young age	old age
Symptom	–	+ or –	+ or –
Esophagitis	–	+ or –	+
Ulcer or Scar	–	+ or –	+ or –
Hiatal Hernia	–	–	+ or –
Aberrant organ around columnar cell	+ or –	+ or –	–
Inflammatory cell	–	+ or –	+
Parietal cell	+ or –	+ or –	+ or –
Squamous islets in Barrett's Esophagus	–	–	+ or –
History of laparotomy	–	–	+ or –

hiatal hernia. In the literature, two cases of 9 year-old boy and 10 year-old girl were reported [3, 4]. Both children had experienced dysphagia since infancy.

References

1. Barrett NR (1950) Chronic peptic ulcer of the oesophagus and oesophagitis. Br J Surg 38: 175–182
2. Allison PR, Johnstone AS (1953) The esophagus lined with gastric mucous membrane. Thorax 8: 87–101
3. Postlethwait RW, Sealy WC (1961) Surgery of the esophagus. Springerfield, 3, ed Thomas CC
4. Wyndham N (1956) The significance of gastric mucosa in the oesophagus. Brit J Surg 23: 409–412

Experimental Barrett's esophagus leads to conclude that this lesion is almost constantly acquired

C. G. Bremner (Johannesburg)

Early attempts to reproduce an experimental columnar lined esophagus (CLE) failed because the process of columnar replacement is a slow one. The process was accelerated in the experimental reflux dog model by stripping the squamous epithelium and stimulating acid secretion with histamine in beeswax [1].

Reflux Model (25 dogs)

The lower esophageal sphincter was destroyed by an anterior longitudinal incision through the wall of the esophagus and proximal 1–2 cm of stomach. The distal esophageal mucosa was dissected away from the muscle for a distance of 6–10 cm. A transverse 2-layer closure was made, and the diaphragmatic hiatus was sutured to the gastric fundus making a hiatal hernia 2–3 cm long. Histamine in beeswax was given to 11 of these dogs by intramuscular injection for periods of up to 12 weeks.

Control Model

The distal 6–8 cm of esophageal mucosa was excised as in the previous model, leaving the lower esophageal sphincter intact, and without the addition of a hiatal hernia.

Cinefluoroscopy demonstrated reflux in the reflux model, but not in the control model. The pattern of epithelium replacement was studied by potential difference measurements, biopsy and pathology of the whole organ.

Results

Columnar epithelium replaced part of, or in some cases, the entire length of the denuded esophagus only in the reflux models. The replacement was greatest in the histamine in beeswax group. Animals without reflux had a rapid replacement of squamous epithelium only.

These results lent support to the concept that the columnar-lined esophagus may be acquired, but did not exlude the possibility of a congenital group.

Models with Intact epithelium

Further reflux models in the dog and baboon were less successful when the mucosa was not stripped and histamine was omitted: Up to 6 mm of columnar replacement resulted after several months in the dog model, but not in the baboon. This is probably related to the fact that the baboon never lies down.

Pollara [2] also reproduced a columnar-lined esophagus in dog experiments. He stripped the squamous mucosa for a 4 cm length, and did not use histamine stimulation: after 30 days, he measured an area of 46 sq mm of columnar replacement, and after 60 days an area of 60 sq mm. Several ulcers also developed in his models.

Human Models (Fig.)

Gastroesophageal reflux which follows esophago-gastrectomy may result in a columnar-lined segment above the esophago-gastric anastomosis, and we have seen this 14 and 21 years following resection for a benign reflux stricture. Naef et al. [3] and Hamilton and Yardley [4] have described similar cases who developed extensive columnar metaplasia following subtotal esophagectomy many years previously. Columnar replacement has also been described following esophagomyotomy for achalasia, and in scleroderma patients.

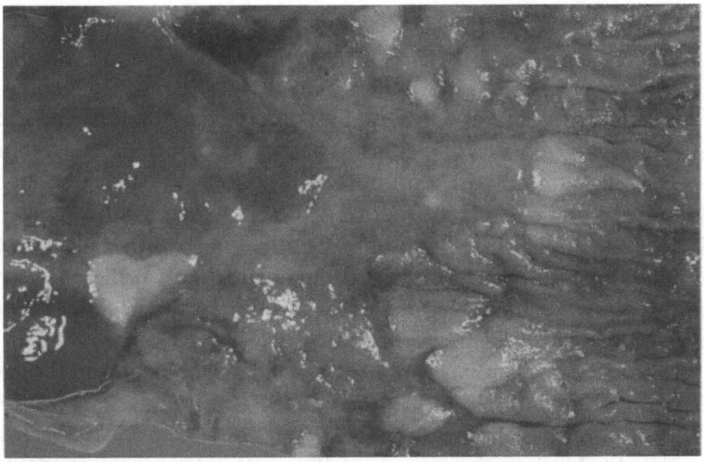

Fig. 1. Three authors have described a columnar replacement above the anastomotic site many years after esophago-gastrectomy, and this figure shows such a case. This could be called a "human" model

These models all support the concept that long-continued gastroesophageal reflux can result in a replacement of denuded squamous epithelium by columnar epithelium derived from the gastric cardia. The models do not exclude the possibility of a congenital columnar-lining. Manometric and pH tests in CLE have demonstrated a poor lower esophageal sphincter and gastroesophageal reflux in most patients tested [5, 6].

References

1. Bremner CG, Lynch VP, Ellis F, Henry Jr. (1970) Barrett's esophagus: Congential or Acquired? An experimental study of esophageal mucosal regeneration in the dog. Surgery 68(1): 209–216
2. Pollara W (1981) An experimental study of mucosal regeneration in the presence of gastroesophageal reflux. Thesis presented to University of Sao Paulo Brazil
3. Naef AP, Savary M, Ozzello L, Pearson FG (1975) Columnar-lined lower esophagus. Surgery 70: 826–834
4. Hamilton SR, Yardley JH (1977) Regeneration of cardial type mucosa and acquisition of Barrett's mucosa after esophagogastrectomy. Gastroenterol 72: 669–675
5. Bremner CG, (1982) Benign stricture of the Esophagus. Current Problems in Surgery. 19(8): 402–492
6. Bremner CG (1977) The columnar-lined (Barrett's) Esophagus. Surg Ann 9: 103–124

H. W. Pinotti, W. M. Pollara, I. Cecconello, and *B. Zilberstein* (Sao Paulo)

The interpretation and origin of columnar epithelium in the lower esophagus secondary to reflux esophagitis has been variously debated by many authors [2, 3, 7].

The first attempts to reproduce this condition experimentally were unsuccessful [4, 8]. Bremner et al. [6] reported the first successful attempt: they were able to induce the appearance of columnar epithelium after surgical resection of squamous epithelium with procedures provoking esophageal reflux. However, it was difficult in this study to characterize the real position of this regenerated epithelium because a reference point in the esophagus was lacking.

In the present study the inferior esophageal sphincter in the esophageal wall, that is perfecty individualized in the dog [10, 15], was used as a reference point.

Twelve dogs of both sexes, weighing from 16 to 23 kilograms, were used in this study. At the time they were sacrificed, the dogs were randomly divided into two groups of six. Group 1 was sacrificed 30 days after operation and Group 2 60 days postoperatively.

The dogs were operated on under general anesthesia. A thoracotomy through the seventh intercostal space was performed and an incision made through the wall of the esophagus and stomach for about 4 centimeters, including the lower esophageal sphincter, three centimeters on the esophageal side and one centimeter on the gastric side. Then, a section four millimeters in width and forty millimeters in length was removed next to one the margins of the incision. It included all the layers of the esophagogastric junction. This specimen was labeled the operative control. An extension of forty millimeters of mucosa, measured from the gross limit of esophagogastric junction was also removed from the distal esophagus, creating a cylindrical region of the esophagus without mucosa. The incision of the esophagogastric junction was sutured transversally, as in a Wendel cardioplasty, and the gastric fundus was sutured to the diaphragm, creating a hiatal hernia with an intrathoracic gastric chamber of about three centimeters.

Gastroesophageal reflux and hiatal hernia were demonstrated by X ray studies of the dogs between the first and second weeks. The removed mucosa was examined.

The distance between the transition of the columnar and squamous epithelium and the superior limit of the inferior sphincter of the esophagus (SLISE), clearly individualized in the dog, were determined in the operative control, that is, in the total specimen of the esophageal wall obtained during surgery.

After the animals were killed, the esophagus, gastric fundus, part of the diaphragm and gastric body were immediately removed. The stomach was opened along the great curvature and the esophagus cut open longitudinally in the same direction as the gastric incision. The appearance of the esophagogastric junction, especially the epithelial lining, was observed.

After gross examination, the entire circumference of the specimen was sliced in longitudinal bands, two millimeters in width, parallel to the major axis of the esophagus. The superior and inferior limits of the incision were grossly determined above and below the reepithelized region, so that segments of about 35 to 40 millimeters in length were obtained.

Table 1. Summary of the statistical comparison of the results and values

	Group I	Group II	(P)
Level of the columnar epithelium in the operative control	$-0.80\,mm^2$ (1.72)	-1.33 mm (1.96)	N.S.
Level of the gastric mucosa in relation to the SLISE during the late postoperative period	-0.67 mm (2.58)	5.17 mm (6.57)	0.05
Regenerated columnar epithelium	$46.00\,mm^2$ (31.94)	$58.66\,mm^2$ (39.79)	N.S.
Ulcer	$131.66\,mm^2$ (42.99)	$89.66\,mm^2$ (75.15)	N.S.
Regenerated squamous epithelium	$54.33\,mm^2$ (39.96)	$19.33\,mm^2$ (22.32)	0.10
Columnar epithelium above the SLISE	$43\,mm^2$ (20.09)	$125.66\,mm^2$ (81.49)	

The microscopic sections were stained with hematoxylin and eosin, alcian-blue, PAS and Masson's trichrome stain. Thus, we were able to study the characteristics of the epithelium, the type of mucus produced and the muscular structure of the esophageal wall.

For a clearer interpretation of the results, the approximate area of each epithelium was calculated:

- the area of reepithelization by columnar and squamous epithelium:
- the ulcerated area in each of the groups;
- the total area of the columnar epithelium above the SLISE (Table 1).

The histologic studies of the operative control show that preoperatively, the transition between the columnar and squamous epithelium was with minor variation at the level of the superior limit of the inferior sphincter of the esophagus. In all cases the esophageal mucosa removed during surgery was composed of squamous epithelium without any sign of columnar epithelium in the resected region.

After the animal was sacrified, the gross specimen in both groups showed that the characteristics of the epithelium lining the region from which the mucosa was removed were different from those of normal esophageal epithelium: the coloration was somewhat orange and the surface slighty depressed in relation to the adjacent mucosa, it was more wrinkled than the esophageal epithelium but smoother than the adjacent gastric epithelium.

The microscopic study of the serial sections of the esophagogastric junction done on the specimen showed that it was lined by simple columnar epithelium with no muscularis mucosae, which was newly formed over inflammatory tissue and located above the SLISE. This epithelium presented varying degrees of differentiation. In some instances it was formed by simple columnar epithelium with a single layer of cells, and in others, it presented a more complex structure, forming crypts and villi. At times resembling gastric or intestinal epithelium.

There were focal areas of regeneration columnar epithelium in the midst of squamous epithelium in two dogs, both in Group 1. Focal areas of squamous regeneration in the midst of columnar epithelium were found in five dogs, three in Group 2 above the SLISE, with the gastric mucosa at the same level as that observed pre-operatively.

Continuity of the regenerated columnar epithelium with ducts of the submucosal glands of esophagus, was observed in three dogs. They grew progressively in the direction of the lumen of the esophagus, actually lining the organ when they reached the surface. This epithelium was similar to staining with alcian-blue-PAS stain, as the submucosal glands of the esophagus.

In two dogs, the presence of squamous epitelium was observed in the neck of the duct of esophageal submucosal glands in the midst of regenerating epithelium.

The microscopic appearance of the esophageal mucosa above the region resected by surgery presented signs of esophagitis, characterized by micro ulcerations and hypertrophy of the papillae of the corium and basal layer. This confirms the action of gastroesophageal reflux on the region in question.

Analysis of the sections of the operative control showed that in the dog, the transition of the squamous and columnar epithelia occurs at the level of the upper limit of the muscular bundle corresponding to the inferior sphincter of the esophagus. A study of the manner by which the region devoid of its epithelial lining is repaired was undertaken by means of histologic sections and with the inferior esophageal sphincter as a limit.

The normal gastric mucosa present in the inferior border and visible in all the sections, underwent scar retraction, proximaly going beyond the SLISE.

The regenerated columnar epithelium was found in all cases with various characteristics. At times it was in the form of simple columnar epithelium, at others presenting glandular aspects or more evolved, acquiring a structure similar to the gastric epithelium.

Microscopic descriptions of columnar epithelium have differed considerably: various authors describe the epithelium as junctional [7, 14], of the gastric fundus [1, 9], intestinal [1], specialized columnar epithelium [5, 16], or all of the above [11, 12]. In this study, we also found the four types of differentiated columnar epithelium, based on the complexity of its structure.

The regenerated columnar epithelium was in continuity with the gastric mucosa most of the time. However, at other times it was found focally in the midst of squamous epithelium: in these cases, it presented clear continuity with the ducts of the submucous glands of the esophagus. This confirms the theories of Pava et al. [13] and Adler [2], who feel that the columnar epithelium that lines the esophagus may under some circumstances originate from the submucous glands of the esophagus, that surface due to the destruction of the squamous epithelium normally lining the esophagus.

Esophagitis was intense in all cases in which existed small areas of squamous epithelization. This fact may also be explained by the probable damaging action of the refluxed digestive secretion. No difference was found between the reepithelized columnar and squamous areas in Group 1. This means that in the initial stages, the rate of growth of both epithelia is similar. However, this difference in the dogs in Group 2 was observed as being due not to the speed of columnar regeneration, but to the retraction of the area of squamous regeneration. The most important point to be considered is the total area of the columnar epithelium above the SLISE, because it is the esophagus itself covered by columnar epithelium, the main reason for this study. This area includes the sum total of the regenerated columnar epithelium and the scar retraction of the gastric mucosa that are found above the SLISE.

The analysis of these results enables us to conclude that in the presence of gastroesophageal reflux, the repair of esophageal epithelium resected surgically resulted in the appearance of columnar epithelium above the inferior sphincter of the esophagus, similar to what occurs in man under certain circumstances. It is also evident that the process is not unique but multiple, and not static, but dynamic, attempting to reestablish the equilibrium of the region, which has been changed by the presence of acid and the loss of mucosa.

References

1. Abrams L, Heath D (1965) Lower oesophagus lined with intestinal and gastric epithelia. Thorax, 20: 66
2. Adler RH (1963) The lower esophagus lined by columnar epithelium. Its association with hiatal hernia, ulcer, structure, and tumor. J Thorac Cardiovasc Surg 45: 13
3. Barrett NR (1950) Chronic peptic ulcer of the oesophagus and oesophagitis. Br J Surg 38: 175
4. Barrett NR (1957) The lower oesophagus lined by columnar epithelium. Surgery, 41: 881
5. Berenson MM, Herbst JJ, Freston JW (1978) Enzyme and ultrastructural characteristics of esophageal columnar epithelium. Am J Dig Dis 19: 895
6. Bremner CG, Lynch VP, Ellis FH Jr (1970) Barrett's esophagus congenital or acquired? An experimental study of esophageal mucosa regeneration in the dog. Surgery 68: 209
7. Hayward J (1961) The lower end of the esophagus. Thorax 16: 36
8. Hennessy TP, Edlich RF, Buchin RJ, Tsung MS, Prevost M, Wangensteen OH (1968) Influence of gastroesophageal incompetence on regeneration of esophageal mucosa. Arch. Surg 97: 105
9. Hershfield, NB, Lind JF, Hildes JA, McMorris LS (1965) Secretory function of Barrett's ephitelium. Gut 6: 535
10. Naef AP, Savary M, Ozzello L (1975) Columnar-lined lower esophagus: an acquired lesion with malignant predisposition. Report on 140 cases of Barrett's esophagus with 12 adenocarcinomas. J Thorac Cardiovasc Surg 70: 826
11. Paull A, Traier JS, Dalton MD, Camp RC, Loeb P, Goyal RK (1976) The histologic spectrum of Barrett's esophagus. N Engl J Med 295: 476
12. Pava S, de la Pickren JW, Adler RH (1964) Ectopic gastric mucosa of the esophagus. A study on histogenesis. N.Y. State J Med 64: 1831
13. Pedersen SA, Hage E, Nielsen PA (1971) Barrett's syndrome. Morphological and physiological characteristics. Scand J Thorac Cardiovasc Surg 6: 191
14. Thier JS (1970) Morphology of the epithelium of the distal esophagus in patients with midesophageal peptic strictures. Gastroenterology 58: 444
15. Van de Kerchhof J, Gahagan T (1963) Regeneration of the mucosal lining of the esophagus. Henry Ford Hosp Med Bull 11: 129

"Diffuse" Barrett's esophagus

Y. Kawaura (Kanazawa)

The Barrett's esophagus is usually recognized as the columnar epithelium lining the lower half or third of the esophagus. When the columnar epithelium was seen over the lower half, including the skip lesion, the author named it "Diffuse Barrett's Esophagus" (Table 1).

Table 1. Diffuse Barrett's Esophagus

Category	Number of Esophagitis	Number of Diffuse Barrett's Esophagus
(1)	715 cases	1 case
(2)	18	0
(3)	44	2
(4)	35	2
(5)	12	2
Total	824 cases	7 cases

Reflux esophagitis was divided into 5 radiologic and endoscopic categories [1].

1. *Diffuse superficial esophagitis*: this type is associated with direct sliding hernia and the length of involvement is usually up to 10 cm of the distal esophagus. In this category, "diffuse Barrett's esophagus" is rare and the author experienced only one case. When a "diffuse Barrett's esophagus" was recognized, in this category the congenital theory of Barrett's esophagus was suspected strongly.
2. *Peptic stricture type*: the stricture is always located between the squamous and the hernia sac and there is often diffuse superficial esophagitis proximal to the stricture. In this category, the author could not recognize Barrett's esophagus.
3. *Localized penetrating ulcer*: gastric epithelium is present along the distal border of the ulcer, while squamous epithelium surrounds the remainder. In this category, the author recognized 2 cases of "diffuse Barrett's esophagus".
4. *Esophagitis or stricture or ulcer associated with columnar epithelial lined esophagus*: this category is noted in the mid or upper portion of the thoracic esophagus. The stricture is seen at the junction of the squamous and columnar lined segments. When the stricture is very severe or several strictures were recognized, diffuse Barrett's esophagus is associated with the lesions. The author experienced "diffuse Barrett's esophagus" in 2 cases in this, category. In these cases the columnar epithelium appears to be the result of metaplasia and the result of recurring reflux esophagitis, or is likely to extend further proximally over a period of time, and the author thinks this type is "probably acquired".
5. *Diffuse severe esophagitis*: radiologically, the distal 10 cm or more of esophagus are markedly narrowed and irregular. This type are usually seen in a patient with laparotomy.

Table 2. Diffuse Barrett's Esophagus

Type of Diffuse Barrett's Esophagus			Number of Diffuse Barrett's Esophagus
Epithelial ⟶ junction	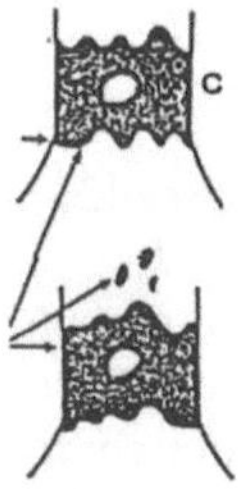	continuous type	6 cases
Esophago ⟶ gastric junction			
Barrett's ⟶ epithelium		scattered type	1 case

The author experienced one case with a history of laparotomy and hiatal hernia was seen. 5 years after laparotomy, the columnar epithelium was seen 4.8 cm from the esophagogastric junction, and after 14 years the columnar epithelium was seen up to 10.3 cm.

Necropsy studies have occasionally shown the columnar epithelium to be scattered in islands throughout the esophagus [2]. In author's experience, in two cases this scattered columnar epithelium was seen. For detection of "diffuse Barrett's esophagus", it is advisable to obtain multiple biopsies (Table 2).

References

1. Roth JLA (1963) Reflux esophagitis and esophageal ulcer. Gastroenterology vol. 1 (Chapter 11), 247–288, Sounders WB company Third Edition (ed Bockus HL), Philadelphia
2. Hershfield NB, Lind JF, Hildes JA et al. (1965) Secretory function of Barrett's epithelium. Gut 6:535–539

Are there specific radiologic signs in Barrett's esophagus?

M. Levesque, P. Legmann, L. Engelhom, F. de Broucker, and *J. Pringot* (Paris and Brussels)

In most cases, columnar lined esophagus (CLE) is a consequence of gastroesophageal reflux. It has been observed in 8 to 20% of patients who undergo endoscopic examinations for esophagitis [9], and in 44% of patients with chronic peptic strictures [8].

The task of the radiologist is to identify the signs of reflux esophagitis, to be aware of circumstances that favor its development [5], and to assess the diagnosis of CLE and its complications (cancerisation).

Radiological signs of peptic esophagitis

- Thickened folds occur in 97% of cases [2, 7].
- A sliding hiatal hernia is found in 65% to 90% of cases [2, 3], often associated with gastroesophageal reflux [5, 6].
- Benign stricture formation is noted in 40% to 86% of patients [2, 3], frequently associated with ulceration [10]. Most of these strictures are confined to the distal esophagus, although a midesophageal stricture is more characteristic. The strictures, which may be short, extensive or thin, are sometimes associated with pseudo-diverticula [2].
- Superficial ulcerations or ulcers (Fig. 1, 2) are seen in 17% to 47% of cases [3, 10]. In squamous epithelium, ulcerations are superficial; whereas in the columnar mucosa they are deep [8]. A deep esophageal ulceration is very suggestive of Barrett's esophagus (Fig. 3).
- A granular pattern of the mucosa, that can be recognized by double contrast examination [7] is present in more than 50% of cases of Barrett's esophagus [1, 4, 10]. This pattern is nearly always present in cases of stricture and may be observed at any level of the esophagus (Fig. 4).
- A reticular pattern [6] is noted in 20% to 25% of cases [1, 3], and is usually found if stenosis [2, 6] or ulceration [10] are present (Fig. 5).

As with reflux esophagitis, most of the findings of Barrett's esophagus occur in the lower esophagus. The appearance of the esophagus in cases of CLE ranges from slightly to grossly abnormal.

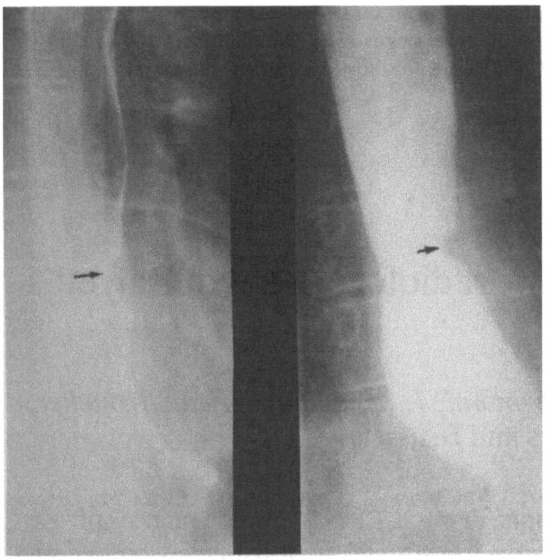

Fig. 1. Hiatal hernia, ulcer and large folds. CLE probable

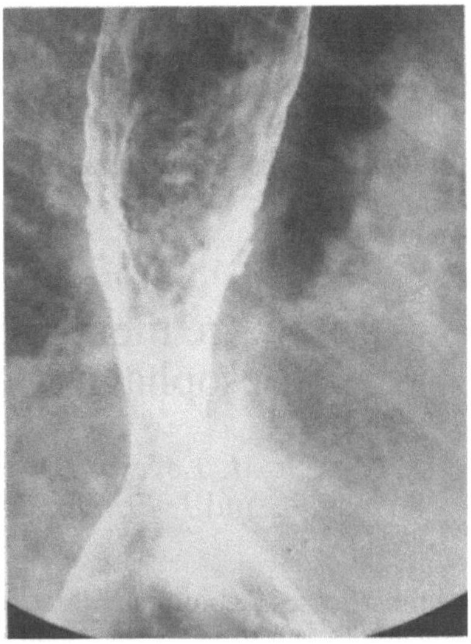

Fig. 2. Superficial ulcer, hiatal hernia with excessive nodularity. CLE probable

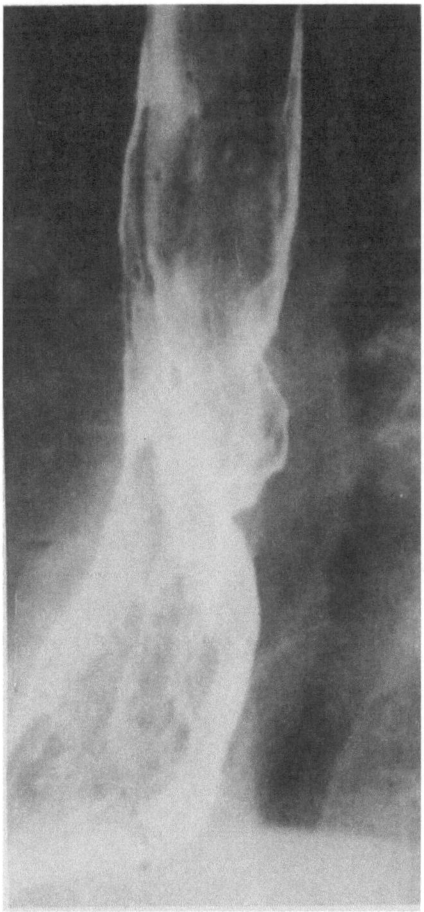

Fig. 3. Large Barrett's ulcer

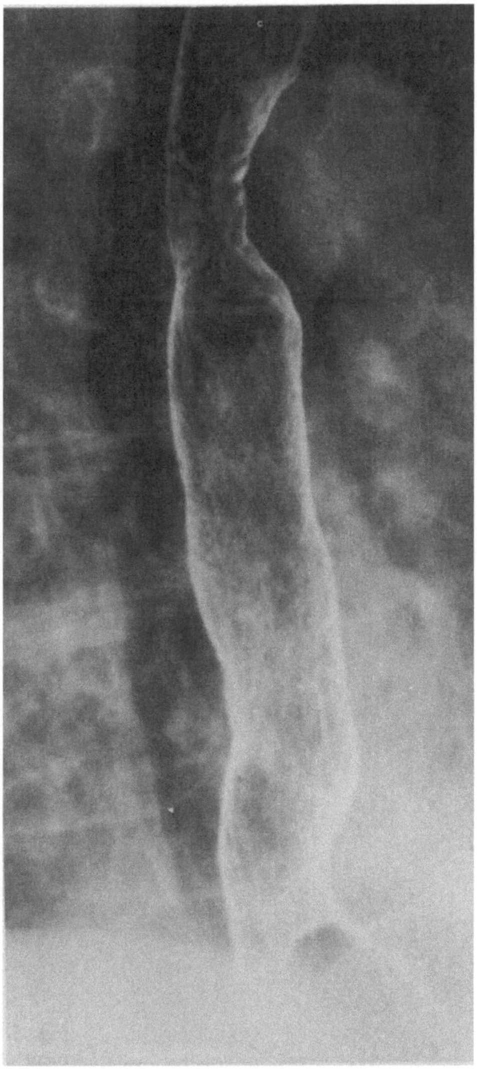

Fig. 4. CLE. Granular-nodular pattern under a stenosis

Nevertheless, certain signs strongly suggest this diagnosis: midesophageal stricture which may or may not be associated with an ulcer, sliding hiatal hernia and gastroesophageal reflux, abnormal granular or reticular pattern [1, 4, 6].

Clinical states that promote secondary lower esophageal sphincter incompetence

A CLE may be observed in circumstances which interfere with the functioning of the inferior esophageal spincter [5], such as:

- scleroderma

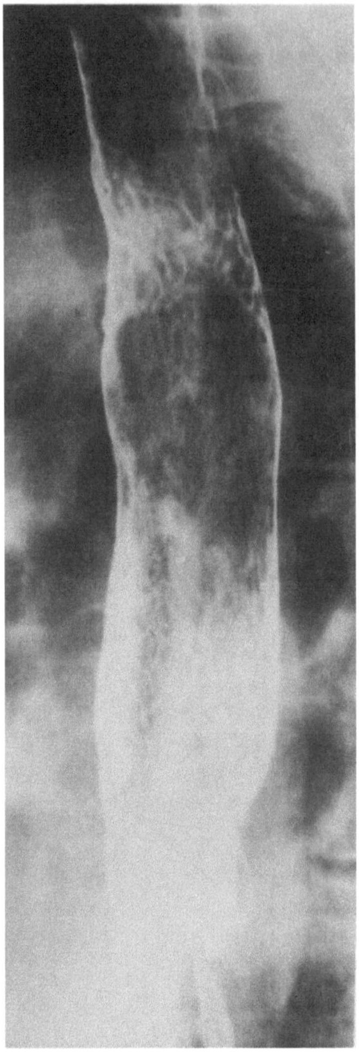

Fig. 5. Nodular and reticular pattern above Barrett's ulcer

- myotomy for achalasia
- gastric surgery
- long continued naso-gastric intubation.

Conclusion

The radiological findings of Barrett's esophagus (CLE) are those of a long standing reflux esophagitis and its sequelae [8, 9]. There is no radiologic sign specific [3, 10] for this condition. However, the association of several signs is sufficient to strongly suggest a diagnosis of CLE, which should be kept in mind whenever are observed radiologic signs of severe esophagitis, particularly if they are accompanied by ulcer or stricture.

References

1. Agha FP (1986) Radiologic diagnosis of Barrett's esophagus. Clinical analysis of 65 cases. Gastro-intest Radiol 11: 128–130
2. Chen YM, Gelfand DW, Ott DJ, Wu WC (1985) Barrett's esophagus as an extension of severe esophagitis. Analysis of radiographic signs in 29 cas. AJR. 145: 275–281
3. Chernin MM, Amberg JR, Kogan FJ, Morgan TR, Sampliner RE (1986) Efficacy of radiologic studies in the detection of Barrett's esophagus. AJR. 147: 257–260
4. Graziani L, Bearzi J, Romagnoni A, Pesaresi A, Montesi A (1985) Significance of diffuse granularity and nodularity of the esophageal mucosa at double-contrast radiography. Gastro Intest Radiol 10: 1–6
5. Halpert RD, Feczko PJ, Chason DP (1984) Barrett's esophagus: radiological and clinical considerations. J Canad Assoc Radiol 35: 120–123
6. Levine MS, Kressel HY, Caroline DF, Laufer I, Herlinger M, Thompson JJ (1983) Barrett's esophagus: reticular pattern of the mucosa. Rad 147: 663–667
7. McDermott P, Wallers KJ, Holden R, James WB (1982) Double contrast examination of the esophagus: the radiological changes of peptic esophagitis. Clin Radiol 33: 259–264
8. Spechler SJ, Goyal RK (1986) Barrett's esophagus. The New Engl J Med 315: 362–371
9. Starnes VA, Adkins RB, Balliner JF, Sawyers JL (1984) Barrett's esophagus: a surgical entity. Arch Surg 119: 563–567
10. Vincent MC, Robbins AH, Spechler SJ, Schwartz R, Doos WC, Schimmel EM (1984) The reticular pattern as a radiographic sign of the Barrett's esophagus: an assessment. Rad 153: 333–335.

A. H. Robbins (Boston)

The more common radiologic signs of the columnar-lined or Barrett esophagus include hiatal hernia, GE reflux, esophageal stricture, mucosal abnormalities (thickening, granularity, nodularity, irregularity, reticular pattern), ulcer niche and distal esophageal widening. Infrequently seen are fixed spiral folds, cricopharyngeal dysfunction, intramural diverticula, and esophagogastric polyp-fold (Table 1).

Most radiologically detectable lesions in Barrett's will be in the distal esophagus and will be generally indistinguishable from findings that would be produced by severe reflux esophagitis uncomplicated by the presence of columnar epithelium. When one detects the presence of a stricture and/or ulcer proximal to the distal esophagus, one should strongly suspect Barrett's esophagus (Table 2).

However, most radiologic signs have been disappointing at best as reliable predictors of the presence of Barrett epithelium. In our experience this includes the reticular pattern that was thought originally to be a specific criterion for the Barrett's esophagus [5]. Subsequent work at several centers has shown such a pattern to be non-specific also (Table 3).

The possibility of Barrett's esophagus [2, 3, 8] should be considered whenever findings of severe esophagitis are found. However, the absence of radiologic

Table 1. Barrett's Esophagus. Common radiologic signs. (percent occurrence)

			n	HH	Reflux	Stric.	Muc. Abn.	Esoph. Ulcer
Robbins	Current	1987	180	85	63	68	77	47
Agha	Gast. Rad.	1986	65	75	58	49	31	18
Chen	AJR	1985	29	90	79	86	97	69
Chernin	AJR	1986	30	83	N/A	47	44	17
Halpert	JACR	1984	30	83	93	80	27	33
Levine	Radiology	1983	29	90	45	83	48	7
Shapir	BJR	1985	19	79	79	58	53	26
Yulish	AJR	1987	32	13	75	38	N/A	31
		Total	414	78	61	64	61	36

Table 2. Barrett's Esophagus Strictures

			(n)	%	% Dist.
Robbins	Current	1987	180	68	83
Agha	Gast. Rad.	1986	65	49	53
Chen	AJR	1985	29	86	44
Chernin	AJR	1986	30	47	N/A
Halpert	JACR	1984	30	80	79
Levine	Radiology	1983	29	83	54
Shapir	BJR	1985	19	58	73
Yulish	AJR	1987	32	38	42
		Total	414	64	66

Table 3. Barrett's Esophagus – Mucosal changes. (percent occurrence)

			(n)	Muc. Abn.	Ret. Patt.
Robbins	Current	1987	180	77	26
Agha	Gast. Rad.	1986	65	31	8
Chen	AJR	1985	29	97	21
Halpert	JACR	1984	30	27	0
Levine	Radiology	1983	29	48	24
Shapir	BJR	1985	19	53	5
Yulish	AJR	1987	32	N/A	N/A
Chernin	AJR	1986	30	44	27
		Total	414	61	19

abnormality does not rule out the presence of Barrett's esophagus because it has been well documented that esophagograms may be normal despite the condition being present.

References

1. Agha FP (1986) Radiologic diagnosis of Barrett's esophagus: critical analysis of 65 cases. Gastrointest Radiol 11: 128–130
2. Chen YM, Gelfand DW, Ott DJ, Wu WC (1985) Barrett esophagus as an extension of severe esophagitis: analysis of radiologic signs in 29 cases. AJR 145: 275–281
3. Chernin MM, Amberg JR, Kogan FJ, Morgan TR, Sampliner RE (1986) Efficacy of radiologic studies in the detection of Barrett's esophagus. AJR 147: 257–260
4. Halpert RD, Feezko PJ, Chason DP (1984) Barrett's esophagus: radiological and clinical considerations. Journal de l'Association Canadienne des Radiologistes 35: 120–123
5. Levine MS, Kressel HY, Caroline DF, Laufer I, Herlinger H, Thompson JT (1983) Barrett esophagus: reticular pattern of the mucosa. Radiology 147: 663–667
6. Robbins AH, Vincent ME, Saini M, Schimmel EM (1978) Revised radiologic concepts of the Barrett esophagus. Gastrointest Radiol 3: 377–381
7. Shapir J, DeBrow R, Frank P (1985) Barrett oesophagus: analysis of 19 cases. The British Journal of Radiology 58: 491–493
8. Vincent ME, Robbins AH, Spechler SJ, Schwartz R, Doos WG, Schimmel EM (1984) The reticular pattern as a radiographic sign of the Barrett esophagus: an assessment. Radiology 153: 333–335
9. Yulish BS, Rothstein FC, Halpin TC Jr. (1987) Radiographic findings in children and young adults with Barrett's esophagus. AJR 148: 353–357

Is post-prandial pH measurement an adequate method of diagnosis?

G. Cargill, and *M. Duché* (Paris)

It is not conventional to include post-prandial pH measurement in the range of techniques for the diagnosis of endobrachyesophagus and we are unaware of any studies on the subject. Schlesinger [1] has recently shown that pH measurement does not allow identification of patients exhibiting risks of developing endobrachyesophagus, finding no difference in 24 hour pH measurement between the reflux of endobrachyesophagus and that of erosive esophagitis. The parameters studied on this occasion were the mean age of patients, the inferior sphincteric pressure, esophageal emptying, the time passed at pH 4 in decubitus and vertical positions and the number of episodes exceeding 5 minutes.

However, this study is inconsistent with that of DeMeester [2], who clearly shows that endobrachyesophagus is the ultimate stage of reflux disorder. The sphincteric pressure is significantly lower than in esophagitis and the proportion of time spent at pH 4 significantly greater, as is the number of longer episodes; finally, clearance is of less good quality.

However, considering the question asked us, we reviewed the pH measurement scores of 30 cases of uncomplicated reflux esophagitis, 30 cases of esophagitis complicated with ulceration and 30 of endobrachyesophagus.

The technique used for this short study was the standard technique described by Kaye, with post-prandial recording over 3 hours, after a test meal. The only parameter studied here was the global Kaye score. This was as follows:

- 188/333±145,892 in the first series (uncomplicated GER)
- 344.8±207.444 in the second series (GER with ulcerated esophagitis)
- 883.06±234.264 in the third series (EBE)

This last very high value was significantly higher than that noted in uncomplicated reflux ($\alpha < 0.001$) or in GER complicated by esophagitis ($\alpha < 0.001$). However, there exists a zone of overlap of considerable degree between these different series, which does not allow of diagnosis by means of pH measurement. The pH measurement data obtained here, while imprecise, are consistent with the manometric and pH data reported by DeMeester. On the other hand, these are markedly opposed to the work of Schlesinger cited above, and we are unable to explain this major difference.

The possible explanation of the very high Kaye scores observed in endobrachyesophagus is the presence of gastric mucosa close to the sound. In fact, in this study the sounds were positioned in terms of the manometric data and not in relation to the potential difference which marks passage of the line Z.

In sum, while pH measurement cannot be considered a diagnostic factor in endobrachyesophagus, this short study, currently in progress and contradictory to certain current data, does clearly show that this examination is an important element in assessment.

References

1. Schlesinger PK, Schmid B (1987) Esophageal pH profiles fail to identify patients at risk for development of Barrett's esophagus Digestive Disease Week, Chicago May 10–13
2. Iascone CL, DeMeester TR, et al. (1983) Barrett's esophagus. Arch Surg 118: 543–549

H. F. Weiser (Munich)

Reported series showed that 24 h pH monitoring is an accurate test with high sensitivity, specificity and of great validity for the diagnosis of reflux disease (Table 1).

Nevertheless the 24 hr period of esophageal pH-monitoring is unpleasant for the patients and sometimes requires overnight admission to hospital. It would therefore be more convenient for the patient if shorter periods of pH-monitoring could be achieved in a more practical test, without losing its diagnostic accuracy [2, 4].

Table 1. pH-metry compared to endoscopy. Own results on 163 patients

	stage 1	stage 2	stage 3–4
sensitivity	94%	52%	72%
specificity	85%	88%	97%
pos. pred. value	90%	50%	86%
neg. pred. value	91%	89%	93%
validity	91%	82%	91%

In recent studies, good correlations between different pH-monitoring phases and reflux complaints were demonstrated, so that a reduction of long-term pHmetry to the postprandial phase for diagnosis of reflux disease seems possible. But it is important to notice that these results were obtained under standardized conditions without regard to a patient-specific nutritional and behavioristic reflux profile [1, 3].

The aim of this study was therefore to find out whether the diagnosis of reflux disease under physiologic conditions, obtained by a pH-profile that is specific to different monitoring phases, is possible and would correlate with endoscopic findings.

For this reason the findings in 163 patients, 102 male, 61 female, with a mean age of 50.1 years were analyzed retrospectively. All patients showed a reflux esophagitis endoscopically and had a pathological long-term pH-metry. During statistical analysis the results of the different measuring phases were compared with each other and also correlated with the stages 1–4 of reflux esophagitis Fig. 1.

In our patients we found; with regard to the total number of patients with endoscopically proven reflux disease of different stages, that the best correlation was between the profiles of the 18 h total phase and the 8 hr awake phase.

Sufficient correlation coefficients would be demonstrated between total and sleeping phase, total and empty stomach phase, empty stomach and awake phase.

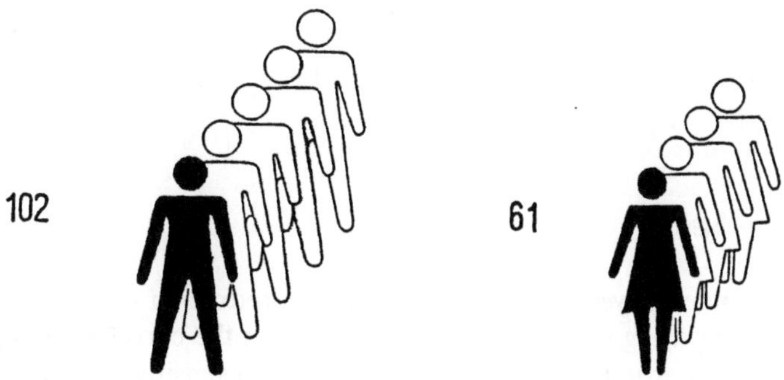

		$\bar{X}$=48.3 years		$\bar{X}$=51.3 years
esophagitis stage	1	63% ($\bar{X}$=47.2 years)	1	58% ($\bar{X}$=47.0 years)
	2	15% ($\bar{X}$=46.3 years)	2	21% ($\bar{X}$=45.8 years)
	3–4	22% ($\bar{X}$=60.2 years)	3–4	21% ($\bar{X}$=58.0 years)

Fig. 1. Age distribution of 163 patients with esophagitis stage 1–4; average age: $\bar{X}$=50.1 years

Table 2. Long-term pHmetry. Correlation between different measuring periods under physiological conditions

total	– awake	r=0.92
total	– sleep	r=0.89
total	– postprandial	r=0.58
total	– empty stomach	r=0.84
empty stomach	– awake	r=0.87
awake	– sleep	r=0.69

There was a moderate correlation between awake phase and sleeping phase, caused by a significantly higher reflux in the awake phase of the clearly more strongly represented patients with moderate reflux disease; the mild-moderate ratio in our patients was 1:4 ($p < 0.01$) Table 2.

Trying to demonstrate a correlation of pH-profiles of different measuring phases at different endoscopic stages of reflux esophagitis, we found that this was best for the total phase.

For stage 2 (moderate) reflux esophagitis only, the postprandial phase seems to offer the best diagnostic value, since 70% of the cases could be pointed-out in this group correctly Table 3.

Table 3. Different phases of pH-metry and correlating endoscopic findings in %

	stage 1	stage 2	Stage 3–4	stage 1–4
Total measuring period (18 h)	93	52	72	79
Awake phase (8 h)	72	53	50	64
Empty stomach phase (5 h)	69	30	47	57
Postprandial phase (3 h)	31	70	53	63
Sleeping phase (8 h)	83	40	62	71

Conclusions

1. Under physiological conditions, the reduction of long-term pHmetry to single measuring phases leads to a decrease in the correlation between endoscopic and pH-metric findings and to a decrease in sensitivity and specificity of pHmetry.
2. In order to be able to differentiate between the stages of reflux disease as accurately as possible, and for the deduction of therapeutic consequences from the reflux profile, it is absolutely necessary to evaluate the 18 h total phase.
3. In patients with moderate reflux disease only, an improvement of the diagnostic score can be achieved by looking at the postprandial phase separately.

References

1. Branicki FJ, Evans DF, Jones JA, Hardcastle JD (1986) A short term radiotelemetric reflux provocation test for the diagnosis of gastro-esophageal reflux (GER) disease Intern Esophageal Week, Sept. 14–19, Munich
2. DeMeester TR, Johnson LF, Joseph GJ, Toscano MS, Hall AW, Skinner DB (1976) Patterns of gastroesophageal reflux in health and disease. Ann Surg 184: 459–470
3. Rokkas T, Anggiansah A, Uzoechina E, Owen WJ, Sladen GE (1986) The role of shorter than 24-h pH monitoring periods in the diagnosis of gastro-oesophageal reflux. Scand J Gastroenterol 21: 614–620
4. Weiser HF, Lange R, Bollschweiler E (1986) Intraesophageal 24-pH-metry: an indispensible tool for the diagnosis of reflux disorders. Intern Esophageal Week, Sept. 14–19, Munich

What is the importance of the difference of esophageal potentials after manometry in the diagnosis of Barrett's esophagus?

G. Cargill, and *M. Duché* (Paris)

Measurement of potential difference (PD) is not performed after manometry, but during endoscopy or during manometry.

Endoscopically, it suffices to pass a pH-metric sound of small caliber through the operating channel to measure, under visual control, the PD at any given point in the esophagus. To do so, the reference electrode, preferably on glass-calomel, should be connected to the patient by an agar bridge.

However, it is possible to perform measurement directly during manometry (Fig. 1) by perfusing, with the aid of the pneumohydraulic infuser, not water but Ringer's solution. An agar bridge is established between the head of pressure involved and the pH electrode, while a second agar bridge makes a reference connection to the glass-calomel and subcutaneous tissue. Thus, it is possible to measure the intragastric PD in relation to the inferior esophageal sphincter. At passage of the line Z, the potential, which within the stomach is of the order of –30/–40 mV, suddenly changes to –7/–8 mV, which makes it possible to define very precisely the height of extent of the endobrachyesophagus.

The sensitivity, of this method is 0.8 and its specificity 0.7. Though attractive, it is nevertheless tricky to operate because of the technical difficulty of handling. Apart from assessment of the extent of the endobrachyesophagus, it should allow positioning of the pH sounds, not only in relation to the LES but also in relation to the Z electrical line. Other applications may be possible as much in the esophagus as in the colo-anal region.

We thank Dr. Ottignon (Besançon) for his help in devising this technique

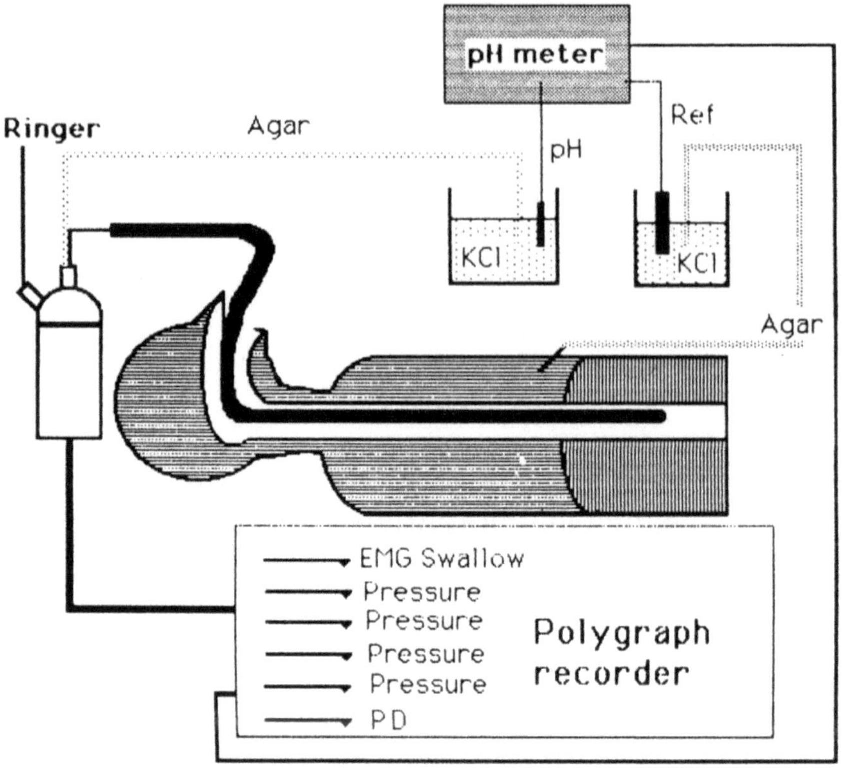

Fig. 1. Direct measurement of PD during manometry

Are the histochemical and immuno-cyto-chemical criteria useful?

B. Dupin, L. Garbe, E. Ragni, R. Giudicelli, P. Fuentes, and *E. Reboud* (Marseilles)

Columnar epithelium-lined esophagus, called Barrett's esophagus is a complication of gastroesophageal reflux (GER) in 20% of cases. Columnar metaplasic mucosa is probably more frequent if limited types of Barrett's esophagus are included.

The most important problem of this epithelium is the risk of cancer. According to Savary [1], adenocarcinoma develops in 15.7% of cases and other authors have reported higher figures up to 46% [2]. Indeed a lot of primary esophageal adenocarcinoma probably involves Barrett's epithelium [4, 5], this epithelium having been missed in histologic study.

It is now generally accepted that adenocarcinoma occurring on Barrett's esophagus evolves through a spectrum of neoplastic changes in the mucosa ranging from low grade dysplasia to high grade and carcinoma in situ. The presence of dysplasia dictates an endoscopic follow up and can be an indication for esophageal resection in the case of persistent high grade dysplasia. Conversely, the frequent regression of moderate grade dysplasia after surgical anti-reflux procedure is an argument for this treatment in Barrett's esophagus but the success of surgical treatment should be assessed by pH monitoring.

Authors have different opinions about the usefulness and the frequency of endoscopic follow up after anti-reflux procedure. It seems difficult to impose an endoscopic examination every year or every 18 months, moreover it is not cost effective.

To gain insight into this problem, we try to ascertain the histologic and especially histochemical profile of high risk patient for the development of adenocarcinoma, requiring regular endoscopic examinations.

Histochemical study in Barrett's esophagus

Columnar epithelium is classified according to Paull's criteria in three distinct categories: the fundic type, the junctional type and the specialized type that resembles intestinal metaplasia. By analogy with gastric cancer, Potet supposed that the presence of intestinal metaplasia secreting sulfomucins must be considered as a precancerous lesion.

The histochemical study [3, 6] of acid mucins, sialo and sulfomucins, is performed after staining with Alcian Blue (AB) pH 1.5 and 2.5 and High Iron Diamine (HID) to differentiate sialomucins and sulfomucins, sulfomucins being stained in dark-brown with HID.

So we have performed this histochemical study in two groups of patients: the first group [7] with adenocarcinoma complicating Barrett's epithelium and the second with Barrett's esophagus without tumor.

Comparison between histologic and histochemical findings in these 2 groups:

Study of Barrett's epithelium associated with adenocarcinoma

Between 1979 and 1986, 56 primary esophageal adenocarcinomas were resected and submitted to histologic study. We can affirm that adenocarcinoma developed from Barrett's esophagus in 20 cases. The histologic and histochemical study of non malignant areas of Barrett's epithelium gave the following results:

- specialized epithelium in 17 cases with association of at least 2 types in 14 patients.
- dysplasia in 14 cases with 7 cases of high grade or in situ carcinoma.
- Sulfomucins on specialized epithelium in 14 cases. (Table 1).

Table 1. Barrett's esophagus with adenocarcinoma: 20 cases

study on resected specimens
specialized=17
dysplasia=14
sulfomucins=14/17
clinical study GER in 16 patients

Table 2. Barrett's Esophagus without tumor: 36 patients

Study on endoscopic biopsy
Savary's classification:
type 1:15
type 2:6
type 3:15
specialized=27
dysplasia=8
sulfomucins=12/27
GER in 35 cases
anti-reflux procedure in 26 patients

Study of Barrett's esophagus without tumor

In 1984, we began a prospective histologic and histochemical study on endoscopic biopsies in patients with barrett's epithelium. Presently, we have 36 cases. In this group, only one patient had no reflux on pHmonitoring and scintigraphic examination, and out of these 36 cases, 26 patients were referred to us for an anti-reflux procedure (Table 2). The results were:

- according to Savary's endoscopic classification, Barrett's esophagus was classified as type 1 in 15 cases, type 2 in 6 and type 3 in 15.
- specialized epithelium was found in 27 cases with association of 2 types in 10 cases.
- dysplasia was present in 8 cases with high grade dysplasia in one patient.
- sulfomucins were present in 12 cases out of the 27 specialized types.

Comments

Our study, although it compares histologic findings from resected specimens and endoscopic biopsies, is interesting for three reasons (Table 3).

1. No significant difference exists between epihelium types in Barrett's esophagus adjacent to the tumor and Barrett's without tumor: the most frequent type is the specialized epithelium: 85% in Barrett's esophagus with tumor and 75% in Barrett's without tumor, according to other authors' findings.

Table 3. Comments

1. no difference between histologic types
2. dysplasia: 70% tumoral group versus 22% non tumoral group
3. sulfomucins: 82.4% tumoral group versus 44.4% non tumoral group

2. Frequency of dysplasia is significant higher in the tumoral group (70%) than the non tumoral group (22%); this difference is even greater for high grade dysplasia (35% versus 2.7%). These results are in agreement with previous reports.
3. Conversely, the histochemical comparative study of sulfomucins in specialized epithelium (unpublished) shows a significant difference between the 2 groups: 82.4% in the tumoral group and 44.4% in the non tumoral group. This latter percentage confirms Potet's [3] findings (53% on biopsy specimens in 17 patients with Barrett's esophagus).

Conclusion

Malignant transformation of Barrett's epithelium is now widely accepted; however contreversy remains over the usefullness of endoscopic surveillance in every case. The presence of dysplasia is a major criteria justifying regular endoscopy and its persistence may be an indication for esophageal resection. In absence of dysplasia, our data suggests that specialized epithelium secreting sulfomucins should be considered as a high risk situation requiring regular endoscopic and histologic examination (12 to 18 months) in order to allow early detection of dysplasia or in situ carcinoma.

We are now pursuing our study to determine firstly, if an anti-reflux procedure leads to regression of columnar epithelium and secondly, if long term secretion of sulfomucins is changed by such a procedure.

References

1. Savary M, Monnier P (1985) Diagnosis, pathophysiology, and adenocarcinogenesis of Barrett's esophagus. Esophageal Disorders: pathophysiology and therapy, edited by DeMeester TR, Skinner DB, Raven Press, New York
2. Haggitt RC, Tryzelaar J, Ellis FH, Colcher H (1978) Adenocarcinoma complicating columnar epithelium-lined (Barrett's) esophagus. Am J Clin Pathol 70: 1–5
3. Peuchmaur M, Potet F, Goldfain D (1984) Mucin histochemistry of columnar epithelium of the esophagus (Barrett's Esophagus): a prospective biopsy study. J Clin Pathol 37: 607–610
4. Skinner DB, Walter BC, Riddell RH, Schmidt H, Iascone C, DeMeester TR (1983) Barrett's esophagus: comparison of benign and malignant cases. Ann Surg 198: 554–566
5. Kalish RJ, Clancy PE, Orringer MB, Appelman HD (1984) A clinical, epidemiologic and morphology comparison between adenocarcinoma arising in Barrett's esophageal mucosa and in gastric cardia. Gastroenteerology 86: 461–467

6. Jass JR (1981) Mucin histochemistry of the columnar epithelium of esophagus. A retrospective study. J Clin Pathol 34: 866–870
7. Dupin B, Garbe L, Fuentes P, Giudicelli R, Reboud E (1986) Adenocarcinoma complicating columnar epithelium-lined (Barrett's) esophagus: a clinical and histological study. International Esophageal Week, Munich, September 14–19

Ch. Fontolliet, J. Hurlimann, and *D. Gardiol* (Lausanne)

Three types of cylinder-cell epithelium lining Barrett's esophagus have been described [5]:
1. an epithelium of gastric fundus type
2. an epithelium of gastric cardiac type
3. an epithelium of specialized type which is probably the precursor of dysplasia [1] and which therefore needs to be identified.

This epithelium is a mosaic of varied cell-types [8, 9], each exhibiting its specific histochemical properties. The mucous cells have a basal nucleus and an apical clear cytoplasm like those lining the normal stomach. The goblet cells are identical to those of the small intestine or colon. The cylinder cells resemble enterocytes, but contain glycoproteins in the apical part of their cytoplasm and do not always exhibit a clearly recognizable brush border. More rarely, neuroendocrine cells and Paneth cells with intracytoplasmic eosinophil granules are found.

Does the specialized epithelium consist of cells with special histochemical and immunohistochemical properties favoring the development of dysplasia? Is histochemistry a useful or indispensable method in the diagnosis of preneoplastic lesions?

Our attempt to answer these questions is based on a personal study of 39 specimens from esophagectomy for Barrett's adenocarcinoma, associated with dysplasia in 36 cases, severe in 21 of these cases.

Staining with hematoxylin-eosin, PAS-Alcian Blue (AB) at pH 2.5, AB at pH 1.5 and High Iron Diamine-AB by Spicer's method [7] was performed on several samples from cases of specialized epithelium, with and without dysplasia. The histochemical results were estimated qualitatively (type of secretion) and quantitatively (number of cells and of positive or negative foci), done subjectively without morphometric analysis. In 12 of these cases we performed histoimmunochemical examination by Pap's method, using 5 lectins (SBA, WGA, VEA, DBA, RCA) and 8 antisera (antikeratin, anti-SC, antiprealbumin, anti-CEA, anti-IgA, antigastrin, antiserotonin, anti-FGM). The immunohistochemical results were compared with those obtained in normal gastric, jejunal and duodenal mucosae. They were assessed quantitatively (intensity of staining) and qualitatively (localization throughout cytoplasm, apical, cuticular, supranuclear).

Our histochemical study confirms the heterogeneity of the mucins of the specialized nondysplastic epithelium [3, 4]. In all the cell types described, even in the mucous cells of gastric type, we were able to demonstrate acid mucins, sulfo- and/or

Table 1. Presence of secretion of acid mucins: relation to dysplasia

	Negative for sialomucins N 3	Negative for sulfomucins N 5	Negative for acid mucins N 1
Without dysplasia N 3	0	0	0
With dysplasia N 8	3	5	1
With severe dysplasia N 6	3	3	1

sialomucins, by staining with HID-AB. The expression of the secretion of all the mucins varied from one specimen to another, both qualitatively and quantitatively. The dysplastic epithelium loses its secretory capacity and this tendency increases in parallel with the degree of dysplasia.

Some authors [2, 6] have asserted that the demonstration of sulfomucins in the alimentary epithelia indicates a predisposition to the development of preneoplastic lesions. Dysplasia was found in 36 of our 39 patients, and assessed as severe in 21 cases. All but one showed secretion of sialo- and/or sulfomucins.

In 19 cases, sialomucin secretion predominated, in 4 cases that of sulfomucins. The two types of secretion were equally represented in 16 cases. The sulfomucins were less abundant than the sialomucins, even in the cases with severe dysplasia (Table 1). 3 cases showed no sialomucin secretion and 5 were negative for sulfomucins. The case without secretion of acid mucins exhibited severe dysplasia. The cases negative for sialo or sulfomucine were associated 6 times with severe dysplasia and twice with moderate dysplasia (Table 2). To sum up, our study does not suggest any relation between the presence of a particular type of acid mucin and that of preneoplastic lesions.

The immunohistochemistry of the specialized epithelium, with and without dysplasia, is nonspecific. In these two categories the pattern is varied both quantitatively and qualitatively. Its appearance is nearly always that of a mosaic, with markedly positive cells or zones adjacent to frankly negative cells or zones. From the immunologic point of view, the nondysplastic specialized epithelium does not differ from the dysplastic epithelium, and no transition from one type of epithelium to the

Table 2. Absence of secretion of acid mucins relation to dysplasia

	Sialomucins predominant N 19	Sulfomucins predominant N 4	Mixed N 16
Without dysplasia N 3	2	0	1
With dysplasia N 36	17	4	15
With severe dysplasia N 21	9	3	9

other was noted. The immunologic aspect of the specialized epithelium is of intestinal type, with positivity of the surface cells for SC and CEA; the glands are positive for lysozyme and there is a predominance of IgA plasmocytes. Numerous cells are positive for serotonin, but none for gastrin. Positivity for the different lectins is mosaic and particularly polarized (cuticle, apical cytoplasm, Golgi apparatus). The intestinal immunologic aspect persists in dysplasia. However, the localization of CEA is more diffuse in the cytoplasm and staining with certain lectins (SBA, DBA) is less abundant.

In conclusion, in our experience neither the histochemistry nor the immunohistochemistry permit the recognition of a particular type of specialized epithelium as a precursor to neoplasia.

References

1. Hamilton SR, Smith RR (1987) The relationship between columnar epithelial dysplasia and invasive adenocarcinoma arising in Barrett's esophagus. Am J Clin Pathol 87: 301–312
2. Jass JR (1980) Role of intestinal metaplasia in the histogenesis of gastric carcinoma J Clin Pathol 33: 801–810
3. Jass JR (1981) Mucin histochemistry of the columnar epithelium of the oesophagus: a retrospective study. J Clin Pathol 34: 866–870
4. Lee RG (1984) Mucins in Barrett's Esophagus: a histochemical study. Am J Clin Pathol 81: 500–503
5. Paull A, Trier JS, Dalton MD, Camp RC, Loeb P, Goyal RK (1976) The histologic spectrum of Barrett's esophagus. N Engl J Med 295: 476–480
6. Penchmaur M, Potet F, Goldgain D (1984) Mucin histochemistry of the columnar epithelium of the esophagus (Barrett's oesophagus): a prospective biopsy study. J Clin Pathol 37: 607–610
7. Spicer SS (1965) Diamine methods for differentiation mucosubstances histochemically J Histochem Cytochem 13: 211–234
8. Thompson JJ, Zinsser KR, Enterline HT (1983) Barrett's metaplasia and adenocarcinoma of the esophagus and gastroesophageal junction. Hum Pathol 14: 42–61
9. Zwas F, Shields HM, Doos WG (1986) Scanning electron microscopy of Barrett's epithelium and its correlation with light microscopy and mucins stains. Gastroenterology 90: 1932–1941.

How long does it take for Barrett's esophagus to develop?

C. G. Bremner (Johannesburg)

Barrett's columnar-lined esophagus (CLE) is the result of a creeping substitution of reflux denuded squamous epithelium by columnar epithelium which is derived from the gastric fundic epithelium. Experimental and clinical evidence has shown that the replacement process is a very slow one. The process is one of repair, and the denuded segment is the stimulus for replacement by acid-resistent columnar epithelium

Table 1. The rate of columnar replacement in the experimental animal is 0,75 – lmm/week

1. Without histamine stimulation: (28 mm in 400 days) = 0,75 mm/week wet specimen
2. With histamine stimulation: (40 mm in 404 days) = 1,0 mm/week wet specimen

Rate of columnar replacement in the experimental model

The replacement was accelerated in the reflux model by mucosal stripping and histamine stimulation (Table 1). After 404 days of reflux, a length of 40 mm of columnar epithelium was measured in the formalinized specimen. The reflux model without stimulation had a slower rate of replacement and after 400 days, a length of 28 mm replacement was measured. Allowing for shrinkage in the formalin, the lengths would be approximately 60 mm and 42 mm.

This gives a replacement rate of approximately 0,15 mm/day in the stimulated model and 0,1 mm/day in the intact unstimulated model. The rate of replacement was very much slower in the dog model when acid was not stimulated. This is not surprising because the dog has an interdigestive mechanism of acid secretion, and the stimulated model of continued acid secretion would be more appropriate as a comparison with the human situation. The fact that the acid stimulated model showed a more rapid regeneration rate is also of interest because in a series of 72 patients tested it was shown that patients with a CLE have had statistically more esophageal acid exposures than patients with esophagitis, and also had a greater number of reflux episodes lasting longer than 5 minutes. Furthermore, the extent of the Barrett's mucosal change was related to the level of the LES pressure and the number of reflux episodes that were five minutes or longer in duration [4].

Rate of Replacement in Humans (Table 2)

It is difficult to assess the rate of replacement in man because the duration of symptoms given is always vague. Borrie and Goldwater [2] documented the rate of replacement on repeat endoscopic studies, and noted a 5 cm replacement in 3 years and 17 cm in 10 years.

Table 2. The rate of columnar replacement on endoscopic follow-up (5 cases) is approx 17 mm/year

	Years	Length (cm)	Rate per year (mm)
Goldman & Beckman 1960	7	11	15,7
Mossberg 1966	2,5	20	80
Halvorsen 1975	9	15	16,6
Borrie & Goldwater 1976	10	17	17
	3	5	1,6

Table 3. The rate of columnar replacement as assessed by the duration of reflux is approx 4,8 mm/year (300 patient-years)

Duration of reflux vs length of Replacement
15 patients
300 patient years of reflux: 1460 mm
4.8 mm/year

We have tried to extrapolate a rate of growth from the duration of reflux as given by the patient and the length of columnar epithelium measured at endoscopy. Three hundred patients-years of reflux resulted in 146 mm of columnar epithelium (i.e. 4.8 mm/year) Table 3. Clearly there is a wide variation in the rate depending on the severity of reflux, acid clearing and epithelial regeneration properties.

The remarkable follow-up observation by Halvorsen and Semb [5] on a single patient over a 9 year period showed a replacement of 15 cm in length. Moosberg [6] gave a very detailed history of a careful follow-up in a single case, and a length of 20 cm of columnar epithelium apparently developed over a 30 month period. A similar follow-up over a 7 year period by Goldman and Beckman [7] documented a 7 cm growth of columnar epithelium in 11 years.

*

There are few records of careful documentation of the rate of growth of columnar epithelium in patients with gastroesophageal reflux. The two longest periods of follow-up suggest that the rate is approximately 17 mm/year Table 4.

Table 4. Summary of Results

		mm/year
A. Experiment:	Unstimulated	38,5
	Stimulated	54,5
B. Endoscopic (5 patients)		17
C. History (15 patients)		4,8

References

1. Bremner CG, Lynch VP, Ellis FH Jr (1970) Barrett's esophagus: Congenital or Acquired? An experimental study of mucosal regeneration in the dog Surgery 68(1): 209–216
2. Borrie J, Goldwater L (1976) Columnar-lined esophagus: assessment of etiology and treatment. J Thorac Cardiovasc Surg 71: 825–834
3. Pollaro W (1982) An experimental study of mucosal regeneration in Barrett's esophagus. Thesis presented to University of Sao Paulo Brazil
4. Iascone C, DeMeester TR, Little AG, Skinner DB (1983) Barrett's esophagus. Functional assessment, proposed pathogenesis, and surgical therapy. Arch Surg 118(5): 543–549
5. Halvorsen JF, Semb BKH (1975) The "Barrett Syndrome" (The columnarlined lower esophagus): An acquired condition secondary to reflux esophagitis. Acta Chir Scand 141: 683–687
6. Mossberg SM (1966) The columnar-lined esophagus (Barrett Syndrome): an acquired condition? Gastroenterology 50: 671–676
7. Goldman MC and Beckmann RC (1960) Barrett Syndrome. Case report with discussion about concepts and pathogenesis. Gastroenterol 39: 104–110

S. Stipa, A. Moraldi, C. Iascone, M. Zerilli, and *R. Arca* (Rome)

Barrett's esophagus (B.E.) is a condition in which the lower esophagus is lined with columnar epithelium instead of the usual stratified squamous epithelium; this condition is now generally accepted as being secondary to gastroesophageal reflux. It is difficult to state how long it takes for Barrett's esophagus to develop. Data from literature vary extremely; in fact the time between the onset of symptoms and diagnosis may range from few months to many years; moreover, at the time of diagnosis, we do not know how long before the Barrett's was already evident.

Herlihy et al. [2] differentiate by endoscopy two distinct types of B. E.: a circumferential-type and an island-type; symptoms duration in 9 pts. with island-type B.E. was 8±3 years, while in 11 pts with circumferential type it was 13±3 years. Symptoms duration in all 20 patients ranged from 9 months to 25 years. The authors suggest that the island lesion, because of its association with less severe esophagitis, may be an earlier stage of B.E. than the circumferential type.

Spechler et al. [5] studied the prevalence of B.E. in 25 pts with chronic peptic esophageal strictures where Barrett's epithelium had not been identified by endoscopic biopsy performed one year or more previously. Patients were regularly followed-up and after a mean time from diagnosis of the stricture of 55.1±11.7 months (range 12–150 months) biopsies became positive for Barrett's epithelium in 11 pts (44%).

40 patients out of 439 with esophagitis documented by endoscopy were found to have B.E. by Starnes et al. [6]; 25 had benign columnar epithelium and 15 had adenocarcinoma associated with the columnar epithelium. The average duration of symptoms in the benign group was 7.2 years (range 4 months to 15 years); it was 7.3 years in the adenocarcinoma group.

The case reported by Mossberg [3] is very interesting because it represents a rare demonstration of the evolution of the disease. The patient was first seen in 1960 at age of 32, when noted heartburn and black stool; one year later for persistence of pyrosis associated with abdominal pain and an episode of hematemesis, he was hospitalized: at esophagoscopy, redness of the distal esophageal mucosa was noted and a biopsy specimen taken at 38 cm revealed squamous epithelium. On June 1962 because of persistence of symptoms and melena an esophagoscopy was repeated and showed at 38 cm a deep, posterior wall crater; a biopsy specimen was reported as acute and chronic inflammation in gastric mucosa. On August 1962, after a brisk hematemesis and melena, the patient was submitted to another esophagoscopy that revealed red, friable, bleeding esophageal mucosa starting at 20 cm from the incisor teeth and extending to the gastroesophageal junction (40 cm). Biopsy specimens taken at 22, 30 and 37 cm revealed columnar epithelium lining the esophagus, whereas tissue obtained at 18 cm was covered by squamous epithelium. In this case of particular interest is the demonstration that B.E. developed over a 30-month period.

Also Goldman and Beckman [1], documented the onset and the ascent of columnar mucosa in the esophagus over a 7 year period in a 66 year old man with symptoms duration of 13 years for recurrent esophagitis. Savary and Monnier [4] identified columnar epithelialization in the esophagus proximal to an esophagogastric anastomosis in a patient who had undergone esophagectomy and esophagogastrostomy for a lye stricture 15 years before. In another patient columnar epithelialization was observed over the course of one year and a half.

Our experience on Barrett's esophagus is very limited because of the rarity of this pathology in our area.

We want just to report a typical case of B.E. in a 35 year old woman that we have observed in November 1981. Since infancy the patient was complaining of mild dysphagia, heartburn and occasional vomiting; at six years of age, because of the persistence of symptoms, she underwent an esophagoscopy that showed an esophageal stricture at the lower third; biopsy specimen was not taken at that time. The patient was dilated few times and she did relatively well, under medical treatment, with recurrent symptoms of gastroesophageal reflux. In November 1981 the patient experienced daily episodes of epigastric and burning retrosternal pain with severe dysphagia. She was admitted in our hospital and the endoscopy performed showed a stricture at 32 cm from the incisor teeth; the mucosa proximal to the stenosis was normal, but just below it was friable, reddened and easly bleeding. Multiple biopsies were taken at the level and below the stricture and revealed columnar epithelium with interspersed goblet cells.

What we just reported is a typical case of B.E., with symptoms increasing during the years and the final diagnosis of BE, even though we do not know how long the Barrett's epithelium has been present.

*

With the exception of those rare congenital cases in which more properly we should talk about ectopy of gastric mucosa islands, Barrett's Esophagus should be considered as an acquired lesion due to chronic gastroesophageal reflux.The severity of reflux and the individual response will determine how long the B.E. takes to develop; at present, it is difficult to assess this because we diagnose the B.E. only when we observe the patient, without knowing whether the lesion was already present for few months or many years at the time of clinical observation.

References

1. Goldman MC, Beckman RC (1960) Barrett syndrome: case report with discussion about concepts of pathogenesis. Gastroenterology 39: 104
2. Herlihy KS, Orlando RC, Bryson JC, Bozymski EM, Carney CN, Powell DW (1984) Barrett's esophagus: clinical, endoscopic, histologic, manometric, and electrical potential difference characteristics. Gastroenterology 86: 436
3. Mossberg SM (1966) The columnar-lined esophagus (Barrett Syndrome). An acquired condition? Gastroenterology 50: 671
4. Savary M, Monnier P (1985) Diagnosis, pathophysiology, and adenocarcinogenesis of Barrett's esophagus. Esophageal disorders: pathophysiology, and therapy, edited by DeMeester TR, Skinner DB, Raven Press, New York
5. Spechler SJ, Sperber H, Doos WG, Schimmel EM (1983) The prevalence of Barrett's esophagus in patients with chronic peptic esophageal strictures. Digestive diseases and Sciences 28: 769
6. Starnes VA, Adkins RB, Ballinger JF, Sawyers JL (1984) Barrett's esophagus: a surgical entity. Arch. Surg 119: 563

Can the pathogenesis of this lesion be defined?

C. G. Bremner (Johannesburg)

The answer to this question is in the affirmative. The dog experimental model [1, 2] has clearly shown that in the presence of acid reflux, there is a columnar replacement of denuded squamous epithelium. There are many studies showing that Barrett's esophagus patients have a poor LES pressure, increased acid reflux and poor acid clearing [3, 4]. Sarr et al. [5] found a hypotensive lower esophageal sphincter in all of 84 patients tested. Acid reflux is also greater and acid clearing slower in patients with Barrett's when compared to normals and to patients with esophagitis in the absence of columnar lining [6]. An upward extension of the level of squamo-columnar change has also been observed by serial endoscopy in patients who were treated medically.

Hiatal hernia is also present in the majority of cases, supporting reflux, but in many of those without a hiatal hernia, including children, reflux has also been demonstrated [7]. Finally, in patients who have had esophago-gastrectomy, chronic gastro-esophageal reflux may result in a columnar replacement above the gastroesophageal anastomotic site [8].

*

The pathogenesis of Barrett's esophagus may be defined as follows: Excessive gastro-esophageal acid reflux resulting from incompetence of the lower esophageal sphincter in the presence or absence of a hiatal hernia and poor acid clearing, will denude the squamous epithelium which will be replaced by a process of creeping substitution of the columnar epithelium derived from the gastric cardia. These cells are mucous secreting but totipotent, in that gastrin, pepsin, neuroendocrine and acid secreting cells, enterochromafin and somastostatin cells are present in some specimens [9].

It is possible that duodenogastric reflux acid "alkaline" reflux results in the complication of ulceration, stricture formation and adenocarcinoma. This is more likely in smokers and in males.

References

1. Bremner CG, Lynch VP, Ellis FH Jr (1970) Barrett's esophagus: Congenital or Acquired? An experimental study of esophageal mucosal regeneration in the dog. Surgery 68(1): 209–216
2. Pollara W (1982) An experimental study of mucosal regeneration in Barrett's Esophagus. Thesis presented to University of Sao Paulo, Brazil
3. Bremner CG (1984) Barrett's esophagus. In Disorders of the oesophagus. Advances and Controversies. Ed Watson A, Celestin LR (Pitman) Pp 94: 104
4. Iascone C, DeMeester TR, Little AG, Skinner DB (1983) Barrett's esophagus. Functional assessment, proposed pathogenesis and Surgical therapy. Arch Surg 118: 543–549
5. Sarr MG, Hamilton SR, Marrone GC, Cameron JL (1985) Barrett's esophagus: Its prevalence and association with adenocarcinoma in patients with symptoms of gastroesophageal reflux. Amer J Surg 149: 187–193

6. Borrie J Goldwater L (1976) Columnar cell-lined esophagus. Assessment of etiology and treatment. J Cardiovasc Thorac Surg 71: 825–834
7. Dahms BB, Rothstein FC (1984) Barrett's esophagus in children: a consequence of chronic gastroesophageal reflux. Gastroenterology 86(2): 318–323
8. Hamilton SR, Yardley JH (1977) Regeneration of cardiac type mucosa and acquisition of Barrett's mucosa after esophago-gastrectomy. Gastroenterol 72: 669–675
9. Thompson JJ, Zinsser KK, Enterline HT (1983) Barrett's metaplasia and adenocarcinoma of the esophagus and gastroesophageal junction. Human Path 44(1): 42–61

Barrett's esophagus (2)

President: *Guo J. Huang* (Peking)

Free Commentators: *J. A. Borges d'Almeida* (Lisbon)
Y. Kawaura (Kanazawa)
H. Larrieu (Paris)
R. W. McCallum (Charlottesville)
W. J. Pories (Greenville)
E. Reboud (Marseilles)

Classifications of Barrett's esophagus

M. Savary, Ph. Monnier, J. B. Ollyo, D. Gardiol, Ch. Fontolliet, and *J. Wellinger* (Lausanne)

Endoscopy exploration with biopsy sampling is the principal means to study the columnar epithelial lining in the esophagus because of the abundance of clinical material and the precision of the macroscopic and microscopic observation that it provides and because of the possibility to repeat observations during the evolution of a living organ.

The sum of the clinical observations available at the present time form the basis for the definition of the different morphological aspects of this phenomenon. But the physiopathological and epidemiological data (prevalence and incidence) remain incomplete. When biopsies are not routinely performed at endoscopy, there are numerous false positive and false negative diagnosis of columnar epithelium lining of the esophagus, even in spite of vital colorations [3, 4].

Columnar epithelium not in continuity with the Z-line

Islands, bands, or sleeves of columnar epithelium can be found throughout the esophagus and they are characterized *by not displaying any continuity with the Z-line* (Fig. 1).

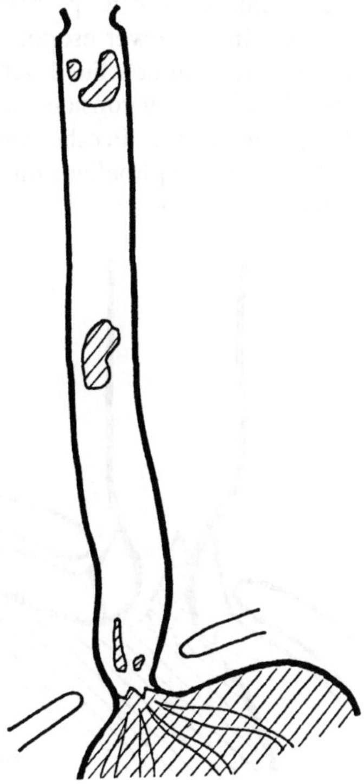

Fig. 1. Columnar epithelium lining without continuity with the Z-Line

These areas of columnar epithelium are most often found at the superior part of the cervical esophagus and are shaped as islands. Lateral as well as bilateral mirror localizations are well known. More rare are the semicircular and sleeve shapes.

The same phenomenon can be observed at the inferior part of the esophagus, shaped as longitudinal bands or islands. It is rarely found in the thoracic esophagus [4, 5].

In the majority of cases the histology of the epithelium is fundic (cervical esophagus) or cardiac (lower esophagus). Microcysts are found in half of the cases [1]. These ectopic islands are found at all ages of life. Their origin is thought to be congenital and without relation to gastroesophageal reflux [5].

It is possible that some islands and longitudinal bands in the lower esophagus, not in continuity with the Z-line, are an exception and are secondary to esophagitis.

The most unobtrusive form of columnar epithelium lining in the lower esophagus is shaped as islands, bands or epithelial areas which are not circumferential and without continuity with the Z-line [2].

Columnar epithelium in continuity with the Z-line

To confirm the presence of a columnar epithelium lined lower esophagus (CLLE), the endoscopist must be able to recognize and localize the various elements of the esophagogastric junction: the sphincter segment, Z-line, and diaphragmatic hiatus. This endoscopic anatomy is known and the Z-line, as a rule, is located within the sphincter segment, usually in it's lower third [2]. However, it is accepted that occasionally the entire sphincter segment can be totally or partially lined with gastric mucosa. In the lower esophagus a tubular segment of about 3 cm proximal to the junction tube-pouch lined with columnar epithelium must be considered normal. The CLLE is only considered pathological if it extends above the superior limit of the sphincter zone. In other words, the tubular segment of the lower esophagus lined with columnar epithelium must exceed a length of 3 cm in order to be considered pathological (Fig. 2).

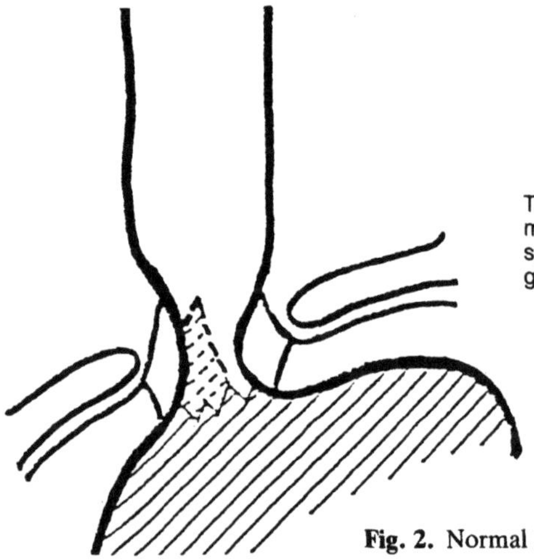

The Z-line is normally located within the sphincter segment, usually in the lower third. Occasionally the sphincter segment can be lined totally or in part by gastric mucosa

Fig. 2. Normal Esophagogastric junction: Position of the Z-Line

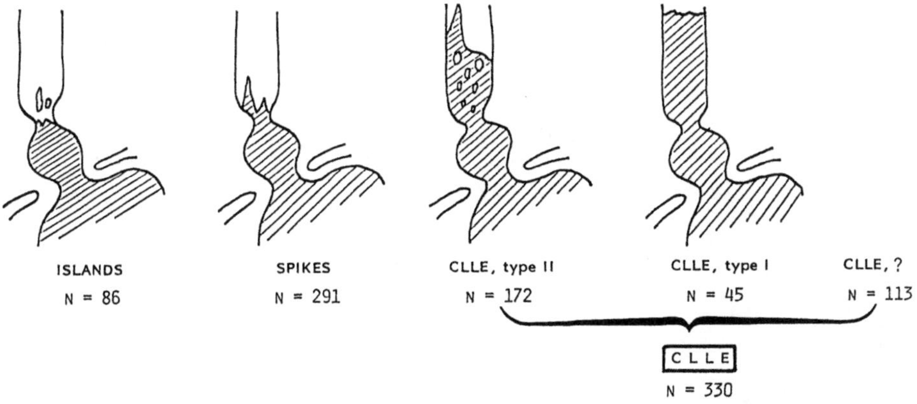

Fig. 3. Columnar epithelial lining of the lower esophagus: Topographic aspects

According to this endoscopic definition, the different pathological aspects of the CLLE are as follows [2]:

a) linear extensions, single or multiple, confluent or not at their base, shaped as tongues or spikes, but never circumferential.
b) circumferential sleeve with scattered islands of squamous epithelium with a columnar-squamous junction which is asymmetric, irregular and not segmental (=CLLE type 2).
c) circumferential sleeve, widespread, continuous with a circular superior edge (=CLLE type 1).

In addition to these 3 forms, we have the islands or bands of columnar epithelium lining not continuous with the gastric mucosa (Fig. 3).

These different topographies of the columnar lining in the lower esophagus call to mind the topography and morphology of erosive reflux esophagitis in its different stages (Fig. 4).

From an epidemiological point of view, non circumferential extensions in the shape of tongues, bands or spikes, as well as circumferential sleeves with squamous islands are found only exceptionally in the child and are found with the highest incidence in the sixties. The pathogenesis is acquired [4, 5].

On the contrary, columnar islands of the lower esophagus as well as widespread sleeves with segmental upper edges are found in the child as well as in the adult. The pathogenesis could be partly a malformation and congenital [5].

Barrett's ulcer as well as adenocarcinoma are usually associated with a CLLE type 2 (columnar cuff with residual squamous cell islands and an irregular non segmental upper edge). In a series of 34 cases of Barrett's ulcer, 24 were associated with a type 2 CLLE, 10 with a CLLE of an undetermined type and none with a type 1 CLLE.

Of 40 intraesophageal adenocarcinomas associated with a columnar epithelial lining, 31 adenocarcinomas were associated with a type 2 CLLE, 9 with an CLLE of an unknown type and none with a type 1 CLLE.

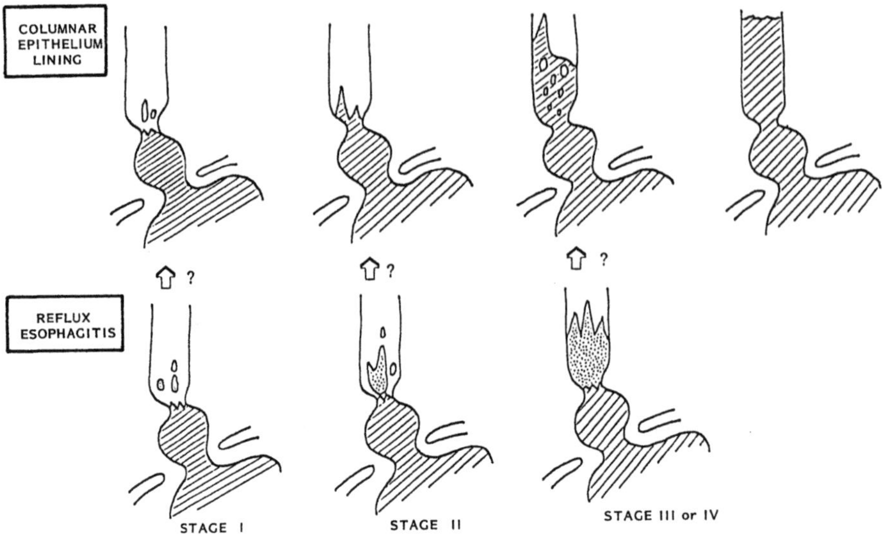

Fig. 4. The topography of the columnar lined lower esophagus is similar to that of reflux esophagitis lesions

To be accepted as final, the differentiation of the topographic aspect of the columnar epithelium lining requires a *follow-up endoscopy after the healing of the reflux lesions*. Of 17.023 endoscopies performed between 1963 and 1986, we have found 707 pathological CLLE, 330 as sleeves, 291 in the shape of tongues or spikes, and 86 as islands. Of the 330 sleeve linings, the differentiation between type 1 and type 2 was only possible in 217 cases and remained undetermined in 113 cases because of the associated peptic lesions (Fig. 3).

References

1. Ollyo JB, Fontolliet Ch, Gonvers JJ, Levi F, Savary M (1987) "Ectopic gastric mucosa of the upper and middle esophagus: a study of 194 cases" Gastroenterology (in Press)
2. Savary M, Miller G (1977) "L'oesophage: manuel et atlas d'endoscopie" Ed Gassmann, Soleure
3. Savary M, Miller G, Roethlisberger B (1981) "Spezielle Probleme des Endobrachy-ösophagus" In: Reflux-Therapie-Herausgegeben Ed Siewert JR, Blum AL, Springer-Verlag, Berlin, Heidelberg, New-York, 437–461
4. Savary M, Monnier Ph (1980) "Le reflux gastro-oesophagien: l'apport de l'endoscopie dans l'indication opératoire et les contrôles post-opératoires" Helv Chir Acta 47:693–706
5. Savary M, Monnier Ph (1985) "Diagnosis, Pathophysiology, and Adenocarcinogenesis of Barrett's Esophagus" In: Esophageal Disorders. Pathophysiology and Therapy. Ed TR DeMeester, DB, Skinner Raven Press, New-York 101–108

Can motility studies be of use in the classification of these lesions?

G. G. Jamieson (Adelaide)

Esophageal manometry gives us information about motility in the body of the esophagus and the tone and function of the lower esophageal sphincter. Are there manometric differences between patients with gastroesophageal reflux disease (GERD) with an esophagus-lined normally with squamous mucosa and patients with GERD who have an esophagus partly lined with columnar mucosa (Barrett's esophagus).

Esophageal body function: there have been several reports of abnormalities of esophageal body motor function in patients with Barrett's esophagus; for example, increased tertiary contractions in four of seven patients [1] and abnormalities such as aperistalsis, double peaked contractions and decreased peristaltic amplitude in six of eight patients [2], and similar abnormalities in four of eighteen patients [3]. However similar abnormalities have also been detected in the esophageal body in patients with severe esophagitis without columnar lining [4]. Detailed studies comparing esophageal body motility in patients with GERD with and without Barrett's esophagus have yet to be reported.

Lower esophageal sphincter: in general patients with Barrett's esophagus tend to have a low basal tone in their lower esophageal sphincter (LES) [2, 5, 6].

Iascone et al. [7] in a very careful study demonstrated that in an unequivocal Barrett's esophagus with columnar mucosa extending proximal to 30 cm from the incisor teeth all ten of their patients had LES pressures of less than 6 mm Hg. Furthermore, in comparison with a group of 31 patients with endoscopic esophagitis without Barrett's esophagus, the Barrett's patients had a basal tone which was significantly lower (–5 mm Hg mean), compared to 9 mm Hg mean or to 17 mm Hg in 33 normal volunteers.

However Herlihy et al. [3] found only five of ten patients with Barrett's esophagus who had a low basal tone.

Therefore it seems that esophageal manometry is not capable of distinguishing between patients with GERD with and without Barrett's esophagus. However, the studies show that the columnar lining is associated with patients who are at the severe end of the reflux disease spectrum.

Localization of proximal extent of columnar lining: the major objective use of manometry in the diagnosis of Barrett's esophagus may be in those cases which Iascone et al. called "limited Barrett's" – that is those patients in whom the columnar lining was found closer to the esophago-gastric junction than in the patients with "extended Barrett's".

For a patient to be clearly identified as having a Barrett's esophagus the columnar lined mucosa should extend above the LES [8]. This is true, even though most clinicians would accept complete columnar lining within the LES region as abnormal. The difficulty is in providing objective evidence for lesser degrees of columnar lining which have not risen above the lower esophageal sphincter level.

Manometry can be used to determine the proximal extent of the LES and its distance from the incisor teeth. Endoscopy can then be undertaken, with biopsies of the columnar mucosa under vision above the previously established lower esophageal sphincter level. Whilst esophageal movement means that even this technique leaves room for error, it is probably the most practical approach to objectively documenting columnar lined esophagus at the present time.

References

1. Burgess JN, Payne WS, Andersen HA, Weiland LH, Carlson HC (1971) Barrett's esophagus. The columnar-epithelial lower esophagus. May Clin Proc 46: 728–734
2. Burbidge EJ, Radigan JJ (1979) Characteristics of the columnar cell lined (Barrett's) esophagus. Gastrointest Endosc 25: 133–136
3. Herlihy KJ, Orlando RC, Bryson JC, Bozymski EM, Carney CN, Powell DW (1984) Barrett's esophagus: clinical, endoscopic, histologic, manometric and electrical potential difference characteristics. Gastroenterology 86: 436–43
4. Heddle R, Dent J, Toouli J, Lewis I (1984) Esophageal peristaltic dysfunction in peptic esophagitis. Gastroenterology 85: 1109
5. Heightmann P, Strauszer P, Sapunar J, Larrain A (1967) Lower esophagus lined with columnar epithelium morphologic and physiological correlation. Gastroenterology 53: 611–624
6. Robbins AH, Hermos JA, Schimmel EM, Friedlander DM, Messian RA (1977) The columnar lined esophagus–analysis of 26 cases. Diagnostic Radiol 123: 1–7
7. Iascone C, DeMeester TR, Little AG, Skinner DB (1983) Barrett's esophagus. Functional assessment, proposed pathogenesis and surgical therapy. Arch Surg 118: 543–549
8. Goyal RK (1985) Columnar cell lined (Barrett's) esophagus. A historical perspective. Chapter 1 In: Barrett's Esophagus, pathophysiology, diagnosis and management. Eds. Spechler SJ, Goyal RK, Elsevier ER, New York

How should one interpret the histologic changes observed during the endoscopic surveillance of these patients?

Ch. Fontolliet, D. Gardiol, Ph. Monnier, M. Savary, and *J. B. Ollyo* (Lausanne)

Adenocarcinoma is an acknowledged complication of Barrett's esophagus [1, 7, 8]. The marked dysplasia often associated with carcinoma is regarded by some as the precursor of an invasive lesion and its histologic discovery as an indication for esophagectomy [3, 4]. However, the dysplasis-carcinoma sequence is not generally recognized and the monitoring of patients suffering from Barrett's esophagus is not currently well organized.

In the attempt to answer certain undecided questions, such as the incidence of malignancy and frequency and severity of the dysplasia, also to establish a model for monitoring Barrett patients, we shall rely on two personal studies. One is retrospective and consists of 42 esophagectomy specimens with adenocarcinoma arising in Barrett's esophagus. The other is prospective and relates to biopsies of 37 patients with Barrett's esophagus without carcinoma, monitored endoscopically.

The dysplasia has been classified as slight, moderate and severe on the basis of preneoplastic cytologic and structural modifications according to the international classification used for gastric dysplasia [5].

Our first group consists (Table 1) of 35 men and 7 women, with a mean age of 62 years. In 4 cases only the diagnosis of Barrett's esophagus preceded that of adenocarcinoma. 29 cases formed the basis for an extensive cartographic study. Dysplasia was found in 38 of the 42 cases and in all the cases studied extensively. There was no macroscopic substrate. This dysplasia was severe in 23 cases. In 60% of cases the dysplasia was a mixture of all grades of severity. It was present 26 out of 29 times throughout the territory showing metaplasia of specialized type.

Table 1. Barrett's epithelium Dysplasia

Results, Retrospective study

		Extensive study
	n=42	n=29
Dysplasia	38/42	29/29
Severe dysplasia	23/42	20/29
Dysplasia throughout metaplastic territory		26/29

Our second series (Table 2) consists of 25 men and 12 women with a mean age of 63 years. These patients have undergone multiple staged biopsies throughout the metaplastic territory. 8 patients have had repeated biopsies at an interval of from 1 to 4 years (Table 3). 12 patients present slight dysplasia, always situated on a specialized type of epithelium. One man developed a slight dysplasia on the

Table 2. Barrett's epithelium

Dysplasia
Series
Prospective study
37 patients with Barrett's without carcinoma, monitored histologically
25 M 12 F Mean age 63 years
8 patients with repeated biopsies

Table 3. Barrett's epithelium Dysplasia

Results. Prospective study 12×slight dysplasia
Repeated biopsies (8×)

∅ D	1 year →	∅ D (2)	∅	Absence of
∅ D	2 years →	∅ D	D	Dysplasia
∅ D	1 year →	SD	S	Slight
∅ D	4 years →	SD	M	Moderate
SD	2 years →	SD		
SD	3 years →	SD		
SD	2 years →	SD to MD		

Barrett's epithelium after a 4 year course, and another after one year. In one male patient the dysplasia changed from slight to moderate after an interval of 2 years. Two patients present a slight dysplasia that has not advanced, one over 2 years and one over 3 years. No severe dysplasia was recorded in our series.

To sum up, the incidence of carcinoma in Barrett's esophagus is probably not as great as some have claimed [2, 6]. Nevertheless, our study is evidence of the prevalence of this association. Our observations do not allow us to specify the latent period required for the development of a carcinoma arising from cylinder-cell metaplasia of the lower esophagus. However, our second study suggests that development towards neoplasia is a long-term process. The extensive cartographic study demonstrated the presence of dysplasia associated with the cancer in virtually all the cases, and thereby argues in favor of the relation between dysplasia and invasive carcinoma. It likewise makes it possible to specify the topography of the preneoplastic changes, which generally extend throughout the metaplastic epithelium. In both our studies this epithelium was of specialized type, and this is therefore the type of metaplasia we consider as a risk type, unlike the metaplasia of gastric fundus or cardiac type also reported in endobrachyesophagus.

These several conclusions allow us to advance the following proposals:

1. In cases where the biopsy diagnosis is one of severe dysplasia the biopsy should first be repeated after a short interval, and then, if the diagnosis is confirmed, immediate esophagectomy should be performed even in the absence of an invasive lesion.
2. Patients suffering from Barrett's esophagus, especially of specialized type, should be submitted to regular endoscopic monitoring. The interval between two endoscopies is difficult to define, but it seems reasonable to perform endoscopy about once a year. Monitoring should be done at closer intervals after the discovery of a dysplastic focus, at least of moderate degree.
3. As preneoplastic transformation often occurs invisibly and in multicentric fashion, we feel it is very important to proceed to biopsies for histologic examination in the course of every endoscopy. Any macroscopically recognizable lesion must be removed.

Moreover multiple staged biopsies should be made throughout the metaplastic territory at intervals of 1 cm, starting from the inferior esophageal sphincter, along a vertical line determined in relation to the maximal extent of the lesion.

References

1. Enterline HT, Thompson JJ (1984) Barrett's metaplasia and adenocarcinoma. Pathology of the esophagus. New York, Springer Verlag, 109–126
2. Haggitt RC, Tryzelaar J, Ellis E, Colcher H (1978) Adenocarcinoma complicating columnar epithelium-lined (Barrett's) esophagus. Am J Clin Pathol 70: 1–5
3. Hamilton SR, Smith RR (1987) The relationship between columnar epithelial dysplasia and invasive adenocarcinoma arising in Barrett's esophagus. Am J Clin Pathol 87: 301–312
4. Lee RG (1985) Dysplasia in Barrett's esophagus. Am J Surg Pathol 9: 845–852
5. Morson BC, Sobin LH, Grundman NE, Johansen A, Nagayu T, Serck-Hansson A (1984) Precancerous conditions and epithelial dysplasia in the stomach J Clin Pathol 33: 711–721
6. Naef AP, Savary M, Ozzello L (1975) Columnar-lined esophagus: an acquired lesion with malignant predisposition. Report on 140 cases of Barrett's esophagus with 12 adenocarcinomas. J Thorac Cardiovasc Surg 70: 826–835
7. Skinner DB, Walther BC, Riddell RH, Schmidt H, Iascone C, DeMeester TR (1983) Barrett's esophagus comparison of benign and malignant cases. Ann Surg 198: 554–565
8. Thompson JJ, Zinsser KR, Enterline HT (1983) Barrett's metaplasia and adenocarcinoma of the esophagus and gastroesophageal junction. Hum Pathol 14: 42–61

T. Lerut, G. Leman, C. Aelvoet, Y. Leclef, and *J. A. Grüwez* (Leuven)

It is generally conceived that patients with a Barrett's esophagus and an uncontrolled reflux have a higher risk of malignant degeneration. This idea is mainly based on the fact that in a number of series dealing with adenocarcinoma of the esophagus and the cardia a high percentage of Barrett's esophagus, usually 10 to 15%, was noticed [6]. In other series it was found that out of the total number of treated benign and malignant Barrett's esophagus the proportion of malignant cases was very high, even as high as 46% in one series [5]. Those figures however only describe the prevalence of malignancy in Barrett's esophagus, which means the number of malignant cases at the moment of the initial diagnosis of Barrett's esophagus [5].

The incidence is however the number of new cases that develop during some specified time interval and not well known, but is clearly lower than the prevalence shown in the series of Cameron [5]. In this study 104 patients were followed up and only two of the patients who were free of cancer at the time of diagnosis developed an adenocarcinoma during the follow-up period. This represented an incidence of only one case for 441 patient-years. The available data indicate that the risk of esophageal cancer in such patients appears to be 30 fold to 40 fold higher than in the general population. So the discussion on whether or not Barrett's esophagus is a precancerous lesion goes on and consequently some other questions remain unanswered. Does the higher risk of deterioration justify the risk and cost of regular endoscopic follow-up? How should endoscopic changes during follow-up be judged? Are there any sub-groups that would include the higher risk of degeneration?

In Barrett's esophagus, three types of epithelium are commonly found [1]:

the fundic type where parietal cells and chief cells are present,

the junctional or cardia type, including the mucous secreting columnar cells and often also pyloric type of glands.

The intestinal type of metaplasia, characterized by the presence of goblet cells, with sometimes the presence of pyloric glands. Between those three types of metaplasia, different combinations are possible, but in case of degeneration the intestinal type of metaplasia is practically always present and therefore seems to be in itself an indicator of a possible risk of degeneration.

Even more important is the presence of dysplasia, that is to say unequivocal neoplastic changes in the columnar epithelium [3]. Dysplasia is an ominous finding, not only because it can in itself be a precursor of malignancy, but also because this dysplastic epithelium can be malignant and invasive.

This dysplasia can be graded as:

Negative: when nuclear changes within the metaplastic epithelium are similar to those found in the same epithelium in its normal anatomic localization.

If the dysplastic nuclei are mainly limited to the basal side of the cells it is called low grade dysplasia. All severe changes with the nuclei coming close to the upper pole of the cell, and all changes including carcinoma in situ are called high grade dysplasia.

The interpretation of these different grades is often very difficult, as for instance in case of active regeneration in the immediate neighbourhood of a Barrett's ulcer, and one can frequently find substantial interobserver variations in the classification of dysplastic changes. Because of the important clinical implication, certainly in the case of high grade dysplasia and carcinoma in situ, multiple biopsies and the opinion of at least two expert anatomopathologists is recommended to make a decision [6].

Dysplasia has been found in degenerated Barrett's esophagi in 68% to 100% of the cases. In patients with Barrett's esophagus who have no adenocarcinoma, the incidence of dysplasia is only about 5 to 10%.

It seems that the high grade dysplasia is often, although not always, associated with invasive adenocarcinoma. There are few data on the incidence of low grade dysplasia leading to invasive carcinoma.

Material and Methods

Taking into account these facts we have analysed our own material. From 1979 till 1986 50 patients were treated for a Barrett's esophagus: 26 benign cases and 24 malignant cases, giving a prevalence of 48%. The analysis of malignant cases provides interesting information concerning the incidence. Out of these 24 carcinoma cases, 10 patients (Table 1) had a biopsy-proven history of Barrett's esophagus but developed a carcinoma during the follow-up. In other words "the

Table 1

M.R. 51 Y. ♂	12. 1979	: Intestinal metaplasia
	05. 1980	: Ulcer : adenoca
		R/Resection: Well-differ. adenoca
		Invasion tunica musculosa
		Intestinal metaplasia
		Severe dysplasia
		N –
C.A. 58 Y. ♂	11. 1980	: Severe esophagitis – resection hyperplastic polyp
	06. 1981	: Intestinal metaplasia – severe dysplasia
	07. 1982	: Resection polyp : adenoca.
		R/Resection: transmur. well diff. adenoca. N –
G.H. 58 Y. ♀	1979	: Barrett+stenosis – intestinal metaplasia no dysplasia
	07. 1983	: Adenoca intestinal metaplasia
		R/Resection: transmur. well diff. adenoca.
		N – intestinal metaplasia
H.L. 69 Y. ♂	1969	: Intestinal metaplasia
	05. 1984	: Adenoca intestinal metaplasia
		R/Resection: transmur. undiff. adenoca
		N + intestinal metaplasia
D.G. 76 Y. ♂	04. 1985	: Ulcer – intestinal metaplasia – severe dysplasia
	07. 1985	: Ulcer: adenoca-intestinal metaplasia
		R/Resection: transmur, well diff.
		N + intestinal metaplasia
V.M.E. 65 Y. ♂	1982	: Reflux esophagitis
		R/Medical therapy – 6 monthly endoscopy
	1984	: Ulcer
		Severe dysplasia – intestinal metaplasia
		R/Medical therapy – persistant ulcer nuclear atypical
	10. 1986	: Substenosis + infrastenotic ulcer
	12. 1986	: Ulcer : adenoca.
		R/Resection: ca. intramucosal
		N –
B.M. 61 Y. ♀	10. 1984	: Ulcer: Intestinal metaplasia no dysplasia
	07. 1985	: Ulcer: Adenoca-intestinal metaplasia
		R/Resection: intramucosal well diff. adenoca
		N –
		intestinal metaplasia
V.M.E. 64 Y. ♂	1979	: Esophagitis – intestinal metaplasia
	05. 1986	: Ulcer: intestinal metaplasia
	06. 1986	: Healed ulcer – intestinal metaplasia ca in situ-severe dysplasia
		R/Resection: Adenoca in situ N –
		intestinal metaplasia – severe
		dysplasia
V.D.V.H.	03. 1979	: Longstanding history of reflux
48 Y. ♂		Ulcer – intestinal metaplasia
		Severe dysplasia
	05. 1979	: Ulcer: Adenoca
		R/Resection: Adenoca intramucosal undiff.
		severe dysplasia
		N –

Table 1. Continued

C. A. 35 Y. ♂	04. 1979	: Longstanding history of reflux intestinal metaplasia – dysplasia
	06. 1979	: Severe dysplasia
	08. 1979	: Severe dysplasia
	10. 1979	: Ca in situ
		R/Resection: Ca in situ Junctional metaplasia Severe dysplasia N –

incidence" of degeneration in this retrospective series is 20%. On top of this, in the series of benign Barrett's esophagus, 1 patient had severe dysplasia zones, highly suspicious of carcinoma in situ, around an ulcer located within a Barrett's esophagus with the intestinal type of metaplasia.

In 6 out of 10 above-mentioned cases degeneration occurred within 1 year after the initial diagnosis of Barrett's esophagus. All 10 cases were patients presenting intestinal metaplasia.

In our patients no systematic search for dysplasia with vital staining techniques was performed, but nevertheless there were 4 patients, all with intestinal metaplasia, showing severe dysplasia in the biopsies taken in the period preceding the degeneration. In two other patients severe dysplasia was present at the time of diagnosis of carcinoma or in the resected specimen. In six patients the diagnosis of malignancy was made on a biopsy taken in ulcer. In 5 cases the ulcer was not initially diagnosed as being malignant but in 3 out of these five patients severe dysplasia was present in the period preceding the onset of carcinoma.

Reviewing the resection specimens, we found in two patients a carcinoma in situ, a T_1 tumor three times and a T_2 tumour once. All these patients had no lymph node involvement. Out of the four patients with transmural tumors, two patients had no lymph node involvement.

Conclusions

Although this series is a retrospective one and so in no way representing the real incidence of degeneration in Barrett's esophagus, there is to our knowledge no series in the literature demonstrating so clearly and in such a high percentage the evolution from benign Barrett's esophagus towards an adenocarcinoma. These figures clearly exceed the data of Cameron and Goyal [6] confirming the already existing impression that Barrett's esophagus has to be considered as a premalignant condition and that any patient with this pathology should be endoscopically followed on a regular basis even after successful conservative medical or surgical treatment.

Multiple biopsies with a systematic search for dysplastic zones are mandatory. Our data confirm that especially patients with intestinal metaplasia should be followed-up.

Certainly the combination of intestinal metaplasia containing an ulcer should be regarded as a highly suspicious. In the endoscopic follow-up of these cases treated on a medical basis, it is of paramount importance not to lose too much time if the ulcer fails to heal, since in the vast majority of these cases degeneration can occur within 1 year or even within 6 months. In these cases the question rises whether an antireflux procedure or a resection has to be performed. The frequent presence of severe dysplasias (60%) in this series is an indicator for potential degeneration, confirming the data from the literature [1, 4]. Some authors even pretend that in cases of high grade dysplasia there will always be a concommitant carcinoma in situ [2]. The major problem with this phenomenon however is the rather difficult differentiation between this dysplasia and regenerative processes after healing of the mucosa and regeneration in or around the ulcer. Therefore multiple and repeated biopsies are imperative in cases of high grade dysplasia and if possible the biopsies should be reviewed by at least two expert pathologists before deciding to perform a resection.

References

1. Goyal RK (1985) Columnar cell-lined (Barrett's) esophagus. In: Barrett's esophagus Pathophysiology, diagnosis and management. Spechler SJ, Goyal RK (eds), New York, Elsevier Science 1–17
2. Peuchmour M, Potet F, Goldfain D (1984) Mucin histochemistry of the columnar epithelium of the oesophagus (Barrett's oesophagus): a prospective biopsy study. J Clin Pathol 37: 607–610
3. Riddell RH (1985) Dysplasia and regression in Barrett's epithelium. In: Barrett's esophagus Pathophysiology, diagnosis and management. Spechler SJ, Goyal RK (eds) New York, Elsevier Science 142–152
4. Skinner DB, Walther BC, Riddell RH, Schmidt H, Iascone C, DeMeester TR (1983) Barrett's esophagus. Comparison of benign and malignant cases. Ann Surg 198: 554–565
5. Spechler SJ (1985) The risk of cancer in Barrett's esophagus. In: Barrett's esophagus Pathophysiology, diagnosis and management. Spechler SJ, Goyal RK (eds) New York, Elsevier Science 189–197
6. Spechler SJ, Goyal RK (1986) Barrett's esophagus. New Engl J Med 315: 362–371

What is the role of alkaline reflux in the development of complications?

C. G. Bremner (Johannesburg)

Gastric columnar epithelium is resistant to ulceration unless the mucosal barrier is destroyed [1], and there is much evidence to show that bile can destroy this barrier [1–3].

The same mechanism may be responsible for the breakdown of the new columnar lining in a Barrett's esophagus. The columnar epithelium in a Barrett's esophagus has developed because it is acid resistant. Why should this epithelium ulcerate, stricture or degenerate to an adenocarcinoma? It is well known that bile may contaminate gastric juice and participate in the genesis of severe reflux esophagitis [4, 5]. In 1972 the author suggested that the submucosal inflammatory infiltrate seen in biopsy and resected specimens of Barrett's epithelium could be due to bile reflux [6]. Subsequently we have postulated that the complications seen in Barrett's esophagus could also be due to bile contaminated gastric juice [7].

Support for a bile reflux hypothesis

1. We have measured total bile acids in 15 patients with a columnar-lined esophagus. Gastric juice was aspirated in the fasting state and 1 hour after a standard milk meal. In 7 of these patients the bile acids were in excess of normal, and all had a stricture at the squamo-columnar junction. However, 2 patients with strictures had normal bile acids.
2. If bile and acid refluxes from the stomach, the gastric epithelium would also be subject to irritation of this mixture and there would be an expected occurrence of gastritis or gastric ulcer. We therefore took multiple gastric biopsies in 17 patients with CLE and found evidence of gastritis in 16 (chronic active gastritis in 9; mild gastritis in 3; atrophic gastritis in 4). Bile introduced into the stomach of experimental animals produces a similar gastritis [3].
5. There is an incidence of gastric ulceration following the Nissen fundoplication operation for gastroesophageal reflux [8, 9]. Although the pathogenesis of this complication is controversial, we have given evidence implicating duodeno-gastric bile reflux [9, 10]. Following a Nissen fundoplication for Barrett's esophagus 4 of 24 patients in our series have developed gastric ulcers.
4. Duodeno-gastric reflux has been assessed by HIDA scanning in 11 of our patients with Barrett's esophagus. To date, of 7 scans on patients with strictures, 5 have been positive, and 4 scans on uncomplicated Barrett's have been negative.

Further clinical support

A very rapid ascent of 15 cm of columnar epithelium was reported by Halvorsen and Semb [11] in a patient who had a previous vagotomy and pyloroplasty. Bile-contamination was evident on esophagoscopy and gastroscopy. This patient developed an ulcer in a columnar segment 10 years later. A Roux-en-Y bile diversion cured the esophageal ulceration and gastritis. On follow-up 18 months later the columnar segment was still 15 cm in length.

"Alkaline" reflux is associated with up to a half of patients with gastroesophageal reflux. Alkaline reflux causes a more severe esophagitis than acid reflux. There is some evidence that alkaline reflux is associated with some cases of Barrett's esophagus, and may be the cause of the complications.

References

1. Davenport HW (1968) Destruction of the gastric mucosal barrier by detergents and urea. Gastroenterol 54: 175
2. Ivey KJ (1971) Gastric mucosal barrier. Gastroenterol 61: 247
3. Lawson HH (1966) Gastritis and gastric ulceration Br J Surg 43: 493
4. Gillison EW, De Castro VAM, Nyhus LM, Kusakari K, Bombeck CT (1972) The significance of bile in reflux esophagitis. Surg Gynec Obstet 134: 119
5. Henderson RD, Mugashe F, Jeejeebhoy KN, Cullen J et al (1972) The role of bile and acid in the production of esophagitis and the motor defect of esophagitis. Ann Thor Surg 14: 465
6. Bremner CG (1977) The Columnar-lined (Barrett's) Esophagus Surgery Annual. Ed LM Nyhus Appleton-Century Crofts
7. Bremner CG, Hamilton DG (1985) Barrett's Esophagus: Controversial Aspects. In Esophageal Disorders: Pathophysiology and Therapy: Ed DeMeester TR, Skinner DB. Raven Press New York
8. Bushkin FL, Woodward ER, O'Leary JP (1976) Occurrence of gastric ulcer after Nissen Fundoplication. Am Surg 42: 821
9. Bremner CG (1979) Gastric ulceration after a Fundoplication operation for gastroesophageal reflux. Surg Gynec Obstet 148: 62–64
10. Bremner CG (1977) Gastric ulcer after the Nissen fundoplication. S Afr Med J 51: 791
11. Goldman MC, Beckman RC (1960) Barrett syndrome. Case report with discussion about concepts of pathogenesis. Gastroenterology 39: 104

Are clinical symptoms of reflux a necessary indication for antireflux surgery in Barrett's esophagus?

D. B. Skinner (Chicago)

Symptoms bring the patient to the physician. The diagnosis of Barrett's esophagus in an asymptomatic person is an unlikely event. Unfortunately the severity of the symptoms in Barrett's esophagus cases does not correlate to the severity of the reflux or the likelihood of complications.

In our population of benign Barrett's esophagus patients , heartburn is an almost universal complaint, but the severity of heartburn when scored quantitatively is not as severe in Barrett's patients as in a matched group of patients with reflux-caused ulcerative esophagitis [1]. Similarly, regurgitation is less severe symptomatically in Barrett's patients compared to the ulcerative esophagitis group. On the other hand, the Barrett's patients tend to complain of more dysphagia than do ulcerative esophagitis patients without a well-developed stricture.

In the matched group of patients with Barrett's epithelium and those with ulcerative esophagitis, the distal esophageal sphincter pressures were significantly lower in the Barrett's group. Those with more proximal squamo-columnar junctions 6 or more cm above the cardia had even less tension in the distal esophageal segment. The Barrett's patients had greater frequency and duration of reflux and more abnormalities in acid clearing than did the ulcerative esophagitis group.

Here we have a difficult clinical paradox wherein those patients with more severe reflux acquiring a Barrett's epithelium have fewer symptoms than do patients whose response to reflux is ulceration without Barrett's epithelium. This lack of symptomatic correlation is particularly disturbing because of the premalignant nature of the Barrett's epithelium. As the Barrett's progresses the symptoms appear to be less severe, and the patient is less likely to seek medical evaluation for symptomatic relief.

Among patients with adenocarcinoma arising in a Barrett's esophagus, the incidence and severity of heartburn and regurgitation are less than in those with benign Barrett's disease. In fact dysphagia is the symptom which brings the patient to the clinician once the carcinoma has developed. When the patient is asked whether he or she has heartburn the answer may be "no." But if the clinician asks whether there is a past history of heartburn and ingestion of antacids, the patient frequently says "yes, but it went away several years ago". There is often a quiet interlude when symptoms lessen before the dysphagia of the carcinoma begins. For this reason symptomatic response to medical or surgical treatment for reflux in Barrett's patients cannot be taken as a satisfactory guideline to the success of treatment. Antireflux therapy of medical or surgical nature in patients with Barrett's esophagus must be documented by objective pH studies, and the patient must remain under lifelong surveillance to detect early premalignant or malignant changes in the metaplastic epithelium.

In spite of this hazard of the premalignant epithelium, the decision as to whether to perform antireflux surgery is still guided to some degree by the severity of symptoms: in a patient with documented Barrett's esophagus but minimal symptoms and no complications of stricture or a penetrating ulcer, an antireflux repair is hard to justify. The evidence that the antireflux repair will provide complete protection against future malignancy is simply not available, although it is proposed theoretically.

In fact, the indications for antireflux surgery in Barrett's esophagus are the same as for other types of reflux esophagitis: patients having strictures, persisting ulcerations, aspiration, bleeding, or symptoms which are intractable to medical therapy are selected for antireflux surgery. Those with less severe symptoms and no complications are usually treated medically. Both groups of patients remain under long-term surveillance for metaplastic and dysplastic mucosal changes.

Reference

1. Iascone C, DeMeester TR, Little AG, Skinner DB (1983) Barrett's esophagus. Arch Surg 118:543–549

Can the ectopic epithelium regress after antireflux surgery?

A. E. Badaloni (Buenos Aires)

The reversibility of the metaplasia is implicit in the definition made by Robbins and Cotran, mentioned by Pope II [2]: "in an epithelium metaplasia is a reversible change in which one adult cell type is replaced by another cell type".

The regression of Barrett's epithelium is feasible after successful antireflux surgery. The literature is limited and reveals isolated cases [1–4]. Pope II [2] presented one series with 10 patients who had been controlled with pre and postoperative vacuum biopsies made with manometric control. Preoperative biopsies were made, and the sub-sequent follow-up revealed four cases that receded. Riddell [3] presents one case operated with an antireflux surgery at the University of Chicago in which the biopsy revealed squamous epithelium apparently growing over Barrett's epithelium. This finding was never seen in medically treated patients in resection specimens of Barrett's esophagus.

*

The partial regression of columnar metaplasia has been observed in three of 21 cases with Barrett's esophagus that underwent antireflux surgery at the Pirovano General Hospital in Buenos Aires in the years 1980 to 1985, with a follow-up of one or more years.

Five years after antireflux surgery, patient number one showed large patches of squamous epithelium arising on columnar-lined areas, that were not observed at the preoperative esophagoscopy and continued to grow in the following controls.

Patient number two presented a ring-shaped stricture after surgery and several dilatations, but while at the preoperative time the stricture was found to coincide with the squamo-columnar mucosal junction (SCMJ), four years later this area is completely covered with squamous epithelium: and the SCMJ is found to be three cm lower than the persistent stricture.

Two years after antireflux surgery, our third patient revealed great increase in size and joining of the pre-existing squamous patches, and the SCMJ descended four cm related with the first post-operative esophagoscopy.

Patients number 1 and 2 had a stricture with a marginal ulcer on admission. The third patient had only a superficial marginal ulcer. The SCMJs were at 30, 36 and 27 cm respectively, taking the incisor teeth as a landmark. All patients were treated by freeing the lower esophagus by dissection, including high vagotomy by steps to elongate the esophagus, narrowing the hiatus, Nissen's procedure and pyloromyotomy. The two patients with strictures underwent pre, peri and postoperative dilatations. There were no signs of postsurgical reflux with the standard acid reflux test, and they are all free of symptoms. On the other hand, we have not observed metaplastic regression in four cases treated medically; they did not undergo surgery because of high surgical risk.

Discussion

None of our three cases show a complete regression of Barrett's epithelium, and although endoscopic controls are not sufficiently accurate, we believe this to be the best procedure to demonstrate regression: assuming that it can be caused by dissection, mobilization and lengthening of the esophagus during the surgical procedure. This is called "pseudoregression" by Riddell [3] this mistake is obviated if we employ the basis length with endoscopic control 30 days after surgery and not the length checked before.

Charles E. Pope II [2] employs as reference in his study all the lower esophageal sphincter manometric level and takes vacuum blind biopsies in an oral direction. The area where the biopsy is taken is generally "folded" during the preoperative examination and "lengthened" after the surgery, caused by lowering the esophagus gastric junction into the abdomen and sometimes it's anchorage to the arcuate ligament. This item, in addition to the fact that the biopsies are taken in a blind fashion, makes this method less reliable than the one proposed by us with direct visualization endoscopy, intravital iodine staining, targeted biopsies and endoscopy 30 days after antireflux operation.

References

1. Brand DL, Ylvisaker JT, Gelfand M, Pope CE II (1980) Regression of columnar esophageal (Barrett's) epithelium after antireflux surgery. New Engl J Med 302: 844–848
2. Pope CE II (1985) Regression of Barrett's epithelium. "Barrett's Esophagus: Pathophysiology, Diagnosis and Management". Spechler and Goyal (eds), 223–229
3. Riddell RH (1985) Dysplasia and regression in Barrett's epithelium. "Barrett's Esophagus: Pathophysiology, Diagnosis and Management". Spechler and Goyal (eds), 151–152
4. Skinner DB, Walther BC, Riddell RH, Schmidt H, Iascone C, DeMeester TR (1983) Barrett's esophagus. Comparison of benign and malignant cases. Ann Surg 198: 554–565

A. H. Hölscher (Munich)

A regression of Barrett's esophagus means a replacement of ectopic columnar epithelium in the esophagus by squamous cell epithelium.

The review of the literature shows that 7 authors have reported a regression of Barrett's esophagus after antireflux surgery, whereas another 7 did not observe this phenomenon (Tables 1, 2).

In total 163 patients were followed up by endoscopy to prove regression of Barrett's esophagus. Only in 17 cases, that means 10.4%, a regression could be stated (Table 3). The mean duration of follow-up was 4.3 years: the mean time till regression was observed took 2.9 years. A proved success of antireflux surgery in case of regression of Barrett's esophagus was reported in 12 of 17 cases (70%). The regression was partial in 14 cases and complete in 3 cases.

Table 1. Compilation of studies with persistence of Barrett's esophagus after antireflux surgery (Hölscher 1985)

Author	Year	n	Anti-reflux-operation	Time of follow up (years)	Success on anti-reflux-operation
Endo	1974	1	?	5	?
Naef	1975	?	fundoplication	5	?
Desbaillets	1976	2	?	?	?
Burke	1976	2	?	?	?
Mangla	1976	3	fundoplication	1–3	?
Mangla	1980	24	fundoplication	?	?
Starnes	1984	8	PVG* and fundoplication (n=7) Hill-operation (n=1)	?	?
Wellinger	1987	39	anti-reflux-operation	$\bar{x}$5.4	?
total		79		1–5.4	

* proximal gestion vagotomy

Table 2. Compilation of studies with (partial) regression of Barrett's esophagus after antireflux surgery (Hölscher 1985)

Author	Year	n	Patients with (partial) regression	Anti-reflux operation	Time of follow-up (years)	Time till regression (years)	Success of anti-reflux operation
Radigan	1977	13	1	fundoplication	1	0.33	+
Zamora	1980	1	1	fundoplication	?	0.75	?
Brand	1980	10	4	fundoplication (n=2)	2–11	2	+ (pH-metry)
				Hill-operation (n=2)		2	+ (pH-metry)
						5	+ (pH-metry)
						11	+ (pH-metry)
Ransom	1982	6	4	fundoplication	$\bar{x}$ 5.7	?	+ (n=4)
Skinner	1983	10	2	Belsey Mark IV	$\bar{x}$ 4(2–7)	2	+ (pH-metry)
						2	+ (pH-metry)
Pollara	1987	22	4	part. fundoplication	2–12	?	?
Perniceni	1987	22	1	TV, antrectomy, Roux-en-Y	$\bar{x}$ 2.8	1	+ (pH-metry)
total		84	17 (20%)		$\bar{x}$ 4.9	$\bar{x}$ 2.9	

Table 3. Joint evaluation of all studies about changement of Barrett's esophagus after antireflux surgery (review of literature 1975–1987)

n	Regression of Barrett's esophagus*	Time of follow-up (years)	Proved success of anti-reflux operation in case of regression (pH-metry)
163	10% (17/163)	$\bar{x}$4.3	70% (12/17)

* partial regression in 14 cases
complete regression in 3 cases

The best documented reports are those from Brand et al. [1] and Skinner et al [13]. These studies show that after a successful antireflux operation a regression of columnar epithelium seems to be possible. In those series the patients who developed a regression of Barrett's esophagus postoperatively had no reflux or only physiologic reflux proved by pH-metry. Brand et al. have drawn the conclusion that a regression of columnar epithelium correlates with the success of antireflux surgery. However, their studies have been severely criticized because the biopsies have been obtained by suction capsules without knowledge of the precise location of the biopsy and its relationship to the squamocolumnar junction (Mangla, [7]).

The study of Skinner et al. showed that after a successful antireflux operation a regression of Barrett's epithelium is not mandatory. Only in 2 of their 10 patients with regular follow-up a regression was stated although in all patients a good prevention of reflux after operation could be proved by pH-metry. It is interesting that in 2 other patients of this group there has been a regression of dysplasias in Barrett's esophagus after successful antireflux surgery.

Two facts have to be taken into consideration for the interpretation of the different results in literature: it is very difficult to do an exact measurement of the extent of Barrett's esophagus as the points of reference are difficult to define, especially after antireflux surgery. If one chooses the incisors it has to be considered that after an antireflux operation the cardia is often dislocated because of the removal of a hiatal hernia. The safest point of reference still seems to be the manometrically localized lower esophageal sphincter. Another problem has to be taken into account: if reflux esophagitis heals up after a successful operation, this can result in a so-called pseudo-regression at the oral edge of Barrett's esophagus. By endoscopic examination it is often very difficult to differentiate between circular erosions and columnar epithelium of Barrett's esophagus. If the erosions have healed, only the real columnar epithelium remains and a regression of Barrett's esophagus is simulated.

Summarizing the results in the literature, a regression of columnar epithelium in Barrett's esophagus after successful antireflux surgery seems to be possible but it is an exception. Only in 10% of all cases a partial regression has been observed. There are only few well documented cases in which the regression of Barrett's esophagus seems to be definitely proved. Most of the reports have to be doubted either because of the technique of esophageal biopsies or with regard to the phenomenon of pseudoregression respectively topographic change of the cardia after antireflux surgery.

*

In conclusion, Barrett's esophagus generally is an irreversible condition. A regression of ectopic epithelium after antireflux operations is possible, but it happens in less than 10% of the cases. A correlation between the success of antireflux surgery and the regression of Barrett's epithelium is not proved.

References

1. Brand DL, Ylvisaker JT, Gelfand N, Pope II CE (1980) Regression of columnar esophageal (Barrett's) epithelium after antireflux surgery. N Engl J Med 302: 844
2. Burke BI, Mullen ST (1976) Barrett's esophagus: A multifaced condition. South Med J 69: 331
3. Desbaillets LG, Mangla JC (1976) Endoscopic diagnosis of Barrett's esophagus. Endoscopy 8: 65–70
4. Endo M, Kobayashi S, Kouzu T, Takimoto T, Nakayama K (1974) A case of Barrett's epithelisation followed up for 5 years. Endoscopy 6: 48–51
5. Hölscher AH, Bader M, Siewert JR (1985) Kann Antirefluxchirurgie eine maligne Entartung des Endobrachyoesophagus verhindern? Dtsch Med Wschr 110: 551–555
6. Mangla JC, Schenk EA, Desbaillets L, Guarasci G, Kubasik NP, Turner MD (1976) Pepsin secretion, pepsinogen, and gastrin in Barrett's esophagus. Clinical and morphologic characteristics. Gastroenterology 70: 669
7. Mangla JC (1980) Reply to Brand DL: Barrett's epithelium: Regression or no regression? N Engl J Med 303: 529
8. Naef AP, Savary M, Ozzello C (1975) Columnar lined lower esophagus: An acquired lesion with malignant predisposition. Report of 140 cases of Barrett's esophagus with proved adenocarcinoma. J Thoracic Cardiovasc Surg 70: 826
9. Pollara WM, Zilberstein B, Cecconello I, Venco SE, Parada AA, Pinotti WH (1987) Barrett's esophagus. Late results of conservative treatment. In: Siewert JR, Hölscher AH (eds): Diseases of the Esophagus 1986. Springer, Berlin Heidelberg New York Tokyo
10. Perniceni T, Fekete F (1987) Endobrachyesophagus after antireflux surgery with truncal vagotomy, antrectomy and Roux-en-Y diversion. 6th Meeting of the Geemo, March 14, Lisbon
11. Radigan LR, Glover JL, Shipley FE, Shoemaker RE (1977) Barrett's esophagus. Arch Surg 112: 486
12. Ransom JM, Patel GK, Clift SA, Wombel NE, Read RC (1982) Extended and limited types of Barrett's esophagus in the adult. Ann Thorac Surg 33: 19
13. Skinner DB, Walther BC, Riddell RH, Schmidt H, Iascone C, DeMeester TR (1983) Barrett's esophagus. Comparison of benign and malignant cases. Ann Surg 189: 554
14. Starnes VA, Atkins RD, Bellinger JF, Sawyers JL (1984) Barrett's esophagus. A surgical entity. Arch Surg 119: 563
15. Wellinger J, Savary M (1987) Endobrachyesophagus after antireflux surgery. 6th Meeting of the Geemo March 14 Lisbon
16. Zamora JL, Donahue PE (1980) Columnar epithelium in the esophagus. Curr Surg 37: 372

K. Jeyasingham (Bristol)

When the question of regression after antireflux surgery is considered, one has to take into account the modes of study that have been employed, the sites of biopsy and their mapping in the pre and postoperative examinations, the incidence of response and correlation to documented effectiveness of the anti reflux surgery. Two other considerations are, the incidence of adenocarcinomatous change in the epithelium with or without anti reflux surgery, and what are the alternatives to anti reflux surgery.

Accurate localization and mapping of the sites of biopsy can only be done by direct visualization of the area at the time. Hence, the use of the suction technique is not reliable. Even when direct visual techniques are employed the changes produced

Table 1. Positive regression

Brand et al. (1980) – 4/10
Correlation to
1. Effectiveness of surgery
2. Age of onset of symptoms
3. Time interval for total regression – may be >2 years
Skinner et al. (1983)
1. Epithelial overgrowth (detached islets)
2. All three types can regress
3. No regression with high grade dysplasia

by surgical fixation as part of an anti reflux procedure, is bound to introduce an element of error. Therefore, in pre and postoperative comparative studies, only total regression can be interpreted as regression and not partial regression in particular areas. The shift of the Z line can be totally artefactual and does not necessarily have any bearing on the changes of regression.

Brand [1] in drawing our attention to regression of columnar epithelium after anti reflux surgery, presented four such patients out of a series of ten (Table 1). There was a significant correlation of the regression to subjective and objective responses to the surgery. A further point was that those who showed regression were the ones in whom symptoms set in in their teens, whereas the ones that did not show regression were in a higher age group at the time of onset of symptoms. The time taken for regression could be as long as two years.

Skinner's observations [2] of squamous epithelial overgrowth over intestinal type of columnar epithelium is interesting, but this phenomenon cannot in itself protect against adenocarcinoma transformation in such sunken epithelial remnants. Although the intestinal type of epithelium has been most associated with malignant change, all three sub types have been known to be associated with the regression except for columnar epithelium showing dysplasia. High grade dysplasia has never been shown to regress and has been considered pre-malignant [2, 3].

Other investigators have not been so fortunate as to see regression in their follow up of columnar celled esophageal patients [4, 5] (Table 2). In my own series of ten patients with columnar lined esophagus with no dysplasia, who underwent antireflux surgery, two returned after a variable interval of two to three years with an adenocarcinoma in the lower esophagus.

Table 2. Negative regression

Endo et al. 1974
Bremner 1984
Personal experience – 1986 (non dysplastic)
Adenocarcinoma in 2/10
After anti reflux surgery

Table 3. Suggested management

Medical measures – no good persisting
Close surveillance with systematic biopsies

No dysplasia ↙ ↘ Dysplastic

Antireflux surgery *Resection*

and
continued surveillance

Regression ↙ ↘ Persistence after surgery almost certainly will become malignant

Resection

How does one manage a patient who has columnar epithelium in his esophagus? It is known that medical regime by itself does not cause regression, even with the use of potent H_2 receptor blockers [6]. Therefore persistence with medical measures alone is pointless. However, if there is symptomatic improvement and close surveillance can be maintained, then in the absence of dysplasia there is justification in continuing with the program.

With increasing reports of regression with anti reflux surgery, one would strongly advocate surgical repair provided dysplasia has not been seen, and continued surveillance can be maintained. If, however, there is high grade dysplasia or carcinoma in situ, then surgical resection should be strongly advised and carried out.

My personal practice is to advise resection, not only for carcinoma in situ and high grade dysplasia, but also in intestinal metaplasia not showing regression or if there is any doubtful feature in the histopathology (Table 3).

References

1. Brand DL, Ylvisaker JT, Gelfand M, Pope CE (1980) Regression of columnar esophageal (Barrett's) epithelium after anti-reflux surgery. The New England Journal of Medicine 302: 844–848
2. Skinner DB, Walther BC, Riddell RH, Schmidt H, Iascone C, DeMeester TR (1983) Barrett's Esophagus: Comparison of benign and malignant cases. Ann Surg 198(4): 554–566
3. Saubier EC, Gouillat C, Samaniego C, Guillaud M, Moulinier B (1985) Adenocarcinoma in columnar-lined Barrett's Esophagus: analysis of 13 esophagectomies. Am J Surg 150: 365–369
4. Bremner CG, In Watson A, Celestin LR, editors (1984) Disorders of the oesophagus. Advances and Controversies. London Pitman 94–104
5. Endo M, Kobayashi S, Kozu T et al (1974) A case of Barrett's epithelialization followed up for five years. Endoscopy 6: 48–51
6. Wesdorp ICE, Bartelsen J, Schipper MEI, Offerhaus J, Tytgat GN (1981) Malignancy and premalignancy in Barrett's esophagus: a clinical endoscopical and histological study. Acta Endoscopica 11: 317–326

Can esophageal mucosa return to a malpighian configuration?

A. H. Hölscher (Munich)

The return to a malpighian configuration in Barrett's esophagus means a change of columnar epithelium into stratified squamous epithelium. In contrast to the question of regression of Barrett's esophagus, this special question is, if within the columnar epithelium islands of squamous epithelium may develop? The histogenesis of the change of the columnar epithelium to a malpighian configuration is not known.

In his study about Barrett's esophagus, Skinner has observed that after antireflux surgery in 2 of his patients an extension of patchy zones of squamous epithelium into regions of previously columnar lined esophagus developed [2]. By endoscopy this regenerating squamous epithelium appeared as distinct thin patches of opaque epithelium overlying the reddened residual columnar epithelium. This observation was confirmed by multiple biopsies which showed superficial normal squamous epithelium with residual glandular epithelium beneath.

A similar report was given by Ransom [1]. He saw that one patient showed islands of squamous epithelium below the previous level of the squamo-columnar junction after fundoplication.

These reports state that it is basically possible that squamous epithelium with malpighian configuration is possible to develop within the columnar epithelium of Barrett's esophagus after antireflux surgery. Other observations concerning this change of epithelium are not available. These rare findings again demonstrate that in Barrett's esophagus a return of esophageal mucosa to malpighian configuration is an extremely rare condition.

References

1. Ransom JM, Patel GH, Clift SA, Wombel ME, Read RC (1982) Extended and limited types of Barrett's esophagus in the adult. Ann Thorac Surg 33: 19–27
2. Skinner DB, Walther BC, Riddell RH, Schmidt H, Iascone C, DeMeester TR (1983) Barrett's esophagus. Comparison of benign and malignant cases. Ann Surg 198: 554–566.

F. Potet (Paris)

This question may relate to 4 different fields; those of regression of the columnar epithelium of dysplasia and that of regression of the histochemical aspects. Sampling is essential for evaluating any feature of response, and depends on the number of biopsies, usually very inadequate. Again, the distance from the dental arches and the distance from the LES are also involved, and must be exactly comparable before possible regression can be truly confirmed.

Regression of dysplasia is one of the important points already raised, but here again it is clear how important the problem of sampling error may be. The dysplasia is not actually diffuse over the entire columnar zone, and if the biopsy site is a little to one side of the dysplastic zone, this will be enough to give a false appearance of regression.

As for the histochemical type of regression, no valid study on this subject has been made, and it seems necessary to organize prospective studies on this aspect.

What is the outcome of esophageal fibrosis after correction of reflux?

Th. H. Gouge (New York)

Our experience with peptic stricture associated with Barrett's esophagus suggests that fibrosis will resolve following correction of reflux by a complete, loose fundoplication.

We have operated on 48 patients with esophageal stricture from gastroesophageal reflux in our service at the New York University Medical Center since 1975. Thirty-six patients had strictures from gastroesophageal reflux alone (Table 1); twelve patients had strictures from gastroesophageal reflux and Barrett's esophagus. All the patients with Barrett's esophagus and 18 of the patients with simple esophagitis required pre-operative dilation.

We eliminated from analysis those patients with lesser strictures which did not require preoperative dilation, those patients operated recently and one patient who developed adenocarcinoma in Barrett's mucosa. The remaining 16 patients (Table 2) with esophagitis and stricture and 9 patients with Barrett's esophagus and stricture were compared. All were followed for at least 2 years.

The age and sex distribution of the groups were comparable. All had histologic confirmation of the diagnosis and all were treated by intraoperative dilation and complete, loose fundoplication. Postoperative dilations were done as required to relieve dysphagia. Periodic follow-up examinations with endoscopy were done. Symptomatic patients were further evaluated for evidence of reflux.

Table 1. N.Y.U. Experience. General series

	Esophagitis and Stricture	Barrett's Esophagus and Stricture
Number of patients	36	12
Pre-operative dilations	50%	100%
Multiple pre-operative dilations	12.5%	67%

Table 2. N.Y.U. Experience. Cases studied

	Esophagitis and Stricture	Barrett's Esophagus and Stricture
Number of patients	16	9
Post-operative dilations	75%	78%
Multiple post-operative dilations	6.25%	33%

Results

Comparison of the two groups revealed minor differences consistent with the subjective impression that Barrett's strictures were firmer and higher than those with esophagitis alone. Only 12.5% of esophagitis patients required multiple preoperative dilations; 67% of Barrett's patients had more than one pre-operative dilation. Post-operatively, 75% of the esophagitis patients required dilation during the first six months, 50% were dilated once; only one patient (6.25%) required more than two dilations. That patient was dilated 4 times in six months. No patient required dilation after six months and all were able to eat a regular diet without radiographic evidence of stricture or dysphagia thereafter (Table 3).

Among the patients with Barrett's esophagus, 78 % required postoperative dilation and 67% required more than one dilation. Two patients (22%) were dilated for over a year, and although no patient had recurrent or persistent stricture radiographically, 22% still had mild dysphagia at 2 years.

None of the patients with Barrett's mucosa had regression to normal epithelium and no patient had a decrease in the length of the Barrett's mucosa following the initial correction for post-operative change. No patient required resection for stricture. All patients had effective control of reflux.

Discussion and conclusion

These results parallel those reported by Mercer and Hill [1] and others [2, 3, 4] who reported that conservative treatment of benign strictures will yield good results in most patients. In strictures associated with esophagitis alone, complete resolution of

Table 3. N.Y.U. Experience. Follow-up study

	Esophagitis and Stricture	Barrett's Esophagus and Stricture
Number of patients	16	9
Duration of Dilations		
<6 months	100%	78%
>1 year	0	22%
Duration of Dysphagia		
6 months	6.25%	33%
1 year	0	22%
2 years	0	22%

fibrosis is the rule even if dilation is not done [4]. In the firmer strictures associated with Barrett's esophagus, excellent results can still be anticipated and following dilation and reflux control, fibrosis will resolve completely in 78% of patients.

We presume that the reflux which led to Barrett's esophagus has sufficiently damaged the esophagus that enough mural fibrosis remains to cause mild dysphagia without radiographic evidence of stricture.

References

1. Mercer CD, Hill LD (1986) Surgical management of peptic esophageal stricture. Twenty-year experience. J Thor Cardiovasc Surg 91: 371
2. Starnes VA, Adkins B, Ballinger JF, Sawyers JL (1984) Barrett's esophagus: A surgical entity. Arch Surg 119: 563
3. Berardi RS, Devaiah KA (1983) Barrett's esophagus. Surg Gynecol Obstet 156: 521
4. Watson A (1984) The role of antireflux surgery combined with fiberoptic endoscopic dilation in peptic esophageal stricture. Am J Surg 148: 346

Malignant degeneration of benign lesions (1)

Experimental cancers of the esophagus

G. Castrini, and *F. S. Correnti* (Rome)

Several epidemiologic and experimental studies have been done around the esophageal cancer (E.C.), nevertheless the exact etiology is still unknown like most of the cancers.

A greater geographic variation is apparent for the incidence of E.C. than for any other cancer with endemic regions (Caspian littoral of Iran, Northeastern China, Hong Kong, New Zealand, Japan, South Carolina, Northern France, etc.) where the E.C. seems to be significantly related to the dietary habits [1, 2, 4, 7, 21].

Variations in such high risk areas are usually relatively stable and therefore should provide clues to causation. A lot of dietary staples as result of improper processing and/or storage (salted fish, dried shrimp, chinese sausage, liver sausage, chinese bacon, preserved oyster, preserved duck, pickled turnip, wheat, maize and millet from the high incidence Linxian area, mouldy cornmeal, bracken fern, red and birdproof sorghum, etc.) contain chemical or organic carcinogens [1, 11] whose effect on esophageal carcinogenesis is modified by dietary deficiences and/or abuse of alcohol, tobacco, etc.

The two most studied groups of carcinogens are Mycotoxins, Aflatoxin in particular, and N-Nitrosamines. Mycotoxins are elaborated by some strains of fungi (Fusarium, Geotricum and, especially, Aspergillus) and frequently isolated in preserved food. These are steroid compounds with an immunosuppressive action and cause irritation and ulceration followed by basal hyperplasia of the squamous epithelium of the esophagus leading to E.C. [38]. In laboratory animals they produce cancers in different organs (liver, colon, kidney, stomach, esophagus and tongue) [24].

Mouldy preserved foods are also responsable for the synthesis of N-Nitroso compounds and/or their precursors (Nitrites, Nitrates, etc.). Experimentally, rats fed F. Moniliforme-Contaminated cornbread, where it was demonstrated the presence of mycotoxins and nitrosamines, developed E.C. in 43% of the cases besides other papillary hyperplastic lesions of the remaining animals that did not develop cancer [11]. In further studies, in 100% of mice fed with crude extracts from cultures of strains of Fusaria, the lining of the esophagus become ulcerated, keratinised and desquamated with microscopical disorganised architecture [38].

Regarding the N-Nitrosamines, carcinogenic in more than 80% of cases [1, 24], the most interesting property is their organ specificity: the N-Nitrosomethyl-benzylamine (MBN), in particular, has carcinogenic effects against the esophageal mucosa; squamouscell E.C. develops in 90% of the laboratory animals fed these nitroso compounds by whatever route they are administered (enteral or parenteral [1, 7, 9, 11, 12, 24, 31]. The mechanisms by which nitrosamines induce E.C. is not completely understood yet, it is known that to exert their biological effect they require enzymatic conversion to intermediates (06 Alkyl-2-deoxyguanosines) which subsequently react with cellular macromolecules including DNA [8].

Epidemiologic evidence has increasingly indicated that dietary excesses and deficiences play important roles in the etiology of many forms of human cancers. Various studies in the Caspian littoral of Iran and in China suggest that the high frequency of the tumor is strongly associated with a low intake of fresh vegetables, fruit, and animal products, accompanied by simultaneous low intake of several vitamines (A, Riboflavin, C, etc.), animal proteins and minerals (Zinc, Molybdenum, Iron, Copper, Chrome, Manganese, Nickel Selenium, etc.) [1, 19, 21, 22, 25, 26, 27, 29].

Dietary vitamin A deficiency increases carcinogenic effects of aflatoxins [26, 27]. Riboflavin deficient mice developed hyperkeratosis, hyperplasia and tumors in the upper alimentary tract, and the supply of nitroso-compounds produced more cancers than in animals fed with them but with normal riboflavin diet [1, 21]. Vitamin C supply seems to be able to prevent the growth of esophageal carcinoma in 100% of rats fed nitrite and methylbenzylamine, antagonizing perhaps the formation of nitrosamines [1, 28].

Among the trace elements, it is interesting to note the effect of molybdenum, an important constituent of certain enzymes such as nitrate-reductases and other oxydases: its deficiency leads to the accumulation of nitrates in plants and to the gastric synthesis of nitrosamines [1, 11, 20].

Anyway, the most important of these minerals is zinc, essential for the normal development of many species. Dietary zinc deficiency alone has been shown to produce extensive mucosal lesions in the esophagus of the rat (hyperplasia, parakeratosis, hyperkeratosis), and to cause athrophy of limphoid tissues leading to derangements in both humoral and cellular immunity [1, 10, 21, 22, 31].

How zinc deprivation affects immunodepression remains largely unknown: data from literature suggest that zinc is required by enzymes involved in DNA synthesis and plays an important role in maintaining the integrity and function of lymphocite membrane [10]. All such conditions might enhance the susceptibility of the esophageal epithelium to chemical carcinogens and promote the subsequent growth of tumors, such as proved by rats maintained on a zinc deficient diet who exhibit a significant increased incidence of MBN-induced E.C. (79% of the cases) when compared to rats on a control diet (29% of the cases) [10]. 83% of these MBN-induced E.C. in zinc deficient rats were invasive carcinoma, and also the multiplicity of the tumors was greater in the deficient group. Zinc deficiency seems also to be able to modifie the organ-specificity of some nitrosamines such as nitrosodimethylamine (DMN), usually liver carcinogenic compound [9]. Recently Barch et al. [31] demonstrated in rats maintained on a zinc-deficient and MBA diet a significantly $p<0.001$) larger number (28.75 ± 1.95) of E.C. greater than 1 mm in diameter than in the animals on the control zinc diet (13.96 ± 1.23). Histologic examination of the esophagus from MBA treated animals also revealed microinvasive carcinoma in 62% of the rats on the zinc-deficient diet vs 40% of those on the zinc-control diet ($p<0.01$). The same authors observed an increased esophageal microsomal metabolism of MBA in rats on zinc-deficient diet which could then form more active metabolites (Benzaldehyde), and lead to the increased incidence of esophageal carcinoma.

Further experimental studies proved also that when a zinc-deficient dietary group of animals was switched to a control diet after the end of carcinogen treatment, a significantly reduced tumor incidence from the level of the zinc-deficient group was observed (75.7 vs 51%, $p < 0.05$) [22].

All these findings suggest a possible mechanism by which zinc-deficiency enhances E.C. incidence.

Although in most of the high incidence areas (Asia, Africa, etc.) the drinking of alcohol as a risk factor is not considered important, epidemiological studies indicate that the consumption of alcoholic beverages entails an increased risk for E.C. in Western countries [4, 13, 17] with a relative risk for developing tumors 8.47 times greater for heavy drinkers than for non drinkers [2].

However pure alcohol per se has been proved to be noncarcinogenic in laboratory animals [2, 13] but it works as enhancing factor promoting, for example, the carcinogenic activity of cigarette smoke condensate when applied to the skin of rats [2, 13]. Benzopyrene has been shown to penetrate esophageal mucosa when diluted in ethanol [2, 17, 18]. Anyway, benzopyrene has been demonstrated to be able to induce squamous-cell carcinoma in no more than 37% of hamsters, and only if there is a concomitant distal esophageal constriction [37]. An indicative hypothesis is that alcohol may increase the permeability of the esophagus, perhaps to carcinogens, and may allow the carcinogens to reach the basal premitotic layer of the esophageal epithelium [24]. Moreover, in humans, studies of alcoholics have shown many of them to be serum zinc deficient (increased zincuria in 50% of noncirrhotic alcoholics [22] and studies on rats fed alcohol showed a significantly lower absorption of dietary zinc [22, 23, 24, 31]. Moreover, the addition of chronic alcohol consumption to the zinc deficient diet of laboratory animals further enhances tumor incidence (85.3 vs 75.7%) [22].

If such an effect of alcohol on zinc status does exist, it suggests a connection between these two factors in the etiology of E.C. Authors suggest chronic consumption of alcohol favors reflux esophagitis and transformation into columnar-type epithelium of different types which could explain the increased prevalence of E.C. in alcohol consumers [34]. The risk for cancers of the esophagus is increased significantly when the use of tobacco is combined with heavy alcohol intake [2, 12, 13, 18]: The precise mechanism by which alcohol and tobacco act synergistically remains to be specified but, whatever the mechanism, abstinence from alcohol would greatly reduce the rate of E.C. among smokers [13].

The widespread use of opium and its recycled pyrolytic products, particularly in high incidence regions (Iran), seems to be associated with the development of E.C. Their mechanism is not clear yet, but functional studies proved that opium decreases esophageal peristalsis and inhibits the relaxation of the lower esophageal sphincter; the consequent stasis might allow potential swallowed carcinogens to have prolonged contact with the esophageal mucosa and enhance neoplasia [32]. This would be particularly true if the mucosa is vulnerable as a result of chronic malnutrition: recent experimental studies proved that, with carcinogen exposure, rats with operatively induced esophageal stenosis had 43% more E.C. than control group without stenosis ($p < 0.002$) [3].

Radiation can be another causa of esophageal carcinoma even if only 10 cases have been reported since 1957. Radiation induced cancer can be a consequence of the typical progression of acute radiation esophagitis to chronic changes [35]. Radiation induced E.C. perhaps is less rare than the literature shows; in fact the prolonged interval following radiotherapy before the growth of E.C., with an average latent time of 20–30 years [35], may lead to ignore this important past history: in our experience we had a 37 year old patient with invasive squamous-cell carcinoma of the middle esophagus 25 years after massive radiotherapy for hyperplasia of the thymus. Gates and Warren [36] were able experimentally to induce squamous-cell E.C. in 15% of mice irradiated with Cobalt-60 implants, and the incidence of radiation induced cancer was dependent upon both the total dosage and intensity of radiation exposure.

The recent literature report of the first demonstration of herpes virus in association with E.C. and the frequently observed association of herpes viruses and esophagitis, with the presumptive relationship between esophagitis and E.C. (at least in Iran), beside the known role of these viruses in certain cancers, suggested that herpes virus could initiate malignant change in the esophagus [39]. More intense investigations are needed to demonstrate such a hypothesis.

In conclusion, although a great deal of information on E.C. has been obtained, the causative factors and the mechanisms by which they enhance E.C. incidence remain to be established. However, epidemiological and laboratory investigations proved that E.C. is a multifactorial event where the primary suspects in causing the cancer are likely to be chemical carcinogens and dietary deficiences. In particular nitroso-compounds and zinc deficiency have been seen to be associated with an increased incidence of esophageal carcinoma.

References

1. Yang CS (1980) Research on esophageal cancer in China: a review Cancer Res 40: 2633–2644
2. Winder EL, Bross IJ (1961) A study of etiological factors in cancer of the esophagus. Cancer 14: 389–413
3. Sons HU, Borchard F, Muller-Jaak K, Sandmann H (1985) Acerebral tumor induction by distal esophageal construction in the rat under the influence of N-Ethyl-N-Butyl-Nitrosamine. Cancer 56: 2617–2621
4. Warwick GP (1973) Some aspects of the epidemiology and etiology of the esophageal cancer with particular emphasis on the transkey, South Africa. Adv Cancer Res 17: 81–229
5. Shimkin MB (1984) Environmental carcinogenesis in "Surgical Oncology" by Pilch YH, Ed McGraw-Hill Book Co 7–22
6. Pradhan SH, Chung EB, Ghosh B, Paul BD, Kapadia GY (1974) Potential carcinogens. I – Carcinogenicity of some plant extracts and their tannin-containing fractions in rats. J Nat Cancer Inst 52: 1579–1582
7. Preussmann R, Stewart BW (1984) In: Searle CE (Ed), Chemical carcinogens. 2nd Ed 643–828, Am Chem Soc Washington DC
8. Goth R, Rajewsky MF (1974) Persistence of O-ethylguanine in rat brain DNA: correlation with nervous system-specific genesis by ethylnitrosourea. Proc Nat Acad Sci (Washington) VI: 639–643
9. Magee PN, Montesano R, Preussmann R (1976) N-nitroso compounds and related carcinogens. Chemical carcinogens ACS monograph 173: 491–625, CE Searle Am Chem Soc Press

10. Fong LYY, Sivak A, Newberne PM (1978) Zinc deficiency and methyl-benzylnitrosamine-induced esophageal cancer in rats. J Nat Cancer Inst 61: 145–150
11. Li MH, Li P, Li PJ (1980) Recent progress in research on esophageal cancer in China. Adv Cancer Res 33: 173–249
12. Mirvish SS, Salmasi S, Lawson TA, Pour P, Sutherland D (1985) Test of cathecol, Tannic Acid, Bidens Pilosa, Croton Oil, and Phorbol for cocarcinogenesis of esophageal tumors induced in rats by Methyl-n-amylnitrosamine. J Nat Cancer Inst 74, 6: 1283–1289
13. Tuyns AJ (1983) Oesophageal cancer in non-smoking drinkers and in non-drinking smokers. Int J Cancer 32: 443–444
14. Mahboubi E, Ghadirian P (1976) Tea drinking habits and esophageal cancer in adjacent low and high incidence areas in Iran. Proc Am Ass Cancer Res 17: 87
15. Segi M (1975) Tea-gruel as a possible factor for cancer of the esophagus. Gann 66: 199–202
16. Morton JF (1973) Plant products and occupational materials ingested by esophageal cancer victims in South Carolina. QJ Crude Drug Res 13: 2005–2022
17. Kuratsune M, Kohchi S, Horie A (1965) Carcinogenesis in the esophagus. I – Penetration of benzo (a) prine and other hydrocarbons into the esophageal mucosa. Gann 56: 177–187
18. Horie A, Kohchi S, Kuratsune M (1965) Carcinogenesis in the esophagus. II – Experimental production of esophageal cancer by administration of ethanolic solution of carcinogens. Gann 56: 429–441
19. Berra B, Rapelli S (1986) Aspetti biochimico-funzionali degli oligoelementi in traccia. Rass Clin Scient 5, 6, 7: 104–120
20. Cohen HJ, Fridovich E, Rajagopalan KV (1971) Hepatic sulfite oxidase. A functional role for molybdenum. J Biol Chem 246: 374–382
21. Newberne PM (1983) Dietary factors affecting biological responses to esophageal and colon chemical carcinogenesis. Proceedings of the "2nd Int Cong of ISDE, 163–171
22. Gabrial GN, Schrager TF, Newberne PM (1982) Zinc deficiency alcohol and a retinoid: association with esophageal cancer in rats. J Nat Cancer Inst 68: 785–789
23. Mobarhan S, Dowlatshahi K, Diba YY (1980) Hair zinc levels from normal population of Northeast Iran with high incidence of esophageal cancer. Clin Res 28: 598 A
24. Fong LY, Julin H, Lee CLH (1979) Methylation of DNA in target and non target organs the rat with methylbenzyl nitrosamine and dimethylnitrosamine. Int J Cancer 23: 679–682
25. Joint-Iran-International Agency for Research on Cancer Study Group (1977) Esophageal cancer studies in thye Caspian Littoral of Iran: results of population studies. A prodrome. J Nat Cancer Inst 59: 1127–1132
26. Hormozdiari H, Day NE, Aramesh B, Nahboubi E (1975) Dietary factors and esophageal cancer in the Caspian Littoral of Iran. Cancer Res 35: 3493–3498
27. Kaplan SC, Tsuchitani PJ (1978) Cancer in China. Alan R Liss, New York, Chap 4
28. Coordinating Group for research on the etiology of esophageal Cancer of North China: The epidemiology of esophageal cancer in North China and preliminary results in the investigation of its etiological factors. Paper presented at the 11th Int Cancer Congress
29. Diamond I, Hurley LS (1970) Histopathology of zinc-deficient fetal rats. J Nutr 100: 326–331
30. Diamond I, Swenerton H, Hurley LS (1971) Testicular and esophageal lesions in zinc-deficient rats and their reversibility. J Nutr 101: 77–81
31. Barch DH, Kummerle SC, Hollenberg PF, Iannaccone PM (1984) Esophageal microsomal metabolism of N-Nitrosomethylbenzylamine in the zinc-deficient rat. Cancer Res 44: 5629–5633
32. Dowlatshahi D, Miller RJ (1985) Role of the opium in esophageal cancer: a hypothesis. Cancer Res 45: 1906–1907
33. Spence IM (1985) Electron microscopic evidence of herpes-virus in association with esophageal carcinoma. Samy 68: 103–105
34. Martini GA (1976) Ethanol and Barrett's esophagus. N Engl J Med 2: 1322
35. O'Connell EW, Seaman WB, Gharhemani GG (1984) Radiation-induced esophageal carcinoma. Gastroent Radiol 9: 287–291
36. Gates O, Warren S (1968) Radiation-induced experimental cancer of the esophagus. Am J Pathol 53: 667–685
37. Dunham LJ, Sheets RH (1974) Effects of esophageal constriction on Benzopyrene carcinogenesis in Hamster esophagus and forestomach. J Nat Cancer Inst 53, 3: 875–878

38. Schoental R, Joffe AZ (1974) Lesions induced in radents by extracts from cultures of Fusarium and F Sporotrichioides. J Pathol 112: 37–42
39. Spence IM (1985) Electron microscopic evidence of herpesvirus in association with oesophageal carcinoma. Samt Deel, 68: 103–105
40. Ohshima H, Mahon GAT, Wahrendorf J, Bartsch H (1983) Doseresponse study of N-Nitrosoproline formation in rats and a deduced kinetik model for prolicting carcinogenic effects caused by endogenous nitrosation. Cancer Res 43: 5072–5076
41. Van Rensburg SJ, Hall JM, Bruyn DB (1985) Effects of various staples on esophageal carcinogenesis induced in rats by subcutaneously administered N-Nitrosomethylbenzylamine. JNCI 75, 3: 561–566

W. J. Pories (Greenville)

Basic research in carcinoma of the esophagus has been primarily based on the epidemiologic studies in man which have demonstrated that this malignancy is primarily environmental and therefore a preventable disease.

Epidemiologic clues

As noted by Mannell in her excellent monograph [6], "one of the most striking features of carcinoma of the esophagus is the extraordinary variation in its geographic distribution". As she points out, the regional variations within countries provide important clues for further research: In China's mountainous Henan, Hubei, and Shanxi provinces, for example, cancer of the esophagus is the most common cause of death in men and women with an incidence of 130/100.000 population. Yet nearby, in areas only short distances from these mountains, the mortality from this disease falls to less than 2/100.000.

Similarly demarcated areas exist in Iran (Caspian littoral: M/F=93/110/100.000), Africa (Transkei: 47% of all tumors in men and 36% in women are esophageal), France (Western Brittany, Normandy: 60/100.000) and the U.S. (Washington, DC; San Francisco; the eastern Carolinas). Other high risk regions include the Moslem Soviet Republics, Gur'evsk province in the USSR, the mountains of Japan, central Kenya, southern Zimbabwe, and the mountains of Iraq.

The epidemiologic studies of these regions clearly indicate that the causes of esophageal cancer in man include chronic irritation, alcohol, tobacco, dietary carcinogens, and malnutrition. Well recognized examples of *chronic irritation* which are considered premalignant include scarring from corrosives, chronic esophagitis, achalasia, scleroderma, and Barrett's esophagus.

Similarly, a heavy intake of *alcohol* has been shown to be a major factor in esophageal malignancies. Whether the damage is due to the physiologic effects of the alcohol per se, to malnutrition associated with alcoholism, to the contaminants frequently seen in alcoholic beverages (fusel oils, benzopyrene, and volatile nitrosoamines) or to a combination of these factors, is not clear.

Tobacco may also be a carcinogen due to several effects: the swallowing of tars; nitrosoamines in smoke, the potentiation by alcohol of the penetration of carcinogens into the esophageal mucosa, or the absorption from smoke of such toxic trace elements as cadmium and nickel.

Tobacco and alcohol, however, do not explain the majority of cases seen in the world. Although these two toxins may explain the high incidence of cancer of the esophagus in France and the coastal Carolinas, they are clearly not a cause among the orthodox Moslems of Iran and the USSR who neither smoke or drink.

A number of *dietary carcinogens* have been identified by the regional variations: nitrates, nitrites and nitrosoamines in food and water in China; fungal contaminants in Asian foods; chilis and spices in India; bracken fern in Japan; cereal contaminated by Fusarium species in Transkei; and silica fibers in wheat flour in Iran.

The common denominator for cancer of the esophagus, however, in all of the regions and with the various carcinogens is *malnutrition*. The victims are almost invariably poor and malnourished. The deficiencies identified in the populations at risk include protein, trace elements, and such vitamins as riboflavin, thiamine, nicotinic acid, and vitamins A and C.

Basic research in animals

Research in animals has therefore focused on malnutrition, exposure to carcinogens, or a combination of both: Newbern and his associates [9] have demonstrated that *zinc deficiency* in rats is associated with decreased zinc levels in esophageal tissue and enhances the induction of esophageal tumors by methylbenzylnitrosamine. Thirteen-retinoic acid combined with alcohol further enhanced the carcinogenic effect of zinc deficiency. They further demonstrated that putting the rats back on a control diet after exposure to the carcinogen during zinc deficiency, i.e. restoring some of the zinc deficit, significantly reduced the tumor incidence.

Our researches [10] in zinc nutrition have also documented that zinc deficiency, in a variety of species, interferes with epithelization and healing of injured squamous epithelium and that zinc supplementation prevents these defects.

These reports are supported by the findings of van Rensburg [11] who observed, in a large study in South African esophageal cancer areas that those at high risk consumed dietary staples which result in deficiencies of riboflavin, nicotinic acid, magnesium and zinc.

Newbern's group [5] also showed that Chinese patients with esophageal cancer in the Hong Kong area have reduced levels of zinc in hair, serum and esophageal tissue, compared to healthy controls or patients with other types of cancer.

Retinoids are another family of nutrients which appear to have a protective effect against the development of esophageal cancer in rats. Postcarcinogen administration of 13-cis-retinoic acid to N-methyl-N-benzylnitrosamine (MBzN) treated rats significantly reduced tumor related mortality compared with a nonretinoid group [8].

The roles of zinc and vitamin A (a retinoid) together were assessed in man by Mellow [7] and his coworkers. They found that plasma zinc and vitamin A were both significantly less in esophageal carcinoma than in age-matched healthy controls.

Although the evidence appears to be good that zinc and vitamin A deficiency may play a role in the development of esophageal cancer, it must be remembered that most patients with esophageal cancer are already malnourished at the time of diagnosis due to their dysphagia. There is little question that these patients are nutritionally deficient but that is not adequate evidence to conclude that the deficiency either caused or helped to cause the cancer. In addition, it is likely that zinc and vitamin A are not the only two missing dietary factors.

A large variety of *carcinogens* have been shown to induce carcinoma of the esophagus in animals: nitrosopiperidine and derivatives of that molecule in rats [3]; methyl-benzylnitrosamine (NMBzA) in rats [1], nitrosomethylbenzylamine and nitromethylethylamine in rats [4] are good examples. Goodall and Lijinski [2] emphasized the strong differences in the effect of these agents in different species: for example, rats differ considerably from hamsters in their sensitivity to these agents and in which organs the tumors develop. Accordingly, caution needs to be exercised before assuming that the dramatic findings made in animals really pertain also to man.

Although additional animal studies may prove useful in delineating the underlying mechanismus of carcinogenesis, it would appear that the most productive area of research would be in the field of prevention: such studies might include prospective randomized trials in which high risk populations are supplemented with proteins, trace elements, and vitamins and then tested periodically with such screening techniques as the blind abrasive cytology currently practiced in China. Although such studies would be expensive, they would be far cheaper than our current approaches to this dreadful disease.

References

1. Craddock VM, Sparrow S, Henderson AR (1986) The effect of the trichothecene mycotoxin diacetotoxyscirpenol on nitrosoamineinduced esophageal cancer in the rat. Cancer Letters 31: 197–204
2. Goodall CM, Lijinski W (1984) Strain and sex differences in N-nitrosohexamethyleneimine carcinogenesis in NZB, NZC, NZO and NZ:Y mice. JNCI 73: 1215–1218
3. Lijinski W, Singer GM, Reuber MD (1981) The effect of 4-substitution on the carcinogenicity of nitrosopiperadine. Carcinogenesis 2: 1045–1048
4. Lijinski W, Saavedea JE, Reuber MD, Singer SS (1982) Esophageal carcinogenesis in f344 rats by nitrosomethylethylamines substituted in the ethyl group. JNCI 68jj: 681–684
5. Lin HJ, Chan WC, Fong YY, Newbern PM (1977) Zinc levels in serum, hair, and tumors from patients with esophageal cancer. Nutr Repts Intern 15: 635–643
6. Mannell A (1982) Carcinoma of the Esophagus. Current Problems in Surgery 19: 555-647
7. Mellow MH, Layne EA, Lipman TO, Kaushik M, Hostetler C, Smith JC (1983) Plasma zinc and vitamin A in human squamous carcinoma of the esophagus. Cancer 51: 1615–1620
8. Moon RC, McCormick DL (1982) Inhibition of chemical carcinogenesis by retinoids. J Am Acad Dermatology 6: 809–814
9. Newbern PM, Schrager T (1983) Promotion of gastrointestinal tract tumors in animals: Dietary Factors. Environmental Health Perspectives 50: 71–83
10. Pories WJ, Strain WH, Hsu JM, Woosley RL (1974) RL: *Clinical Applications of Zinc Metabolism.* CC Thomas Pub Springfield, Ill. pp 301
11. van Rensburg SJ (1978) Epidemiologic and dietary evidence for a specific nutritional predisposition to esophageal cancer. J Natl Cancer Inst 61: 145–150

T. Lehnert, S. Ivankovic, K. Junghanns, and *N. Yioris*
(Heidelberg)

Having a dismal prognosis with a 5 year survival hardly exceeding 10% [1, 2], much would be gained if pathogenetic factors of esophageal carcinoma could be identified. In human pathology a number of conditions such as achalasia [3], Plummer-Vinson syndrome [4] or tylosis [5] have been identified as bearing an increased risk of esophageal malignancy. Such conditions are rare, however, and cannot be related to the majority of esophageal cancers detected.

Based on studies conducted in a high-incidence area of esophageal carcinoma, it has been suggested that esophageal cancer may develop via a sequence of chronic esophagitis, atrophy and subsequent dysplasia [6]. We have, therefore, studied the effect of chronic reflux esophagitis on esophageal tumorigenesis in an experimental model using a nitrosamide as carcinogen.

Material and Methods

Experimental animals were inbred Wistar rats (250–300 g) supplied by Ivanovas Kiesslegg, FRG. Animals were housed in plastic cages in a temperature- and humidity-controlled environment with a 12 hour day and night cycle. Animals were fed with a commercial laboratory rat feed (Altromin) and tap water.

Animals were divided into three experimental groups: first: 2.5 mg carcinogen/kg body weight, second: 2.5 carcinogen/kg body weight plus reflux, third: reflux alone. A concurrent group of untreated animals with a strain-specific tumor incidence of 2% (mainly fibroadenoma of the breast) served as control.

Chronic reflux of all duodenal contents into the esophagus was achieved by means of an esophagojejunostomy end-to-side (Fig. 1). Carcinogen-treatment with N-

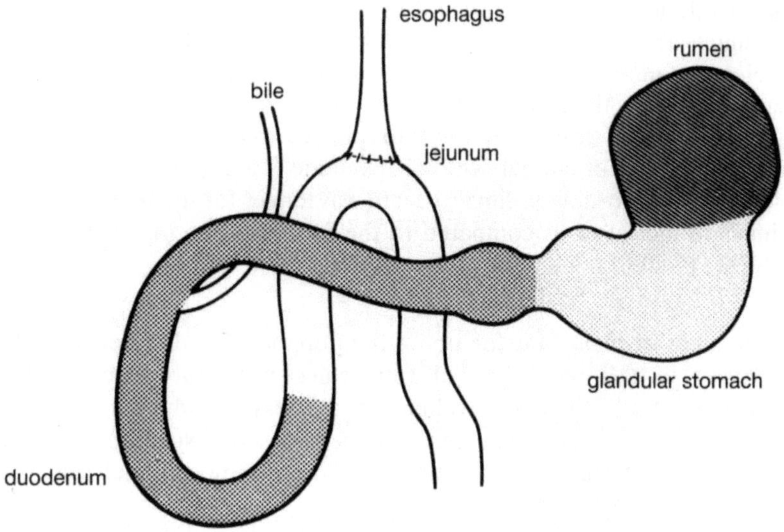

Fig. 1. Surgical preparation to induce chronic reflux of duodenal contents into the esophagus

Methyl-N-Nitro-N-Nitrosoguanidine (MNNG; CAS 70–25–7) was started 4 weeks postoperatively at a daily dose of 2.5 mg per kilogram initial weight. The carcinogen was administered in drinking water.

All animals were followed until spontaneous death. At autopsy specimens of the esophagus were removed for histologic examination. Tissues were fixed in 10% neutral formalin, dehydrated in graded alcohols and embedded in paraffin. Sections were cut at 5 μ and stained with hematoxylin-eosin. Only animals surviving 50 days postoperatively were included in the statistical analysis to account for early death. For statistical analysis the Student's t-test and Fisher's exact test were used.

Results

Chronic reflux of duodenal contents into the esophagus resulted in severe ulcerative esophagitis. Such changes were more pronounced in the distal esophagus regardless of the addition of carcinogen treatment. No pathologic changes were observed in the esophagus of animals without reflux surgery. Histologically, hyperplasia of basal layers of squamous epithelium with hyperkeratosis and ingrowth of epithelial cell buds into the submucosal layer were noted.

The first malignant tumor of the esophagus was observed in an animal with reflux plus carcinogen treatment on day 130 of the study. Histologically this tumor was determined to be a polymorphocellular sarcoma (Fig. 2). The first epithelial tumor of the esophagus in this group was seen on day 154 of the study. Histologically this was a squamous cell carcinoma (Fig. 3, Table 1).

The first malignant tumor in the group that was subjected to chronic reflux alone was a squamous cell carcinoma detected on day 280. The first mesenchymal tumor was detected on day 300. In addition to these malignant tumors, a number of benign papillomas were noted in the esophagus of animals subjected to reflux alone. The first such lesion was seen on day 236.

Animals receiving treatment with the carcinogen, but without reflux surgery, developed a number of malignant tumors in the stomach and colon, but no lesions were detected in the esophagus.

The survival of animals with reflux plus carcinogen treatment was significantly shorter than that of animals with reflux alone (160±17 vs. 280±22 days; x±SEM; $p < 0.0005$). Accordingly, time to death was longer for squamous carcinoma bearing animals in the latter as compared to the former group (420±70 vs. 233±44 days, x±SEM; $p < 0.05$).

*

A number of malignant tumors of both epithelial and mesenchymal origin have developed in the esophagus of rats which were subjected to chronic reflux esophagitis. Such tumors developed regardless of whether animals had been exposed to additional carcinogen treatment or not. No esophageal tumors were noted in animals that were treated with the carcinogen, but that had not been operated.

Mean survival was shorter in animals with chronic reflux when they were exposed to additional carcinogen treatment as compared to animals with reflux but without

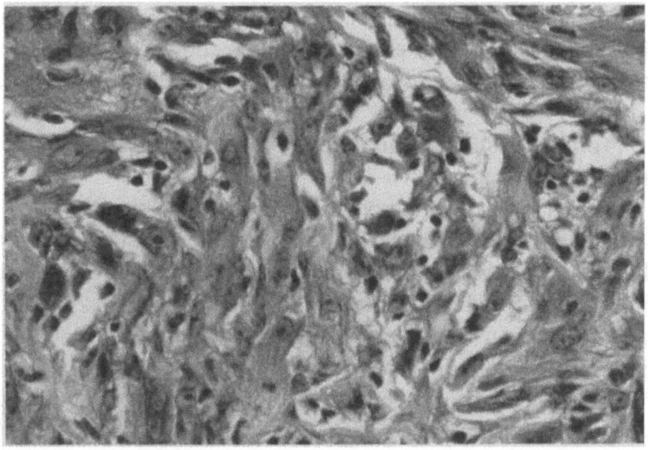

Fig. 2. Polymorphocellular sarcoma of the esophagus (H & E, 250×)

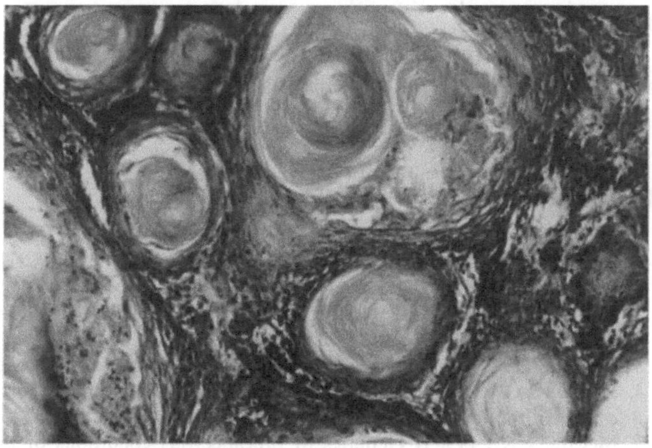

Fig. 3. Squamous cell carcinoma of the esophagus (H & E, 250×)

Table 1. Malignant Tumors of the GI-Tract

I	Carcinogen alone	n=30	stomach	2 adeno-ca
				1 leiomyo-sa
			colon	1 adeno-ca
II	Carcinogen plus reflux	n=23	esophagus	4 squamous-ca
				4 sarcoma
III	Reflux alone	n=30	esophagus	3 squamous-ca
				2 sarcoma
				4 papilloma
IV	Control	n=10	none	

I vs. II all esophageal malignancies $p < 0.0006$ (Fisher's exact test) carcinogen treatment. This may indicate toxicity of the carcinogen even though a low dosage had been chosen. Tumors, however, developed significantly earlier in this group. This points at a cocarcinogenic effect of MNNG in this setting.

From the results of this study, a carcinogenic effect of diverted duodenal contents must be concluded.

Such a notion is supported by other observations on the effects of diverted duodenal contents in the upper gastrointestinal tract in rats. Several investigators have reported gastric adenocarcinoma in rats following surgical procedures resulting in reflux of duodenal contents into the stomach [7, 8, 9, 10], even in the absence of any carcinogen treatment. Bile has been shown to enhance gastric carcinogenesis induced by MNNG [11].

Constituents of duodenal secretions such as bile and trypsin have been shown to play an important role in the development of esophagitis [12, 13, 14]. Such reflux esophagitis has also been examined with respect to its proliferative characteristics: labelling studies using ^{3}H-thymidine have shown that epithelial proliferation is increased, and that such cell kinetic changes are accompanied by a thickening of the basal layer of esophageal squamous epithelium and increasing papillary length [15, 16].

Our study therefore supports the concept that esophageal carcinoma develops via a state of chronic reflux esophagitis.

References

1. Earlam R, Cunha-Melo JR (1980) Oesophageal carcinoma: A critical review of surgery. Br J Surg 67: 381–390
2. Earlam R, Cunha-Melo JR (1980) Oesophageal carcinoma: A critical review of radiotherapy. Br J Surg 67: 457–461
3. Cohen S (1979) Motor disorders of the Oesophagus. N Engl J Med 301: 184–192
4. Larsson LG, Sandstrom A, Westling P (1975) Relationship of Plummer-Vinson disease to cancer of the upper alimentary tract in Sweden. Cancer Res 35: 3308–3316
5. McConell RB (1983) Genetics of precancerous conditions of the gastrointestinal tract. In: Sherlock P, Morson BC, Barbara L, Veronesi U (eds) Raven Press, New York 23–42
6. Munoz N, Crespi M, Grassi A et al. (1982) Precursor lesions of oesophageal cancer in high-risk populations in Iran and China. Lancet I, 876–879
7. Langhans P, Heger RA, Hohenstein J et al. (1981) Operation sequel carcinoma of the stomach. Experimental studies of surgical techniques with and without resection. World J Surg 5: 595–605
8. Dittrich S, Theuring F, Heinrich P, Wolter FH (1984) Das Karzinom im operierten Rattenmagen – ein Tumormodell. Arch Geschwulstforschung 54: 33–40
9. Kondo K, Suzuki H, Nagayo T (1984) The influence of gastrojejunal anastomosis on gastric carcinogenesis in rats. Jpn J Cancer Res 75: 362–369
10. Salmon RJ, Merle S, Zafrani B et al. (1985) Gastric carcinogenesis induced by MNNG: Role of gastrectomy and duodenal reflux. Jpn J Cancer Res 76: 167–172
11. Kobori O, Shimizu T, Maeda M et al. (1984) Enhancing effect of bile and bile acid on stomach tumori genesis induced by MNNG in Wista rats. JNCI 73: 853–861
12. Mud H, Kranendonk SE, Obertop H, Van Houten H, Westbroek DL (1982) Active trypsin and reflux oesophagitis: An experimental study. Br J Surg 69: 269–272
13. Salo JA, Kivilaakso E (1982) Role of bile salts and trypsin in the pathogenesis of experimental alkaline esophagitis. Surgery 93: 525–532

14. Cross FS, Wangensteen OH (1951) Role of bile and pancreatic juice in production of esophageal erosions and anemia. Proc Soc Exp Biol Med (N.Y.) 77: 862–866
15. Johnson LF, DeMeester TR, Haggitt RC (1978) Esophageal epithelial response to gastroesophageal reflux. Dig Dis 23: 498–509
16. Livston EM, Sheahan DG, Behar J (1977) Studies on esophageal epithelial cell proliferation in patients with reflux esophagitis. Gastroenterology 73: 1315–1319

What are the histologic criteria of developing carcinoma in biopsies of benign lesions?

F. Potet (Paris)

The problem that may prove difficult is that of malignant degeneration in a Barrett's mucosa, i.e. a preceding columnar cell type of lesion, and the interpretation to be given to lesions of dysplastic appearance.

Riddell et al. insist on a very precise definition of the dysplasia, as an unequivocally neoplastic change in a columnar cell mucosa. They classify the appearances of the mucosa under three heads: a mucosa negative for dysplasia; a mucosa of indeterminate dysplasia (with regenerative lesions); and a mucosa positive for dysplasia. It is this last that poses the most difficult problems, especially when dealing with high-grade dysplasias.

It is therefore essential in examining the biopsies to look for rupture of the basal layer and invasion of the lamina propria by carcinomatous formations which would confirm the presence of cancer, and not to hesitate to review the sections carefully and to repeat them at several levels before deciding that the lesion is malignant.

In the presence of such appearances of severe dysplasia, the prospect of surgery should not be raised without a totally assured diagnosis of cancer, which entails the possibility of several repeated biopsies during regular supervision of the patient.

What is the value of retrograde biopsies?

J. Baulieux, and *P. Maillet* (Lyons)

All the publications about benign peptic stenosis of the esophagus mention a certain percentage of dubious lesions (between 2 and 4%) for which the security indication remains for a long time the exeresis.

It is obvious nowadays that the conjunction of biopsy and cytology (wich may be repeated) also bring a huge security. But sometimes the uncertainty comes from the anatomo pathologic answer itself. However, it is essential to have absolute certainty in the diagnosis, for deliberate purpose is today preferable to conservative methods.

Some years ago, we underlined the interest of surgical exploration which in some cases allows confirmation or correction of the diagnosis: the method consists of performing a high gastrotomy after investigation of the hiatus and the juxtacardiac nodules. This is done by using endoesophageal palpation to explore the inferior pole of the lesion, its rigidity, the existence of friable buds, and finally its degree of fixation, which shows the malignancy.

On the other hand, the axial size of the stenosis, the possibility of digital dilatation, and its regularity indicate its being benign.

The use of flexible biopsy forceps, eventually guided by a rectoscope introduced into the gastrotomy allows biopsies in areas that have not been correctly explored.

So, we can report a series of 14 cases where such a procedure had been performed preoperatively (3.6% of the total experiment).

This series allows:

- confirmation of an uncertain diagnostic of peptic stenosis (7 cases),
- correction of a mistaken diagnosis (6 cases),
- with only one mistake by excess (resection for benign stenosis).

We are conscious of the effectiveness of this method. We acknowledge that during the last five years the combination of present fiberoscopic methods, for instance the use of the pediatric fiberoscope after dilatation of the stenosis, gave us all the necessary information on what course to take. This possibility must be known, and in some cases, can be helpful.

Reference

1. Maillet P, Boulez J, Baulieux J, Peix JL, Donne R (1980) Sténose peptique ou cancer de l'œsophage. Difficultés diagnostiques et valeur de l'exploration per-opératoire. Chirurgie, 106: 719-721

Malignant degeneration of benign lesions (2)

President: *Marcel Savary* (Lausanne)

Free Commentators: *G. Friehs* (Graz)
Th. H. Gouge (New York)
T. Orlowski (Wroclaw)
Cl. A. Richard (Paris)
G. H. Willital, K. H. Dietl (Münster)

Degeneration of megaesophagus. Is there a particular symptomatology?

F. H. Ellis (Boston)

It is now generally accepted that achalasia is a pre-malignant condition. However, the prevalence and incidence of malignant degeneration in achalasia are not well defined and certain features of its symptomatology and precise etiology are unclear.

While the precise mechanism responsible for the development of carcinoma in the achalasic esophagus is not known, it is generally thought to be due to chronic irritation secondary to stasis. There are certain features peculiar to this lesion that support this view: it occurs in the dilated portion of the thoracic esophagus, usually the lower half to two thirds, rather than in the distal narrowed segment, after many years of dysphagia (20 on average) [1] and usually develops at an earlier age than is true of other esophageal cancers. Successful treatment either by dilation or surgery does not protect against the subsequent development of carcinoma, suggesting that since neither form of therapy restores normal function to the esophagus, persistent stasis after treatment due to lack of peristalsis may continue to play an etiologic role in the development of cancer in esophageal achalasia.

The prevalence rate of cancer varys in esophageal achalasia. It has been reported in 0–7.7% of clinical cases and 20 to 29% in autopsy series [2]. The risk of developing cancer for the achalasic patient is harder to define. The data from the Mayo Clinic presented by Wychulis and associates is the best available [3]. 1.018 patients with the diagnosis of achalasia were followed for an average of 13 years per patient; carcinoma developed in 7, for an incidence of 41 cases per year per 100.000, a rate approximately 7 times that reported in the general population. In addition to these seven patients, there were since then six others with carcinoma and achalasia available for study.

Difficulty in swallowing was present in all but one of the patients and was characterized by a recent increase in severity in the majority. Of importance to this discussion, a history of bleeding was present in five of the thirteen patients, hematemesis in four, and melena in two, one patient exhibiting both phenomena. Pain was present in eight of the thirteen patients.

Thus, a history of dysphagia recently increasing in severity coupled with symptoms of gastrointestinal bleeding and/or pain may be useful in diagnosing malignant degeneration of the achalasic esophagus.

The Lahey Clinic experience with carcinoma of the thoracic esophagus between January 1970 and January 1987 includes 143 surgical patients. Five developed carcinoma after a prior diagnosis of esophageal achalasia, a prevalence of 3.5% (Table 1). Of these five surgical patients, three had been treated successfully in the past by esophagomyotomy, one of them 23 years earlier and this patient has been reported in detail elsewhere [4].

Two of these patients were found to be nonresectable. These patients were treated by intubation with a (Celestin) tube with survival of one and a half and two

Table 1. Carcinoma in achalasia (Lahey Clinic)

Age	Sex	Symptoms	Treatment	Location	Treatment	Result
63	M	30 yrs.	Dilation	Upper	Celestin Tube	D 2½ mos.
57	F	52 yrs.	Myotomy × 2	Upper	Resection	D 6 mos.
69	M	2½ yrs.	Myotomy	Lower	Celestin Tube	D 1½ mos.
67	F	28 yrs.	Myotomy	Upper	Resection	D 7 mos.
67	M	13 yrs.	None	Lower	Resection	D 22 mos.

and a half months respectively. None of the three patients having resection were cured, survival being 6, 7, and 22 months respectively after resection.

*

Whether post-treatment stasis is a factor in the development of carcinoma in these patients, remains unclear. My personal opinion is that the total duration of stasis, whether pre-treatment or post-treatment, is the important factor in the subsequent development of carcinoma. Since stasis is more profound before treatment than after, pre-treatment stasis probably is a more important contributing factor to the development of carcinoma than is post-treatment stasis. More importantly, treatment whether surgical or by forceful dilation that successfully relieves the patient's symptoms of distal obstruction does not protect against the subsequent development of carcinoma. Accordingly, all such patients should receive long term regular endoscopic and histologic surveillance.

References

1. Hankins JR, McLaughlin JS (1975) The association of carcinoma of the esophagus with achalasia. J Thorac Cardiovasc Surg 69: 355–360
2. Bolivar JC, Herendeen TL (1970) Carcinoma of the esophagus and achalasia. Ann Thorac Surg 10: 81–89
3. Wychulis AR, Woolam GL, Andersen HA, Ellis FH Jr (1971) Achalasia and carcinoma of the esophagus. JAMA 215: 1638–1641
4. Heiss FW, Tarshis A, Ellis FH Jr (1984) Carcinoma associated with achalasia. Occurrence 23 years after esophagomyotomy. Dig Dis and Sci 29: 1066–1069

M. Endo (Tokyo)

There is no particular symptomatology in the early stages of esophageal cancer associated with achalasia. The cancer is commonly diagnosed at an advanced stage. Dysphagia worsens when the tumor becomes bigger in size. We sometimes recognize the carcinoma through the accompanying back pain and hoarseness. Retrosternal pain or compression is also an accompanying feature.

We have observed 11 cases of accompanying esophageal carcinoma among 153 cases of achalasia in our hospital, that is, a prevalence of 7.2%. One of the 11 cases of carcinoma was superficial cancer, the infiltration of which reached the submucosa. There was no particular symptom specific to esophageal carcinoma. Some of the tumors were diagnosed by periodic X-ray examination.

An analysis of 11 cases of carcinoma associated with achalasia revealed a long history of achalasia, with 70% having a history of 10 years or more, of whom 40% had a history of 30 years or more. Moreover, esophageal carcinoma was observed in three cases that had had a radical operation for achalasia.

Good results were obtained in cases in which curative resection was performed. Periodic examinations once or twice a year are considered necessary in order to diagnose malignant lesions at an early stage.

Malignant change in megaesophagus: has it a specific clinical picture?

R. Giuli (Paris)

The incidence of malignant degeneration in megaesophagus is not low; it amounted to 8.6% (26 cases) in our series of 302 operations for megaesophagus. The correlation between the two disorders seems to be genuine rather than simple coincidence, taking into account that the mean incidence of cancer in a normal population is only 15.5 per 100.000 men. On the other hand, in our series of 26 cases, we noted a relative frequency of this degeneration in women (5 cases).

Localization of the cancer was very often at the lower third (11 cases) or middle third (12 cases) of the esophagus. Without drawing any formal conclusion from this observation, such distribution by level is an argument that may be advanced to support the view that esophagitis due to stasis may play a part in malignant change. Infection of the esophagus at this stage and chemical irritation due to decomposition of nutrients certainly promote esophagitis; small submucous ulcerations then form which are eventually covered by the growth of fibrous tissue. Hyperplasia of this epithelium leads to the formation of small papillomata, one of which may be the site of malignant change, a phenomenon that may be analogous to that observed during the course of ulcerative colitis.

On the other hand, it seems equally possible to imagine that repeated dilatations over long periods of time, as observed in virtually all of our patients, may promote irritation of the mucous membrane with possible secondary malignant change.

In nearly all of these 26 patients the disease history was very long, going back 15–20 years on average. Before cancer was discovered, 11 of these had undergone a Heller's operation, on average 14 years previously, but 8 of these procedures had had a definitely poor result. The other 15 patients had not been operated and adapted to their symptoms at the price of repeated dilatations. It is clear that in such patients, with little relief from their Heller's operation or long subject to dilatation, the diagnosis of malignant change may often be very difficult to make and may only be made very late.

Aggravation of the dysphagia will attract attention and in half of our cases this change was recent, of less than 6 months' duration. In the other half, changes in the symptomatology had developed 1 to 2 years previously but had not disturbed the patient. However, loss of weight by 10 kg or more was a virtually constant feature. The relative frequency of regurgitation of food, sometimes bloodstained, should also be noted, in some cases (5 patients) amounting to actual hematemesis. Although such incidents may not greatly distress a patient suffering from dilatation, they should nevertheless call for new investigations as they are practically always indicative of serious complications. More rarely (2 cases), the first signs of malignancy were respiratory complications, due to tracheal compression or fistulization of the growth into the lung, with symptoms of a communication between the esophagus and the airway. Here again, these symptoms may not routinely suggest malignant degeneration, given the relative frequency of respiratory disorder due to alimentary regurgitation in the course of development of uncomplicated mega-esophagus.

Thus, it is mainly changes in the dysphagia or the appearance of hemorrhage that should arouse suspicion of malignant change during the course of a mega-esophagus. Radiography is an essential examination, but may be a source of error if poorly performed or interpreted. In 18 cases the films gave evidence of malignant change (Fig. 1), but the appearances were those of an already very advanced tumor and this, for the greater part (12) in patients who had had a series of radiographs staged over a year without the diagnosis having been confirmed. However in 6 cases the diagnosis had been suggested at one point and yet, in two of these patients, the biopsy revealed no abnormal features.

The errors in radiographic interpretation are often secondary to technical causes, due to the existence of fluid associated with stasis and of food debris (Fig. 2) which may create false tumor images. Again, the esophageal dilatation prevents good display of the passage of the barium in contact with the walls; it pools in the lower part of the organ and blurs the contours, whereas in the upper part the absence of contrast medium does not allow a perfect grasp of the parietal outlines. It is therefore necessary to repeat these examinations after proper esophageal lavage and evacuation, and it may also be advisable to make these films using viscous media combined with effervescent agents, which sometimes favors a more definite opinion. In all these cases, present-day ability to resort to a CT scan provides an essential adjunct to diagnosis.

Fiberoscopy encounters the same difficulties in interpretation as radiography because of the alimentary stasis, and should be repeated after proper esophageal evacuation while realizing that this incurs a considerable risk of perforation.

The delayed nature of the discovery of the cancer explains why this may have so developed that its excision has become impossible. In fact, in this series ablation of the tumor was possible in only 9 patients, 5 of whom underwent total excision of the esophagus. 4 of these patients died in the postoperative period and none of the others survived for a year. The 17 other patients in this series were unable to

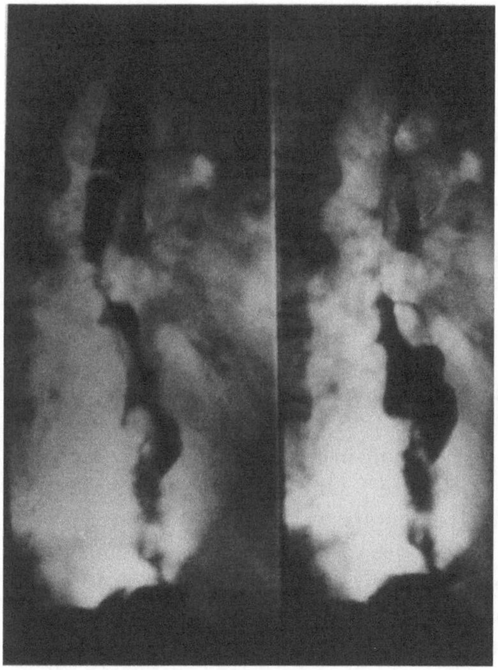

Fig. 1. Advanced tumor developped on megaescophagus

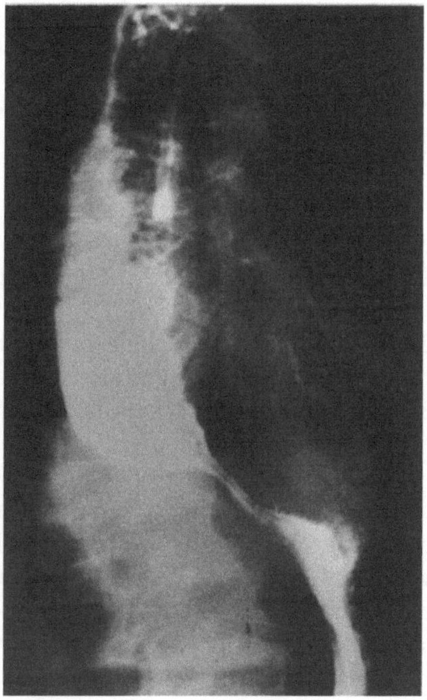

Fig. 2. Difficult radiographic interpretation due to stasis and food debris

undergo radical treatment, either because the cancer was judged inoperable due to the presence of liver or spinal metastases or because operation was denied by a state of cachexia or tracheobronchial invasion.

The gravity of these figures, certainly in relation to the very long and stealthy evolution of the growth, argues in favor of the absolute necessity of regular radiologic monitoring of all these patients and of the early performance of Heller's operation when such long-term surveillance is not feasible.

Is the incidence of this degeneration known?

K. Jeyasingham (Bristol)

The entire controversy concerning the incidence of malignant degeneration in achalasia cardia can squarely be put on the shoulders of the late Dr. Fagge of Hythe in Kent who in 1872 suggested that an epithelioma that he as a pathologist diagnosed in a patient of his father's, was a recent development in an esophagus with longstanding narrowing of the cardiac end [1]. Dr. Fagge did not even say one caused the other, but merely drew attention to the association of one with the other. Over the past 115 years, an increasing array of published papers has accumulated "evidence" that will lend itself to continued discussion by clinicians, pathologists, epidemiologists and statisticians for a true appraisal of the "incidence" of carcinoma of the esophagus in achalasia cardia.

The numerous reports available to us of carcinoma in achalasia cardia have been derived from three types of series,

1. Retrospective analysis of individual series of achalasia patients in whom carcinoma developed.
2. Autopsy series of achalasia patients in whom carcinoma of the esophagus was seen at the time of autopsy.
3. The number of achalasia patients in any one series of carcinoma of the esophagus.

All these categories of malignant degeneration in achalasia can only truly be described as "prevalence" and not as "incidence". One of the largest reviews of published case reports in the first half of the century was that of Williams [2] who was able to collect 26 such cases and added one of his own, but concluded that achalasia cardia does not appear to predispose to cancer of the esophagus, but should it occur it does so at a much younger age.

Of the three types of "prevalence" literature available to-day, the figures quoted for carcinoma of the esophagus seen in achalasia patients coming to autopsy vary from 20 to 29% [3]. In achalasia patients being followed up, the number of carcinomas of the esophagus over a period ranges from one to 7.7% [3]: the prevalence of achalasia cardia patients amongst esophageal carcinoma patients has been estimated at one per cent over a 25 year span [4]. When compared to some of the other esophageal conditions that are often thought to predispose to malignant degeneration, achalasia does not reach the top of the table, e.g. an esophageal web increases the chances by 91 times, a lye stricture by 22 times, achalasia 7 times, and peptic stricture 6 times [5] (Tables 1, 2).

Table 1. "League table" of predisposition to carcinoma of the esophagus

Esophageal WEB	91 times
Lye stricture	22 times
Achalasia cardia	7 times
Peptic stricture	6 times

(Carter & Brewer 1975)

Table 2. Prevalence of carcinoma in esophageal disease

Esophageal WEB	21%
Lye stricture	3.5 to 5.2%
Achalasia cardia	1.7%
Peptic stricture	1.3%
Short esophagus	5.5%

(Joske & Benedict 1959)

The average age at which esophageal carcinoma occurs in achalasia patients appears to be nearly 10 to 14 years younger than in the general population. In achalasia the average age is between 48 and 52 years whilst in the general population the average age is 62 years [6]. Although achalasia is commoner in females, like esophageal carcinoma in the general population, malignant degeneration occurs to a higher proportion in males (male: female ratio being 3:1) [6] (Table 3).

Table 3. Evidence for predisposition

For	– age	– occurs 10 to 14 years younger than in general population
Against	– sex	– in achalasia F:M 2:1 in esophageal carcinoma F:M 1:3

The main duration of symptoms up to the time of appearance of malignant change is estimated at 17.7 years [6, 7], although the shortest interval excluding the case reported by Rock [8] appears to be 22 months [9] whereas the longest interval reported is 23 years after esophagomyotomy in a patient who had symptoms for 6 years, a total of 29 years from the onset of symptoms [10].

An attempt at defining the incidence of carcinoma in achalasia cardia will require a prospective study of the type suggested by Chuong et al. [11] applied on a national or controlled population level for a period of not less than 17 years, more likely extending over the entire life expectancy of each individual patient in the defined population (Table 4).

Table 4. Prospective epidemiological study

1. Controlled population – all achalasia patients over 10–20 years
2. Follow-up for > 20 years or whole survival of every patient

References

1. Fagge CH (1872) A case of simple stenosis of the oesophagus followed by epithelium. Guy's Hospital Rep 17: 413
2. Williams JL (1956) Carcinoma of the oesophagus as a complication of achalasia of the cardia. Thorax 11: 268–274
3. Camara-Lopes CH (1961) Carcinoma of the esophagus as a complication of mega esophagus: an analysis of seven cases. J Dig Dis 6: 742–756
4. Norton GA, Postlethwait RW, Thompson WM (1980) Esophageal carcinoma: a survey of the population at risk. South Med J 73: 23–27
5. Carter R, Brewer LA (1975) Achalasia and esophageal carcinoma. Studies in early diagnosis for improved surgical management. Am J Surg 130: 114–120

6. Just-Viera JO, Haight C (1969) Achalasia and carcinoma of the esophagus. Surg Gyn Obstet 128:1081–1095
7. Ellis FH Jr, Crozier RE, Gibb SP (1986) Re-operative achalasia surgery. J Thorac Cardiovasc Surg 92:859–865
8. Rock LA, Latham PS, Hankins JR, Nasrallah SM (1985) Achalasia associated with squamous cell carcinoma of the esophagus: a case report. Am J Gastroenterol 80:526–528
9. Lamb RK, Edwards CW, Pattison CW, Matthews HR (1985) Squamous carcinoma in situ of the oesophagus in a patient with achalasia. Thorax 40:795–796
10. Heiss FW, Tarshis A, Ellis RF Jr (1984) Carcinoma associated with achalasia: occurrence 23 years after esophagomyotomy. Dig Diseases & Sciences 29:1066–1069
11. Chuong JJH, DuBovik S, McCallum RW (1984) Achalasia as a risk factor for esophageal carcinoma: a reappraisal. Dig Dis & Sciences 12:1105–1108

M. Rossetti (Liestal)

Out of the 67 "surgical megaesophagus" operated between 1960–1986 and out of which 39 deserve the name megaesophagus, we observed 2 malignant degenerations, respectively 3 and 5 years after the transabdominal myotomy and fundoplication. In both cases the operations improved the passage without change in the caliber and tonus (the peristalsis always remains disturbed even with a spectacular diminution of the dilatation). One other patient was hospitalized with cancerization of a non-operated megaesophagus with cerebral metastasis.

The 3 cases were squamous-cell carcinoma located in the middle third of the esophagus. The incidence is then 3 cases out of 40 megaesophagus (7.5%) and out of 67 operated achalasias (4.4%).

Cancerous degeneration is a recognized complication of achalasia and it is not known if an early dilatation or a functional surgical procedure prevent the degeneration. We thus don't advocate any preventive excision, when not motivated by one of the rare absolute indications or, by the same attitude adopted by our Brazilian colleagues regarding Chagas disease.

Verrucous cancers of the esophagus

R. Fiasse, J. Wallon, J. Pringot, and *J. B. Otte* (Leuven)

This is a rare type of well-differentiated squamous cell carcinoma, characterized by slow growth and extension to local structures rather than metastatic spreading [1, 2].

We observed four cases related to a chronic esophageal disease (caustic esophagitis:2, achalasia:2) (Table 1).

Table 1. Verrucous squamous cell carcinoma of the esophagus

Patient, sex, age	Chronic disease of the esophagus	Latency (months) 1st Biopsies-diagnosis	Complications	Surgical treatment	Outcome
V. ♂ 59	Caustic stenosis	12	Esophagobronchial fistula	Esophagectomy + left pneumonectomy	Death
A. ♂ 39	Caustic stenosis		Esophagotracheal fistula		Death
S. ♂ 64	Achalasia with upper third strictures	5	Esophagobronchial fistula		Death
B. ♀ 65	Achalasia	18	Intramural fistulae	Esophagectomy	Survival >5 years

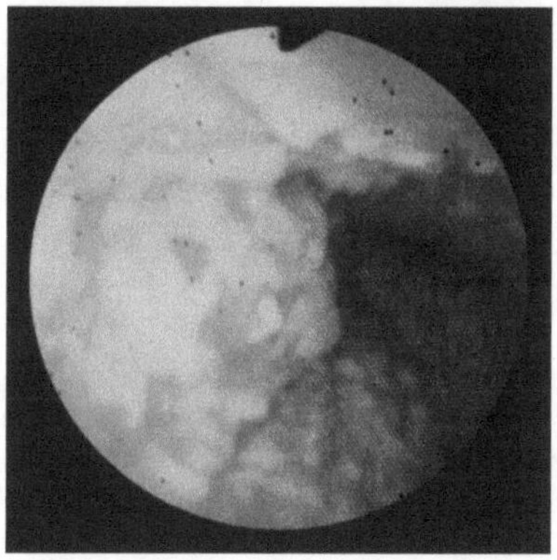

Fig. 1. Endoscopic aspect of the lower third of the esophagus in the first patient, treated for caustic stricture. Multilobulated tumor with a warty, whitish surface

- The first patient, a 59 year old man, was treated by dilatations for a lower esophageal lye stricture since age 4. A verrucous tumor above the stenosis was discovered at endoscopy (Fig. 1) and, despite the absence of malignancy at repeated biopsies, an esophageal resection was proposed, but refused by the patient. One year later, an esophagobronchial fistula occurred and a verrucous squamous cell carcinoma was diagnosed by cytologic and histologic analysis through bronchoscopy. The patient died after esophagectomy and left pneumonectomy.
- The second patient, a 39 year old man, with a lye stenosis since age 4, was admitted with a esophagotracheal fistula, rapidly fatal.
- The third patient, a 64 year old man, had an achalasia since age 7. Two benign strictures of the upper third were found in 1968. After pneumatic dilatation of the cardia, he underwent mechanical dilatations of the upper strictures with endoscopic surveillance. In 1984, dysplasia was found but not confirmed by subsequent biopsies. He died in 1985 of an esophagobronchial fistula caused by a verrucous squamous cell carcinoma.
- The fourth patient, a 65 year old woman, had symptoms of achalasia since more than 20 years. A small verrucous tumor of the middle third was discovered but without signs of malignancy at repeated histology and cytology. After 18 months evolution characterized by tumor growth and development of intramural fistulae (Fig. 2), a total esophagectomy with coloplasty was performed, with a survival now exceeding 5 years.

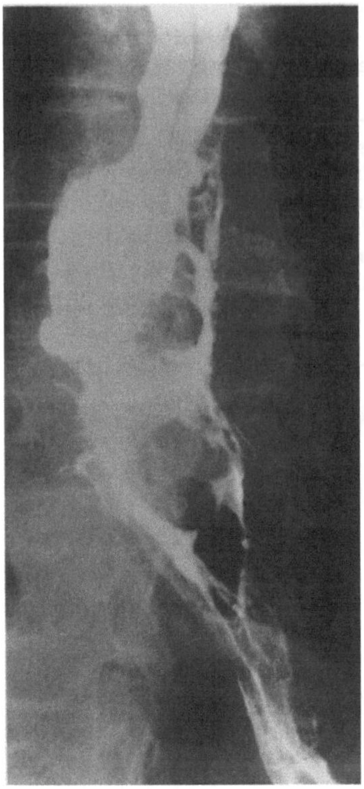

Fig. 2. Baryum swallow in the fourth patient, 18 months after discovery of a benign tumor, following repeat biopsies. Large extension of the tumor, which is infiltrating the left inferior wall of the esophagus with development of intramural fistulae

We confirm that this type of carcinoma is associated with chronic esophageal diseases and that its natural history is different from that of common squamous cell carcinoma, with a better prognosis. This type of carcinoma is however difficult to diagnose, because of cytologic characteristics close to benign lesions [3].

References

1. Minielly JA, Harrison EG, Fontana RS, Payne WS (1967) Verrucous squamous cell carcinoma of the esophagus. Cancer 20: 2078–2087
2. Meyerowitz BR, Shea LT (1971) The natural history of squamous verricose carcinoma of the esophagus. J Thorac Cardiovasc Surg 61: 646–649
3. Wallon J, Libotte B, Fiasse R, Haot J Verrucous carcinoma of the oesophagus. Pathological features. (in preparation)

Degeneration of caustic stenosis

C. G. Bremner (Johannesburg)

Because there is a risk of developing squamous carcinoma in a caustic strictured esophagus, resectional surgery would theoretically be preferable to bypass surgery. However, resectional surgery carries a higher mortality and morbidity than bypass surgery, and these risks must be considered.

What, therefore, is the risk of carcinomatous degeneration of a caustic stenosis? Carcinomatous degeneration has not been documented in a caustic stenosis in the Johannesburg group of hospitals (approx 2 million population), despite the fact that caustic accidents and suicide attempts have been common in the last 50 years.

Marchand [1] had never seen a case of malignant change developing in a series of 133 patients with caustic burns, and his 30 years experience subsequent to that publication still verifies this situation. Nakayama et al. [2] reported on a total of only 8 cases in Japan, and 100 other cases in the literature. Bigelow [3] reported on 1 case of carcinoma and reviewed the reported cases prior to 1953: the average age of these patients was 52 years. In the larger series of 63 cases described by Appelquist [4], the average age was 48 years. Hopkins [5] recently added 12 cases (average age 52.8 years), and noted that the interval from injury to the development of carcinoma was 45.8 years.

In reported series of squamous carcinoma of the esophagus, a history of caustic injestion was noted in 1–4% of patients.

In a further series [6], nine of 381 caustic injuries developed carcinoma (1000 fold possibility of developing carcinoma in patients aged 25–64 who had injested caustic 24 years previously). In a further large series the overall occurrence of carcinoma in caustic strictures was 7.2%. The interval between the caustic burn was 46.1 years. Of interest the interval was 14 years less for those who drank lye in adulthood [7].

There is a 1–4% risk of developing a squamous carcinoma in a previous caustic injury to the esophagus, and the time interval from the initial injury to the malignant degeneration is 24–45 years. There may be a geographic relationship because of the low occurrence in Japan and South Africa.

References

1. Marchand P (1955) Caustic strictures of the esophagus. Thorax 10: 171–181
2. Nakayama R, Aoki A, Tshiro Y, Kuramochi S (1983) Carcinoma of the esophagus engrafted on corrosive stricture of the esophagus. Nippon Geka Gakkai Zasshi 84(10): 1094–1194
3. Bigelow NH (1953) Carcinoma of the esophagus developing at the site of lye stricture. Cancer 6: 1159
4. Appelquist TP, Salmo M (1980) Lye corrosion carcinoma of the esophagus. Cancer 45: 2655
5. Hopkins RA, Postlethwait RW (1981) Caustic burns and carcinoma of the esophagus. Ann Surg 194: 146–148
6. Kiviranta UK (1952) Corrosion carcinoma of the esophagus. Acta Oto-Laryngol 42: 89
7. Csiikos M, Horvath O, Petri A, Petri L, Imre J (1985) Late malignant transformation of chronic corrosive esophageal strictures. Langenbecks Arch Chir 365(4): 231–238

R. Giudicelli, P. Fuentes, L. Garbe, B. Dupin, P. Heurte, V. Fulachier, J. F. Dumon, and *E. Reboud* (Marseilles)

Malignant transformation after caustic esophageal injury is widely recognized. A review of the literature shows that it is a rare complication.

Over the last thirteen years we treated fifty four patients for caustic lesions. Five of these developed esophageal cancer.

We would like to emphasize three points which in our opinion are very important:

- Etiologic factors,
- Conditions of diagnosis,
- Therapeutic attitude.

Etiologic factors

The kind of caustic agent is not important in the development of malignant transformation.

The grade of caustic injury is important: esophageal stenosis occurs in about 50% of patients with third degree burns, and these patients run a great risk of malignant transformation.

Malignant transformation often occurs "on old burned esophagus" and the average interval between injury and diagnosis of cancer is 30 years [3]. In all cases patients had undergone repeated forceful esophageal dilatations [4].

These last two factors are present without exception in each observation.

Conditions of diagnosis

Patients with malignant transformation can be divided into three groups.

- The first group includes cases in which cancer is already clinically evident. The biopsy confirms the diagnosis.
- The second group includes patients with barium transit study typical of a caustic stenosis. The diagnosis of cancer is made by endoscopic examination after esophageal dilatation. We wish to underscore the important diagnostic role of esophageal dilatation which allows endoscopic examination of the full length of the stenosis and staged biopsies. In one of our observations the cancer was located just below the stenosis so that without dilatation the endoscopist would not have been able to see and biopsy the lesion.

Clinically, in this group, when observe a worsening of the dysphagia occurs in spite of dilatation, a malignant transformation is to be suspected [1, 2].

- The third group includes patients with infra-radiologic and infra-endoscopic cancer. The diagnosis is made by biopsy. Histologic examination shows the presence of several zones of severe dysplasia with invasive and in situ carcinoma foci in the dysplasic zones.

When biopsy does not show direct evidence of carcinoma, the therapeutic attitude is not very easy: some authors advise further staged biopsy and close surveillance, while other recommend immediate surgical resection because in many cases dysplasia and in situ carcinoma coexist.

The therapeutic attitude

All caustic stenosis must be resected after 20 years.

Severe dysplasia occurring many years after caustic esophageal injury is an absolute indication for esophagectomy, as because it should be considered as a precancerous lesion with a high risk for malignant transformation [5]. In many cases, on histologic examination, it is difficult to distinguish between severely dysplastic cells and cancerous cells.

Currently, many surgeons perform a long colonic interposition without resection of the esophagus three months after the acute phase of injury. They believe that there is pratically no risk of malignant transformation if the burned esophagus is immediately inactivated.

References

1. Garcia Bengoechea, Cosme A, Arriola J, Lopez P, Arena J (1980) Esofagitis caustica y cancer de esofago. Aportacion de dos casos. Rev Esp Enferm Apar Digest ESP Vol 57, N° 5, Pages 573–576
2. Dor J, Depieds R, Humbert P, Boulaya JM, Guerinel J (1960) La cancérisation des retrécissements cicatriciels de l'œsophage par caustiques. Ann chir vol 14, N° 19–20; Pages 1193–1203
3. Gaillard J, Bouchayer M, Haguenauer JP (1970) Le risque de dégénérescence cancéreuse tardive dans les sténoses caustiques de l'œsophage. Ann Oto-Laryng tome 87; N° 10–11; Pages 637–644
4. Hopkins. Caustic burns and carcinoma of the esophagus. Ann Surg (1981) 194–2 (146–148).
5. Tcherveniakov P (1986) Malignant transformation of corrosive strictures.Symposium international sur les brûlures caustiques du tractus digestif supérieur. Décembre – Marseille (France)

M. Csikos, Ö. Horváth, A. Petri, I. Petri, and *J. Imre* (Szeged)

Attention was first drawn last century to the possibility of carcinoma arising in a corrosive esophageal stricture [7, 18].

Several publications have since appeared suggesting that malignancy may develop in a narrowed part of the gullet due to the swallowing of lye or acid [2, 4, 5, 6, 10, 14, 17, 19, 22]. The first Hungarian paper on this topic was published in 1904 [23], and was subsequently followed by others [8, 11, 12, 13, 20]. Considerable numbers of cases were reported by Benedict [3], Dubecz [8], Kiviranta [15] and Wurning [25].

The number of such cases in our material seems to have been rising more rapidly in the last two decades. This is by no means due only to the improved diagnostic procedures. Our team has already published its experiences in this field in three papers [11, 12, 13]. Nevertheless, there are many unsettled questions concerning the treatment of this condition. The rising number of new cases and our changing policy toward its treatment on the basis of the cumulated experience have led us to report our results again, now completed with the late survival investigations.

*

Between January 1965 and January 1984, 502 patients with esophageal cancer were admitted to the 1st Surgical Clinic of Medical University of Szeged, Hungary. Among them, 36 patients had suffered earlier from long-standing esophageal stricture due to corrosive burn.

The interval between the ingestion of the corrosive agent and the admission for carcinoma averaged 46.1 years (the shortest period was 23, and the longest 66 years).

The mean age of these patients was 54.1 years, nearly 6 years lower than that of the overall cancer patients. Sex distribution: 19 males and 17 females. The ratio is 10:1 in the total material. No significant difference can be observed in the localization of tumors compared with the total material – with the exception of the upper third of the esophagus (Table 1).

Table 1. Patients with scar carcinoma (1965–1984) at the Department of Surgery of the Medical University of Szeged, Hungary

	Corrosion carcinomas	All esophageal carcinomas
Resecability rate	60%	64.8%
Localization		
upper third	6 (16.6%)	49 (9.7%)
middle third	23 (64.0%)	355 (70.7%)
lower third	7 (19.4%)	98 (19.5%)

The resecability rates in the two groups were almost the same. In one instance endoscopy revealed signs of inoperability on bronchoscopy: the carina and part of the right main bronchi were found to be infiltrated by the growth.

21 resections and 14 explorations were performed. There was no mortality among the inoperable group. The mortality was 10% after resection (14.3% in the total material). The types of operation can be seen in Table 2. Table 3 contains the data on the long-term survival investigations.

Carcinoma may develop in the gullet as a complication of a lesion of long-standing duration [6]. Pathologic alterations of the mucosa and muscle wall of the esophagus may be followed by malignant transformation [22]. Scar cancer always occurs in the stenosed part [9, 15]. The corrosive lesion is the most severe at the physiologically stenosed parts of the gullet in most of the cases, so it is a straightforward conclusion that scar carcinoma predominantly develops in the physiologic narrowing [13].

Table 2. Types of operation performed for scar carcinoma of the esophagus

1. Resection		2. Palliation	
Op. Torek	9	Expl. thoracotomy	2
No substitution	4	Expl. thoracotomy + Tygon intubation	5
Substernal colon substitution	4	Laparotomy+gastrostomy	4
Antethoracal jejunum+skin tube	1	Laparotomy+gastrostomy + Tygon intubation	2
Esophago-gastrostomy	5	Thoraco-laparotomy+gastrostomy	1
Esophago-jejuno-gastrostomy	5	Irradiation only	1
Primary colon subst.	2		
	21		15

Table 3. Comparison of survival of patients resected for esophageal scar cancer and for all malignancies of the gullet according to the "life table method" of Cutler and Ederer

	Scar carcinomas n=21	All esophageal carcinomas n=210
Per cent or radical resections	45%	32.3%
Survival rates		
1 year	84.2±1.8%	70.9±8.3%
2 years	68.4±2.4%	31.1±13.2%
5 years	45.6±1.7%	15.4±3.1%
10 years	14.4±1.6%	10.3±1.0%

It seems to be possible to state on the basis of cumulated experience that it is not just an accidental coincidence to find carcinoma in a corrosive stricture. Malignancies occurring after corrosion at a young age are strong evidence of this: our youngest patient was 31 years old, but there is an observation in the literature of a 12-year-old boy with esophageal cancer after a lye burn (Baló and Korpássy cit. 8). Schmidt-Baumler and Fahr [21] called attention in 1970 to the fact that esophageal carcinoma develops later in childhood and sooner in adults after a corrosive lesion. In our material the latency period was 50.9 years when the corrosive injury took place under 12 years of age (29 cases), while it was only 36.1 years in 7 cases in which it happened in adults.

The connection between scars and the development of malignancy is accepted: scar carcinoma of the lung, and carcinoma in the scar of the skin and in lesions due to lupus disease [6, 22, cit. 8].The role of the bad nutritional state of scar-tissue is also a possible factor in the pathomechanism of carcinogenesis.

Esophageal carcinoma was found in 7 out of 200 patients with corrosive burn (3.5%) in the material of Bigger and Vinson [5], in 9 out of 381 (2.4%) in that of Kiviranta [15], and in 2 cut of 50 corrosive cases in that of Kay [14].

Carcinoma developing on these basis of a previous corrosive stricture was demonstrated in 5.5% of the esophageal cancer cases by Benedict [3], in 1.2% by Kiviranta [15], in 6% by Dubecz [8], in 0.8% by Lawler [17] and in 1.4% by Hopkins and Postlethwait [10].

Appelquist and Salmo reported the largest series of esophageal scar cancer in the literature in 1930, with 63 patients [2]. Our material is the second largest, with 36 patients. The incidence of scar carcinoma varies between 0.8 and 7.2% according to the different authors. The data of the well-known authors are listed in Table 4.

Table 4. Occurrence of scar carcinoma in the literature material on esophageal malignancy

Wurning	1955	3.7%	(7/198)
Lawler	1969	0.8%	(2/265)
Appelquist	1972	7.2%	(2/375)
Appelquist and Salmo	1980	2.6%	(63/2414)
Hopkins and Postlethwait	1981	1.4%	(12/846)
Our material	1984	7.2%	(36/502)

Our 7.2% incidence is at present the highest of all in the literature known by us. A similar frequency was reported by Appelquist in 1972 [1], but by 1980 Appelquist and Salmo [2] described an incidence of only 2.6% in their cumulative series of cases. Our high percentage is by no means due only to the rising effectivity of the diagnostic procedures; it also means that the delayed results of attempted suicide by lye or acid swallowing (frequently done 40–50 years ago) are now appearing.

Examination of the data on our patients with scar cancer revealed the following characteristics: their mean age is lower than that of those who had not suffered from lye corrosion (54.1 vs. 59.8 years). In the literature data, the mean age of esophageal cancer patients is 62-69 years [8]. However, the mean age of our patients with scar carcinoma is higher than that in other reports [4, 15].

The latency period between the corrosive burn and the diagnosis of scar carcinoma is essentially longer than in the (30-35 years) corresponding literature [4, 8, 19, 24]: (46.1 years). In our material, this period is longer by 3 years among the resected patients than the inoperable cases.

The long-term survival of our patients with scar carcinoma is significantly better than with other esophageal malignancies. This is understandable in view of the fact that the operation was radical in a great proportion of our cases. Most authors consider that the prognosis of scar carcinoma is better than that of other forms of esophageal malignancies [1, 2, 16]. The better prognosis can be attributed to several factors:

1. Scar carcinoma can generally be diagnosed earlier, because the tumor grows only intramurally due to the surrounding scarring; thus, even a smaller lesion can increase dysphagia in a given narrow space.

2. For the same reason, metastases can only develop in a later phase.
3. Radical operation can therefore be performed in a considerable percentage of the cases.

According to Kiviranta [15], the risk of development of scar cancer is 1000 times higher in a corrosive stricture than in the normal population of the same age, provided that more than 24 years has passed since the injury. This risk can be regarded as 2–3000 times according to our data. (3–4 esophageal carcinoma cases can be expected for 100 000 inhabitants in Hungary, but among the 250 cases with corrosive stricture at our institute who had sustained the chemical injury more than 10 years previously 36 suffered from scar cancer, i.e. 14.4%).

Teleky [23] published the first case of esophageal scar carcinoma in Hungary in 1904. Dubecz and co-workers [8] and Imre and Kopp [13] later drew attention to the danger of scar cancer appearing in post-burn esophageal stenosis.

Several factors together may lead to the development of carcinoma in the event of a corrosive stricture:

1. scarring,
2. repeated traumatic injuries during esophagoscopy and dilatations,
3. slow passage of food (stasis) due to stricture (physical and chemical noxae caused by food are manifested more intensively at the narrowed parts),
4. reflux due to a traction-type hiatal hernia, almost always occurring in connection with corrosive strictures (Imre, Wooler cit. 13).

Because of the possible malignant transformation, Imre and Gergely [12] recommended resection for corrosive esophageal strictures as the surgical method of choice, instead of the conservative dilatations and by-pass procedures. According to Rubányi and E. Szabó [20], the danger of malignant transformation decreases after by-pass operations.

Removal of only the stenosed part of the gullet in the case of corrosive esophageal stricture does not offer full protection for the prevention of scar carcinoma, as two of our cases show. This is why patients whose gullet has been resected for corrosive stricture need regular control.

Two questions arise in connection with the surgical treatment of corrosive esophageal strictures: first, the timing of the operation of a proved benign corrosive stricture, and secondly, which type of intervention to choose, resection or by-pass.

In our opinion, the answer to the first question is that every corrosive esophageal stricture should be operated on which does not respond properly to repeated dilatations during a limited period, and if increasingly tight stenosis develops in a chronically diseased esophagus originating from caustic injury.

To answer the second question is not so easy, and this is where our standpoint has partially changed during the past few years: we initially thought that resection was the method of choice in this condition, because removal of the stenosed part of the corroded gullet is the best prevention against scar carcinoma too.

Our two cases mentioned above, where carcinoma developed in the remaining part of the esophagus many years after resection, altered our opinion. The solution can be either to perform total esophagectomy and to put the anastomosis on the pharynx, if the organ for replacement reaches this level, or, in contrast with the views held by our team previously [11, 12, 13], carry out a by-pass operation with the colon in the case of a corrosive esophageal stricture. In proved benign cases we have tended to choose the by-pass recently, but is must be pointed out that if X-ray and esophagoscopy (including biopsy and histology) give the slightest uncertainty on benignancy, resection should be chosen.

In the case of a benign corrosive stricture of not too long duration, but which does not respond well to dilatations, by-pass with left or right colon can be done high up to the cervical part of the esophagus. With the food not passing down in the diseased gullet, and therefore not able to cause physical and chemical irritation, scar carcinoma will presumably not develop in it.

Another change in the operative principles and practice is that we do not perform Torek operation in the already malignized cases, but carry out replacement at the same time. This change was introduced since almost half of our patients previously operated on by this method did not survive to reach the second phase.

References

1. Appelquist P (1972) Carcinoma of the oesophagus and gastric cardia. A retrospective study based on statistical and clinical material from Finland. Acta Chir Scand Suppl 430: 1–92
2. Appelquist P, Salmo M (1980) Lye corrosion carcinoma of the esophagus: a review of 63 cases. Cancer 45: 2655–2658
3. Benedict EB (1941) Carcinoma of the esophagus developing in benign stricture. New Engl J Med 224: 408–412
4. Bigelow NH (1953) Carcinoma of the esophagus developing at the site of the lye stricture. Cancer 6: 1159–1164
5. Bigger IA, Vinson PP (1950) Carcinoma secondary to burn of the esophagus from ingestion of lye; report of a case. Surgery 28: 887-889
6. Boyd W (1961) Textbook of Pathology, Structure and Function in Diseases. 7th ed 717. Lea and Febiger, Philadelphia
7. Catell HW (1896) Cancer of the esophagus following a stricture due to taking of lye with recent metastasis to the liver. Trans Path Soc Philadelphia 17: 18–20
8. Dubecz S, Dávid Gy, Juhász J (1959) Lúgmérgezés utáni heges nyelöcsöszükületben keletkezett rákról. Magy Seb 13: 301–304
9. Gowing NFC (1961) Miscellaneous lesions associated with carcinoma of the esophagus. Neoplastic disease at various sites. Vol IV E and S Livingstone Ltd Edinburgh and London
10. Hopkins RA, Postlethwait RW (1981) Caustic burns and carcinoma of the oesophagus. Ann Surg 194: 146–148
11. Imre J, Gergely M (1969) Cancer arising from cicatricial esophageal stenosis. Orv Hetil 110: 1480–1484
12. Imre J, Gergely M (1971) Cicatricial esophageal carcinomas. Thoraxchirurgie 19: 181–187
13. Imre J, Kopp M (1972) Arguments against long-term conservative treatment of oesophageal strictures due to corrosive burns. Thorax 27: 594–598
14. Kay EB, Cross FS (1956) Chronic esophagitis – a possible factor in production of carcinoma of esophagus. Arch Int Med (Chic) 98: 475–481
15. Kiviranta UK (1952) Corrosion carcinoma of the esophagus, 381 cases of corrosion and nine cases of corrosion carcinoma. Acta Otolaryngol 42: 89–95
16. Lansing PS, Ferrante WA, Ochsner JL (1969) Carcinoma of the oesophagus at the site of lye stricture. Amer J Surg 118: 108–111
17. Lawler MR, Gobbel WG, Killen DA, Daniel RA (1969) Carcinoma of the oesophagus. J Thor Cardiovasc Surg 58: 609–613
18. Neumann E (1861) Virchows Arch 20: 142
19. Parkinson AT, Haidak GL, McInerney RP (1970) Verrucous squamous cell carcinoma of the esophagus following lye stricture. Chest 57: 489–492

20. Rubányi P, Szabó EL (1971) A nyelöcsö marásos és peptikus szükületeinek sebészi kezelése. Magy Seb 24: 145–151
21. Schmidt-Baumler V, Fahr K (1970) Karzinom des Ösophagus nachw Laugenverätzung. Z Laryng Rhinol Otol 49: 827–832
22. Stout AP, Lattes R: Tumors of the esophagus. In: Atlas of Tumor Pathology Sect V Fasc 20. pp. 44, 46, 50. American Registry of Pathology AFIP Washington DC
23. Teleky L (1904) Die Laugenverätzungen der Speiseröhre. Ein Beitrag zur Kentniss ihrer Verbreitung, ihrer Prognose und Therapie. Ztschr f Heilk 5: 1–50
24. Vantsian EN, Chernousov AF, Stranadko EF, Posudnevsky VI (1976) Malignization of post burn esophageal strictures. Khirurgiia (Mosk) 1: 113–119
25. Wurning P (1955) Über krebsdisponierende Zustände an Oesophagus und Kardia. Langenbecks Arch Chir 280: 504–515

What are the indications of conservative surgery in caustic stenosis?

L. Kotsis, F. Kulka, and *Z. Krisár* (Budapest and Oradea)

Concerning the management of caustic strictures, the first question may be the indication for surgery. We agree with Daly and Cardoua [4] that these are:
- complete stenosis, long irregularity or pocketing of the esophagus,
- failure to establish a lumen or to maintain above a 40 French bougie or consequent mediastinitis,
- leak of patient cooperation,
- developed fistula,

together with 3 other conditions, associated gastric or hypopharyngeal lesions, previous iatrogenic perforation, and a long history of more than 10 years.

Opinions about the question of whether resection or by-pass is justified are not uniform (Table 1). The hazard of one-stage esophageal resection replacement is higher than that of possible malignant transformation of the scarred tissue: therefore, in young patients, with a relatively short history (less than 10 years) we prefer –

Table 1. Substernal by-pass or resection + replacement?

characteristics	
– low mortality (4–6%)	– higher, not justified risk
– malignancy never seen after by-pass	
indications	
– usually young patients	1st stage: by-pass
– relatively short history	2nd stage: resection
– extensive lesions	– long history, regardless of the level

Table 2. Undilatable corrosive esophageal strictures (n=137)

1. Untractable esophageal strictures	89
2. associated with:	
a./ gastric or hypopharyngeal strictures	32
b./ esophago-tracheal-or-bronchial fistula	4
c./ or both	3
d./ artificial perforation	9
	137
mortality: 5.1%	

Thoracic Surgical Clinic, Budapest, Hungary, and Dept. of Surgery Hospital Oradea, Rumania 1962–1982

in concordance with the majority of authors [2, 3, 8, 13, 14] – a lower-risk procedure: a simple substernal by-pass with isoperistaltic transverse colon. Our mortality is 5.1% for 137 patients (Table 2) and, like Dubost [5] and others, we have never seen malignant degeneration in the follow-up (4–20 years) of the patients we have managed in this way. In contrast, the danger of malignancy of long-standing corrosive lesions, leads to avoid long-term dilatational therapy, as stressed by Imre [7], and demands resection, as a second-stage operation after by-pass.

The third question is the type of reconstruction (Table 3): lower esophageal strictures should be dealt with by Roux-en-Y loop by-pass, as the morbidity of Merendino or Belsey type interposition with a short colon segment [1] is higher.

For total esophageal by-pass, the graft of choice is a transverse colon pedicled exceptionally on the middle and left [9] or usually on the left colic artery, which is a more constant artery than the middle one [6, 10, 11, 15, 16, 17, 18], and whose mobilized long trunk permits a preferable high gastric anastomosis. Moreover, the multihaustral propulsive contractions of this more active colonic segment, achieved by isoperistaltic interposition, prove to be basic factors of gastro-colic reflux prevention.

In cases of caustic esophageal strictures associated with an extensively burned stomach, implantation of the colonic segment into the antro-pyloric region is more physiological than a Montenegro [12] or Petrov type by-pass. Successive developed gastro-esophageal strictures required first a limited gastric (usually Billroth I type)-resection, followed by a second-stage colonic by-pass (9 obs. in this study).

In concomitant esophago-gastric outlet obstruction, in young, good-risk patients, addition of an economic Billroth I resection to the esophagoplasty does not increase the risk, but decrease the duration of alimentary tract reconstruction. To avoid gastric emptying disturbance, even after gastric resection, the nutritive pedicle must be placed retrogastrically. No patient was lost in our 11 operations.

Table 3. Type of by-pass

lower third:	by-pass with Roux-en-Y loop (alternative procedure: Merendino or Belsey op. with "short" colon graft)
all other levels:	substernal by-pass with isoperistaltic transverse colon segment (± flexures)

In our 4 cases with associated esophago-respiratory fistulas, exclusion with by-pass of the lesions proves to be sufficient for both. In circumstances of previously perforated strictures, the recommanded time for coloesophagoplasty is 2–3 months later.

References

1. Belsey R (1965) Reconstruction of the esophagus with left colon. J Thorac Cardiovasc Surg 49: 33–55
2. Chien KY et al. (1974) Esophagoplasty for corrosive stricture of the esophagus: an analysis of 60 cases. Ann Surg 175: 510–515
3. Chrysospathis P (1967) Large bowel as substitute for the esophagus. Pacif Med Surg 75: 141–147
4. Daly JF, Cardoua JC (1957) Corrosive esophagitis. Am J Surg 93: 242–247
5. Dubost Cl et al. (1976) Les grands brulures caustiques œso-gastriques de l'adulte. J Chir 112: 385–408
6. Giuli R et al. (1972) Valeur de l'œsophagoplastie dans le traitement des sténoses caustiques de l'œsophage. Ann Chir 26: 1273–1282
7. Imre J, Kopp A (1972) Arguments against long term conservative treatment of esophageal strictures due to corrosive burns. Thorax 27: 594–598
8. Kirsh MM, Ritter F (1976) Caustic ingestion and subsequent damage to the oropharyngeal and digestive passages. Ann Thorac Surg 21: 74–82
9. Kotsis L (1973) Esophagoplasty with isoperistaltic transverse colon. Thesis Bucuresti
10. Kotsis L et al. (1972) Angiological basis of the coloesophagoplasty. Digest Surg 1: 63–65
11. Lortat-Jacob JL, Giuli R (1973) Esophageal replacement. Prog Surg 12: 77–95
12. Montenegro EB, Cutait DE (1958) Construction of a new esophagus by means of the transverse colon and its application for caustic atresia, carcinoma, and varices of the esophagus. Surgery 44: 785–794
13. Nardi G (1957) Surgical treatment of lye stricture of the esophagus by mediastinal colon transplant without resection. New Engl J Med 75: 141–147
14. Petrov BA (1964) Retrosternal artificial esophagus created from colon; 100 operations. Surgery 55: 520–523
15. Postlethwait RW (1983) Colonic interposition for esophageal substitution. Surg Gynecol Obstet 156: 377–383
16. Reboud E et al. (1968) Les transplants coliques gauches en chirurgie œsophagienne. Mem Acad Chir 94: 324–329
17. Sonneland J et al. (1958) Surgical anatomy of the arterial supply to the colon from the superior mesenteric artery, based upon a study of 600 specimens. Surg Gynecol Obstet 106: 385–396
18. Wilkins EW (1980) Long segment colon substitution for the esophagus. Ann Surg 192: 722–725

Degeneration in peptic esophagitis

R. Giuli (Paris)

Whether coincidence or causal relationship, peptic esophagitis and cancer are associated in a not negligible proportion of cases. In 240 operations for esophagitis, we found 41 cancers, i.e., 17%. It is said that chronic irritation of the esophageal mucosa may favor the development of an epithelioma at that site, a hypothesis often advanced during the course of caustic esophagitis or certain cases of longstanding mega-esophagus, and which may apply equally to peptic esophagitis. When this association is not recognized, the consequences may be catastrophic, as in the following cases:

A patient aged 25, known to have had a cardiac malposition from the age of 4 years, became dysphagic and lost 10 kg in a few months. A diagnosis of ulcerated peptic stricture was made and confirmed by biopsies. A suggested operation was refused for 9 months, during which dilatations were performed. At the end of this period the patient agreed to operation, but it was only possible to carry out a palliative excision which provided only a few months of temporary improvement.

Another patient (Fig. 1) suffered from an endobrachyesophagus (Barrett's esophagus) associated with an ulcer. The presence of an embedded niche on the films put the diagnosis in doubt and several biopsies were performed, none of which yielded evidence of any neoplastic process. 7 years later, there was an enormous cancer at the gastro-esophageal junction (Fig. 2), requiring the performance of a palliative excision which was followed by death after a few months.

Apart from disorders of the pyloric sphincter, isolated hiatus hernia only seldom causes severe esophagitis, as the reflux is intermittent and diluted in the alimentary bolus. On the contrary, in brachyesophagus, the close and permanent contact of the two mucosae allows prolonged stagnation of the gastric fluid and certainly favors the development of peptic ulcer. In our series, it was this type of esophagitis that was associated with cancer of the esophagus.

The patients were classified in two groups: those with an adenocarcinoma of the esophagus, and those with a malpighian epithelioma. In interpreting the figures, there is no question of the prevalence, still less of the incidence, of malignant degeneration. The only factor we wish to emphasize, for each of these patients, is

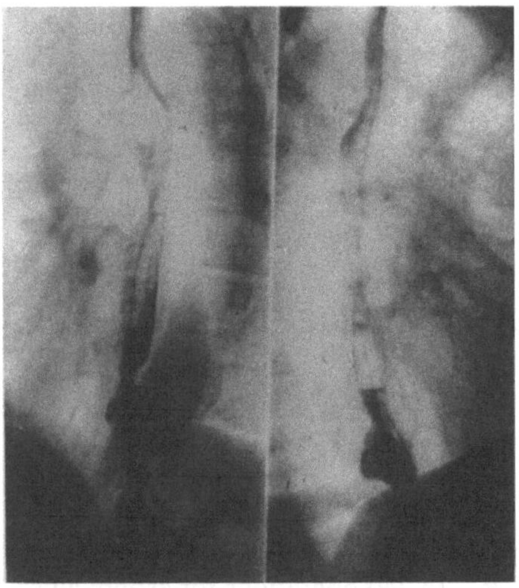

Fig. 1. Ulcer on Barrett's esophagus

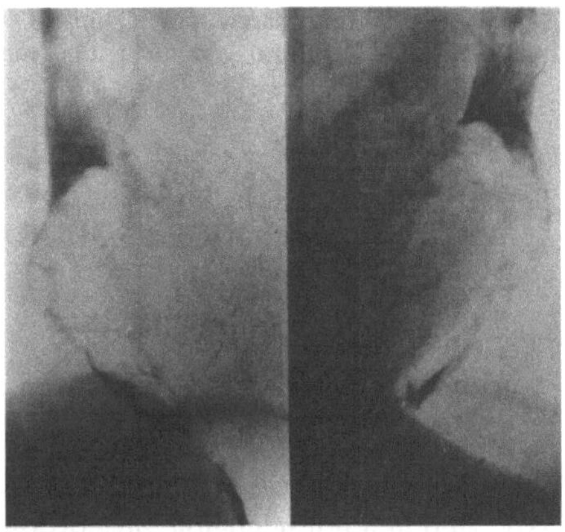

Fig. 2. Adenocarcinoma 7 years later

the true preliminary history of esophagitis, monitored by endoscopy, over a period of from 2 to 10 years.

- The first group comprises 29 *adenocarcinomas*, and in all cases, the constant element was the *sudden* transformation of the clinical picture, with major exacerbation of the dysphagia and rate of weight-loss. In patients suffering from peptic stricture damaging the esophageal mucosa, it is known that the cylindrical epithelium may be regarded as a mode of cicatrization of the esophageal mucosa. This cylindrical ascent along the esophagus (Fig. 3) is evidence of the acquired nature of endobrachyesophagus and may possibly include the histologic type of the majority of carcinomas associated with peptic esophagitis.

On the other hand, in 3 of these patients, pathologic examination revealed very well-marked submucous sclerosis (Fig. 4) such as is found in peptic esophagitis, with loss of muscle substance that appears to be due to a true preexisting ulcer and not to the tumor. In such tissues, it may be thought that the persistent irritation of a chronic reflux might favor secondarily the development of a cancer.

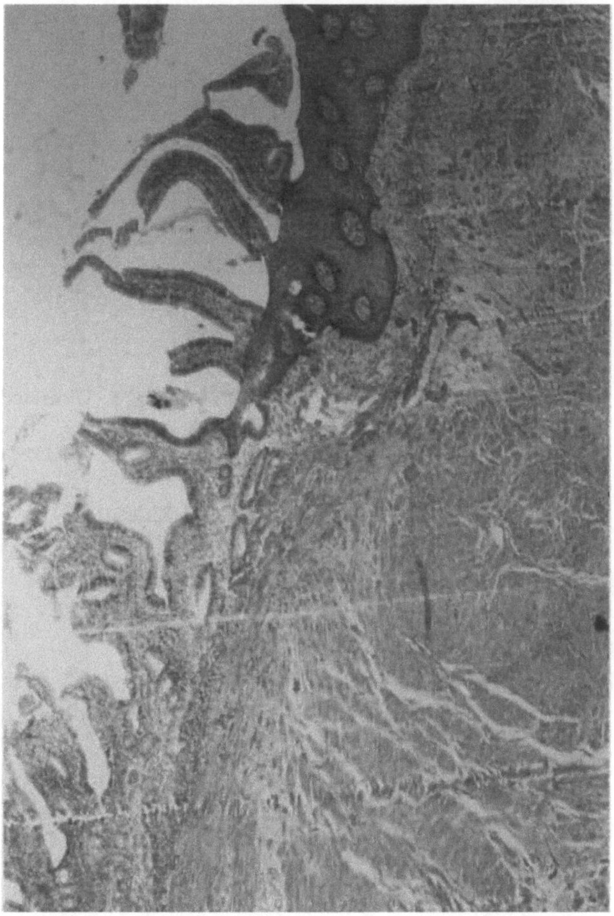

Fig. 3. Cylindrical ascent on the esophageal mucosa

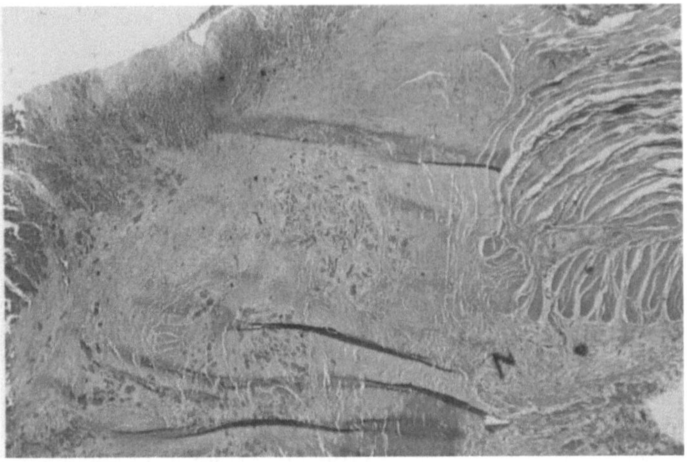

Fig. 4. Submucous sclerosis underlying the tumor

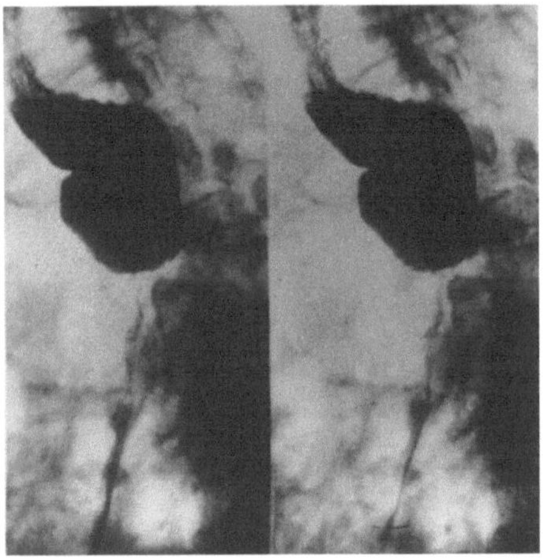

Fig. 5. Ulcerated peptic esophagitis

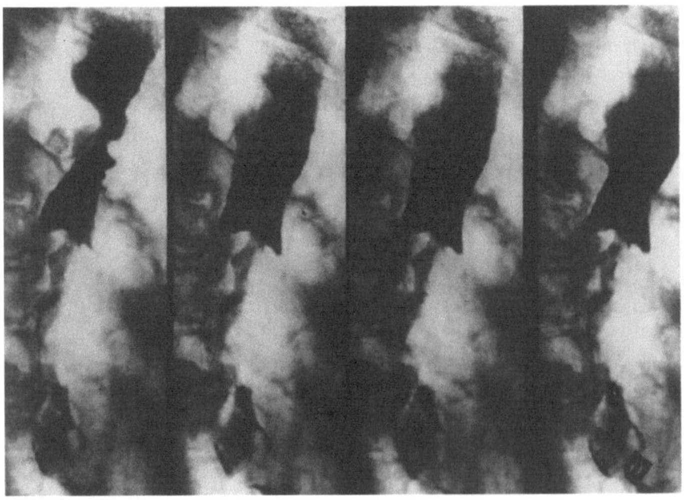

Fig. 6. Malpighian carcinoma 2,5 years later

- The second and smaller group of patients includes those in whom the histologic type of cancer was *malpighian*: a man aged 70 suffered from an ulcerated peptic esophagitis (Fig. 5), confirmed by biopsies, and underwent dilatations over 2 years. 6 months after cessation of treatment the radiograph (Fig. 6) showed a bulky cancer of the middle third of the esophagus, of epidermoid malpighian type at biopsy, and surgically inoperable.

This group includes 12 similar cases, 2 of which were histologically epidermoid epitheliomas associated with a glandular epithelioma. While, in the first group, the anomaly consisted in the development of a glandular cancer on a gastric type of mucosa, the development of a malpighian cancer on an esophagitis may lay stress, if not on the absolute connection of two pathologic processes, at least on the great possibility of their linkage.

*

The considerable rate of 17% of cancers observed by us in a population of 240 patients followed-up for peptic esophagitis, and operated after a period varying from 2 to 9 years, should in no way be regarded as any indication of the true incidence of neoplastic degeneration in peptic esophagitis. This is because these figures are those derived after the event from a population of patients operated for the same lesion in the same department drawing on a very special intake, without similar attention having been paid to a global population of patients suffering from the same benign lesion. Still less can this be regarded as an estimate of the prevalence of this degeneration, since the different cancers we are dealing with developed at different times during the years of monitoring of these patients.

Such figures only permit an emphasis on the frequency of the coexistence of peptic esophagitis and of a cancerous lesion at the site of this abnormal tissue. Despite the absence of positive proof of a developmental change, it may be allowed that the risk of error in biopsy interpretation justifies the further pursuit of operative treatment in these patients when conservative medical treatment has not been obviously successful.

*

Only the results of a multicenter polydisciplinary study, such as OESO is undertaking (see p. 839), bringing together on a wide scale the same criteria of surveillance and systematic detection, would be likely to clarify the uncertainties still existing in the natural history of this disease.

J. B. Ollyo, A. P. Naef, M. Savary, Ph. Monnier, Ch. Fontolliet, J. Wellinger, J. J. Gonvers, and *F. Levi* (Lausanne)

A relationship between squamous cell carcinoma of the esophagus and hiatal hernia or reflux esophagitis has often been mentioned [1, 2, 4]. Objective data to substantiate this relationship are missing in the literature.

Table 1. Malignant change in esophagitis complicated by reflux (OCR)

OCR	Prevalence of Cancer		Incidence of Cancer		mean following
Savary grade IV	EPI*	A/EBE*	EPI*	A/EBE*	months
Cylindrical Metaplasia "Sleeves" (n=330) "Tongues" (n=291)	 3/330 6/291	 35/330 25/291	 0 0	 5/264*** 3/241	 58 61
Peptic Strictures without Cylindrical Metaplasia (n=196)	0	–	2**	–	84
Single Esophageal Ulcers (n=73)	0	–	0	–	72
Total	9/890	60/621	2/890	8/505	65

* EPI: Epidermoid A/EBE adenocarcinoma on Barrett's Epithelium
** Only one of these 2 cancers situated in the lower ⅓ of the Esophagus
*** Patients without cancer at long-term follow-up

In our experience (Table 1) the risk of malignant evolution of reflux esophagitis is primarily limited to the malignant transformation of columnar epithelium of the esophagus (Barrett's esophagus). Erosive, ulcerated and stenosing reflux lesions are not at a risk for direct transformation to squamous carcinoma, as might be expected since these lesions are located within squamous epithelium [3, 5, 6].

In our opinion the principal arguments against a relationship between reflux esophagitis and the development of epidermoid carcinoma are the following:

1. the usual absence of documented reflux esophagitis prior to the development of epidermoid carcinoma.
2. epidermoid carcinomas are rare in patients with reflux esophagitis with complications (11/230, 4.8%, Table 2) whereas the prevalence of extraesophageal tumors is very high [7, 8].
3. reflux esophagitis almost always involves the distal third of the esophagus whereas the majority of epidermoid carcinomas are in the middle third of the esophagus (Table 3).

In conclusion the risk of malignant evolution of reflux esophagitis is primarily the risk of malignant transformation of metaplastic columnar epithelium of the lower esophagus.

References

1. Kuylenstierna R, Munck-Wikland E (1985) Esophagitis and cancer of the oesophagus. Cancer 56: 837–839
2. Moghissi K (1977) Carcinoma of the cardia and thoracic oesophagus coexisting with and following sliding hiatal hernia and peptic stricture. Thorax 32: 342–345

Table 2. Esophagitis complicated by reflux and cancers other than adenocarcinomas in endobrachy-esophagus

	Cylindrical Metaplasias (CM)		Peptic Strictures without CM	Single Esophageal Ulcers	Total
	Sleeves	Tongues			
Patients	330	291	196	73	890
Carcinomas	90 (27%)	72 (24%)	56 (28%)	12 (16%)	230 (26%)
• Sphere E.N.T	32	31	7	2	72
• Esophagus	3	6	2	0	11
• Lungs	8	7	6	1	22
• Colon	8	6	6	1	21
• Other	39	22	35	8	104

Chuv, Lausanne, Switzerland (01. 01. 1963–31. 12. 1986)

Table 3. Epidermoid cancers, adenocarcinomas in endobrachyesophagus (A/EBE) and reflux esophagitis: epidemiologic and endoscopic data

	Epidermoid Cancers	A/EBE	Reflux Esophagitis
Patients	724	68	3102
Men (%)	82%	85%	69%
Mean age	72 years	67 years	55 years
Hiatus hernia (%)	?	75%	86%
Sites			
– Upper ⅓	127 (17.5%)	0	29 (1%)
– Middle ⅓	344 (47.5%)	9 (13.3%)	341 (11%)
– Lower ⅓	253 (35 %)	59 (86.7%)	2732 (88%)

Chuv, Lausanne, Switzerland (01. 01. 1963–31. 12. 1986)

3. Ollyo JB, Savary M, Fasel J (1986) L'ulcère de Barrett: mythes et réalités. Schweiz Med Wschr 116: 958–959
4. Oettle GJ, Paterson AC, Leiman G, Segal I (1986) Esophagitis in a population at risk for esophageal carcinoma. Cancer 57: 2222–2229
5. Savary M, Monnier P (1985) Diagnosis, pathophysiology and adenocarcinogenesis of Barrett's esophagus, in: DeMeester TR, Skinner DB: esophageal disorders. Pathophysiology and therapy. Raven Press, New-York 101–108
6. Savary M, Ollyo JB. L'œsophagite par reflux et ses complications: ulcère, sténose, endobrachy-œsophage. Encycl Med Chir (Paris, France), ORL 20822 A[10], 10–1986 (16 p)
7. Sontag SJ, Schnell TG, Chejfec G et al (1985) Barrett's esophagus and colonic tumors. Lancet I, 946–949
8. Spechler SJ, Robbins AH, Bloomfield Rubins H et al (1984) Adenocarcinoma and Barrett's esophagus. An overrated risk? Gastroenterology 87: 927–933

Must the risks of degeneration be taken into consideration in the choice of treatment for a caustic or peptic stenosis in an infant or a child?

G. H. Willital, and *K. H. Dietl* (Münster)

Diagnosis of reflux in children

Reflux in children is physiological till the age of one year. *The pathological picture* is clinically characterized by:

- vomiting mucus at the beginning, later on if there are ulcerations with blood
- anemia
- painful swallowing
- respiratory distress (Fig. 1)

The diagnosis is performed furthermore by *X-ray* studies demonstrating either a sliding hiatal hernia, a paraesophageal hernia or an upsidedown stomach.

An *endoscopy* is necessary in order to classify the reflux, to determine whether a stenosis is present or not and decide which therapy is necessary.

The longtime *pH-metry* over a 12 hours period of time today is the most reliable method to distinguish between a pathological from a physiological reflux. By this method, not only the number of refluxes but also the duration can be determined very accuratly. At a 12 hours interval of time, no more than 10 refluxes of a time lapse of 3 min each should occur.

Manometry should be performed before pH-metry; it is important to determine the reflux mechanism of the esophagus. The pressure of the so-called lower sphincter is normally about 20 mm Hg [11].

Reasons of reflux in children

As mentioned before, there is a physiologic maturation of the esophageal gastric junction with a physiologic reflux within the first 6–12 months of life. Further

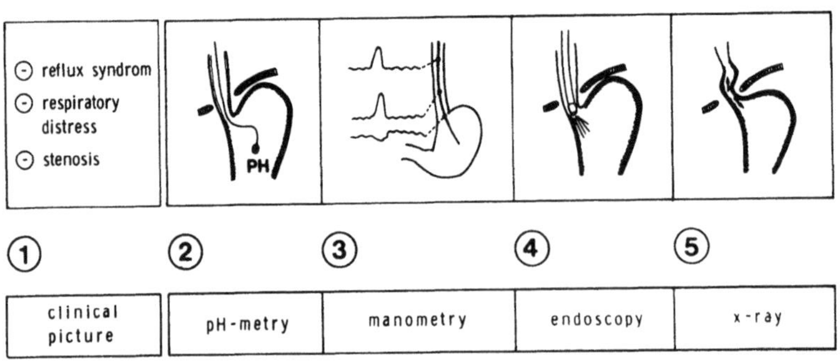

Fig. 1. Methods for Diagnosis of reflux in children

1. hiatus hernia
2. physiological maturation of the esophageal gastric junction
3. recurrent bougienage in esophageal atresia (sequelae of TOF)
4. diaphragmatic hernia
5. diaphragmatic relaxation

Fig. 2. The 5 most important reasons for reflux in children

reasons for reflux are the different types of hiatus hernia and paraesophageal hernia, a recurrent bougienage procedure in esophageal atresias following esophageal reconstruction, large diaphragmatic hernia repair and subsequent alterations of the anatomy and the physiology of the gastroesophageal junction [15] (Fig. 2).

Classification of reflux

In all symptomatic children, an endoscopy should be performed in order to determine which type and which degree of reflux is present. This endoscopic classification of alterations of the esophagus in the reflux disease – performed by Savary and Miller – is important for the indication of further treatment [16]: the endoscopic criteria are defects of the esophageal epithelium either isolated, closed together or circular with or without stenosis. The sequelae of longterm reflux esophagitis that are not treated medically can lead to a progressive stadium with esophageal stenosis, ulcerations of the esophagus and severe bleeding [8, 17, 18] (Fig. 3).

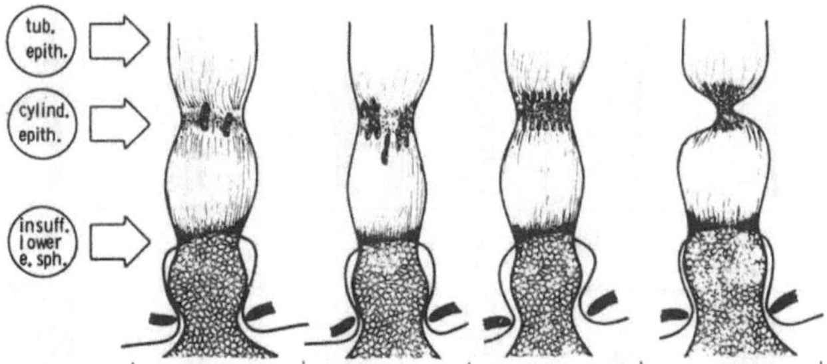

Stadium	I	II	III	IV
epithelium defect	+	+	+	+
multiple defects		+	+	+
circular defects			+	+
scars + stenosis				+

Fig. 3. Survey of the classification of reflux

Esophageal stenosis – morphological findings and therapy

Esophageal stenosis in children can be congenital or acquired 12% of the congenital esophageal stenosis are caused by extraluminal or intraluminal alterations. The acquired esophageal stenosis have a frequency of 88%. The reasons are:

- postoperative after esophageal atresia repair
- esophageal perforations
- caustics of the esophagus and
- reflux [1, 2, 3, 7, 19] (Fig. 4)

There are 14 different anatomical variations of congenital esophageal stenosis in children (Fig. 5)

The most frequent causes of postoperative esophageal stenosis that have a frequency of 44% after esophageal repair for esophageal atresias are:

a) the big difference of diameter of the upper and lower segment
b) scar formation at the anastomotic line because of the high tension
c) ischaemia at the border line of the anastomosis because of too many stitches and
d) insufficiency of the anastomosis itself (Fig. 6)

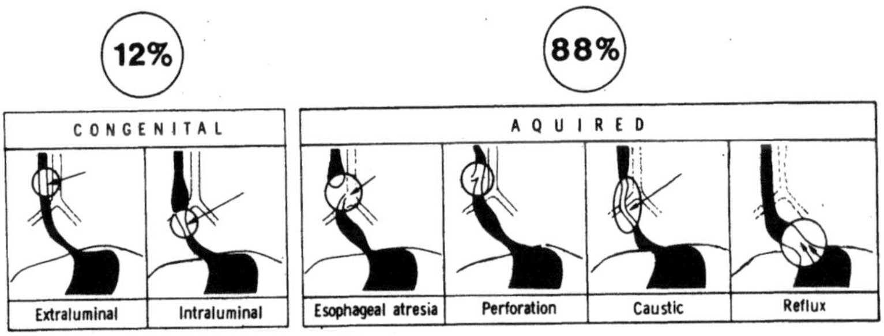

Fig. 4. Reasons and types of esophageal stenosis in children (n=240)

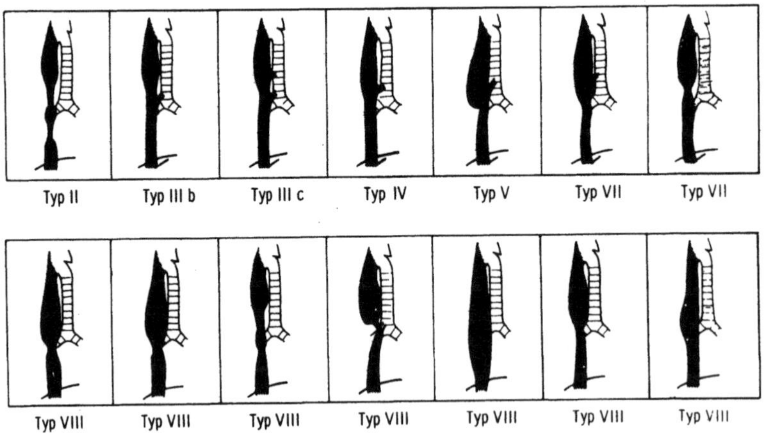

Fig. 5. The 14 different types of congenital esophageal stenosis

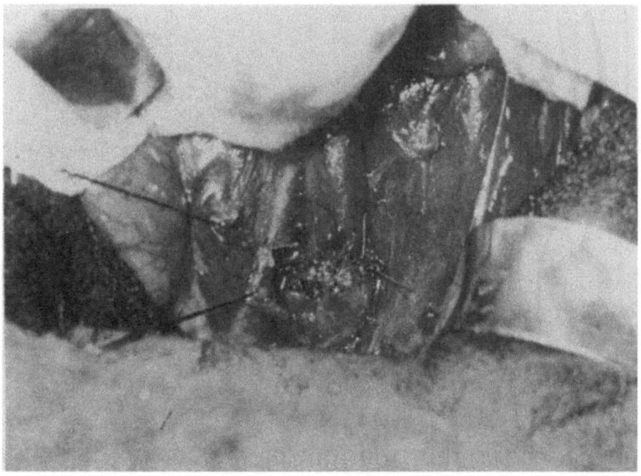

Fig. 6. Reconstruction of the esophagus in an esophageal atresia by a one layer anastomosis of the proximal and distal segment

There are different methods of treatment for esophageal stenosis in children. First of all one has to distinguish between esophageal stenosis with a long segment and those who have a short extension. Long esophageal stenosis are best treated by Rehbein bougienage procedure [5, 6, 10].

For the short segment stenosis four different methods are available:

- If the stenosis can be dilated easily with a pneumatic dilatation under pressure control this will be the best way [12].
- If the stenosis cannot be treated successfully by pneumatic dilatation the Rehbein bougienage is indicated.
- In those children who have a persistent thick scar formation causing an esophageal stenosis, an endoscopic intraluminal laser resection is indicated for a few cases.
- A small esophageal segment resection is only indicated if conservative treatment is unsuccessful, and the wall of the esophagus is too thin for laser resection (Fig. 7).

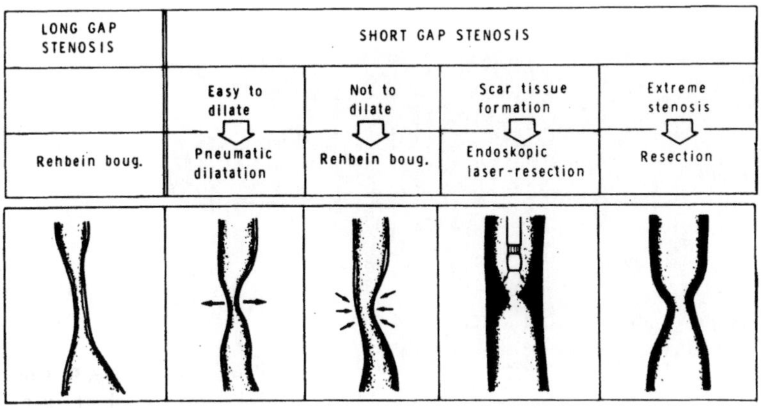

Fig. 7. Indication for different methods of treatment in esophageal stenosis in children depending on the anatomical morphological situation

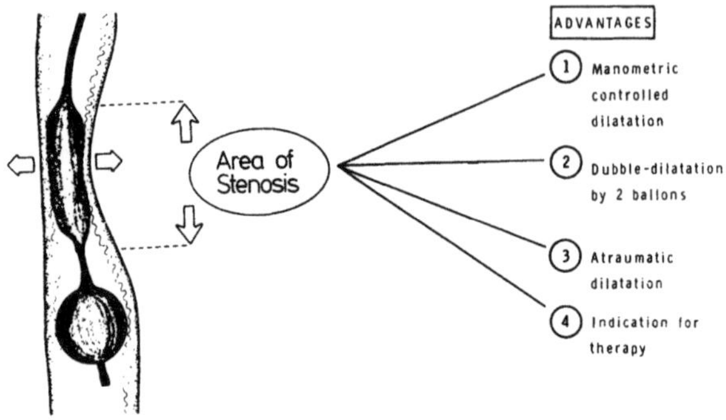

Fig. 8. Technique and advantages of pneumatic dilatation

Fig. 8 shows the principle of pneumatic dilatation. The advantage is that the pressure inside the esophagus can be determined manometrically. Using a double balloon system a double dilatation can be performed. The dilatation is much more smooth and not so traumatic compared to those with flexible bougies. The configuration of the compression of the balloons gives an idea how flexible the stenosis is. This is important for the indication for a further pneumatic dilatation therapy (Fig. 8).

Fig. 9 shows a child with a postoperative esophageal stenosis after an esophageal repair in the neonatal period. A pneumatic dilatation was not successful. In this baby a 7 months dilatation with the flexible bougies over a gastrostomy has been performed successfully.

Fig. 10 demonstrates the survey of our results of an interval of 10 years.

- The treatment by Rehbein bougies in 19 cases for the long esophageal stenosis took on average 2½ years.
- 42 children with a short segment stenosis could be treated successfully by pneumatic dilatation over a period of 6 months, whereas the Rehbein bougienage procedure for the short segment stenosis which could not be treated by pneumatic dilatation took an average 8–12 months.

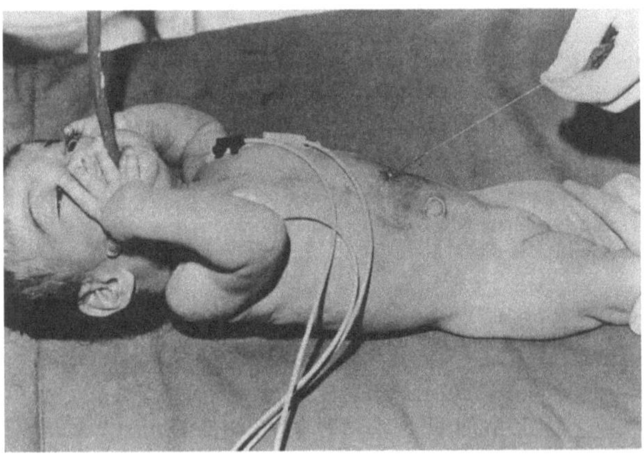

Fig. 9. Continous dilatation of short gap stenosis of the esophagus by the Rehbein dilatation procedure

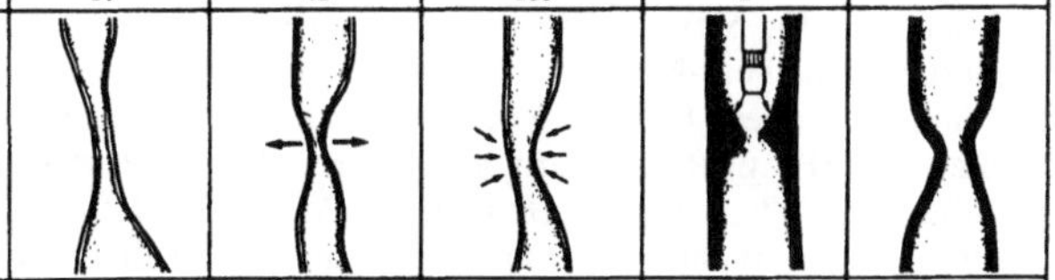

n	19	42	166	2	11
Time of treatment	2 1/2 yrs.	1/2 yrs.	3/4 yrs.	No stenosis normal function	Op.
Results after	15%	86%	76%		9/2
2 yrs.	41%	95%	81%		10/1
3 yrs.	56%	95%	83%		10/1
4 yrs.	61%	96%	89%		11/0
5 yrs.	76%	96%	96%		11/0
10 yrs.	83%	96%	99%		11/0

Fig. 10. Results of treatment in esophageal stenosis with a long gap and with a short gap that can be treated by pneumatic dilatation; a short gap stenosis, that could not be treated by pneumatic dilatation, needed a Rehbein bougienage procedure; an esophageal stenosis with a localized scar formation needed a small resection

We followed up our patients after 1, 2, 3, 4, 5 and after 10 years.

- After 5 years, for example, the long segment stenosis that underwent the Rehbein bougienage procedure, are successfully treated in 76%, whereas for the short segment stenosis successful treatment could be achieved in 96% – the same rate as for the children with pneumatic dilatation.
- We have just begun to use the endoscopic laser resection, so no reliable statement can be given.
- In the 11 children where we had to perform a small resection of the esophagus, the operative treatment was successful in all 11 cases (Fig. 10).

Children who suffer for a long time period from reflux disease should be followed up by clinical investigations regularly.

If the reflux is based on a severe anatomical morphological alteration of the esophageal gastric junction, for example by hiatus hernia [9, 13, 14, 20], a surgical repair is necessary if the reflux persists over a year with increasing symptoms and alterations diagnosed by endoscopic investigations [1, 2].

This is necessary especially in elder children, in whom, with time, a metaplasy of the epithelium can occur [4].

References

1. Behar J, Sheahan DG, Biancani P (1975) Medical and surgical management of reflux esophagitis. New Engl J Med 193:263

2. Blum A, Siewert J (1976) Pathogenese, Diagnostik und konservative Therapie der Refluxkrankheit. In: Siewert JR, Blum A (Hrsg.) Funktionsstörungen der Speiseröhre. Springer, Berlin-Heidelberg-New York
3. Blum A, Siewert J (1981) Notwendige Diagnostik: Klinische Symptomatologie. In: Blum A, Siewert J (Hrsg) Refluxtherapie. Springer, Berlin-Heidelberg-New York
4. Brand DL, Ylvisaker JT, Gelfand M, Pope CE 2 (1980) Regression of columnar esophageal (Barrett's) epithelium after anti-reflux surgery. N Engl J Med 302: 844
5. Buntain WL, Payne WS, Lynn HB (1980) Esophageal reconstruction for benign disease: a longterm appraisal. Am Surg 46: 67
6. Burkhardt K, Bahners W (1975) Therapie peptischer Oesophagusstenosen im Kindesalter. Chirurg 46: 507
7. Carcassonne M, Gregoire A, Magalon G (1974) Les reflux gastrocesophagiens du nourrisson. Pédiatrie 29: 815
8. Cohen S (1974) Developmental characteristics of lower esophageal sphincter function: a possible mechanism for infantile chalasia. Gastroenterology 67: 252
9. Harrel G (1974) The importance of Hiatal Herniae in Children. Gastroenterology 67: 1075
10. Hasse W (1975) Bougierung des oberen und unteren Oesophagussegmentes bei der Oesophagusatresie Typ 2. Z Kinderchir 17: 170
11. Kehrer B, Oesch A, Bettex M (1972) Manometric studies of esophageal motility in infants with hiatus hernia. J Pediatr Surg 7: 499
12. McAdam WAF, Morgan AG, Darnborough A (1980) Eder-Puestow esophageal dilatation. Brit J Surg 67: 898
13. Nissen R, Rossetti M, Siewert R (1981) Fundoplicatio und Gastropexie bei Refluxkrankheit und Hiatushernien. Thieme-Verlag Stuttgart
14. Prinsen J (1975) Hiatus hernia in infants and children: A long term follow-up of medical treatment. J Pediat Surg 10: 97
15. Randolph J, Lilly J, Anderson K (1974) Surgical treatment of gastroesophageal reflux in infants. Ann Surg 180: 479
16. Savary M, Miller G (1977) Der Ösophagus. Lehrbuch und endoskopischer Atlas. Gassmann, Solothurn
17. Schumpelick V (1981) Duodenogastraler Reflux und Ösophagitis. In: Blum A, Siewert J (Hrsg) Refluxtherapie. Springer, Berlin-Heidelberg-New York
18. Siewert JR (1981) Refluxkrankheit der Speiseröhre. In: Heberer G, Schweiberer L: Indikation zur Operation. Springer-Verlag Berlin-Heidelberg-New York
19. Siewert J, Blum A Endobrachyesophagus und peptische Stenose. In: Allgöwer M, Harder F, Hollender V, Peiper HJ, Siewert RJ (Hrsg) Gastroenterol Chirurgie, Kap 23.3 Springer, Berlin-Heidelberg-New York
20. Siewert J, Blum A (1981) Stellenwert der axialen Hiatushernie. In: Blum A, Siewert J (Hrsg) Refluxtherapie, Springer, Berlin-Heidelberg-New York Kap 34, 424–429
21. Willital GH (1982) Oesophagusatresie. In: Encke A, Kremer K (Hrsg) Husemann B. Chirurgie der Speiseröhre, Enke, Bd 94: 63

Degeneration of Barrett's esophagus

F. H. Ellis (Boston)

The columnar epithelium-lined distal esophagus, to which Norman Barrett's name has become attached because of his 1950 report [1], constitutes a ripe source of controversy today. Barrett described peptic ulceration in what he considered to be an intra-thoracic extension of the stomach in the presence of a congenitally short esophagus. This impression was later corrected by Allison and Johnstone who identified the location of the ulcer as in the esophagus [2]. Although Barrett considered the condition as "rare and of little clinical significance", it is now recognized as a relatively common entity. However, many aspects of its development, management and precancerous nature remain controversial. Its propensity for malignant degeneration is what concerns us here and by way of introducing the topic, let me make a few general comments based on both the literature and my own personal experience.

There are a number of features of the disease that are now widely accepted: all agree that the columnar epithelium lines the lower esophagus and does not represent a tubular extension of the stomach. The condition is always associated with a hypotensive lower esophageal sphincter and gastroesophageal reflux with or without a hiatus hernia, which clearly establishes its acquired nature in the vast majority of cases. The disease may or may not be associated with a stricture which develops at the squamocolumnar junction and not the esophagogastric junction, so that the stricture usually lies at a relatively high level. An ulcer may develop in the columnar epithelium, the so-called Barrett ulcer. As experience has grown, the association of Barrett's mucosa with malignant degeneration has been widely appreciated so that it is generally considered to be a pre-malignant lesion.

Controversial Topics

The prevalence of Barrett's esophagus in the general population is not known. However, approximately 10% of patients who have endoscopic evidence of esophagitis are found to have a columnar epithelium-lined lower esophagus [3]. The reported prevalence of carcinoma in patients with Barrett's esophagus varies widely from 8.6% [4] to 46% [5], presumably reflecting the different types of patients seen in different clinics and this will be a question that will receive more detailed attention later in this conference.

The risk of malignant degeneration occurring in a given patient with Barrett's esophagus is also not known. A report from the Mayo Clinic suggests that this is extremely rare, occurring once in 440 patient years of follow-up. In a recent study by Spechler and Goyal [7], 105 patients with Barrett's esophagus were followed for 350 person years, and only two developed cancer for an incidence of one case per 176 person years of follow-up representing a 42.5% increase in incidence as compared to that of the general population.

There is also little agreement on the fate of the abnormal mucosa following treatment. With the exception of the report by Patel and associates [8], who described resolution of carcinoma in situ in one patient and regression of the columnar epithelium in two, medical treatment has failed to lead to mucosal regression. Antireflux surgery is more successful in this regard, regression of the abnormal epithelium being recorded as occurring in from ⅓ to ½ the cases studied, though in no instance has regression been complete [5, 9].

The therapeutic implication of the presence of mucosal dysplasia is also controversial. The high incidence of dysplasia in association with carcinoma in Barrett's esophagus suggests a strong etiologic relationship, but the natural history of mild dysplasia remains to be determined. In view of the fact that high grade dysplasia occurs in the vast majority of patients who have cancer in Barrett's mucosa, there is increasing support for recommending esophagectomy in such cases. In contrast to its frequent association with cancer, the finding of dysplasia is relatively rare in patients with Barrett's epithelium without cancer, estimated as occurring in only 5% to 10% [7].

*

The Lahey Clinic experience with Barrett's esophagus has already been presented in a preliminary form elsewhere [10, 11]. I will summarize briefly here certain aspects of that report that bear on some of these controversial issues.

From 1973 to 1984, 18450 endoscopies were done at the Lahey Clinic of which 2167 (11,7%) demonstrated esophagitis. 108 of these (5%) had a diagnosis of Barrett's esophagus based on endoscopic biopsies. This is a lower prevalence rate than others have reported, probably because strict criteria for the diagnosis were used: extension of the columnar epithelium 3 cm or more proximal to the esophagogastric junction and circumferential involvement of the esophagus were required for the diagnosis to be made.

Twenty-four of these patients had adenocarcinoma for a prevalence of 22%. Nine other patients exhibited varying degrees of dysplasia, six with either mild or moderate dysplasia and three with a severe form of this cellular abnormality. All were treated medically: five of the six with mild or moderate dysplasia were re-endoscoped and four showed reversion to non-dysplastic epithelium while none of the two with severe dysplasia who were studied showed any change in the severity of the cellular abnormality.

The risk of malignant degeneration of the columnar epithelium was estimated by reviewing 41 patients with the disease without cancer who were endoscoped and biopsied yearly and were followed for from one to 11 years. Adenocarcinoma developed in two patients 3½ and 4½ years after diagnosis, for an incidence of one case per 81 years of patient follow-up, a somewhat higher incidence than reported by others.

*

Although Barrett's esophagus is known to be a premalignant lesion, controversy persists regarding the prevalence and incidence of carcinoma in Barrett's. The prevalence of Barrett's esophagus in patients with endoscopically diagnosed esophagitis at the Lahey Clinic between 1973 and 1984, was 5%, a somewhat lower rate than is usually reported. Of the 108 patients with Barrett's esophagus identified during this period, adenocarcinoma was present in 24 for a prevalence of 22%. The risk of malignant degeneration in patients with Barrett's esophagus was estimated as one case per 81 years of patient follow-up, somewhat higher than that reported by others.

Four of fifteen patients unresponsive to medical therapy, who underwent antireflux surgery by a Nissen fundoplication exhibited evidence of mucosal regression

(27%), yet in no case was regression complete. Furthermore, carcinoma developed in two patients in spite of a successful antireflux operation performed 3½ years previously.

Because treatment, whether medical or surgical, does not result in complete regression of the abnormal epithelium nor does it protect against the subsequent development of carcinoma, all patients with Barrett's esophagus should be placed under close surveillance with periodic endoscopic examination of the esophagus.

References

1. Barrett NR (1950) Chronic peptic ulcer of the oesophagus and "oesophagitis". Brit J Surg 38: 175–182
2. Allison PR, Johnstone AS (1953) The oesophagus lined with gastric mucous membrane. Thorax 8: 87–101
3. Winters C Jr, Spurling TJ, Chobanian SJ et al (1987) Barrett's esophagus: a prevalent, occult complication of gastroesophageal reflux disease. Gastroent 92: 118
4. Haggitt RC, Tryzelaar J, Ellis FH Jr et al (1978) Adenocarcinoma complicating columnar epithelium-lined (Barrett's) esophagus. Amer Journ Clin Path 70(1): 1–5
5. Herlihy KS, Orlando RC, Bryson JC et al (1984) Barrett's esophagus – clinical, endoscopic, histologic, manometric and electrical potential difference characteristics. Gastroent 86: 436–443
6. Cameron AJ, Ott BJ, Payne WS (1985) The incidence of adenocarcinoma in columnarlined (Barrett's) esophagus. N Eng J Med 313: 857–859
7. Spechler SJ, Goyal RK (1986) Barrett's esophagus. N Eng J Med 315: 362
8. Patel GK, Clift SA, Schaefer RA et al (1982) Resolution of severe dysplastic (CA in situ) changes with regression of columnar epithelium (CE) in Barrett's esophagus (BE) on medical treatment (MT) (abst) Gastroent 22: 1147
9. Brand DL, Ylvisakes JT, Gelfand M et al (1980) Regression of columnar esophageal (Barrett's) epithelium after anti-reflux surgery. N Eng J Med 302: 844–848
10. Sprung DJ, Ellis FH Jr, Gibb SP (1984) Incidence of adenocarcinoma in Barrett's esophagus. (abst) Am J Gastroent 79: 817
11. Ibid (1984) Regression of Barrett's epithelium after antireflux surgery (abst) Amer J Gastroent 79: 817

Can the delay in this degeneration be defined?

J. B. Ollyo, M. Savary, F. Levi, J. J. Gonvers, J. Wellinger, Ch. Fontolliet, and *Ph. Monnier* (Lausanne)

Adenocarcinoma can only be described as a malignant evolution of the columnar epithelium of Barrett's esophagus if the two following conditions are fulfilled:

1. documentation of the presence of columnar epithelium in the absence of carcinoma and high-grade dysplasia proven by multiple biopsies at various levels of the esophagus. In our experience an adenocarcinoma can be present at a distance from high-grade dysplasia.
2. Appearance of an adenocarcinoma at least one year after diagnosis of Barrett's esophagus.

Table 1. Malignant change in endobrachyesophagus (EBE) at Lausanne (1963–1986)

	HGER* Duration years	Diagnosis of EBE E*	H*	T*	Dysplasia	Diagnosis of Adenocarcinoma / EBE year	Interval
B.M., ♀ 1923	36	1964	SE	M*	–	1980	186 months] mean
B.E., ♂ 1913	10	1976	SE	M*	1985	1986	124 months] interval
C.L., ♂ 1912	3	1970	SE	S*	–	1973	31 months]
P.J., ♂ 1912	5	1975	SE	S*	–	1980	58 months] 98 months
T.A., ♂ 1921	7	1978	SE	M*	–	1986	91 months] (8.1 years)

* HGER: History of gastro-esophageal reflux: E: endoscopy H: histology
SE: specialized epithelium T: treatment M: medical
S: surgery (Nissen)

Thirty-five of the 318 cases of circumferential Barrett's esophagus diagnosed by endoscopy at Lausanne from 1963 to 1986 were initially associated with an adenocarcinoma which was totally within the esophagus. Five of the remaining 283 patients later developed an adenocarcinoma (Table 1). Two of these five patients had a functioning Nissen fundoplication without any reflux esophagitis at endoscopy. The columnar epithelium of Barrett's esophagus does not seem to disappear and continues to maintain a malignant potential after correction of reflux [8, 13, 14].

We found 752 cases of adenocarcinoma complicating Barrett's esophagus reported in the English, French, German, Italian and Spanish literature from 1952, date of the first report by Morson and Belcher, to 1986. This represents 6 times as many cases as Sjøgren [19], and 4 times as many cases as Hölscher [11]. In only 35 cases was the diagnosis of adenocarcinoma made after the diagnosis of Barrett's esophagus [1–18, 20–23]. The intervals ranged from 18 months [1, 23] to 18 years [6] and averaged 5.9 years. Table 2 shows the average ages at the diagnosis of the various stages of reflux esophagitis, Barrett's esophagus and adenocarcinoma: we see that the age is progressively greater as the stages of esophagitis become more severe. This may be interpreted as meaning that the 4 stages of reflux esophagitis

Table 2. Reflux esophagitis: Mean ages related to Savary's 4 stages.
Mean ages of endobrachyesophagus (EBE) and adenocarcinoma (A)

	Grade 1 (n=1564)	Grade 2 (n=420)	Grade 3 (n=160)	Grade 4 (n=925)	EBE (n=278)	A (n=40)
Men (≥16 years) (n=2140)	49.7	56.1	59.8	60.3	62.1	65.4
Women (≥16 years) (n=929)	56.3	62.7	63.1	64.7	67.3	69.6
Total (n=3069)	51.7	57.8	60.8	61.7	63.7	66.4

CHUV, Lausanne, Switzerland (01.01.1963–31.12.1986)

described by Savary and Miller represent stages of increasing severity of the same disease, and that adenocarcinoma represents the ultimate complication of reflux disease.

At the present time, it is impossible to determine for a particular patient what the risk of carcinoma is at various time intervals after the diagnosis of Barrett's esophagus. This means that all patients with columnar epithelium of the lower esophagus, whether treated by antireflux surgery or not, should be followed on a very long-term basis by annual endoscopies with multiple biopsies.

References

1. Adler RH (1963) The lower esophagus lined by columnar epithelium. J Thorac Cardiosvasc Surg 45: 13–34
2. Aprigliano F (1977) Cited in: Bremner CG The Columnar-lined (Barrett's) esophagus. Surg Annual 9: 103–123
3. Brand DL, Ylvisaker JT, Gelfand M, Pope CE II. (1980) Regression of columnar esophageal (Barrett's) epithelium after anti-reflux surgery. N Engl J Med 302: 844–848
4. Cameron AJ, Ott BJ, Payne WS (1985) The incidence of adenocarcinoma in columnar-lined (Barrett's) esophagus. N Engl J Med 313: 857–859
5. Crabb DW, Berk MA, Hall TR et al (1985) Familial gastroesophageal reflux and development of Barrett's esophagus. Ann Intern Med 103: 52–54
6. DenBesten L (1984) In discussion Starnes VA, Adkins RB, Ballinger JF, Sawyers JL. Barrett's esophagus. A surgical entity. Arch Surg 119: 563–567
7. Haggitt RC, Tryzelaar J, Ellis H, Colcher H (1978) Adenocarcinoma complicating columnar epithelium-lined (Barrett's) esophagus. Am J Clin Pathol 70: 1–5
8. Hamilton SR, Hutcheon DF, Ravich WJ, Cameron JL, Paulson M (1984) Adenocarcinoma in Barrett's esophagus after elimination of gastroesophageal reflux. Gastroenterology 86: 356–360
9. Harle IA, Bondy DC, Finley RJ et al (1985) Management of adenocarcinoma in a columnar-lined esophagus. Ann Thorac Surg 40: 330–336
10. Hershfield NB, Lind JF, Hildes JA, McMorris LS (1985) Secretory function of Barrett's epithelium. Gut 6: 535–539
11. Hölscher AH, Bader M, Siewert JR (1985) Kann Antireflux-Chirurgie eine maligne Entartung des Endobrachyösophagus verhindern? Dtsch Med Wschr 110: 551–555
12. Hureau J, Bourdais JP, Delavierre Ph, Vayre P (1979) Œsophagite peptique et cancer du tiers inférieur de l'œsophage. A propos de sept observations. J Chir (Paris) 116: 167–174
13. Luna L (1983) Endoscopic therapy of benign esophageal stricture. Endoscopy 15: 203–206
14. Naef AP, Savary M, Ozzello L (1975) Columnar-lined lower esophagus: An acquired lesion with malignant predisposition. J Thoracic Cardiovasc Surg 70: 826–835
15. Payne WS (1973) Cited in: Hawe A, Payne WS, Weiland LH, Fontana RS: Adenocarcinoma in the columnar epithelial lined lower (Barrett's) oesophagus. Thorax 28: 511–514
16. Rosenberg JC, Buden H, Edwards RC et al (1985) Analysis of adenocarcinoma in Barrett's esophagus utilizing a staging system. Cancer 55: 1353–1360
17. Sampliner RE, Kogan FJ, Morgan TR, Tripp M (1985) Progression – Regression of Barrett's esophagus. Gastroenterology 88: 1567
18. Saubier EC, Gouillat C, Samaniego C, Guillaud M, Moulinier B (1985) Adenocarcinoma in columnar-lined Barrett's esophagus. Analysis of 13 esophagectomies. Am J Surg 150: 365–369
19. Sjogren RW, Johnson LF (1983) Barrett's esophagus: A review. Am J Med 74: 313–321
20. Spechler SJ, Robbins AH, Rubins HB et al (1984) Adenocarcinoma and Barrett's esophagus. An overrated risk? Gastroenterology 87: 927–933
21. Sprung J, Ellis FH, Gibb P (1984) Incidence of adenocarcinoma in Barrett's esophagus. Am J Gastroenterol 79: 817
22. Starnes VA, Adkins RB, Ballinger JF, Sawyers JL (1984) Barrett's esophagus. A surgical entity. Arch Surg 119: 563–567
23. Watson A (1984) The role of antireflux surgery combined with fiberoptic endoscopic dilatation in peptic esophageal stricture. Amer J Surg 148: 346–349

What are the means of early detection of malignant degeneration?

C. G. Bremner (Johannesburg)

The means of early detection of malignant degeneration in an established columnar-lined esophagus (CLE) are far from satisfactory. The methods available are as follows:

1. Clinical presentation

Continued reflux symptoms or the development of dysphagia demand repeated endoscopic, histologic and cytologic evalutation. The risk is higher in smokers [1].

2. Endoscopic techniques

Any stricture, ulcer, mucosal irregularity or polyp must have adequate histologic and cytologic material taken for evaluation.

3. Dye-spraying techniques

Lugol's iodine has been used to define the area of the columnar lining but indigo carmine is reported to detect dysplastic epithelium, and highlights small areas of abnormalities where biopsy should be performed [2].

4. Histology and Cytology

Every patient with a CLE must have adequate material reviewed both histologically and cytologically. Any erosion, stricture, polypoidal or other suspicious area must be biopsied. If no such area is present, biopsies at 2 cm intervals of the columnar epithelial segment should be taken.

If a high grade dysplasia is detected on biopsy, resection is probably indicated [1, 3]: Saubier et al. [3] reviewed 13 esophagectomy specimens and found variable degrees of intestinal metaplasia, and several foci of intramucosal carcinoma, suggesting that the adenocarcinoma develops in dysplasia. Invasive carcinoma probably develops through a sequence of epithelial dysplasia and carcinoma-in-situ, and this can be detected by biopsy and cytology [4].

Lee [5] resected the esophagus in 4 patients with a high-grade dysplasia but no detectable carcinoma, and in three of the four specimens invasive carcinoma was found to be present. A further 2 patients had low-grade dysplasia and had not developed carcinoma.

Schmidt et al. [6] considered that dysplasia may be a marker for co-existing carcinoma: in 23 specimens resected for adenocarcinoma, dysplasia was found in 18, whilst dysplasia was only found in 2 of 38 patients without carcinoma in Barrett's esophagus.

5. Histochemical studies

Berenson et al. [7] have suggested that serial determinations of Beta-glucuronidase may serve as a marker for neoplastic degeneration. This enzyme appears to be greater in tissues which are undifferentiated. No further studies on this aspect have been reported. Jass [8] found an incompletely differentiated variant of intestinal metaplasia secreting sulphomucins associated with well-differentiated carcinomas, but Rothery et al. [9] showed that the presence of sulphomucins was not helpful.

6. Labelling Index

Herbst [10] suggested that surface labelling of cells using tritiated thymidine may herald malignant change. We have labelled cells in the CLE and did not detect surface labelling in a patient who developed adenocarcinoma while on surveillance.

7. Surveillance

The optimal frequency of repeat endoscopic, cytologic and biopsy surveillance is unclear. We have re-examined our patients yearly and two of our patients have developed a carcinoma, one in a pre-existing Barrett's ulcer, and the other 1 year after diagnosis of a CLE. Sjogren and Johnson [11] have evaluated their patients at 6 monthly intervals and Mangla [12] has suggested a one-year interval.

However, the risk of developing adenocarcinoma is low, and Cameron et al. [13] reviewed the Mayo Clinic experience in which only 2 of 104 patients with CLE developed adenocarcinoma 6 and 10 years after the inital diagnosis had been made (882 patient-years follow-up). In Spechler's series [14] of 105 patients followed for 350 person-years only 2 developed adenocarcinoma. Despite the low frequency of adenocarcinoma in the CLE, it is felt that annual surveillance is still advisable on all patients, 4 times a year in cases of dysplasia and monthly if an ulcer is present.

At present, the only way of detecting early malignant change in Barrett's esophagus is by biopsy. Evidence strongly suggests that a high-grade dysplastic epithelium is a precursor of malignancy. Greater use of dye-spraying techniques should be encouraged to detect dysplastic epithelium. If a high grade dysplastic epithelium is diagnosed on biopsy, the esophagus should be resected.

References

1. Skinner DB, Walther BC, Riddell RH, Schmidt H, Iascone C, DeMeester TR (1983) Barrett's esophagus: comparison of benign and malignant cases. Ann Surg 198: 554–566
2. Kawai K, Takemoto T, Suzuki S, Ida K (1979) Proposed nomenclature and classification of the dye-spraying techniques in endoscopy. Endoscopy 1: 23–25
3. Haggitt RC, Tryzelaar J, Ellis FH Jr, Colcher H (1978) Adenocarcinoma complicating columnar epithelium-lined (Barrett's) Esophagus. Amer J Clin Path 70(1): 1–5
4. Saubier EC, Gouillat C, Samaniego C, Guillaud M, Moulinier B (1985) Adenocarcinoma in columnar-lined Barrett's esophagus. Analysis of 13 esophagectomies. Amer J Surg 150 :365–369

5. Lee RG (1985) Dysplasia in Barrett's esophagus. A clinico-pathologic study of six patients. Am J Surg Path 9(12): 845–852
6. Schmidt HG, Riddell RH, Walther BC, Skinner DB, Riemann JF (1985) Dysplasia in Barrett's esophagus. J Amer Res Clin Oncol 110(2): 145–152
7. Berenson MM, Herbst JJ, Freston JW (1975) Esophageal columnar epithelial B-galactosidase and B-glucuronidase. Gastroenterol 68(6): 1417–1419
8. Jass JR (1981) Mucin histochemistry of the columnar epithelium of the esophagus: a retrospective study. J Clin Path 34: 866–870
9. Rothery GA, Patterson JE, Stoddard CJ, Day DW (1986) Histological and histochemical changes in the columnar-lined (Barrett's) esophagus. Gut 27(9): 1062–1068
10. Herbst JJ, Berenson MM, McCloskey DW, Wiser WC (1978) Cell proliferation in esophageal columnar epithelium (Barrett's esophagus). Gastroenterol 75: 683–687
11. Sjogren RW, Johnson LF (1983) Barrett's esophagus: A review. Am J Med 74: 313–321
12. Mangla JC (1981) Barrett's esophagus: an old entity rediscovered. J Clin Gastroenterol 3: 347–356
13. Cameron AJ, Ott BJ, Payne WS (1985) The incidence of adenocarcinoma in columnar-lined (Barrett's) esophagus. N Engl J Med 313(14): 857–859
14. Spechler SJ, Robbins AH, Rubins HB, Vincent HE, Heerer et al (1984) Adenocarcinoma and Barrett's esophagus: an overrated risk? Gastroenterol 87: 927–933

A. J. Cameron (Rochester)

Patients with Barrett's esophagus have an increased risk of developing adenocarcinoma in the columnar lined epithelium. When a tumor mass or malignant stricture has caused symptoms and is visible on a barium X-ray, the chance of a surgical cure is small: the 5-year survival in two series of operated patients was 22% and 14.5% (Skinner et al, [1], Sanfey et al [2]). In other types of malignancy such as cancer of the colon, cancer of the breast and melanoma, prognosis is related to the extent of spread at the time of surgical resection. It is therefore assumed, but not proven, that early diagnosis of cancer in Barrett's esophagus will also improve the chance of cure.

Endoscopy is required for early detection of carcinoma. An early cancer may be impossible to recognize by looking down the gastroscope: carcinoma has been found when biopsies have been taken of small nodules, benign appearing ulcers and areas of mucosa that looked "different". Carcinomas have also been found in biopsies of flat, smooth, dark red columnar mucosa where there was nothing to suggest malignancy on the endoscopic appearance (Hamilton and Smith [3]).

Biopsies from the columnar lined esophagus may be obtained through the normal endoscope channel. It is my practice to biopsy any abnormal looking area, and also to take four-quadrant biopsies every 2 cm along the entire length of columnar mucosa (Fig. 1). Reid and Rubin in Seattle [9] have taken larger biopsies with a large forceps and a wide bore channel endoscope.

Esophageal cytologic specimens have been obtained using endoscopic washings (Maimon et al [4]), a sponge in a capsule attached to a thread (Nabeya [5]) and a net covered balloon inflated in the esophagus (Korsten et al [6]). These methods have not been evaluated in Barrett's esophagus.

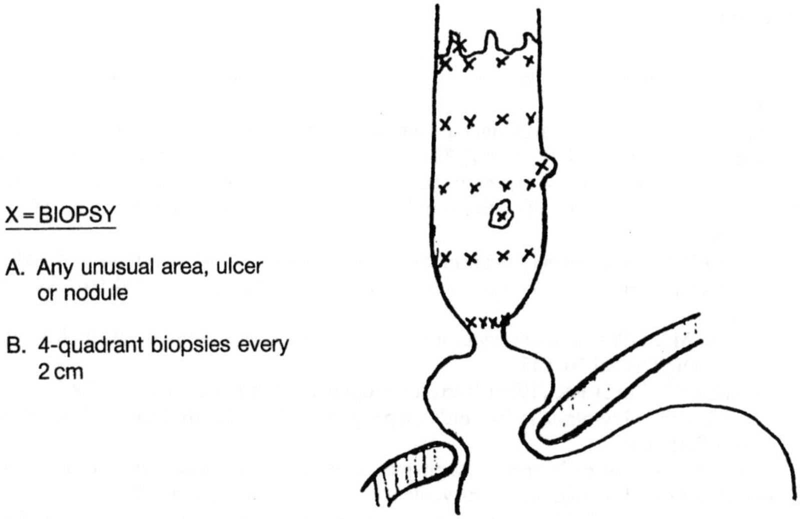

Fig. 1. *X* = *Biopsy* a) Any unusual area, ulcer or nodule; b) 4-quadrant biopsies every 2 cm

Even if biopsy does not show invasive carcinoma, the finding of dysplasia may lead to the diagnosis: dysplasia has been reported in the mucosa adjacent to gross tumor in 68 to 100% of cases with carcinoma, but only in 0 to 10% of other patients with Barrett esophagus (Spechler and Goyal [7]). When high grade dysplasia was found on biopsies, surgical resection revealed early invasive carcinoma in three of four patients (Lee [8]), one of seven patients (Reid et al [9]) and three of five patients (Hamilton and Smith [3]).

Endoscopy with multiple biopsies is recommended at one year intervals for early detection of dysplasia and carcinoma in patients known to have a Barrett's esophagus. We can expect to pick up about one carcinoma in every 300 yearly examinations. By doing this, we may help a few of our patients, but will have little impact on the incidence of adenocarcinoma of the esophagus: in most of our patients with carcinoma, the Barrett's esophagus is found at the same time the carcinoma is diagnosed.

About 10% of the population have esophageal reflux symptoms once a week or more (Nebel et al [10]) and a prospective study showed that about 10% of persons with these symptoms have a Barrett's esophagus (Winters et al [11]). Therefore, about 1 in 100 of the adult population should have a Barrett's esophagus.

Work in progress has confirmed this estimate, but a population survey in progress shows that only about 1 in 20 cases of Barrett's esophagus in the general population has been diagnosed. At present, early cancer detection can only be applied to the 5% of Barrett patients whose diagnosis is established. Most people with a Barrett's esophagus do not know it.

References

1. Skinner DB et al. (1983) Barrett's esophagus. Comparison of benign and malignant cases. Ann Surg 198: 554
2. Sanfey M et al. (1985) Carcinoma arising in Barrett's esophagus. Surg Gynecol Obstet 161: 570
3. Hamilton SR, Smith RRL (1987) The relationship between columnar epithelial dysplasia and invasive adenocarcinoma arising in Barrett's esophagus. Amer J Clin Path 87: 301
4. Maimon HN et al. (1974) Positive esophageal cytology without detectable neoplasm. Gastroint Endosc 20: 156
5. Nabeya K (1983) Markers of cancer risk in the esophagus and surveillance of high-risk groups. In: Precancerous lesions of the gastrointestinal tract. Sherlock P et al (ed) Raven Press New York
6. Korsten MA (1985) Balloon cytology in screening of asymptomatic alcoholics for esophageal cancer. Dig Dis Sci 30: 845
7. Spechler SJ, Goyal RK (1986) Barrett's esophagus. N Engl J Med 315: 366
8. Lee RG (1985) Dysplasia in Barrett's esophagus: A clinical pathologic study of six patients. Am J Surg Pathol 9: 845
9. Reid BJ et al. (1986) Barrett's esophagus: High grade dysplasia and intramucosal carcinoma detected by endoscopic biopsy surveillance. Gastroenterology 90: 601
10. Nebel OT et al. (1953) Symptomatic gastroesophageal reflux: Incidence and precipitating factors. Am J Dig Dis 21: 953
11. Winters C et al. (1987) Barrett's esophagus. A prevalent, occult complication of gastroesophageal reflux disease. Gastroenterology 92: 118

R. E. Condon (Milwaukee)

Although there is some disagreement [1, 2, 3], most knowledgeable surgeons accept that Barrett's mucosa in the esophagus is a precancerous lesion. Indeed, some authorities view most cases of adenocarcinoma arising in the body of the esophagus as originating in Barrett's mucosa, contending that the subsequent growth of the cancer destroys the evidence of the pre-existing Barrett's mucosa [4].

Among our recently reported series of 37 patients with adenocarcinoma of the esophagus [5], there were 10 patients who had Barrett's mucosa. Of the Barrett's patients, a majority (6/10) had a history of reflux esophagitis and 2/6 had had a previous Nissen fundoplication. But, 4 of these 10 patients were completely asymptomatic until obstructive symptoms secondary to their adenocarcinoma appeared. There seems to be no clinically practicable means of early detection of degenerating Barrett's mucosa presently available for such asymptomatic patients.

Our patients with Barrett's mucosa and adenocarcinoma of the esophagus had less extensive disease when surgically treated than did patients without Barrett's mucosa, but their postoperative survival was shorter (Table 1).

To assist in early detection of degeneration of Barrett's mucosa among symptomatic (reflux) patients, we currently recommend endoscopic observation of the lesion every six months with biopsy of any suspicious (white dot) areas, and blind biopsy of a representative area of the Barrett's mucosa. The biopsies are graded for dysplasia, particularly seeking Barrett's mucosa in which dysplasia is progressive over time.

Table 1. Esophageal adenocarcinoma Barrett's mucosa

	No of Patients	Clinical Stage (AJCC) II	III	IV	Mean Survival (Mos.)
Barrett's	10	3	3	4	9,3
No Barrett's	27	1	11	15	16,9

The program has been functioning for six years: two patients with adenocarcinoma among 150 patients with Barrett's mucosa have been identified so far.

References

1. Spechler JS, Robbins AH, Rubins HB et al (1984) Adenocarcinoma and Barrett's esophagus: An overrated risk? Gastroenterol 87: 927–933
2. Sarr MG, Hamilton SR, Marrone GC, Cameron JL (1985) Barrett's esophagus: Its prevalence and association with adenocarcinoma in patients with symptoms of gastroesophageal reflux. Amer J Surg 185; 149: 187–193
3. Cameron AJ, Ott BJ, Payne WS (1985) The incidence of adenocarcinoma in columnar-lined (Barrett's) esophagus. N Engl J Med 313: 857–859
4. Soergel K personal communication
5. Mahoney JL, Condon RE (1987) Adenocarcinoma of the esophagus. Ann Surg 205: 557–562

J.-P. Favre, P. Rat, O. Haas, and *H. Viard* (Dijon)

Frequency of Barrett's esophagus malignant degeneration is difficult to determine because of the variety of patients referred to surgical unit. However, the most common frequency estimation is 10% degeneration risk.

1. If we consider that Barrett's esophagus is due to gastroesophageal reflux (GER), most commonly acid, is it possible to compare the importance and risk of Barrett's esophagus with age and the importance of such reflux?

Age of reflux does not seem to be of any value: no study says what reflux age is required to develop a Barrett's esophagus, or a cancer on Barrett's esophagus. Some Barrett's esophagus are acquired, some others may be congenital. Reflux quantity is difficult to appreciate. Clinically, Barrett's mucosa is less sensitive to GER, so clinical signs are of less value.

We studied 5 patients with adenocarcinoma developed on a Barrett's esophagus: 24 hour pHmetry was done using DeMeester criteria and Kaye score. All patients had a GER corresponding, at least, to esophagitis grade 2 or 3 (Kaye's Score between 120–230).

2. If we stop reflux, do we allow a regression of Barrett's esophagus and do we avoid malignant degeneration?

In patients with Barrett's esophagus, suppression of GER by medical treatment does not show any regression of Barrett's esophagus [2, 3, 8].

Surgical correction of GER leads to various regressions of Barrett's esophagus, but successful antireflux surgery does not suppress the risk of malignant degeneration. Some cases of cancer developed on Barrett's esophagus after successful antireflux surgery have been reported [4, 5, 6].

3. Do we have any possibility of treating Barrett's esophagus before malignant degeneration?

The one possibility is to prove the presence of a specialized mucosa (Columnar epithelium showing intestinal type metaplasia). Coloration of a specimen of cancer on Barrett's esophagus with orthotoluidin blue, a nucleus dye, shows dysplastic areas and microinvasive cancer [4]. This is not possible in vivo. So one possibility is to find dysplasia by multiple biopsies, or intestinal metaplasia. Multiple biopsies must be guided by dye spraying esophagoscopy with Lugol or Indigo carmin, as described by Savary and Naef [7]. Discovery of intestinal metaplasia could be helped by histochemical study, and the finding of a sulphated mucus in such mucosa. They could be considered a premalignant state [9].

The importance of GER is not a predictive factor of degeneration. Suppression of GER by medical treatment or surgery does not avoid degeneration. Biopsies guided by dye spraying allow the finding of dysplastic lesions that must be considered as degeneration. In lesions of intestinal metaplasia, the finding of sulphated mucus in the nucleus will show which mucosa is degenerated.

References

1. Brand DL, Ylvisaker JT, Gelfand M, Pope CE II (1980) Regression of columnar esophageal (Barrett's) epithelium after anti-reflux surgery. New Engl J Med 302: 844–846
2. Delpre G, Kadish U, Glanz I, Avidor L (1984) Prolonged cimetidine therapy in ulcerated Barrett's columnar-lined esophagus. Amer J Gastroent 79: 8–11
3. Everhart CW, Humphries TJ (1978) Medical treatment of Barrett's esophagus with betanechol. Report of three cases with prolonged follow-up. Gastroenterology 74: 1033–1035
4. Favre JP, Sala JJ, Haas O, Gouillat C, Viard H, Saubier EC Adenocarcinoma of lower esophagus and Barrett's esophagus. Sous presse Digestive Surgery
5. Hamilton SR, Hutcheon DF, Ravich WJ, Cameron JL, Paulson M (1984) Adenocarcinoma in Barrett's esophagus after elimination of gastroesophageal reflux. Gastroenterology 86: 356–359
6. Hölscher AH, Bader M, Siewert JR (1985) Kann Antireflux-chirurgie eine maligne Entartung des Endobrachyösophagus verhindern? Dtsch med Wschr 10: 551–555
7. Naef AP, Savary M, Ozzelo C (1975) Columnar-lined lower esophagus: an acquired lesion with malignant predisposition. Report on 140 cases of Barrett's esophagus with 12 adenocarcinomas. J Thorac Cardiosvasc Surg 70: 826–835
8. Patel GK, Clift SA, Schaefer RA, Read RC, Texter EC (1982) Resolution of severe dysplastic (Ca in situ) changes with regression of columnar epithelium (CE) in Barrett's esophagus (BE) on medical treatment. Gastroenterology 82: 1147–1150
9. Potet F, Peuchmaur M (1984) Etude histochimique des mucines dans l'endobrachyœsophage. Archives d'Anatomie et de Cytologie Pathologie 32: 59
10. Skinner DB, Walther BC, Riddell RH, Schmidt H, Iascone C, DeMeester TR (1985) Barrett's esophagus. Comparison of benign and malignant cases. Ann Surg 198: 554–566

Does the symptomatology of cancer differ when occurring in Barrett's esophagus?

M. B. Orringer (Ann Arbor)

In order to answer this question, the clinical characteristics of adenocarcinoma arising in Barrett's esophagus must be defined (Table 1). Patients with such adenocarcinoma generally have an average age of 61 years. Barrett's esophagus is predominantly a disease of white males, and I have been unable to find a single case report of esophageal adenocarcinoma in a black patient. This is a striking contrast to the predominance of black males among patients with squamous cell carcinoma of the esophagus. The male to female ratio in patients with adenocarcinoma in Barrett's esophagus is about 4–5 to 1.

Table 1. Adenocarcinoma in Barrett's esophagus. Clinical characteristics

Age: 60 yrs. (AVG)
Male: female ratio 4–5:1
Race: rare (if ever) in blacks
Hiatal Hernia: 50–70%
History of reflux symptoms: 65%
Epigastric pain: 59%
Cigarette smoking: 36–50%
Alcohol ingestion: 45%

All patients with Barrett's esophagus and cancer do not have a history of reflux symptoms. The reported incidence of heartburn is about 65%, with an average duration of 5 years, and that of regurgitation about 35%.

On careful questioning, however, many of these patients will recall having experienced reflux symptoms in the distant past, but then these symptoms seemed to resolve spontaneously. Clearly, the columnar-epithelial lined lower esophagus is frequently not as acid sensitive as normal squamous epithelium, and spontaneous remission of reflux symptoms may occur as the Barrett's esophagus develops. Epigastric pain is a symptom in 59% of our patients, and is often indicative of celiac plexus invasion by the tumor.

The relationship between cigarette smoking and carcinoma in Barrett's esophagus has been questioned. Skinner [4] has reported that 80% of his patients with carcinoma in Barrett's esophagus have a history of cigarette smoking compared to only 43% of those with Barrett's esophagus without carcinoma. Others reported incidence of cigarette smoking that ranges from 36–50%.

Forty-five percent of our patients with carcinoma in a Barrett's esophagus also had a history of regular alcohol ingestion. A hiatal hernia has been present in 50–70% of these patients.

By far the most common presenting symptom in 80–90% of patients with carcinoma in a Barrett's esophagus is dysphagia, due in about 70% to a tumor mass and in the remainder to a stricture. Basically, patients with carcinoma in Barrett's esophagus, when compared with those with typical squamous carcinoma, are more likely to be Caucasian and to have a history of reflux symptoms. The role of alcohol seems less prominent in patients with Barrett's carcinoma, and the contribution of cigarette smoking remains to be established.

References

1. Kalish RJ, Clancy PE, Orringer MB, Appelman HD (1984) Clinical epidemiologic, and morphologic comparison between adenocarcinomas arising in Barrett's esophageal mucosa and in gastric cardia. Gastroenterology 86: 461
2. Haggitt RC, Dean PJ (1985) Adenocarcinoma in Barrett's epithelium. Chapter 14 in Barrett's Esophagus – Pathophysiology, Diagnosis, and Management. Spechler SJ, Goyal RK (eds) Elsevier Science Publishing Co, New York, pp 153–165
3. Sjogren RW, Johnson LF (1983) Barrett's esophagus: A review. Am J Med 74: 313
4. Skinner DB, Walther BC, Riddell RH et al (1983) Barrett's esophagus: comparison of benign and malignant cases. Ann Surg 198: 554

How to differentiate cancers of the cardia from those occurring in Barrett's esophagus?

H. D. Appelman (Ann Arbor)

These two carcinomas may usually be separated by a combination of gross, microscopic and epidemiologic features. We define Barrett's carcinomas as adenocarcinomas arising within the esophagus in a field of Barrett's mucosa which, ideally, is dysplastic at the margin of the carcinoma. Similarly, cardiac carcinomas are adenocarcinomas arising within the most proximal stomach in cardiac mucosa which, ideally, is dysplastic at the margin of the carcinoma.

Adenocarcinoma occurring about the region of the cardioesophageal junction presumably all arise from either esophageal Barrett's mucosa superiorly or from gastric cardiac mucosa inferiorly. However, the definition of this junction is not clear-cut in many cases. The squamocolumnar junction is not always the same as the cardioesophageal junction because of two phenomena: first, in Barrett's mucosa, the squamocolumnar junction moves proximally, whereas the cardioesophageal junction remains in place. Second, in normal people, the cardiac mucosa may extend irregularly into the distal 2 cm of the esophagus. Thus, the definition of Barrett's mucosa must begin with columnar mucosa situated above this 2 cm point.

Gross

Assuming that we have the ability to determine the location of the true cardioesophageal junction, then the simplest distinction between Barrett's and cardiac

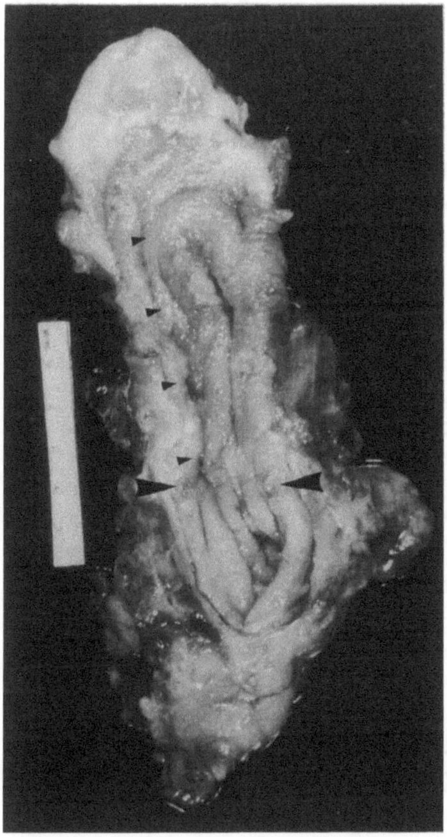

Fig. 1. This longitudinally oriented Barrett's carcinoma (small arrowheads) is totally above in the cardioesophageal junction (large arrow heads)

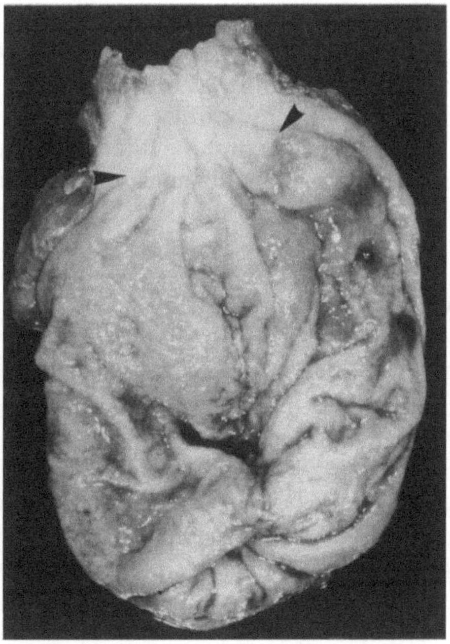

Fig. 2. The cardioesophageal junction (arrowheads) is above this nodular carcinoma of the gastric cardia, seen best below the arrowhead on the right

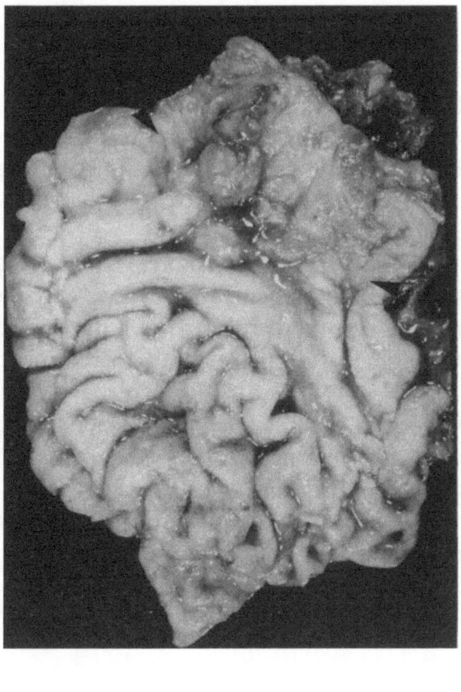

Fig. 3. The arrowheads identify the cardioesophageal junction. A nodular carcinoma is present both above and below the junction. Grossly, it is impossible to determine if this is a Barrett's or a cardiac carcinoma

carcinomas is by examination of the junction regions either endoscopically, radiologically, or in the resected specimen. Those carcinomas obviously above the junction are considered to be Barrett's, whereas those clearly below the junction must be considered cardiac.

The problem with this definition is that a number of carcinomas actually straddle and even obliterate the junction with roughly equal components above and below it so that determination of site of origin becomes impossible (Figs. 1, 2, 3).

Microscopic

To separe Barrett's from cardiac carcinomas microscopically, we look for changes designated either as *in situ* carcinoma or high grade dysplasia in the mucosa next to the carcinoma. It is presumably from such intramucosal abnormalities that the carcinomas arise. Fastidious sampling of the mucosa adjacent to these tumors often yields such intramucosal changes. The liklihood of detecting such changes may be proportional to the number of marginal microscopic samples analyzed. Actually, such dysplasias are more likely to be seen in Barrett's mucosae, because they can extend for considerable distances above the tumor.

The finding of *in situ* carcinoma or high-grade dysplasias in the mucosa next to cardiac carcinomas is more difficult because the cardiac mucosa itself tends to be quite limited. Presumably such changes were there at one time, but they were overgrown by the advancing tumor.

From a histologic standpoint these two adenocarcinomas are identical. They tend to be generally well differentiated lesions with papillary or tubular growth patterns.

Clinical and Epidemiologic

There is no difference in terms of age and sex distribution. Male predominance is most impressive for both neoplasms. Patients with Barrett's carcinomas are more likely to have hiatal hernias and long term symptoms attributable to gastroesophageal reflux. After all, that is the milieu in which Barrett's mucosa and Barrett's carcinomas evolve.

On the other hand, there is a suggestion in the data from the University of Michigan that patients with cardiac carcinomas are more likely to be heavy smokers and drinkers than are those with Barrett's carcinomas [1]. This background becomes increasingly impressive with increasing tobacco exposure. Much the same risk factors apply for cardiac adenocarcinoma as for squamous cell carcinoma of the esophagus. At the same time, in our series, almost half of the patients with Barrett's carcinoma had no alcohol or smoking history. It must be emphasized that not all studies confirm this data.

Whether or not it is important to distinguish between Barrett's and cardiac carcinomas is not clear. From the standpoint of extent of the carcinoma when detected and the results of treatment, there appears to be no difference.

Reference

1. Appelman HD, Kalish RJ, Clancy PE, Orringer MB (1985) Distinguishing features of adenocarcinoma in Barrett's esophagus and in the gastric cardia. Ch 15 in Barrett's Esophagus Pathophysiology, Diagnosis and Management, Spechler SJ, Goyal RK (eds) Elsevier, New York

May squamous cell carcinoma occur in Barrett's mucosa?

H. D. Appelman (Ann Arbor)

Barrett's mucosa can occasionally undergo regression with regrowth of squamous epithelium over the columnar epithelium. This then becomes a squamous metaplasia occurring in an area of columnar metaplasia.

There is no reason why squamous cell carcinomas might not occur in such a milieu, but this must be an extremely unusual circumstance. At the same time there is absolutely no reason to suspect that Barrett's mucosa is at high risk for the development of squamous cell carcinoma. Finally, there does not appear to be anything intrinsic about the development of Barrett's mucosa that protects the esophagus from developing squamous cell carcinoma. I don't know of any data which has studied the occurrence of Barrett's mucosa in patients with routine or more mundane forms of squamous cell carcinoma, but we might expect that this incidence would be comparable to that in the general population at large.

Malignant degeneration of benign lesions (3)

President: *David B. Skinner* (Chicago)

Free Commentators: *H. D. Appelman* (Ann Arbor)
G. Champault (Paris)
P. B. Desai (Bombay)
M. B. Orringer (Ann Arbor)
H. Sancho-Garnier (Villejuif)
J. R. Siewert (Munich)

The incidence of cancer in Barrett's esophagus vary according to series

M. Endo (Tokyo)

In the literature, the reported incidence of cancer in Barrett's esophagus varies from 0 to 46%: the higher figures probably reflect a selection bias in favour of carcinoma. The cancer prevalence of 8.1%–8.8% reported from four different institutions appears to be the best available estimate of the risk of adenocarcinoma in Barrett's esophagus (Table 1).

Table 1. Prevalence of adenocarcinoma in Barrett's esophagus [1]

Reference		Cases with Barrett's esophagus	Cases with carcinoma	Percent with carcinoma
Borrie and Goldwater	(1976)	45	0	0
Hawe et al.	(1973)	85	2	2,4
Messian et al.	(1978)	26	1	3,8
Bremner	(1982)	49	4	8,1
Naef et al.	(1975)	140	12	8,6
Menguy	(1979)	35	3	8,6
Ransom	(1982)	34	3	8,8
Radigan et al.	(1977)	19	5	26,3
Skinner et al.	(1983)	43	20	46,5
Total		476	50	10,5

We have had experience with more than 1300 patients in whom esophageal carcinoma had been resected; there were 52 cases (4%) of adenocarcinoma. Most of these were advanced cases in which it was impossible to determine satisfactorily the exact site of origin. However, in 12 cases this was possible. Barrett's esophagus was the site of origin in six cases of adenocarcinoma; five of these developed from the submucosal esophageal gland and the remaining one developed from the ectopic gastric mucosa. Concomitant dysplasia was observed in only one of the six patients, and was located in the middle esophagus.

A total of 17 cases (including ours) of adenocarcinoma in Barrett's esophagus in the Japanese literature were analyzed. Of these, 15 were located in the lower third of the esophagus, one was in the middle third and the remaining one was in the upper third. The size of the cancers was most frequently 4–6 cm.

As regards cancer depth, five were superficial cancers within the submucosa, in three cases the invasion had reached the muscle layers, in six cases the invasion had reached the adventitia and in three cases the extent of the cancer was unknown. Lymph node metastasis was observed in seven cases. There were metastases to secondary and tertiary groups of lymph nodes in all of these.

In Japan, Barrett's esophagus is uncommon. Since a complete follow-up did not take place it is not possible to draw conclusions here about the risk of adenocarcinoma in Barrett's esophagus.

Reference

1. Haggitt RC, Dean PJ (1985) Adenocarcinoma in Barrett's epithelium. In: Spechler JS, Goyal RK Eds. Barrett's Esophagus: Pathophysiology, Diagnosis and Management. Elsevier, New York

M. Ribet, E. Mensier, and *F. R. Pruvot* (Lille)

Adenocarcinoma in a Barrett's esophagus must be accurately described: to admit the tumor as being in the esophagus in at least 75% of its length and associated with a columnar mucosa above its upper limit, does not exclude cases of cancer of the cardia that can spread up into the esophagus. The following criteria must be observed:

1. a detailed description of resected esophagus and exact topography of the specimen;
2. an identification of esophageal mucosa with its characteristic glands;
3. the existence of a Barrett's esophagus next to and above the tumor;
4. the presence of pavimentous mucosa or of Barrett's esophagus between the tumor and gastric mucosa.

Material

Between 1970 and 1986 (Table 1), we operated 62 Barrett's esophagus on a total of 707 hiatal hernias (8.7%); the sex ratio was 6 males to 2 females; mean age was 50 years with extremes of 5 and 72 years. Mean duration of symptomatology had been 5.7 years before operation (extremes: 3 months and 25 years). Endoscopy showed esophagitis in 56 cases (1 stage 1, 18 stage 2, 37 stage 3), a stricture in 33 cases (30 at the border of pavimentous and columnar epitheliums, 1 in columnar epithelium, 2 with a double localization), an ulcer eroding the columnar mucosa in 7 cases.

During the same length of time, we operated 10 adenocarcinomas associated with a Barrett's esophagus, i.e. a prevalence of 10/12 (13.8%). The sex ratio was 4 males to 1 female; mean age was 56 years with extremes of 37 and 67 years. Mean preoperative duration of disease had been 12.5 years. In 5 cases we observed a decrease of heart burns and pain with development of dysphagia.

Table 1

	Barrett's esophagus (62)	Adenocarcinoma (10)	Comparisons
Mean age	50 years	56 years	N.S.
Sex ratio	5,88 M./1F.	4 M. / 1F.	N.S.
Reflux	87 p. cent	90 p. cent	N.S.
Mean duration	5,7 years	12 years	S.D. $p<0.001$
Dysphagia	60 p. cent	60 p. cent	N.S.
Loss of weight	16 p. cent	60 p. cent	S.D. $p<0.01$
Distance from dental arch	33,3 cm	32.2 cm	N.S.
Epithelium: intestine	14 p. cent	80 p. cent	S.D. $p<0.001$
cardia	40 p. cent	30 p. cent	N.S.
fundus	55 p. cent	50 p. cent	N.S.
Dysplasia	14,5 p. cent	50 p. cent	S.D. $p<0.01$

NS: non significant difference
SD: significant difference

Methods

We operated on Barrett's esophagus with an anti-reflux operation in 51 cases and a resection in 11 cases (3 wrong diagnosis of cancer, 4 narrow strictures, 2 relapses after a Thal's cardioplasty, 2 ulcers).

We did a resection for the 10 adenocarcinomas: 5 Lewis-Santy procedures, 1 Sweet operation, 1 coloplasty with Belsey's technique, 2 esogastrectomies with esojejunal anastomosis, and 1 closed esophageal resection with coloplasty.

Results

There was 1 death after antireflux surgery, by rupture of a peroperative esophagotomy for biopsy during acute post-operative dilatation of the stomach; 48 patients were followed up with 37 good results where endoscopy showed disappearance of 9 stage III esophagitis, and 3 stage II out of 4. Good results after antireflux surgery were present in 72.5% of cases.

There was 1 death after resection, due to colic transplant necrosis. Two patients died later from extraesophageal causes. Eight patients were followed up with 5 good clinical results.

Considering the entire surgery for Barrett's esophagus, the results were good in 42/62 patients (67.7%) with a mortality of 3.2%. Those results have been evaluated on an average of 4.72 years on 56 patients.

As for adenocarcinomas, there was 1 postoperative death from esophagobronchial fistula. Six patients are alive with a follow-up of 6 months to 5 years; 3 died from relapse (12 months, 18 months, 42 months).

Pathology specimens of the 10 tumors showed an intestinal type mucosa in 8 cases; there was severe surrounding dysplasia (grade 3) in 5 cases. Sulfomucins were shown to be present in 7 cases.

Discussion

Adenocarcinoma represents 4% of the malignant esophageal tumors (21/534 observed in 15 years).

On 62 Barrett's esophagus operated during the same period after a mean clinical evolution of 5.7 years, and 56 followed up after operation for a mean duration of 4.72 years, which adds up to a mean total time of clinical observation of more than 10 years, we observed one malignant transformation, i.e. an incidence of 1/274 patient-years or 1.72%. This proportion is opposed to a prevalence of 10/72, i.e. 13.8%. Indeed, in cases of associated cancer:

- only symptomatic Barrett's esophagus are concerned;
- chances of discovering an unknown Barrett's esophagus are increased with the presence of dysphagia, endoscopy, surgical resection or autopsy;
- cancers of the cardia are included in the series if the definitions are not strict.

Table 1 summarizes the characteristics of Barrett's esophagus and those of adenocarcinoma associated with Barrett's esophagus. Practically any reflux esophagitis should be efficiently corrected to avoid the production of a Barrett's esophagus. When this exists, we propose anti-reflux surgery in the absence of complications, when there is an easily dilatable stricture, when an ulcer is healed after 3 months of medical treatment, and when dysphagia decreases with medical treatment. In other cases we propose resection with coloplasty.

Does columnar epithelium regress after anti-reflux surgery? On 15 controlled cases we observed only 3 decreases of length and 1 disappearance of that epithelium: one must take into account anatomical modifications brought on by the operation. In all cases endoscopy should be repeated according to the same rules, with a planimetric scheme, to resolve the double problem of the possibility of Barrett's esophagus regression after anti-reflux surgery, and the possibility of a malignant transformation of the columnar epithelium after the disappearance of reflux.

Conclusion

Barrett's esophagus is secondary to reflux esophagitis in the majority of cases. It may degenerate. If the prevalence of malignancy is 13.8%, the incidence is 1 case for 274 patients/year (1.72%). A clinical duration of more than 10 years, a modification of symptoms, a loss of weight, the presence of intestinal epithelium, of sulfomucins and of dysplasia are alarming factors. Conservative entireflux surgery seems indicated for the majority of cases but its preventive effect on degeneration is not yet established. A prospective standardized and multicentric study on Barrett's esophagus pursued over several years will be the only way to define the risk and the best preventive treatment of malignancy.

J. R. Siewert (Munich)

I have some problems in understanding the data published in the last few years dealing with the incidence of carcinoma in the esophagus.

There are a great number of retrospective analyses which state an average of 14% incidence of carcinoma in the endobrachyesophagus (Fig. 1). On the other hand, there are 4 prospective trials stating the incidence of carcinoma in the endobrachyesophagus much lower (Table 1).

How can this contradiction be explained?

From our point of view the prospective studies on hand have the great disadvantage of mixing up retrospective analyses with prospective observations of the course.

As a rule, a collective of patients with endobrachyesophagus is compared retrospectively, the first step being to analyse how many patients have developed an adenocarcinoma till now, according to all authors. In the second phase, the patients

Table 1. Incidence of Adeno-Ca in Barrett's esophagus-Prospective Studies

Authors/year	n	meantime of follow-up	Adeno-Ca.	Incidence per patient years	risk in comparison to normal population
Spechler 1984	105	3,3 years	2	1/175	× 42
Sprung 1984	108	4,0 years	2	1/ 81	⁒
Cameron 1985	104	8,5 years	2	1/441	× 30
Savary 1987	402	3,8 years	5	1/305	⁒

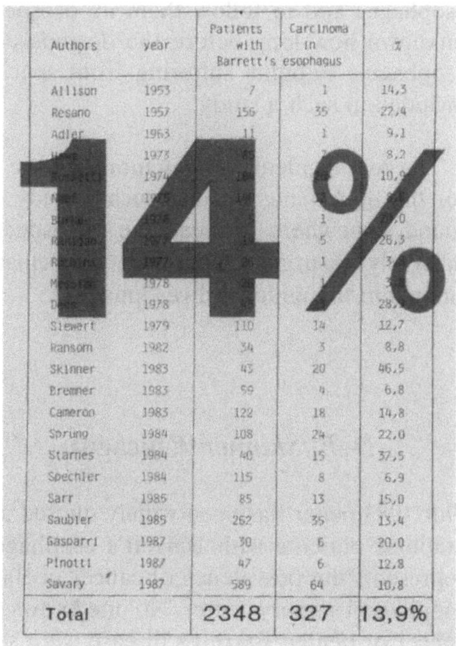

Authors	year	Patients with Barrett's esophagus	Carcinoma in Barrett's esophagus	%
Allison	1953	7	1	14,3
Resano	1957	156	35	22,4
Adler	1963	11	1	9,1
[illegible]	1973	[illegible]	[illegible]	8,2
[illegible]	1974	[illegible]	[illegible]	[illegible]
[illegible]	[illegible]	[illegible]	[illegible]	[illegible]
[illegible]	[illegible]	[illegible]	1	[illegible]
[illegible]	[illegible]	[illegible]	5	26,3
[illegible]	1977	[illegible]	1	[illegible]
[illegible]	1978	[illegible]	1	[illegible]
[illegible]	1978	[illegible]	[illegible]	[illegible]
Siewert	1979	110	14	12,7
Ransom	1982	34	3	8,8
Skinner	1983	43	20	46,5
Bremner	1983	59	4	6,8
Cameron	1983	122	18	14,8
Sprung	1984	108	24	22,0
Starnes	1984	40	15	37,5
Spechler	1984	115	8	6,9
Sarr	1985	85	13	15,0
Saubier	1985	262	35	13,4
Gasparri	1987	30	6	20,0
Pinotti	1987	47	6	12,8
Savary	1987	589	64	10,8
Total		2348	327	13,9%

Fig. 1. Prevalence of Adeno-Ca in Barrett's Esophagus

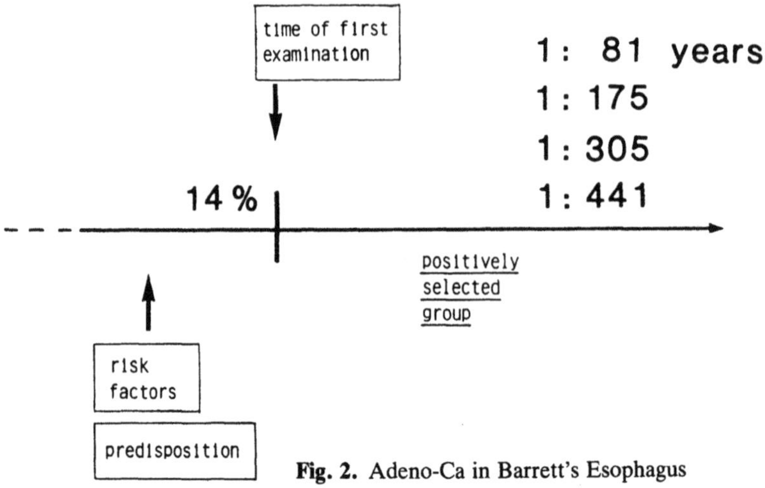

Fig. 2. Adeno-Ca in Barrett's Esophagus

with endobrachyesophagus but without carcinoma will be followed prospectively: this group of patients (Fig. 2) represents however a positively selected group, because most of the patients with typical risk factors have already developed a carcinoma at the time of registration. The continuous prospective observation of this selected patient group results, as expected, in the published low incidence rate of malignancy.

In other words, the prospectively found incidence rates are too low because the patients with risk factors concerning carcinoma have been eliminated. The right way would be to include all casually newly diagnosed patients with an endobrachyesophagus and to follow them up prospectively. In this case of course it remains unknown how long before the diagnosis the patient already had the endobrachyesophagus. Patients suffering from specific symptoms as dysphagia may not be included in such a study.

The real incidence of carcinoma in the endobrachyesophagus cannot be defined for the time being because such a study does not yet exist. Presumably it will be found somewhere between the retrospective and prospective data. Till then, we must rely on surgical experience. This clearly indicates a high incidence of adenocarcinoma in the endobrachyesophagus.

D. B. Skinner (Chicago)

Our 1983 paper has been widely quoted as showing a 47% incidence of carcinoma amongst patients with Barrett's esophagus [1]. This is clearly not accurate as it represents the prevalence of cancer in Barrett's patients referred specifically to an esophageal surgery center. No one knows the pool of patients from which those with cancer or benign Barrett's disease were selected.

In more recent years, the numbers of patients with benign Barrett's epithelium as well as malignant Barrett's epithelium referred to our center have increased. The prevalence of carcinoma is now 35 out of 104 patients with Barrett's esophagus seen between 1974 and July 1986. Risk factors remain unknown but it is a disease of white males.

Several centers have attempted to arrive at an estimate of the incidence of cancer developing among patients with a prior diagnosis of Barrett's epithelium. In other series the estimated incidence of carcinoma developing in a patient with known Barrett's epithelium is stated to be between 1 in 175 to 1 in 400 patient years of follow-up [2, 3].

In a recent survey of a personal series of 45 patients with benign Barrett's epithelium followed for 1 to 10 years (mean and median 3 years), three patients developed adenocarcinoma in a total of 145 patient years of follow-up for an incidence of 1 per 48 years. One of these patients had the diagnosis of Barrett's esophagus made prior to subsequent referral to us for treatment of high-grade dysplasia and early carcinoma. Even if this case is excluded and only those patients in whom we made the primary diagnosis of Barrett's epithelium and undertook the initial therapy, the incidence is still approximately 1 carcinoma in 72 patient years of follow-up.

There is no significant difference amongst these several studies, and all of them point out that this condition is the highest known risk for developing malignancy of any acquired condition of the digestive tract.

Lifetime surveillance seems clearly indicated. Our experience with brush cytologies indicates that this is an effective and inexpensive means of performing the surveillance program.

References

1. Skinner DB, Walther BC, Riddell RH, Schmidt H, Iascone C, DeMeester TR (1983) Barrett's esophagus: comparison of benign and malignant cases. Ann Surg 198:554–565
2. Spechler SJ (1985) The risk of cancer in Barrett's esophagus. In Barrett's Esophagus: Pathophysiology, Diagnosis, and Management. SJ Spechler, RK Goyal (eds) New York: Elsevier
3. Cameron AJ, Ott BJ, Payne WS (1983) Barrett esophagus: incidence of adenocarcinoma during long-term follow up. Gut 24: A1007–1008

Is their prevalence in patients with Barrett's esophagus overestimated?

J. B. Ollyo, M. Savary, Ph. Monnier, J. Wellinger, J. J. Gonvers, and *Ch. Fontolliet* (Lausanne)

The prevalence of adenocarcinoma in patients with Barrett's esophagus ranges from 7% to 40% in patients undergoing endoscopy (Table 1) [2], and from 37% up to 85% in patients undergoing surgery [9, 12, 13].

Table 1. Prevalence and incidence of adenocarcinoma in endobrachyesophagus (A/EBE)

	Cameron (1)	Sampliner (6)	Spechler (10)	Sprung (11)	Savary (*)
Number of patients	122	52	115	108	318
Prevalence of A/EBE	15%	?	7%	22%	11%
Number of patients without cancer followed up	104	25	105	41	264
Mean follow-up** (ranges)	8.5 (3->15)	2.1 (0.4–6.6)	3.3 (0.1–20)	4.0 (1–11)	4.8 (0.1–22.5)
Developed A/EBE	2	1	2	2	5
Interval before appearance**	6 and 10	?	5.3 and 8.0	3.5 and 4.3	2.5 and 15.5
Incidence of A/EBE (cases/persons/years)	1/441	1/92	1/175	1/81	1/253

* Unpublished data (*CHUV, Lausanne*, Switzerland, 01. 01. 1963–31. 12. 1986)
** years

The majority of patients with Barrett's esophagus without carcinoma are treated medically, either because of the absence of complications such as stenosis or ulcer, or because they are too great an operative risk [5, 7]. The prevalence of adenocarcinoma complicating Barrett's esophagus is therefore clearly overestimated in surgical series because of the initial selection of cases [9]. Many cases without carcinoma do not come to surgery.

The prevalence of adenocarcinoma may also be overestimated in the medical series due to the following reasons:

1. Columnar epithelium of the lower esophagus may be very easily missed, even by an experienced endoscopist, especially if biopsies are not routinely performed [8]. On the other hand an adenocarcinoma, even in the early stages, will not usually be missed by the endoscopist.
2. A given case may or may not be diagnosed as Barrett's esophagus because of very different definitions of the disease. Some authors will only diagnose Barrett's esophagus if the columnar epithelium is circumferential and measures at least 3 cm [9] or even 5 cm [3] in length. Others will diagnose Barrett's in the presence of any columnar epithelium in the esophagus of less than 3 cm in length and whether circumferential or not [4].
3. Patients with Barrett's esophagus may be asymptomatic and are therefore not endoscoped. In contrast, patients with adenocarcinoma become symptomatic and are usually all endoscoped [9]

In conclusion, the prevalence of adenocarcinoma in patient's with Barrett's esophagus is most probably overestimated in the majority of the reported endoscopic and surgical series.

References

1. Cameron AJ, Ott BJ, Payne WS (1985) The incidence of adenocarcinoma in columnar-lined (Barrett's) esophagus. N Engl J Med 313: 857–859
2. Dees J, van Blankenstein M, Frenkel M (1978) Adenocarcinoma in Barrett's esophagus: a report of 13 cases. Gastroenterology 1978; 74: 1119
3. Henrion J, Heller F (1983) Endobrachyoesophage (Oesophage de Barrett). Etude clinique et endoscopique de 22 cas. Acta Gastro-Enterol Belg 46: 207–219
4. Herlihy KJ, Orlando RC, Bryston JC et al (1984) Barrett's esophagus: clinical, endoscopic, histologic, manometric and electrical potential difference characteristics. Gastroenterology 86: 436–443
5. Ollyo JB, Savary M, Gonvers JJ, Levi F (1985) L'endobrachy-oesophage: Etude rétrospective de 258 cas. Schweiz Med Wschr 115: 996–997
6. Sampliner RE, Kogan FJ, Morgan TR et al (1986) Progression-regression of Barrett's esophagus. Gastroenterology 88: 1567
7. Savary M, Ollyo JB L'esophagite par reflux et ses complications: ulcère, sténose, endobrachy-oesophage. Encycl Med Chir (Paris, France) ORL 20822 A 10, 10–1986 (16 p)
8. Sarr MG, Hamilton SR, Marrone GC, Cameron JL (1985) Barrett's esophagus: Its prevalence and association with adenocarcinoma in patients with symptoms of gastroesophageal reflux. Am J Surg 149: 187–193
9. Skinner DB, Walther BC, Riddell RH et al (1983) Barrett's esophagus. Comparison of benign and malignant cases. Ann Surg 198: 554–566
10. Spechler SJ, Robbins AH, Rubins HB et al (1984) Adenocarcinoma and Barrett's esophagus. An overrated risk? Gastroenterology 87: 927–933
11. Sprung DJ (1984) Incidence of adenocarcinoma in Barrett's esophagus. Am J Gastroenterol 79: 817
12. Starnes VA, Adkins RB, Ballinger JF et al (1984) Barrett's esophagus. A surgical entity. Arch Surg 119: 563–567
13. West AB, Sheahan DG, Stephens RB, Hennessy TP (1982) Barrett's mucosa: incidence and association with primary oesophageal adenocarcinoma in surgical patients with oesophageal symptoms. Brit J Surg 69: 281.

S. J. Spechler (Boston)

Reported prevalence rates for esophageal adenocarcinoma in series of patients with Barrett's esophagus range from 0% to almost 50%, with a mean rate of approximately 10%. These reports describe primarily the frequency with which cancer and Barrett's epithelium are discovered simultaneously, not the rate with which adenocarcinoma develops in cancer-free patients. Therefore, it is not appropriate to conclude on the basis of these data that 10% of all patients with Barrett's esophagus will develop an esophageal malignancy. Such an extrapolation of prevalence data is likely to exaggerate the risk of cancer development. That risk is better estimated using incidence, rather than prevalence, data.

Only a few reports provide data on the incidence of adenocarcinoma in Barrett's esophagus. Based on those reports, it appears that cancer develops in these patients at the rate of approximately 500 cases per 100.000 patients per year. This incidence rate is some 30 to 40-fold higher than that for esophageal cancer in the general population of the United States. Cancer of the esophagus is an uncommon malignancy in the general population of the United States, however; when that low incidence rate is increased by a factor of 30 to 40, the resulting rate (500:100.000) still represents a small risk for the *individual* patient with Barrett's esophagus. Clinicians who treat these patients need a method for gauging the importance of that risk. One method is to compare the incidence of cancer in patients with Barrett's esophagus with that of a common malignancy in the general population: Lung cancer is the most common malignancy in the general population of the United States. Based on data from the Surveillance, Epidemiology, and End Results (SEER) program of the National Cancer Institute, incidence rates for cancer of the lung in older white American males during 1983 were:

Ages	*Incidence of Lung Cancer*
55–64	227:100.000
65–74	459:100.000
75+	539:100.000

Most series of patients with Barrett's esophagus are comprised of older white males. Thus, the incidence of esophageal cancer in Barrett's esophagus (500:100.000) is similar to the incidence of lung cancer in men of the same age group in the general population of the United States.

Cancer of the esophagus is a disease that exhibits dramatic geographic variations in its incidence rate. For example, that rate is so high in some areas of China that the government has sponsored mass esophageal cancer screening programs. One such area is Linxian County of Henan Province where the incidence rate for cancer of the esophagus in men is approximately 160:100.000. Thus, the incidence of cancer for patients with Barrett's esophagus is greater than that for residents of this high-risk area of China.

Based on the above comparisons, the risk of cancer in Barrett's esophagus is formidable, although smaller than that suggested by many earlier prevalence studies. Appropriate management of these patients requires that their risk of cancer development be neither overestimated nor underestimated.

How can the risk of degeneration be distinguished from the associated epidemiologic risk?

M. Crespi, and *N. Muñoz* (Rome and Lyons)

From all the research performed in high incidence areas for esophageal cancer no specific risk factors seem to be associated with the main one: to be born and grow up in a high incidence area. Well known risk factors for such neoplasia, like smoking and drinking, are of negligible importance in such areas.

Table 1. Vitamin levels at initial investigation

	Placebo		Vitamins	
	Male	Female	Male	Female
No	146	156	153	150
Retinol (μg/l)	418·8±108·3	334·4±94·6	421·8±109·5	336·3±105·6
Retinol ≥400 μg/l	74 *(50·7%)*	35 *(22·4%)*	84 *(54·9%)*	29 *(19·3%)*
β-carotene (μg/l)	128·6±69·6	195·6±104·5	129·6±66·1	178·7±86·7
β-carotene ≥200 μg/l	*24 (16·4%)*	65 *(41·7%)*	19 *(12·4%)*	51 *(34·0%)*
No.	138	153	146	147
RAC*	1·60±0·23	1·63±0·26	1·60±0·25	1·62±0·28
RAC ≤1·3	9 *(6·5%)*	14 *(9·2%)*	16 *(11·0%)*	17 *(11·6%)*

* Riboflavine Activation Coefficient

An interesting finding was the high prevalence of riboflavin deficiency in those populations (around 90% of subjects) and that of retinol, as established by the basal results in a group of 610 subjects later randomized for a double blind intervention study (Table 1).

In that group no difference in the prevalence of esophageal lesions were encountered after a 13.5 months vitamin supplementation [1] except, perhaps, a slightly lesser prevalence of the lesions in those with higher levels of retinol [2].

References

1. Muñoz N et al (1985) No effect of Riboflavine, Retinol and Zinc on prevalence of precancerous lesions of esophagus. Lancet II: 111–114
2. Wahrendorf J et al: Precancerous lesions of esophagus: logistic regression analysis of data from an intervention trial in the People's Republic of China – Cancer Research, in press

Must scleroderma, a factor of Barrett's esophagus, be considered as a precancerous lesion?

M. B. Orringer (Ann Arbor)

Scleroderma is a disease of unknown etiology characterized by induration of the skin, fibrous replacement of smooth muscle of internal organs, and progressive loss of visceral and cutaneous function.

Table 1. Scleroderma esophageal involvement

Fibrinoid degeneration of smooth muscle
Loss of progressive peristalsis
Loss of HPZ tone
Gastroesophageal reflux
Reflux esophagitis

Disruption of normal esophageal peristalsis is so common in scleroderma that it is regarded as a major diagnostic sign of the disease: with progressive fibrosis of esophageal smooth muscle, the distal esophageal high pressure zone (HPZ) loses its tone and normal response to swallowing. The resultant gastroesophageal reflux [3], coupled with impaired ability of the atonic lower esophagus to clear refluxed gastric contence back into the stomach, sets the stage for accelerated reflux esophagitis.

Typical symptoms of gastroesophageal reflux are experienced by approximately 75–95% of patients with scleroderma. Similarly, the standard acid reflux test using an intraesophageal pH electrode demonstrates abnormal gastroesophageal reflux in more that 70% of patients. At autopsy, at least 40% of patients with scleroderma, have been found to have reflux esophagitis, (Table 1).

Because of the relationship between severe reflux esophagitis and the subsequent development of Barrett's mucosa, it has been suggested that scleroderma, which predisposes to gastroesophageal reflux, is a potentially pre-malignant condition: in the English medical literature in the past 25 years (through 1985), only 13 patients with scleroderma and esophageal carcinoma have been reported (Table 2). Only four had adenocarcinoma, seven had squamous cell carcinoma, one an adenoacanthoma, and one an undifferentiated carcinoma. Of the four reported esophageal adenocarcinomas associated with scleroderma, two were definitely associated with Barrett's epithelium.

Medsger and Masi [2] reported 18 malignant neoplasms of various types in 504 men with scleroderma. There were *no* esophageal carcinomas. Duncan and Winkelmann [1] reported 87 malignancies in 2141 patients with scleroderma. Gastrointestinal malignancies were no more common in the scleroderma patients than the nationwide average in America. Only one of the 2141 patients developed esophageal carcinoma. Segel and associates [4] carefully reviewed the medical records of 680 patients with scleroderma followed over a ten year period. Only one case of undifferentiated esophageal carcinoma was found, an incidence well within the expected range for the normal population.

Table 2. Scleroderma and esophageal carcinoma

13	reported cases
4	adenocarcinoma (2 Barrett's)
7	squamous cell
1	adenoacanthoma
1	undifferentiated

The incidence of Barrett's esophagus in scleroderma is simply unknown, but it is reasonable to expect that with the high incidence of reflux esophagitis in these patients, Barrett's epithelium may be a common finding. It appears from available data that esophageal carcinoma is *rare* in this patient population. It is possible, however, that the small number of reported cases may reflect either under reporting or be a function of reduced survival and limited follow-up in these patients.

From the available data, however, there is no justification for increased surveillance of the patient with scleroderma for Barrett's mucosa and esophageal adenocarcinoma: such surveillance is neither warranted nor cost effective. There is no objective evidence that either the incidence of Barrett's mucosa or of esophageal adenocarcinoma is increased in the patient with scleroderma.

References

1. Duncan SC, Winkelmann RK (1979) Cancer and scleroderma. Arch Dermatol 115: 950
2. Medsger TA Jr, Masi AT (1978) The epidemiology of systemic sclerosis (scleroderma) among male US veterans. J Chron Dis 31: 73
3. Orringer MB, Dabich L, Zarafonetis CJD, Sloan H (1976) Gastroesophageal reflux in esophageal scleroderma, diagnosis and implications. Ann Thorac Surg 22: 120
4. Segel MC, Campbell WL, Medsger TA Jr, Roumm AD (1985) Systemic sclerosis (Scleroderma) and esophageal adenocarcinoma: is increased patient screening necessary? Gastroenterology 89: 485

Does aperistalsis, in certain cases, lead to abandon a Nissen type procedure on behalf of a direct resection?

J. W. Maher (Iowa City)

Esophagitis in patients with aperistalsis, most commonly scleroderma or achalasia following myotomy, is a perplexing problem. These patients have defects in both major components of the body's defense mechanism against gastroesophageal reflux, i.e. the lower esophageal sphincter is unable to prevent gastroesophageal reflux, and aperistalsis renders the esophagus incapable of clearing gastroesophageal reflux in an efficient manner. This produces a particularly severe form of reflux that often results in transmural esophageal strictures. Fundoplication prevents reflux by augmenting lower esophageal sphincter pressure; however, this increase in sphincter pressure works both ways; reflux is prevented, but there is also an increase in resistance to the antegrade passage of food. This is no problem in patients with normal peristalsis, since this slight increase in resistance may be easily overcome. These unfortunate patients with aperistalsis, however, have only the hydrostatic pressure of the column of fluid in the esophagus to promote emptying.

Table 1. Thal-Nissen poor results

Early Recurrence	1 Patient	(1-achalasia following Heller)
Late Recurrence	3 Patients	(1-scleroderma (2 years)) (1-achalasia (6 years)) (1-DES (11 years))

Table 2. Current preference

	Primary Treatment	*Recurrence*
Achalasja	Heller Myotomy	Resection with cervical esophagogastrostomy of visceral interposition
Scleroderma	Medical	Resection with interposition

Many have tried making a floppy short wrap in these patients to minimize this problem; however, the long-term effects of this strategy are unknown at present.

As with many other endeavors, the author and his colleagues have learned more from their failures than their successes. On examination of patients undergoing Thal-Nissen procedures (Table 1), and intrathoracic fundoplications, it became evident that nearly all poor results had been obtained in patients with aperistalsis: three of these patients had originally been considered to have good results; however, over periods ranging from two to eleven years they developed esophageal obstruction from the wrap and ultimately required resection with either colon interposition, jejunal interposition, or esophagogastrectomy. It is the author's personal opinion that the former two are preferable to the latter because of the risk of recurrent esophagitis in the long term. If stomach is chosen for the reconstruction, the anastomosis should be done in the neck to try and minimize reflux.

We would now choose resection with visceral interposition for patients with aperistalsis who require surgical intervention (Table 2).

Does the presence of an associated stenosis modify the principle of the operation proposed?

A. Watson (Lancaster)

Whilst the precise incidence of associated stenosis in Barrett's esophagus is unclear, it is known that approximately 75% of all high strictures are associated with columnarisation [1, 2] and tend to occur at the squamo-columnar junction. The observation that strictures frequently occur in the most florid refluxers with predominantly supine reflux [3], in the presence of motility disorders [4] and in the presence of alkaline reflux [5] emphasize the need for careful pre-treatment evaluation, the results of which may modify the management policy.

Endoscopy, biopsy and cytology are necessary to exclude malignancy and to assess the degree of dysplasia, esophageal shortening and dilatability of the stricture. Manometry is essential to assess motility disturbances and exclude primary motility problems, e.g. scleroderma. Simultaneous intra-esophageal and intra-gastric 24 hour pH monitoring should be performed to quantify the degree and pattern of acid exposure, and to assess the relative contribution of acid and alkaline refluxate.

A careful general assessment for operative risk factors is important, as approximately half the patients with reflux stricture will be over 70 [6], and many will be unsuitable for surgical treatment and best managed by intermittent dilatation and anti-reflux medication. A controlled trial on our Unit has shown, however, that medical reflux control is less effective than anti-reflux surgery in reducing dilatation requirements [7].

In those patients suitable for surgery, since 95% of strictures are dilatable [8, 9], the preferred management is dilatation, anti-reflux surgery and regular surveillance, which will give good results in approximately 75 to 80% of patients [10, 11] (Table 1). We, in common with Belsey, Hill and Pearson, prefer a partial fundo-plication procedure, in view of the frequency of impaired motility in these patients. We have used a procedure based on a long intra-abdominal segment and restoration of the flap valve mechanism, which requires only a 120° fundo-plication to restore LES characteristics close to physiological levels, and allows total LES relaxation on swallowing [12].

Others, such as Orringer, and Ellis prefer a total fundo-plication procedure, although the results may be less satisfactory, with a higher incidence of residual dysphagia [13].

Table 1. Results of anti-reflux surgery and dilatation

No residual dysphagia in 79% (Hill, 1970)
Mean stricture diameter increased from 6.3 mm to 13.0 mm (Larrain, Csendes and Pope, 1975) [16]
No further dilatations required in 75% (Watson, 1985)

Modification of the usual technique for anti-reflux surgery is indicated in the presence of significant esophageal shortening, when either a trans-thoracic approach or a lengthening procedure such as a Collis gastroplasty or Thal patch are necessary, and where there is significant alkaline reflux, when a Roux-en-Y biliary diversion procedure should be added [5].

A more radical approach involving resection is indicated when the stricture is undilatable, when significant dysplasia exists and when grossly disordered motility e.g. scleroderma precludes an adequate functional result. In these circumstances, colon interposition gives the best functional result and can be achieved with a low mortality [14, 15].

References

1. Hill LD, Gelfand M, Bauermeister D (1970) Simplified management of reflux esophagitis with stricture. Ann Surg 172: 638–646
2. Siewert R (1980) Surgical therapy of peptic stenoses. In: Stipa S, Belsey RHR, Moraldi A eds. Medical and surgical problems of the esophagus. New York Academic Press 146–154
3. DeMeester TR (1980) Management of benign esophageal strictures. In: Stipa S, Belsey RHR, Moraldi A eds. Medical and surgical problems of the esophagus. New York Academic Press 173–176
4. Henderson RD (1983) Management of the patient with benign esophageal stricture. Surg Clin North Am: 63: 885–903
5. Bremner CG (1982) Benign strictures of the esophagus. Curr Probl Surg 19: 406–89
6. Watson A (1984) The role of anti-reflux surgery combined with fibreoptic endoscopic dilatation in peptic esophageal stricture. Am J Surg 148: 346–349
7. Watson A (1985) Randomized study comparing medical and surgical reflux control in the management of peptic esophageal stricture treated by intermittent dilatation. Gut 26: 553–554
8. Orringer MB (1980) Surgical treatment of esophageal strictures resulting from gastro-esophageal reflux. In: Stipa S, Belsey RHR, Moraldi A eds. Medical and surgical problems of the esophagus. New York Academic Press: 165–169
9. Watson A (1985) Dilatation of benign esophageal strictures. Br. J Surg 72: 153–154
10. Russel CO, Hill LD (1983) Gastro-oesophageal reflux. Curr Probl Surg 20: 209–277
11. Watson A (1987) Reflux stricture of the oesophagus. Br J Surg 74: In press
12. Watson A (1975) Lower oesophageal sphincter characteristics after a simplified anti-reflux procedure. Br J Surg 72: 1028
13. Ellis FH, Garabedion M, Gibb SP (1973) Fundoplication for gastro-oesophageal reflux. Arch Surg 107: 186–192
14. Belsey RHR (1980) Esophageal reconstruction with colon for benign disease. In: Stipa S, Belsey RHR, Moraldi A eds. Medical and Surgical problems of the esophagus. New York Academic Press 195–200
15. Skinner DB (1980) Functional effects of colon interposition in reconstruction of the esophagus. In Stipa S, Belsey RHR, Moraldi A eds. Medical and Surgical problems of the esophagus. New York Academic Press 193–194
16. Larrain A, Csendes A, Pope CE (1975) Surgical correction of reflux and effective therapy of esophageal strictures. Gastroenterology 69: 578–583

Is it logical to treat a Barrett's type lesion by a simple antireflux operation?

R. Belsey (Chicago)

What type of Barrett's lesion? What type of "simple" antireflux operation?

The consensus of surgical opinion now supports the contention of Savary and Monnier that there are two etiological factors responsible for the development of the columnar lined esophagus.

In Type 1 where the mucosal junction is regular in outline and situated in the region of the aortic arch, an anomaly in the development of the primitive foregut may be responsible. The lesion is frequently encountered in children and adults who present no history suggestive of prior esophagitis. The indications for antireflux surgery in this type are:

1. Peptic esophagitis proximal to the mucosal junction, resistent to medical treatment, and frequently complicated by a dilatable stricture.
2. "Early", superficial Barretts ulcers in the columnar lined segment. A debatable indication.
3. Recurring aspiration pneumonitis.
4. "Minor degrees" of dysplasia may warrent a "speculative" antireflux procedure and periodic biopsy examination to detect any possible changes in the severity of the dysplasia. Also a debatable indication, as no two pathologists will agree on the criteria for diagnosing dysplasia.

In cases where the dominant symptoms are of recurring aspiration pneumonitis, and the cell population in the columnar lined segment suggests no peptic activity, a "speculative" antireflux procedure is justified, assuming control of the reflux can be guaranteed. Failure to control the pneumonitis may indicate resection and reconstruction of the Barrett's segment, in view of the crippling sequelae of continuing aspiration.

There are contraindications to antireflux surgery:

1. Asymptomatic, uncomplicated, Barrett's anomaly observed as an incidental finding on routine esophagoscopy performed on other indications, in spite of the incompetence of the cardia normally present in most cases of the Barrett's anomaly, irrespective of type.
2. Chronic, deep, penetrating "Barrett's ulcers" are unlikely to respond. Malignancy cannot be eliminated with confidence on endoscopie biopsy alone. The risks of perforation or severe hemorrhage can be prevented only by resection.
3. Undilatable peptic strictures above the musocal junction.
4. Severe, indisputable, degrees of dysplasia. There is scant evidence that this premalignant condition can be reversed by control of the reflux alone, even when successful on pH testing.
5. Adenocarcinoma.

*

In the Type 2 Barrett's anomaly, an obvious response to chronic peptic esophagitis, antireflux surgery is indicated irrespective of symptomatology and assuming medical treatment has failed, to limit further extension of the columnar epithelialisation and hopefully prevent later complications.

The contraindications are similar to those already enumerated in discussing the management of the Type 1 lesion.

The problem of malignant degeneration and its possible prevention persist as a major cause of anxiety. Currently there is no recorded evidence on which of the two types is more prone to adenocarcinomatosis, nor on the true incidence in view of the varying criteria for the designation of a Barrett's esophagus: opinions vary between a 3 cm and 7 cm upward extension of the columnar mucosa. Chronic esophagitis is regularly complicated by some degree of acquired shortening which can confuse the relationship of the irregular mucosal junction to the anatomical esophagogastric junction. In the Type 1 lesion, the relationship of a tumour to the abnormal mucosa is relatively easy to determine. In the Type 2 lesion, the upward extension of a coincidental gastric carcinoma cannot be excluded with certainty. The problem is of more than academic interest: if in fact the Type 2 lesion is prone to malignant degeneration, the claim may be advanced that every case of reflux, irrespective of symptomatology, should be treated surgically "to prevent a subsequent malignancy". The current spate of failed antireflux surgery would undoubtedly be aggravated were this philosophy to be universally adopted.

*

The logical answer to the opening question must therefore be a qualified "no". Were Barrett with us today the ongoing discussion on the definition and etiology of Barrett's esophagus, sometimes emotional rather than rational would have appealed to his sardonic sense of humour. Barrett believed wholeheartedly in the developmental theory of etiology for the anomaly he initially described. The possibly acquired Type 2 lesion was not recognized by Barrett, and this may be yet another situation where the use of eponymous terminology has led to unnecessary confusion. Barrett's interest was stimulated by the study of the chronic penetrating Barrett's ulcer and peptic stricture rather than the incidence of adenocarcinoma.

What should be the approach to surveillance of these patients?

C. A. Hiebert (Portland)

Any plan or surveillance, especially expensive surveillance, must take into account the incidence of malignant degeneration of Barrett's epithelium and the probability that early identification of such change can favorably affect the outcome.

While published *prevalence* rates show adenocarcinoma in approximately 10% of patients with Barrett's esophagus [1], this is not at all the same thing as saying 10% of patients with Barrett's esophagus will develop cancer. Indeed cancer is the trigger for tests leading to a discovery of the Barrett's epithelium in many of these patients. We must look rather to the *incidence* of cancer in a population of patients with esophagi lined with columnar epithelium to ascertain what surveillance is meaningful.

The *incidence* of malignant degeneration is of the order of magnitude of one cancer in several hundred patient years. In the Mayo Clinic series [2], (with a mean surveillance period of 8.5 years) only two individuals developed cancer during 441 patient years. Overall survival for patients with Barrett's was as good as for the general population. The experience of the Boston VA Center was similar with one cancer case in 175 patient years [3]. Survival was not improved by early discovery.

Hence, when one weighs the risks and costs of esophagoscopy plus the anxiety imposed on these patients, it would appear that surveillance should be determined by the patient's reflux symptoms and not out of concern for detection of early cancer. The sole exception is the patient whose original biopsies show low-grade dysplasia where a trial of antireflux treatment should be followed up in three to six months by repeat endoscopy and biopsy.

References

1. Spechler SJ, Stuart JS, Raj KG (1986) Barrett's esophagus N Engl J Med 315: 362–371
2. Cameron AJ, Ott BJ, Payne WS (1985) The Incidence of adenocarcinoma in columnar-lined (Barrett's) Esophagus. N J Med 313: 857–859
3. Spechler SJ, et al (1984) Adenocarcinoma and Barrett's Esophagus: an overrated risk? Gastroenterology 87: 924–933

E. Reboud (Marseilles)

Observations

In our personal experience we have encountered a total of 90 cases of columnar epithelium lined esophagus, or Barrett's esophagus. This study includes 56 of these 90 patients. These 56 patients underwent:
- endoscopy;
- 24 h pH monitoring;
- biopsy or histologic study of surgical specimens;
- detection of sulfomucins.

Out of these 56 patients, 36 had only Barrett's esophagus and 20 had Barrett's esophagus associated with a tumor.

1. Histologic Type of Barrett's Esophagus

In the 36 cases of Barrett's Esophagus without carcinoma (endoscopic biopsy) 27 patients, i.e. 75%, exhibited specialized metaplasia associated with patches of fundic or junctional metaplasia in 14.

In the 20 cases of Barrett's Esophagus with carcinoma (histologic study of surgical specimens), 17 patients, i.e. 85%, displayed specialized metaplasia associated with fundic or junctional metaplasia in 14.

2. Dysplasia

Dysplasia was observed in 14 of the 20 cases of Barrett's Esophagus with tumor, i.e. 70% of cases. It was severe in 7.

Dysplasia was observed in 8 of the 36 cases of Barrett's Esophagus without tumor, i.e. 22%. It was mild in 5 cases, moderate in 2 and severe in 1. In the non malignant group, mild dysplasia disappeared within in 3 months after antireflux surgery in 2 out of 5 of the cases and in 1 case it disappeared later after adjunction of drug therapy. Surgery has not yet been performed in the remaining two cases. In the moderate group, dysplasia disappeared 3 months after surgery in 1 case and persisted after failure of surgery in 1 case.

3. Sulfomucins

Sulfomucin detection is an applicable study only in cases involving specialized metaplasia. Out of the 20 cases of Barrett's Esophagus with carcinoma. 17 had specialized metaplasia and sulfomucin secretion was detected in 14 i.e. 82%. Out of the 36 cases of Barrett's Esophagus without carcinoma, 27 had specialized metaplasia and sulfomucin secretion was detected in 12, i.e. 44%.

4. Follow-up of Barrett's Esophagus after Anti-Reflux Surgery

Follow-up is longer than 1 year in 13 of the 26 patients who underwent surgery. In 3 of these cases grade 3 Barrett's Esophagus regressed to grade 2 and in 1 grade 2 regressed to grade 1. In the remaining 9 cases surgery lead to no change in the grade of Barrett's Esophagus. Follow-up after antireflux surgery is too short to allow assessment in the 13 other cases. It should be stated that one patient who was contraindicated for surgery and received only drug treatment went from grade 1 to grade 3 Barrett's Esophagus.

Proposed Guidelines

1. Barrett's Esophagus with dysplasia

When Barrett's esophagus is accompanied by mild or moderate dysplasia, multiple biopsies are necessary to rule out the presence of patches of severe dysplasia or in situ carcinoma. If severe dysplasia or in situ carcinoma are not found, then an antireflux procedure should be carried out followed by endoscopic surveillance and pH monitoring every 3 months. Normally dysplasia regresses after surgery. If sulfomucin were detected before surgery, particularly strict surveillance is called for.

When Barrett's Esophagus with severe dysplasia is observed in a young patient amenable to regular surveillance, an antireflux procedure should be peformed followed by careful surveillance. If dysplasia does not disappear within 6 months, esophageal resection is needed. In older patients presenting Barrett's Esophagus and severe dysplasia, the risk of in situ carcinoma is high. Furthermore these patients usually have a long history of reflux and are often less amenable to surveillance. For these reasons immediate esophageal resection is the most appropriate treatment.

2. Barrett's Esophagus without Dysplasia

In patients without dysplasia or in those in whom surgery brings complete resolution of dysplasia, endoscopy should be carried out yearly at first. If sulfomucins were detected, then follow-up endoscopy must be carried out more frequently and for a longer period.

Conclusions

With regard to malignant transformation of Barrett's Esophagus, three factors seem especially important. The first is the presence of specialized metaplasia. The second is the degree of dysplasia and its evolution. The third is more hypothetical; it is the detection of sulfomucin secretions. It is also important to stress the importance of patient psychology, i.e. his aptitude to submit to regular surveillance, in choosing the type of surgical treatment.

Symposium on the anatomic pathology of esophageal neoplasia

President: *Henry D. Appelman* (Ann Arbor, Michigan)

Free Commentators: *J. Chomé* (Versailles)
J. Hemet (Rouen)
H. Ide (Tokyo)
W. S. Payne (Rochester)
J. Wong (Hong-Kong)

Introduction to the classification of esophageal neoplasms

H. D. Appelman (Ann Arbor)

This OESO Congress is a forum for the exchange of information about neoplasms of the esophagus, both benign and malignant, as well as the abnormalities associated with or predisposing to them. Throughout this Congress, pathologists are presenting different morphologic aspects of these conditions, but this information darts in and out of the more clinically oriented discussions which concentrate on symptoms, physical status of the patients, various treatment programs, and, ultimately, survival statistics.

This symposium has been organized to consolidate all of the anatomic pathology aspects into one session. The participants are pathologists who have worked extensively in one area of esophageal neoplasia or another.

Since the OESO triple-armed study covers squamous cell carcinomas, our discussions emphasize the morphologic features of the usual squamous cell carcinomas, its limited or superficial variants, what we know of the morphologic precursor lesions, and the perspective of the animal models.

In the second part of the program, all the other tumors of the esophagus will be considered, beginning with Barrett's carcinomas, including precursors and high risk lesions, unusual esophageal neoplasms, and stromal and lymphoid tumors.

Squamous cell carcinoma of the esophagus

What are the morphologic features of usual squamous cell carcinoma?

H. D. Appelman (Ann Arbor)

Usual or typical or characteristic squamous cell carcinoma of the esophagus is really not a single tumor, but a collection of tumors which vary in the ways that they express their gross and microscopic characteristics.

It is amazing how little published information is available on the morphologic natural history of squamous cell carcinoma of the esophagus [1]. Much of the information that is available is end result: for instance, in several recently published autopsy studies on squamous cell carcinoma of the esophagus from France in 1981 [2], the United States in 1982 [3], Germany in 1984 [4] and Hong Kong in 1986 [5], it

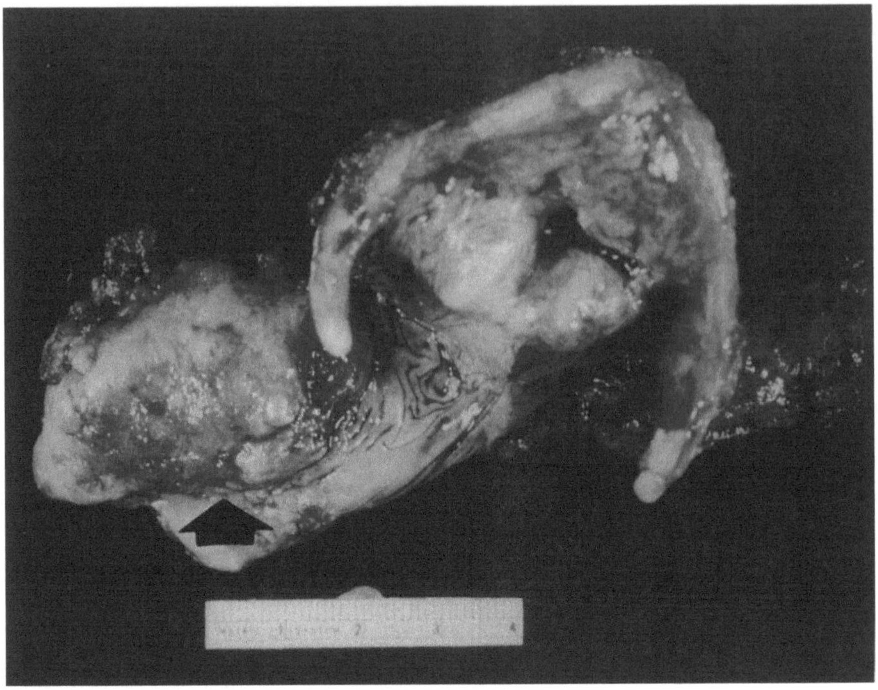

Fig. 1. An exophytic (polypoid) squamous carcinoma of the upper esophagus (arrowhead). The larynx is on the right

is clear that one half to two thirds occur in the middle esophagus, about a quarter to a third in the lower part and about 10–15% in the upper or cervical esophagus. In these same studies, the patients were treated by various mixtures of resection and irradiation: about two thirds to three quarters of the cases had lymph node metastases no matter what treatment was used. Visceral metastases, mainly to liver and lungs, were found at autopsy in 30–75% of the patients, but the reasons for this wide variation are unknown.

Obviously, these data are not controlled, and the studies are not comparable, since some contained undifferentiated carcinomas or adenocarcinomas with the squamous and treatments were different.

Grossly, some esophageal squamous cell carcinomas are exophytic forming lumps growing into the lumen (Fig. 1); terms used for such a growth pattern are "polypoid" or "fungating". Other tumors are mainly infiltrative and tend to confine their bulk to the esophageal wall, producing thickening of a segment with obliteration of the normal anatomic layers (Fig. 2).

Complicating either of these primary patterns are ulcers of varying depths and strictures secondary to lateral expansion (Fig. 3). Furthermore, mixtures of patterns occur, so it is common to have an infiltrative constricting tumor with a polypoid surface that is secondarily ulcerated.

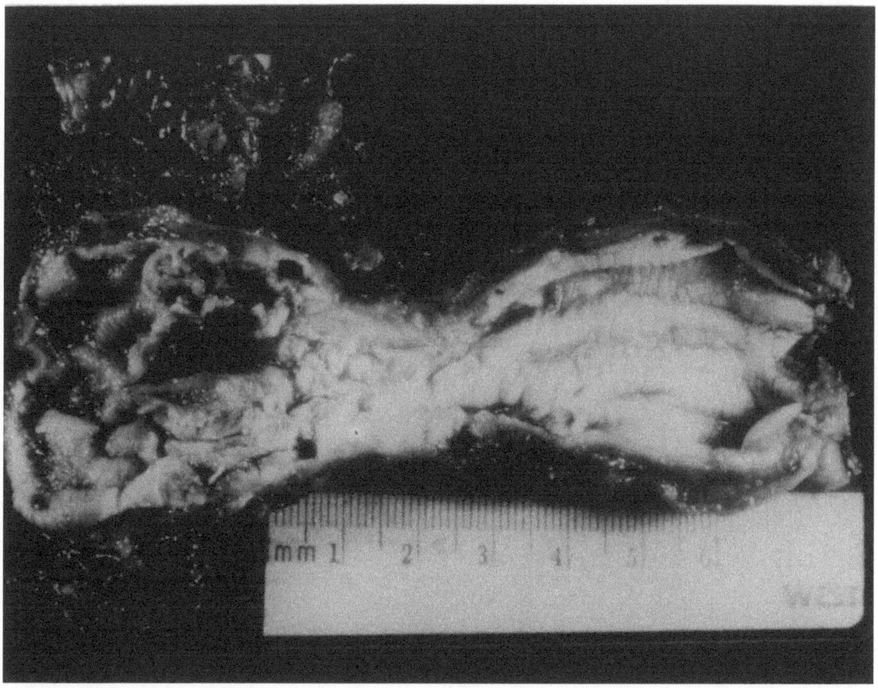

Fig. 2. This is a constricting squamous carcinoma of the lower esophagus which thickens the wall circumferentially

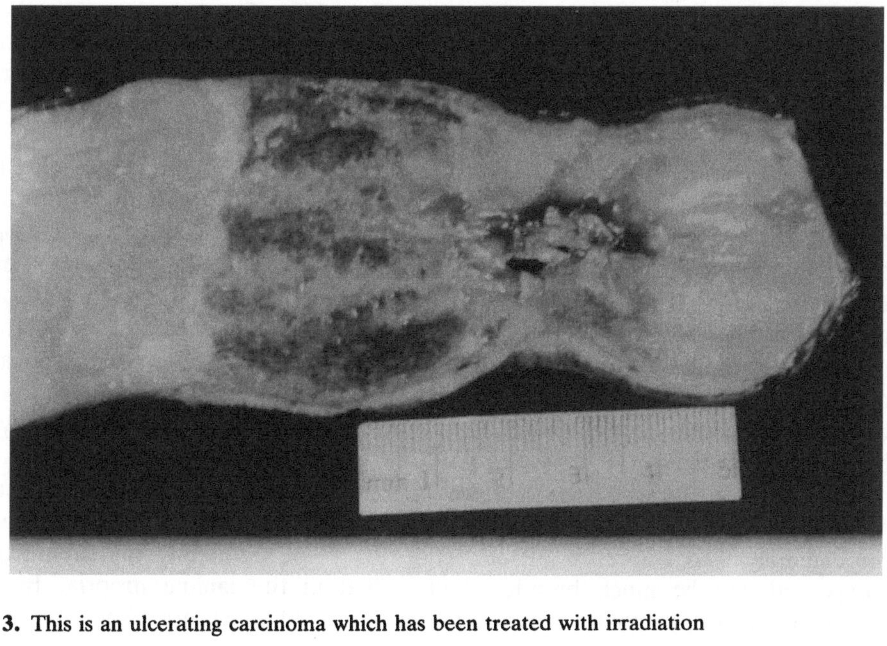

Fig. 3. This is an ulcerating carcinoma which has been treated with irradiation

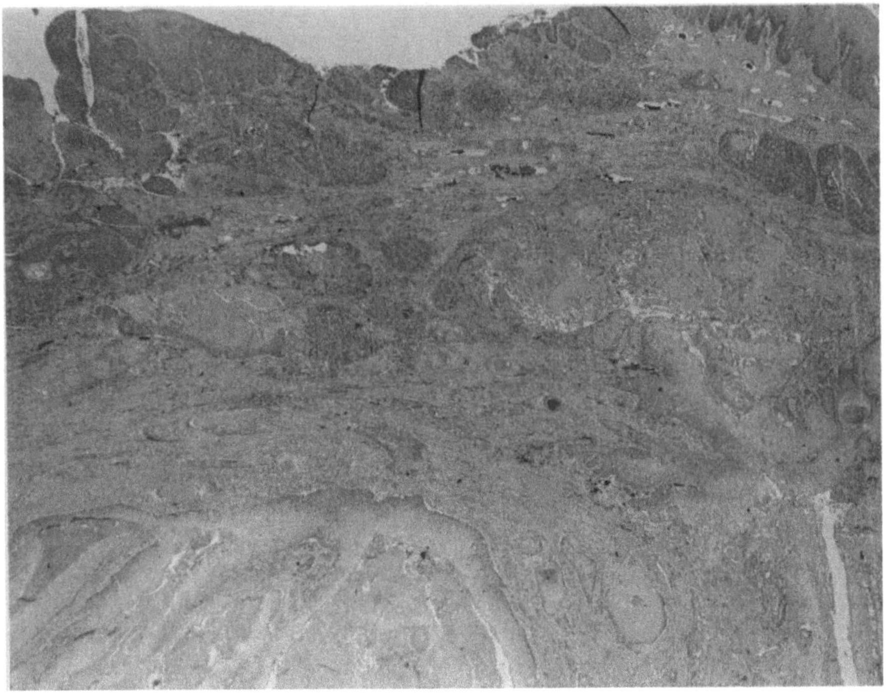

Fig. 4. This invasive squamous cell carcinoma of esophagus has poorly differentiated dark-staining tumor nests on the surface (top) and well-differentiated, keratin-forming masses deeply (bottom) x13

Some tumors orient themselves longitudinally, while others are transverse. Why this happens is enigmatic. Finally, these carcinomas come in all sizes: the limiting width is the esophageal circumference. There is no limit to the length, since esophageal carcinomas are not likely to cover the entire 25 cm length of the viscus.

From the *in situ* stage, tongues of squamous cell carcinoma penetrate the epithelial basement membrane and extend into the lamina propria, where, apparently, a rich lymphatic plexus exists; this is in contrast to the puny lymphatic supply of the gastric lamina propria which is non-existent except at the very base. Thus, tumors invading into the esophageal lamina propria, a basic part of the mucosa, have a readily available mode of metastasis through the mucosal lymphatics; nevertheless, tumors of this limited infiltration rarely metastasize. As with squamous carcinoma in other sites, such as the uterine cervix, the invasive component may be better differentiated than the *in situ* component which may be predominantly of basal or parabasal type (Fig. 4).

Gradually, the tumors penetrate the muscularis mucosae and extend into the submucosa, where lateral or circumferential spread is common with orientation of the carcinomatous trabecula outward (Fig. 5). Thus, frequently the submucosal component will be much broader than is that in the lamina propria. In the submucosa, more lymphatic channels are encountered which drain superiorly and

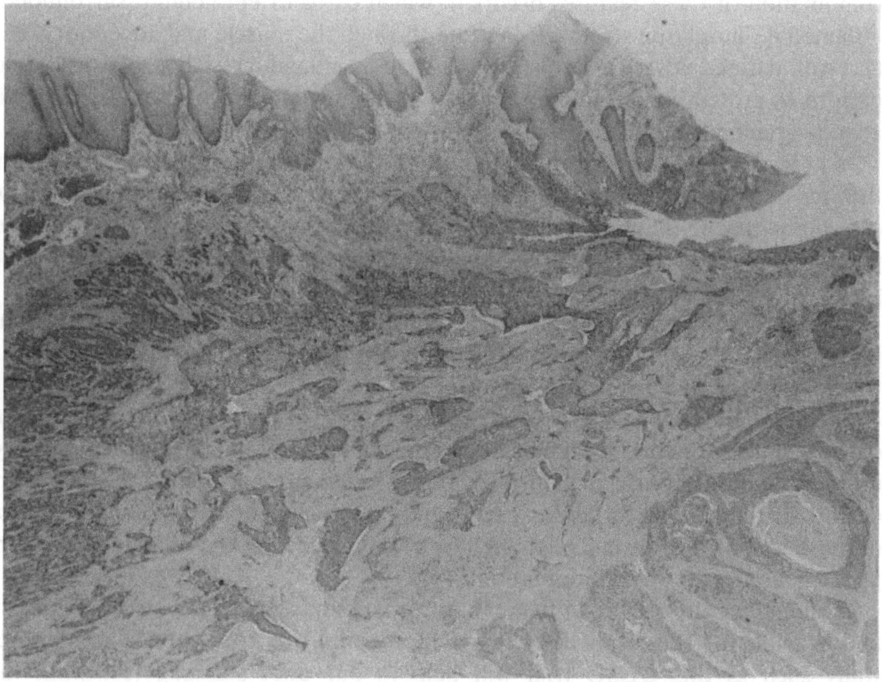

Fig. 5. This squamous carcinoma extends outward in the submucosa, undermining the mucosa (top) x13

inferiorly. Carcinomatous penetration of these channels can lead to extensive lymphatic embolization of tumor cells at a considerable distance from the primary neoplasm and even formation of satellite nodules, some of which may ulcerate the mucosa and look like additional primary tumors.

On occasions, the extension of tumor through the mucosa into the submucosa is characterized by the production of a crater which communicates with the esophageal lumen and which is often filled with carcinomatous keratin.

The pattern of growth in the submucosa is quite variable. Many tumors will form interconnecting thick trabecula in which there is variable central differentiation, including keratin production. At the periphery of these trabecula, in general, are the proliferating or generating cells. Other tumors form thin cords surrounded by desmoplastic stroma; sometimes, such cords interconnect. At other times, they seem to spread out from the central neoplastic focus.

The intramuscular component often has a narrower cross-section than does the submucosal. In the muscularis, the tumors develop several patterns of interface growth with the adjacent non-neoplastic tissues. Sometimes, large lumps are formed which appear to push the stroma away. In other situations, fine fingers or tongues of carcinomatous epithelium seem to slither between muscle fibers. The keratin-filled craters formed in the submucosa may enlarge as the tumor invades the muscularis propria, producing huge chasms full of cancerous keratinous debris. A common combination of these features occurs in which cords of epithelium, surrounded by inflamed desmoplastic stroma, penetrate through the muscle and adventitial tissues as a well defined advancing edge, rather than as individual islands. This is a unique pattern of growth for carcinomas of the gastrointestinal tract. The gastrointestinal adeno-carcinomas tend to insinuate in a more irregular fashion.

Also in the muscularis propria, the cords of carcinoma may change direction as they move from the inner circular to the outer longitudinal muscle. In an occasional case there may be peripheral growth in the junction between the two muscle layers, possibly along the myenteric plexus, thus producing a larger cross-section at this point.

Finally, as the adventitia is involved, dense desmoplasia often occurs. From here invasion of adjacent organs may occur with secondary complications such as trachoesophageal or bronchoesophageal fistulae.

This is a basic outline or skeleton of the anatomy of the squamous cell carcinoma of the esophagus. Now, if each of these alterations is accompanied by the variety of differentiations, patterns of growth, and associated stromal events, then it becomes clear that tremendous variability exists, and that there is no common microanatomy of these lesions. For instance, at any level, the carcinoma may change its pattern of growth and degree of differentiation.

Presumably, all or some of these characteristics have some behavioral correlation and account for the relatively late symptoms and the poor prognosis. Perhaps a study such as this OESO trial will help in our understanding just what these characteristics mean.

References

1. Enterline H Thompson J (1986) Pathology of the Esophagus, Ch 9: Squamous cell carcinoma. Springer-Verlag, New York
2. Mandard AM, et al (1981) Autopsy findings in 111 cases of esophageal cancer. Cancer 48: 329–335
3. Anderson LL and Lad TE (1982) Autopsy findings in squamous-cell carcinoma of the esophagus. Cancer 50: 1581–1590
4. Sons HU and Borchard F (1984) Esophageal cancer: autopsy findings in 171 cases. Arch Pathol Lab Med 108: 983–988
5. Chan KW et al (1986) Carcinoma of the esophagus. An autopsy study of 231 cases. Pathology 18: 400–405

Superficial squamous cell carcinoma

W. V. Bogomoletz (Reims)

Superficial esophageal squamous carcinoma (SESC) can be defined as invasive squamous carcinoma confined to the mucosa and submucosa. Although some authors use the term SESC regardless of the absence or presence of lymph node metastasis, cases of SESC with lymph node involvement should preferably be excluded from the above definition [1]. Terminology confusion also exists between SESC and the strictly non invasive carcinoma in situ (intraepithelial carcinoma).

Most published series of SESC have originated from China and Japan [4]. But with advances in fiberoptic endoscopy, an increasing number of cases have been reported from the Western hemisphere [1, 3, 5].

Dysphagia is a common symptom in Western patients with SESC, but many cases from high-risk areas in the East are asymptomatic. Conventional radiology is often negative, but double-contrast studies may be helpful. Early diagnosis of SESC relies on endoscopy and biopsy. Mass cytology screening, using the abrasive balloon technique, has been used successfully in China, but this is probably inapplicable in Western countries. Several different endoscopic classifications of SESC have been proposed.

Four macroscopic types of SESC are commonly recognized in surgical specimens: plaque-like, erosive, papillary and occult, the first 2 types accounting for about 80% of cases. The plaque-like and occult types are best identified after partial fixation of specimens or with the use of dyes. Microscopically, the degree of differentiation and keratinization of SESC is variable. Regarding the depth of invasion, cases of SESC strictly confined to the mucosa ("intramucosal") should be distinguished from those involving the submucosa ("submucosal"), and also separated from cases encroaching on the muscularis mucosae.

Detailed studies of surgical specimens have shown that SESC often merges with carcinoma in situ or dysplasia. Furthermore, multicentric lesions including SESC, carcinoma in situ and dysplasia have also been described. Hence, the need for performing frozen sections from the margins of resected specimens during surgery.

Although a presumptive diagnosis of SESC is sometimes possible on biopsy material, accurate diagnosis and pathologic staging can only be made after a thorough macroscopic and microscopic examination of the surgical specimen.

Alcohol and tobacco, as well as co-existing orolaryngopharyngeal squamous carcinoma, appear to be frequently associated with SESC in Western cases. On the other hand, epidemiological studies in high risk areas (Northern parts of China and Iran) have suggested a somewhat different pathogenesis [2]. In particular, endoscopic surveys of these Eastern populations have demonstrated the prevalence of an atrophic form of chronic esophagitis, unrelated to gastroesophageal reflux and probably representing a precancerous phase of SESC.

Following screening programs, early diagnosis and prompt surgery, data from Northern China and Japan have indicated a 5 year survival of 90% for patients with SESC (without lymph node involvement). However, the survival rate in Western patients has been reported as somewhat lower (about 60%).

Considering the poor prognosis of the advanced stage of invasive squamous carcinoma of the esophagus, its superficial variant deserves continuing attention from pathologists and clinicians. Early diagnosis and treatment of SESC can provide hope for curative resection. In that respect, SESC can be considered as the esophageal counterpart of early gastric cancer.

References

1. Barge J, Molas G, Maillard JN, Fekete F, Bogomoletz WV, Potet F (1981) Superficial oesophageal carcinoma: an oesophageal counterpart of early gastric cancer. Histopathology 5:499–510
2. Crespi M, Muñoz N, Grassi A, Qiong S, Jing WK, Jien LJ (1984) Precursor lesions of oesophageal cancer in a low-risk population in China: comparison with high risk populations. Int J Cancer 34:599–602
3. Froelicher P, Miller G (1986) The European experience with esophageal cancer limited to the mucosa and submucosa. Gastrointest Endosc 32:88–90
4. Liu FS, Li L, Qu SL (1982) Clinical and pathological characteristics of early oesophageal cancer. Clin Oncol 1:539–557
5. Schmidt LW, Dean PJ, Wilson RT (1986) Superficially invasive squamous cell carcinoma of the esophagus. Gastroenterology 91:1456–1461

What is known about precursor and squamous cell carcinoma? Are there different nomenclatures in different parts of the world for these lesions?

D. Gardiol, J. Hurlimann, and *P. Anani* (Lausanne)

It is currently assumed that before their invasive stages most squamous cell carcinomas of the esophagus (ESCC) are preceded by dysplastic changes and an in situ carcinomatous phase. Whereas the latter is bound to progress to invasiveness, dysplasia, graded into mild, moderate and severe, is possibly still reversible, the reversibility being inversely related to the grade.

In fact the evidence in favor of a dysplasia-carcinoma sequence in the esophagus is still scanty and mostly circumstantial.

Compared with controls there is a higher prevalence of dysplasia (moderate to severe) in subjects from regions or ethnic groups at high risk for ESCC (some provinces of northern China, litoral zone around the Caspian sea, some black populations around the city of Durban and from Transkei in South Africa) [1, 5, 7]. However, the results of an autopsy study from Japan showed the same high rate of dysplasia among subjects from both high risk and low risk prefectures [14].

The strongest evidence comes from the results of mass surveys done in Chinese provinces where there is a high incidence of ESCC. Groups of subjects initially diagnosed by abrasive esophageal cytological techniques as having mild or severe dysplasia have been followed during several years [1]. Among 105 cases of mild dysplasia 16 progressed to severe dysplasia, 42 remained mildly dysplastic and 47 reverted to normal. Out of 79 patients with severe dysplasia 21 progressed to carcinoma, 26 showed the same cytology and 32 regressed to normal or mild dysplasia. Among 11011 individuals having a normal cytology at first screening and not regularly followed up, 13 presented with an esophageal carcinoma (EC) within

2.5 to 7 years. The risk of developing EC can thus be calculated as 224x higher in subjects with severe dysplasia compared to normal. It was also established in China that the mean age of patients with severe dysplasia on cytological examination was 7 to 8 years younger than that of cancer patients [22].

The interpretation of the results obtained from these Chinese studies must take into account the fact that they are based on cytology. Cytologic grading of dysplasia may not be equivalent to histologic grading. The Chinese authors equate cytologic mild dysplasia with histologic parabasal hyperplasia and cytologic severe dysplasia with atypical hyperplasia [1]. The latter, according to the published illustrations, should correspond to dysplastic changes of moderate degree. Some cases classified cytologically as carcinoma in situ seem to correspond rather to histologic severe dysplasia.

Facts pointing to the probability of a dysplasia-carcinoma sequence can be gathered from extensive histologic studies of esophagi either surgically resected or taken out at autopsy. In an extensive study of autopsy specimens without gross malignancy, Mukada et al. [14] found high rates of dysplastic changes. Their findings could be interpreted as suggesting that dysplasia does not appear or progress haphazardly but conforms to a trend of stepwise progression from mild dysplasia to higher grade dysplasia and to carcinoma in situ with each step resulting from the merging of multiple small foci of lower grade dysplasia before the appearance of higher grade foci; thus, progression in severity goes along with progression in extension.

In order to remove extraneous factors when studying associated dysplastic or other changes in esophagi resected for carcinoma, preference should be given to cases of microinvasive cancer without preoperative irradiation or chemotherapy. The study should attempt to obtain a mapping of the lesions. Very few studies, if any, conform to these requirements.

Areas, often extensive, of carcinoma in situ (i.s.) can usually be observed around early carcinomas [3]. Transition from carcinoma i.s. to normal epithelium is often gradual through a series of dysplastic changes, but abrupt transition is not rare [19]. The deeper the tumor invasion, the rarer seems to be the finding of carcinoma i.s. adjacent to the main lesion [11]. On the whole, carcinoma i.s. is associated with invasive carcinoma in about 70 to 80% of the cases and to severe dysplasia in 50 to 65% [11, 12, 17]. Depending somewhat on the gross appearance of the main tumor the distribution of intraepithelial (i.e.) neoplasia (moderate or severe dysplasia or carcinoma i.s.) could be categorized into extensive, multifocal or scanty [17].

Immunocytochemical studies have shown that preneoplastic esophageal epithelium may contain markers associated with malignancy and not detected in normal epithelium [4]. In the oral epithelium, dysplasia and carcinoma show similar staining patterns with antikeratin antibodies in contrast to normal controls [18].

Our experience [10] is based on study of 28 cases of EC (undifferentiated or differentiated squamous cell) associated with dysplastic changes including carcinoma in situ. Using various antibodies, mostly monoclonal, directed against keratins, involucrin, various glycosylated proteins, blood group antigens, TPA (tissue polypeptide antigen), as well as a monoclonal anti-epithelial antibody (Lu5), we have

Table 1. Immunocytochemical study of dysplastic changes in 28 esophagi resected for squamous cell or undifferentiated carcinoma

Markers*	Lu 5, EAB 903	TPA	EAB 902	Involucrin
Normal (surface epithelium)	+ throughout	± basal and parabasal	± parabasal	+ superficial
High-grade dysplasia**: transepithelial n 21	+ throughout	±	0	+ superficial
High-grade dysplasia**: deep n 7	0	±	+	0

* See text for abbreviations
** Severe dysplasia and carcinoma in situ

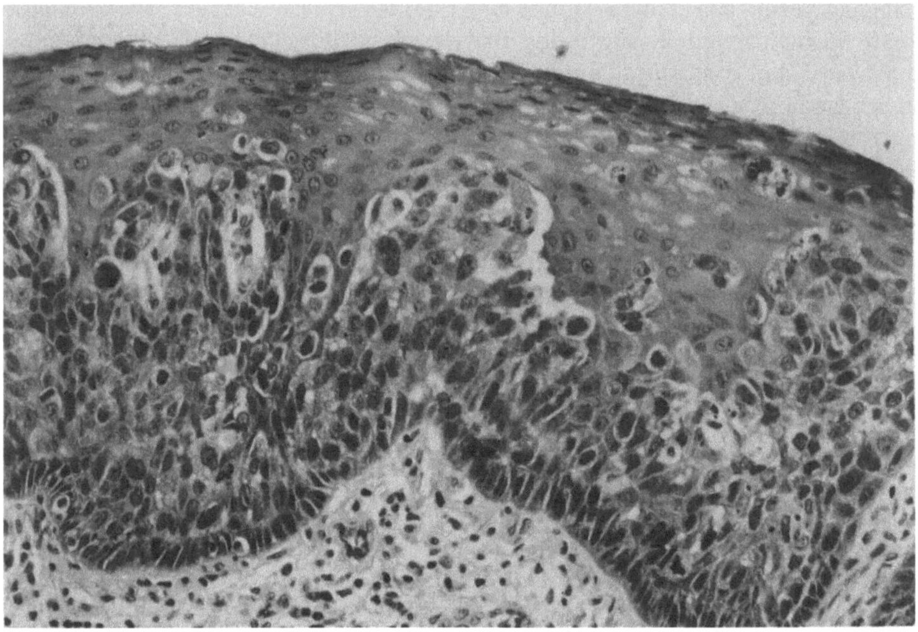

Fig. 1. High-grade dysplasia (carcinoma in situ) of the "deep" subtype. Malignant-appearing cells occupy the basal half of the epithelium leaving intact the major part of the basal layer, some parabasal cells and the whole of the upper layers (x206)

found, as preliminary results, that there are two main types of high-grade dysplasia (severe dysplasia or carcinoma i.s.) differing in phenotype, histologic appearance and differentiating capability (Table 1). In the first type, abnormal undifferentiated cells occupy the basal third or half of the epithelium, leaving intact part of the basal layer, occasional parabasal cells and the whole of the superficial layers (Fig. 1). A pagetoid appearance of the abnormal cells may also be observed. The dysplastic

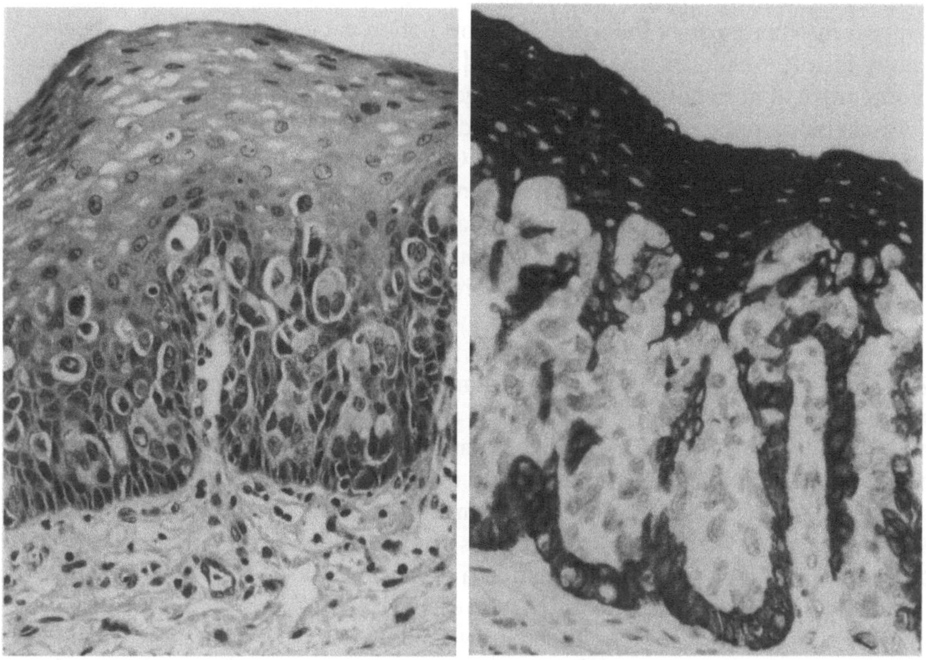

Fig. 2a, b. High-grade dysplasia (same case as on Fig. 1): **a)** pagetoid appearance of the abnormal cells; **b)** immunostaining with a monoclonal anti-keratin antibody (EAB 903) negative for the abnormal cells, positive for the normal-appearing epithelial cells (x206)

cells are phenotypically distinct from normal epithelial cells (Fig. 2) as well as from the cells of the main invasive tumors. The latter are mostly undifferentiated. The second type of high grade dysplasia shows transepithelial changes originating in basal cells that have better preserved their differentiating potential. The associated invasive carcinoma is mostly of a fairly well differentiated squamous cell type.

Whereas there is fairly strong evidence that most esophageal carcinomas have developed through stages of progressive dysplasia, the carcinogenic significance of other associated lesions, such as esophagitis, atrophy, hyperplasia, has not been ascertained.

One promising candidate seems to be human papilloma virus (HPV) infection. Signs of it were found in 33% to 40%, of biopsy or esophagectomy speci-mens from patients with invasive ESCC [9, 20]. A persistent HPV infection associated with depressed MALT (mucosal-associated lymphoid tissue) in the presence of co-factors such as nutritional deficiency, chronic alcoholism or tobacco smoking, might cause dysplastic changes leading to carcinoma [13].

Comparative endoscopic surveys made on adult subjects in Iran and China have shown diffuse chronic esophagitis. If one takes into account only cases which are moderate or severe, chronic esophagitis is almost entirely restricted to individuals from regions at high risk for EC, the lesion being more frequent in Iran than in China (21.5% versus 8.3%) [6]. In Iran it has a high prevalence even in young individuals. Its significance from a carcinogenic point of view is unknown. Such a diffuse esophagitis is apparently not observed during endoscopies made on high risk patients in other parts of the world. No correlation could be made in Iran between family history of cancer and esophagitis [5] or in China between esophagitis and proliferative abnormalities of the esophageal epithelium [16].

Epithelial atrophy (defined as a reduced thickness down to 10 cell layers or less) has been mentioned in association with EC. It has been observed in about 10% of subjects during endoscopic mass surveys in high risk regions of Iran and China [6]. In esophagectomy specimens with cancer, atrophy were noted in 79% of the cases in a well-conducted French study [12]. Although its significance is unknown atrophy is proposed by some authors as a possible preliminary step in the development of EC [2, 15].

Hyperplasia, defined as an expansion of the basal cell layer up to the basal half or 2/3, without accompanying atypia, is almost synonymous with mild dysplasia in which there is, in addition, slight cellular atypia. In this respect it is interesting to note that authors using the terms hyperplasia or basal cell hyperplasia or parabasal cell hyperplasia do not use the term mild dysplasia [7, 17, 21]. For them dysplasia signifies a higher grade disorder in the range of moderate to severe.

Granting that hyperplasia is more or less synonymous with mild dysplasia, what is the evidence, if any, for considering it as a precursor lesion of EC? Chinese follow-up studies have demonstrated that subjects with cytologic mild dysplasia, i.e. histologic hyperplasia, show an unequivocal tendency toward more malignant lesions (16 out 105 cases) [1]. On the other hand hyperplastic changes have commonly been observed in controls during comparative studies [7, 17].

Gland duct hyperplasia, metaplasia, dysplasia and carcinoma i.s. are not infrequently observed in association with similar changes of the superficial epithelium [2, 12, 21].

The current definitions of esophageal dysplasia, including carcinoma i.s., are mainly based on those in use for the cervix uteri and are inadequate in two respects:
- many of them do not take into consideration that intraepithelial neoplasia can display various grades of differentiation [11, 17];
- most of them undeservedly equate intraepithelial level of changes with grade of dysplasia [11, 12, 14].

For our part, we are convinced that carcinoma i.s., with its potential for microinvasion, can be localized in the basal third or half of the epithelium, leaving intact part of the basal layer and the whole of the upper layers. This type of lesion, which does not seem to have gained recognition, is not are and, as we have shown, is phenotypically distinct and commonly associated with undifferentiated carcinomas.

Our proposition for defining dysplasia includes two components:
1. The grading system is based on the following assumptions: basal cell hyperplasia does not differ from mild dysplasia; severe dysplasia and carcinoma i.s. are synonymous; an intermediate grade is necessery from a practical point of view, a two grade-system being too rigid. We have thus low-grade, intermediate-grade and high-grade dysplasia (Fig. 1, 3, 4, 5, 6).
2. The grading of dysplastic lesions is the end-result of an integrated observation of various histologic signs that may develop independently from each other. These signs are: expansion of the basal cell layer; nuclear characteristics such as size,

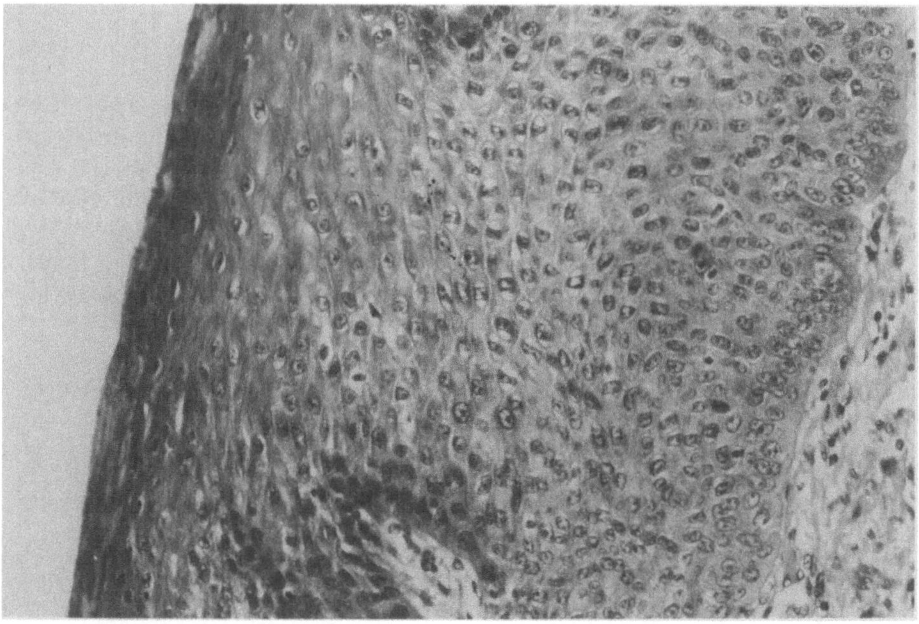

Fig. 3. Low-grade dysplasia. Expansion of the basal cell layer with slightly atypical cells in the basal 2/3 of the epithelium (x206)

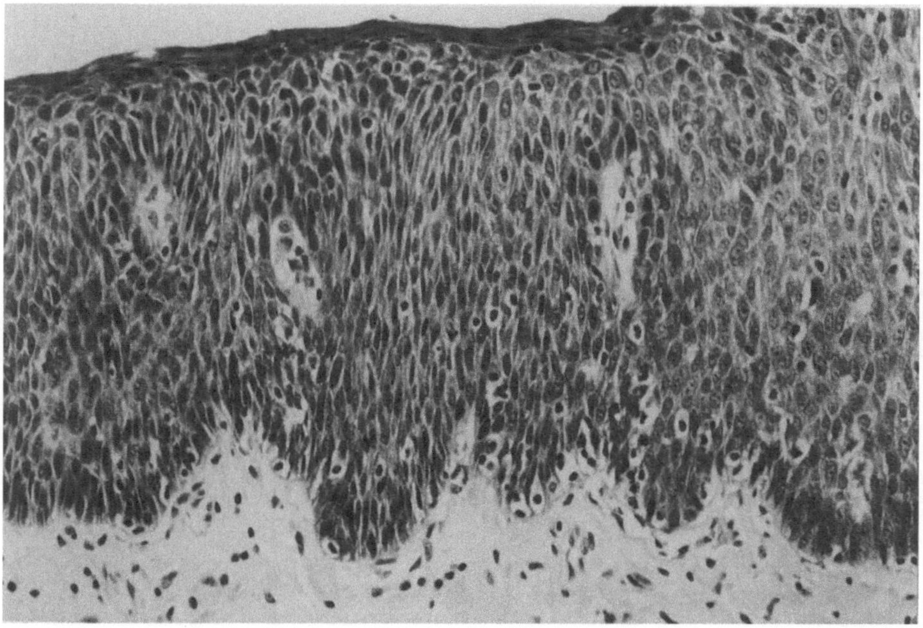

Fig. 4. Intermediate-grade dysplasia. Poorly differentiated cells with higher nuclear-cytoplasmic ratio occupy the major part of the epithelium. The general epithelial structure is preserved (x206)

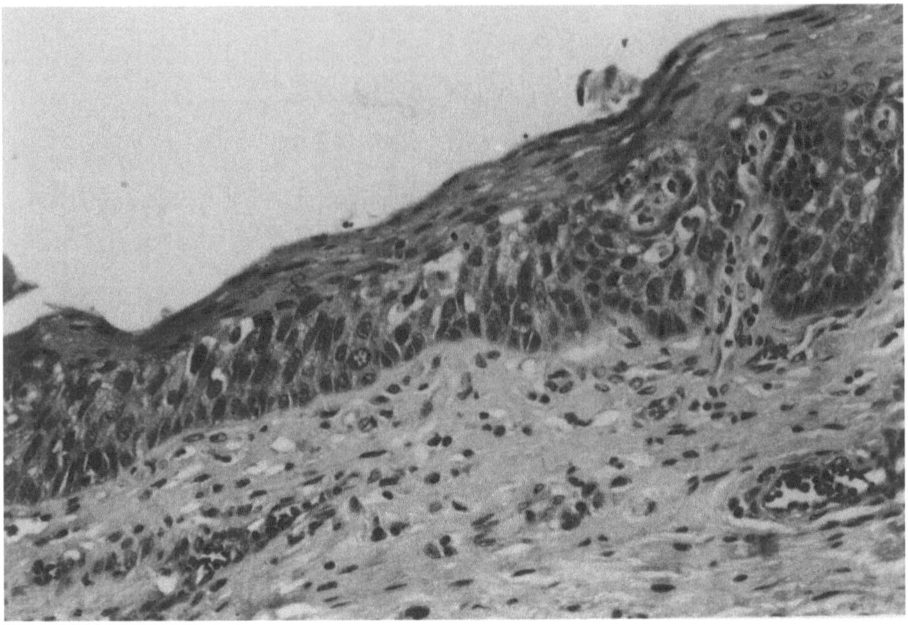

Fig. 5. High-grade dysplasia (severe dysplasia) of the "deep" subtype. Highly abnormal cells in the basal 2/3 of the atrophic epithelium leaving intact part of the basal layer (x206)

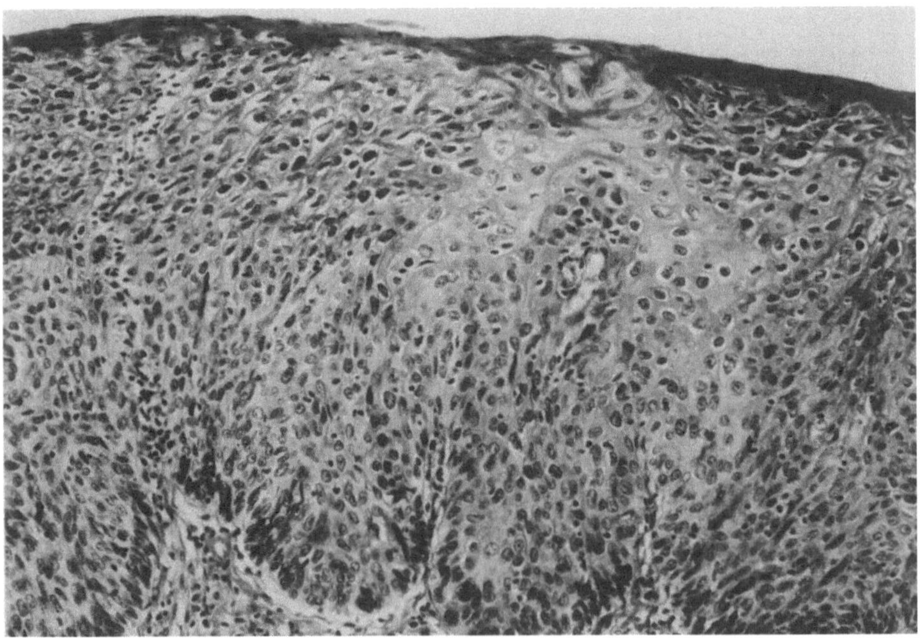

Fig. 6. High-grade dysplasia (carcinoma in situ) of the "transepithelial" subtype. Marked structural disarrangement with rather severe atypia and fairly preserved differentiation (x165)

hyperchromatism, pleomorphism, mitotic figures; abnormal pattern of maturation; structural disarrangement. Inflammatory reaction or previous irradiation may cause changes that have to be distinguished from true dysplasia. When in doubt one should use terms like indefinite or suspicious for dysplasia [8]. The diagnosis of dysplasia is a challenge to the pathologist who must globally evaluate the observed histological abnormalities with respect to malignancy without invasion.

References

1. The Coordinating Groups for the Research of Esophageal Carcinoma, Honan Province and Chinese Academy of Medical Sciences: Studies on relationship between epithelial dysplasia and carcinoma of the esophagus. Chin Med J 1:110–116 (1975)
2. Tumor Prevention, Treatment and Research Group, Chengchow, Honan; Esophageal Cancer Research Group, Chinese Academy of Medical Sciences, Peking; and Linhsien County People's Hospital, Honan: Pathology of early esophageal squamous cell carcinoma. Chin Med J 3:180–192 (1977)
3. Barge J, Molas G, Maillard JN, Fekete F, Bogomoletz WV, Potet F (1981) Superficial oesophageal carcinoma: an oesophageal counterpart of early gastric cancer. Histopathology 5:499–510
4. Burg-Kurland CL, Purnell DM, Combs JW, Hillman EA, Harris CC, Trump BF (1986) Immunocytochemical evaluation of human esophageal neoplasms and preneoplastic lesions for beta-chorionic gonadotropin, placental lactogen, alpha-fetoprotein, carcinoembryonic antigen, and nonspecific cross-reacting antigen. Cancer Res 46:2936–2943
5. Crespi M, Munoz N, Grassi A, Aramesh B, Amiri G, Mojtabai A, Casale V (1979) Oesophageal lesions in northern Iran: a premalignant condition? Lancet ii:217–221
6. Crespi M, Munoz N, Grassi A, Qiong S, Jing WK, Jien LJ (1984) Precursor lesions of oesophageal cancer in a low-risk population in China: comparison with high-risk populations. Int J Cancer 34:599–602
7. Dreyer L (1980) The incidence of dysplasia and associated epithelial lesions in the esophageal mucosa of South African blacks. S Afr Med J 58:406–408
8. Goran DA, Shields HM, Bates ML, Zuckerman GR, Deschryver-Kecskemeti K (1984) Esophageal dysplasia. Assessment by light microscopy and scanning electron microscopy. Gastroenterology 86:39–50
9. Hille JJ, Margolius KA, Markowitz S, Isaacson C (1986) Human papillomavirus infection related to oesophageal carcinoma in black South Africans. A preliminary study. S Afr Med J 69:417–420
10. Hurlimann J, Gardiol D Immunocytochemical study of human premalignant esophageal epithelium and squamous cell carcinoma. To be published.
11. Kuwano H, Matsuda H, Matsuoka H, Kai H, Okudaira Y, Sugimachi K (1987) Intra-epithelial carcinoma concomitant with esophageal squamous cell carcinoma. Cancer 59:783–787
12. Mandard AM, Marnay J, Gignoux M, Segol P, Blanc L, Ollivier JM, Borel B, Mandard JC (1984) Cancer of the esophagus and associated lesions: detailed pathologic study of 100 esophagectomy specimens. Hum Pathol 15:660–669
13. Morris H, Price S (1986) Langerhans' cells, papillomaviruses and oesophageal carcinoma. A hypothesis. S Afr Med J 69:413–417
14. Mukada T, Sato E, Sasano N (1976) Comparative studies on dysplasia of esophageal epithelium in four prefectures of Japan (Miyagi, Nara, Wakayama and Aomori) with reference to risk of carcinoma. Tohoku J Exp Med 119:51–63
15. Munoz N, Crespi M, Grassi A, Qing WG, Qiong S, Cai LZ (1982) Precursor lesions of oesophageal cancer in high-risk populations in Iran and China. Lancet i:876–879
16. Munoz N, Lipkin M, Crespi M, Wahrendorf J, Grassi A, Shih-Hsien L (1985) Proliferative abnormalities of the oesophageal epithelium of Chinese populations at high and low risk for oesophageal cancer. Int J Cancer 36:187–189

17. Ohta H, Nakazawa S, Segawa K, Yoshino J (1986) Distribution of epithelial dysplasia in the cancerous esophagus. Scand J Gastroenterol 21: 392–398
18. Reibel J, Clausen H, Dabelsteen (1985) Staining patterns of human premalignant oral epithelium and squamous cell carcinomas by monoclonal anti-keratin antibodies. Acta pathol microbiol immunol scand (A) 93: 323–330
19. Soga J, Tanaka O, Sasaki K, Kawaguchi M, Muto T (1982) Superficial spreading carcinoma of the esophagus. Cancer 50: 1641–1645
20. Syrjänen KJ (1982) Histological changes identical to those of condylomatous lesions found in esophageal squamous cell carcinoma. Arch Geschwulstforsch 52: 283–292
21. Takubo K, Tsuchiya S, Fukushi K, Shirota A, Mitomo Y (1981) Dysplasia and reserve cell hyperplasia-like change in human esophagus. Acta Pathol Jpn 31: 999–1013
22. Yang CS (1980) Research on esophageal cancer in China: a review. Cancer Res 40: 2633–2644

Are there animal models in non-human primates of precursor lesions and squamous cell carcinoma of the esophagus?

P. Correa, S. M. Sieber, R. H. Adamson, D. W. Dalgard, E. Rodriguez, and *C. Santamaria* (New Orleans)

Although esophageal cancer has been induced experimentally in rodents [1–5], the findings are difficult to extrapolate to humans in a way that could have applicability to clinical medicine. This report briefly describes, a model of experimental induction of squamous cell carcinoma in non-human primates, emphasizing the precursor stages and discussing similarities and differences from human experience.

Material and Methods

A total of 42 subhuman primates (38 rhesus, cynomolgus or rhesus x cynomolgus hybrids and 4 African greens) were given 1-Methyl-1-nitrosourea (MNU) daily for 5 days each week at doses of 10, 20 or 40 mg/kg body weight, starting approximately one week after birth and continuing indefinitely. For oral administration to newborn monkeys, MNU was added to the Similac formula at the time of feeding. When the monkeys were six months old, the carcinogen was incorporated into a vitamin-molasses mixture given to monkeys as a sandwich on a half slice of bread. The other components of the sandwich are powdered milk, folic acid and vitamin C. The animals received Purina monkey chow and half an apple daily. The experimental procedures have been described previously [6]. In the 31 animals who died or were sacrificed a complete autopsy was performed with special attention to the upper alimentary tract. Eleven animals remain on study as of March, 1987.

Results

The following esophageal lesions were observed in the nonhuman primates that lived or were sacrificed.

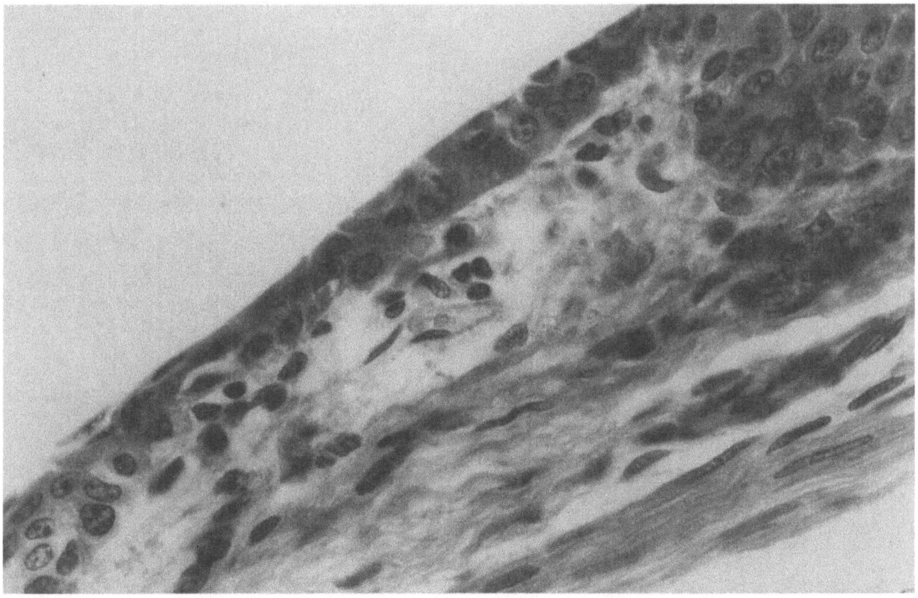

Fig. 1. Focal area of atrophy of the esophageal squamous epithelium in animal 585G who died because of an accident at the age of 27 months. Only 2–3 layers or keratinacytes cover the area of atrophy. A mild superficial inflammatory infiltrate is observed. The right of the section shows the edge of the atrophic area

1. *Chronic multifocal esophagitis* consisting of lympho plasmocytic infiltrate in the lamina propria and the submucosa, most prominent in the middle and lower esophagus. With a few exceptions this lesion was accompanied by other lesions described below.
2. *Multifocal atrophy*, mostly suprapapillary. In our series this appears to be the first detectable pathologic change, observed in its early stages in animal 585G which died at the age of 27 months after having received a total of 3.70 gm of MNU. Fig. 1 shows one of the many foci of atrophy of the esophageal epithelium whose supra-papillary portion is reduced to one or two layers of keratinocytes. The lamina propria shows scanly inflammatory leucocytic infiltrate. Animals Nos. 549G, 615H and 580G died at an early age from causes apparently unrelated to MNU treatment and showed similar multifocal suprapapillary atrophy and esophagitis. Animal No. 563G showed similar findings, but death may have been due to bone marrow depression, which could be related to MNU administration.
3. *Acanthosis*: this lesion was not prominent but had a prevalence of approximately 20%. When present, acanthosis was local, as shown in Fig. 2 in which the two central rete pegs show expansion and hypercellularity when compared to the neighboring rete pegs. Supra papillary atrophy is also apparent in the area of acanthosis. Acanthosis was sometimes associated with hyperkeratosis and para-keratosis, as illustrated in Fig. 3.

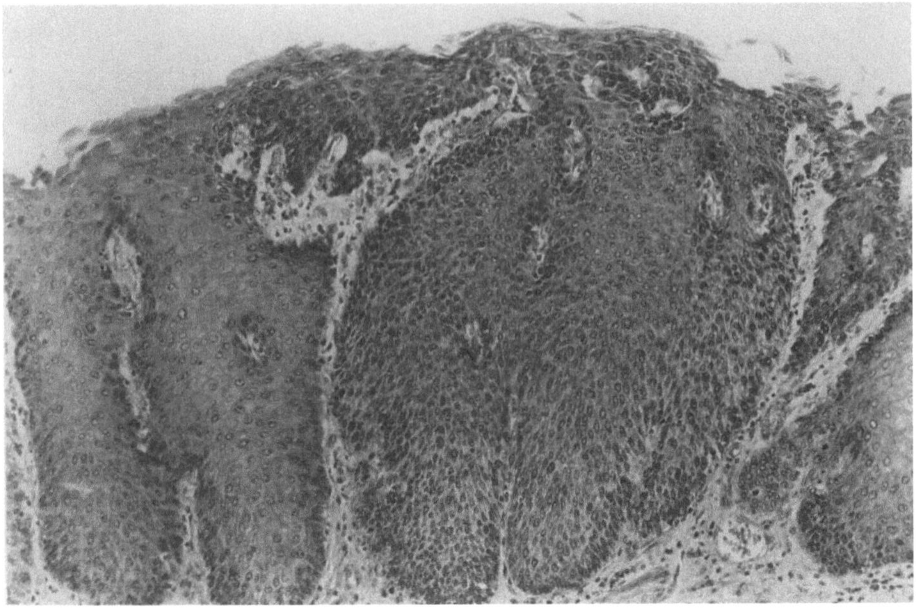

Fig. 2. The central portion of the esophageal mucosa shows atrophy of the suprapapillary layers and hypertrophy (acanthosis) of the two central rete pegs. The increased cellularity of the central rete pegs (hyperplasia) contrasts with the normal architecture of the surrounding rete pegs

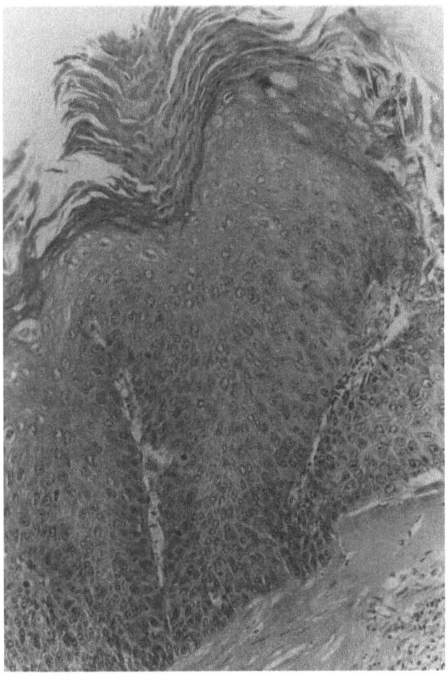

Fig. 3. Focal acanthosis and hyperkeratosis

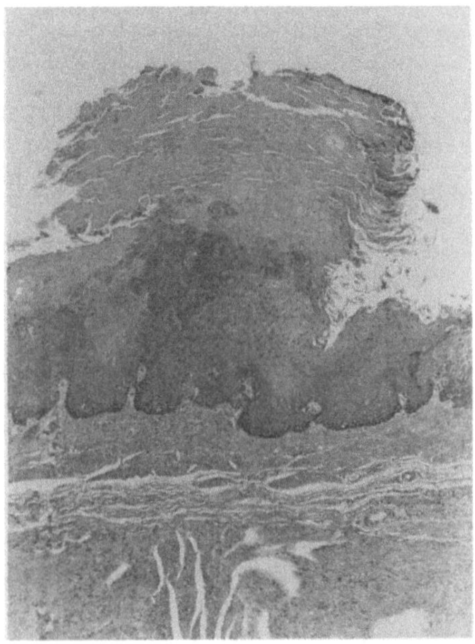

Fig. 4. Parakeratotic micropapilloma resulting from excessive keratin layers which conserve their nuclei and their intercellular adhesions

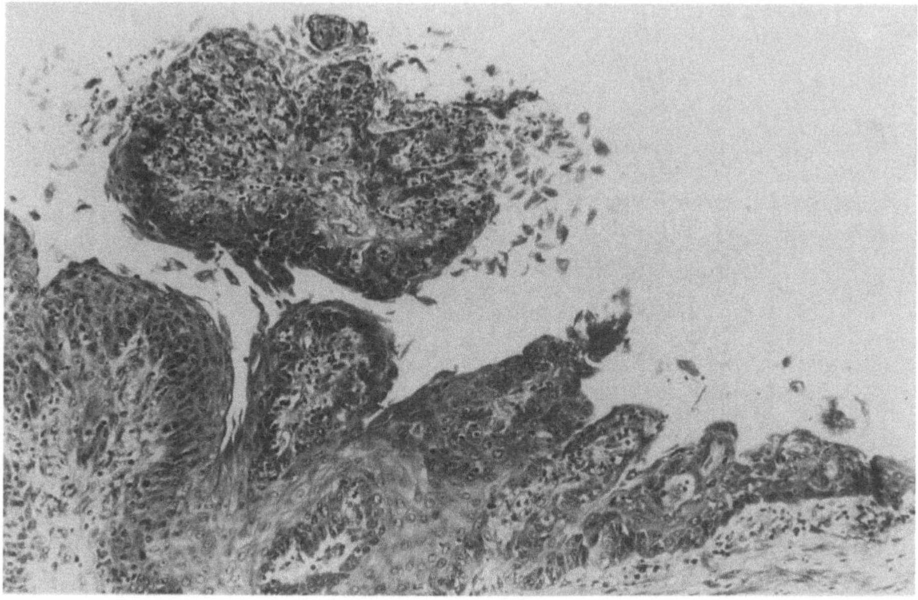

Fig. 5. Squamous papilloma with central connective-vascular core lined by hyperkeratotic epithelium with ulceration and inflammation. Hyperkeratosis and acanthosis are also observed at the base of the papilloma. Atrophy is observed laterally outside the papilloma base

4. *Parakeratotic micropapilloma*: this lesion was observed in 4 of the 30 autopsied animals. It represents a small verruciform micropolyp made of parakeratotic layers which remain attached to the original mucosa, as illustrated in Fig. 4.
5. *Squamous papilloma*: these are intraluminal projections of tissue with a central connective-vascular core lined by hyperkeratotic epithelium, as illustrated in Fig. 5. They can be associated with dysplastic or carcinomatous changes in the neighboring mucosa but are not seen in most carcinomas.
6. *Dysplasia*: these changes, characterized by nuclear atypism and architectural distortion, were observed very frequently in our material. However, in only 3 cases was the lesion identified in the absence of an overt squamous cell carcinoma somewhere else in the esophagus. Most foci of dysplasia were associated with atrophy rather than hypertrophy of the mucosa and appeared grossly as somewhat depressed areas, as shown in Fig. 6. The change from normal maturing to dysplastic epithelium was often abrupt, as shown in Fig. 7.
7. *Carcinoma in situ*: this was a frequent lesion in this series, but in all cases it was found accompanied by invasive carcinoma in other areas of the esophagus. These tumors were frequently at the base of an erosion, or a depressed area near an ulcer (Fig. 8).
8. *Invasive squamous cell carcinoma*: this tumor was found in 50% of our autopsied cases but since there are still 11 living monkeys, the overall prevalence at the time of this report is approximately 36%. Most tumors were well differentiated and penetrated the submucosa, muscularis propria and adventitia. It is remarkable

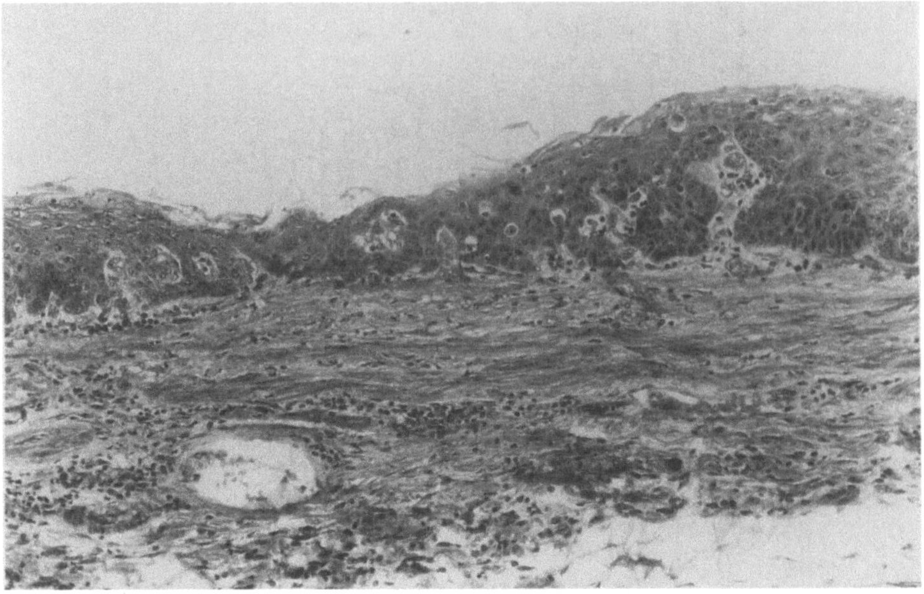

Fig. 6. Dysplastic epithelium showing hyperchromasia, loss of polarity and individual cell keratinization, most prominent in the atrophic epithelium and the center of the microphotograph. Chronic inflammation is also present

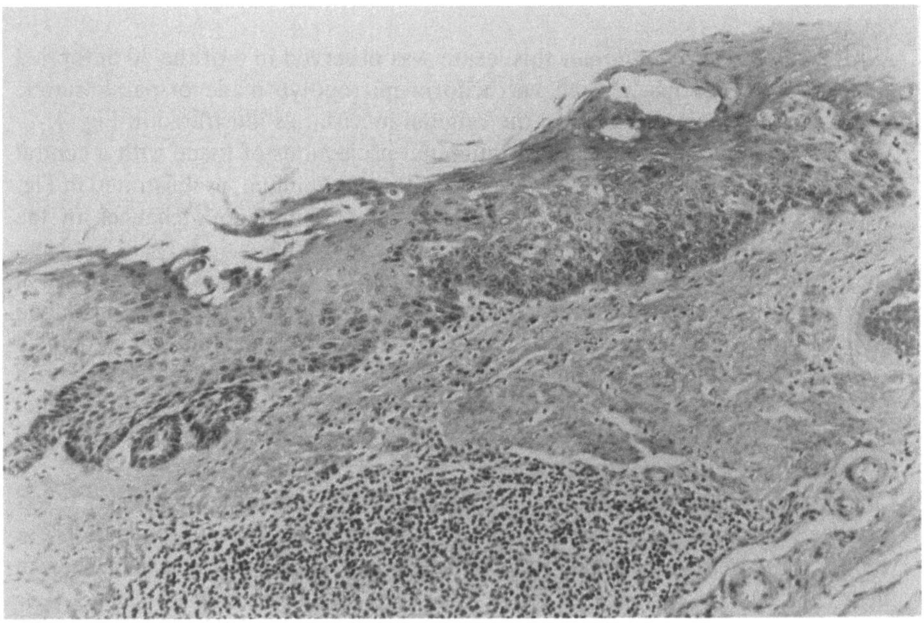

Fig. 7. Well circumscribed focal area of dysplasia resulting in an expansion of the epithelial layer. On both sides of the dysplastic focus normal maturation of the epithelium is observed. Chronic esophagitis is also observed

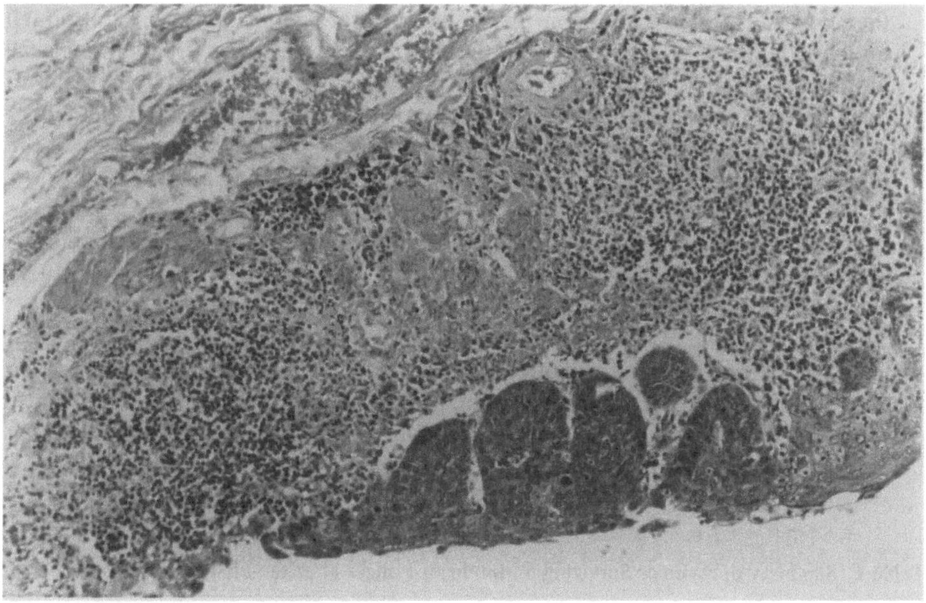

Fig. 8. Carcinoma in situ partially covering an ulcerated area of the esophageal mucosa. Marked inflammatory reaction is present

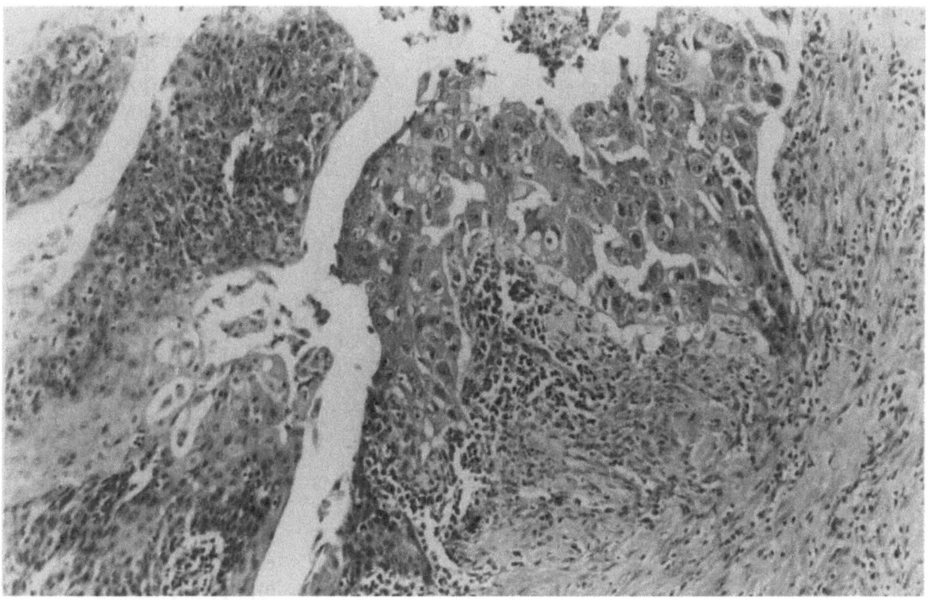

Fig. 9. Well differentiated squamous cell carcinoma involving the submucosa at the base of a squamous papilloma

that no distant metastasis from these tumors were found at autopsy although direct extension of the tumor to neighboring organs was frequent. Fig. 9 illustrates a carcinoma found at the ulcerated base of a squamous papilloma. Ten out 15 animals had multiple invasive tumors. One animal (624H) had 9 independent invasive esophageal carcinomas. Tumors were found in all segments of the esophagus but were more predominant in the lower third.

The earliest invasive carcinoma was observed in animal 617H who developed two independent invasive tumors after receiving a total dose of MNU of 53.21 gm (9.96 gm/kg) over a period of 62 months.

The most frequent extraesophageal tumors observed were in the oropharyngeal and laryngeal mucosa, found in 8 out of 15 animals with esophageal carcinoma. Also observed were two gastric carcinomas, one gastric adenomatous polyp, one leiomyosarcoma of the colon and one atypical rhabdomyoblastic lesion of the heart. Bone marrow depression and hypercellularity were also observed.

Table 1. Summary of Animals Surviving 6 Months or Longer after the First Dose of MNU

Animal No.	Species	Sex	Cum. Dose (gm)*	Cum. Dose (gm/kg)*	Latent/Obs. Pd. (mo)	Histopath. Findings
Surviving Animals						
541G	Hybrid	F	259.09	55.27	234	N/A
561G	Rh	F	266.70	54.13	233	N/A
565G	Cyno	M	360.53	54.33	232	N/A
574G	Hybrid	F	251.45	54.29	232	N/A
583G	Cyno	F	142.26	51.33	231	N/A
584G	Cyno	F	211.96	80.32	231	squamous papilloma, tongue
616H	Rh	M	251.36	44.87	224	N/A
621H	Cyno	F	138.51	43.80	223	N/A
626H	Rh	M	224.35	27.94	222	N/A
630H	Cyno	F	113.92	24.90	221	N/A
631H	Rh	F	174.25	27.17	221	N/A
Dead Animals Without Tumor						
585G	Cyno	F	3.70	4.88	20	multifocal atrophy & esophagitis
549G	Cyno	M	21.48	6.42	25	TH; colitis; BM hyperplasia
615H	Cyno	F	9.04	5.03	27	multifocal atrophy & esophagitis
580G	Green	F	10.63	7.49	29	esophagitis
563G	Rh	M	7.37	11.74	30	BM atrophy
550G	Green	M	19.11	13.75	39	Severe multifocal esophagitis with atrophy, acanthosis, dyskeratosis, erosions, micropapilloma & mild dysplasia
564G	Rh	F	63.53	20.25	58	normal esophagus visceral congestion
559G	Rh	M	201.40	37.94	125	multifocal esophagitis & dysplasia
586G	Cyno	F	177.39	44.32	169	esophagitis; atypical acinar hyperplasia pancreas
575G	Cyno	M	258.71	53.96	185	cardiomyopathy
581G	Cyno	F	205.95	48.32	185	endometriosis; hydronephrosis & -ureter

Table 1. Continued

Animal No.	Species	Sex	Cum. Dose (gm)*	Cum. Dose (gm/kg)*	Latent/Obs. Pd. (mo)	Histopath. Findings
632H	Cyno	F	136.06	25.14	184	diabetes; endometriosis; normal esophagus
634H	Green	M	118.33	24.89	184	systemic varicella; pustules upper digestive mucosa
578G	Rh	F	260.75	29.61	213	esophagitis & focal atrophy; endometriosis
577G	Rh	F	297.59	53.89	219	endometriosis; multifocal atrophy, esophagus
614H	Cyno	M	361.19	19.63	216	multifocal esophagitis, atrophy dysplasia & squamous papillomas. Chronic gastritis; acute meningitis
	Dead animals with tumors					
617H	Cyno	M	53.21	9.96	62	two SCA, upper & lower esophagus
622H	Rh	M	64.80	10.29	64	multiple SCA, tongue, palate & esophagus
539G	Rh	F	108.15	28.26	71	SCA, esophagopharynx; dysplasia, CIS & micropapilloma, esophagus
540G	Rh	M	129.28	28.09	72	multiple SCA, middle & lower esophagus
627H	Rh	M	129.91	13.98	134	multiple SCA, upper & middle esophagus; multifocal atrophy & dysplasia
538G	Rh	M	133.81	23.08	67	multiple SCA, larynx, pharynx & esophagus. Adenoma of stomach
569G	Green	M	137.20	30.17	124	SCA, lower esophagus; oral & esophageal papillomas
624H	Rh	F	142.33	30.17	134	multiple SCA & dysplasia, gingiva & esophagus
566G	Cyno	F	146.33	42.68	167	SCA, lower esophagus; tongue papilloma; endometriosis
579G	Rh	M	180.64	37.74	67	multiple SCA, pouches & distal esophagus; multifocal dysplasia
560G	Cyno	M	246.43	45.93	169	SCA, esophagus; ACA, stomach; rhabdomyoblastoma, heart
625H	Rh	F	84.77	20.29	161	multiple SCA, esophagus, upper & lower
633H	Rh	M	136.80	15.84	178	multiple SCA, esophagus & epiglottis; multiple ACA, stomach. Gastric atrophy & dysplasia
613H	Cyno	F	149.05	32.99	210	SCA, lower esophagus; CIS upper esophagus; leiomyosarcoma; LI; endometriosis
623H	Cyno	M	151.61	33.49	200	SCA, lower esophagus. Multiple dysplasia

* at death or as of 9/30/86. Abbrevations are: IL, islets of Langerhans; TH, toxic hepatitis; BM, bone marrow; N/A, no specific abnormalities; SOS, Sertoli-only syndrome; SCA, squamous cell carcinoma; ACA, adenocarcinoma; CA=carcinoma; LI=large intestine; CIS=carcinoma in situ

A wide spectrum of susceptibility versus resistance to the action of this carcinogen is evident in the present experiment. Eleven animals remain alive after more than 18 years of treatment. Animal No. 584G has received the highest cumulative dose (211.96 gm total dose, 80.32 gm/kg), had a squamous papilloma removed from the tongue in 1981 and is still alive while animal 617H developed two carcinomas with a dose approximately 8 times smaller in terms of gm/kg of body weight. At least three monkeys died without tumors after receiving cummulative doses around 50 gm/kg (Table 1).

Table 1 is a summary of the present findings (as of March, 1987). Eighteen were rhesus (Macaca mulatta), 19 were cynomolgus (Macaca fascicularis), 4 were African green (Cercopithecus aethiops) and 2 were rhesus × cynomolgus hybrids.

Table 2 shows the esophageal lesions encountered in monkeys fed MNU in the vitamin sandwich, with the exception of monkey No. 634H whose esophagus could not be adequately evaluated for precancerous lesions because it was massively involved with pustules resulting from a systemic varicella infection.

Table 2. Esophageal lesions in monkeys receiving MNU orally

Lesions	*Cumulative dose, gm/kg* 4.88–9.96	10.29–24.9	25.14–30.17	32.99–48.32	51.33–80.32	Total	Prevalence in 30 autopsied monkeys %
Unknown (living)		1	2	2	6	11	-
Normal		1	1	1		3	10
Multifocal chronic esophagitis	5	8	5	7	2	27	90
Multifocal suprapapillary atrophy	4	8	3	5	1	21	70
Focal acanthosis	1	4	1			6	20
Parakeratotic micro-papilloma	1	2	1			4	13
Squamous papilloma		3	2			5	17
Dysplasia							
low grade		2	1	2		5	17
high grade		5	3	3		11	37
Carcinoma in situ		2	3	2		7	23
Invasive carcinoma							
upper	1	2	2			5	17
middle		4	2			6	20 50
lower	1	3	3	5		12	50

Discussion

Before drawing any conclusions on differences and similarities between the human situation and the simian model described in this paper, it should be stressed that the carcinogen in our series was given on a vitamin sandwich contained vitamin C, a substance which could potentially have a protective effect against carcinogenicity by MNU. The monkeys were well fed, received a balanced diet and were not exposed to tobacco or alcohol, which is contrary to the situation of many esophageal cancer patients. Consequently, the carcinogenic dose of MNU for simians under these circumstances may be higher than that required for humans.

Our observations in general conform to the previously proposed model of esophageal carcinogenesis [7] in that esophagitis, atrophy and dysplasia may precede invasive cancer. However, several observations in the presently reported experiment may throw further light into the model. The earliest and most persistent and pervasive change observed is that of multifocal suprapapillary atrophy, implying that the carcinogen interferes with the process of differentiation of the esophageal epithelium. Inflammation, erosion, ulceration and invasion by bacteria and fungi would appear to be consequences of this loss of the capacity to differentiate. Acanthosis basically represents proliferation without adequate differentiation, which might be interpreted as a response to the incapacity to differentiate. After this point, dysplastic and neoplastic cells come into play, which require mutagenic events eventually leading to invasion.

If the simian model applies to the human situation, several observations can be made.

1. The carcinogenesis process is multifocal and very extensive, which implies that primary or secondary prevention measures need to be systemic or at least cover the whole upper digestive mucosa.
2. Most dysplastic and early carcinomatous lesions are associated with multifocal atrophy and therefore would appear endoscopically as depressed areas. Polypoid and papillomatous lesions are not the frequent precursors of invasive carcinoma and in many instances appear to be epiphenomena of the carcinogenic process.
3. When dysplasia is found, the great majority of subjects will have invasive carcinoma somewhere else in the upper digestive mucosa. In this simian model all carcinomas in situ were found in animals with other invasive neoplasms.
4. There is a large spectrum of susceptibility – resistance to esophageal carcinogens, so far totally unexplored and unexplained. Males appear more susceptible than females: the male/female ratio was 3/8 in surviving monkeys, 7/9 in monkeys dead without tumors and 9/6 in monkeys dead with tumors.
5. High risk of esophageal cancer may imply high risk of other cancers, most notably the oral cavity, pharynx and larynx.
6. The latency time between initiation to carcinogen exposure and clinically detectable tumor is very prolonged: 5 to 17 years in monkeys exposed soon after birth. This offers hope for chemoprevention in humans in whom the latency should be expected to be even longer.

The simian model appears much closer to the human situation than the rodent models. The Reuber model in BUF rats results mostly in poorly differentiated carcinomas of the proximal esophagus [3]. The Napalkov model in non-inbred albino rats develops mostly in hyperkeratotic and papillomatous lesions [1]. The Stinson model based in F344 rats receiving injections of carcinogen develops mostly in squamous papillomas [4]. The Ito model on Wistar rats is also frequently associated with squamous papillomas [2]. Barch and others have developed models incorporating zinc deficiency, which may play a role in humans [5].

Systematic studies of precancerous lesions carried out in high-risk populations show close morphologic similarities with the simian model [8].

One thing in common to most animal models is that the most effective carcinogens are the N-nitroso compounds. In humans these compounds may be found in the diet. It is also possible that they may be formed in situ by the interaction of NO and appropriate substrates, a situation that has been investigated experimentally in animals [9].

The simian model of esophageal cancer described in this report is similar to esophageal cancer as it develops, in that it is a neoplasm characterized by accompanying early lesions it is multifocal, carries a high risk for other cancers especially in the oral cavity, and there is a long latency for tumor development. This model may also be useful for testing the effectiveness of chemopreventive or chemotherapeutic agents.

References

1. Napalkov NP, Kazymir M, Pozharis SKI (1969) Morphogenesis of experimental tumors in the esophagus. J Nat Cancer Inst 42: 922–940
2. Ito N, Kamamoto Y, Hiasa Y, Makiura S, Marugami M, Yokota Y, Sugihara S, Hirao K (1971) Histopathological and ultrastructural studies of esophageal tumors in rats treated with N-nitrosopiperidine. Gann 62: 445–451
3. Reuber MD (1977) Histopathology of preneoplastic and neoplastic lesions in the esophagus in BUF rats ingesting methylnitrosamine. J Nat Cancer Inst 58: 313–334
4. Stinson SF, Squire RA, Sporn MB (1978) Pathology of esophageal neoplasms associated with proliferative lesions induced in rats by N-methyl-N-benzilnitrosamine. J Nat Cancer Inst 61: 1471–1475
5. Barch DH, Walloch J, Hedvegi D, Iannaccone PM (1986) Histopathology of methylbenzilnitrosamine induced esophageal carcinoma in the rat: comparison with cytomorphology. JNCI 77: 1145–1153
6. Adamson RH, Krolikowski FJ, Correa P, Sieber SM, Dalgard DW (1977) Carcinogenicity of 1-methyl-nitrosourea in non-human primates. J Nat Cancer Inst 59: 415–422
7. Correa P (1982) Precursors of gastric and esophageal cancer. Cancer 50: 2554–2565
8. Munoz N, Wahrendorf J, Bang LJ, et al (1985) No effect of riboflavin, retinol and zinc on prevalence of precancerous lesions of the esophagus. The Lancet 2: 111–114
9. Sander T, Burkle G, Schweinberg F (1969) Induktion malignen tumoren bei ratten durch gleichzertge verfütterung von nitrit und sekundären aminen. Z. Krebsforsch 73: 54–66

What are the morphologic predictors of behavior of squamous cell carcinoma of the esophagus? The OESO malignancy index and histologic staging

H. D. Appelman (Ann Arbor)

A malignancy index identifies a group of morphologic features that have some validity as predictors of survival, separates each of them into subsets to which are given numbers, and then derives a numerical total of all the numbers of all the morphologic subsets for each case. This is predicated upon the supposition that all morphologic features carry the same weight, so that their variable subsets will define a series of valid measurements. The index is also predicated upon the supposition that the numerical designations given to each morphologic aspect are given in the proper order. Unfortunately, these features may not be equal, and we may not know how to put them in proper sequence.

Fortunately, within the OESO study and its statistical capabilities, we can measure each parameter separately against outcome, and we can measure clusters of parameters against outcome. Superimposed upon all this, is the fact that the available data in each case may necessitate limiting the index as published, because the complete data subsets are not available for every case.

For many cases, the biopsies of the carcinomas will be the only available material from which to derive data. The treatments may destroy any residual tumor within the esophageal wall. Similarly, treatments may modify the neoplasm within the wall to such an extent that data derived from morphologic analysis is no longer valid.

*

We are attempting to develop a malignancy index, or at least to identify important prognostic factors, because this is a multidirectional therapeutic study. Any individual pieces of data that can be tabulated may have importance. We may find, for instance, that certain morphologic parameters are important in patients treated in a certain way, whereas similar parameters are unimportant when other treatment programs are used. Our surgical, radiotherapeutic and chemotherapeutic colleagues hope to accomplish something therapeutically important in this study. We, pathologists, are simply adding our part by searching for morphologic markers which may correlate with the prognosis in the face of one of the three treatment modalities.

The morphologic features potentially important in predicting behavior of these carcinomas may be separated into those which are derived from gross analysis of the specimen, and those which are derived from the microscopic appearances of the tumor. The gross features include size, the orientation of the tumor in regard to the esophageal axis, its topographical appearances, or shape, and finally, the gross depth of penetration, although the microscopic evaluation of depth will be much more accurate.

The microscopic features include differentiation, pattern of growth, appearance at the advancing edges, depth, blood vessels or lymphatic permeation and stromal characteristics. Added to this, will be other microscopic features, mainly whether there is tumor at the resection margins, including the deep margins, whether there are metastases in lymph nodes, and whether there are any other lesions in the esophagus.

Not all of these parameters may be useful in the establishment of a malignancy index. At the same time, additional features of which we are not currently aware may be incorporated into such an index. Therefore, the index as it currently exists must be considered a fluid collection of data which may be modified dramatically or even done away with completely. The initial choice of these parameters is to a great extent guesswork: many of them may be closely interrelated, and thus not independent variables. It must be emphasized that gross analysis will be performed by the contributing pathologists, not by the Pathology Panel. The Panel will mainly deal with the microscopic features in submitted slides.

Size of malignant neoplasms is usually considered to be an important prognosticator. On the other hand, size often relates to extent of spread or stage.

At the moment, it is not clear if size is important for squamous cell carcinoma of the esophagus. Similarly, whether the carcinoma is *oriented* parallel to the axis of the esophagus, perpendicular to it or is circumferential, may not be an important prognosticator. This is one of the features included in the preoperative TNM staging system of the American Joint Committee on Cancer and the International Union Against Cancer [1].

The way the tumor looks *topographically,* in other words, whether it mainly protrudes into the lumen, mainly invades the wall, or both, is really a stage related phenomena. For instance, we know that the pseudosarcomatous squamous cell carcinoma can often achieve a huge size and be almost entirely exophytic and thus, of low stage, and it is probably this peculiarity of growth which accounts for its unusually favorable prognosis compared to other squamous cell carcinomas.

There is conflicting data about whether cytologic *differentiation* correlates with prognosis: the disagreement may center about how various levels of differentiation are defined, and this is one of the benefits of having a Pathology Panel which, hopefully, will determine the differences among well, moderately, and poorly differentiated squamous carcinomas. Differentiation refers to how closely a tumor caricatures the normal structures from which it presumably arises (Figs. 1, 2, and 3). These tumors have the tremendous capability of differentiating differently in different areas of the esophageal wall. As mentioned earlier, quite often the mucosal aspect of the tumor will be much more poorly differentiated than the deeper.

We hope to look at differentiation, not only in the dominant areas of the tumor, but at the advancing edge. We might suspect that those parts of the tumor which are invading may be the important growth areas, and, therefore, what they look like may be critical for survival.

One microscopic feature offers quantitative information, and that is the *mitotic counts.* Theoretically, all highly trained, sophisticated pathologists should be able to recognize mitotic figures: amazingly enough, there have been a number of studies indicating that there is individual variability from one pathologists to another in

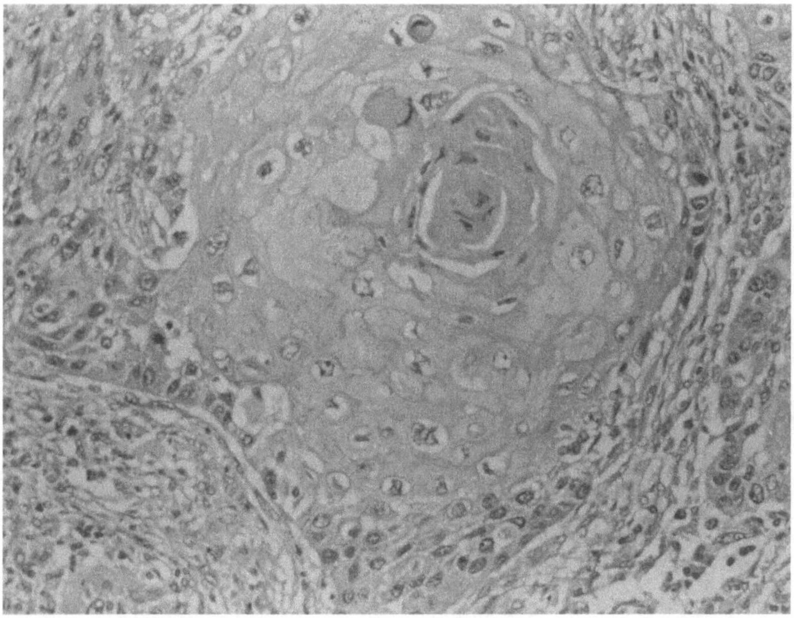

Fig. 1. Well differentiated squamous cell carcinoma with a central keratin pearl (x208)

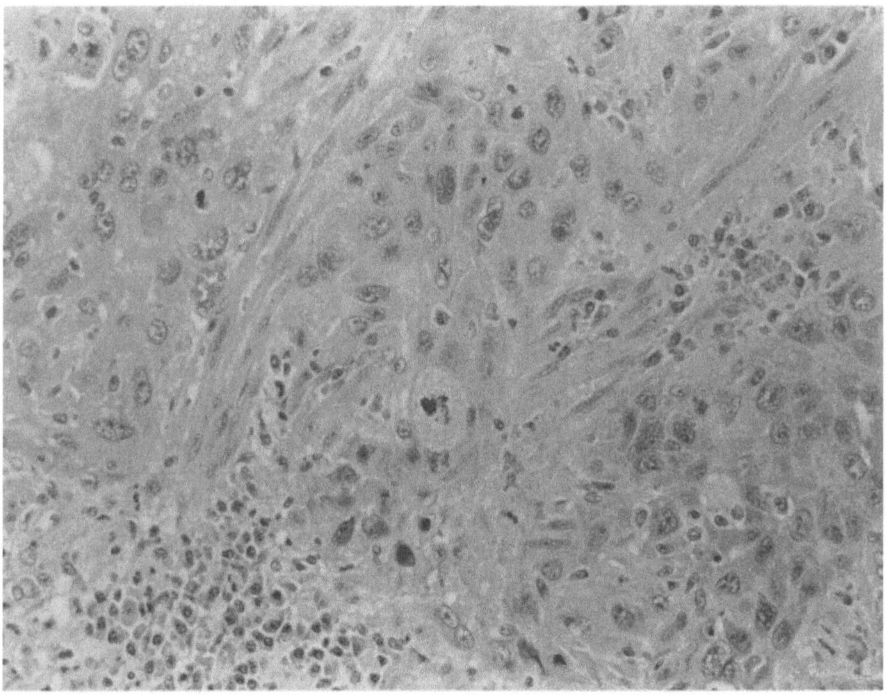

Fig. 2. Moderately differentiated squamous cell carcinoma. The large polygonal cells resemble squamous cells (x208)

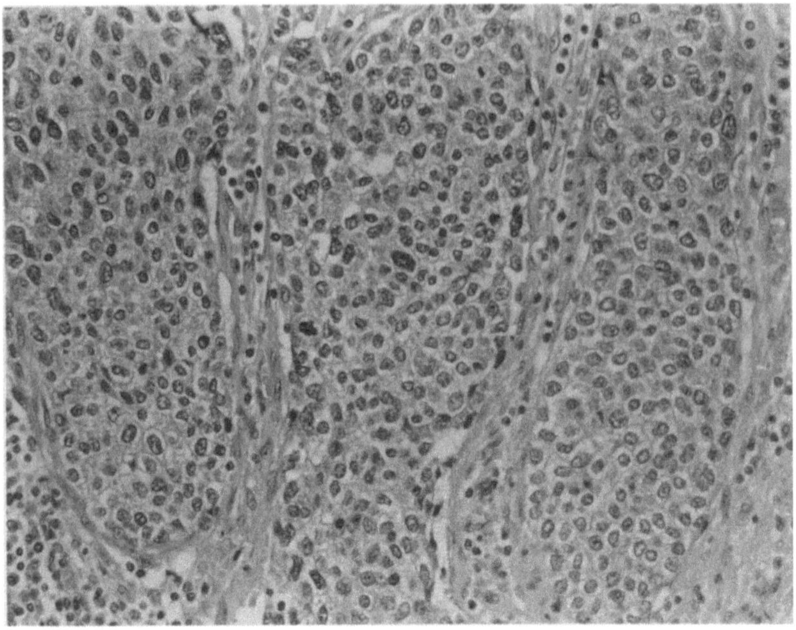

Fig. 3. Poorly differentiated squamous cell carcinoma. The cells are small and resemble basilar cells (x208)

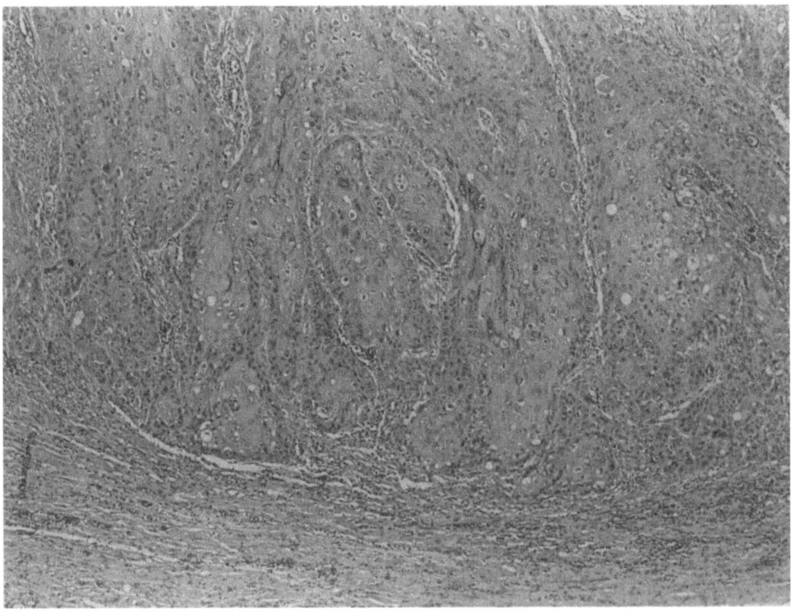

Fig. 4. Expansile growth pattern: the advancing edge of the carcinoma seems to push the peripheral tissues (x53)

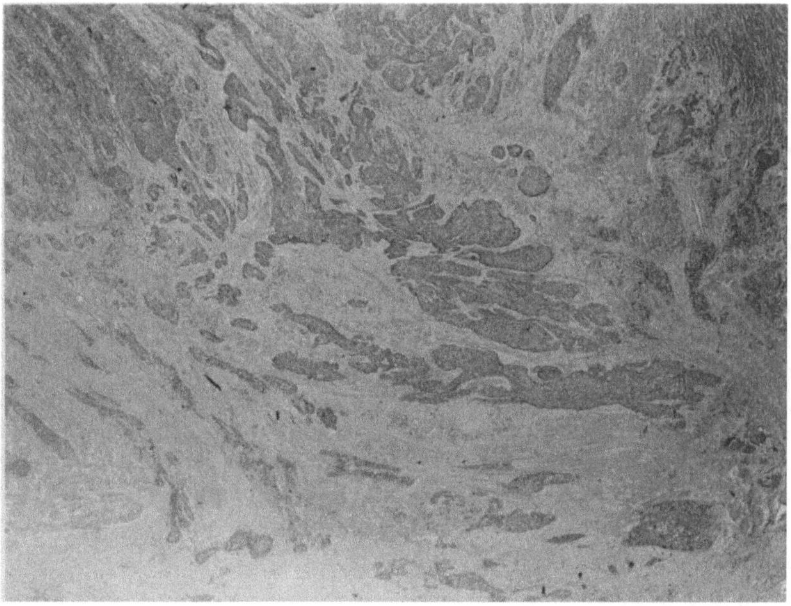

Fig. 5. Infiltrative margins in which nests and cords of tumor penetrate the marginal tissues in an irregular fashion (x13)

terms of recognition of mitotic figures in a microscopic field. We may find that this variability is so great that this parameter might be useless.

These tumors grow in many *patterns*. They make thin cords or thick trabeculae or big clumps or little nests or form cysts or cavitations communicating with the surface. Perhaps we will wish to examine what these different patterns mean, if anything.

Not only is differentiation of the tumor at the advancing margin a potentially useful marker of behavior, but so is the way the tumor interacts with the normal marginal tissue. Therefore, as mentioned in the earlier discussion, we will look at this advancing edge to determine if it has a circumscribed or *expansile* pattern, an *infiltrative* pattern, or a mixture of the two (Figs. 4 and 5).

The *depth of invasion* really is what defines the extent of the primary tumor, the T of the TNM system. We are avoiding any TNM designation, instead subdividing invasion by layers of the wall involved. Data presented at the last OESO Congress indicates there is clear interrelation between depth of invasion and other parameters, such as vascular permeation, lymph node metastases, and short term survival [2].

The presence of *tumor thromboemboli in intramural blood vessels or lymphatic vessels* seems to be an important index of tumor behavior for most malignant neoplasms, so we will evaluate this feature. Of course, finding this is often dependent upon the number and type of samples of the tumor that are available for review. Therefore, this is clearly one parameter that may have to be modified.

Furthermore, it is quite difficult to tell lymphatic from blood vascular channels with routine light microscopy.

The importance of the interaction between the carcinoma and its *stroma* has yet to be analyzed: for some tumors, an immunologic reaction with lymphocytes and plasma cells may indicate a better prognosis, whereas large amounts of collagenous or desmoplastic stroma may indicate just the opposite. Clearly, it is important to evaluate *lymph nodes* for metastases. Ideally, at the time of resection, large numbers of lymph nodes covering the entire areas of potential metastases, would be harvested by the surgeons and submitted to the pathologists, appropriately labeled by sites. Practically, this will not happen, except in a very few institutions where these tumors are studied in exquisite detail. In fact, there are procedures being used by many surgeons which do not involve lymph node resection at all. Therefore, although nodes are important in defining stage, they may not be available in many cases for us to utilize lymph node metastases as an important piece of information.

A few other things that we will want to evaluate is what is going on at the *margin of resection*. The status at the deep margin of resection is an index of whether any tumor remains locally. The margins of resection of the esophageal wall are a different issue. Carcinoma of the esophagus is one of the gastrointestinal carcinomas which may spread submucosally, and, as a result, may extend well beyond the gross boundaries of the tumor. It shares this feature with carcinoma of the stomach. Colonic carcinoma, on the other hand, virtually never grows in this way, and the gross tumor margins almost always identify the microscopic margins as well.

Finally, we will look for *other lesions in the esophagus,* such as dysplasias or other foci of carcinoma, in an attempt to define the milieu in which the carcinoma has developed. Of course with chemotherapy and radiation, many of the changes that we see are going to be related to those treatment programs, and, as a result, will not be intrinsic to the esophagus in which the squamous cell carcinoma evolved.

References

1. Beahrs OH, Myers MH eds (1983) Manual for Staging of Cancer JB Lippincott Co, Philadelphia, 2nd Ed., p 61–64
2. Gardiol D, Saraga P, Anani P, Fontolliet CH (1984) Answer to question: "Can common staging criteria be adopted?" Cancer of The Esophagus in 1984: 135 Questions. Proceedings of the First Polydisciplinary International Congress, OESO, Maloine publ. Paris, p 359–360

The role of the pathology panel in the OESO study

H. D. Appelman (Ann Arbor)

The OESO triple-armed study is a multicentered, multinational study of squamous cell carcinoma of the esophagus, including all stages of growth, as well as all gross and histologic variations. Five hundred carcinomas of the esophagus are to be included within this study, split evenly into three treatment groups.

These carcinomas initially will be analyzed by many different pathologists throughout the world, most of whom have their own built-in biases in terms of defining pattern of growth, degrees of differentiation and levels of invasion. Therefore, the OESO Pathology Panel has been assembled to deal with these variabilities in interpretation and nomenclature for all cases entered into the OESO study. The following is a summary of the role of the pathology panel:

1. Establish *uniformity in definition* and morphologic criteria.
   a) Evaluate the reproducibility of morphologic criteria: is agreement on morphologic criteria among the panel members necessary for useful data to be generated? If not, can the panel arrive at a consensus, subjugating in the process the prejudices of the panel members? If the members of the panel can agree mong themselves on the criteria and the name or label for a particular parameter in a given tumor, then this may be an optimal result for that parameter.
   b) Exclude non-reproducible criteria: the panel must determine if it should discard those morphologic criteria that do not lend themselves to reproducability.
   c) Standardize the nomenclature: the panel must develop a set of rigid definitions so that terms which may be confusing will become clear. Examples of such terms include "undifferentiated", "dysplasia", "intramucosal carcinoma", "superficial carcinoma", and virtually every other term that is used to define any morphologic feature of squamous carcinoma of the esophagus. For instance, the definition of the word "undifferentiated" is complicated: some pathologists use this to refer to tumors with no differentiating features at all, whereas others use this synonymously with poorly differentiated variants which still manifest clear cut differentiating features somewhere.

2. Determine *exclusion criteria*: the panel must decide if a case does not belong in the study. For instance, there may be peculiar forms of carcinoma of the esophagus which initially are classified as squamous cell carcinoma but which, on review, the panel determines are other types of carcinoma. Such lesions obviously do not fulfill the basic requirement for the study, namely that a tumor be squamous cell carcinoma:

   Similarly, a tumor that is truly undifferentiated, in other words, one that has absolutely no squamous features, should not be included in the study. A corollary to this is how fastidious or energetic we should become in deciding on the differentiation of an otherwise undifferentiated tumor. Under ideal circumstances, we could resort to immunohistochemistry or to electron microscopy to determine if a questionable tumor has squamous characteristics. Obviously, such activities would make the study ponderous and impossibly expensive.

3. Establish both *minimal* and *optimal* morphologic data bases: the panel must determine what morphologic data base is feasible, given the difficulties in compliance by the various contributing pathologists throughout the world. There

are recommended samples for microscopic analysis to be be submitted to the pathology panel for all specimens; however, it is clear from the specimens submitted to date that obtaining this ideal sampling in all cases is impossible. Pathologists throughout the world are busy people. They have multiple responsibilities and generally limited finances and personnel. If were are asking too much of them, then we will have to settle for less than the ideal.

4. Determine the relation between biopsy and resection specimens. In some cases treated by chemotherapy, the tumor may be entirely or almost entirely destroyed so that all histologic data for the study would, by necessity, be biopsy derived. The panel must determine if it is possible to utilize both biopsy derived data and resection derived data in this study and weigh them equally. Similarly, does chemotherapy alter morphology so as to exaggerate the discrepancies between biopsy and resection features?
5. Study the issue of whether squamous cell carcinoma of esophagus is a single disease throughout the world or a relatively common morphologic manifestation of a number of different diseases. Is the low frequency disease encountered in Western societies the same as the high frequency disease encountered in certain parts of China and Iran?
6. As the study progresses, additional factors may surface that the Panel may wish to evaluate.

Barrett's esophagus and adenocarcinoma

What are the general morphologic features of Barrett's esophagus and the carcinomas arising in it? Can Barrett's carcinoma be differentiated from carcinoma of the gastric cardia?

R. H. Riddell (Hamilton)

The columnarlined esophagus (CLE) often referred to as Barrett's esophagus is a condition where the squamous epithelium normally lining the distal esophagus becomes replaced by columnar epithelium with features of either gastric or intestinal mucosa or both. It is almost certainly the result of acid gastro-esophageal reflux. Complications include peptic ulceration, stricture, dysplasia and adenocarcinoma. Although commonly referred to as Barrett's esophagus, the condition probably most recognized by Tileston in 1906 [1], while Lyall described the condition well in 1937 [2]. It should be pointed out that residual islands of gastric type mucosa can be found at endoscopy in about 4% of the population in the cervical esophagus. This is excluded from further discussions of the columnar-lined esophagus.

Morphological features of CLE

The columnar lined esophagus may be lined by a variety of different types of epithelium, none of which is in itself absolutely specific or diagnostic because they represent a combination of cell types found either in the normal stomach, intestine or a combination of both. Epithelium may therefore resemble or be indistinguishable from gastric cardiac mucosa (junctional type epithelium), it may contain specialized cells such as parietal cells (gastric fundic-type epithelium), or there may be incomplete or complete intestinal metaplasia (specialized columnar epithelium) [3].

- *Junctional type epithelium:* This may be completely indistinguishable from normal gastric cardiac mucosa. Superficial foveolar cells each contain an apical mucin vacuole that does not have the flask shape so characteristic of intestinal type goblet cells. There may be a hint of a villous pattern superficially. Specialized cells such as chief or parietal cells as seen in the normal gastric fundus, or goblet and Paneth cells as found in intestinal epithelium are not present.
- *Gastric fundic type epithelium:* The same superficial foveolar mucinproducing epithelium that is seen in junctional type epithelium and superficially in the entire stomach is present. However, occasional parietal and chief cells may be present. However, these are present in far fewer numbers than in normal gastric fundic epithelium and much more resemble the transitional mucosa between the gastric body/fundus and either cardiac or antral mucosa.
- *Specialized columnar epithelium:* The characteristic of this type of epithelium is the presence of incomplete or complete intestinal metaplasia. This is recognized

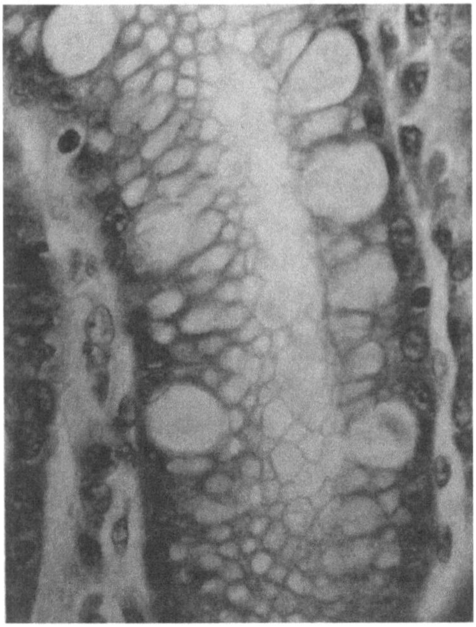

Fig. 1. Incomplete intestinal metaplasia characteristic of that seen in the columnar-lined esophagus. Note that admixture of gastric foveolartype mucin secreting cells, where each cell has an apical mucin goblet, interspersed with intestinal type goblet cells

primarily by the presence of intestinal type goblet cells admixed with foveolar mucin producing cells (incomplete intestinal metaplasia) (Fig. 1). Intestinalization is considered to be complete when absorptive cells replace gastric foveolar cells, and although only the merest hint of a superficial villus configuration may be present, cell types present are essentially those found in the small or large intestine. Paneth cells may sometimes be found in the crypts, while argentaffin and other enteroendocrine cells, of a variety of types, may also be present. The most frequently found enteroendocrine cell types are enterochromaffin cells and somatostatin containing cells but other hormones can be demonstrated immunocytochemically usually in small numbers.

In patients with severe reflux and ulcer disease, typical regenerative epithelium may be present. This typically is low cuboidal, nuclei may be relatively widely spaced, be opened and vesicular, have prominent eosinophilic nuclear-like and therefore can be confused with dysplasia. In addition, architectural abnormalities with back-to-back glands may also occur in regenerated epithelium (Fig. 2).

Distribution of epithelial subtypes

There has been a suggestion that the types of epithelium described above do have a distinct distribution early in the course of the disease. In children, intestinalized epithelium seems to be relatively uncommon with junctional mucosa predominating [4]. In Paull's paper describing epithelial subtypes, there is a suggestion that

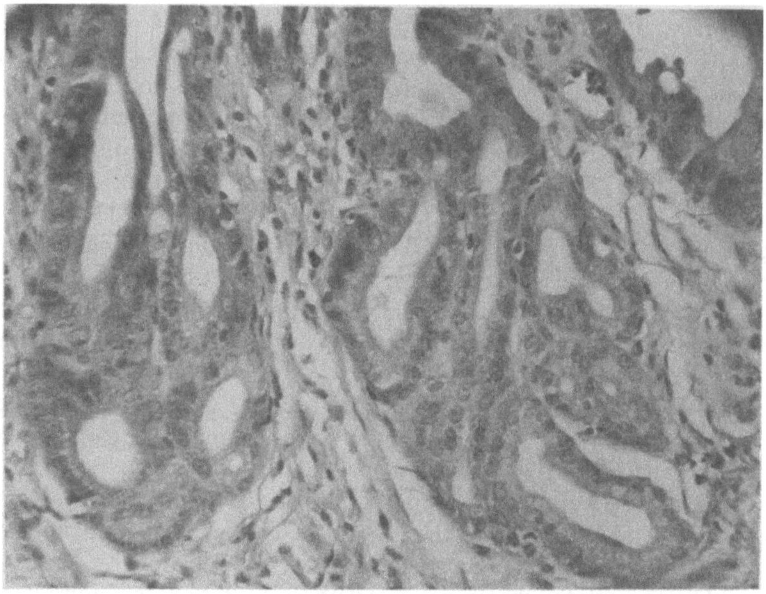

Fig. 2. Regenerated CLE. Note the regenerated features in the epithelium and also the structural abnormality, a back-to-back arrangement of the glands being present in the absence of dysplasia. Such architectural changes could cause problems when accompanied by a little dysplasia

intestinalized mucosa is always the most proximal, and that junctional and fundic mucosa proceed more distally [3]. However, in autopsy studies there seems to be much more of a mosaic [5], pattern with admixtures of these epithelial patterns.

Diagnosis

The diagnosis of Barrett's esophagus can be difficult because it requires the demonstration of a proximal shift of the squamo-columnar junction relative to the lower esophageal sphincter. It should be remembered that the distal 1–2 cm of the tubular esophagus are normally lined by gastric cardiac mucosa, and that the Z-line is within the lower esophageal sphincter representing the squamo-columnar junction. Although anatomically the stomach and esophagus are supposed to be separated by the former having a serosal and mesenteric investment, this can clearly only be demonstrated in resected specimens, but even then is somewhat variable. Measurements in centimeters from the incisor teeth can be of value, the Z-line usually being between 38 and 40 cm from them. Biopsies showing glandular epithelium less than 35 cm from the incisors are therefore very likely to come from Barrett's esophagus. The use of the "sniff test" to demarcate the crura of the diaphragm can be useful in suggesting where the lower esophageal sphincter should be, but in patients with a hiatal hernia, the entire lower esophageal sphincter and Z-line may be moved proximally together.

Because of this, it may be very difficult or impossible to make a diagnosis of Barrett's esophagus in the absence of intestinal metaplasia. Interestingly, in the absence of a CLE it is most uncommon for patients to have isolated intestinal metaplasia at the gastric cardia and also a columnar-lined esophagus. For this reason, the diagnosis is best established by taking a series of biopsies beginning in the stomach on the lesser curve side where intestinal metaplasia is most likely to be present if it is extending up from the gastric antrum, and then to take a biopsy every centimeter or two until obvious endoscopic squamous epithelium is reached. This should yield a series of biopies in which the lowest is clearly of gastric origin. Subsequent biopsies from the cardia, and if present, intestinalized epithelium in the esophagus which are demonstrably not associated with intestinal metaplasia in the stomach can be demonstrated.

Histologically, this is virtually diagnostic of the columnar-lined esophagus. This works well for tubular extensions of the glandular mucosa proximally, but may work less well if small tongues of possible columnar epithelium are present, such as may be seen in a very irregular Z-line. Under these circumstances a similar series of biopsies in a direct line immediately beneath the tongue of epithelium and extending into the squamous epithelium again are most likely to yield the correct diagnosis. It should be appreciated that in patients with severe reflux, the entire lower esophagus may appear red and the squamous-columnar junction very indistinct.

Use of mucin stains in making the diagnosis of Barrett's esophagus

Mucin stains which demonstrate intestinal metaplasia, such as alcian blue at pH 2.5 (Fig. 3), or mucicarmine stain may be of value in highlighting rare goblet cells in esophageal biopsies. An intesting feature of these biopsies is that histologically-

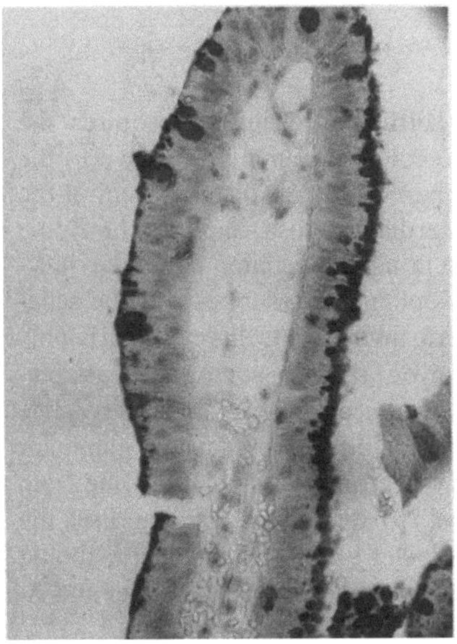

Fig. 3. CLE in a biopsy state with alcian blue at pH 2.5. Note the positive staining of the epithelium in the absence of intestinal type goblet cells

normal gastric foveolar type epithelium in the CLE may produce acidic mucins abnormally in the absence of metaplasia. It is unclear whether this represents a "form fruste" of intestinal metaplasia and whether such patients inevitably go on to develop CLE.

Carcinoma in Barrett's esophagus

It has been estimated that between 5 and 10% of all esophageal cancers are associated with Barrett's esophagus [6]. While it has been estimated that approximately 10% of patients presenting at hospitals with symptoms of reflux have CLE, the prevalence and incidence of esophageal cancer in CLE suffers from the lack of data. However, it appears that the prevalence in patients presenting with Barrett's esophagus is between 6 and 20%, but the incidence of esophageal cancer is between 1/80 and 1/450 cases per person per year [7].

Predisposing factors include being male, being white, a long history of reflux and smoking [7, 8]. Factors such as the extent of CLE, the length of time that it has been present and the presence of persistent reflux have not yet been established as predisposing factors. Carcinomas can certainly arise following anti-reflux surgery, but seem to be quite uncommon, particularly if reflux is prevented. It should be remembered that with time many patients redevelop evidence of reflux.

Gross pathology (Fig. 4, 5, 6)

Endoscopically and in resected specimens, adenocarcinomas of the esophagus may be indistinguishable from most other types of adenocarcinoma, with polypoid, ulcerated and fungating variants. Many are circumferential or almost so. A distinct variant may present as a raised plaque or slight mucosal irregularity, thereby resembling early gastric carcinoma. These varieties may be particularly difficult to recognize endoscopically when visualized end on. They are usually associated with relatively limited spread of tumor and it is in this subgroup that long-term survivors occur. This is because virtually all patients with tumor that infiltrates through the muscularis propria of the esophagus, or who have a lymph node metastasis, die of disease. This is less likely to be the case with plaque-like or finely nodular tumors.

Microscopic pathology

The range of carcinomas that may be seen accompanying Barrett's esophagus is very similar to that encountered in the stomach, there is perhaps an excess of intestinal-type tumors. Well recognized variants resemble so-called pylorocardiac gland cell carcinoma [9, 10]. In addition, it is apparent that squamous differentiation within adenocarcinomas associated with CLE is not uncommon. The adjacent CLE invariably shows intestinal metaplasia, but this is of no value in predicting patients who will develop carcinoma because of its frequency in patients with CLE but without adenocarcinoma. We have also been impressed by the frequent association in the

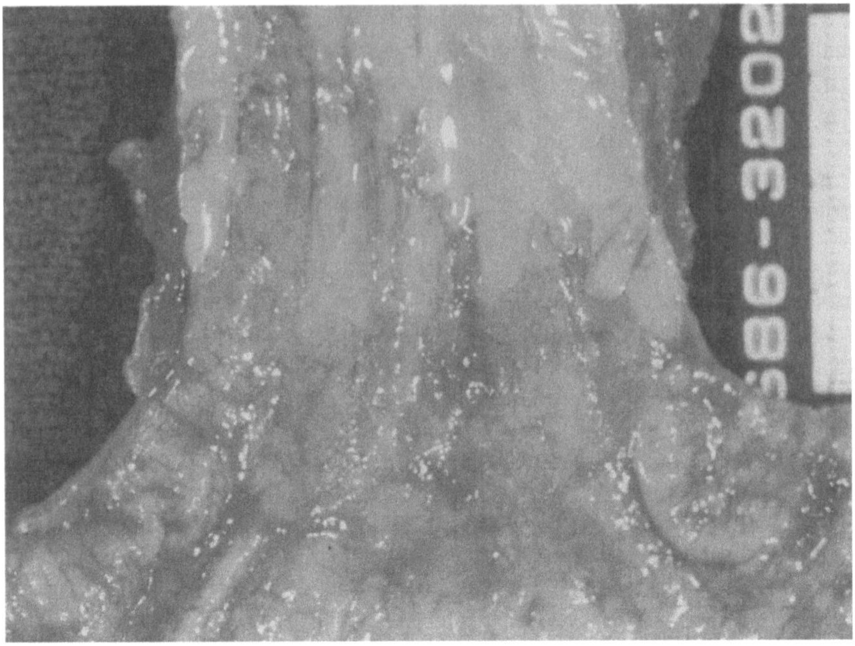

Fig. 4. Gross appearance of Barrett's esophagus with a high irregular Z-line but also a mucosal irregularity just above the anatomic junction of esophagus and stomach "right" which represented an early invasive adenocarcinoma

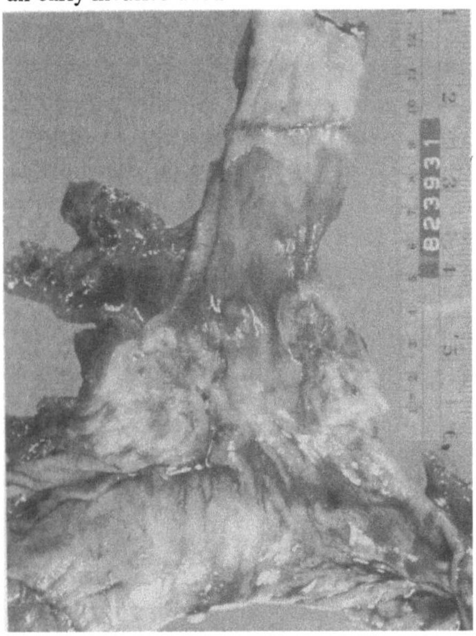

Fig. 5. Typical adenocarcinoma arising within Barrett's mucosa which can usually be seen above the tumor. The transition between non-dysplastic, dysplastic and carcinomatous epithelium was readily demonstrated

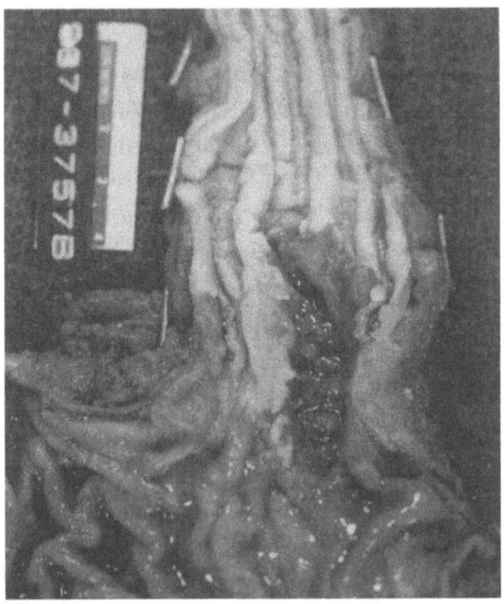

Fig. 6. Photograph of adenocarcinoma at gastroesophageal junction. A small zone of dysplastic intestinalized mucosa was found and entered this tumor beneath which was some mucosal esophageal glands, suggesting strongly that this tumor arose within a columnar-lined esophagus

adjacent mucosa not only of intestinal metaplasia with typical adenomatous dysplasia, but of a second type of dysplasia characterized by a single layer of markedly enlarged hypochromatic nuclei. When both types of dysplasia are present the invasion tends to be associated with the latter rather than the former. Interestingly, but perhaps not surprisingly, there are increasing numbers of mitoses, and abnormal mitoses in the transition from non-dysplastic through dysplastic to carcinomatous mucosa [11].

Differential diagnosis: distinction from gastric carcinoma

The differential diagnosis of adenocarcinoma within the esophagus is shown in Table 1.

Table 1. Differential Diagnosis of Adenocarcinoma of Esophagus

Adenocarcinoma associated with CLE
Adenocarcinoma of gastric cardia extending into the esophagus
Adenocarcinoma of esophageal submucosal glands and duct
Adenocarcinoma associated with heterotopic gastric mucosa
Poorly differentiated squamous carcinoma
Enteroendocrine carcinoma (Oat cell type with glands)

It should be noted that carcinoma associated with submucosal glands tends to resemble salivary gland tumors, but these behave much more aggressively. Overlying mucosa is invariably squamous and not glandular, although it may be ulcerated. The carcinoma associated with heterotopic gastric mucosa is rare and involves the cervical esophagus. The more distal esophagus is entirely squamous and then this is therefore not a problem of differential diagnosis.

Poorly differentiated squamous carcinomas may at times be very difficult to separate from poorly differentiated adenocarcinomas, and traditional techniques including the use of special stains, electron microscopy and immunocytochemistry may be necessary to make this distinction. The most difficult distinction is in the adenocarcinomas of the lower esophagus. The clinical history is unlikely to be of value in that both tumors tend to have occurred primarily in white males with a smoking history [12]. When adjacent (and usually proximal or lateral) epithelium is clearly columnar-lined and contains metaplastic epithelium, similar changes are not demonstrated in the gastric cardia, and the tumor is within the intestinalized epithelium, a reasonable deduction can be made that the tumor has arisen within the CLE of the esophagus. This statement can be strengthened if dysplastic mucosa is found in the adjacent epithelium (see chapter by Potet). The presence of submucosal esophageal glands with overlying glandular mucosa is diagnostic of CLE as these glands do not occur in the stomach. Finally, the lack of dysplasia in gastric cardiac mucosa is negative evidence of a primary gastric tumor, but may not be useful if a pre-existing dysplastic lesion, if it was present, was destroyed by the tumor.

Ultimately, there remains a small group of tumors which straddle the gastroesophageal junction, where it may be impossible to be certain whether the tumor arose in the gastric cardia or lower esophagus. If the epicenter is clearly above the Z-line, or more than about 3 cm above the anatomical junction of esophagus and stomach, this is at best presumptive evidence of an origin in CLE.

References

1. Tileston W (1906) Peptic ulcer of the esophagus. Am J Med Sci 132: 240–265
2. Lyall A (1937) Chronic peptic ulcer of the esophagus: a report of 8 cases. J Surg 24: 534–547
3. Paull A, Trier JS, Dalton MD, Kemp RC, Loeb P, Goyal RK (1976) The histological spectrum of Barrett's esophagus. N Engl J Med 295: 476–480
4. Dahms BB, Rothstein FC (1983) Barrett's esophagus in children: a consequence of chronic gastroesophageal reflux Gastroenterology 18: 318
5. Thompson JJ, Zinsser KR, Enterline HT (1983) Barrett's metaplasia and adenocarcinoma of the esophagus and gastroesophageal junction. Human Pathol 14: 42–61
6. Haggitt RC, Dean PJ (1985) Adenocarcinoma in Barrett's epithelium. In: Spechler JS, Goyal RK, Eds Barrett's Esophagus: Pathophysiology, Diagnosis and Management. New York Elsevier, 153–166
7. Spechler JS, Goyal RK (1986) Barrett's esophagus. N Engl J Med 315: 366–371
8. Skinner DB, Walther BC, Riddell RH, Schmidt H, Iascone C, DeMeester TR (1983) Barrett's esophagus: a comparison of benign and malignant cases. Ann Surg 198: 554–566
9. Teglebjaerg PS, Vetner M (1977) Gastric Carcinoma 1. Acta Pathol Microbiol Scand 85: 519–527
10. Teglebjaerg PS, Vetner M (1977) Gastric Carcinoma 2. Acta Pathol Microbiol Scand; 85: 528–534
11. Rubio C, Riddell RH (1987) Submitted for publication
12. Kalish RJ, Clancy PE, Orringer MB, Appelman HD (1984) A clinical, epidemiologic and morphologic comparison between adenocarcinoma arising in Barrett's esophageal mucosa and in the gastric cardia. Gastroenterology 86: 461–477

What is the status of our understanding of the morphologic predictors of cancer risk in patients with Barrett's mucosa? How do histochemistry and immunohistochemistry help in the prediction of this risk?

F. Potet, V. Duchatelle, and *A. Souqué* (Paris)

Barrett's esophagus or columnar epithelial lined esophagus (CELE) is usually an acquired disorder complicating prolonged reflux esophagitis. CELE consists of several types of columnar epithelium, one of them being a very distinctive epithelium, the "specialized columnar type", resembling intestinal metaplasia (IM) of the stomach. This condition is of considerable interest because several authors have reported a high incidence of adenocarcinoma arising in CELE. In several series, the premalignant character of CELE was established by a 10 to 15% prevalence of adenocarcinomas. In our experience in Beaujon hospital, we found a 10% prevalence in a biopsy series of 44 cases.

An attempt should be made to identify structural and functional changes preceding the development of adenocarcinoma in CELE. Among the changes studied, most involve epithelial differentiation. In order to define the precancerous lesions in CELE, it is possible to study:

1. the different types of dysplasia;
2. the mucus secretion using different methods such as histochemistry and immunohistochemistry.
3. The detection of tumor markers, embryonal antigens or differentiation antigens;
4. the measure of the cell kinetics in the columnar epithelium, using for example incorporation of ^{3}H-thymidine.

Dysplastic lesions

Dysplasia is rarely found in CELE without carcinoma: Skinner noted low grade dysplasia in only 3 cases. In contrast, high grade dysplasia often occurs adjacent to adenocarcinoma. In our experience, we found only 2 cases of moderate dysplasia in 40 cases of CELE without carcinoma and never high grade dysplasia. Because of the low incidence of low grade dysplasia in CELE, we have studied other markers.

Histochemical study in intestinal metaplasia

Jass showed that mucin histochemistry was helpful in further classifying the specialized columnar epithelium. Jass found an incompletely differentiated variant of IM secreting sulfomucins called, type 3, which was associated with well differentiated adenocarcinoma in CELE in surgical specimens. This variant had been previously described in the stomach by other authors. We attempted to define the same profile on biopsy material. 79 patients with symptoms of reflux esophagitis were included in this prospective study. The mean age was 56 years. 53 patients were men and 26 women. The endoscopic examinations and biopsies were performed from January 1981 to January 1986 in the same endoscopic center. The number of biopsy samples taken from each patient ranged between 2 and 12 (mean 3.8). CELE was found in 38 patients 2 of fundic type, on of cardiac type, and 35 with specialized type. The 39 remaining patients had no CELE and normal gastric cardias on biopsy. All the samples were fixed in 3.6% neutral buffered formalin (modified Millonig's phosphate buffer) for 48 hours and paraffin embedded. Serial sections, 5 μ thick, were cut from each sample, and stained with the following: hematoxylin and eosin, Alcian blue-PAS pH 2.5 to differentiate acid from neutral mucins, High iron diamine-alcian blue pH 2.5 to differentiate sulfomucins from sialomucins.

The results showed one IM tpye 1, 12 IM type 2 and 22 IM type 3. Thus, 22 of the 38 CELE cases (57.9%) had IM type 3. Our results, as well as those of other studies, show a higher incidence of type 3 IM in CELE. Among the 39 control (reflux esophagitis without CELE), 29 showed a normal mucin profile of the gastric cardiac mucosa with PAS positivity and alcian blue negative features. In 10 cases, without IM, the columnar cells of the cardia were partly alcian blue positive with AB-PAS and HID positive with HID-AB, demonstrating the presence of sulfomucins in some cells: we called this pattern the "modified mucosa".

With regard to a possible precancerous connotation of type 3 IM, our findings are consistent with the hypothesis that patients, with CELE comprise a very high risk group for adenocarcinoma of the lower esophagus. Moreover, in 10 biopsy specimens taken from the gastroesophageal junction of patients with reflux esophagitis, but without CELE, we found the presence of sulfomucins in columnar cells; we suspect that pattern maybe an intermediate state before the evolution to the IM type 3 in CELE. Finally, it would be of considerable interest to obtain a complete follow-up of patients whose biopsy specimens contained IM type 3 in order to see if this IM type is a useful marker of a precancerous condition in reflux esophagitis.

Immunohistochemical study of mucins

We have used four antibodies against mucins: these antibodies were anti-M_1, and anti-M_3 from Dr Bara, anti-LIMA (large intestin mucus antigen) and anti-SIMA (small intestin mucus antigen) from Dr Ma.

- Anti-M_1 is a monoclonal antibody raised against normal gastric mucins.
- Anti-M_3 is a polyclonal antibody raised against intestinal and colonic mucins.
- Anti-LIMA is a monoclonal antibody raised against normal colonic mucins.
- Anti-SIMA is a monoclonal antibody raised against normal small intestinal mucus.

  Because of the formalin fixation we had to pretreat the slides with pronase (Merck) diluted 0,020% in tris HCl 0.05M pH 8, during 7 minutes.

Indirect 3 step method was employed for monoclonal antibodies, PAP (peroxidase anti peroxidase)method for polyclonal. DAB (diaminobenzidine, Sigma) was used as the developer. Normal gastric and colonic mucosa, formalin fixed, were used as controls.

With anti-M_1, the labelling is localised between the nuclei and the drop of mucus, in the Golgi region. The fixation probably modifies the molecular structure of the mucus. With anti-M_3, labelling is intense and affects all the goblet cells of IM. Intermediate cells are negative with anti-M_3.

Anti-LIMA labels all the goblet cells of IM, and also the intermediate cells in IM 2 and 3. Some of the mucus cells of modified cardiac mucosa are also positive with anti-LIMA. Anti-SIMA, like anti-M_3, labels only goblet cells; the intermediate cells are negative.

Comparison between histo-chemistry and immuno-histo-chemistry

- Anti-M_1 is always positive with normal mucosa, fundic or cardiac, as was expected.
- Types 2 and 3 IM have similar antigenic profiles, with positivity for nearly all the antibodies; all the modified cardiac mucosae are anti-LIMA positive.

The immunohistochemical method couldn't identify a special group within the type 3 IM. It is interesting that types 2 and 3 IM have a close antigenic profile, but some of the type 2 IM are anti-LIMA negative. In contrast all type 3 IM are anti-LIMA positive. The most interesting positivity is that of the intermediate cells. We suggest that the positivity of intermediate cells in IM could reduce IM to two subtypes: anti-LIMA positive and anti-LIMA negative. We emphasize also the labelling in "modified cardiac mucosa", using histochemistry, there are sulfomucins in a few mucus cells, and in immunohistochemistry some of the cells are anti-LIMA positive, resembling the positivity of intermediate cells in type 2 and 3 IM. These features confirm the results of the histochemistry in the modified mucosa.

Finally, the histochemical and immunohistochemical profiles of mucins in CELE resemble the mucin profile in adenocarcinoma arising in CELE. They are also similar to the fetal esophagus where it is possible to find on the surface of the squamous epithelium several mucus cells that have the same characteristics as the cells in CELE.

Other directions of research

Garewall et al. (1986), measuring ornithine decarboxylase (ODC) levels in biopsy specimens from 21 patients with CELE, have found an ODC activity markedly higher than in the control tissues in 15 (71%) of the 21 patients.

Schimamoto et al. (1985), using fluorescent lectins have studied the glycoconjugate expression in CELE. Minor changes in GC expression are seen in the specialized epithelium, but much more distinctive alterations are observed in high grade dysplastic epithelium and in carcinoma arising on CELE.

Conclusion

Several technics are available to detect the functional changes preceding the development of adenocarcinoma in CELE.

One of the best is probably histochemical studies of the mucins.

Unusual and rare epithelial tumors of the esophagus

W. V. Bogomoletz (Reims)

This group of esophageal tumors include a variety of unusual and rare neoplasms [1]. The majority are primary malignant tumors; polypoid carcinoma, malignant melanoma, oat cell carcinoma, etc. Squamous papilloma is a benign tumor. Metastatic carcinoma to the esophagus is also a rare occurrence. Different histogenetic origins have been attributed to these uncommon tumors: squamous epithelial for polypoid carcinoma, neuroendocrine for oat cell carcinoma or melanocytic for malignant melanoma. The relevant literature consists essentially of single case reports, with few published series, the latter mainly from Japan [5, 6, 8]. Hence, it is often difficult to meaningfully assess data on the incidence, clinical aspects, histopathological features, response to treatment and patients survival. The classification, cell origin and terminology of these rare tumors of the esophagus have also been the subject of much controversy.

Squamous Papilloma

Squamous papilloma of the esophagus is a very rare lesion, mostly described in females and considered as benign. It usually arises as a single lesion, but instances of multiple squamous papillomas have been reported. Squamous papilloma tends to be asymptomatic and can be located in any portion of the esophagus. Endoscopically, it presents as a fairly small and warty lesion. Microscopy is characterized by many finger-like projections of connective tissue covered by stratified squamous epithelium. Squamous papilloma should be differentiated from inflammatory fibrous polyp. The etiology of esophageal squamous papilloma is unknown, but a viral origin has been suggested. There is no evidence that squamous papillomas have any significant malignant potential.

Polypoid Carcinoma

Polypoid carcinoma of the esophagus is a rare variant of conventional squamous cell carcinoma and is characterized by spindle cell metaplasia. For many years, cases of polypoid carcinoma were described as either “carcinosarcomas” or “pseudosarcomas”, thus reflecting controversial opinions about the origin and nature of this tumor.The unifying concept of polypoid carcinoma has been established in the last decade, on the basis of clinicopathological studies [3, 5].

The incidence of polypoid carcinoma is difficult to assess because of the varying terminology applied to this tumor, prior to the emergence of its unifying concept. Patients are mostly males, aged 50 to 75 and present with dysphagia and weight loss. Polypoid carcinoma arises as a large and pedunculated mass, from the middle or lower thirds of the esophagus. The prognosis of polypoid carcinoma differs little from that of conventional squamous carcinoma.

Histologically, the tumor includes a localized area of conventional in situ or invasive squamous carcinoma (usually found near the base), rarely of adenocarcinoma or undifferentiated carcinoma. The bulk of the tumor consists of spindle cells mimicking a sarcomatous proliferation. The squamous nature of this spindle cell metaplasia has been demonstrated by electron microscopy or immunocytochemistry.

Oat Cell Carcinoma

Oat cell carcinoma of the esophagus is a highly malignant tumor, morphologically indistinguishable from typical oat cell of the bronchus [2]. It often shows electron microscopy and histochemical evidence of being related to the APUD system. Over 70 cases have been reported, mostly from Japan. The incidence has been variously recorded from 0.05% to 7.6% of all carcinomas of the esophagus. Patients are aged 50 to 60, with a male predominance. Oat cell carcinoma of the esophagus usually occurs as a single and large polypoid tumor, arising in the middle or lower third and causing dysphagia. Like its counterpart in the bronchus, oat cell carcinoma of the esophagus is an aggressive tumor. Patients die rapidly with widespread metastases, despite surgery, radiotherapy or chemotherapy.

Microscopically, oat cell carcinoma of the esophagus resembles its bronchial counterpart, with characteristic sheets of small anaplastic cells. Other growth patterns can be encountered: nests, anastomosing cords or ribbons. "Rosettes" can also be found. Squamous or glandular differentiation may be present. Necrosis is frequent. Argyrophilic stains (Grimelius) usually demonstrate positive granules in tumor cells; however, some cases are entirely negative. Ultrastructural studies have shown the presence of neurosecretory granules in 3% to 50% of tumor cells. Ectopic hormone production (ACTH, calcitonin) has been noted in a few cases. The histogenesis of oat cell carcinoma of the oesophagus has not been entirely resolved. The tumor could arise from argyrophilic cells present in the esophageal mucosa or from totipotential "reserve" cells.

"Pure" cases of oat cell carcinoma should be separated from "combined" cases, the latter containing oat cells admixed with squamous or glandular elements. Rare instances of tumors lacking evidence of neuroendocrine features or squamous differentiation, should be best classified as "non-oat cell anaplastic (undifferentiated) carcinoma" [4].

Adenoid Cystic Carcinoma

Adenoid cystic carcinoma of the esophagus is a fairly rare tumor (about 50 cases reported) [7]. Histologically, it resembles adenoid cystic carcinoma of salivary gland origin, but shows greater aggressiveness (patients dying with widespread metastases). Its incidence has been reported as 0.75% to 5% of all esophageal carcinomas. Patients are mostly males, in their sixties, and present with dysphagia. The tumor arises as a large and fungating growth, from the middle or lower portion of the esophagus.

Adenoid cystic carcinoma shows a characteristic microscopic cribriform pattern; solid and basaloid patterns have also been described. Mucin secretion can be identified in cystic spaces. Focal areas of necrosis, nuclear pleomorphism and increased mitotic rate are often noted. Adenoid cystic carcinoma should be distinguished from adenocarcinoma arising in Barrett's esophagus.

Adenosquamous and Mucoepidermoid Carcinomas

Adenosquamous and mucoepidermoid carcinomas are characterized by an admixture of squamous and glandular elements [6]. These tumors constitute a small subgroup of primary adenocarcinoma of the esophagus. Adenosquamous and mucoepidermoid carcinomas usually arise in the lower portion of the esophagus, close to the esophagogastric junction or cardia. The degree of differentiation of both squamous and glandular elements is variable, from poorly differentiated examples ("adenosquamous") to well differentiated instances ("mucoepidermoid"), the latter closely resembling identical tumors from salivary gland origin. Cases reported as "mucoepidermoid" have shown a distinctive aggressive tumor behaviour. It has been suggested that mucoepidermoid carcinoma could arise from submucosal esophageal glands and ducts.

Malignant Melanoma

Over 100 cases of primary malignant melanoma of the esophagus have been published, at least half from Japan [8]. The incidence has been quoted from 3% to 3.9% of all primary malignant esophageal tumors other than conventional squamous cell carcinoma. Patients are aged 60 to 80, with males outnumbering females; they generally present with symptoms resulting from esophageal obstruction. The tumor usually arises as a single, large and polypoid growth (pigmented or not), from the middle or lower portion of the esophagus. Prognosis is poor and most patients die with disseminated metastases, despite surgery, chemotherapy or radiotherapy.

The tumor tends to be nodular and is histologically identical to mucosal malignant melanoma arising in other sites. It consists of diffuse sheets of pleomorphic cells. Melanin pigment can be identified by conventional histochemical methods (Masson Fontana silver method, bleaching by oxidising agents, DOPA). The presence of melanosomes in tumor cells has been confirmed by ultrastructural studies. Junctional activity is found adjacent to the tumor in about 40% of cases. The tumor may also be associated with patchy or diffuse melanosis of the esophageal mucosa; melanosis is characterized by melanin-laden melanocytes in the basal cells of the squamous epithelium. When a malignant melanoma arising in the esophagus is also found associated with adjacent junctional activity and mucosal melanosis, this is good evidence of its primary origin.

The histogenesis of both melanosis and primary malignant melanoma of the esophagus remains controversial. Two possibilities can be envisaged: embryonic migration of melanocytes from the neutral crest or in situ differentiation from totipotential "reserve" cells (located in the basal layer of the squamous epithelium).

Metastatic Carcinoma of the Esophagus

Metastatic spread of carcinoma to the esophagus is blood-borne. Furthermore, and by definition, the primary site should not be contiguous with the esophagus. Hence, direct extension of carcinoma from the stomach, hypopharynx, thyroid or tracheobronchial tract should not be considered as metastatic carcinoma.

The incidence of genuine metastatic carcinoma in the esophagus is estimated has 1% to 3% of all patients dying with carcinoma, particularly from lung and breast. Clinical and radiological findings are usually suggestive of primary malignant disease.

References

1. Bogomoletz WV Rare tumours of the esophagus. In Whitehead R, ed. Gastrointestinal Pathology. Edinburgh: Churchill Livingstone, in press
2. Briggs JC, Ibrahim NBN (1983) Oat cell carcinoma of the oesophagus: a clinicopathological study of 23 cases. Histopathology 7: 261–277
3. Du Boulay CEH, Isaacson P (1981) Carcinoma of the oesophagus with spindle cell features. Histopathology 5: 403–414
4. Ho KJ, Herrera GA, Jones JM, Alexander CB (1984) Small cell carcinoma of the esophagus: evidence for a unified histogenesis. Hum Pathol 15: 460–468
5. Osamura RY, Shimamura K, Hata J et al (1978) Polypoid carcinoma of the esophagus. A unifying concept for "carcinosarcoma" and "pseudosarcoma". Am J Surg Pathol 2: 201–208
6. Suzuki H, Nagayo T (1980) Primary tumors of the esophagus other than squamous cell carcinoma – Histologic classification and statistics in the surgical and autopsied material in Japan. Int Adv Surg Oncol 3: 73–109
7. Sweeney EC, Cooney T (1980) Adenoid cystic carcinoma of the esophagus. A light and electron microscopic study. Cancer (1980) 45: 1516–1525
8. Takubo K, Kanda Y, Ishii M et al (1983) Primary malignant melanoma of the esophagus. Hum Pathol 14: 727–730

Stromal and lymphoid tumors of the esophagus

H.D. Appelman (Ann Arbor)

In the most recent (1977) World Health Organization classification of esophageal tumors, the non-epithelial benign tumors are designated as leiomyomas and others, and the malignant tumors, as leiomyosarcomas and others [1]. In fact, the two most common stromal tumors of the esophagus are the leiomyoma and the granular cell tumor [2]. Everything else is so rare that most of us have not even encountered examples.

The number of reported cases of leiomyosarcoma of the esophagus is quite small. It appears that many of the tumors designated as leiomyosarcoma are probably the spindle cell aspects of the pseudosarcomatous squamous cell carcinoma. We know that this spindle cell component can assume a variety of differentiating features. It is always important to look carefully for malignant epithelium in any lumpy polypoid tumor of the esophagus that resembles sarcoma. Fastidious sampling of such tumors are quite likely to yield carcinomatous foci. In fact, there even have been reported cases of leiomyosarcoma of the esophagus with adjacent squamous cell carcinomas, further evidence that many such tumors are really pseudosarcomas.

Probably at least one of every other kind of stromal tumor has been reported in the esophagus, and there is no reason to doubt that at least one of everything will occur here. For instance, there have been a half dozen reported cases of esophageal rhabdomyosarcomas and recently two cases of synovial sarcoma. The bulk of this discussion will be limited to those tumors which we tend to see relatively frequently, namely the leiomyomas and the granular cell tumors.

*

Most *leiomyomas* of esophagus arise in the muscularis propria, although, on occasions, a microscopic tumor of the muscularis mucosae is discovered serendipitously. Over half occur in the lower third with about a third in the middle and the rest in the upper esophagus. This is a somewhat different distribution than that for squamous cell carcinoma, a predominantly middle third lesion. Actually, this distribution probably only refers to the clinically apparent or solitary lesions. There is a group of small intramuscular leiomyomas, the "seedling leiomyomas", which are probably much more common, and at present, we are not certain of their distribution, although they seem to be mostly in the cardioesophageal junction area [3]. Most of the clinically apparent leiomyomas are small, but, occasionally, monstrous tumors have been reported, weighing a kilogram or more. The gross and microscopic appearances of esophageal leiomyomas are exactly the same as for leiomyomas arising in the uterus. They are firm, white, whorled and bulge above the cut surface. The constituent cells are typical smooth muscle cells in whorls and fascicles. Variable amounts of secondary changes such as liquefaction, fibrosis and calcification occur. Occasional cases of circumferential leiomyomas have been reported; these may not be leiomyomas at all, but examples of diffuse leiomyomatosis which produces a multinodular thickening of the muscularis propria of the lower esophagus and proximal stomach. This looks like a collection of circumferential confluent leiomyomas, but it may simply be a nodular muscular hypertrophy [4].

The *granular cell tumors* are small, rarely symptomatic, intramural lesions. In most studies, the tumor cells appear to be ultrastructurally and immunohistochemically variants of Schwann cells filled with granules which are giant phagolysosomes, containing granular and membranous debris. The tumor cells are spindled and arranged in fascicles which involve submucosa and lamina propria, often obliterating the muscularis mucosae and extending immediately up to the basilar epithelium. Therefore, a full thickness biopsy of the squamous epithelium will likely contain the tumor cells at the very base. The overlying epithelium may be hyperplastic or normal or thinner than normal. The distribution of these tumors tends to be much the same as that for leiomyomas. With the increased use of upper endoscopy, more and more of these are being found incidently in asymptomatic patients.

There is very little published information about *lymphomas* of the esophagus because there are so few cases [4, 5]. In a compendium of primary gastrointestinal lymphomas reported in nine series between 1969 and 1985, covering almost 1.500

cases, only three lymphomas of the esophagus were included, an incidence of 0.2%. Review of the English language literature over the past ten years produced a scattering of case reports and a series of eight patients in the radiologic literature. This latter reference indicated that the most common radiologic abnormality was continuous involvement of the distal esophagus and proximal stomach, so many, if not most, of these cases probably were not primary esophageal lymphomas, but were gastric primaries with secondary extension to the esophagus. In both the hospital based and referral case load of the Department of Pathology at the University of Michigan, not a single primary esophageal lymphoma was found among a total of over 300 primary gastrointestinal lymphomas, but we did find a few secondary lymphomas which involved the esophagus as part of systemic spread. Even fewer cases of localized nodular lymphoid hyperplasia or pseudolymphoma have been uncovered in the esophagus.

One recent minor change in the characteristics of esophageal nonepithelial tumors involves the acquired immunodeficiency syndromes. A few lymphomas and patches of Kaposi's sarcoma in the esophagus occur in patients with AIDS, but at the moment, there are only sporadic case reports. We shall see whether this becomes more of a significant issue and if esophageal neoplasia becomes more important in this syndrome as larger numbers of cases are evaluated.

References

1. Oota K, Sobin LH (1977) Histological typing of gastric and oesophageal tumors. World Health Organization, Geneva
2. Appelman HD (1984) Stromal tumors of the esophagus, stomach and duodenum, Ch 7, in Pathology of the Esophagus, Stomach and Duodenum, Appelman HD, ed Churchill-Livingstone, New York
3. Takubo K, Nagawa H, Tsuchiya S et al (1981) Seedling leiomyoma of the esophagus and esophagogastric junction zone. Hum Pathol 12: 1006
4. Enterline H, Thompson J (1984) Pathology of the Esophagus. Ch 10: Non-epithelial tumors. Springer-Verlag, New York
5. Platz CE (1984) Lymphoid proliferations of the stomach. Ch 8 in Pathology of the Esophagus, Stomach and Duodenum, Appelman HD, ed Churchill-Livingstone, New York

Current state of the various surveys and therapeutic trials conducted by the group OESO

Robert Giuli (Paris)

After the first stage of our joint work, shown in a *retrospective* study dealing with 2400 resected cancers published in 1980 [1], a second stage was achieved by the *prospective* study presented at our 1984 Congress and later published [2]. Today, the growth of OESO, comprising working sections of such different specialties as surgery, intensive care, ENT, pathology, endoscopy, radiotherapy and chemotherapy, has enabled the Group to enter the third stage.

*

It is a matter, this time, of *a randomized therapeutic trial* on **cancer of the esophagus**, that I am coordinating in collaboration with David Kelsen (Sloan Kettering Cancer Center of New York) and Dr Sancho-Garnier. Professor Appelman (Ann Arbor) has accepted the very heavy responsibility of unifying the different anatomo-pathologic aspects relating to each of the patients in this study.

The needed number of cases is quite important: **500**, affected by a potentially curable disease.

This trial is aimed at comparing, at threefold level, the effects of post-operative radiotherapy or peri-operative chemotherapy in relation to surgical resection alone.

On the basis of existing publications, we have chosen *postoperative* radiotherapy, administered to the patient 6 to 8 weeks after the operation in a dose of 45 Grays over 3 months, in 5 sessions of 1.6 Grays per week (P^r = F. Baillet, Paris).

The chemotherapy protocol is that developed by Kelsen: *preoperatively*, it comprises a combination of Cis-platinum (2 cycles), Vindesine (7 cycles) and Bleomycin (8 cycles), the collective treatment being halted about 3 weeks before operation.

6 to 8 weeks after operation, chemotherapy is resumed using a combination of Cis-platinum (3 cycles) and Vindesine (12 cycles) this time without Bleomycin. This *postoperative* regime lasts 7 months.

*

38 teams* from 16 different countries in Europe, America and Asia have accepted the major discipline involved in this collaborative trial of surgery, chemotherapy and radiotherapy by different teams of specialists in these fields, and the completion of complex forms accepted by each team. For each patient, the collection of the reports is done mainly at the Institut Gustave Roussy at Villejuif. Today (June 1987), a little over a year after the start of this trial, 209 of the 500 patients required have already been randomized.

* Participating countries: Europe: Belgium, Spain, France, Hungary, Italy, Poland, West Germany, Turkey, Yugoslavia. America: Argentina, Brazil, Chile, United States. Asia: China, India, Japan

Among these, 65 have been randomized in the surgical group, 73 in the radiotherapy group and 71 in the chemotherapy group**. In this last group, the need for long-term treatment, extending over 9 months, clearly explains why we were unable so far to give any result for a trial that began only a little more than a year ago. The only information that we can as yet provide is that the age limit of 75 years fixed for the inclusion of our patients does not seem, as far as the records received indicate, to require an attenuation of the doses. Only one accident has been recorded, due to renal failure following the hyperhydration necessary after Cisplatinum treatment.

For the totality of operations performed, the operative mortality is still 14%. Despite the requirement that each patient included be a priori radically operable, 14 purely exploratory operations have been performed.

Among the other patients, the size of the total esophagectomy group (47 cases) is noteworthy. In nearly 80% of cases lymph-node eradication was combined with the surgical procedure, achieved in a little more than half the cases by a mainly right-sided approach; the other half were divided almost equally between blunt dissections, without thoracotomy, and left-sided thoracotomy. Finally, as already noted in our first prospective study, not all surgeons seem to have adopted the mechanical method of anastomosis since 64% of patients were dealt with by manual anastomosis.

Two parallel investigations are being conducted during this therapeutic trial. One of these, already discussed by Dr Appelman (see p. 809), concerns the evaluation of a **prognostic anatomo-pathologic index** of resected tumors: it involves the different morphologic features of the removed tumor besides its specifically histologic nature; this relates to the main axis of the tumor, the state of the tumor margins and the general form of the lesion.

At the same time, in an attempt to discover the reasons for the very considerable differences existing between the statistics published by the different teams, a **preoperative clinical evaluation** of the patients is currently being tested, using 4 different scores. The clinical features that may help in assessing a more or less favorable prognosis before operation include: age, pulmonary insufficiency, chronic infection, wasting, evidence of malnutrition, length of history of symptoms and patient cooperation.

*

On the first day of this Congress, I presented important figures provided by Professor Huang during our first meeting (1984) that noted an incidence of malignant degeneration of 66% for severe dysplasias discovered by routine investigation in Chinese patients. OESO has therefore supplied the more important endoscopic centers in the different countries collaborating in this study with a protocol for

---

** As regards chemotherapy, we wish to thank the following firms: Logeais and Roger-Bellon (France), Eli Lilly (France and Great Britain) and Nippon Kayaku (Japan), who help us to carry out this study and supply chemotherapeutic drugs to certain foreign countries routine endoscopic detection of **dysplastic lesions** of the esophagus. Its aim is to test by randomization the long-term effect of their treatment by retinoid substances, in relation to specific monitoring (see p. 94).

Finally, apart from these trials, the OESO Group is currently trying to carry out a very large-scale epidemiologic enquiry: for this, we have contacted the Mutualité Française, which has agreed to supply several hundreds of thousands of its clients with a questionnaire we have prepared in order to discover the exact incidence, in a million persons, of clinical symptoms of **esophageal reflux** and of **caustic burns** of the esophagus.

All these factors form an essential element of our investigations, allowing us to envisage the early detection of lesions liable to malignant degeneration and therefore our intervention in the prevention of cancer of the esophagus.

*

During the organization of this Congress I had the idea of suggesting to teams, that so desired, that they might actively participate in our clinical research studies by forwarding to us their own protocol plan. The response far exceeded our expectations, and has placed Mme Sancho-Garnier and myself in an impossible situation of choice. 16 different protocols were sent to us:

• In the *cancer field,* Dr Philippe Bernard (Centre de Forcilles) has developed in his dietetic center a project for assessing the nutritional status of patients according to the stage of the neoplastic disease, tested mainly by administration of histamine. At the same time, Dr Elman, anesthetist and intensive care specialist at the Hôpital Beaujon, has developed a project in an attempt to establish a correlation between malnutrition, respiratory muscular fatigue and the respiratory complications of the operations proposed for these patients.

• Another project, submitted by Dr Pinotti of São Paulo, deals with a comparison of treatment of *megaesophagus* by surgical and nonsurgical procedures.

• Dr Lerut (Leuwen) suggests the very interesting morphologic and histochemical enzyme comparison of the anomalies presented by the cricothyroid muscle in patients with a pharyngoesophageal *diverticulum.*

But most of the protocols put forward deal with **peptic esophageal disease.** Two come from Dr DeMeester (Omaha, Nebraska) and are of a more *physiologic* nature: one on the role of hypersecretion in the harmfulness of reflux, the other on the differences between peptic and drug-induced strictures. At the same time, and on the same lines, Dr Bremner of Johannesburg suggests an interesting study on the role of alkaline reflux in the columnar-lined esophagus.

The treatment of gastroesophageal reflux has also been the subject of many protocols:

• one, also proposed by Dr DeMeester, is on the future of anti-reflux operations in terms of preoperative manometry.

• The other, also from Dr Bremner, deals with the role of the type of operation performed in the development of the columnar lined esophagus towards late complications.

• At the same time, Dr Obertop (Maestricht) suggests a postoperative comparison of Nissen's operation and a cardiopexy procedure, while Dr Henderson, of Toronto, wishes to define the criteria to be used in choosing an effective procedure for peptic stricture of the esophagus.

*

The problems of **Barrett's esophagus** are particularly important:

- Dr Lerut (Leuwen) and Husemann (Erlangen) suggest evaluation of the true incidence of malignant degeneration of these lesions by long-term surveillance of patients subjected to esophago-gastroduodenoscopy.
- Similarly, Dr Conio (Genoa) proposes to define the real incidence of adenocarcinoma in Barrett's esophagus by long-term follow-up of these patients.
- In this context, we were very interested in the proposal of Dr McCallum (Charlottesville, Virginia), suggesting evaluation of the true incidence of Barrett's esophagus and its long-term surveillance using a protocol currently developed by the American College of Gastroenterology. Dr Young of Melbourne also suggests an extensive study on this subject.

*

It the refere appears to us, as a normal manifestation of a certain continuity, since the inaugural thesis of 1950 signed by Madame Lortat-Jacob [3], that already at that time dealt with the problems of esophageal ulceration, to proceed with a vast world therapeutic trial with different interested teams devoted to the lesion described al most simultaneously nearly 40 years ago by *Barrett* in Great Britain and *Lortat-Jacob* in France under the name of endobrachyesophagus.

A trial of such extent should involve surgeons as well as epidemiologists, anatomo-pathologists and gastroenterologists. A start up meeting will be organized on March 12, 1988 with all the teams involved, to effectively develop a protocol for this multidisciplinary multicenter study, an international effort that is consistent with the vocation of the OESO Group.

References

1. Giuli R, Gignoux M (1980) Treatment of Carcinoma of the Esophagus. Retrospective study of 2400 patients. Ann Surg 192, 1: 44–52
2. Giuli R, Sancho-Garnier H (1986) Diagnostic, therapeutic and prognosis features of Cancers of the Esophagus: results of the International prospective study conducted by the OESO group (790 patients). Surgery 99, 5: 14–622
3. Smaith, Lortat-Jacob, Madeleine (1950) Cinq observations d'ulcère peptique de l'œsophage Thèse pour le Doctorat en médecine, Paris

General conclusions and future outlook

Ronald Belsey (Chicago)

Seeking a consensus from this wide ranging symposium is complicated by the diversity of opinions expressed. A few outstanding problems have been clarified; others have been doubly confused.

*

Achalasia

With one notable exception, it is generally agreed that a synchronous antireflux proceedure following myotomy is advisable. The type of antireflux proceedure is critical: any proceedure involving a 360° fundoplication is too aggressive in the presence of the dyskinaesia characteristic of the anomaly.

The persisting problem is the early detection of malignancy, before or after myotomy. Successful palliative surgery does not reduce the risk of subsequent malignancy. The problem of long term monitoring without reducing the patient to a psychological wreck from chronic anxiety has yet to be addressed.

*

Corrosive strictures

There is still no proof that any form of emergency treatment can limit the extent of the trauma and discourage subsequent undilatable stenosis. Any prospective study is hardly feasable. Aggressive attempts to dilate potentially undilatable strictures, adding trauma to trauma, can result in fatal mediastinitis or compromise subsequent definitive surgery by rendering resection technically impossible.

The major problem: resection or bypass? The statistical risk of malignant degeneration has been obscured by the average interval of 40 years after the initial chemical trauma, but there are other indications for resection, such as acquired reflux esophagitis and haemorrhage.

*

Peptic esophagitis

The medical treatment of esophagitis has been discussed at length: no more convincing proof of the success of drug and non-operative therapy can be documented than the dramatic decline in the observed incidence of undilatable peptic strictures. Early prophylactic antireflux surgery may have contributed to the decline, but the gastroenterologists remain sceptical of the value of surgery as currently performed.

Many questions on this program referred to the histological diagnosis of esophagitis has been discussed at length but confuses the relative incidence of this complication, and has been rejected by the majority of surgeons, in the absence of irrefutable endoscopic evidence, as an indication for surgical treatment.

We had proof, during this symposium, that evidence is accumulating on the contribution of delayed gastric emptying to the severity of esophagitis and the surgical control; radionucleide transit studies are now a necessary routine element in the investigation of every case of reflux. Radiological studies have proved less informative.

Bile reflux mainly, following gastric surgery, may be a significant factor but the diagnosis and management of alkaline reflux remain debatable.

*

Peptic stenosis

With earlier diagnosis, this complication is now preventable. Previous discussion on management has been most often rendered largely sterile by the current tendancy to designate any radiological zone of luminal narrowing as a "stricture", ignoring the fact that acute and subacute inflammatory changes such as oedema and localised spasm can result in these radiological changes. Any such narrowing that responds permanently to one or two dilatations is not a stricture and should not be designated as such. The non-operative treatment of "strictures" has thus acquired a spurious reputation for effectiveness: For practical purposes, the classification of such radiological manifestations as dilatable or undilatable will prove of greater value.

The management of undilatable strictures, including those that fail to respond with adequate relief following multiple dilatations over a prolonged period, could have been the subject of longer discussions; two further problems arise in this context: the dangers of dilatation cannot be ignored. A negative endoscopic biopsy examination of a stricture does not rule out cancer.

*

Antireflux surgery

During these four days, we could note that the "merry-go-round" of surgical antireflux techniques continues unabated, embellished by enthusiastic claims for success and counter claims of failure; attempts to prove that the techniques of others are useless or downright dangerous have acquired international condonation.

The early results of all techniques, in terms of immediate reflux control, are comparable. Postoperative complications are glossed over or forgotten; these claims have to be viewed in perspective against a background of the current spate of "redo" surgery for recurrent reflux following the failure of prior surgical adventures.

After 30 years and many thousands of such proceedures, there are few objective assessments of the long term results and late complications; it will be a sad day for the organisers of surgical symposia and the editors of journals if we ever agree on a "best" antireflux technique, however such an eventuality appears extremely unlikely – fortunately.

The disenchantment of the gastroenterologists with so much surgical success and clinical failure can be appreciated. Certain techniques have undergone annual modifications, involving the inevitable revision of claims for the success of prior versions. Other techniques have survived without the "benefits" of repeated modifications.

As was pointed out, the only recent technical advances have been the advocacy of intraoperative manometry and endoscopy in an attempt to refine certain techniques, but the necessity for such time consuming interference is not generally accepted by surgeons.

*

Dysplasia

In the view of this author, the discussions on the pathology and diagnosis of dysplasia have proved the most illuminating topics on the program.

The prior confusion concerning the criteria for the histological diagnosis may be responding to attempts to correlate with clinical prognosis: there is still no convincing evidence that dysplasia can be reversed by successful antireflux surgery, nor has the statistical risk of adenocarcinoma been finally agreed.

The finding of carcinoma-in-situ in association with severe dysplasia has been advanced as justification for resection: the prognosis in such cases, with or without resection, has yet to be clarified by long term follow-up; the concept of resection has been raised repeatedly during these discussions, ignoring the probable operative mortality of 10%, possibly comparable to the ultimate mortality from adenocarcinoma in untreated cases.

*

Reconstruction for benign disease

Indications and surgical techniques have been reviewed briefly. The emphasis has been on the early results. However the operative survivors can reasonably be expected to live for many years and the incidence of the late complications will probably parallel the duration of survival.

The little information offered on the late functional results of various reconstructive techniques led to the concensus that replacement with isoperistaltic segments of left colon incurs the least risk of disabling late sequelae. The futility and dangers of antiperistaltic interposition proceedures have finally been accepted.

*

Barrett's esophagus

It was confirmed that the true incidence of the anomaly is unknown. Confusion arises partly from the lack of general agreement on the extent of columnar epithelialisation that can justify a diagnosis of "Barrett's esophagus", another instance of the fallacy of eponymus terminology: In the condition originally described by Barrett, the mucosal junction was situated at the level of the aortic arch, there was no doubt about that. Currently 3 cm or more of acquired columnar epithelialisation is so designated.

The anomaly can occur as an incidental finding in an asymptomatic subject, not infrequently a child, and the debate on etiology, congenital or acquired as the end stage of ulcerative esophagitis, has tended to become emotional rather than rational. But does it matter which theory ultimately prevails?

The theory of Savary and Monnier that both etiological factors may play a role will probably be accepted when all the available evidence is collated. Histological examination, rarely reported, of the full thickness of the wall of the Barrett's segment in specimens resected from children with no history of esophagitis, for undilatable strictures, does not suggest the end stage of a chronic ulcerative esophagitis with progressive mucosal regeneration. And where are the intermediate stages approaching the aortic arch?

Evidence produced by the various contributors of this symposium reveals the cell population of the columnar epithelium to be far more complex than was previously assumed. There is scant corroborated evidence that regression can follow successful antireflux surgery, nor is there any evidence that the risk of adenocarcinoma can be reduced in the same way.

The indications for antireflux surgery are now generally agreed, but resection may ultimately be necessary if the Barrett's epithelium continues to secrete erosive acid pepsin above the restored sphincter.

Those surgeons who claim that all cases result from ulcerative esophagitis are morally bound to recommend antireflux surgery, even in the asymptomatic subject, to limit further progression of the process and hopefully deter major complications. Barrett's esophagus is a premalignant condition so again antireflux surgery might be advocated "to prevent a subsequent malignancy": the imagination bogles at the consequences of such a policy.

The major persisting problem relates to the incidence, diagnosis and evaluation of severity of dysplasia in the columnar epithelium. Severe dysplasia may be an indication for resection, again with a probable operative mortality of 10%. The incidence of adenocarcinoma varies widely in series reported in this symposium.

In the management of cases with moderate dysplasia, it has been suggested that antireflux surgery should be followed by long term monitoring with frequent endoscopic biopsy examination. Hiebert has pointed out that in North America alone such a program would cost the state billions of dollars annually and incur the risk of several hundred instrumental perforations.

The whole problem of the early diagnosis of malignant degeneration in benign disease, often in the asymptomatic patient, and long term monitoring, demand cool headed debate and objective review of the possible incidence, relative risks, the economic and psychological implications.

*

Future outlook

A survey of the numbers of papers devoted to the major topics on this program indicates the current state of play and may suggest future developments.

Esophageal function

The contribution of the "lower sphincter" to the control of reflux has been largely debunked to the status of a sheep in wolf's clothing. The main contribution of the esophageal lab has been the objective assessment of reflux and the elucidation of dyskinaesia, apart from the employment of an army of gastroenterologists, technicians, research fellows, and others.

It must be recalled that all current antireflux surgical techniques were perfected long before the facilities of the esophageal lab were available, and the contribution of these sophisticated investigations to the improvement of surgical technique has been therefore negligible; the suspicion that the human subject is the most sensitive instrument for diagnosing reflux and indicating the need for surgical treatment may be on the threshold of revival. Esophageal function is so labile that a single study may be grossly misleading and a further source of error and confusion is the current tendancy to base dogmatic conclusions on solitary studies in individual cases. It is suggested in all sincerity that any further discussion on the "LES" be banned for the next 5 years.

Criteria

During this Congress, emphasis was placed on the urgent need today for the establishment of universally acceptable criteria for the indications for surgical treatment in benign disease and for the objective assessment and documentation of the long term results. Despite Earlam's theory, long term follow-up is possible and should be accorded more than the customary lip service.

Failures

The high incidence of late surgical failure is unacceptable, and we observed the spate of "redo" surgery for recurrent reflux and the poor functional results of some reconstructive techniques can be cited; there has certainly been not enough attempt to analyse the causes of failure and relate them to the initial technique. The bottom line is the simple equation: "no follow-up, no failures".

Operative risks

Throughout this symposium, not enough attention has been directed to the outstanding problems of postoperative morbidity and mortality, and their prevention. The major killers are still anastomotic failure and pulmonary complications. A cynic may claim that in spite of highly sophisticated postoperative intensive care the patients continue to die just as frequently but rather more mysteriously. This subject, already the theme of several sessions during the first Congress of OESO on cancer of the esophagus, must be accorded top priority in any future symposia on esophageal surgery.

Experimental surgery

The potentially most rewarding experimental laboratory at our disposal is the operating room. The animal laboratory may afford confirmation of data that has already been proven in the OR: however, this potential goldmine of essential data has been largely negated by the abysmal quality of operation reporting. Any surgeon confronted by the problems of "redo" surgery will testify to the uselessness of the available records of prior proceedures. Any operation report dictated by other than the operating surgeon, or delayed 24 hours or longer, is sterile as a source of valid information.

Regrettably, many surgical publications are based on this misinformation, and can be grossly misleading. This is a further problem which must be addressed with determined aggression.

Pediatric surgery

Although pediatric surgeons participated in this symposium, the future productivity of the specialty demands much closer cooperation between them and "adult" esophageal surgeons. Both disciplines can benefit materially from the interchange of experience and philosophy.

The choice of subjects for examination at future meetings is relevant to audience appeal and to further progress of the long term work undertaken by OESO.

Thanks to Giuli's original formula, we this time avoided a conference emasculated by repetition, with the presentation "ad nauseam" of quite similar papers.

The work of the Group must continue to relate to practical problems we all face and discuss, thus commanding sustained interest and audience participation.

Among those topics recently suggested, the multicenter international study, now to be undertaken by OESO on Barrett's esophagus, seems to me of foremost importance: it is likely to elicit a working consensus on definition and diagnosis, on etiology, on the relationship of subsequent malignant disease, and on the treatment as dictated by the wide variations on the physiopathology of the syndrome.

Such an efficient attempt at placing an embargo on the current loose talk on the syndrome must prove, for all of us, to be of the greatest practical benefit.

In conclusion I wish, on behalf of the assembled company, to pay a most sincere tribute to my friend Professor Lortat-Jacob, the President of Honour of OESO, "éminence grise" and doyen of esophageal surgery, who for many years has been a constant source of inspiration to surgeons throughout the whole world.

Conclusions of the Congress

Jean-Louis Lortat-Jacob (Paris)

Only a very brief commentary is required from me at the conclusion of such a very successful Congress. Once again, I emphasize the value of the multicenter statistical enquiries to which OESO has been devoted by definition since its creation. Similarly, I record how the multidisciplinary nature of the participants, with which we were not familiar in our traditional congresses, has yielded so much diagnostic and therapeutic information, and so many efficient approaches to problems of common interest which can only be usefully dealt with by this original approach.

Certainly, the knowledge acquired over the last 40 years by means of clinical studies, rigid esophagoscopy and classical radiology has today, thanks to the modernization of paraclinical investigations, led to important discoveries.

This applies to esophageal manometry, pH measurement, fiberoscopy and videoendoscopy. These have added to our understanding of the physio-pathology, and these gains daily improve our diagnostic precision and the essential therapeutical indications, now discussed at a different and more precise level.

Similarly, these studies allow increasingly improved conclusions as to the true incidence of malignant degeneration in so-called “benign” disorders of the esophagus.

*

The original design of our Congresses, as laid down by Robert Giuli, therefore seems to me exceptionally satisfactory, knowing that there are going to be valuable statistical extensions to all the replies given here to 210 questions by all those personalities from the 5 continents who have succeeded in crystallizing the fruits of their experience for us during 4 days of exceptional interest.

* *

Our task is not completed. Robert Giuli reminds us of this by the choice of the marvellous emblem of OESO, representing this unconquerable white horse, the “Cheval de Marly”, an image of the drive of an entire group and of its efforts to attempt to master all the problems still remaining in esophageal pathology.

MIX
Papier aus verantwortungsvollen Quellen
Paper from responsible sources
FSC® C105338

If you have any concerns about our products,
you can contact us on
ProductSafety@springernature.com

In case Publisher is established outside the EU,
the EU authorized representative is:
Springer Nature Customer Service Center GmbH
Europaplatz 3, 69115 Heidelberg, Germany

Printed by Libri Plureos GmbH
in Hamburg, Germany